HANDBOOK OF PERSONALITY

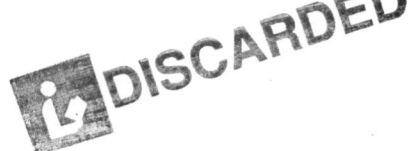

Handbook of
Personality

Theory and Research

THIRD EDITION

edited by
**Oliver P. John
Richard W. Robins
Lawrence A. Pervin**

THE GUILFORD PRESS
New York   London

© 2008 The Guilford Press
A Division of Guilford Publications, Inc.
72 Spring Street, New York, NY 10012
www.guilford.com

Paperback edition 2010

Printed in the United States of America

This book is printed on acid-free paper.

Last digit is print number: 9   8   7   6   5   4   3   2

Library of Congress Cataloging-in-Publication Data

Handbook of personality : theory and research / edited by Oliver P. John, Richard W. Robins,
Lawrence A. Pervin. — 3rd ed.
     p. cm.
Includes bibliographical references and index.
ISBN 978-1-59385-836-0 (hardcover)
ISBN 978-1-60918-059-1 (paperback)
1. Personality. I. John, Oliver P. II. Robins, Richard W. III. Pervin, Lawrence A.
BF698.H335 2008
155.2—dc22

2008006659

About the Editors

Oliver P. John, PhD, at the University of California, Berkeley, since 1987, is both Professor in the Department of Psychology, where he was recently recognized as the most cited faculty member, and Research Psychologist at the Institute of Personality and Social Research, where he has twice served as Acting Director. Dr. John has won the Distinguished Teaching Award from Berkeley's College of Letters and Science (2004), the Theoretical Innovation Prize from the Society for Personality and Social Psychology (2002), the Best Paper of the Year Award from the *Journal of Research in Personality* (1998, 2003), and the Cattell Award for Early Career Contributions from the Society of Multivariate Experimental Psychology (1996). He has served as Associate Editor of *Personality and Social Psychology Bulletin*, as an Honorary Gast Professor at the University of Heidelberg in Germany, and as Kurt Lewin Fellow at the University of Groningen in The Netherlands. In more than 90 articles and three books, Dr. John has examined personality structure and processes, emotion expression and regulation, self and self-perception processes, and methodological issues; his Big Five Inventory and Emotion Regulation Questionnaire have each been translated into more than 15 languages.

Richard W. Robins, PhD, is Professor of Psychology at the University of California, Davis. His research focuses on personality, emotion, and the self. Dr. Robins is coeditor of two books, *Handbook of Research Methods in Personality Psychology* and *The Self-Conscious Emotions* (both published by Guilford in 2007), and served as Associate Editor of the *Journal of Personality and Social Psychology*. He has won the Distinguished Scientific Award for Early Career Contribution to Psychology from the American Psychological Association and the Theoretical Innovation Prize from the Society for Personality and Social Psychology.

Lawrence A. Pervin, PhD, is Professor Emeritus at Rutgers University, where he served as Professor of Psychology from 1971 to 2004. In addition to editing the first edition of this handbook (Guilford, 1990), he is the original author of the textbook *Personality: Theory and Research*, now in its 10th edition (with Daniel Cervone; Wiley, 2008); the author of three editions of *Current Controversies and Issues in Personality*; and the founding editor of the journal *Psychological Inquiry*. His books have been translated into eight foreign languages.

Contributors

Nicole B. Barenbaum, PhD, Department of Psychology, University of the South, Sewanee, Tennessee

Justin L. Barrett, PhD, Institute of Cognitive and Evolutionary Anthropology, School of Anthropology and Museum Ethnography, University of Oxford, Oxford, United Kingdom

Roy F. Baumeister, PhD, Department of Psychology, Florida State University, Tallahassee, Florida

Verónica Benet-Martínez, PhD, Department of Psychology, University of California, Riverside, California

Jennifer K. Bosson, PhD, Department of Psychology, University of South Florida, Tampa, Florida

David M. Buss, PhD, Department of Psychology, University of Texas at Austin, Austin, Texas

Turhan Canli, PhD, Social, Cognitive, and Affective Neuroscience Center, Graduate Program in Genetics, and Department of Psychology, Stony Brook University, Stony Brook, New York

John P. Capitanio, PhD, Department of Psychology, University of California, Davis, California

Charles S. Carver, PhD, Department of Psychology, University of Miami, Coral Gables, Florida

Avshalom Caspi, PhD, Social, Genetic and Developmental Psychiatry Research Centre, Institute of Psychiatry, King's College London, London, United Kingdom, and Department of Psychology and Neuroscience, Duke University, Durham, North Carolina

Lee Anna Clark, PhD, Department of Psychology, University of Iowa, Iowa City, Iowa

Paul T. Costa, Jr., Biomedical Research Center, National Institute on Aging, National Institutes of Health, Baltimore, Maryland

Edward L. Deci, PhD, Department of Psychology, University of Rochester, Rochester, New York

Ed Diener, PhD, Department of Psychology, University of Illinois at Urbana–Champaign, Champaign, Illinois

Robert A. Emmons, PhD, Department of Psychology, University of California, Davis, California

R. Chris Fraley, PhD, Department of Psychology, University of Illinois at Urbana–Champaign, Champaign, Illinois

Howard S. Friedman, PhD, Department of Psychology, University of California, Riverside, California

Daniel Fulford, MS, Department of Psychology, University of Miami, Coral Gables, Florida

David C. Funder, PhD, Department of Psychology, University of California, Riverside, California

Glen O. Gabbard, MD, Department of Psychiatry and Behavioral Sciences, Baylor College of Medicine, Houston, Texas

Matthew T. Gailliot, PhD, Faculty of Social and Behavioural Sciences, University of Amsterdam, Amsterdam, The Netherlands

Samuel D. Gosling, PhD, Department of Psychology, University of Texas at Austin, Austin, Texas

James J. Gross, PhD, Department of Psychology, Stanford University, Stanford, California

Sarah E. Hampson, PhD, Oregon Research Institute, Eugene, Oregon, and Department of Psychology, University of Surrey, Guildford, United Kingdom

E. Tory Higgins, PhD, Department of Psychology, Columbia University, New York, New York

Oliver P. John, PhD, Department of Psychology and Institute of Personality and Social Research, University of California, Berkeley, California

Wendy Johnson, PhD, Department of Psychology, University of Minnesota, Minneapolis, Minnesota

John F. Kihlstrom, PhD, Department of Psychology, University of California, Berkeley, California

Robert F. Krueger, PhD, Department of Psychology, University of Minnesota, Minneapolis, Minnesota

Richard E. Lucas, PhD, Department of Psychology, Michigan State University, East Lansing, Michigan

Dan P. McAdams, PhD, Department of Psychology, Northwestern University, Evanston, Illinois

Robert R. McCrae, PhD, Biomedical Research Center, National Institute on Aging, National Institutes of Health, Baltimore, Maryland

Nicole L. Mead, MSc, Department of Psychology, Florida State University, Tallahassee, Florida

Walter Mischel, PhD, Department of Psychology, Columbia University, New York, New York

Laura P. Naumann, MA, Department of Psychology, University of California, Berkeley, California

Shigehiro Oishi, PhD, Department of Psychology, University of Virginia, Charlottesville, Virginia

Kile M. Ortigo, MA, Department of Psychology, Emory University, Atlanta, Georgia

Delroy L. Paulhus, PhD, Department of Psychology, University of British Columbia, Vancouver, British Columbia, Canada

Eva M. Pomerantz, PhD, Department of Psychology, University of Illinois at Urbana–Champaign, Champaign, Illinois

Brent W. Roberts, PhD, Department of Psychology, University of Illinois at Urbana–Champaign, Champaign, Illinois

Richard W. Robins, PhD, Department of Psychology, University of California, Davis, California

Richard M. Ryan, PhD, Department of Clinical and Social Psychology, University of Rochester, Rochester, New York

Carol D. Ryff, PhD, Institute on Aging and Department of Psychology, University of Wisconsin, Madison, Wisconsin

Michael F. Scheier, PhD, Department of Psychology, Carnegie Mellon University, Pittsburgh, Pennsylvania

Sarah A. Schnitker, MA, Department of Psychology, University of California, Davis, California

Abigail A. Scholer, MA, Department of Psychology, Columbia University, New York, New York

Oliver C. Schultheiss, PhD, Department of Psychology and Sport Sciences, Friedrich-Alexander University, Erlangen, Germany

Phillip R. Shaver, PhD, Department of Psychology, University of California, Davis, California

Yuichi Shoda, PhD, Department of Psychology, University of Washington, Seattle, Washington

Dean Keith Simonton, PhD, Department of Psychology, University of California, Davis, California

Gregory T. Smith, PhD, Department of Psychology, University of Kentucky, Lexington, Kentucky

Christopher J. Soto, PhD, Department of Psychology, University of California, Berkeley, California

William B. Swann, Jr., PhD, Department of Psychology, University of Texas at Austin, Austin, Texas

Ross A. Thompson, PhD, Department of Psychology, University of California, Davis, California

Jessica L. Tracy, PhD, Department of Psychology, University of British Columbia, Vancouver, British Columbia, Canada

Paul D. Trapnell, PhD, Department of Psychology, University of Winnipeg, Winnipeg, Manitoba, Canada

Kali H. Trzesniewski, PhD, Department of Psychology, University of Western Ontario, London, Ontario, Canada

David Watson, PhD, Department of Psychology, University of Iowa, Iowa City, Iowa

Tamara A. R. Weinstein, PhD, Department of Psychology, University of California, Davis, California

Drew Westen, PhD, Department of Psychology, Emory University, Atlanta, Georgia

Thomas A. Widiger, PhD, Department of Psychology, University of Kentucky, Lexington, Kentucky

David G. Winter, PhD, Department of Psychology, University of Michigan, Ann Arbor, Michigan

Dustin Wood, PhD, Department of Psychology, University of Illinois at Urbana–Champaign, Champaign, Illinois

Preface

This third edition of the *Handbook of Personality* follows almost two decades after the inaugural volume and a decade after the second edition. It thus chronicles the substantial advances and growth in the field. Indeed, the field of personality psychology, as a unified discipline distinct from clinical and social psychology, has come of age, and the third edition of this book is testimony to its increasing maturation.

To accommodate these changes in the field, we have expanded and completely restructured the *Handbook*; 17 of the now 32 chapters are entirely new and the remaining chapters have been thoroughly updated and revised. The *Handbook* is now organized into seven sections. The first two sections include an introductory chapter on the history of the field followed by a section with seven chapters summarizing the most important theoretical approaches. The remainder of the volume is now organized around five broad content areas of personality theory and research: biological bases; development; self and social processes; cognitive and motivational processes; and emotion, adjustment, and health. This new and expanded format has enabled us to substantially update and deepen our coverage of core topics and to include additional chapters on topics such as aging, identity, relationships and attachment, implicit motives, spirituality and religion, animal personality, and happiness and well-being.

Conceiving and overseeing publication of the third edition of the *Handbook* also provided many opportunities to reflect on the past and present state of the field. Handbooks generally serve to provide an up-to-date summary and evaluation of the current state of knowledge in a scientific discipline; thus, each edition of the *Handbook of Personality* provides a snapshot of our discipline at a particular point of time. However, when published with some regularity, handbooks also serve to chronicle the history and development of a field. When we look back to the original 1990 edition, it becomes clear that the pace of change has been rapid and remarkable.

Much has changed in the past two decades. Several important conferences featuring the next generation of personality psychologists, such as that organized by Nancy Cantor and David Buss at the University of Michigan in 1988, eventually led to the founding of the Association for Research in Personality. This new society provides a single organizational base for all researchers interested in personality psychology as well as a yearly conference that offers much-needed opportunities for contact and exchange. The *Handbook of Personality* reflects these historical and generational changes as well. The 1990 edition featured the influence and continued presence of the "pioneer generation" of personality researchers that has since retired, such as Albert Bandura, Jack Block, Raymond Cattell, Seymour Epstein, Hans Eysenck, Lewis Goldberg, Richard Lazarus, John Loehlin, David Magnusson, Bernard Weiner, and the founding editor of this *Handbook*, Larry Pervin. Only five of the 28 chapters from the first edition remain in the third edition today. The change of interest and focus in the literature are also plainly apparent; topics that seem indispensable from today's perspective were not yet sufficiently developed or important to be included in the first edition, such as the evolutionary basis of personality, self-regulation processes, or well-being and happiness.

These historical shifts are also reflected in the editorship of the *Handbook*. At the time of the inaugural edition in 1990, the now senior and second editors of this edition were just an Assistant Professor and a graduate student at the University of California at Berkeley. With increasing specialization in the field and the larger number of chapters in the *Handbook*, we have also instituted a new review process for this third edition. Each chapter was reviewed by the first or second editor, with the additional input from an anonymous external reviewer with particular expertise in the subject at hand. We gratefully acknowledge the enthusiastic support and careful reviews provided our many colleagues; they have importantly contributed to the quality and relevance of all the chapters in this edition.

Finally, we would like to thank the team at Guilford Press for their efforts and dedication to this *Handbook*: Editor-in-Chief Seymour Weingarten, who knew the field was ready for the next edition before we were quite ready to take on that challenge and provided input and support all along the way, as well as Carolyn Graham, Judy Grauman, Laura Specht Patchkofsky, and Katherine Lieber for their thoughtful and patient work on our behalf.

OLIVER P. JOHN, PhD
RICHARD W. ROBINS, PhD
LAWRENCE A. PERVIN, PhD

Contents

PART III. BIOLOGICAL BASES

PART IV. DEVELOPMENTAL APPROACHES

PART V. SELF AND SOCIAL PROCESSES

PART VI. COGNITIVE AND MOTIVATIONAL PROCESSES

PART VII. EMOTION, ADJUSTMENT, AND HEALTH

PART I

Introduction

CHAPTER 1

History of Modern Personality Theory and Research

Nicole B. Barenbaum
David G. Winter

In my judgment ... you should issue [an] entire Handbook on personality; the subject cannot be treated surreptitiously as a subdivision of a subdivision of social psychology.

—ALLPORT (1934)

Readers of this third edition of the *Handbook of Personality* may be surprised to learn that Gordon Allport's call for such a handbook went unheeded some 75 years ago. Having agreed to prepare a chapter on "Attitude Patterns (Character)" for the first *Handbook of Social Psychology* (Murchison & Allee, 1935), Allport (1934) objected that he could not cover the "vast field of personality"— the term he preferred to "character"—in a chapter on attitudes (Allport, 1935). But in 1934, personality had yet to be recognized as a separate subfield of psychology, and the first *Handbook of Personality* (Borgatta & Lambert, 1968) would not appear for several decades. Despite Allport's early efforts to promote a "field of personality" (e.g., Allport & Vernon, 1930, p. 677), psychologists generally continued to view personality as a topic of abnormal psychology or of social psychology—at that time broadly construed as encompassing what later became separate subfields of clinical, developmental, industrial, personality, and social psychology—until the late 1930s, when the texts by Allport (1937), Stagner (1937), and Murray (1938) signaled the consolidation of the new subfield (Barenbaum, 2000). Yet this gradual emergence of "personality psychology" was far from an indicator of indifference toward the topic of personality. The early 20th century saw the growth of a lively popular interest in personality as well as increasing attention from scholars in many disciplines, each laying claim to personality while proposing different definitions of the concept and promoting different methods of study (Barenbaum & Winter, 2003; Danziger, 1990; Nicholson, 2003).

This diversity of theoretical and methodological approaches has contributed a number of themes and controversies that have persisted, or emerged periodically in different forms, throughout the history of personality psychology. In particular, we examine the distinction between research on common dimensions and processes of personality, usually conducted with groups of participants, and research on unique persons that attempts to understand the thematic coherence of individual lives. We consider more briefly the question of consistency and the person–situation debate, the relative contributions of biological and environmental factors to personality, and the search for a model of personality that integrates multiple units of analysis. An analysis of the historical roots of personality psychology can provide insights into these issues and into approaches currently prominent in the field. We begin with a look at the multidisciplinary study of personality in the United States that preceded the establishment of personality psychology.

MULTIDISCIPLINARY APPROACHES TO PERSONALITY

To understand the history of American personality psychology, it is important to examine the broader cultural and institutional contexts that influenced the emergence of psychological approaches to personality in the early decades of the 20th century (Danziger, 1990, 1997; Nicholson, 2003; Parker, 1991). These contexts included developments not only in psychology, but also in the larger culture and in neighboring disciplines that adopted different investigative practices and perspectives on personality. We discuss first the popular "culture of personality" (Susman, 1979, p. 216), then consider psychiatry and sociology, two disciplines recognized for their use of case study and life history methods in personality research. In contrast, we consider several factors that interacted to promote and maintain psychologists' interest in personality, their emphasis on psychometric methods, and their ambivalence toward studies of individual personalities.

The "Culture of Personality"

Experiencing rapid societal changes associated with industrialization, urbanization, immigration, and mass education early in the 20th century, many Americans responded with fears of depersonalization. Captivated by popular press reports of dramatic cases of

psychopathology, these Americans consulted self-improvement manuals that emphasized the cultivation of a unique "personality"—a term that soon "became an important part of the American vocabulary" (Susman, 1979, p. 217). By the 1920s the "mass market for popularized personal documents" (Burnham, 1968, p. 368) included such magazines as *True Story* (Krueger, 1925), and biography—dubbed "the literature of personality"—enjoyed a "wide vogue" (Johnston, 1927, p. x). The "new psychology" (Burnham, 1968, p. 352) became a fad, illustrated by the first appearance of Freud on the cover of *Time* magazine in 1924 (Fancher, 2000).

Personality became a central concern in business (Susman, 1979) and a focus in such academic and professional fields as psychopathology and psychiatry, sociology, education, and social work, and in the mental hygiene movement as well as in psychology. These fields also began to reflect the influence of psychoanalysis following Freud's visit to America in 1909 (Danziger, 1997; Hale, 1971). Although boundaries between psychology and disciplines such as psychiatry and sociology were somewhat unclear during this period, representatives of these disciplines differed in their methodological choices regarding the study of personality.

Psychiatry and Psychopathology

Before the 1920s, the term "personality" was used in the United States first in religious and ethical writings and somewhat later in discussions of abnormal psychology, which was considered a province of the medical specialty of psychiatry rather than an area of psychology (Parker, 1991). The later usage reflected the influence of a tradition of personality study from 19th-century France (Lombardo & Foschi, 2003). Personality appeared as a topic of American psychiatry in journals such as the *Journal of Abnormal Psychology*, founded in 1906 by Morton Prince. Originally oriented toward medical psychopathologists, the journal featured personal accounts and case studies; between 1906 and 1916, nearly all of the empirical studies presented data on individuals rather than groups (Shermer, 1985). Case studies held central status as investigative practices and pedagogical tools in medical and psychiatric research and in psychoanalysis (e.g.,

Forrester, 1996; S. Freud, 1910/1957); they appeared regularly in psychiatric and psychoanalytic journals throughout the 1920s and 1930s. Psychopathologists also proposed general physiological theories of personality (e.g., Berman, 1921).

Sociology

During the 1920s and 1930s personality was an important focus among sociologists, whose research on social adjustment and social roles drew on their close collaboration with social workers (Platt, 1996). In 1921, "personality" appeared as a main category used to classify abstracts published in the *American Journal of Sociology*, as did subcategories for biography, case studies, and life histories and psychoanalysis ("Recent Literature," 1921). Inspired by *The Polish Peasant in Europe and America* (Thomas & Znaniecki, 1918–1920), prominent sociologists promoted case studies and life histories into the 1940s (Bulmer, 1984) in their own research and through their involvement with the Social Science Research Council (SSRC). Interest in quantitative methods, prompted in part by psychologists' "heroic efforts to become more scientific, that is to say, statistical" (Burgess, 1927, p. 108), resulted in an extended debate on the relative merits of case study and statistical methods, with some participants advocating both approaches (Bulmer, 1984). In the 1930s, the Chicago sociology department held student–faculty baseball games featuring "case study" versus "statistics" teams (pp. 45–46).

American Psychology

The 1920s and 1930s were years of intense psychological research on personality. Attempting to claim personality as an appropriate psychological topic and to establish their professional expertise, psychologists differentiated their own research not only from the popular literature on personality but also from personality research in other disciplines. The first American review of psychological literature on "personality and character" appeared in 1921 (Allport, 1921). Many of the sources cited by Allport involved the *trait* concept, which by then had already achieved a theoretical dominance (Parker, 1991). Allport emphasized the distinction

between "personality" and "character," two concepts that had been used interchangeably by American psychologists up to that time (e.g., Warren, 1920). In agreement with behaviorist John B. Watson, Allport suggested that "character," defined as "the personality evaluated according to prevailing standards of conduct" (1921, p. 443), was not an appropriate psychological topic (see Nicholson, 2003). He continued to advocate the use of "personality" as a more objective, scientific term (e.g., Allport, 1927); this soon became standard practice.

By the late 1920s, reviewers of the multidisciplinary personality literature recognized the distinctive contributions of psychologists. Unlike sociological and psychiatric studies, early psychological research devoted little attention to social roles, to cases of psychopathology, or to methods of investigating individual persons; instead, it featured psychometric and statistical studies of groups (e.g., Young, 1928). Several closely interacting factors influenced the emergence of personality psychology and promoted the development of psychometric approaches, as well as psychologists' skepticism regarding studies of individuals, throughout the early decades of the 20th century.

Scientific Ethos

Psychometric studies of personality reflected psychologists' efforts to follow in the footsteps of the prestigious "exact sciences" that had developed rapidly in the late 19th century. Drawing on "the work of Galton, Pearson, Cattell, Thorndike and Terman with their investigations of individual differences" (Young, 1928, p. 431), psychologists created paper-and-pencil "tests" of personality based on the IQ test model of adding "scores" on discrete individual "items" to get a total. The first such test was probably Woodworth's (1919) Personal Data Sheet. Later on, personality psychologists expanded their measurement technology to include ratings and behavioral observations. Psychologists were particularly concerned with producing "objective" knowledge and eliminating sources of "subjectivity." For example, Thurstone, who thought "the center of psychology probably was the study of personality," turned to other interests that seemed to promise more "experimental leverage" (1952, p. 318).

From this perspective, case studies and life histories, relying on subjective reports or interpretations, appeared unscientific, and many psychologists hesitated to use them.

Institutional Support

The 1920s saw increasing institutional support in the form of journals, textbook chapters, courses, and conference sessions devoted to personality. In 1921, social psychologist Floyd Allport joined psychopathologist Morton Prince as coeditor of the newly expanded *Journal of Abnormal Psychology and Social Psychology*. In a joint editorial, Prince and Allport noted the shared interest of psychopathologists and social psychologists in the "dynamics of human nature" and invited contributions on a number of topics, including "the foundation-study of human traits" and "the personality of the individual" (1921, p. 2). The issue began with a study of personality traits by the Allport brothers (F. H. Allport & G. W. Allport, 1921). Seven years later, in a special issue of the renamed *Journal of Abnormal and Social Psychology* devoted to personality, Prince and Moore (1928) commented on the "extraordinary" increase in studies of "temperament, character and personal traits"—a topic "which until quite recently numbered but a few brief pages in any standard textbook of psychology." They called for "more manifold studies" and concluded with a prophetic reference to "the complex task that faces the author of a Psychology of Personality ten years hence" (p. 117). Coverage of personality in general psychology texts increased dramatically in the 1920s, and by the early 1930s many psychology departments were offering courses in personality (Parker, 1991).

Between 1923 and 1928, the American Psychological Association scheduled convention sessions on "character" and "personality," sometimes in the practical context of vocational guidance or selection (Parker, 1991). Several private foundations also supported personality research. During the 1930s, psychologists joined anthropologists and sociologists in research, seminars, and conferences sponsored by the SSRC's committees on personality and culture (Bryson, 2002). Other signs of recognition included the founding of *Character and Personality* (later renamed *Journal of Personality*) in 1932 and the addition of "personality" as a category in the *Psychological Index*, in 1929, and in *Psychological Abstracts* in 1934 (Parker, 1991).

In contrast with psychiatry and sociology (and, somewhat later, anthropology), institutional support for case study and life history methods was generally lacking in psychology. For example, the proportion of case studies published in the *Journal of Abnormal Psychology and Social Psychology* decreased dramatically following the transfer of the journal, renamed *Journal of Abnormal and Social Psychology*, to the American Psychological Association in 1925. Many authors of psychological texts and reference works echoed the views of Woodworth, who considered the "case history method" primarily a clinical one and judged it "the least rather than the most preferred" method, albeit one that "can give us … some indication of the topics that are deserving of closer examination" (1929, p. 19).

Practical Demands

Psychologists' success with mental tests during World War I promoted their interest in developing efficient "scientific" tests for selection, diagnosis, and placement to meet practical needs of industries, educational institutions, and social agencies (e.g., Danziger, 1990). Critics of the predictive utility of intelligence tests suggested the need for measures of personality or character traits (e.g., Fernald, 1920). Although early trait measures took various forms, the less "efficient" methods were soon replaced by tests modeled on mental tests (Parker, 1991). Another important influence on the psychometric approach in the 1920s and 1930s was the mental hygiene movement, a well-funded alliance of psychiatrists, educationists, and social workers who viewed individual maladjustment as the root cause of a wide variety of social and personal problems (Cohen, 1983). The movement enlisted psychologists to supply a "scientific" basis for the therapeutic efforts of mental hygiene workers (Danziger, 1990).

Professional Concerns

Although psychologists recognized the value of multidisciplinary perspectives on personality (e.g., Murphy & Jensen, 1932), they were also concerned with claiming personality as an object especially suitable for *psychological* study and with asserting their particular expertise in developing scientific and technological methods of assessment. For example, Allport (1935) argued that "the personality of each man is a unique integration, and as such is a datum for psychology, and for psychology only" (p. 838) and that social scientists (e.g., sociologists) were interested in personality only as "the subjective side of culture" (p. 837) or in "common social attitudes" (p. 838). Psychometric methods served to bolster the scientific status of psychologists competing with other "experts" who offered solutions for practical problems. During the 1920s and 1930s, psychologists were particularly eager to distance themselves from psychoanalysts and from "pseudopsychologists" working in applied settings to serve a public fascinated with personality (e.g., Crider, 1936; Hornstein, 1992). In this context, case studies not only appeared unscientific but also recalled the "true confessions" of abnormal behavior that were appearing in the popular media (Burnham, 1968, p. 368).

THE TWO TASKS OF PERSONALITY PSYCHOLOGY

Science ... is not interested in the unique event; the unique belongs to history, not to science.
—Guilford (1936, p. 676)

The object of our study is a single human being.
—Stagner (1937, p. viii)

As we have seen, early reviewers of the personality literature (e.g., Young, 1928) described two related but contrasting endeavors: (1) the *study of individual differences*, or the dimensions along which people differ from each other, and (2) the *study of individual persons as unique, integrated wholes*. They identified the first approach with the work of psychologists and the second with the work of psychiatrists, psychoanalysts, and sociologists. However, from the beginning, in keeping with an intellectual climate of individualism, some psychologists were drawn to the study of individual persons, and since the "official" emergence of personality psychology, reviews of the field have

identified both approaches, variously labeled as "analytic" versus "structural," or "quantitative" versus "qualitative," as tasks of personality psychology itself (see, e.g., McAdams, 1997). Much of the difference between these two approaches is also captured by the *nomothetic–idiographic* dichotomy—terms first used by Windelband (1894/1904), later adopted by Allport (1937; see also Stern, 1911), and still a lively topic today (e.g., Grice, Jackson, & McDaniel, 2006). In this section we describe briefly each approach, and then discuss the work of Allport and Murray, who were particularly vocal advocates of the whole-person approach, and of Raymond B. Cattell, who became known somewhat later for his efforts to advance the psychometric approach.

The Psychometric "Analysis" Approach

According to Murphy (1932), psychologists using the analytic or *quantitative* (i.e., psychometric) approach defined personality as the "sum of all of an individual's traits" (p. 386). The practical goal of their research, which measured and studied the intercorrelations of separate personality traits, was to predict, modify, and control behavior, with individual differences conceived as coefficients to be supplied to linear, additive prediction equations. The psychometric approach reflected the influence of intelligence testing and of the mental hygiene movement, which promoted psychologists' expertise in constructing, administering, and analyzing the results of tests designed to meet practical demands.

The Psychiatric and Historical "Interpretation" Approach

The interpretative approach focuses on understanding the underlying thematic coherence of an individual life, typically using biographical and case study methods. Early psychologists generally ignored or criticized this approach, associating it with an "old-fashioned and unscientific" medical tradition (Hale, 1971, p. 115). With these concerns in mind, Allport and Vernon (1930) echoed the prevailing view that the case studies of psychiatrists, psychoanalysts, and sociologists were "unsatisfactory" but suggested that "the concrete individual has eluded study by any other approach" (p. 700) and that in the future psychologists might standardize case studies to improve their scientific status.

For the past 80 years, the two approaches to personality psychology—the study of individual personality *differences* through psychometric methods and the study of individual *persons* through biographical and case study methods—have existed in an uneasy coalition or truce. As part of their efforts to define, systematize, and broaden personality psychology, Allport (1937) and Murray (1938) tried to correct the field's overemphasis on psychometric research and group studies by promoting the study of individual persons, but with few exceptions (e.g., White, 1952), personality psychologists avoided studies of individual lives through most of the 20th century (see, e.g., Carlson, 1971; McAdams & West, 1997; Runyan, 1997).

In the following sections, we examine the work of Allport and Murray, as well as that of another pioneer of personality psychology, Raymond Cattell. Although Murray and Allport are best known as advocates of the study of individual lives and Cattell as an advocate of the psychometric approach to personality, in fact, all three conducted research on both individuals and groups, but with different emphases.

Gordon Allport: Defining, Systematizing, and Separating the Field of Personality

In his biography of Gordon Allport, Nicholson (2003) argued that Allport pursued two contradictory goals in attempting to define and systematize the field of personality psychology. Measuring personality with tests of "traits," he sought to define it as a devaluated natural object of scientific control. At the same time, he attempted to preserve personality as a unique spiritual essence that could be captured only incompletely by scientific methods. In his doctoral dissertation on "the traits of personality," Allport (1922) adopted a behavioristic definition of traits as systems of habits and designed measures of those traits he saw as basic components of personality. But as a postdoctoral student in Germany (1922–1923), Allport encountered a whole-person, interpretive approach to personality that "converted" him from his "semifaith in behaviorism" (1967, p. 12). Influenced by philosopher Wilhelm Dilthey's

view of psychology as a "human science" (*Geisteswissenschaft*), this approach emphasized the organization or patterning of personality characteristics and other psychological processes within the unique individual: "More fundamental than differential psychology [i.e., the psychometric focus on dimensions of difference among people], by far, is the problem of the nature, the activity, and the unity of the *total personality*" (Allport, 1923, p. 614; original emphasis). From that time onward, Allport advocated structural approaches such as Gestalt psychology, Eduard Spranger's intuitive method, and William Stern's personalistic emphasis on the uniqueness and unity of personality (e.g., Allport, 1923, 1924, 1929). He was especially influenced by Stern's "repudiation" of his earlier view of "personality as a sum-total of traits" in favor of emphases on "the total personality" (Allport, 1924, p. 359) and on the organization of the individual's traits (Allport, 1967; Nicholson, 2003). Stern's influence is reflected in many of Allport's later (1937) views (e.g., the very definition of "trait," the concept of functional autonomy of motives, and the distinction between idiographic and nomothetic methods).

Allport taught what he considered "probably the first course on the subject [of personality] offered in an American college" (Allport, 1967, p. 9) in the Department of Social Ethics at Harvard in 1924 (in fact, Kimball Young began teaching "Personality and Character" at the University of Oregon in 1920; see Barenbaum, 2000). During his time at Dartmouth (from 1926 to 1930) and later at Harvard (in the psychology department), Allport taught courses on personality, refined his definition of traits (1931), and attempted to synthesize analytic and interpretive methods of studying personality. He experimented with case methods in teaching (1929) and developed the Study of Values, an instrument based on Spranger's sixfold conception of value (Vernon & Allport, 1931).

Allport's 1937 text, like his early reviews, attempted to define and systematize the field of personality psychology in order to provide "co-ordinating concepts and theories" (p. ix). Defining "the psychology of personality" as a "new field of study" (p. vii) that focused not on "the factors *shaping* personality" but on "personality *itself*" (p. viii), Allport continued his efforts to separate the field from social psychology and sociology. His survey of existing definitions of personality and methods of studying it led to a renewed emphasis on *trait* as the fundamental unit of study for personality. Traits, Allport suggested, were neuropsychic systems with dynamic or motivational properties. At the same time, Allport's focus throughout was on "the manifest individuality of mind" (p. vii), which implied both idiographic and nomothetic methods. Although some critics considered his focus on the individual unscientific, even reviewers who took issue with his approach recognized his text as a pioneering contribution to the field (e.g., Guilford, 1938).

Working within Harvard's scientifically oriented department of psychology, Allport opted for a moderate, eclectic approach that included both analytic and interpretive methods (see Nicholson, 2003; but also Pandora, 1997), and he exercised caution in advocating case studies. He published only one case study (Allport, 1965), late in his career, and much of his research involved nomothetic trait studies (Allport, 1928; Vernon & Allport, 1931). Yet his unpublished record reveals extensive efforts to develop scientific case study methods and promote case studies "behind the scenes" in his teaching and editorial activities (see Barenbaum, 1997; Barenbaum & Winter, 2003). Unable to interest a publisher in a book on case studies, Allport eventually used some of his work in an SSRC monograph on the use of personal documents in psychology (1942).

Allport's influence on the emerging field of personality psychology is well known (see, e.g., Craik, Hogan, & Wolfe, 1993). Noting his "uncanny ability to comprehend the major issues in the field," Cohler (1993) observed that even in his earliest work,

> Allport was aware of the fundamental problems confronting those who wished to study persons, such as the problem of distinguishing between text and interpretation, the advantages and drawbacks of individual difference formulations in the study of personality structure, the fact that traits as well as environments were ever-changing, and the challenges of accounting for continuity and change in lives over time. (p. 142)

We have discussed Allport's efforts to reconcile analytic and interpretive approaches and his emphasis on the structure and organization of the individual personality. Considering both his pioneering contribution to the lexical study of traits (Allport & Odbert, 1936) and his insistence that "a theory of personality requires more than a descriptive taxonomy" of traits, John and Robins (1993) claim Allport as "father and critic of the Five-Factor Model" (pp. 225, 215). Furthermore, Allport's critique of the situationist "doctrine of specificity" (1937, p. 249) anticipated the persistent person–situation debate (e.g., Funder, Chapter 22, this volume). His suggestion that factors derived from group data may not "resemble the dispositions and traits identified ... when the *individual* is studied intensively" (Allport, 1937, p. 244, original emphasis) foreshadowed recent critiques concerning the applicability of the Big Five traits to individuals' constructions of self and others (e.g., Grice et al., 2006).

Henry Murray: Organismic Science, Depth Psychology, and Literature

Henry Murray came to the study of personality by way of psychoanalysis and abnormal psychology. Trained originally in medicine and in biochemistry, Murray chose a career in "depth psychology" after encountering the work of Jung and Freud. Only after accepting a position as assistant director of Morton Prince's Harvard Psychological Clinic in 1926 did he realize that the academic psychology of the time had very little in common with psychoanalysis (Murray, 1940, 1967). At a time when psychologists were struggling to define and delimit the disciplinary boundaries of their field, Murray's unorthodox and divergent interests were not acceptable to proponents of a strictly scientific psychology; in fact, they almost cost him his position at Harvard (Triplet, 1983).

Murray's eclectic, multimethod approach reflected his medical training as well as the holistic philosophy of science of Alfred North Whitehead and Lawrence J. Henderson, the theories of Freud and Jung, and his passion to understand the creative works of such authors as Herman Melville and Thomas Wolfe (Barenbaum, 2006; Laughlin, 1973; Robinson, 1992). At the same time, Murray's background in biochemistry permeated his work, for example, in the explicit analogy between his classification of the "variables of personality" and the periodic table of chemistry (1938, pp. 142–143). The difficulty of such an eclectic and ambitious enterprise is perhaps indicated by Murray's numerous revisions of his system of multiple interacting personality variables and by the tentative titles he used for these works (e.g., Murray, 1959).

In *Explorations in Personality*, Murray (1938) and his collaborators described an intensive interdisciplinary study of 51 young men that combined techniques developed by psychoanalysts and by academic psychologists. Although Murray's efforts to bring the two disciplines together were praised, academic psychologists remained skeptical, criticizing psychoanalysis as unproven and unscientific. One reviewer (Elliott, 1939), for example, was impressed with the new tests and procedures (especially the Thematic Apperception Test; TAT) and with Murray's analysis of the variables of personality and environment but considered the book's single case study too speculative and criticized Murray for insufficient use of statistics and for overlooking existing work in experimental and differential psychology.

Murray's work had a profound effect on the expansion of the disciplinary boundaries of personality psychology (Triplet, 1983). By demonstrating the use of experimental techniques to investigate psychoanalytic concepts, teaching courses on abnormal and dynamic psychology in a prestigious academic psychology department, and inspiring a large number of graduate students, Murray played an important part in expanding the definition of personality psychology to include psychoanalytic theories that had earlier "had pariah status in academia" (M. B. Smith, 1990, p. 537). Situated as a maverick in opposition to the "scientistic" Harvard department (Robinson, 1992), Murray advocated the interpretive study of lives and considered case histories "the proof of the pudding" as tests of personological theory (1938, p. 606). Still, he needed to justify his financial support from the Rockefeller Foundation on the basis of the "scientific" status of his work (Triplet, 1983). Murray's research group developed elaborate procedures for the intensive study of individual persons, culminating in the "diagnostic council," a case conference of researchers who reached a consensus

in interpreting each participant's personality. Yet their book (Murray, 1938) included only one case, and several of Murray's biographical and case studies remained unpublished (Barenbaum, 2006; Robinson, 1992). Murray's most enduring legacy was probably his catalog of "variables of personality" (1938, Ch. 3; see Danziger, 1997) and the Thematic Apperception Test (Morgan & Murray, 1935). His diagnostic council method was generally overlooked, however (McLeod, 1992). Although variants of the approach were used in later assessment settings such as the Office of Strategic Services (OSS Assessment Staff, 1948), the Institute for Personality Assessment and Research (IPAR) at the University of California (MacKinnon, 1975), and organizations such as AT&T (Bray, 1982), the practical demands of assessment even in those well-financed settings led assessors to base decisions "on statistical averages of ratings, rather than on discussion" (McLeod, 1992, p. 10).

Raymond Cattell and the Measurement Imperative

Another major figure in the formative years of American personality psychology was Raymond Cattell. Known for his work in multivariate techniques and intelligence testing, Cattell prefaced his first major book on personality by asserting that "it is on measurement that all further scientific advance depends" (1946, p. iv). Most of his professional career was spent at the University of Illinois, where he introduced many conceptual refinements and elaborated methodological developments, especially concerning the use of correlation, factor analysis, and other multivariate techniques, into the field of personality.

The Search for Personality Structure through Factor Analysis of Traits

Like Allport, Cattell adopted *traits* as the fundamental conceptual unit of personality, arguing that "the ideal of a science of personality description [is] to build its traits upon a foundation of objective test measurements, as has been done to a very large extent in the analysis of abilities" (1946, p. 210). Believing that the essence of a trait was *co-variation* or correlation, he concluded that the "most potent method of attacking the tangle is to work out correlation coefficients between the inconveniently multitudinous variables abounding in the subject and to seek some smaller number of 'behind the scenes' or underlying variables, known as factors" (p. 272). On the basis of factor analyses of trait ratings, he concluded that 12 factors represented "the established primary traits" (Cattell, 1946, Chs. 10–12). Using different statistical procedures and building on different assumptions, later researchers (e.g., Eysenck & Eysenck, 1985, and followers of the five-factor model; see John, Naumann, & Soto, Chapter 4, this volume, and McCrae & Costa, Chapter 5, this volume) have argued for a smaller number of basic traits.

Psychometric Technology

The prestige and apparent success of intelligence testing early in the 20th century convinced many personality psychologists that personality could (and should) also be measured by scales of "items." Although factor analysis was the apotheosis of this ideal, the same conviction guided the construction of numerous other scales, inventories, and questionnaires not based on factor analysis: omnibus instruments such as the Bernreuter Personality Inventory, Minnesota Multiphasic Personality Inventory (MMPI), California Personality Inventory (CPI; Gough, 1987), Adjective Check List, and Personality Research Form (PRF; Jackson, 1974), and countless scales designed to measure particular personality characteristics.

As statistical methods of scale construction and refinement became increasingly sophisticated, the psychometric rule book expanded to include matters such as test–retest reliability, internal and cross-situational consistency (Cronbach, 1951), convergent–discriminant validity (Campbell & Fiske, 1959), and the distinction between "trait" and "state." Some psychologists protested that psychometric rules unduly constrain personality theorizing and research because they do not take account of nonlinear, interactive, or functionally substitutable (but not correlated) relationships among components of a concept. At the turn of the 21st century, the increased popularity of chaos theory and associated mathematical concepts (e.g., Barton, 1994) suggested possible alternatives to the classic psychometric rules.

SPECIALIZATION: THE FLOWERING OF PERSONALITY PSYCHOLOGY

By 1946, shortly after the end of World War II, the main concepts and issues of personality psychology were established. Although most personality psychologists, like Allport and Cattell, considered traits a major element of personality, some, like Murray, argued for the distinctiveness and importance of motives as well (see Winter, John, Stewart, Klohnen, & Duncan, 1998). Rating scales and questionnaires were firmly established as the preferred method of measurement, especially for traits. During the postwar era of specialization, personality psychologists turned from developing grand theoretical systems focused on the whole person to the elaboration of specific elements of personality (McAdams, 1997; Runyan, 1997). Our account of this turn is framed in terms of the four elements or classes of variables and theories introduced by Winter (1996): traits, motives, cognitions, and social context (for a similar scheme, see Emmons & McAdams, 1995). After discussing each of these elements, we consider the study of biological bases of personality, a perspective that has flourished in recent years.

PERSONALITY TRAITS

In personality psychology, the concept of *trait* has been used to denote consistent patterns of behavior, especially expressive or stylistic behavior (see Winter et al., 1998). Theorizing and research about traits have focused most on questions regarding the number, nature, and organization of "basic" traits, using three different strategies. In approximate order of popularity, they are (1) factor analysis and related mathematical techniques, typically used in nomothetic research to identify trait dimensions applicable to people in general; (2) rational or a priori theorizing, often involving the construction of typologies applicable to subgroups of people; and (3) the idiographic approach, which essentially rejects the attempt to identify "basic" traits, focusing instead on an individual's unique traits or pattern of traits.

Factor-Analytic Study of Traits

Each individual is ... represented as a point in a multidimensional common factor space. [The individual's] position is unique for no other individual possesses exactly the same combination of the amounts of the various factors.
—GUILFORD (1936, p. 675)

The factors ... represent only *average* tendencies. Whether a factor is really an *organic* disposition in any one individual life is not demonstrated. All one can say for certain is that a factor is an empirically derived component of the *average* personality, and that the average personality is a complete abstraction.
—ALLPORT (1937, p. 244)

Recent historical accounts of the "Big Five" (see John et al., Chapter 4, this volume) note Cattell's (1943) pioneering efforts to reduce Allport and Odbert's (1936) list of 4,500 traits to a manageable set of clusters or factors. However, the search for personality factors began much earlier, with Webb's (1915) study using a precursor of factor analysis to find a general factor relating to character. By the mid-1930s, psychologists were showing a lively interest in factor-analytic studies of personality (Odbert, 1936). Exchanges between critics (e.g., Allport & Odbert, 1936) and proponents (e.g., Guilford, 1936) of this approach anticipated contemporary debates concerning the number of factors sufficient to describe personality and the applicability of group factors to individual personalities. By the 1990s, many personality psychologists had reached a working consensus that the trait domain could be described, at least at the broadest and most abstract level, by five orthogonal (i.e., uncorrelated) factors or clusters of traits (see McCrae & Costa, Chapter 5, this volume; John et al., Chapter 4, this volume), measured in a variety of ways: extraversion or surgency, agreeableness, conscientiousness, neuroticism, and openness (often called the five-factor model or Big Five). Nevertheless, Eysenck and his followers (Eysenck & Eysenck, 1985) continued to argue that three factors—extraversion, neuroticism, and psychoticism—are sufficient (see the exchange between Costa & McCrae, 1992a, 1992b; and Eysenck, 1992a, 1992b).

Block (1995) challenged many of the underlying assumptions of factor-analytic techniques in general as well as the five-factor model in particular. Recent research has examined stability and change in Big Five traits over the lifespan (Caspi, Roberts, & Shiner, 2005) and has underscored the success of these traits in predicting consequential outcomes at individual, interpersonal, and social institutional levels (Ozer & Benet-Martínez, 2006).

Alternative Analyses of Traits

Rationally and Theoretically Derived Constructs

In contrast to the factor-analytic approach to identifying essential traits, some personality researchers have studied traits or trait-like characteristics derived from personality theories or from folk concepts. Often, these researchers develop personality inventories that reflect their conceptualization of the important units of personality. Jackson (1974) developed the PRF to measure characteristics based on needs from Murray's theory, although these appeared to function essentially as traits (factor analyses of this measure reveal six factors; see Jackson & Tremblay, 2002). Gough (1957) used contrasting groups to construct the CPI scales for positive lay or "folk" concepts such as "achievement," "sociability," or "dominance." Later (Gough, 1987), he used clustering techniques to construct three "vectors" that bore some resemblance to Eysenck's three factors.

Typologies

Other personality psychologists have proposed certain syndromes or types, or coherently organized bundles of trait-like characteristics that define interesting patterns. The Myers–Briggs Type Indicator (Myers, 1962), until recently one of the most widely used personality tests, was based on Jung's (1923/1971) typological combination of "attitudes" (extraversion–introversion) and "functions" (thinking, feeling, sensing, and intuiting). Jung's typology and Gough's vectors are presumed to cover all people. Other types and typologies are used in a more limited way, to formalize observations about interesting cases or summarize complex data patterns. For example, Sigmund Freud wrote about the anal type (1908/1959) and various character types (1916/1957). Murray (1938, 1955/1981) described an "Icarus" type. Combining typological and factor-analytic approaches, some psychologists have used Q-sort methods and inverse (P) factor analysis to define types—for example, Block's (1971) account of how personality develops over time, Wink's (1992) description of different forms of narcissism, and York and John's (1992) use of Rank's theory to interpret patterns of adult women's lives. The utility and replicability of personality types continue to be topics of debate (e.g., Asendorpf, Caspi, & Hofstee, 2002).

The Idiographic Approach

Despite the popularity and prestige of factor analysis, the idiographic approach, which rejects the search for underlying "basic" traits and instead draws upon the broad lexicon for whatever trait adjectives fit a particular person, has survived (West, 1983; Winter, 1996, Ch. 11). Researchers who adopt this approach (e.g., Allport, 1965) may search for the individualized traits or combinations of traits most relevant to a particular person, identify central themes in an individual life, describe the patterning or organization of an individual's traits, or use such patterns to make predictions about an individual's behavior. Recent research on individuals' assessments of self and others (e.g., Cervone, 2005; Grice et al., 2006) suggests that the Big Five may not capture the full range of idiographic trait ratings.

MOTIVATIONAL CONCEPTS IN PERSONALITY

The personality construct of "motive" is based on the fundamental postulate that most behavior is oriented toward a *goal* and shows intelligent variation in moving toward the goal and responding to incentives, circumstances, opportunities, obstacles, and other current goals. Thus motives contrast with traits; as Murray (1938, pp. 56–58) pointed out, a given motive may be associated with an indefinitely large number of quite different actions; correspondingly, the same action may serve multiple and varied goals (see also Little, 1999; Pervin, 1989). In one form or another, the distinction between

motives and traits appears in the theorizing of many personality psychologists (Winter et al., 1998).

Motive Concepts in the Psychoanalytic Tradition

Nature and Organization of Motives

Freud placed motivation at the center of personality. He argued that all behavior was motivated, and he grouped human motives into two broad classes: life instincts (including self-preservation and the libidinal or sexual motives) and aggressive motives or "death instinct" (S. Freud, 1916–1917/1961–1963, 1920/1955, 1933/1964).

Many post-Freudian theorists rephrased Freud's dualistic motivational theory. For example, Bakan's (1966) concepts of "agency" and "communion" stimulated a good deal of empirical research (Helgeson, 1994; Wiggins & Trobst, 1999), and Winter (1996, Ch. 5) linked Freud's libidinal and aggressive motive groupings to the TAT-measured affiliation and power motives.

Drawing eclectically on psychoanalytic theory and its neo-Freudian variants in an intensive study of a group of normal adult males, Murray (1938) constructed an empirically based catalog of 20[1] "needs" or motives that was widely accepted by later personality psychologists, either as a general list measured by questionnaires such as the PRF, or as the basis for elaborate research programs measuring particular motives (see C. P. Smith, 1992).

Related Concepts Deriving from Psychoanalytic Motivational Theory

Freud believed that many human motives (represented as the id mental system) conflict with external reality, parental demands, and social mores (represented by the superego); this conflict is mediated by the ego. Unacceptable motives, which would arouse anxiety, are transformed and/or rendered unconscious by defense mechanisms so as to make them "safe," thereby reducing anxiety. Anna Freud (1937/1946) elaborated the nature and operation of the defense mechanisms more fully.

Over the years, psychologists have carried out a good deal of experimental research to evaluate psychoanalytic theory and especially defense mechanisms such as repression (e.g., Fisher & Greenberg, 1977). To positivist, behaviorist psychologists such as Skinner (1953), the notion of an "unconscious" was suspect.[2] However, the study of sophisticated mechanisms of information processing (Erdelyi, 1985; see also Kihlstrom, Chapter 23, this volume) and research on "implicit" psychological mechanisms and processes (Greenwald et al., 2002) have made the notion of processes that operate out of conscious awareness scientifically respectable (see Westen, Gabbard, & Ortigo, Chapter 3, this volume).

Modern Concepts of Motivation

As a reaction against what he considered to be the excessive psychoanalytic (and behaviorist) search for childhood motivational origins of adult behavior, Allport introduced the notion of the "functional autonomy" of motives (1937), by which he meant that the motives actually influencing here-and-now adult behavior are not (or are not any longer) derived from original "primitive" or "primary" drives such as libido or childhood experiences. More formally, functional autonomy presumes an "acquired system of motivation in which the tensions involved are not of the same kind as the antecedent tensions from which the acquired system developed" (Allport, 1961, p. 229).

From the beginning, the concept of functional autonomy was criticized, and it is fair to say that personality psychologists have not accepted it. On the other hand, Allport's argument certainly anticipated several important motivational developments in the last half-century: (1) Rogers's (1959) concept of actualization as a motivational force—that capacities can create their own motivation—which is manifest in recent work on self-determination theory and intrinsic motivation (Ryan & Deci, 2000); (2) the contrast between motivational orientations toward "process" versus "results" (phrased as "mastery" versus "performance" in the case of achievement; Elliot & Church, 1997); (3) the difference between motives to approach desired goals and motives to avoid aversive states of affairs (e.g., Elliot, Gable, & Mapes, 2006); and (4) the notion that age-graded tasks derived from cultural imperatives create "motivation" through mechanisms such

as "life tasks," "goals," or "personal projects" (Little, 1999, 2005).

In recent years, terror management theory (Pyszczynski, Greenberg, & Solomon, 1997), drawing on the work of Becker (1973) and Rank (1931/1936), asserted that fear of death and annihilation is a fundamental human motive. When mortality is made salient through a variety of cues both obvious and subtle, people engage in a wide variety of actions intended to reinforce their fundamental values. So far, terror management research has concentrated on situations that arouse mortality salience; yet it seems likely that although fear of death may be a universal human motive, it assumes different forms and drives different actions in different people.

Measuring Motives through Thematic Apperception

Among the many novel assessment procedures introduced in Murray's (1938) *Explorations in Personality*, the TAT (Morgan & Murray, 1935) is undoubtedly the most famous and widely used. Although psychologists developed many ways to interpret and score the TAT (see Gieser & Stein, 1999), the empirically derived motive measures pioneered by McClelland are noteworthy (see C. P. Smith, 1992; Winter, 1998), because they were based on changes in thematic apperception actually produced by experimental arousal of motives.

Application to Cognate Fields

Using thematic apperceptive measures, McClelland expanded the application of personality psychology to other social sciences. Achievement motivation, for example, is a major personality impetus to entrepreneurship and economic growth (McClelland, 1961; Spangler, 1992), whereas power motivation is related to charisma and management success (House, Spangler, & Woycke, 1991), and high power combined with low affiliation motivation predict aggression and war (Winter, 1993).

McClelland (1989) linked TAT-measured motives to physiological mechanisms, immune system functioning, and vulnerability to infectious diseases. In recent years, Schultheiss and his colleagues have demonstrated several complex relationships between particular motives and specific hormones—for example, between power motivation and testosterone, and between affiliation and progesterone (see Schultheiss, Chapter 24, this volume).

Psychometric Issues

The early popularity of TAT-based motive measures diminished in reaction to criticisms about low internal consistency and temporal reliability, as well as the consistent lack of correlation between TAT measures and questionnaire measures of the presumed "same" constructs. Because motives wax and wane, and because a given motive can drive a variety of quite different actions, many traditional methodological principles and rules, such as internal consistency and coefficient alpha, are not fully appropriate to motive concepts and thematic apperceptive measures (see Winter & Stewart, 1977). McClelland, Koestner, and Weinberger (1989) argued that TAT and direct questionnaire measures reflect two fundamentally different motive systems—one unconscious or "implicit," the other conscious and self-attributed. Recent research suggests that congruence between these two independent motivational systems is associated with psychological well-being (see also Brunstein & Maier, 2005).

COGNITIONS AND PERSONALITY

The "cognitive revolution" of the late 1950s and early 1960s had major effects on the field of personality (see Blake & Ramsey, 1951, for an early review). Early research on cognitive style reflected the influence of Witkin (e.g., 1949) and Kelly (1955), whose theory of personal constructs dispensed completely with motivation. Kelly's ideas inspired several measures of cognitive complexity (e.g., Bieri, 1955; Suedfeld, Tetlock, & Streufert, 1992). Although drawn from psychoanalysis, ego development (Loevinger & Blasi, 1976) as concept and measure shares substantial construct and empirical validity with cognitive complexity measures. Bandura (e.g., 2001) and Mischel, a former student of Kelly, used cognitive concepts to broaden learning theories of personality (Mischel & Shoda, Chapter 7, this volume). The development of causal attribution theory in social psychology led to a concern with attributional or explanatory style as a personality variable (see Weiner & Graham, 1999). Explanatory style has been linked to depression, performance, health, and other significant life outcomes (e.g., Wise & Rosqvist, 2006). Cognitive strategies have generated considerable research (e.g., Norem & Chang, 2002).

"Self"-Related Personality Variables

While personality psychologists had long recognized the importance of the self (e.g., Allport, 1937), the cognitive revolution brought a proliferation of "self-" related variables (see Higgins & Scholer, Chapter 6, this volume; Robins, Tracy, & Trzesniewski, Chapter 16, this volume): self-concept (Wylie, 1974–1979), self-schema (Markus, 1977), self-esteem (Rosenberg, 1979), self-monitoring (Snyder, 1987), and self-regulation (Gailliot, Mead, & Baumeister, Chapter 18, this volume; Carver, Scheier, & Fulford, Chapter 29, this volume). Classic early 20th-century concepts of the role of the "generalized other" (George Herbert Mead) and the "looking-glass self" (Charles Horton Cooley) influenced the symbolic interactionism approach (see Gordon & Gergen, 1968), which suggests that our self-concepts reflect our views of others' perceptions of, and responses to, us. With the advent of postmodernism and the notion of multiple selves (Gergen, 1991) came the concept of a "dialogical self" (e.g., Hermans, 2001).

Erikson's (1950/1963) psychosocial elaboration of psychoanalysis was most fully developed around the concept of ego identity (Erikson, 1959/1980), which involved congruence between people's inner sense of self and the external social definition they receive. Using the identity concept, Erikson analyzed the lives of historical figures such as Luther (Erikson, 1958) and Gandhi (Erikson, 1969). Marcia and his colleagues (Marcia, Waterman, Matteson, Archer, & Orlofski, 1993) developed methods for measuring different aspects of identity. As a conceptual bridge between the individual and society, identity also proved particularly useful in analyzing *social identity*, or the role that social variables such as gender, race, class, and nationality play in the formation of personality (e.g., Postmes & Jetten, 2006). McAdams (Chapter 8, this volume) has suggested a "life story" model of identity. Coincident with "self psychology" (Kohut & Strozier, 1985) and perhaps Lasch's (1979) analysis of the "culture of narcissism" came increased research interest in the psychoanalytic concept of narcissism (Ames, Rose, & Anderson, 2006; Wink, 1992). Epstein's (2003) cognitive–experiential self theory suggested the interaction of rational and unconscious information-processing systems.

THE SOCIAL CONTEXT OF PERSONALITY

In many different (though apparently unrelated) ways, personality psychologists have long been concerned about context. Early in the 20th century, the study of personality came under the sway of behaviorism and the prestige of experimental research on learning. Later, the culture and personality movement stressed the broader social–cultural matrix in which personality is formed. In the late 1960s and 1970s, the situationist critique of personality caused a major crisis in the field and led to a reexamination of fundamental postulates and research methods. Finally, at the turn of the century, the rise of "cultural psychology" and the influence of feminist and other critical perspectives from the humanities, as well as a more global perspective, generated new interest in the social and cultural macro-contexts of personality.

The Influence of Behaviorism

Even as the early personality psychologists were measuring certain socially important traits, early behaviorists such as Watson were trying to reduce personality to conditioning and instrumental learning processes. Watson and Rayner's (1920) famous "Little Albert" demonstration had an enduring influence, despite its many methodological faults and lack of consistent replication (see Harris, 1979). At Yale University during the 1930s and 1940s, the Institute of Human Relations, under the leadership of Hull, tried to bring about a synthesis of psychoanalytic theory and an experimental psychology that was self-consciously striving for immaculate purity of method (see Morawski, 1986). At the behaviorist extreme, Skinner (1953) proposed to dispense with personality theory and constructs altogether.

The Rise and Fall of Culture and Personality

Beginning in the 1930s, as anthropologist and psychoanalysts became interested in on another's disciplines, the field of "culture and personality" tried to connect a culture's distinctive patterns of childrearing with modal adult personalities and cultural themes. (Benedict's 1946 study of Japan is a classic example.) During World War II, culture and personality research contributed to the U.S. war effort with studies of enemies—and allies (see Herman, 1995, Ch. 2).

After the war, the domain of culture and personality inspired interdisciplinary edited volumes (e.g., Kluckhohn & Murray, 1953) and interdisciplinary programs such as Harvard's Department of Social Relations. The Human Relations Area Files (Murdock, 1982) facilitated systematic cross-cultural research on personality (e.g., Whiting & Child, 1953). By the late 1950s, however, the intellectual climate had clearly changed. The methodological and conceptual critiques leveled by Inkeles and Levinson (1954) met with no real response; meanwhile, the Cold War climate of suspicion about the social sciences, recognition of the complexity of culture, the "cognitive revolution," and the prestige of experimentation (e.g., Milgram, 1974) all combined to bring psychologists in from the social–cultural field to the laboratory. Nevertheless, personality researchers have continued to develop new methods for cross-national personality research (e.g., Hofer, Chasiotis, Friedlmeier, Busch, & Campos, 2005; McClelland, 1961; McCrae, Terracciano, & Personality Profiles of Cultures Project, 2005).

Mischel's Critique and Personality's Response

Although its title, *Personality and Assessment*, was innocent enough, Mischel's book (1968) had the effect of a bombshell. Reviewing the field, Mischel claimed that the usefulness of broad dispositional personality variables had been seriously overstated, because they did not show cross-situational or temporal consistency and were not highly correlated with behavioral outcomes. In place of the usual array of personality variables, Mischel advocated use of a highly specific, almost idiographic, version of social learning eory. Later, Mischel and Shoda (Chapter 7, this volume) emphasized cognitive variables, so that Mischel's theory, along with that of Bandura (e.g., 2001), became known as social-cognitive theory.

After some initial disorientation, personality psychologists replied (see Winter, 1996, Ch. 16): some with improved measurement techniques (Epstein, 1979); others with longitudinal studies showing impressive consistency of personality; still others demonstrated the effects of moderator variables or interaction between personality and situational variables (Magnusson & Endler, 1977; see also Caspi, Elder, & Bem, 1987). Influenced by feminist theory, personality researchers have adapted the notion of "intersectionality" to personality research, especially research involving gender (Stewart & McDermott, 2004).

Cultural and Cross-Cultural Psychology

During the 1990s, perhaps as a response to the increasing globalization of economic, social, and intellectual life, personality psychology began to be influenced by the perspectives of cultural psychology (Benet-Martínez & Oishi, Chapter 21, this volume; Shweder, 1991). Some researchers studied psychological processes in particular cultures; others (Nisbett, 2003) made more sweeping claims about psychological differences between "East" and "West." Hofstede (2001) identified five dimensions along which cultures can be compared: individualism–collectivism, power distance, orientation to uncertainty, gendering of male–female relations, and long-term future time perspective. So far, though, the first dimension has received the most attention from personality psychologists interested in culture (e.g., Markus & Kitayama, 1991).

BIOLOGICAL BASES OF PERSONALITY

From the time of Galen's famous theory of humors, people have speculated about links between personality, or mind, and biology, or body. For example, Freud anchored his theory in biology, Allport referred to "psychophysical systems" underlying personality (1937, p. 48), and Murray defined needs as "physico-chemical" forces in the brain (1938, p. 124). Largely forgotten today, Sheldon's early research linking physique and personality types (e.g., Sheldon, Stevens, & Tucker, 1940) appeared so promising that his Harvard colleagues agreed to have their own "somatotypes" measured (Allport, 1940; Boring, 1952). In the mid-20th century, Eysenck began a sustained effort to link the trait factors of extraversion, neuroticism, and psychoticism to individual differences in nervous system structures and functioning. From an early focus on excitation and inhibition (Eysenck, 1957, 1967), he turned to arousal and brain structures such as the reticular formation and the limbic system (Eysenck, 1990; Eysenck & Eysenck, 1985). Alternative models of the biological bases of traits include those proposed by Gray (e.g., Pickering & Gray, 1999) and Cloninger (e.g., 1998).

Biological approaches to personality have flourished in recent years (e.g., Canli, Chapter 11, this volume; Zuckerman, 2005), as has evolutionary psychology, which has expanded from a general focus on human nature to questions of individual differences (Buss, Chapter 2, this volume; Nettle, 2005). Indeed, Funder (2001) labeled evolutionary theory and biology "new paradigms" for personality (p. 197). Regarding the latter, he noted that "two very different methodologies, behavioral genetics and physiology/anatomy, converge on the inescapable conclusion that stable individual differences in personality are to a large extent biologically based" (p. 201). Reviewing limitations of these approaches, however, Funder also noted the dangers of going "beyond the data" (p. 207) and jumping to "simplistic, one-cause → one-effect conclusions" (p. 206) about what are actually complicated multi-directional relationships among biological factors and behavioral patterns.

PUTTING THE PERSON BACK TOGETHER

The postwar flowering of personality psychology was marked by debates between researchers who emphasized one of the elements of personality—traits, motives, cognitions, contexts, or biological factors—and their opponents who emphasized other elements. Some of these debates revived controversies that had first emerged much earlier in the history of the field. In this section we discuss examples of these recurrent issues and then consider more recent trends, including the emergence, around the turn of the 21st century, of calls for more integrative models of personality and the revival of interest in studies of individual lives.

One example of a debate that revived an earlier controversy was the "person–situation" debate of the 1970s and 1980s, sparked by Mischel's (1968) critique of personality variables as poor predictors of cross-situational and temporal consistency in behavior. Many of the issues raised in response to Mischel's challenge echoed Allport's defense of traits against the situationist "doctrine of specificity" (1937, p. 249) some 40 years earlier. Interestingly, both sides of the later person–situation debate tended to overlook Allport's (1931, 1937) suggestion that apparently inconsistent behaviors in different situations might still indicate an *underlying* trait. As Funder (Chapter 22, this volume) notes, the persistence of this debate, despite general agreement with an interactionist view, suggests that deeper values may be at stake.

Personality theory and research have also been the site of many skirmishes regarding the relative contributions of biological and environmental factors. For example, over the past hundred years the "nature–nurture" controversy—whether our personalities are the result of genes or of rearing and environment—has appeared in various guises, often generating more argumentative heat than intellectual illumination. Extreme statements on one side or the other continue to appear, despite general endorsement of interactionist views. This bitterness and persistence suggest that the controversy may have been a surrogate or proxy for the clash of deeper social and political views (see Pervin, 2003). Thus as the American population (and especially its power structure) diversified from its original northern European base, personality psychologists debated the importance of genetic inheritance versus environment and training. Was it really possible for these "new" groups to develop the intelligence, skills, and "manners" of the American elite groups? In personality psychology, this position (usually identified with the political left) was identified with behaviorists, learning theorists, and scholars inclined toward sociology and anthropology. Or did their genes (in earlier decades, "blood" or "bloodlines") set limits to their potential and thereby boundaries to their status and opportunities? This politically conservative position was identified with psychological researchers who were first-born, of higher status, and who had ancestors that were born in the United States (see Sherwood & Nataupsky, 1968). In the end, serious scholars of genetics demonstrated that "heritability" is a complex concept, that genes always interact with environments, and that sweeping conclusions about "nature" versus "nurture" are not really scientific questions. Recent work has focused on identifying specific genes that moderate individuals' responses to environmental stresses (Krueger & Johnson, Chapter 10, this volume).

Darwin's discoveries and his theory of evolution suggest that our genetic inheritance, in turn, has been shaped and is continually being reshaped by environmental forces—albeit at a pace that is usually impossible to detect by simple observation. In the decades between the publication of Darwin's *On the Origin of Species* in 1859 and the First World War, some social theorists reworked his ideas into "social Darwinism," a naive and crude ideology that seemed to justify the position of elite groups. This philosophy influenced early psychological research on the heritability of intelligence and the psychology of sex differences (see Pervin, 2003). In recent decades, many personality psychologists have used neo-Darwinian ideas to construct an evolutionary psychology of personality (e.g., Buss, Chapter 2, this volume; McAdams & Pals, 2006; see also Funder, 2001).

While few would doubt that in a general sense, human beings possess a wide variety of adapted and adaptive mechanisms, the relatively brief span of recorded history (and the tiny "blink" of personality research data) in relation to the vast stretches of evolutionary time make it difficult to draw firm conclusions about the precise ways in which personality—and differing individual *personalities*—may be shaped by evolutionary forces (see Buller, 2005; Gowaty, 2001). As a result, evolutionary accounts often draw upon the subjunctive mode (this "might have happened") and employ metaphorical concepts such as "tactics" and "strategy" to refer to physical forms and behaviors that Darwin described as the result of the blind, unintelligent force of natural selection. Some critics suggest that the surplus connotative meaning in these metaphors is a sign of the intrusion of interests into science and scholarship; for example, they connect the concern to establish an evolutionary basis for sex differences and male dominance with the threat to male status resulting from the transformation in gender roles in the last third of the 20th century (e.g., Segal, 2000). Others question the universality of behaviors explained by evolutionary psychology and test alternative explanations that emphasize social and cultural factors. For example, some evolutionary personality psychologists have examined male–female differences in "reproductive strategies" and the personality processes that underlie them (see, e.g., Buss & Schmitt, 1993), arguing that these reflect universal patterns of evolved personality differences between women and men. However, a reanalysis of typical findings from this research (Eagly & Wood, 1999) showed cross-cultural variation, with smaller sex differences in mate preferences in cultures with greater gender equality; thus cultural and social factors—stratification, power, and roles—may better account for the observed results (see also Gowaty, 2001; Pervin, 2003). In the long run—and the evolutionary run is surely "long"—personality research guided by evolutionary theory is likely to produce complex and nuanced results that integrate contributions from both evolutionary and cultural determinants.

Like the person–situation and biology–environment controversies, the more general question of what units to employ (see Pervin, 2003), or what elements are essential to an understanding of personality, has arisen repeatedly throughout the history of personality psychology, often beginning with exchanges of one-sided arguments and moving toward more interactionist positions. For example, noting the longstanding "rivalry" between traditions emphasizing either traits or motives, Winter and colleagues (1998, p. 230) have shown that traits and motives interact in predicting behavior. Similarly, social cognitive theory has expanded to include dispositions and affects (see Mischel and Shoda, Chapter 7, this volume).

Each of these trends suggests the importance of recognizing the complexity of personality, which involves interactions of factors ranging from biology to history (Winter & Barenbaum, 1999)—putting the person back together, rather than emphasizing one element or another. Following the postwar elaboration of specific constructs and the ensuing debates, personality psychologists began to call for more integrative approaches to understanding the person. Such calls have increased since the turn of the 21st century (e.g., Funder, 2001; McAdams & Pals, 2006; McAdams, Chapter 8, this volume; Mischel & Shoda, Chapter 7, this volume) and include the application of dynamical systems theory to the personality domain (e.g., Vallacher, Read, & Nowak, 2002) as well as a renewed emphasis on within-person structures and processes (e.g., Cervone, 2005). As many of the chapters in this volume suggest, personality psychologists continue to develop multidimensional models and multidisciplinary approaches to the study of personality.

An important aspect of "putting the person back together" is the resurgence of interest in the study of individual lives, increasingly apparent since the 1980s (e.g., Runyan, 1982; see Barenbaum & Winter, 2003). By the turn of the 21st century, studies of lives by a broad range of personality psychologists had appeared (e.g., Elms, 1994; Franz & Stewart, 1994; McAdams & Ochberg, 1988; Nasby & Read, 1997). Recent studies have drawn on developments in disciplines ranging from neurobiology (e.g., Ogilvie, 2004) to political science (e.g., Post, 2003). Examples of works signaling more general acceptance of this approach include a series on narrative studies of lives published by the American Psychological Association (e.g., McAdams, Josselson, & Lieblich, 2006), a comprehensive *Handbook of Psychobiography* (Schultz, 2005), and a chapter on psychobiographical methods in a handbook of research methods in personality psychology (Elms, 2007). We see both of these trends—the recent efforts toward integration and the revival of interest in studies of individual personalities—as hopeful steps toward fulfilling the historical mission of personality psychology: "to provide *an integrative framework for understanding the whole person*" (McAdams & Pals, 2006, p. 204, original emphasis).

NOTES

1. Murray studied several additional needs less formally.
2. Some behaviorists simply ridiculed concepts such as the unconscious, whereas others tried to translate them, for example, as "behavior that has become unverbalizable, due to conflicting reinforcement contingencies."

REFERENCES

Allport, F. H., & Allport, G. W. (1921). Personality traits: Their classification and measurement. *Journal of Abnormal Psychology and Social Psychology, 16*, 6–40.

Allport, G. W. (1921). Personality and character. *Psychological Bulletin, 18*, 441–455.

Allport, G. W. (1922). *An experimental study of the traits of personality, with application to the problem of social diagnosis.* Unpublished doctoral dissertation, Harvard University.

Allport, G. W. (1923). The Leipzig Congress of Psychology. *American Journal of Psychology, 34*, 612–615.

Allport, G. W. (1924). The standpoint of Gestalt psychology. *Psyche, 4*, 354–361.

Allport, G. W. (1927). Concepts of trait and personality. *Psychological Bulletin, 24*, 284–293.

Allport, G. W. (1928). A test for ascendance–submission. *Journal of Abnormal and Social Psychology, 23*, 118–136.

Allport, G. W. (1929). The study of personality by the intuitive method: An experiment in teaching from *The Locomotive God. Journal of Abnormal and Social Psychology, 24*, 14–27.

Allport, G. W. (1931). What is a trait of personality? *Journal of Abnormal and Social Psychology, 25*, 368–372.

Allport, G. W. (1934). [Letter to C. A. Murchison, 1 January]. G. W. Allport Papers, Harvard University Archives, Cambridge, MA.

Allport, G. W. (1935). Attitudes. In C. A. Murchison & W. C. Allee (Eds.), *A handbook of social psychology* (pp. 798–844). Worcester, MA: Clark University Press.

Allport, G. W. (1937). *Personality: A psychological interpretation.* New York: Henry Holt.

Allport, G. W. (1940). [Letter to W. H. Sheldon, 23 July]. G. W. Allport Papers, Harvard University Archives, Cambridge, MA.

Allport, G. W. (1942). *The use of personal documents in psychological science.* New York: Social Science Research Council.

Allport, G. W. (1961). *Pattern and growth in personality.* New York: Holt, Rinehart & Winston.

Allport, G. W. (1965). *Letters from Jenny.* New York: Harcourt, Brace, & World.

Allport, G. W. (1967). Gordon W. Allport. In E. G. Boring & G. Lindzey (Eds.), *A history of psychology in autobiography* (Vol. 5, pp. 1–25). New York: Appleton-Century-Crofts.

Allport, G. W., & Odbert, H. S. (1936). Trait-names: A psycho-lexical study. *Psychological Monographs, 47*(1), 1–171, No. 211.

Allport, G. W., & Vernon, P. E. (1930). The field of personality. *Psychological Bulletin, 27*, 677–730.

Ames, D. R., Rose, P., & Anderson, C. P. (2006). The NPI-16 as a short measure of narcissism. *Journal of Research in Personality, 40*, 440–450.

Asendorpf, J. B., Caspi, A., & Hofstee, W. B. K. (Eds.). (2002). The puzzle of personality types [Special issue]. *European Journal of Personality, 16.*

Bakan, D. (1966). *The duality of human existence: An essay on psychology and religion.* Chicago: Rand McNally.

Bandura, A. (2001). Social cognitive theory: An agentic perspective. *Annual Review of Psychology, 52*, 1–26.

Barenbaum, N. B. (1997). The case(s) of Gordon Allport. *Journal of Personality, 65*, 743–755.

Barenbaum, N. B. (2000). How social was personality?: The Allports' "connection" of social and personality psychology. *Journal of the History of the Behavioral Sciences, 36*, 471–487.

Barenbaum, N. B. (2006). Henry A. Murray: Personology as biography, science, and art. In D. A. Dewsbury, L. T. Benjamin, & M. Wertheimer (Eds.), *Portraits of pioneers in psychology* (Vol. VI, pp. 169–187). Washington, DC: American Psychological Association.

Barenbaum, N. B., & Winter, D. G. (2003). Personality. In D. K. Freedheim (Ed.), *Handbook of psychology: Vol. 1. History of psychology* (pp. 177–203). New York: Wiley.

Barton, S. (1994). Chaos, self-organization, and psychology. *American Psychologist, 49*, 5–14.

Becker, E. (1973). *The denial of death.* New York: Free Press.

Benedict, R. (1946). *The chrysanthemum and the sword: Patterns of Japanese culture.* Boston: Houghton Mifflin.

Berman, L. (1921). *The glands regulating personality: A study of the glands of internal secretion in relation to the types of human nature.* New York: Macmillan.

Bieri, J. (1955). Cognitive complexity–simplicity and predictive behavior. *Journal of Abnormal and Social Psychology, 51*, 263–268.

Blake, R. R., & Ramsey, G. V. (1951). *Perception: An approach to personality.* New York: Ronald Press.

Block, J. (1971). *Lives through time.* Berkeley, CA: Bancroft Books.

Block, J. (1995). A contrarian view of the five-factor approach to personality description. *Psychological Bulletin, 117*, 187–215.

Borgatta, E. F., & Lambert, W. W. (1968). *Handbook of personality theory and research*. Chicago: Rand McNally.

Boring, E. G. (1952). Edwin Garrigues Boring. In E. G. Boring, H. S. Langfeld, H. Werner, & R. M. Yerkes (Eds.), *A history of psychology in autobiography* (Vol. 4, pp. 27–52). New York: Russell & Russell.

Bray, D. W. (1982). The assessment center and the study of lives. *American Psychologist, 37*, 180–189.

Brunstein, J. C., & Maier, G. W. (2005). Implicit and self-attributed motives to achieve: Two separate but interacting needs. *Journal of Personality and Social Psychology, 89*, 205–222.

Bryson, D. R. (2002). *Socializing the young: The role of foundations, 1923–1941*. Westport, CT: Bergin & Garvey.

Buller, D. J. (2005). *Adapting minds: Evolutionary psychology and the persistent quest for human nature*. Cambridge, MA: MIT Press.

Bulmer, M. (1984). *The Chicago school of sociology: Institutionalization, diversity and the rise of sociological research*. Chicago: University of Chicago Press.

Burgess, E. W. (1927). Statistics and case studies as methods of sociological research. *Sociology and Social Research, 12*, 103–120.

Burnham, J. C. (1968). The new psychology: From narcissism to social control. In J. Braeman, R. H. Bremner, & D. Brody (Eds.), *Change and continuity in twentieth-century America: The 1920's* (pp. 351–398). Columbus: Ohio State University Press.

Buss, D. M., & Schmitt, D. P. (1993). Sexual strategies theory: An evolutionary perspective on human mating. *Psychological Review, 100*, 204–232.

Campbell, D. T., & Fiske, D. W. (1959). Convergent and discriminant validity by the multitrait–multimethod matrix. *Psychological Bulletin, 56*, 81–105.

Carlson, R. (1971). Where is the person in personality research? *Psychological Bulletin, 75*, 203–219.

Caspi, A., Elder, G. H., & Bem, D. J. (1987). Moving against the world: Life-course patterns of explosive children. *Developmental Psychology, 23*, 308–313.

Caspi, A., Roberts, B. W., & Shiner, R. L. (2005). Personality development: Stability and change. *Annual Review of Psychology, 56*, 453–484.

Cattell, R. B. (1943). The description of personality: Basic traits resolved into clusters. *Journal of Abnormal and Social Psychology, 38*, 476–506.

Cattell, R. B. (1946). *Description and measurement of personality*. Yonkers-on-Hudson, NY: World Book.

Cervone, D. (2005). Personality architecture: Within-person structures and processes. *Annual Review of Psychology, 56*, 423–452.

Cloninger, C. R. (1998). The genetics and psychobiology of the seven-factor model of personality. In K. R. Silk (Ed.), *Biology of personality disorders* (pp. 63–92). Washington, DC: American Psychiatric Association.

Cohen, S. (1983). The mental hygiene movement, the development of personality and the school: The medicalization of American education. *History of Education Quarterly, 23*, 123–149.

Cohler, B. J. (1993). Describing lives: Gordon Allport and the "science" of personality. In K. H. Craik, R. Hogan, & R. N. Wolfe (Eds.), *Fifty years of personality psychology* (pp. 131–146). New York: Plenum Press.

Costa, P. T., Jr., & McCrae, R. R. (1992a). Four ways five factors are basic. *Personality and Individual Differences, 13*, 653–665.

Costa, P. T., Jr., & McCrae, R. R. (1992b). "Four ways five factors are not basic": Reply. *Personality and Individual Differences, 13*, 861–865.

Craik, K. H., Hogan, R., & Wolfe, R. N. (Eds.). (1993). *Fifty years of personality psychology*. New York: Plenum Press.

Crider, B. (1936). Who is a psychologist? *School and Society, 43*, 370–371.

Cronbach, L. J. (1951). Coefficient alpha and the internal structure of tests. *Psychometrika, 16*, 297–334.

Danziger, K. (1990). *Constructing the subject: Historical origins of psychological research*. New York: Cambridge University Press.

Danziger, K. (1997). *Naming the mind: How psychology found its language*. Thousand Oaks, CA: Sage.

Darwin, C. (1859). *On the origin of the species by means of natural selection: or, The preservation of favoured races in the struggle for life*. London: J. Murray.

Eagly, A. H., & Wood, W. (1999). The origins of sex differences in human behavior: Evolved dispositions versus social roles. *American Psychologist, 54*, 408–423.

Elliot, A. J., & Church, M. A. (1997). A hierarchical model of approach and avoidance achievement motivation. *Journal of Personality and Social Psychology, 72*, 218–232.

Elliot, A. J., Gable, S. L., & Mapes, R. R. (2006). Approach and avoidance motivation in the social domain. *Personality and Social Psychology Bulletin, 32*, 378–391.

Elliott, R. M. (1939). The Harvard *Explorations in Personality* [Review of the book *Explorations in personality: A clinical and experimental study of fifty men of college age*]. *American Journal of Psychology, 52*, 453–462.

Elms, A. C. (1994). *Uncovering lives: The uneasy alliance of biography and psychology*. New York: Oxford University Press.

Elms, A. C. (2007). Psychobiography and case study methods. In R. W. Robins, R. C. Fraley, & R. F. Krueger (Eds.), *Handbook of research methods in personality psychology* (pp. 97–113). New York: Guilford Press.

Emmons, R. A., & McAdams, D. P. (Eds.). (1995). Levels and domains in personality [Special issue]. *Journal of Personality, 63*(3).

Epstein, S. (1979). The stability of behavior: I. On predicting most of the people much of the time. *Journal of Personality and Social Psychology, 37*, 1097–1126.

Epstein, S. (2003). Cognitive–experiential self-theory of personality. In T. Millon & M. J. Lerner (Eds.), *Handbook of psychology: Vol. 5. Personality and social psychology* (pp. 159–184). New York: Wiley.

Erdelyi, M. H. (1985). *Psychoanalysis: Freud's cognitive psychology*. New York: Freeman.

Erikson, E. H. (1958). *Young man Luther*. New York: Norton.

Erikson, E. H. (1963). *Childhood and society* (2nd ed.). New York: Norton. (Original work published 1950)

Erikson, E. H. (1969). *Gandhi's truth*. New York: Norton.

Erikson, E. H. (1980). *Identity and the life cycle: Selected papers*. New York: Norton. (Original work published 1959)

Eysenck, H. J. (1957). *The dynamics of anxiety and hysteria: An experimental application of modern learning theory to psychiatry*. London: Routledge & Kegan Paul.

Eysenck, H. J. (1967). *The biological basis of personality*. Springfield, IL: Thomas.

Eysenck, H. J. (1990). Biological dimensions of personality. In L. A. Pervin (Ed.), *Handbook of personality: Theory and research* (pp. 244–276). New York: Guilford Press.

Eysenck, H. J. (1992a). Four ways five factors are not basic. *Personality and Individual Differences, 13*, 667–673.

Eysenck, H. J. (1992b). A reply to Costa and McCrae: P or A and C—the role of theory. *Personality and Individual Differences, 13*, 867–868.

Eysenck, H. J., & Eysenck, M. W. (1985). *Personality and individual differences: A natural science approach*. New York: Plenum Press.

Fancher, R. E. (2000). Snapshots of Freud in America, 1899–1999. *American Psychologist, 55*, 1025–1028.

Fernald, G. G. (1920). Character vs. intelligence in personality studies. *Journal of Abnormal Psychology, 15*, 1–10.

Fisher, S., & Greenberg, R. P. (1977). *The scientific credibility of Freud's theories and therapy*. New York: Basic Books.

Forrester, J. (1996). If *p*, then what?: Thinking in cases. *History of the Human Sciences, 9*(3), 1–25.

Franz, C. E., & Stewart, A. J. (1994). *Women creating lives: Identities, resilience, and resistance*. Boulder, CO: Westview.

Freud, A. (1946). *The ego and the mechanisms of defense*. New York: International Universities Press. (Original work published 1937)

Freud, S. (1955). Beyond the pleasure principle. In J. Strachey (Ed. & Trans.), *The standard edition of the complete psychological works of Sigmund Freud* (Vol. 18, pp. 7–64). London: Hogarth Press. (Original work published 1920)

Freud, S. (1957). Five lectures on psycho-analysis. In J. Strachey (Ed. & Trans.), *The standard edition of the complete psychological works of Sigmund Freud* (Vol. 11, pp. 7–55). London: Hogarth Press. (Original work published 1910)

Freud, S. (1957). Some character types met with in psycho-analytic work. In J. Strachey (Ed. & Trans.), *The standard edition of the complete psychological works of Sigmund Freud* (Vol. 14, pp. 309–333). London: Hogarth Press. (Original work published 1916)

Freud, S. (1959). Character and anal erotism. In J. Strachey (Ed. & Trans.), *The standard edition of the complete psychological works of Sigmund Freud* (Vol. 9, pp. 169–175). London: Hogarth Press. (Original work published 1908)

Freud, S. (1961–1963). Introductory lectures on psycho-analysis. In J. Strachey (Ed. & Trans.), *The standard edition of the complete psychological works of Sigmund Freud* (Vols. 15 and 16). London: Hogarth Press. (Original work published 1916–1917)

Freud, S. (1964). New introductory lectures on psycho-analysis. In J. Strachey (Ed. & Trans.), *The standard edition of the complete psychological works of Sigmund Freud* (Vol. 22, pp. 5–182). London: Hogarth Press. (Original work published 1933)

Funder, D. C. (2001). Personality. *Annual Review of Psychology, 52*, 197–221.

Gergen, K. J. (1991). *The saturated self: Dilemmas of identity in contemporary life*. New York: Basic Books.

Gieser, L., & Stein, M. I. (1999). *Evocative images: The Thematic Apperception Test and the art of projection*. Washington, DC: American Psychological Association.

Gordon, C., & Gergen, K. J. (Eds.). (1968). *The self in social interaction*. New York: Wiley.

Gough, H. G. (1957). *California Psychological Inventory: Manual*. Palo Alto, CA: Consulting Psychologists Press.

Gough, H. G. (1987). *California Psychological Inventory: Administrator's guide*. Palo Alto, CA: Consulting Psychologists Press.

Gowaty, P. A. (2001). Women, psychology, and evolution. In R. K. Unger (Ed.), *Handbook* of the psychology of women and gender (pp. 53–65). Hoboken, NJ: Wiley.

Greenwald, A. G., Banaji, M. R., Rudman, L. A., Farnham, S. D., Nosek, B. A., & Mellott, D. S. (2002). A unified theory of implicit attitudes, stereotypes, self-esteem, and self-concept. Psychological Review, 109, 3–25.

Grice, J. W., Jackson, B. J., & McDaniel, B. L. (2006). Bridging the idiographic–nomothetic divide: A follow-up study. Journal of Personality, 74, 1191–1218.

Guilford, J. P. (1936). Unitary traits of personality and factor theory. American Journal of Psychology, 48, 673–680.

Guilford, J. P. (1938). [Review of the book Personality: A psychological interpretation]. Journal of Abnormal and Social Psychology, 33, 414–420.

Hale, N. G. (1971). Freud and the Americans: The beginnings of psychoanalysis in the United States, 1876–1917. New York: Oxford University Press.

Harris, B. (1979). Whatever happened to Little Albert? American Psychologist, 34, 151–160.

Helgeson, V. S. (1994). Relation of agency and communion to well-being: Evidence and potential explanations. Psychological Bulletin, 116, 412–428.

Herman, E. (1995). The romance of American psychology: Political culture in the age of experts, 1940–1970. Berkeley: University of California Press.

Hermans, H. J. M. (2001). The dialogical self: Toward a theory of personal and cultural positioning. Culture and Psychology, 7, 243–281.

Hofer, J., Chasiotis, A., Friedlmeier, W., Busch, H., & Campos, D. (2005). The measurement of implicit motives in three cultures: Power and affiliation in Cameroon, Costa Rica, and Germany. Journal of Cross-Cultural Psychology, 36, 689–716.

Hofstede, G. H. (2001). Culture's consequences: Comparing values, behaviors, institutions, and organizations across nations (2nd ed.). Thousand Oaks, CA: Sage.

Hornstein, G. A. (1992). The return of the repressed: Psychology's problematic relations with psychoanalysis, 1909–1960. American Psychologist, 47, 254–263.

House, R. J., Spangler, W. D., & Woycke, J. (1991). Personality and charisma in the U. S. presidency: A psychological theory of leader effectiveness. Administrative Science Quarterly, 36, 364–396.

Inkeles, A., & Levinson, D. J. (1954). National character: The study of modal personality and sociocultural systems. In G. Lindzey (Ed.), Handbook of social psychology (Vol. 2, pp. 977–1020). Cambridge, MA: Addison-Wesley.

Jackson, D. N. (1974). The Personality Research Form. Port Huron, MI: Research Psychologists Press.

Jackson, D. N., & Tremblay, P. F. (2002). The six factor personality questionnaire. In B. de Raad & M. Perugini (Eds.), Big Five assessment. Ashland, OH: Hogrefe & Huber.

John, O. P., & Robins, R. W. (1993). Gordon Allport: Father and critic of the five-factor model. In K. H. Craik, R. Hogan, & R. N. Wolfe (Eds.), Fifty years of personality psychology (pp. 215–236). New York: Plenum Press.

Johnston, J. C. (1927). Biography: The literature of personality. New York: Century.

Jung, C. G. (1971). The collected works of C. G. Jung: Vol. 6. Psychological types (H. Read, M. Fordham, G. Adler, & W. McGuire, Eds.). Princeton, NJ: Princeton University Press. (Original work published 1923)

Kelly, G. A. (1955). The psychology of personal constructs. New York: Norton.

Kluckhohn, C., & Murray, H. A. (Eds.). (1953). Personality in nature, society, and culture (2nd ed.). New York: Knopf.

Kohut, H., & Strozier, C. B. (1985). Self psychology and the humanities: Reflections on a new psychoanalytic approach. New York: Norton.

Krueger, E. T. (1925). Autobiographical documents and personality. Unpublished doctoral dissertation, University of Chicago.

Lasch, C. (1979). The culture of narcissism: American life in an age of diminishing expectations. New York: Norton.

Laughlin, C. D. (1973). Discussion: The influence of Whitehead's organism upon Murray's personology. Journal of the History of the Behavioral Sciences, 9, 251–257.

Little, B. R. (1999). Personality and motivation: Personal action and the conative evolution. In L. A. Pervin & O. P. John (Eds.), Handbook of personality: Theory and research (2nd ed., pp. 501–524). New York: Guilford Press.

Little, B. R. (2005). Personality science and personal projects: Six impossible things before breakfast. Journal of Research in Personality, 39, 4–21.

Loevinger, J., & Blasi, A. (1976). Ego development: Conceptions and theories. San Francisco: Jossey-Bass.

Lombardo, G. P., & Foschi, R. (2003). The concept of personality in 19th-century French and 20th-century American psychology. History of Psychology, 6, 123–142.

MacKinnon, D. W. (1975). IPAR's contribution to the conceptualization and study of creativity. In I. A. Taylor & J. W. Getzells (Eds.), Perspectives in creativity. Chicago: Aldine.

Magnusson, D., & Endler, N. S. (1977). Personality at the crossroads: Current issues in international psychology. Hillsdale, NJ: Erlbaum.

Marcia, J. E., Waterman, A. S., Matteson, D. R., Archer, S. L., & Orlofsky, J. L. (Eds.). (1993).

Ego identity: A handbook for psychosocial research. New York: Springer-Verlag.

Markus, H. R. (1977). Self-schemata and processing information about the self. *Journal of Personality and Social Psychology, 35*, 63–78.

Markus, H. R., & Kitayama, S. (1991). Culture and the self: Implications for cognition, emotion, and motivation. *Psychological Review, 98*, 224–253.

McAdams, D. P. (1997). A conceptual history of personality psychology. In R. Hogan, J. Johnson, & S. Briggs (Eds.), *Handbook of personality psychology* (pp. 3–39). San Diego, CA: Academic Press.

McAdams, D. P., Josselson, R., & Lieblich, A. (2006). *Identity and story: Creating self in narrative*. Washington, DC: American Psychological Association.

McAdams, D. P., & Ochberg, R. L. (Eds.). (1988). *Psychobiography and life narratives*. Durham, NC: Duke University Press.

McAdams, D. P., & Pals, J. L. (2006). A new Big Five: Fundamental principles for an integrative science of personality. *American Psychologist, 61*, 204–217.

McAdams, D. P., & West, S. G. (1997). Introduction: Personality psychology and the case study. *Journal of Personality, 65*, 757–783.

McClelland, D. C. (1961). *The achieving society*. Princeton, NJ: Van Nostrand.

McClelland, D. C. (1989). Motivational factors in health and disease. *American Psychologist, 44*, 675–683.

McClelland, D. C., Koestner, R., & Weinberger, J. (1989). How do self-attributed and implicit motives differ? *Psychological Review, 96*, 690–702.

McCrae, R. R., Terracciano, A., & Personality Profiles of Cultures Project. (2005). Personality profiles of cultures: Aggregate personality traits. *Journal of Personality and Social Psychology, 89*, 407–425.

McLeod, J. (1992). The story of Henry Murray's diagnostic council: A case study in the demise of a scientific method. *Clinical Psychology Forum, 44*, 6–12.

Milgram, S. (1974). *Obedience to authority: An experimental view*. New York: Harper & Row.

Mischel, W. (1968). *Personality and assessment*. New York: Wiley.

Morawski, J. (1986). Organizing knowledge and behavior at Yale's Institute of Human Relations. *Isis, 77*, 219–242.

Morgan, C. D., & Murray, H. H. (1935). A method for investigating fantasies: The Thematic Apperception Test. *Archives of Neurology and Psychiatry (Chicago), 34*, 289–306.

Murchison, C. A., & Allee, W. C. (1935). *A handbook of social psychology*. Worcester, MA: Clark University Press.

Murdock, G. P. (1982). *Outline of cultural materials* (5th ed.). New Haven, CT: Human Relations Area Files.

Murphy, G. (1932). *An historical introduction to modern psychology* (4th ed.). New York: Harcourt, Brace.

Murphy, G., & Jensen, F. (1932). *Approaches to personality: Some contemporary conceptions used in psychology and psychiatry*. New York: Coward-McCann.

Murray, H. A. (1938). *Explorations in personality: A clinical and experimental study of fifty men of college age*. New York: Oxford University Press.

Murray, H. A. (1940). What should psychologists do about psychoanalysis? *Journal of Abnormal and Social Psychology, 35*, 150–175.

Murray, H. A. (1959). Preparations for the scaffold of a comprehensive system. In S. Koch (Ed.), *Psychology: A study of a science* (Vol. 3, pp. 7–54). New York: McGraw-Hill.

Murray, H. A. (1967). Henry A. Murray. In E. G. Boring & G. Lindzey (Eds.), *A history of psychology in autobiography* (Vol. 5, pp. 283–310). New York: Appleton-Century-Crofts.

Murray, H. A. (1981). American Icarus. In E. S. Shneidman (Ed.), *Endeavors in psychology* (pp. 535–556). New York: Harper & Row. (Original work published 1955)

Myers, I. (1962). *The Myers–Briggs Type Indicator*. Princeton, NJ: Educational Testing Service.

Nasby, W., & Read, N. W. (1997). The life voyage of a solo circumnavigator: Integrating theoretical and methodological perspectives. *Journal of Personality, 65*, 785–1068.

Nettle, D. (2005). An evolutionary approach to the extraversion continuum. *Evolution and Human Behavior, 26*, 363–373.

Nicholson, I. A. M. (2003). *Inventing personality: Gordon Allport and the science of selfhood*. Washington, DC: American Psychological Association.

Nisbett, R. E. (2003). *The geography of thought: How Asians and Westerners think differently and why*. New York: Free Press.

Norem, J. K., & Chang, E. C. (2002). The positive psychology of negative thinking. *Journal of Clinical Psychology, 58*, 993–1001.

Odbert, H. S. (1936). Trends in the study of personality. *Character and Personality, 5*, 149–154.

Ogilvie, D. M. (2004). *Fantasies of flight*. New York: Oxford University Press.

OSS Assessment Staff. (1948). *Assessment of men: Selection of personnel for the Office of Strategic Services*. New York: Rinehart.

Ozer, D. J., & Benet-Martínez, V. (2006). Personality and the prediction of consequential outcomes. *Annual Review of Psychology, 57*, 401–421.

Pandora, K. (1997). *Rebels within the ranks: Psychologists' critique of scientific authority and democratic realities in New Deal America.* Cambridge, UK: Cambridge University Press.

Parker, J. D. A. (1991). *In search of the person: The historical development of American personality psychology.* Unpublished doctoral dissertation, York University, North York, Ontario, Canada.

Pervin, L. A. (Ed.). (1989). *Goal concepts in personality and social psychology.* Hillsdale, NJ: Erlbaum.

Pervin, L. A. (2003). *Current controversies and issues in personality* (3rd ed.). New York: Wiley.

Pickering, A. D., & Gray, J. A. (1999). The neuroscience of personality. In L. A. Pervin & O. P. John (Eds.), *Handbook of personality: Theory and research* (2nd ed., pp. 277–299). New York: Guilford Press.

Platt, J. (1996). *A history of sociological research methods in America 1920–1960.* Cambridge, UK: Cambridge University Press.

Post, J. M. (Ed.). (2003). *The psychological assessment of political leaders: With profiles of Saddam Hussein and Bill Clinton.* Ann Arbor: University of Michigan Press.

Postmes, T., & Jetten, J. (Eds.). (2006). *Individuality and the group: Advances in social identity.* Thousand Oaks, CA: Sage.

Prince, M., & Allport, F. H. (1921). Editorial announcement. *Journal of Abnormal Psychology and Social Psychology, 16,* 1–5.

Prince, M., & Moore, H. T. (1928). Editorial: The current number. *Journal of Abnormal and Social Psychology, 23,* 117.

Pyszczynski, T., Greenberg, J., & Solomon, S. (1997). Why do we need what we need? A terror management perspective on the roots of human social motivation. *Psychological Inquiry, 8,* 1–20.

Rank, O. (1936). *Will therapy: An analysis of the therapeutic process in terms of relationship.* New York: Knopf. (Original work published 1931)

Recent literature. (1921). *American Journal of Sociology, 27,* 128–144.

Robinson, F. G. (1992). *Love's story told: A life of Henry A. Murray.* Cambridge, MA: Harvard University Press.

Rogers, C. R. (1959). A theory of therapy, personality, and interpersonal relationships, as developed in the client-centered framework. In S. Koch (Ed.), *Psychology: A study of a science* (Vol. 3, pp. 184–256). New York: McGraw-Hill.

Rosenberg, M. (1979). *Conceiving the self.* New York: Basic Books.

Runyan, W. M. (1982). *Life histories and psychobiography: Explorations in theory and method.* New York: Oxford University Press.

Runyan, W. M. (1997). Studying lives: Psychobi-

ography and the conceptual structure of personality psychology. In R. Hogan, J. Johnson, & S. Briggs (Eds.), *Handbook of personality psychology* (pp. 41–69). San Diego, CA: Academic Press.

Ryan, R. M., & Deci, E. L. (2000). Self-determination theory and the facilitation of intrinsic motivation, social development, and well-being. *American Psychologist, 55,* 68–78.

Schultz, W. T. (2005). *Handbook of psychobiography.* New York: Oxford University Press.

Segal, L. (2000). Gender, genes and genetics: From Darwin to the human genome. In C. Squire (Ed.), *Culture in psychology* (pp. 31–43). New York: Routledge.

Sheldon, W. H., Stevens, S. S., & Tucker, W. B. (1940). *The varieties of human physique: An introduction to constitutional psychology.* New York: Harper.

Shermer, P. (1985). *The development of research practice in abnormal and personality psychology: 1906–1956.* Unpublished master's thesis, York University, North York, Ontario, Canada.

Sherwood, J. J., & Nataupsky, M. (1968). Predicting the conclusions of Negro–White intelligence research from biographical characteristics of the investigator. *Journal of Personality and Social Psychology, 8,* 53–58.

Shweder, R. A. (1991). *Thinking through cultures: Expeditions in cultural psychology.* Cambridge, MA: Harvard University Press.

Skinner, B. F. (1953). *Science and human behavior.* New York: Macmillan.

Smith, C. P. (Ed.). (1992). *Motivation and personality: Handbook of thematic content analysis.* New York: Cambridge University Press.

Smith, M. B. (1990). Personology launched [Review of the book *Explorations in personality: A clinical and experimental study of fifty men of college age*]. *Contemporary Psychology, 35,* 537–539.

Snyder, M. (1987). *Public appearances, private realities: The psychology of self-monitoring.* New York: Freeman.

Spangler, W. D. (1992). Validity of questionnaire and TAT measures of need for achievement: Two meta-analyses. *Psychological Bulletin, 112,* 140–154.

Stagner, R. (1937). *Psychology of personality.* New York: McGraw-Hill.

Stern, W. (1911). *Die differentielle Psychologie in ihren methodischen Grundlagen* [Differential psychology in its methodological foundations]. Leipzig: Barth.

Stewart, A. J., & McDermott, C. (2004). Gender in psychology. *Annual Review of Psychology, 55,* 519–544.

Suedfeld, P., Tetlock, P. E., & Streufert, S. (1992). Conceptual/integrative complexity. In C. P. Smith (Ed.), *Motivation and person-*

ality: Handbook of thematic content analysis (pp. 393–400). New York: Cambridge University Press.

Susman, W. I. (1979). "Personality" and the making of twentieth-century culture. In J. Higham & P. K. Conklin (Eds.), *New directions in American intellectual history* (pp. 212–226). Baltimore: Johns Hopkins University Press.

Thomas, W. I., & Znaniecki, F. (1918–1920). *The Polish peasant in Europe and America* (Vols. 1–5). Chicago: University of Chicago Press.

Thurstone, L. L. (1952). L. L. Thurstone. In E. G. Boring, H. S. Langfeld, H. Werner, & R. M. Yerkes (Eds.), *A history of psychology in autobiography* (Vol. 4, pp. 295–321). New York: Russell & Russell.

Triplet, R. G. (1983). *Henry A. Murray and the Harvard Psychological Clinic, 1926–1938: A struggle to expand the disciplinary boundaries of academic psychology.* Unpublished doctoral dissertation, University of New Hampshire, Durham, NH.

Vallacher, R. R., Read, S. J., & Nowak, A. (2002). The dynamical perspective in personality and social psychology. *Personality and Social Psychology Review*, 6, 264–273.

Vernon, P. E., & Allport, G. W. (1931). A test for personal values. *Journal of Abnormal and Social Psychology*, 26, 231–248.

Warren, H. C. (1920). *Human psychology.* Boston: Houghton Mifflin.

Watson, J. B., & Rayner, R. (1920). Conditioned emotional reactions. *Journal of Experimental Psychology*, 3, 1–14.

Webb, E. (1915). Character and intelligence. *British Journal of Psychology Monographs*, 1(3), 1–99.

Weiner, B., & Graham, S. (1999). Attribution in personality psychology. In L. A. Pervin & O. P. John (Eds.), *Handbook of personality: Theory and research* (2nd ed., pp. 605–628). New York: Guilford Press.

West, S. G. (Ed.). (1983). Personality and prediction: Nomothetic and idiographic approaches [Special issue]. *Journal of Personality*, 51(3).

White, R. W. (1952). *Lives in progress.* New York: Holt, Rinehart, & Winston.

Whiting, J. W. M., & Child, I. L. (1953). *Child training and personality: A cross-cultural study.* New Haven, CT: Yale University Press.

Wiggins, J. S., & Trobst, K. K. (1999). The fields of interpersonal behavior. In L. A. Pervin & O. P. John (Eds.), *Handbook of personality: Theory and research* (2nd ed., pp. 653–670). New York: Guilford Press.

Windelband, W. (1904). *Geschichte und Natur-* *wissenschaft* [History and natural science] (3rd ed.). Strassburg: Heitz. (Original work published 1894)

Wink, P. (1992). Three types of narcissism in women from college to mid-life. *Journal of Personality*, 60, 7–30.

Winter, D. G. (1993). Power, affiliation, and war: Three tests of a motivational model. *Journal of Personality and Social Psychology*, 65, 532–545.

Winter, D. G. (1996). *Personality: Analysis and interpretation of lives.* New York: McGraw-Hill.

Winter, D. G. (1998). "Toward a science of personality psychology": David McClelland's development of empirically derived TAT measures. *History of Psychology*, 1, 130–153.

Winter, D. G., & Barenbaum, N. B. (1999). History of modern personality theory and research. In L. A. Pervin & O. P. John (Eds.), *Handbook of personality: Theory and research* (2nd ed., pp. 3–27). New York: Guilford Press.

Winter, D. G., John, O. P., Stewart, A. J., Klohnen, E. C., & Duncan, L. E. (1998). Traits and motives: Toward an integration of two traditions in personality research. *Psychological Review*, 105, 230–250.

Winter, D. G., & Stewart, A. J. (1977). Power motive reliability as a function of retest instructions. *Journal of Consulting and Clinical Psychology*, 45, 436–440.

Wise, D., & Rosqvist, J. (2006). Explanatory style and well-being. In J. C. Thomas, D. L. Segal, & M. Hersen (Eds.), *Comprehensive handbook of personality and psychopathology: Vol. 1. Personality and everyday functioning* (pp. 285–305). Hoboken, NJ: Wiley.

Witkin, H. A. (1949). The nature and importance of individual differences in perception. *Journal of Personality*, 18, 145–170.

Woodworth, R. S. (1919). Examination of emotional fitness for warfare. *Psychological Bulletin*, 15, 59–60.

Woodworth, R. S. (1929). *Psychology* (rev. ed.). New York: Henry Holt.

Wylie, R. C. (1974–1979). *The self-concept* (rev. ed.). Lincoln: University of Nebraska Press.

York, K. L., & John, O. P. (1992). The four faces of Eve: A typological analysis of women's personality at midlife. *Journal of Personality and Social Psychology*, 63, 494–508.

Young, K. (1928). The measurement of personal and social traits. *Journal of Abnormal and Social Psychology*, 22, 431–442.

Zuckerman, M. (2005). *Psychobiology of personality* (2nd ed.). New York: Cambridge University Press.

PART II

Theoretical Perspectives

CHAPTER 2

Human Nature and Individual Differences

Evolution of Human Personality

David M. Buss

Personality psychology aspires to be the broadest, most integrative, branch of the psychological sciences. Its content is not restricted to particular subsets of psychological phenomena, such as information processing, social interaction, or deviations from normality. Personality psychologists historically have attempted to synthesize and integrate these diverse phenomena into a larger unifying theory that includes the whole person in all myriad modes of functioning (McAdams, 1997; Pervin, 1990). Moreover, personality theorists have attempted to conceptualize the place of whole persons within the broader matrix of groups and society. The central argument of this chapter is that these theoretical goals cannot be attained without an explicit consideration of the causal processes that gave rise to the mechanisms of mind that define human nature.

Although there has been much debate about the definition of personality, two major themes have pervaded nearly all efforts at grand personality theorizing: human nature and individual differences (Buss, 1984). Human nature comprises the common characteristics of humans—the shared motives, goals, and psychological mechanisms that are either universal or nearly universal. Proposed species-typical motives range from the sexual and aggressive instincts postulated by Freud (1953/1905) to the motives to get along and get ahead postulated by Hogan (1983). A proper conceptualization of human nature, however, is much larger than the forces that impel people out of bed in the morning and motivate them in their daily quests. Human nature also includes the species-typical ways in which humans make decisions (e.g., selection of mates and habitats), the ways in which humans respond to environmental stimuli (e.g., fears of snakes and heights are more typical than fears of cars or electrical outlets), and even the ways in which people influence and manipulate the world around them. No branch of psychology except personality psychology aspires to this broad conceptualization of human nature.

Personality psychology is also the central branch of psychology for which individual differences play a prominent role. Indeed, some leading personality psychologists define the field of personality psychology as that branch of psychology concerned with identifying the most important individual differences (e.g., Goldberg, 1981; Norman, 1963; Wiggins, 1979). Individuals differ in an infinite number of ways that either go unnoticed or are not sufficiently noteworthy to warrant much discussion. Some individuals have belly buttons turned in, others have belly buttons turned out. Some lead with their left foot, others with their right. Some prefer blondes, others prefer brunettes. One key function of personality theory is to identify the most important ways in which individuals differ from among the infinite dimensions of possible difference.

These two themes—human nature and individual differences—ideally should not occupy separate and isolated branches of the field of personality psychology (Buss, 1984). Most grand theories of personality have incorporated propositions about ways in which human nature and individual differences are systematically linked. In Freud's (1953/1905) theory of psychoanalysis, for example, all humans are presumed to progress through the universal stages of oral, anal, phallic, latency, and genital development. Different environmental events occurring during these stages, however, produce systematic individual differences. Overindulgence at the oral stage might lead to an oral fixation that shapes an adult who talks a lot, chews gum, and feels "hungry" for the attention of others. An overly strict mode of toilet training might lead to a different personality, such as an adult who is compulsively neat. In this manner, the theory's specification of human nature—the universal progression through the psychosexual stages—is coherently linked with the major ways in which individuals are proposed to differ.

Over the past few decades, the field of personality has retreated somewhat from its grander goals. Most actual research on personality psychology deals with individual differences, not with human nature or with the links between human nature and individual differences (e.g., McCrae & John, 1992). In this sense, personality may have ceded the study of human nature to other branches of psychology, such as cognitive and social psychology, which typically concentrate on shared characteristics of human nature and neglect individual differences.

One of the central arguments of this chapter is that the grand goals of personality psychology should be reclaimed. An analogy might help to clarify this argument. Suppose that invisible Martian scientists were assigned the task of studying the large metallic vehicles that earthlings use for transportation. One group of scientists was assigned the task of figuring out "car nature"—the basic design that is common to all cars. They might conclude that all cars have tires, a steering mechanism, a method of braking, and an engine that provides propulsion. The second group of scientists, in contrast, was assigned the task of determining the major ways in which cars differ from one another. They conclude that some have large tires, others small tires; some have rack-and-pinion steering, others do not; some have antilock brakes, others do not; some have a six-cylinder engines, whereas others make due with four cylinders.

The second group of scientists is faced with the task of determining which individual differences are the really important ones and separating these from the trivial ones. Cars differ in the color of the engine wires, for example, but are these differences really important (Tooby & Cosmides, 1990a)? The Martian scientists who study car differences conclude that they cannot really accomplish their task—identifying in a nonarbitrary fashion the most important individual differences—without talking to the first group of scientists that is responsible for developing a theory of "car nature." From a collaboration between these two groups, they arrive at a nonarbitrary criterion for determining which car differences are really important: those differences that affect the basic functioning of the car, that is, those that affect the component parts that contribute to what cars are designed to do. Using this criterion, they decide that "differences in the colors of the engine wires" are really trivial, because these differences have no impact on the functioning of the car's engine. But they include differences in engine cylinder number, tire size, and breaking mechanism because these differences have a profound effect on what the car is designed to do, affecting its power, propulsion, ability to "hug" the road, and ability to stop. The key point is that it would be illogical to have two entirely separate "car theorists," one dealing with car nature and one dealing with car differences. The two are inextricably bound, and their integration provides the basis for a nonarbitrary theory that includes both car nature and the major ways in which cars differ.

People are not cars, and the analogy breaks down at a certain point. Cars are designed by humans, for example, but humans were designed by a different causal process. Nevertheless, the central point of the analogy can be expressed as a syllogism: (1) If humans have a human nature, and (2) if the components of that nature were "designed" to perform certain functions, then (3) a nonarbitrary means for identifying the most important individual differences involves discovering those differences that affect the performance of those functions. In order to establish the veracity of the first two premises, we must examine the causal processes that "designed" humans and ask whether these processes have produced a human nature with an identifiable set of functions.

THE EVOLUTIONARY PROCESS

Scientists over the past two centuries have proposed a delimited set of theories about the causal processes responsible for the design of humans and other life forms. One theory is that of "divine creation," the idea that a deity created humans in all of their glorious nature. Another theory is that extraterrestrial organisms planted the seeds of life on earth, and that these seeds were transformed by some evolutionary process, over millions of years, into humans. Neither divine creation nor seeding theory have many proponents among modern scientists. Indeed, only one theory of origins, albeit with modifications and extensions, has had held sway among scientists over the past century and a half: the theory of evolution by selection.

Natural and Sexual Selection

Although it is widely misunderstood, the theory of evolution by selection is remarkably simple as applied to all organic forms. First, individuals differ in a variety of ways. Second, some of these variants are heritable, that is, reliably passed down from parents to children. Third, some of these variants are recurrently correlated with survival and reproduction over generations. Fourth, those variants that contribute to greater reproduction, however indirectly, are passed down to succeeding generations in greater numbers than those that do not lead to greater relative reproduction. Fifth, over generations, those variants that contribute to greater reproduc-

tion displace those that do not, eventually spreading to most or all members of the species. This selective process, occurring over vast expanses of time and space, is responsible for the origins of the basic "design" of all organisms.

Selection, of course, is not the only causal process that produces change over time. Genetic drift, sudden catastrophes such as a meteorite hitting the earth, and other processes certainly produce change and must be included in any complete history of the evolution of species. Natural selection, however, is generally regarded as the most important causal process, because it is the *only known causal process* that can produce *complex functional design*. A meteorite may have caused the extinction of dinosaurs and perhaps even opened up new niches for the explosive evolution of mammals, but such catastrophic events cannot create the complex functional design that characterized dinosaurs or any other organisms. Whereas unpredictable catastrophes are important in understanding the evolution of life on earth, no known causal process other than natural selection can produce the complex functional design that characterizes each species (see Buss, Haselton, Shackelford, Bleske, & Wakefield, 1998, for a more detailed discussion of these issues).

Darwin envisioned two classes of evolved variants—one playing a role in survival and one playing a role in reproductive competition (Darwin, 1859/1958). Among humans, for example, our sweat glands help us to maintain a constant body temperature and thus presumably help us to survive (or more accurately, helped our ancestors to survive). Our tastes for sugar and fat presumably helped to guide our ancestors to eat certain foods and to avoid others, and thus helped them to survive. Other inherited attributes aid more directly in reproductive competition and were said to be sexually selected (Darwin, 1871/1981). The elaborate songs and brilliant plumage of various bird species, for example, help to attract mates, and hence to reproduce, but do nothing to enhance the individual's survival. In fact, these characteristics may be detrimental to survival by carrying large metabolic costs or by alerting predators.

In summary, although differential reproductive success as a consequence of heritable variants is the crux of Darwin's theory of natural selection, he conceived of two classes of variants that might evolve—those that help organisms to survive (and thus indirectly help them to reproduce) and those that more directly help organisms in mate competition. The theory of natural selection unified all living creatures, from single-celled amoebas to multicellular mammals, into one grand tree of descent. It also provided, for the first time, a scientific theory to account for the exquisite design and functional nature of the component parts of each of these species.

In its modern form, the evolutionary process of natural selection has been refined to reflect inclusive fitness theory (Hamilton, 1964). Hamilton reasoned that classical fitness—a measure of an individual's direct reproductive success in passing on genes through the production of offspring—was too narrow to describe the process of evolution by selection. He proposed that natural selection will favor characteristics that cause an organism's genes to be passed on, regardless of whether the organism produces offspring directly. If a person helps his or her brother, sister, or niece to become an ancestor, for example, by sharing resources, offering protection, or helping in times of need, then he or she contributes to the reproductive success of genes "for" brotherly, sisterly, or niecely assistance (assuming that such helping is partly heritable). In other words, parental care—investing in one's own children—is merely a special case of caring for kin who carry copies of one's genes in their bodies. Thus, the notion of classical fitness was expanded to one of inclusive fitness.

Technically, inclusive fitness is not a property of an individual organism but rather of its actions or effects (Hamilton, 1964; see also Dawkins, 1982). Inclusive fitness can be viewed as the sum of an individual's own reproductive success (classical fitness) plus the effects the individual's actions have on the reproductive success of his or her genetic relatives, weighted by the degree of genetic relatedness.

It is critical to keep in mind that evolution by natural selection is not forward looking or intentional. The giraffe does not notice the juicy leaves stirring high in the tree and "evolve" a longer neck. Rather, those giraffes that happen to have slightly longer necks than other giraffes have a slight advantage in getting to those leaves. Hence, they survive better and are more likely to live to pass on genes for slightly longer necks to offspring. Natural selection acts only on those variants that happen to exist. Evolution is not intentional and cannot look into the future to foresee distant needs.

Products of Evolutionary Processes

In each generation, the process of selection acts as a sieve (Dawkins, 1996). Variants that interfere with successful solutions to adaptive problems are filtered out; variants that are tributary to the successful solution to an adaptive problem pass through the selective sieve. Iterated over thousands of generations, this filtering process tends to produce characteristics that interact with the physical, social, or internal environment in ways that promoted the reproduction of the individuals who possess the characteristics or the reproduction of the individuals' genetic relatives (Dawkins, 1982; Hamilton, 1964; Tooby & Cosmides, 1990b; Williams, 1966). These characteristics are called *adaptations*.

There has been much debate about the precise meaning of adaptation, but a provisional working definition can be offered. An adaptation can be defined as an inherited and reliably developing characteristic that came into existence through natural selection because it helped to solve a problem of reproduction during the period of its evolution (after Tooby & Cosmides, 1992). An adaptation must have genes "for" that adaptation. Those genes are required for the passage of the adaptation from parents to offspring. Adaptations, therefore, are, by definition, inherited.

An adaptation must develop reliably among species members in all "normal" environments. Environmental events during ontogeny always have the potential to disrupt the emergence of an adaptation in a particular individual, and thus the genes "for" the adaptation do not invariably result in its intact phenotypic manifestation. To qualify as an adaptation, the characteristics must reliably emerge in reasonably intact form at the appropriate time during an organism's life, however, and be characteristic of most or all members of a species (with some exceptions, e.g., characteristics that are sex-linked or exist in only a subset of members of a species due to frequent-dependent selection—topics taken up later in this chapter).

Adaptations, of course, need not be present at birth. Many adaptations develop long after birth. Bipedal locomotion is a reliably developing characteristic of humans, but most humans do not begin to walk until a year after birth. The beards of men and the breasts of women are reliably developing, but do not start to develop until puberty.

The characteristics that make it through the filtering process in each generation generally do so because they contribute to the successful solution of adaptive problems— solutions that are either necessary for reproduction or that enhance relative reproductive success. Solutions to adaptive problems can be direct, such as a fear of dangerous snakes, which solves a survival problem, or a desire to mate with fertile members of one's species, which helps to solve a reproductive problem. They can be indirect, as in a desire to ascend a social hierarchy, which many years later might give an individual better access to more desirable mates. Or they can be even more indirect, such as when a person helps a brother or sister, which eventually helps that sibling to reproduce.

Each adaptation has its own period of evolution. Initially, a mutation occurs in a single individual. Most mutations hinder reproduction, disrupting the existing design of the organism. If the mutation is helpful to reproduction, however, it will become integrated into the existing design of the organism and passed down to the next generation in greater numbers. In the next generation, therefore, more individuals will possess the characteristic that was initially a mutation in a single individual. Over many generations, if it continues to be successful, the characteristic will spread to the entire population, so that every species member will have it.

An adaptation's *environment of evolutionary adaptedness* (EEA) refers to the cumulative selection processes that constructed it, piece by piece, until it came to characterize the species. There is no single EEA that can be localized in time and space for all the adaptations that characterize a species. The EEA is best described as a statistical aggregate of selection pressures responsible for the emergence of an adaptation over a particular period of time (Tooby & Cosmides, 1992).

Each adaptation, therefore, has its own EEA. The human eyes, for example, have an EEA that is distinct from the EEA of concealed ovulation or of male sexual jealousy.

The hallmarks of adaptation are features that define *special design*: complexity, economy, efficiency, reliability, precision, and functionality (Williams, 1966). These features are conceptual criteria subject to empirical testing and potential falsification for a particular hypothesis about an adaptation. Because, in principle, there are an infinite number of alternative hypotheses to account for a particular constellation of findings, the evaluation of a specific hypothesis about an adaptation is a probability statement about the likelihood that the complex, reliable, and functional features of special design could not have arisen as an incidental byproduct of another characteristic or by chance alone (Tooby & Cosmides, 1992). As more and more functional features of special design are predicted and subsequently documented for a hypothesized adaptation, each pointing to the successful solution of a specific adaptive problem, the alternative hypotheses of chance and incidental byproduct become increasingly improbable.

Although adaptations are generally considered to be the primary products of the evolutionary process, they are not the only products (see Buss et al., 1998; Tooby & Cosmides, 1992). The evolutionary process also produces *byproducts of adaptations*. Byproducts are characteristics that do not solve adaptive problems and tend not to have functional design. They are carried along with characteristics that do have functional design because they happen to be coupled with those adaptations.

Consider the humanly designed light bulb. A light bulb is designed to produce light. Light production is its function. The design features of a light bulb—the conducting filament, the vacuum surrounding the filament, and the glass encasement—are all tributary to the production of light and part of its functional design. Light bulbs, however, also produce heat. Heat is a byproduct of light production. It is carried along not because the bulb was designed to produce heat, but rather because heat tends to be a reliable incidental consequence of light production.

A naturally occurring example of a byproduct of adaptation would be the human belly button. There is no evidence that the belly button, per se, helped human ancestors to survive or reproduce. A belly button is not good for catching food, detecting predators, avoiding snakes, locating good habitats, or choosing mates. It does not seem to be involved directly or indirectly in the solution to an adaptive problem. Rather the belly button is a byproduct of something that is an adaptation—namely, the umbilical cord that formerly provided the food supply to the growing fetus. The hypothesis that something is a byproduct of an adaptation requires the identification of the adaptation of which it is a byproduct and the cause for it being coupled with that adaptation (Tooby & Cosmides, 1992). In other words, the hypothesis that something is a byproduct, just like the hypothesis that something is an adaptation, must be subjected to rigorous standards of scientific confirmation and potential falsification.

The third and final product of the evolutionary process is *noise* or *random effects*. Noise can be produced by mutations that neither contribute to, nor detract from, the functional design of the organism. The glass encasement of a light bulb, for example, often contains perturbations from smoothness due to imperfections in the materials and the process of manufacturing that do not affect the functioning of the bulb. In self-reproducing systems, these neutral effects can be carried along and passed down to succeeding generations, as long as they do not impair the functioning of the mechanisms that are adaptations.

In summary, the evolutionary process produces three products: adaptations, byproducts of adaptations, and a residue of noise (see Table 2.1). In principle, we can analyze the component parts of a species and conduct empirical studies to determine which parts are adaptations, which are byproducts, and which represent neutral noise. Evolutionary scientists differ in their estimates of the relative sizes of these three categories of products. Some argue that even uniquely human qualities such as language are merely incidental byproducts of large brains (e.g., Gould, 1991). Others argue that qualities such as language show evidence of special design that render it highly improbable that it is anything other than a well-designed adaptation for communication and conspecific manipulation (Pinker, 1994). It is equally incumbent on both sides of this argument to formulate hypotheses in a precise, testable, and potentially falsifiable manner so that the different positions can be adjudicated empirically.

EVOLUTIONARY CONSEQUENCES FOR HUMAN NATURE

One important consequence of a careful consideration of the products of the evolutionary process is an understanding that the core of human nature largely consists primarily of adaptations and byproducts of those adaptations, along with a residue of random noise. This section addresses the core of human nature from an evolutionary psychological perspective. First, I argue that all species, including humans, have a nature that can be described and explained. Second, I provide a definition of *evolved psychological mechanisms*—the core units that comprise human nature. Third, I explore two illustra-

TABLE 2.1. Three Products of the Evolutionary Process

Three products	Brief definition
Adaptations	Inherited and reliably developing characteristics that came into existence through natural selection because they helped to solve problems of survival or reproduction during the period of their evolution. Example: umbilical cord.
Byproducts	Characteristics that do not solve adaptive problems and do not have functional design. They are "carried along" with characteristics that do have functional design because they happen to be coupled with those adaptations. Example: belly button.
Noise	Random effects produced by forces such as chance mutations, sudden and unprecedented changes in the environment, or chance effects during development. Example: particular shape of a person's belly button.

tions of evolved psychological mechanisms. And fourth, I suggest some ways in which evolutionary thinking can provide a nonarbitrary foundation for a personality theory that specifies the core of human nature.

Humans Have a Human Nature

All species have a nature. It is part of lion's nature to walk on four legs, display a large furry mane, hunt other animals for food, and live on the savannah. It is part of butterfly nature to enter a flightless pupae state, wrap itself in a cocoon, and emerge to soar, fluttering gracefully in search of food and mates. It is part of a porcupine's nature to defend itself with quills, a skunk's nature to defend itself with a spray of acrid liquid smell, a stag's nature to defend itself with antlers, and a turtle's nature to defend itself by withdrawing into a shell. All species have a nature, but that nature is different for each species. Each species has faced at least somewhat unique selection pressures during its evolutionary history, and therefore has evolved at least some unique adaptive solutions.

Humans also have a nature—qualities that define us as a species—and all psychological theories imply the existence of a human nature. For William James, human nature consists of dozens or hundreds of instincts. For Freud, human nature consists of raging sexual and aggressive impulses. Even the most ardently environmentalist theories, such as Skinner's theory of radical behaviorism, assume that humans have a nature—in this case, consisting of a few highly general learning mechanisms (Symons, 1987). All psychological theories require as their core a specification of, or fundamental premises about, human nature.

Since evolution by selection is the only known causal process that is capable of producing the fundamental components of that human nature, all psychological theories are implicitly or explicitly evolutionary (Symons, 1987). Although many psychologists fail to specify their assumptions about the evolution of human nature (hence keeping those assumptions implicit), not one has ever proposed a psychological theory that has presumed some other causal process to be responsible for creating human nature.

If humans have a nature and if evolution by selection is the causal process that

produced that nature, then the next question is: What insights into human nature can be provided by examining our evolutionary origins? Can examining the *process* of evolution tell us anything about the *products* of that process in the human case? Can evolutionary theory provide *heuristic value*, guiding personality researchers to important domains that have been neglected, unexamined, or downplayed? Can `it yield specific psychological hypotheses that are capable of being tested empirically, hence confirmed or falsified?

Whereas the broader field of evolutionary biology is concerned with the evolutionary analysis of grandly integrated parts of an organism, evolutionary psychology focuses more narrowly on those parts that are psychological: the analysis of the human mind as a collection of evolved mechanisms, the contexts that activate those mechanisms, and the behavior generated by those mechanisms. And so the next section explores the subclass of adaptations that make up the human mind: evolved psychological mechanisms.

The Nature of Evolved Psychological Mechanisms

An *evolved psychological mechanism* is a set of processes inside an organism that has the following properties (see Buss, 1991, 1995a, 2008; Tooby & Cosmides, 1992):

An evolved psychological mechanism exists in the form that it does because it solved a specific problem of survival or reproduction recurrently over evolutionary history. This means that the form of the mechanism—its set of *design features*—is like a key made to fit a particular lock (Tooby & Cosmides, 1992). Just as the shape of the key must be coordinated to fit the internal features of the lock, the shape of the design features of a psychological mechanism must be coordinated with the features required to solve an adaptive problem of survival or reproduction. Failure to mesh with the adaptive problem means failure to pass through the selective sieve of evolution.

An evolved psychological mechanism is designed to take in only a narrow slice of information. Consider the human eye. Although it seems as though we open our eyes and see nearly everything, in fact the eye is sensitive only to a narrow range of input from the broad spectrum of electromagnetic waves. We do not see X-rays, which are shorter than those in the visual spectrum. We do not see radio waves, which are longer than those in the visual spectrum. In fact, our eyes are designed to process input from only a very narrow wedge of waves—waves within the visual spectrum.

Even within the visual spectrum, our eyes are designed to process a narrower subset of information (Marr, 1982). Our eyes have (1) specific edge detectors that pick up contrasting reflections from objects; (2) specific motion detectors that pick up movement; and (3) specific cones that pick up specific information about the colors of objects. So the eye is not an all-purpose seeing device. It is designed to process only narrow slices of information—waves within a particular range of frequency, edges, motion, and so on—from among the much larger domain of potential information.

Similarly, the psychological mechanism of a predisposition to learn to fear snakes is designed to take in only a narrow slice of information—slithery movements from self-propelled elongated objects. Our evolved preferences for food, landscapes, and mates are all designed to take in only a limited subset of information from among the infinite array of information that could potentially constitute input.

The input of an evolved psychological mechanism tells an organism the particular adaptive problem it is facing. The input of seeing a slithering snake tells you that you are confronting a particular survival problem, namely physical damage and perhaps death if bitten. The differing smells of potentially edible objects—rancid and rotting versus sweet and fragrant—tell you that you are facing an adaptive survival problem of food selection. The input, in short, lets the organism know what adaptive problem it is addressing. This process occurs, almost invariably, out of consciousness. Humans do not smell a cooking pizza and think "Aha, I am facing an adaptive problem of food selection!" Instead, the smell unconsciously triggers food selection mechanisms, and no consciousness or awareness of the adaptive problem is necessary.

The input of an evolved psychological mechanism is transformed into output through cognitive procedures or decision rules. Upon seeing a snake, you can decide to attack it, run away from it, or freeze. Upon smelling a fragrant pizza just out of the oven, you can devour it or walk away (perhaps, if you are on a diet). The decision rules are a set of procedures—"if–then" statements—for channeling an organism down one path or another.

The output of an evolved psychological mechanism can be physiological activity, information to other psychological mechanisms, or manifest behavior. Upon seeing a snake, you may get autonomically aroused or frightened (physiological output), you may use this information to evaluate your behavioral options such as freezing or fleeing (information to other psychological mechanisms), and the consequence of this evaluation is an action, such as running away (behavioral output).

Consider another example: sexual jealousy. Let's say that you go to a party with your romantic partner and then leave the room to get a drink. When you return, you spot your partner talking animatedly to another person. They stand very close to each other, look deeply into each other's eyes, and you notice that they are starting to touch each other.

These cues might trigger a reaction we can call sexual jealousy. The cues act as input to the mechanism, signaling to you the presence of an adaptive problem—the threat of losing your partner. This input is then evaluated according to a set of decision rules. One option is to ignore them and feign indifference. Another is to threaten the rival. A third option is to get enraged and hit your partner. Still another option would be to reevaluate your relationship. Thus, the output of a psychological mechanism can be *physiological* (arousal), *behavioral* (confronting, threatening, hitting), or serve as *input* to other psychological mechanisms (reevaluating the status of your relationship).

The output of an evolved psychological mechanism is directed toward the solution to a specific adaptive problem. Just as the cues to a partner's potential infidelity signal the presence of an adaptive problem, the output of the sexual jealousy mechanism is geared toward solving that problem. The threatened rival may leave the scene. Your romantic partner may be deterred from flirting with others. Or your reevaluation of the relationship may cause you to cut your losses and move into a potentially better relationship. Any of these might help achieve the solution to your adaptive problem.

Stating that the output of a psychological mechanism leads to solutions to specific adaptive problems does not imply that the solutions will always be optimal or invariably successful. The rival may not be deterred by your threats. Your partner may have a fling with your rival despite your display of jealousy. The main point is *not* that the output of a psychological mechanism *always* leads to a successful solution, but rather that the output of the mechanism, *on average*, tended to solve the adaptive problem in the environment in which it evolved better than outputs from alternative designs present in the population during those periods.

An important point to keep in mind is that a mechanism that led to a successful solution in the evolutionary past may or may not lead to a successful solution now. Our strong taste preferences for fat, for example, were clearly adaptive in our evolutionary past because fat was a valuable source of calories but very scarce (Symons, 1987). Now, however, with hamburger and pizza joints on every street corner, fat is no longer a scarce resource. Thus, our strong taste for fatty substances now causes us to overconsume fat, which leads to clogged arteries and heart attacks and hinders our survival. The central point is that evolved mechanisms exist in the form that they do because *they led to success, on average, during the period in which they evolved*. Whether they are currently adaptive—that is, whether they currently lead to increased survival and reproduction—is an empirical matter that must be determined on a case-by-case basis.

In summary, an evolved psychological mechanism is a set of procedures within the organism that is designed to take in a particular slice of information and transform that information via decision rules into output that historically helped with the solution to an adaptive problem. The psychological mechanism exists in current organisms because it led, on average, to the successful solution of a specific adaptive problem for the ancestors of the current species of organism.

Two Illustrations of Evolved
Psychological Mechanisms:
Fear of Spiders and Landscape Preferences

At this early stage in the development of the field of evolutionary psychology, no psychological mechanism has been completely described. We do not know all of the decision rules, the precise range of events that trigger their activation, or the complete range of outputs of any mechanism. Nonetheless, two illustrations of *possible* psychological mechanisms will help to convey the scientific goals of this enterprise.

Let's consider the fear of spiders and preferences for certain landscapes. An evolved fear of spiders exists in the form that it does because it solved a specific problem of survival in human ancestral environments (Marks, 1987). The fear is triggered only by a narrow range of inputs, such certain shapes and movements associated with spiders. Once a spider is perceived as dangerous and within striking range, this information is transformed via decision rules that might activate physiological arousal and perhaps the implementation of a host of behavioral options. The options—such as stomping on the spider, fleeing, or yelling for help—would presumably have lowered the odds of receiving a deadly spider bite in ancestral environments. Thus, the output of the fear-of-spiders mechanism solves an ancestral adaptive problem. It is not by chance that human fears and phobias tend to be concentrated heavily toward environmental events that threatened human survival. Fears of snakes, spiders, heights, darkness, and strangers provide a window for viewing the survival hazards that our human ancestors faced (Marks, 1987).

Preferences are evolved psychological mechanisms of a different sort than fears. Preferences motivate an organism to seek things rich in the "resource providing potential" needed for survival or reproduction (Orians & Heerwagen, 1992). Landscape preferences are one example. Studies of landscape preferences show that savannah-like environments are consistently preferred to other environments. In particular, people like landscapes that provide food, water, and safety. They like places that offer protection from hazards such as bad weather or landslides. And they like places that offer freedom from predators, parasites, toxic foods, and unfriendly humans (Orians & Heerwagen, 1992). Furthermore, people prefer places where they can see without being seen, places containing multiple views for surveillance, and places containing multiple ways of moving through space for escape.

As a human walks through a variety of areas searching for a place to stay for a while, some particular landscapes will fail to fulfill these evolved preferences. Those that do fulfill our evolved preferences for certain features of landscapes trigger a set of cognitive procedures or decision rules, depending partly on other contextual input such as our state of hunger or thirst, the size of our group, and knowledge about the presence of hostile humans in the vicinity. Eventually, these procedures produce output in the form of a behavioral decision to remain in the habitat or to continue our search for a better habitat. These behavioral decisions presumably led our ancestors to survive and reproduce better than those lacking them, or those who possessed alternative preferences that were less effective at securing resources and reducing risk.

Although psychological mechanisms such as landscape preferences clearly differ in important ways from mechanisms such as spider fears, they share critical ingredients that qualify them as evolved psychological mechanisms: They exist due to a history of natural selection; they are triggered only by a narrow range of information; they are characterized by a particular set of decision rules; and they produce behavioral output that solved an adaptive problem in ancestral times.

Given the infinite courses of action a human could pursue, in principle, evolved psychological mechanisms are necessary for channeling action into the narrow pockets of adaptive choices. Psychological mechanisms are necessary for seeking and extracting particular forms of information. Decision rules are necessary for producing action based on that information.

Describing the Human Mind: Important Properties of Evolved Psychological Mechanisms

This section examines several important properties of evolved psychological mecha-nisms. They provide nonarbitrary criteria for "carving the mind at its natural joints" and tend to be problem-specific, numerous, and complex. These features combine to yield the tremendous flexibility of behavior that characterizes modern humans.

Evolved psychological mechanisms provide nonarbitrary criteria for "carving the mind at its joints." A central premise of evolutionary psychology is that the main nonarbitrary way to identify, describe, and understand psychological mechanisms is to articulate their functions—the specific adaptive problems they were designed by selection to solve.

Consider the human body. In principle, the mechanisms of the body could be described in an infinite number of ways. Why do anatomists identify as separate mechanisms the liver, the heart, the hand, the nose, and the eyes? What makes these divisions nonarbitrary compared with alternative ways of dividing the human body? The answer is function. The liver is recognized as a mechanism that performs functions different from those performed by the heart or hand. The eyes and the nose, although they are close to each other on the face, perform different functions and operate according to different input (electromagnetic waves in the visual spectrum vs. odors). If an anatomist tried to lump the eyes and the nose into one category, it would be seen as ludicrous. Understanding the component parts of the body requires the identification of *function*. Function provides the only sensible nonarbitrary way to understand these component parts.

Evolutionary psychologists believe that similar principles should be used for understanding the mechanisms of the mind. Although the mind could be divided in an infinite number of ways, most of these ways would simply be arbitrary. A powerful nonarbitrary analysis of the human mind is one that rests on function. If two components of the mind perform different functions, then they can be regarded as separate mechanisms (although they may interact with other mechanisms in interesting ways).

Evolved psychological mechanisms tend to be problem-specific. Imagine giving directions to someone to get from New York City to a specific street address in San Francisco. If you gave general directions such as "Head west," the person might end up as far south as Texas or as far north as Alaska. The general direction would not reliably get the person to the right state.

Now let's suppose that the person did get to the right state. The "go west" direction now would be entirely useless, since west of California is ocean. The general direction would not provide any guidance to get to the right city within California, let alone the right street address. To get to the right state, city, street, and location on that street, you need to give more specific instructions. Furthermore, although there are many ways to get to a particular street address, some paths will be far more efficient and time-saving than others.

The search for a specific street address across country is an apt analogy for what is needed to reach a specific adaptive solution. Adaptive problems, like street addresses, are specific—don't get bitten by that snake, select a habitat with running water and places to hide, avoid eating food that is poisonous, select a mate who is fertile, and so on. There is no such thing as a "general adaptive problem" (Symons, 1992). All problems are specific.

Because adaptive problems are specific, their solutions tend to be specific as well. Just as general instructions fail to get you to the correct location, general solutions fail to get you to the right adaptive solution. Consider two adaptive problems: selecting the right foods to eat (a survival problem) and selecting the right mates with whom to have children (a reproductive problem). What counts as a "successful solution" is quite different for these two adaptive problems. Successful food selection involves identifying objects that have calories, particular vitamins and minerals, and do not contain toxic substances. Successful mate selection involves, among other things, identifying a partner who is fertile, a reliable provider, and a good parent.

What might a general solution be to these selection problems, and how effective would it be at solving them? One general solution would be: "Select the first thing that comes along." This approach would be disastrous, however, since it might lead to eating poisonous plants or marrying an infertile person. If anyone ever developed such a general solution to these adaptive problems in human evolutionary history, he or she failed to become one of our ancestors.

In order to solve these selection problems in a reasonable way, individuals need more specific guidance about the qualities of foods and qualities of mates that are important. Fruit that looks fresh and ripe, for example, will signal better nutrients than fruit that looks rotten. People who look young and healthy will be more fertile, on average, than people who look old and unhealthy. Individuals need *specific selection criteria*—qualities that are part of our selection mechanisms—in order to solve these selection problems successfully.

The specificity of mechanisms is further illustrated by errors in selection. If you make an error in food selection, then you still have an array of mechanisms that are tailored to correcting that error. When you place a piece of bad food in your mouth, it may taste terrible, in which case you would spit it out. You may gag on it if makes its way past your taste buds. And if it makes its way all the way down to your stomach, you may vomit—a specific mechanism designed to get rid of toxic or detrimental ingested substances. But if you make an error in mate selection, you do not spit, gag, or throw up (at least, not usually!). You correct your error in other ways—by leaving, selecting someone else, or simply telling the person that you don't want to see him or her anymore.

In summary, problem specificity of adaptive mechanisms is favored over generality because (1) general solutions fail to guide the organism to the correct adaptive solutions; (2) general solutions, even if they do work, lead to too many errors and thus are costly to the organism; and (3) what constitutes a "successful solution" differs from problem to problem (e.g., criteria for successful food selection differ from criteria for successful mate selection). The adaptive solutions, in short, must have dedicated procedures and content-sensitive elements in order to solve adaptive problems successfully.

Humans possess many evolved psychological mechanisms. Humans, like most organisms, encounter a large number of adaptive problems. The problems of survival alone number in the dozens or hundreds—problems of thermal regulation (getting too cold or too hot), avoiding predators and parasites, ingesting life-sustaining foods, and so on. Then there are problems of mating, such as selecting, attracting, and keeping good mates and getting rid of bad mates. There are also problems of parenting, such as breast-feeding, weaning, socializing, deciding on the varying needs of different children, and so on. Then there are the problems of investing in kin, such as brothers, sisters, nephews, and nieces; dealing with social conflicts; defending against aggressive groups; grappling with the social hierarchy, and dozens more.

Because specific problems require specific solutions, numerous specific problems will require numerous specific solutions. Just as our bodies contain thousands of specific mechanisms—a heart to pump blood, lungs for oxygen uptake, a liver to filter out toxins—the mind, according to this analysis, almost surely contains dozens, hundreds, or possibly thousands of specific mechanisms (depending on how finely or grossly the mechanisms are described; e.g., the eye can be seen as one mechanism or as a collection of component mechanisms, such as a pupil that dilates, a cornea, rods, cones, edge detectors, and so on). Since a large number of different adaptive problems cannot be solved with just a few mechanisms, the human mind must contain a large number of evolved psychological mechanisms.

The specificity, complexity, and numerousness of evolved psychological mechanisms give humans behavioral flexibility. The definition of a psychological mechanism, including the key components of input, decision rules, and output, highlights why adaptations are not rigid "instincts" that show up invariably in behavior. Consider the example of callous-producing mechanisms that have evolved to protect the structures beneath the skin. You can design your environment so that you don't experience repeated friction. In this case, your callus-producing mechanisms will not be activated. The activation of the mechanisms is dependent on contextual input coming from the environment. In the same way, all psychological mechanisms require input for their activation.

Psychological mechanisms are unlike rigid instincts for another important reason—the decision rules. Decision rules are "if–then" procedures, such as "If the snake hisses, then run for your life" or "If the person I'm attracted to shows interest, then smile and decrease distance." For most mechanisms, these decision rules permit at least several possible response options. Even

in the straightforward example of encountering a snake, you can attack it with a stick, freeze and hope it will go away, or run away. In general, the more complex the mechanism, the more response options there will be.

Consider a carpenter's toolbox. The carpenter gains flexibility not by having one "highly general tool" that can be used to cut, poke, saw, screw, twist, wrench, plane, balance, and hammer. Instead, the carpenter gains flexibility by having a large number of highly specific tools in the toolbox. These highly specific tools can then be used in many combinations that would not be possible with one highly "flexible" tool. Indeed, it is difficult to imagine what a "general" tool would even look like, since there is no such thing as a "general carpenter's problem." In a similar fashion, humans gain their flexibility from having a large number of complex, specific, functional psychological mechanisms.

With each new mechanism that is added to the mind, an organism can perform a new task that it could not perform previously. A bird has feet that enable it to walk. Adding wings to a bird enables it to fly. Adding a beak to a bird enables it to break the shells of seeds and nuts and get at their nutritious core. With each new specific mechanism that is added, the bird can do a new task that it could not do without it. Having both feet and wings gives the bird the flexibility to both walk and fly.

This analogy leads to a conclusion that is contrary to our intuitions. Most people's intuitions are that having a lot of innate mechanisms causes behavior to be rigid and inflexible. But just the opposite is the case. The more mechanisms involved, the greater the range of behaviors we can perform, and hence the greater the flexibility of behavior.

In summary, an evolutionary perspective provides some broad specifications of human nature. First, it suggests a nonarbitrary foundation for describing the contents of human nature—contents described by the evolved psychological mechanisms of humans. Second, it suggests that human nature is likely to be extremely complex, consisting of a large number of evolved psychological mechanisms rather than one or a few simple drives, motives, or goals. Third, because evolved psychological mechanisms tend to be problem-specific and hence activated only in particular contexts, human nature will likely express itself in variable and context-dependent ways, rather than as invariant impulses, as implied by some personality theories. Fourth, human behavioral flexibility comes not from highly general psychological mechanisms, but rather from a large number of specific psychological mechanisms that are activated and concatenated in varying complex sequences, depending on the adaptive problem being confronted. These implications render the study of human nature a difficult and daunting task, but also one that is tractable.

Progress can be made sequentially and cumulatively by uncovering each evolved psychological mechanism along with the adaptive problem it was designed to solve. Ultimately, of course, the field will have to discover how the mechanisms are connected with each other, how they are sequentially activated depending on circumstances, how the activation of one can preempt or supersede the activation of another, and so on (Buss, 2008).

The Evolution of Motives, Goals, and Strivings

This evolutionary analysis has profound implications for personality theories of human nature. It provides an incisive heuristic that guides theorists to the sorts of motives, goals, and strivings that commonly characterize humans. At the most general level, it suggests that, at some fundamental level of description, the *only* directional tendencies that can have evolved are those that historically contributed to the survival and reproduction of human ancestors. For a variety of reasons, outlined by Symons (1992) and Tooby and Cosmides (1990b), what might seem like the most obvious candidate for a human motive—the goal of maximizing inclusive fitness—cannot have evolved. Because what constitutes fitness differs for different species, sexes, times, and contexts, evolution by selection cannot produce a domain-general motive of fitness maximization. It's not just that people never list "maximization of gene replication" as a personal project when asked to list what they are striving toward in their lives (Little, 1989). It's that no such goal can evolve even in principle, consciously or unconsciously. Stated differently, the *products* of the evolutionary process—the specific adaptations and byproducts that characterize

humans—should not be confused with the evolutionary *process* that fashioned them. Differential gene replication caused by differences in design features is the process by which adaptations get created. But the adaptations themselves do not include a desire to maximize gene replication.

Status Striving

What can evolve are *specific* motives, goals, and strivings, the attainment of which recurrently led to reproductive success over human evolutionary history. Consider one candidate for a universal human motive—*striving for status* (Buss, 1995a; Hogan, 1983; Maslow, 1970). Why would status striving be a universal evolved motive in humans? A variety of sources of evidence can be brought to bear to explain why status striving is a good candidate. First, among closely related species, such as chimpanzees, that form status hierarchies, those who are high in status tend to outreproduce those who are lower. They do so because they gain preferential access to the resources needed for survival, such as choice food, and they also gain preferential access to desirable mates. Among chimpanzees, for example, the dominant males tend to monopolize the matings with females during estrus, whereas the copulations of less dominant males, when they occur, take place outside of the peak period of fecundity (de Waal, 1982).

Second, the cross-cultural and historical evidence suggests that high-status males, such as kings, emperors, and despots, routinely used (and probably still do) their status to gain increased sexual access to females (Betzig, 1986). Kings and despots routinely stocked their harems with young, attractive, nubile women and had sex with them frequently. The Moroccan emperor Moulay Ismail the Bloodthirsty, for example, acknowledged having sired 888 children (actually, the number is probably double this, since only male children were acknowledged). His harem had 500 women. But when a woman reached the age of 30, she was banished from the emperor's harem and sent to a lower-level leader's harem, replaced by a younger woman. Roman, Babylonian, Egyptian, Incan, Indian, and Chinese emperors acted in a similar manner, using their status to enjoin their trustees to scour the land for as many young, pretty women as could be found (Betzig, 1992).

Third, the cross-cultural evidence suggests that the children of high-status individuals tend to receive better health care, and hence they survive longer and are healthier than the children of lower-status individuals. Among the Ache Indians, a hunter-gatherer group residing in Paraguay, tribal members take great pains to remove splinters and thorns from the feet of the children of high-status males (Hill & Hurtado, 1996). Choice food, choice territory, and choice mates all flow with greater abundance to those high in status among hunters and gatherers around the world (e.g., Chagnon, 1983; Hart & Pilling, 1960; Hill & Hurtado, 1996).

If the attainment of high status recurrently led to increased reproductive success over human evolutionary history, then selection would have fashioned a human motive of status striving. The evolutionary analysis, however, does not stop there, because specific and testable hypotheses about status striving can be derived. One key hypothesis pertains to a sex difference in the strength of the status-striving motive. Men and women differ in a fundamental fact of their reproductive biology: Women bear the burdens (and pleasures) of heavy obligatory parental investment, since a minimum of 9 months of pregnancy, with all the metabolic costs entailed, is required to produce a single child. Men, on the other hand, can produce a child from a single low-cost act of sexual intercourse. This fundamental sex difference has led to profound sex differences in sexual strategies (Buss, 1994/2003; Symons, 1979; Williams, 1975). The key difference relevant to status striving is this: The reproductive payoff to men of gaining sexual access to multiple partners historically has been far greater than the reproductive payoff for women. Since status leads to increased sexual access to partners, men are predicted to be higher in status striving than women.

This evolutionary reasoning produces a specific and testable prediction: Men in every culture around the world should have a greater desire for status, on average, than women. Among the many possible empirical tests that could be conducted are these: (1) Men should be more willing to take greater risks than women in order to achieve high status; (2) in the allocation of their effort across various adaptive problems, men should allocate more time and effort to status striving than women; (3) men who lose status should engage in more desperate measures to staunch the loss than women who lose status; and (4) the psychological pain that men experience after a status loss should be greater than the psychological pain women experience after a comparable status loss. These are easily testable predictions, but to my knowledge, none of these predictions has been examined empirically in a systematic fashion across cultures.

Several key implications emerge from this evolutionary analysis of status striving. First, evolutionary psychology provides a heuristic, guiding theorists and researchers toward motives and goals that may form the building blocks of human nature. Second, the evolutionary predictions derived are testable and hence potentially falsifiable, contradicting a common but mistaken idea that evolutionary hypotheses are not testable. Third, this evolutionary analysis suggests that the building blocks of human nature will differ for men and women, principally because the sexes have faced recurrently different adaptive problems over the long expanse of human evolutionary history.

Mating Motivation

A second prime candidate for human nature is a universal mating motivation. At first blush, this may seem so obvious as to hardly warrant much comment, but first blushes can be misleading. Despite the obvious importance of sex and sexuality in the everyday lives of people (Buss, 1994), few personality theories explicitly consider sex. Freud, of course, was a major exception. Indeed, sexual motivation was the primary driving force in psychoanalytic theory, providing the raw energy that fueled nearly all other forms of human activity, from sports to cultural innovation (Freud, 1953/1905). Since Freud's theory, however, personality theories have minimized sexual and mating motivations. Evolutionary personality psychology appears to be the only large theoretical framework that predicts that sexual motivation will be a fundamental component of human nature (Buss, 1991). Even personality frameworks that restrict their focus to individual differences typically exclude individual differences in sexuality, despite their prevalence and importance in the everyday lives of people (Schmitt & Buss, 2000).

Evolutionary analysis provides a compelling rationale for the importance of sexuality. Evolution by selection occurs through differential reproduction caused by differences in design (Symons, 1992). Reproductive differences, in other words, are the engine of the evolutionary process. Therefore, anything that resides in close proximity to reproduction and affects the probability of reproduction is likely to be a special target of the selective process. Perhaps nothing lies closer to the reproductive engine than sexuality and mating.

Consider what it would have taken for human ancestors to succeed in reproduction. The first task is mate attraction: successfully enticing a member of the opposite sex to become one's mate. This task is more difficult than it might seem, for it includes at a minimum selecting the "right" mate (e.g., those that are reproductively valuable rather than sterile) on whom to deploy one's attraction tactics as well as embodying the desires of the targeted member of the opposite sex sufficiently to succeed in attracting him or her (Buss, 1994). Embodying or fulfilling the desires of the targeted other might include a prolonged effort at attaining a modicum of social status, establishing a favorable reputation among one's peers, and displaying physical cues of desirability.

Successful attraction is not enough, however. In order to produce viable offspring, human ancestors would also have had to be motivated to engage in sex with the targeted person. Although having sex may appear to flow naturally and effortlessly for some, it actually entails a complex set of properly sequenced and contingent behaviors in order to culminate in successful merging of the male sperm and female egg. Mating motivation also entails the intricate tasks of besting intrasexual competitors in successful attraction tactics (Buss, 1988a; Schmitt & Buss, 1996), perhaps derogation of intrasexual competitors to make them seem less desirable (Buss & Dedden, 1990), and successful mate retention (Buss, 1988b; Buss & Shackelford, 1997). Mating motivation is a multifaceted venture, entailing a host of subtasks, any of which can result in a failure. As descendants of ancestors who succeeded

in all of these mating tasks, modern humans have inherited the mating motivations and strategies that led to their success. Personality theories that fail to include mating motivation, broadly conceived, must be viewed as woefully inadequate, from the perspective of evolutionary psychology.

Like status striving, however, evolutionary analysis provides a powerful rationale for predicting sex differences in the nature of mating motivation. Due to the asymmetries in obligatory parental investment, for example, men are predicted to have a greater desire than women for a larger number of sex partners, and a large body of empirical evidence supports this prediction (Buss & Schmitt, 1993; Kenrick, Sadalla, Groth, & Trost, 1990). Furthermore, a large body of cross-cultural evidence supports the specific predictions that men will be more motivated to seek young and physically attractive mates, whereas women will more motivated to seek mates who offer a willingness and ability to accrue and commit resources (Buss, 1989b; Kenrick & Keefe, 1992). Personality theories that include mating motivation, in short, must also include specific premises about the ways in which mating motivation is known to differ between the sexes, corresponding to sex differences in the adaptive problems faced over human evolutionary history.

Universal Emotions

Another core feature of human nature proposed by evolutionary psychology involves universal mechanisms of emotion (Buss, 1989a; Nesse, 1990; Tooby & Cosmides, 1990b). A large body of cross-cultural evidence already exists to suggest that certain forms of emotional expression are universal (Ekman, 1973). Evolutionary analysis suggests that certain emotions will be universal, designed to solve specific adaptive problems. One candidate for such a universal emotion is jealousy.

Jealousy has been hypothesized to be a universal emotion that evolved to solve the problem of mate retention (Daly, Wilson, & Weghorst, 1982; Buss, 2000; Buss, Larsen, Westen, & Semmelroth, 1992; Buss & Haselton, 2005). Threats to a valued sexual or romantic mating relationship are hypothesized to activate the emotion of jealousy, which then motivates action designed to reduce the threat. Jealousy may motivate actions that range from vigilance to violence, with three potential goals: to ward off intrasexual competitors, to induce one's mate to stay in the relationship and not stray, and to enhance one's value to one's mate as an induction to remain in the relationship (Buss & Shackelford, 1997). Although jealousy and the mate retention tactics it produces clearly fail in their adaptive function some of the time, the hypothesis is that they succeeded, on average, relative to nonjealous counterparts over evolutionary time.

Like status striving and sexual motivation, evolutionary analysis provides a powerful basis for predicting sex differences. These are not sex differences in the presence or intensity of jealousy, since both sexes have faced the adaptive problem of mate retention. And indeed, the empirical evidence suggests that the sexes do not differ in measures such as the frequency and intensity of jealousy experienced (Buunk & Hupka, 1987).

An evolutionary analysis, however, suggests that the sexes might differ in the events that activate jealousy. Specifically, since fertilization occurs internally within women and not within men, over evolutionary history men have faced the adaptive problem of "paternity uncertainty." Since a partner's sexual intercourse with another man would have been the primary threat to paternity certainty, and hence to successful reproduction, men's jealousy is hypothesized to be specially keyed to signals of sexual infidelity by a partner. Ancestral women, in contrast, faced a different adaptive problem: the loss of a mate's time, energy, effort, attention, investment, and commitment, all of which could get rechanneled to a rival woman and her children. Since a man's emotional involvement with another woman is a leading cue to such redirection of commitments, women's jealousy is predicted to be keyed to signals of emotional involvement more than to sexual infidelity, per se, although the two signals are clearly correlated in nature.

Much empirical evidence supports these predicted sex differences (Buss & Haselton, 2005). In forced-choice dilemmas, men more than women report that they would experience greater distress at a partner's sexual infidelity, whereas women more than men report that they would experience greater distress as a result of a partner's emotional infidelity (Buss et al., 1992). These results have been replicated by different researchers (Weiderman & Allgeier, 1993), across methods that include psychophysiological recordings (Buss et al., 1992), and across Western and non-Western cultures (Buunk, Angleitner, Oubaid, & Buss, 1996). The sex differences have also been found using cognitive methods such as measuring attention to, and recall of, cues to sexual versus emotional infidelity; measures of physiological distress to imagining a partner committing a sexual versus emotional infidelity; and using functional magnetic resonance imaging (fMRI) technology, which has documented different patterns of brain activation in response to sexual versus emotional infidelity (see Buss, 2008, and Buss & Haselton, 2005, for summaries of this evidence). All of these empirical findings suggest that jealousy is a universal and universally sex-differentiated emotion that is a good candidate for inclusion in a personality theory of human nature.

Jealousy is clearly not the only candidate. Others include fear, rage, envy, disgust, and sadness. As Ekman (1994) notes, the empirical evidence suggest that these emotions are universal across human cultures, have been adaptive phylogenetically, occur in common eliciting contexts despite individual differences and cultural differences, are likely to be present in closely related primate species, and can be activated quickly, prior to awareness, mobilizing action designed to respond to specific adaptive challenges. There is no reason why theories of personality should fail to include these emotions as candidates for the core of human nature.

Parental Motivation

From an evolutionary perspective, offspring are vehicles for parents: that is, they are a means by which their parents' genes get transported to succeeding generations. Without these vehicles, an individual's genes would perish forever. Given the supreme importance of offspring as genetic vehicles, it is reasonable to expect that natural selection would favor powerful mechanisms in parents to ensure the survival and reproductive success of their children. Aside from the problems of mating, perhaps no other adap-

2. Human Nature and Individual Differences

tive problems are as paramount as making sure that one's offspring survive and thrive. Indeed, without the success of offspring, all the effort that an organism invested in mating would be reproductively meaningless. Evolution, in short, should produce a rich repertoire of parental mechanisms specially adapted to caring for offspring.

Despite the paramount importance of parental care from an evolutionary perspective, it has been a relatively neglected topic within the field of human personality psychology. When the evolutionary psychologists Martin Daly and Margo Wilson prepared a chapter on the topic for the 1987 *Nebraska Symposium on Motivation*, they scanned the 34 previous volumes in the series in search of either psychological research or theories on parental motivation. Not a single one of the 34 volumes contained even a paragraph on parental motivation (Daly & Wilson, 1995). And despite the widespread everyday knowledge that mothers tend to love their children, the very phenomenon of powerful parental love appears to have baffled psychologists at a theoretical level. One prominent psychologist who has written books on the topic of love noted that "the needs that lead many of us to feel unconditional love for our children also seem to be remarkably persistent, for reasons that are not at present altogether clear" (Sternberg, 1986, p. 133). From an evolutionary perspective, however, the reasons for deep parental love do seem clear, or at least understandable. It is reasonable to expect that selection has designed precisely such psychological mechanisms—parental mechanisms of motivation designed to ensure the survival and reproductive success of the invaluable vehicles that transport an individual's genes into the next generation.

The evolution of parenting motivation has produced in humans mechanisms that are far from unconditional. Empirical evidence suggests than parents invest more in children when they are higher in phenotypic quality, have a high probability of genetic relatedness to parents, and have the ability to convert such aid into reproduction (see Buss, 2008, for a summary of the empirical evidence). Mothers, by virtue of internal fertilization, are 100% sure that the offspring they bear are genetically their own. Fathers, until the last decade, can never be sure. This analy-

sis leads to the prediction that maternal love will tend to be stronger than paternal love, on average. Although there is circumstantial evidence to support this prediction, such as the higher rates of child abandonment by men compared with women, this hypothesis remains to be tested rigorously in studies of parental feeling and behavior. The incidence of physical abuse of children, to take another example, is roughly 40 times higher in stepfamilies compared with genetically intact families, supporting the prediction that genetic relatedness affects feelings of parental love (Daly & Wilson, 1988). Moreover, the evolutionary theory of parent–offspring conflict suggests that children will generally desire a higher level of parental investment than parents are willing to give, since parents are motivated to distribute their investments across offspring (Trivers, 1974).

Parental motivation, as a core feature of human nature, appears to be absent from most or all personality theories, although Freud clearly signaled the importance of relationships with parents in the development of personality. Evolutionary psychology provides a heuristic for the inclusion of this neglected component of human nature.

Other Motivational Candidates for Human Nature

Status striving, mating motivation, jealousy, emotions, and parental motivation are merely a few of the most obvious candidates for a comprehensive theory of human nature. Others include the desire to form friendships or dyadic reciprocal alliances (Bleske & Buss, 2001), the desire to help and invest in kin (Burnstein, Crandall, & Kitayama, 1994), and the motivation to form and join larger coalitions (Tooby & Cosmides, 1988). An evolutionary perspective leads us to anticipate the evolution of many complex psychological mechanisms underlying each of these forms of social relationships. One clear implication is that evolutionary psychology provides a nonarbitrary theoretical foundation for postulating fundamental human motivations, such as "sex and aggression" or "love and power" or "getting along and getting ahead." At the same time, it suggests that the postulation of only one or a few such motivational tendencies will grossly underestimate the complexity of human nature.

THE EVOLUTION OF INDIVIDUAL DIFFERENCES

According to this analysis, individual differences cannot be divorced from, or considered apart from, the foundations of human nature. Just as the fundamental mechanisms of cars yield the major dimensions along which cars differ, the fundamental psychological mechanisms of humans yield the major dimensions along which human personality differs. Personality theories of individual differences, according to this reasoning, must have as a foundation a specification of human nature.

This section offers some suggestions for a nonarbitrary evolutionary framework of individual differences (see Buss & Greiling, 1999; Keller & Miller, 2006; MacDonald, 1995, 1998; Nettle, 2006; Penke, Denissen, & Miller, 2007). First, the major ways of treating individual differences from an evolutionary psychological perspective are discussed. Second, specific examples of adaptive individual differences, stemming from species-typical motives and strivings, are presented to illustrate these conceptions.

Individual differences can emerge from a variety of heritable and nonheritable sources. Evidence from behavioral genetic studies of personality strongly suggests that both are important. Personality characteristics commonly show evidence of moderate heritability, typically ranging from 30 to 50% (Bouchard & McGue, 1990; Loehlin, Horn, & Willerman, 1990; Plomin, DeFries, & McClearn, 1990). All heritable individual differences, of course, ultimately originate from mutations—a point taken up later. Simultaneously, these studies provide the strongest evidence of environmental sources of variance, ranging from 50 to 70%. In the following material a conceptual taxonomy of sources of adaptively patterned individual differences is presented, based on environmental and heritable sources, as well as interactions between these sources (Buss & Greiling, 1999). The routes to adaptively patterned individual differences are presented descriptively with illustrative cases that are sometimes speculative (see Table 2.2).

Early Experiential Calibration

Individuals who share a common evolved psychology may experience different early environmental events that channel them into alternative strategies. According to this conception, each person comes equipped with two or more potential strategies within his or her repertoire. From this species-typical menu, one strategy is selected based on early environmental experiences. These early experiences, in essence, "lock in" a person to one strategy to the exclusion of others that could have been pursued, had the environmental input been different.

Belsky, Steinberg, and Draper (1991), for example, propose the critical event of early father presence versus father absence as a calibrator of alternative sexual strategies. Individuals growing up in father-absent homes during the first 5–7 years of life, according to this theory, develop expectations that parental resources will not be reliably or predictably provided and adult pair bonds will not be enduring. Accordingly, such individuals cultivate a sexual strategy marked by early sexual maturation, early sexual initiation, and frequent partner switching—a strategy designed to produce a large number of offspring with low levels of investment in each. Extraverted and impulsive personality traits may accompany this strategy. Other

---

TABLE 2.2. Sources of Individual Differences in Personality

Environmental sources of individual differences

1. Early experiential calibration
2. Enduring situational evocation
3. Strategic specialization
4. Adaptive self-assessment of heritable qualities

Heritable sources of individual differences

1. Balancing Selection 2: temporal or spatial variation in selection pressures
2. Balancing Selection 1: negative frequency-dependent selection
3. Mutation–selection balance

individuals are perceived as untrustworthy, relationships as transitory. Resources sought from brief sexual liaisons are opportunistically attained and immediately extracted.

Individuals marked by a reliably investing father during the first 5–7 years of life, according to the theory, develop a different set of expectations about the nature and trustworthiness of others. People are seen as reliable and trustworthy, and relationships are expected to be enduring. These early environmental experiences channel individuals toward a long-term mating strategy, marked by delay of sexual maturation, a later onset of sexual activity, a search for long-term securely attached adult relationships, and heavy investment in a small number of children.

All theories of environmental influence, including this one, ultimately rest on a foundation of evolved psychological mechanisms, whether they are acknowledged as such or not (Tooby & Cosmides, 1990a). Contrary to views that perpetuate the false dichotomies of nature–nurture or genes–environment, evolved psychological mechanisms are necessarily entailed by theories of environmental influence (Tooby & Cosmides, 1990a). In this particular case, the implicit psychological mechanisms are specifically designed to take as *input* information about the presence and reliability of paternal resources, *process* that input via an evolved set of decision rules, *develop* one of two possible psychological models of the social world, and pursue one of two alternative mating strategies as *output* of the mechanisms. It is possible, of course, that mechanisms of this sort may permit three or more alternative strategies from a larger menu of options.

There are two key points to draw from Belsky and colleagues' (1991) theory of adaptively patterned individual differences. First, the individual variation lies not on a single dimension or trait, but rather represents a coherent constellation of covarying qualities, including reproductive physiology (e.g., early age of menarche), psychological models of the social world (e.g., others as untrustworthy), and overt behavior (e.g., transitory sexual liaisons).

Second, the individual differences that result from early experiential calibration are adaptively patterned—the result of evolved mechanisms that assess the social environ-

ment and select one strategy from the menu. In one case, reproductive success historically was attained through a high reproductive rate, with perhaps a concomitant decrease in the survival and reproduction of any one offspring. In the other case, reproductive success historically was attained through a lower reproductive rate marked by heavy investment in the survival and reproduction of fewer offspring. The evolution of these environment-contingent strategies presumably resulted from a long and recurrent evolutionary history in which different individuals confronted radically different rearing environments. Environmental variation over human evolutionary history presumably selected for developmentally flexible mechanisms that take as input the nature of the rearing environment as a key cue to the expected adult environment.

Enduring Situational Evocation

Many human adaptations respond to immediately encountered environmental contingencies rather than being "set in plaster" by early environmental events. The physiological mechanism that results in calluses, for example, responds to immediately experienced friction to the skin. Individuals differ recurrently in the degree to which they pursue activities that result in frequent, repeated friction to the skin. The stable individual differences in calluses, in this example, are properly understood as adaptively patterned differences stemming from enduring environmental differences in the evocation of the callous-producing mechanism. These enduring individual differences, like those set by early experiential calibration, are the result of a specific form of interaction between environments and evolved mechanisms.

A similar form of adaptively patterned individual differences can occur with psychological factors. Consider a man who is married to a woman who has higher perceived "mate value" on the mating market than he does (Frank, 1988; Tooby & Cosmides, 1990a; Walster, Traupmann, & Walster, 1978). Even if his social environment is not populated with interested same-sex rivals, his enduring relationship with his wife may lower his threshold for jealousy compared with the man who is equal to, or higher than, his wife in perceived mate value (Tooby &

Cosmides, 1990a). As a consequence, he may get jealous more easily (Tooby & Cosmides, 1990a) and engage in mate guarding efforts such as vigilantly monitoring his wife's activities and striving to sequester her more intensely (Buss, 1988a; Buss & Shackelford, 1997). He may become more easily suspicious about her interactions with others and more enraged when observing her conversing casually with other men. Some empirical evidence supports these suggestions, indicating that the more desirable partner is indeed more susceptible to defecting (Buss, 2000; Hatfield, Traupmann, Sprecher, Utne, & Hay, 1985; Walster et al., 1978). From an adaptationist perspective, a mechanism for adjusting one's threshold for jealousy could have resulted from thousands of selective events in the evolutionary past in which a mate value discrepancy, on average, was statistically associated with a greater likelihood of a partner's infidelity or defection (Tooby & Cosmides, 1990a).

Individual differences in jealousy, in this example, endure over time and are adaptively patterned. They rest on a foundation of evolved psychological mechanisms shared by all but differentially activated in some. Were the enduring environment to change—for example, if the man got divorced and remarried a woman of equal or lower mate value—then the enduring pattern of psychological and behavioral jealousy would presumably change (Tooby & Cosmides, 1990a).

In sum, enduring adaptive individual differences result from evocations produced by the enduring situations inhabited. These relatively enduring situations may include one's overall desirability as a mate on the mating market, age, and the ratio of men to women in the local population (Pedersen, 1991). Future research could profitably explore these and other features of enduring environments as sources of relatively stable individual differences.

Strategic Specialization

From an evolutionary perspective, competition is keenest among those pursuing the same strategy. As one niche becomes more and more crowded with competitors, experiences of success can be hard to achieve, compared with those seeking alternative niches

(Maynard Smith, 1982; Wilson, 1994). Selection can favor mechanisms that cause some individuals to seek niches where the competition is less intense and hence where the average payoff may be higher.

Mating provides some clear examples. If most women pursue the man with the highest status or greatest resources, then clearly many women will be unsuccessful. Some women would achieve more success by courting males outside of the arenas in which competition is keenest. In a mating system in which both polygyny and monogamy are possible, for example, a woman might be better off securing all of the resources of a lower-status monogamous man rather than having to settle for a fraction of the resources of a high-status polygynous man.

The ability to exploit a niche will depend on the resources and personal characteristics an individual brings to the situation, whether environmental or heritable in origin (Buss, 1989b; Gangestad & Simpson, 2000). One variable that is *not* heritable is birth order. It is possible that firstborn and second-born children have faced, on average, recurrently different adaptive problems over human evolutionary history. Sulloway (1996), for example, argues that firstborns occupy a niche characterized by strong identification with parents and other existing authority figures. Second-borns, in contrast, have less to gain by authority identification and more to gain by overthrowing the existing order. According to Sulloway, birth order influences niche specialization. Second-borns develop a different personality marked by greater rebelliousness, lower levels of conscientiousness, and higher levels of openness to new experiences (Sulloway, 1996). Birth-order differences show up strongly among scientists, where second-borns tend to be strong advocates of scientific revolutions (e.g., Copernican, Darwinian); firstborns tend to strenuously resist such revolutions (Sulloway, 1996).

Whether or not the details of Sulloway's arguments turn out to be correct, the example illustrates strategic niche specialization. Individual differences are adaptively patterned, but they are *not* based on heritable individual differences. Rather, birth order, a nonheritable individual difference, provides input (presumably through interactions with family members) into a species-typical mechanism that canalizes strategic niche specialization.

All of the above individual differences are examples of environmentally contingent individual differences. In "early experiential calibration," the developmental environment activates stable individual differences in adulthood. In "enduring situational evocation," the stable occupancy of different environments activates and maintains stable individual differences in personality. And in "strategic specialization," the existence or lack of existence of environmental or social niches to exploit activates and maintains stable individual differences. I now turn to those individual differences that have at least a partial basis in heredity.

Adaptive Self-Assessment of Heritable Qualities

According to Tooby and Cosmides (1990a), selection operates through the attainment of goal states. Any feature of an individual's world—*including that individual's own personal characteristics*—that influences the successful attainment of those goal states may be assessed and evaluated by evolved psychological mechanisms (Tooby & Cosmides, 1990a, p. 59). Evolved mechanisms, in this view, are not only attuned to recurrent features of the external world, such as the reliability of parental provisioning, but can also be attuned to the evaluation of self. Tooby and Cosmides coined the term "reactive heritability" to describe evolved psychological mechanisms designed to take as input heritable qualities as a guide to strategic solutions.

Suppose that all men have an evolved decision rule that states: Pursue an aggressive strategy when aggression can be implemented successfully to achieve goals, but pursue a cooperative strategy when aggression cannot be implemented successfully (modified from Tooby & Cosmides, 1990a, p. 58). Evolved decision rules are undoubtedly more complex than this one, but given this simplified rule, consider that men who happen to be mesomorphic (muscular) in body build will be able to carry out an aggressive strategy more successfully than those who are ectomorphic (skinny) or endomorphic (rotund). Heritable individual differences in body build provide

input into the decision rule, thereby producing stable individual differences in aggression and cooperativeness. In this example, the proclivity toward aggression is not directly heritable, but rather would be "reactively heritable" in the sense that it is a secondary consequence of heritable body build, which provides input into species-typical mechanisms of self-assessment and decision making.

Similar models of heritable adaptive input can be developed for individual differences in mating strategies. One study assessed the physical appearance of teenage boys on two dimensions: the degree to which their faces looked dominant or submissive and physically attractive (Mazur, Halpern, & Udry, 1994). Only photographs were available for the judgments of these features, with a dominant person being defined as someone who "tells other people what to do, is respected, influential, and often a leader" (p. 90). The teenagers who were judged to be more facially dominant and physically attractive were discovered to have had more heterosexual experience with "heavy petting" and sexual intercourse. Furthermore, dominant facial appearance predicted cumulative coital experience, even after statistically controlling for facial attractiveness and puberty development.

Although speculative, these findings may illustrate heritable adaptive input, on the assumption that facial features involved in appearing dominant and attractive are partially heritable. Males could all have an evolved psychological mechanism that takes as input a self-assessment (Tooby & Cosmides, 1990a) of the degree to which one appears dominant and attractive: "If high on these dimensions, pursue a short-term sexual strategy; if low, pursue a long-term sexual strategy." In this example, one cannot rule out third variables, of course, such as testosterone, which may simultaneously produce a more dominant-looking face and a higher sex drive.

According to the conception of adaptive self-assessment of heritable qualities, stable individual differences in the pursuit of short-term and long-term sexual strategies are not directly heritable. But they represent adaptive individual differences based on self-assessment of heritable information.

Balancing Selection: Heritable Frequency-Dependent Adaptive Strategies

In general, the process of directional selection tends to use up heritable variation. Heritable variants that are more successful tend to replace those that are less successful, resulting in species-typical adaptations that show little or no heritable variation in the presence or absence of basic functional components (Williams, 1966).

There are several major exceptions to this trend. One is *mutation–selection balance* (see Penke et al., 2007, for a more detailed discussion). Mutations are introduced in every generation, with one estimate being 1.67 mutations per individual in each generation (Keightley & Gaffney, 2003). Since most mutations are deleterious, harming the functioning of the evolved machinery, selection tends to remove them over time. Harmful mutations that are recessive are likely to persist longer than harmful mutations that are dominant. Each individual human carries a "mutation load" consisting of mildly deleterious recessive mutations (Penke et al., 2007). One estimate is that the average number of such mutations carried by humans is approximately 500 (Fay, Whyckoff, & Wu, 2001). Nonetheless, individuals vary tremendously in the number of mildly harmful mutations they carry. These individual differences in mutation load can, in principle, explain some stable individual differences in humans. After a careful analysis, Penke and his colleagues (2007) conclude that mutation load (and hence mutation–selection balance) is an excellent candidate evolutionary mechanism for explaining individual differences in cognitive traits, such as general intelligence as well as mental disorders (see Keller & Miller, 2006). Those with higher intelligence are presumed to have a lower mutation load, and those with various mental disorders are presumed to have a higher mutation load. Nonetheless, mutation–selection balance is unlikely to explain individual differences in personality such as those captured by the Big Five (Penke et al., 2007).

A more plausible evolutionary mechanism for explaining heritable personality differences, Penke and colleagues argue, is that of *balancing selection*. In this proposed process, genetic variation (originally introduced by mutation) is not weeded out by selection but rather is *maintained* by selection. Balancing selection occurs when heritable individual differences on a trait are positively selected for, to the same degree, and hence maintained in the population. There are several forms of balancing selection, but two are the most plausible candidates for explaining heritable personality traits.

The first is *temporal or spatial variation in selection pressure*. Consider the example of variations over time or place in the scarcity or abundance of food resources. In times and places of food scarcity, selection might favor a bold risk-taking personality that propels an individual to venture out into unknown territory to find food. The more timid, risk-averse individuals are more likely to starve to death. In contrast, in times and places of food abundance, a bold risk-taking strategy might be less successful, because it exposes the individual to predators and other risks needlessly. Under these conditions, selection might favor more timid souls who stay close to home and hence avoid these dangers. In short, variation over time or space in selection pressure can create a form of balancing selection in which heritable individual differences are maintained in the population.

A second type of balancing selection is *negative frequency-dependent selection*. In some contexts, two or more heritable variants can be sustained in equilibrium. The most obvious example is biological sex. In sexually reproducing species, the two sexes represent frequency-dependent "suites" of covarying adaptive complexes. If one sex becomes rare relative to the other, success increases for the rare sex, and hence selection favors parents who produce offspring of the less common sex. Typically, the sexes are maintained in approximately equal ratio through the process of frequency-dependent selection, which requires that the payoff of each strategy decreases as its frequency increases, relative to other strategies, in the population.

Alternative adaptive strategies can also be maintained *within sexes* by frequency-dependent selection. Among the bluegill sunfish, for example, three different male mating strategies are observed: a "parental" strategy that defends the nest, a "sneak" strategy that matures to only a small body size, and a "mimic" strategy that resembles the female form (Gross, 1982). The sneakers gain sexual access to the female eggs by avoiding detection due to their small size, while the mimics gain access by resembling females and thus avoiding aggression from the parental males. As the parasitizing strategists increase in frequency, however, their success decreases—their existence depends on the parentals, who become rarer as the parasites become more common, rendering the parasite strategies more difficult to pursue. Thus, heritable alternative strategies within a sex are maintained by the process of frequency-dependent selection. Theoretically, these heritable individual differences can persist in the population indefinitely through frequency-dependent selection, unlike the process of directional selection, which tends to drive out heritable variation.

Frequency-Dependent Mating Strategies

Gangestad and Simpson (1990) argue that individual differences in women's mating strategies have been caused (and are presumably maintained) by frequency-dependent selection. They start with the observation that competition tends to be most intense among individuals pursuing the same mating strategy (Maynard Smith, 1982). This contingency lays the groundwork for the evolution of alternative strategies.

According to Gangestad and Simpson, women's mating strategies should center on two key qualities of potential mates: the *parental investment* a man could provide and his *genetic fitness*. A man who is able and willing to invest in the woman and her children can be an extraordinarily valuable reproductive asset. Similarly, independent of a man's ability to invest, women could benefit by selecting men who are themselves in good condition and are highly attractive to other women. Such men may carry genes for good health, physical attractiveness, or sexiness, which are then passed on to the women's own sons or daughters.

There may be a tradeoff, however, between selecting a man for his parenting abilities and selecting him for his genetic fitness. Men who are highly attractive to women, for example, may be reluctant to commit to any one woman. Thus, a woman seeking a man for his genetic fitness may have to settle for a short-term sexual relationship without parental investment.

These different selection foci, according to Gangestad and Simpson (1990), produce two alternative female mating strategies. Women seeking a high-investing mate are predicted to adopt a "restricted" sexual strategy marked by delayed intercourse and a prolonged courtship. This strategy would enable a woman to assess the man's level of commitment to her, detect the existence of prior commitments to other women or children, and simultaneously signal to the man her sexual fidelity and hence assure him of his paternity in future offspring.

Women "seeking" a man for the quality of his genes (no consciousness of goal state is implied by this formulation), on the other hand, have less reason to delay intercourse. A man's level of commitment to her is less relevant, prolonged assessment of his prior commitments is less necessary, and so there is less need for delaying intercourse. Indeed, if the man is pursuing a short-term sexual strategy, any delay on her part may deter him from seeking sexual intercourse with her, thus defeating the raison detrê of the mating strategy.

According to this theory, the two mating strategies of women—restricted and unrestricted—evolved and are maintained by frequency-dependent selection. As the number of *unrestricted* females in the population increases, the number of "sexy sons" also increases. As their numbers increase, the competition between these sons increases, and hence the success of the unrestricted strategy decreases. On the other hand, as the number of *restricted* females in the population increases, the competition for men who are able and willing to invest exclusively in them and their children increases, and the fitness of that strategy commensurably declines.

There are many complicating factors with this theory, and the authors recognize that it must be described and tested more formally. Furthermore, the theory requires (1) evidence that the key elements of each strategy must covary in an organized, coherent fashion; (2) the covarying suite of elements must fulfill stringent criteria for adaptation, such as efficiency, economy, and precision for solving the respective adaptive problems; and (3) the adaptive payoff of each strategy must decrease as it becomes more common in the population. Pending these further tests, it remains a viable theory of individual differences produced and maintained by frequency-dependent selection.

Psychopathy as a Frequency-Dependent Strategy

Mealey (1995) proposes a theory of primary psychopathy based on frequency-dependent selection. Psychopathy (sometimes called sociopathy or antisocial personality disorder) represents a cluster of traits marked by irresponsible and unreliable behavior, egocentrism, impulsivity, an inability to form lasting relationships, superficial social charm, and a deficit of social emotions such as love, shame, guilt, and empathy (American Psychiatric Association, 1994; Cleckley, 1982). Psychopaths pursue a deceptive or "cheating" strategy in their social interactions. Psychopathy is more common among men than women, forming roughly 3–4% of the former and less than 1% of the latter (*Diagnostic and Statistical Manual of Mental Disorders—Fourth Edition*; American Psychiatric Association, 1994).

Psychopaths pursue a social strategy characterized by an exploitation of the reciprocity mechanisms of others. After feigning cooperation, psychopaths typically defect. This cheating strategy might be pursued by men who are unlikely to out-compete other men in a more traditional or mainstream status hierarchy (Mealey, 1995).

According to the theory, a psychopathic strategy can be maintained by frequency-dependent selection. As the number of cheaters increases, and hence the average cost to the cooperative hosts increases, mechanisms would presumably evolve to detect cheating and to inflict costs on those pursuing a cheating strategy. As the prevalence of psychopaths increases, therefore, the average payoff of the psychopath strategy decreases. As long as the frequency of psychopaths is not too large, it can be maintained amidst a population composed primarily of cooperators (Mealey, 1995).

There is some evidence, albeit indirect, that is at least consistent with Mealey's theory of psychopathy. First, behavioral genetics studies suggest that psychopathy may be moderately heritable, at least as indicated by the Minnesota Multiphasic Personality Inventory (MMPI) Psychopathic Deviate scale (Willerman, Loehlin, & Horn, 1992).

Second, some psychopaths appear to pursue an exploitative short-term sexual strategy, which could be the primary route through which genes for psychopathy increase or are maintained (Rowe, 1995). Psychopathic men tend to be more sexually precocious, have sex with a larger number of women, have more illegitimate children, and are more likely to separate from their wives than nonpsychopathic men (Rowe, 1995). This short-term, opportunistic, exploitative sexual strategy would be expected to rise in populations marked by high mobility, where the reputational costs associated with such a strategy would be least likely to be incurred (Wilson, 1995).

There are several challenges to this theory, such as whether it represents a type or a continuum (Baldwin, 1995; Eysenck, 1995), whether its frequency is sufficiently large to be maintained by frequency-dependent selection, and whether it represents a recently evolved cluster in modern populations or an ancient evolved strategy (Wilson, 1995; but see Mealey's [1995] response to these challenges).

Despite these complications, Mealey's theory of psychopathy and Gangestad and Simpson's theory of sociosexuality nicely illustrate the possibility that heritable alternative strategies can be maintained by frequency-dependent selection. The concept of frequency-dependent selection offers a potential explanation for integrating the cumulative results from behavioral genetics studies (e.g., Willerman et al., 1992) and the findings on the sexual strategies apparently pursued by psychopaths (Rowe, 1995) with an evolutionary analysis of adaptive individual differences.

The K-Factor

Another effort to identify adaptive individual differences through frequency-dependent selection comes from evolutionary psychologist A. J. Figueredo and his colleagues (Figueredo et al., 2006), who propose that individual differences cluster around a single large dimension called the K-factor (see Rushton, 1985, for an earlier version of this theory). Those high on the K-factor show early attachment to their biological father, a long-term mating strategy, high cooperativeness, and low risk taking. The low end of the K-factor is marked by low levels of attachment, high Machiavellianism, high risk taking, high impulsivity, defection from cooperative relationships, and the pursuit of a short-term mating strategy. Individual differences in the K-factor are hypothesized to be maintained by frequency-dependent selection, much like psychopathy is maintained by frequency-dependent selection. Indeed, there appears to be considerable overlap between psychopathy and a low K-factor.

Two final comments on frequency-dependent strategies. First, frequency-dependent strategies need not occur through heritable differences. They can occur through local situation-dependent shifts, whereby individuals adjust their strategy according to the frequency of those pursuing various strategies. Second, the logic of frequency-dependent selection does not require typological thinking or discrete strategies. It can also produce continuous heritable variation, as is the case with Figueredo's hypothesized K-factor.

Balancing Selection: Environmental Heterogeneity of Selection Pressures over Time and Space

As described above, the key to balancing selection comes from the fact that different pressures select for different heritable variants under different conditions. If environments vary, then selection will not favor a single optimal value for a trait, but rather different optima in the different environmental conditions. Averaged across heterogeneous environments, these heritable variants can have identical fitnesses. If some environments favor the trait of boldness and others favor the trait of cautiousness, for example, then this environmental heterogeneity can maintain both boldness and cautiousness, as well as the range of values in between these ends, as long as the reproductive success of the variants is the same, averaged across these environments.

Kevin MacDonald (1995, 1998) was among the first to argue for balancing selection in explaining the maintenance of individual differences on the Big Five personality dimensions. He argued that the extremes of these traits are likely to be maladaptive. Introversion to the point of totally avoiding

people, for example, would make it difficult to find a mate. One the other hand, "There is a broad range of genetic variation in the middle of the distribution underlying a range of viable strategies" (MacDonald, 2005, p. 229).

Nettle (2006), building on MacDonald's ideas, offered a specific set of hypotheses about the adaptive value of being high or low on each of the Big Five. For extraversion, for example, Nettle argues that being high fosters success in mating, forming social allies, and exploring the environment, but his strategy also entails costs in the form of greater exposure to dangers from the physical environment. When environments are relatively safe, an extraverted strategy may pay off, since the risks incurred from the physical environment are minimal. When environments are hazardous, however, an extraverted strategy may suffer in fitness currencies in favor of a more introverted strategy. The argument is that temporal variation in the strategy favored by an environment can maintain genetic variation on the personality dimension of extraversion–introversion.

Nettle argues that each end of the Big Five carries benefits as well as costs. Neuroticism may give an individual the benefit of added vigilance for dangers, but it carries the cost of increased stress, anxiety, and depression. High agreeableness can lead to excellent social alliances and valued partnerships, but an agreeable strategy may also leave the individual vulnerable to being cheated.

The critical agenda for those pursuing this line of theorizing is to identify the specific costs and benefits of variation in each of the key traits across different environments. Nettle's (2006) hypotheses provide a start, but alternatives could be suggested. For extraversion, for example, although one benefit may be mating success, a key cost may be social or physical retribution from jealous mates, if the extraverted strategy leads an individual to have sex with already mated individuals (Buss, 2000). As Penke and his colleagues aptly conclude, "Even if balancing selection proves to be a good general account of heritable personality traits, much more research would be needed to identify each personality trait's relevant fitness costs and benefits across different environments" (Penke et al., 2007, p. 566).

A fascinating recent study supports the notion that different environments favor different heritable personality traits. Ciani, Capiluppi, Veronese, and Sartori (2006) assessed the Big Five personality traits among individuals who resided either on small islands off the coast of Italy or on the mainland of Italy. They found intriguing differences. People from families that were long-time inhabitants of the islands (at least 20 generations) were significantly lower on extraversion and openness compared to those from the mainland. Interestingly, these islanders were also lower on extraversion and openness compared to recent immigrants to the islands. Although circumstantial, these findings support the notion that different environments select for somewhat different levels of personality traits, and that environmental heterogeneity can maintain heritable personality variation.

ADAPTATIONS FOR DETECTING AND ACTING ON PERSONALITY DIFFERENCES

Other individuals compose one of the primary environments within which humans function (Alexander, 1987). Other individuals are crucial for solving adaptive problems. The presence of large individual differences, whether adaptively patterned or not, defines a major part of the human adaptive landscape (Buss, 1991). Attending to those individual differences can facilitate solutions to adaptive problems. Ignoring those individual differences can be disastrous. Failure to assess differences in whether others are pursuing cooperative or defecting social strategies, for example, can result in resources pilfered, reputations damaged, and pregnancies unwanted.

Over evolutionary time, those individuals who attended to and acted on individual differences in others that were adaptively consequential would have survived and reproduced more successfully than those who were oblivious to adaptively consequential differences in others. Buss (1989a, 1996) proposed that humans have evolved difference-detecting assessment mechanisms that facilitated successful adaptive solutions.

These mechanisms would have been critical in assessing individual differences for the goals of mate selection, coalition formation, and dyadic alliance building. The formation of these different relationships and the attendant adaptive problems entailed by them may require assessment specificity. That is, different individual differences in the social landscape may be relevant to some problems and irrelevant to others. Individual differences in sexual fidelity, for example, are more critical to assessing the viability of a long-term mate than a coalition partner (Shackelford & Buss, 1996). Despite some degree of domain specificity, some dimensions of individual differences, such as those captured by the five-factor model of personality, may be important because they are relevant to a host of different adaptive problems, and hence they transcend the particulars of specific relationships (MacDonald, 1995).

Because individual differences are so critical to solving adaptive problems, individuals often attempt to manipulate others' perceptions and reputations of their own and competitors' standings on relevant dimensions of differences. In mate competition, for example, men tend to impugn the surgency, agreeableness, and emotional stability of their rivals (Buss & Dedden, 1990). Thus, derogation of competitors becomes a verbal form of trait usage as manipulation, exploiting the difference-detecting mechanisms of others in the service of mate competition. Simultaneously, men will exaggerate their own positive traits in self-presentation to a woman, striving to appear to fulfill characteristics that she desires in a mate (Buss, 1988b).

Whatever the origins of individual differences—whether they are adaptively patterned or not—they represent important vectors in the human adaptive landscape. When the individual differences of others in one's social environment are adaptively patterned, however, it may be especially important to detect and act on them because they are more likely to represent coherent and hence predictable suites of covarying qualities rather than randomly varying or single-dimension attributes.

Ultimately, comprehensive theories of personality and individual differences will require accounts of both the adaptive and nonadaptive differences, as well as the difference-detecting mechanisms humans have evolved to grapple with the varying terrain of the human adaptive landscape.

CONCLUSIONS

Comprehensive theories of personality should aspire to include both a specification of human nature and an account of the major ways in which individuals differ. Evolutionary psychology provides a powerful heuristic for the discovery of both. Since the evolutionary process is the only known creative process capable, in principle, of producing complex organic mechanisms, all theories of human nature must, at some level, be anchored in the basic principles of evolution by selection. Theories of personality inconsistent with these evolutionary principles stand little or no chance of being correct (Buss, 1991).

The products of the evolutionary process define the contents of the nature of all species, and human nature is no exception. These products are primarily adaptations, byproducts of adaptations, and a residue of noise. Because byproducts can be understood only by first describing the adaptations from which the byproducts flow, adaptations must form the core nature of all animals, including humans.

For a variety of reasons, many adaptations are species-typical, with important exceptions, such as those that are sex-linked or caused by processes such as frequency-dependent selection or variation in selection pressure over time and space (see also Wilson, 1994). The core of personality theory, therefore, must be defined by the adaptive mechanisms that are characteristic of most members of our species—in other words, a species-typical human nature. The mechanisms of human nature cannot be fully understood without identifying the adaptive problems they were designed to solve. These adaptive solutions exist in the present because in the past they contributed, either directly or indirectly, to the successful reproduction of ancestors who carried them. Modern humans are the end products of a long and unbroken chain of ancestors who succeeded in solving the adaptive problems necessary for, or that enhanced, survival and reproduction. As the descendants of these successful ancestors, modern humans carry with them the adaptive mechanisms that led to their success.

The most obvious candidates for the human nature component of personality theory are those that are closely linked with the engine of the evolutionary process—differential reproductive success. These candidates include status striving, which gives humans access to the resources of survival and reproduction; mating motivations, which propel reproduction; parenting motivations, which increase the survival and success of the "vehicles" produced by mating unions; universal emotions such as jealousy, which protect those reproductive resources already acquired; and a host of others, such as the ability to discern the motives and beliefs of other minds (Haselton & Buss, 1997, 2000).

Personality theories would be incomplete without an account of the major ways in which individuals differ. Theories of individual differences, however, cannot be divorced from theories of human nature, any more than a theory of "car differences" could be divorced from a theory of "universal car nature." Although some individual differences may be random, and hence independent of the basic functioning of human nature, the most important individual differences are those that stem from the workings and nature of the species-typical mechanisms.

Major individual differences can originate, in principle, from environmental sources of variation, genetic sources of variation, or a combination of the two. It may seem ironic to some that the environmentally based individual differences are most easily handled within this evolutionary psychological framework. Individual differences can result from varying environmental input into species-typical mechanisms. All individuals possess callus-producing mechanisms, but differ in the thickness and distribution of calluses because of individual differences in experiences of friction to the skin. Similarly, all individual may possess a psychological mechanism of jealousy, but differ in the degree to which they enduringly occupy an environment filled with threats to their romantic relationships, perhaps because they are mated with someone who is habitually flirtatious or who is higher in "mate value," and so gives off signals of defection (Tooby & Cosmides, 1990a). Stable individual differences in jealousy, in this example, arise from stable individual differences in inhabiting jealousy-evoking environments.

Enduring environments experienced, however, are not the only source of individual differences. Early experience during childhood, for example, can potentially calibrate or set thresholds on species-typical mechanisms. Children growing up without an investing father, for example, may select a short-term mating strategy in adulthood, whereas those with an investing father may opt for a long-term mating strategy. In this example, the species-typical mating mechanism contains a fixed "menu" of alternatives. Which alternative is selected from this menu is influenced by early experience.

Individual differences can also derive from strategic specialization. Indeed, selection will sometimes favor the evolution of strategies whereby organisms seek out niches that contain less competition. These forms of strategic specialization may be influenced by environmental factors such as early training in a particular domain, by heritable factors, such as natural athletic or verbal ability, or by a combination of the two.

Balancing selection, where traits can be maintained as a consequence of differences in selective environments over time or space, is an evolutionary process that can potentially explain personality characteristics that are heritable. Negative frequency-dependent selection is form of balancing selection, an evolutionary process that can create heritable individual differences that are adaptively patterned. Like the other forms of major individual differences, those due to frequency-dependent selection will be most likely to occur in domains that are closely linked with the engine of the evolutionary process, that is, differential reproduction. The proposal by Gangestad and Simpson (1990) for individual differences in sociosexuality is one example. Another, hypothesized by Mealey (1995), proposed that psychopathy has evolved as a frequency-dependent social and sexual strategy that can exist in low levels, essentially parasitizing off of the more common long-term cooperative strategy. A third is hypothesized by Figueredo and his colleagues (2006) in the form of the K-factor. These and other forms of frequency-dependent selection require further empirical documentation, but they represent an exciting and promising form of adaptive individual differences for future personality theory.

Others propose that traits such as those captured by the Big Five are maintained through balancing selection. Nettle (2006), for example, posits that there are adaptive advantages as well as costs to being high and low on personality traits—benefits and costs that vary across environments. High levels of extraversion, for example, can lead to mating success, but at a cost of exposure to physical risks and family stability. High levels of neuroticism can help solve environmental dangers by leading to increased vigilance, but it can also tax the body through high levels of stress. Nettle's suggestions provide a promising framework for identifying and empirically testing the specific costs and benefits of differences on the major dimensions of personality.

Not all individual differences, of course, will be adaptively patterned. Some might occur because of random environmental forces, genetic noise, genetic defects, and other factors. Some individual differences, such as those in intelligence or mental health, may reflect differences in mutation load (Keller & Miller, 2006). The evolutionary psychology framework, however, suggests that the most important individual differences will be those linked with the major adaptive mechanisms that define human nature.

Given this early stage in the development of evolutionary personality psychology, no pretense is made that we have arrived at, or even approximated, the ultimate theory of personality. This chapter has merely offered some suggestions for ingredients that might be contained within a future theory of personality. Evolutionary psychology, however, does offer something lacking in all existing nonevolutionary theories of personality—a nonarbitrary anchoring for a specification of the basic psychological machinery that humans share, as well as for the major ways in which humans differ.

REFERENCES

Alexander, R. D. (1987). *The biology of moral systems*. Hawthorne, NY: Aldine de Gruyter.

American Psychiatric Association. (1994). *Diagnostic and statistical manual of mental disorders* (4th ed.). Washington, DC: Author.

Baldwin, J. D. (1995). Continua outperform dichotomies. *Behavioral and Brain Sciences, 18,* 543–544.

Belsky, J., Steinberg, L., & Draper, P. (1991). Childhood experience, interpersonal development, and reproductive strategy: An evolutionary theory of socialization. *Child Development*, 62, 647–670.

Betzig, L. L. (1986). *Despotism and differential reproduction: A Darwinian view of history.* Hawthorne, NY: Aldine.

Betzig, L. L. (1992). Roman polygyny. *Ethology and Sociobiology*, 13, 309–349.

Bleske, A. L., & Buss, D. M. (2001). Opposite sex friendship: Sex differences and similarities in initiation, selection, and dissolution. *Personality and Social Psychology Bulletin*, 27, 1310–1323.

Bouchard, T. J., & McGue, M. (1990). Genetic and rearing environmental influences on adult personality: An analysis of adopted twins reared apart. *Journal of Personality*, 58, 263–292.

Burnstein, E., Crandall, C., & Kitayama, S. (1994). Some neo-Darwinian decision rules for altruism: Weighing cures for inclusive fitness as a function of the biological importance of the decision. *Journal of Personality and Social Psychology*, 67, 773–789.

Buss, D. M. (1984). Evolutionary biology and personality psychology: Toward a conception of human nature and individual differences. *American Psychologist*, 39, 1135–1147.

Buss, D. M. (1988a). The evolution of human intrasexual competition: Tactics of mate attraction. *Journal of Personality and Social Psychology*, 54, 616–628.

Buss, D. M. (1988b). From vigilance to violence: Tactics of mate retention. *Ethology and Sociobiology*, 9, 291–317.

Buss, D. M. (1989a). Conflict between the sexes: Strategic interference and the evocation of anger and upset. *Journal of Personality and Social Psychology*, 56, 735–747.

Buss, D. M. (1989b). Sex differences in human mate preferences: Evolutionary hypotheses testing in 37 cultures. *Behavioral and Brain Sciences*, 12, 1–49.

Buss, D. M. (1991). Evolutionary personality psychology. *Annual Review of Psychology*, 42, 459–492.

Buss, D. M. (1995a). Evolutionary psychology: A new paradigm for psychological science. *Psychological Inquiry*, 6, 1–49.

Buss, D. M. (1995b, June). *Human prestige criteria.* Paper presented at the annual meeting of the Human Behavior and Evolution Society, University of California, Santa Barbara.

Buss, D. M. (1996). Social adaptation and five major factors of personality. In J. S. Wiggins (Ed.), *The five-factor model of personality* (pp. 180–208). New York: Guilford Press.

Buss, D. M. (2000). *The dangerous passion: Why jealousy is as necessary as love and sex.* New York: Free Press.

Buss, D. M. (2003). *The evolution of desire: Strategies of human mating.* New York: Basic Books. (Original work published 1994)

Buss, D. M. (2008). *Evolutionary psychology: The new science of the mind* (3rd ed.) Boston: Allyn & Bacon.

Buss, D. M., & Dedden, L. A. (1990). Derogation of competitors. *Journal of Social and Personal Relationships*, 7, 395–422.

Buss, D. M., & Greiling, H. (1999). Adaptive individual differences. *Journal of Personality*, 67, 209–243.

Buss, D. M., & Haselton, M. G. (2005). The evolution of jealousy. *Trends in Cognitive Science*, 9, 506–507.

Buss, D. M., Haselton, M. G., Shackelford, T. K., Bleske, A. L., & Wakefield, J. C. (1998). Adaptations, exaptations, and spandrels. *American Psychologist*, 53, 533–548.

Buss, D. M., Larsen, R. J., & Westen, D. (1996). Sex differences in jealousy: Not gone, not forgotten, and not explained by alternative hypotheses. *Psychological Science*, 7, 373–375.

Buss, D. M., Larsen, R., Westen, D., & Semmelroth, J. (1992). Sex differences in jealousy: Evolution, physiology, and psychology. *Psychological Science*, 3, 251–255.

Buss, D. M., & Schmitt, D. P. (1993). Sexual strategies theory: An evolutionary perspective on human mating. *Psychological Review*, 100, 204–232.

Buss, D. M., & Shackelford, T. K. (1997). From vigilance to violence: Mate retention tactics in married couples. *Journal of Personality and Social Psychology*, 72, 346–361.

Buunk, A. P., Angleitner, A., Oubaid, V., & Buss, D. M. (1996). Sex differences in jealousy in evolutionary and cultural perspective: Tests from the Netherlands, Germany, and the United States. *Psychological Science*, 7, 359–363.

Buunk, A. P., & Hupka, R. B. (1987). Cross-cultural differences in the elicitation of sexual jealousy. *Journal of Sex Research*, 23, 12–22.

Chagnon, N. (1983). *Yanomamo: The fierce people* (3rd ed.). New York: Holt, Rinehart & Winston.

Ciani, A. S. C., Capiluppi, C., Veronese, A., & Sartori, G. (2006). The adaptive value of personality differences revealed by small island population dynamics. *European Journal of Personality*, 21, 3–22.

Cleckley, H. (1982). *The mask of sanity.* New York: New American Library.

Daly, M., & Wilson, M. (1988). *Homicide.* Hawthorne, NY: Aldine.

Daly, M., & Wilson, M. (1995). Discriminative parental solicitude and the relevance of evolutionary models to the analysis of motivational systems. In M. S. Gazzaniga (Ed.), *The cog-*

nitive neurosciences (pp. 1269–1286). Cambridge, MA: MIT Press.

Daly, M., Wilson, M., & Weghorst, S. J. (1982). Male sexual jealousy. *Ethology and Sociobiology, 3,* 11–27.

Darwin, C. (1958). *The origin of the species.* London: Murray. (Original work published 1859)

Darwin, C. (1981). *The descent of man and selection in relation to sex.* London: Murray. (Original work published 1871)

Dawkins, R. (1982). *The extended phenotype.* San Francisco: Freeman.

Dawkins, R. (1996). *Climbing mount improbable.* New York: Norton.

de Waal, F. (1982). *Chimpanzee politics: Sex and power among apes.* Baltimore: Johns Hopkins University Press.

Dominey, W. J. (1984). Alternative mating tactics and evolutionary stable strategies. *American Zoologist, 24,* 385–396.

Ekman, P. (1973). Cross-cultural studies of facial expression. In P. Ekman (Ed.), *Darwin and facial expression: A century of research in review* (pp. 169–222). New York: Academic Press.

Ekman, P. (1994). All emotions are basic. In P. Ekman & R. J. Davidson (Eds.), *The nature of emotion* (pp. 15–19). New York: Oxford University Press.

Eysenck, H. J. (1995). Psychopathology: Type or trait? *Behavioral and Brain Sciences, 18,* 355–356.

Fay, J. C., Whyckoff, G. J., & Wu, C. (2001). Positive and negative selection of the human genome. *Genetics, 158,* 1227–1234.

Figueredo, A. J., Vasquz, G., Brumbach, B. H., Schneider, S. M. R., Sefcek, J. A., Tal, I. R., et al. (2006). Consilience and life history theory: From genes to brain to reproductive strategy. *Developmental Review, 26,* 243–275.

Frank, R. (1988). *Passions within reason.* New York: Norton.

Freud, S. (1953). Three essays on the theory of sexuality. In J. Strachey (Ed. & Trans.), *The standard edition of the complete psychological works of Sigmund Freud* (Vol. 7, pp. 126–243). London: Hogarth Press. (Original work published 1905)

Gangestad, S. W., & Simpson, J. A. (1990). Toward an evolutionary history of female sociosexual variation. *Journal of Personality, 58,* 69–96.

Gangestad, S. W., & Simpson, J. A. (2000). The evolution of human mating: Trade-offs and strategic pluralism. *Behavioral and Brain Sciences, 23,* 573–644.

Goldberg, L. R. (1981). Language and individual differences: The search for universals in personality lexicons. In L. Wheeler (Ed.), *Review of personality and social psychology* (pp. 141–165). Beverly Hills: Sage.

Gould, S. J. (1991). Exaptation: A crucial tool for evolutionary psychology. *Journal of Social Issues, 47,* 43–65.

Gross, M. R. (1982). [Sneakers, satellites and parentals: Polymorphic mating strategies in North American sunfishes.] *Zeitschrift fur Tierpsychologie, 60,* 1–26.

Hamilton, W. D. (1964). The genetical evolution of social behavior: I and II. *Journal of Theoretical Biology, 7,* 1–52.

Hart, C. W., & Pilling, A. R. (1960). *The Tiwi of North Australia.* New York: Holt, Rinehart & Winston.

Haselton, M. G., & Buss, D. M. (1997, June). *Errors in mind reading: Design flaws or design features?* Paper presented at the ninth annual meeting of the Human Behavior and Evolution Society, University of Arizona, Tucson.

Haselton, M. G., & Buss, D. M. (2000). Error management theory: A new perspective on biases in cross-sex mind reading. *Journal of Personality and Social Psychology, 78,* 81–91.

Hatfield, E., Traupmann, J., Sprecher, S., Utne, M., & Hay, J. (1985). Equity and intimate relations: Recent research. In W. Ickes (Ed.), *Compatible and incompatible relationships* (pp. 91–117). New York: Springer-Verlag.

Hill, K., & Hurtado, A. M. (1996). *Aché life history.* New York: Aldine de Gruyter.

Hogan, R. (1983). A socioanalytic theory of personality. In M. M. Page (Ed.), *Nebraska Symposium on Motivation* (pp. 55–89). Lincoln: University of Nebraska Press.

Keightley, P. D., & Gaffney, D. J. (2003). Functional constraints and frequency of deleterious mutations in noncoding DNA of rodents. *Proceedings of the National Academy of Sciences of the United States of America, 100,* 13402–13406.

Keller, M. C., & Miller, G. F. (2006). An evolutionary framework for mental disorders: Integrating adaptationist and evolutionary genetic models. *Behavioral and Brain Sciences, 29,* 429–441.

Kenrick, D. T., & Keefe, R. C. (1992). Age preferences in mates reflect sex differences in reproductive strategies. *Behavioral and Brain Sciences, 15,* 75–133.

Kenrick, D. T., Sadalla, E. K., Groth, G., & Trost, M. R. (1990). Evolution, traits, and the stages of human courtship: Qualifying the parental investment model. *Journal of Personality, 58,* 97–116.

Little, B. R. (1989). Personal projects analysis: Trivial pursuits, magnificent obsessions, and the search for coherence. In D. M. Buss & N. Cantor (Eds.), *Personality psychology: Recent trends, emerging directions* (pp. 15–31). New York: Springer-Verlag.

Loehlin, J. C., Horn, J. M., & Willerman, L.

(1990). Heredity, environment, and personality change: Evidence from the Texas Adoption Project. *Journal of Personality*, 58, 221–244.

MacDonald, K. (1995). Evolution, the five-factor model, and levels of personality. *Journal of Personality*, 63, 525–568.

MacDonald, K. (1998). Evolution, culture, and the five-factor model. *Journal of Cross-Cultural Psychology*, 29, 119–149.

MacDonald, K. (2005). Personality, evolution, and development. In R. Burgesss & K. MacDonald (Eds.), *Evolutionary perspectives on human development* (2nd ed., pp. 207–242). Thousand Oaks, CA: Sage.

Marks, I. (1987). *Fears, phobias, and rituals: Panic, anxiety, and their disorders.* New York: Oxford University Press.

Marr, D. (1982). *Vision.* San Francisco: Freeman.

Maslow, A. H. (1970). *Motivation and personality* (2nd ed.). New York: Harper & Row.

Maynard Smith, J. (1982). *Evolution and the theory of games.* Cambridge, UK: Cambridge University Press.

Mazur, A., Halpern, C., & Udry, J. R. (1994). Dominant looking male teenagers copulate earlier. *Ethology and Sociobiology*, 15, 87–94.

McAdams, D. P. (1997). A conceptual history of personality psychology. In R. Hogan, J. Johnson, & S. Briggs (Eds.), *Handbook of personality psychology* (pp. 3–39). New York: Academic Press.

McCrae, R. R., & John, O. P. (1992). An introduction to the five-factor model and its applications. *Journal of Personality*, 60, 175–215.

Mealey, L. (1995). The sociobiology of sociopathy: An integrated evolutionary model. *Behavioral and Brain Sciences*, 18, 523–599.

Nesse, R. M. (1990). Evolutionary explanations of emotions. *Human Nature*, 1, 261–289.

Nettle, D. (2006). The evolution of personality variation in humans and other animals. *American Psychologist*, 61, 622–631.

Norman, W. T. (1963). Toward an adequate taxonomy of personality attributes: Replicated factor structure in peer nomination personality ratings. *Journal of Abnormal and Social Psychology*, 66, 574–583.

Orians, G. H., & Heerwagen, J. H. (1992). Evolved responses to landscapes. In J. Barkow, L. Cosmides, & J. Tooby (Eds.), *The adapted mind* (pp. 555–579). New York: Oxford University Press.

Pedersen, F. A. (1991). Secular trends in human sex ratios: Their influence on individual and family behavior. *Human Nature*, 3, 271–291.

Penke, L., Denissen, J. J. A., & Miller, G. F. (2007). The evolutionary genetics of personality. *European Journal of Personality*, 21, 549–587.

Pervin, L. A. (Ed.). (1990). *Handbook of personality: Theory and research.* New York: Guilford Press.

Pinker, S. (1994). *The language instinct.* New York: Morrow.

Plomin, R., DeFries, J. C., & McClearn, G. E. (1990). *Behavioral genetics: A primer* (2nd ed.). New York: Freeman.

Rowe, D. C. (1995). Evolution, mating effort, and crime. *Behavioral and Brain Sciences*, 18, 573–574.

Rushton, J. P. (1985). Differential K theory: The sociobiology of individual and group differences. *Personality and Individual Differences*, 6, 441–452.

Schmitt, D. P., & Buss, D. M. (1996). Strategic self-promotion and competitor derogation: Sex and context effects on perceived effectiveness of mate attraction tactics. *Journal of Personality and Social Psychology*, 70, 1185–1204.

Schmitt, D. P., & Buss, D. M. (2000). Sexual dimensions of person description: Beyond or subsumed by the Big Five? *Journal of Research in Personality*, 34, 141–177.

Shackelford, T. K., & Buss, D. M. (1996). Betrayal in mateships, friendships, and coalitions. *Personality and Social Psychology Bulletin*, 22, 1151–1164.

Sternberg, R. (1986). A triangular theory of love. *Psychological Review*, 93, 119–135.

Sulloway, F. (1996). *Born to rebel.* New York: Pantheon.

Symons, D. (1979). *The evolution of human sexuality.* New York: Oxford University Press.

Symons, D. (1987). If we're all Darwinians, what's the fuss about? In C. Crawford, D. Krebs, & M. Smith (Eds.), *Sociobiology and psychology* (pp. 121–145). Hillsdale, NJ: Erlbaum.

Symons, D. (1992). On the use and misuse of Darwinism in the study of human behavior. In J. Barkow, L. Cosmides, & J. Tooby (Eds.), *The adapted mind* (pp. 137–159). New York: Oxford University Press.

Tooby, J., & Cosmides, L. (1988). The evolution of war and its cognitive foundations. *Institute for Evolutionary Studies, Technical Report #88-1.*

Tooby, J., & Cosmides, L. (1990a). On the universality of human nature and the uniqueness of the individual: The role of genetics and adaptation. *Journal of Personality*, 58, 17–68.

Tooby, J., & Cosmides, L. (1990b). The past explains the present: Emotional adaptations and the structure of ancestral environments. *Ethology and Sociobiology*, 11, 375–424.

Tooby, J., & Cosmides, L. (1992). Psychological foundations of culture. In J. Barkow, L. Cosmides, & J. Tooby (Eds.), *The adapted mind* (pp. 19–136). New York: Oxford University Press.

Trivers, R. (1974). Parent–offspring conflict. *American Zoologist, 14,* 249–264.

Walster, E., Traupmann, J., & Walster, G. W. (1978). Equity and extramarital sexual activity. *Journal of Personality and Social Psychology, 7,* 127–141.

Wiederman, M. W., & Allgeier, R. R. (1993). Gender differences in sexual jealousy: Adaptationist or social learning explanation? *Ethology and Sociobiology, 14,* 115–140.

Wiggins, J. S. (1979). A psychological taxonomy of trait descriptive terms: The interpersonal domain. *Journal of Personality and Social Psychology, 37,* 395–412.

Willerman, L., Loehlin, J. C., & Horn, J. M. (1992). An adoption and a cross-fostering study of the Minnesota Multiphasic Personality Inventory (MMPI) Psychopathic Deviate scale. *Behavior Genetics, 22,* 515–529.

Williams, G. C. (1966). *Adaptation and natural selection.* Princeton, NJ: Princeton University Press.

Williams, G. C. (1975). *Sex and evolution.* Princeton, NJ: Princeton University Press.

Wilson, D. S. (1994). Adaptive genetic variation and human evolutionary psychology. *Ethology and Sociobiology, 15,* 219–235.

Wilson, D. S. (1995). Sociopathy within and between small groups. *Behavioral and Brain Sciences, 18,* 577.

CHAPTER 3

Psychoanalytic Approaches to Personality

Drew Westen
Glen O. Gabbard
Kile M. Ortigo

Perhaps the greatest challenge in trying to summarize the state of psychoanalysis as a theory of personality more than a century after its inception is to delineate precisely what one means by *psychoanalysis*. A half century ago, such a definition would have been relatively clear. Psychoanalysis was a well-guarded fortress, and most psychologists had little interest in scaling its walls. The password to enter was relatively unambiguous: Those who considered themselves psychoanalytic believed in the importance of unconscious processes, conflicts, defenses, the Oedipus complex, and the centrality of the sexual drive in the development of personality and neurosis; those who did not believed in none of these things.

Psychologists who were caught in the moat—who accepted some of Freud's premises but rejected aspects of theory important to him, such as the centrality of sexuality or the Oedipus complex—would, by and large, leave the fold or be cast off as heretics, and their work would never be cited again in psychoanalytic literature. This ragtag army of the not-quite-analytic-enough came to be identified under the broader rubric of "psychodynamic," which included those who believe in the importance of unconscious processes and conflicting forces within the mind but do not necessarily hold to the theory of libido and the preeminence of the Oedipus complex.

The distinction between psychodynamic and psychoanalytic has virtually disappeared in the past 30 years, as previously "forbidden" ideas have entered the fortress and as mainstream psychoanalytic theorists and clinicians have come to reject many of the propositions that Freud considered defining of the approach to the mind he created, such as the centrality of the Oedipus complex and the sexual drive—or the concept of drive at all. Today most of the major psychoanalytic journals publish papers from radically differing theoretical perspectives. Hence the use of the plural in the title of this chapter, "Psychoanalytic *Approaches* to Personality," reflecting the pluralism that characterizes contemporary psychoanalysis—let alone psychologically inspired theory and research in personality, social, and clinical psychology.

Although one reason psychoanalysis has become less easy to define is because its boundaries are more permeable, another is that contemporary psychology has come to accept many of the postulates that once clearly demarcated psychoanalysis from other points of view. The cognitive revolution ushered in an interest in mental events, which had been largely extinguished by the behaviorists (with occasional spontaneous recoveries). Of particular importance in the last two decades is the literature on unconscious processes (called "implicit processes," largely to ward off any association with the Freudian unconscious) in cognitive and social psychology and neuroscience. This development began with the study of implicit memory and cognition (Bowers & Meichenbaum, 1984; Kihlstrom, 1987; Schacter, 1998) but eventually spread, as we predicted in this handbook nearly 20 years ago (Westen, 1990a), to the realms of affect and motivation as well (e.g., Chartrand, van Baaren, & Bargh, 2006; Ferguson & Bargh, 2004; Hassin, Uleman, & Bargh, 2005).

Indeed, the fall of the Berlin Wall between psychology and psychoanalysis may actually have occurred without notice in 1987 when E. Tory Higgins and Jonathan Bargh, two leading experimental social psychologists, criticized exclusive reliance on the "faulty computer" metaphor for explaining errors in social cognition, and called instead for a conception of mental processes that would have been very familiar to Freud and certainly to contemporary psychoanalytic theorists and clinicians:

> It may be that people are not motivated solely to be accurate or correct. Indeed, people are likely to have multiple and conflicting motivations when processing information such that not all of them can be fully satisfied. ... If one abandons this assumption [that people are motivated to be accurate], then an alternative perspective of people as "creatures of compromise" may be considered, a perspective suggesting that people's judgments and inferences must be understood in terms of the competing motivations that they are trying to satisfy. (p. 414)

The focus today among social psychologists (e.g., T. D. Wilson, 2002) and popular writers (e.g., Gladwell, 2005) on the "adaptive unconscious" has similarly "torn down that wall." Substantial differences remain between the views of many academic psychologists and psychoanalytic theorists, par-

ticularly in the way they speak and write, the kinds of evidence they find more or less compelling, and the focus in psychoanalytic theory and research on *motivated* unconscious processes such as defenses and self-deception (although even there, the burgeoning literature on motivated reasoning is a conspicuous exception; see, e.g., Ditto, Munro, Apanovitch, Seepansky, & Lockhart, 2003; Munro et al., 2002). Nevertheless, mutual dismissal and slinging of epithets require considerably more finesse than was once the case.[1]

What, then, is a psychoanalytic approach? Freud (1923/1961) defined psychoanalysis as (1) a theory of the mind or personality, (2) a method of investigation of unconscious processes, and (3) a method of treatment. In the present discussion we focus on psychoanalysis as a theory of personality. At present, psychoanalytic perspectives on personality are probably best categorized prototypically rather than through any particular set of defining features. Psychoanalytic approaches are those that take as axiomatic the importance of unconscious cognitive, affective, and motivational processes; conflicting mental processes; compromises among competing psychological tendencies that may be negotiated unconsciously; defense and self-deception; the influence of the past, directly or in interaction with genetic predispositions, on current functioning; the enduring effects of interpersonal patterns laid down in childhood; and the influence of sexual, aggressive, attachment-related, self-esteem, and other wishes and fears on thought, feeling, and behavior, whether or not the person is aware of it. The degree to which an approach matches this prototype is the degree to which it can be considered psychoanalytic.

The first section of the chapter provides a brief discussion of the evolution of psychoanalytic theory. The next section turns to current issues and controversies in psychoanalysis, focusing on two central issues of particular relevance to personality theory: the nature of motivation, and how we know when we understand a person. The third section addresses the enduring contributions of psychoanalysis to the study of personality and the state of the empirical evidence for some central psychoanalytic propositions. The fourth describes continuing points of contact and integration with other areas of psychology, focusing on research in cognitive neuroscience and evolutionary psychology. The final section suggests directions for the future.

THE EVOLUTION OF PSYCHOANALYTIC THEORY

Freud's models of the mind, and the early revisionist theories of Adler, Jung, and the neo-Freudians, should be well known to readers of this volume and hence are described only briefly here. Freud developed a series of models and theories that he never attempted to integrate fully. Freud's psychological theorizing was, however, guided from the start by his interest and his database: He was interested, first and foremost, in understanding psychopathology, and his primary data were the things that patients wittingly and unwittingly told about themselves in clinical hours. Of the greatest importance methodologically were free associations (which offered insight into associational networks and mental transformations of ideas and feelings) and transference phenomena (in which patients revealed interpersonal cognitive–affective–behavioral patterns that the analyst could observe directly).

Fundamental to Freud's thinking about the mind was a simple assumption: that if there is a discontinuity in consciousness—something the person is doing but cannot report or explain—then the relevant mental processes necessary to "fill in the gaps" must be unconscious (see Rapaport, 1944/1967). This deceptively simple assumption was at once both brilliant and controversial. Freud was led to this assumption by patients, first described in the *Studies on Hysteria* (Breuer & Freud, 1893–1895/1955), who had symptoms with no organic origin. The patients were making every conscious effort to stop these symptoms but could not. Freud's logic was simple: If the "force" behind the symptom is psychological but not conscious, that only leaves one possible explanation: The source of the symptom must be unconscious. Opposing the conscious will, Freud reasoned, must be an unconscious counterwill of equal or greater magnitude; the interplay of these two forces was what he described as *psychodynamics*. (See Erdelyi, 1985, for a vivid and readable account of Freud's discovery of psychodynamics.)

Freud's Early Models

Freud's first model of the mind, his *topographic model*, divided mental processes into what he called conscious, preconscious, and unconscious. *Conscious* thoughts are those of which the person is immediately aware; *preconscious* thoughts are those of which the person is not currently aware but can readily bring to consciousness (e.g., a phone number); *unconscious* mental processes are those that are actively kept unconscious by repression because of their content. This model was first fully elaborated in *The Interpretation of Dreams* (1900/1953), in which Freud also distinguished the *manifest content* of a dream (the consciously recalled, often seemingly bizarre plot line) from the *latent content* (the underlying unconscious meaning, which Freud argued is an unconscious wish). The concept of the transformation of latent wishes through various mental mechanisms to produce seemingly unintelligible but psychologically meaningful mental products became Freud's paradigm for symptom formation as well.

From his earliest publications onward, Freud was concerned with the nature of human motivation, and he attempted to bring together a psychological theory of adaptive and maladaptive mental processes with materialist conceptions of psychic energy, instinct, and drive rooted in the scientific thinking of his age (see Sulloway, 1979). His *drive*, *instinct*, and *energy models*, which for present purposes we largely describe as a single model, evolved throughout his career, but always preserved their emphasis on (1) the conservation of psychic energy and (2) the biological and animal origins of human motivation. Freud assumed that mental processes must be powered by energy, and that this energy must follow the same laws as other forms of energy in nature. A psychological motive to which energy has been attached can be consciously or unconsciously suppressed, but it cannot be destroyed. The act of suppression will itself require an expenditure of energy (for empirical evidence supporting this hypothesis a century later, see Wenzlaff & Wegner, 2000), and the motive, if fueled by enough force, will likely be expressed in another form no longer under conscious control, as a symptom, a dream, a joke, a slip of the tongue, behavior, political ideology (for empirical data, see Jost, Glaser, Kruglanski, & Sulloway, 2003)—the possible outlets are boundless.[2]

Freud also argued that basic human motivations are little different from those of other animals. The major differences between humans and animals in this respect stem from (1) the capacity of humans to express their motives in symbolic and derivative forms; and (2) the greater capacity of humans either to obtain or to inhibit their desires, based on their capacity to adapt to their environment (particularly their social environment). Freud was dualistic in his instinct theory throughout much of his career, at first juxtaposing self-preservation and preservation of the species (through sex) as the two basic motives (e.g., Freud, 1914/1957), and later asserting that sex and aggression are the basic human instincts from which all other motives ultimately flow. Although Freud's model of motivation had many limitations, perhaps what is most compelling about his theory is the notion that certain motives are rooted in our biology, and that there is nothing we can do but to try to adapt to them, enjoy them, or inhibit them when appropriate, or extrude them from our experience of self when they are too threatening to acknowledge as our own.

Freud's Developmental Model

Although Freud's drive theory was dualistic, his primary focus was on the sexual drive, which at times he equated more generally with psychic energy. In his *Three Essays on the Theory of Sexuality* (1905/1953), in which he articulated his *developmental model*, he argued that the development of personality could be understood in terms of the vicissitudes of the sexual drive (broadly understood, from its roots in Plato's theory of *Eros*, to include pleasure seeking of many forms). From this notion springs his argument that stages in the development of libido are *psychosexual* stages—that is, stages in the development of both sexuality and personality.

Freud's psychosexual stages represent the child's evolving quest for pleasure and realization of the limitations of pleasure seeking. According to Freud, a drive has a source (a body zone), an aim (discharge), and an object (something with which to satisfy it). The sources or body zones on which libido is centered at different periods follow a timetable that is biologically determined, although the various modes of pleasure seeking associated with these zones have profound social implications as well. Freud's stages should be understood both concretely and metaphorically: They relate to specific bodily experiences, but these experiences are viewed as exemplars of larger psychological and psychosocial conflicts and concerns (see Erikson's, 1963, elaborations of Freud's developmental theory).

In the oral stage, the child explores the world with its mouth, experiences considerable gratification and connection with people through its mouth, and exists in a state of dependency. The anal stage is characterized by the child's discovery that the anus can be a source of pleasurable excitation; by conflicts with socialization agents over compliance and defiance (the "terrible twos"), which Freud described in terms of conflicts over toilet training; and by the formation of attitudes toward order and disorder, giving and withholding, and messiness and cleanliness. The phallic stage is characterized by the child's discovery of the genitals and masturbation, an expanding social network, identification (particularly with same-sex parents), Oedipal conflicts, and the castration complex in boys and penis envy in girls. In the latency stage, sexual impulses undergo repression, and the child continues to identify with significant others and to learn culturally acceptable sublimations of sex and aggression. Finally, in the genital stage, conscious sexuality resurfaces, genital sex becomes the primary end of sexual activity, and the person becomes capable of mature relatedness to others.

These are among Freud's most controversial formulations, and many are no longer central to contemporary psychoanalytic thinking. The extent to which one finds them credible depends in part upon whether one has observed such phenomena in a clinical or child care setting and how literally or metaphorically one chooses to take them. That little children tend to be very interested in their and others' private parts, that they masturbate, and that they can be coy or competitive with their parents is manifestly obvious to any parent. Experimental evidence provides surprising support for some of Freud's more classical psychosexual hypotheses as well, such as the Oedipus complex (see Fisher & Greenberg, 1996; Westen, 1998b).

Many of Freud's psychosexual hypotheses have not, however, fared as well, and are better understood metaphorically or discarded altogether. Knowing which ones to discard, however, is not always an easy task, in part because the data are not always available, and in part because of difficulties in designing definitive tests of ideas that may nonetheless have merit. Freud's concept of penis envy, seemingly his most outlandish and gender-biased concept, provides a good example. At its most metaphorical, penis envy can refer to the envy developed by a little girl in a society that privileges male status (see Horney, 1967). Given the concreteness of childhood cognition, it would not be surprising if a 5-year-old symbolized this envy in terms of having or not having a penis. If the reader will forgive an anecdote (we cannot help it—we are psychoanalytic, and we break into anecdotes at the slightest provocation), prior to entering psychology a coworker of one of us (D. W.) told him that her 6-year-old daughter had cried the night before in the bathtub because her younger brother, with whom she was bathing, had "one of those things" and she did not. The author has always wondered about the impact of the mother's tongue-in-cheek reply: "Don't worry, you'll get one someday." The coworker, incidentally, had never heard of penis envy.

The Structural Model

Whereas Freud's first model, the topographic model, categorized mental processes by their quality vis-à-vis consciousness, his last basic model, the *structural model* (see Freud, 1923/1961, 1933/1964b), categorized mental processes by their *functions* or purposes (Jahoda, 1977). With the introduction of this tripartite model of id, ego, and superego, Freud's understanding of conflict shifted from conflict between consciousness and the unconscious to conflict between desires and the dictates of conscience or reality.

The id is the reservoir of sexual and aggressive energy and, like the topographic unconscious, operates on the basis of what Freud called primary process thinking (i.e., associative, wishful, illogical, nonvoluntary). The superego is the conscience and is estab-

lished through identification. The ego is the structure that must somehow balance the demands of desire, reality, and morality. To achieve this balance, the ego marshals mechanisms of defense as well as creative compromises among competing forces. Like the conscious and preconscious of the topographic model, the ego is characterized by the use of secondary process thought (controlled, rational, voluntary, planful thinking). (Contemporary readers will no doubt recognize the similarity to many contemporary dual-process models of thought and memory.) As Bettelheim (1983) observes, in the original German Freud's structural model was phrased in much more colloquial terms—the *I*, the *it*, and the *above-me*—so that Freud could actually speak to his patients about feeling that some moralistic part standing above them was judging them, or that an impulse felt like an impersonal, uncontrolled force, as in "It just came over me."

That many contemporary textbooks continue to teach this model as central to psychodynamic approaches to personality, psychopathology, and treatment is unfortunate, given that even the most stalwart advocates of the structural model have now suggested that it has outlived its usefulness (Brenner, 2003). Nevertheless, what was essential to this model, and remains important, is the description of a mind in conflict, in which conflicts among desires, conscience, reality-based concerns, and social acceptability are central to the human condition.

Developments in Psychoanalysis since Freud

Both during and since Freud's time, psychoanalysis has changed in significant ways. The first challenges to psychoanalysis from within were posed by the early revisionists, Adler and Jung, and by later neo-Freudians, who ultimately became challengers from without. The major developments since Freud's time within psychoanalysis are what was originally called ego psychology (because of its focus on the rational, reality-based ego), object relations theory and related developments (self psychology and relational theories), and evolving concepts of conflict and compromise in classical psychoanalysis (now also called, often somewhat confusingly, "classical" ego psychology, for its focus on the "ego" function of defense; e.g., Busch, 1995, 1999; P.

Gray, 1994). Although increasingly integrated (e.g., Kernberg, 1984; Pine, 1990; Westen, Gabbard, & Blagov, 2006), these approaches offer a number of distinct and often competing propositions about personality.

Early Revisionists and Neo-Freudians

Since Adler, Jung, and later neo-Freudians are not, strictly speaking, psychoanalytic, we touch upon their work only briefly here. Adler (1929, 1939) and Jung (1971) were among the first prominent analysts to split with Freud, largely because they felt, to use Jung's phrase, that Freud viewed the brain "as an appendage to the genital glands." Adler placed a greater focus on more conscious, everyday motives and experiences such as needs for achievement, as well on social motivation and the striving for superiority. Jung took psychodynamics in a number of directions, some of them more mystical, although he also emphasized missing aspects of Freud's theory, such as lifespan development.

For decades after Adler and Jung (until the pluralism that became normative in psychoanalytic circles in the 1990s), the ranks of neo-Freudians became swollen with fallen analysts. Psychodynamic theorists such as Horney (1950), Fromm (1947, 1962), and Sullivan (1953) started with Freud's insights about conflict, defense, and the pervasive influence of unconscious processes. However, they placed much greater emphasis on the role of social forces in the genesis of personality, and they rejected Freud's view of libido as the primary motivational force in human life. Fromm criticized Freud's theory primarily on four interrelated grounds, all of which have considerable merit. First, he argued, Freud underestimated the influence of history and culture on motivation. Second, humans are innately social, and Freud's psychosexual stages are as much reflections of psychosocial dilemmas (giving or receiving, complying or defying) as they are of an unfolding ontogenetic blueprint (see also Erikson, 1963). Third, Freud treated acts of benevolence, altruism, and pursuit of ideals largely as reaction formations against them (i.e., as defensive transformations of the opposite wishes), whereas Fromm proposed that humans have innately prosocial tendencies as well. Finally, Freud's psychology is a psychology of want, that is, of the need to

reduce psychological tensions such as drives. Fromm proposed that humans have other kinds of motivation as well, such as a need for relatedness to others, a need to be active and creative, and a need for a coherent sense of identity and meaning in life. Fromm, like Erikson, stressed conflicts specific to particular historical time periods and economic modes of production. He argued, foreshadowing Margaret Mahler and her colleagues (Mahler, Pine, & Bergman, 1975), that particularly in the present age a central conflict is between autonomy and individuation, on the one hand, and the fear of aloneness and loss of connectedness on the other. Today, many theorists within mainstream psychoanalysis would agree with Fromm's criticisms.

Ego Psychology

Although psychoanalytic theory evolved considerably during Freud's lifetime, in many ways it remained an "id psychology," focusing on the vicissitudes of the libidinal drive and the person's attempts to deal with impulses. A significant shift in psychoanalytic theory began at about the time of Freud's death, with the development of ego psychology, which focused on the functions and development of the ego (see Blanck & Blanck, 1974, 1979). During the same period in which Anna Freud (1936) was delineating various mechanisms of defense postulated to be used by the ego to cope with internal and external forces, Heinz Hartmann (1939/1958) and his colleagues were beginning to describe the interaction of motivational processes with ego functions such as perception, cognition, and impulse regulation. Hartmann argued that alongside drive development, as described by Freud, is the development of a "conflict-free ego sphere" that may become entangled in conflicts but is primarily an evolutionary endowment that subserves adaptation. Hartmann and his colleagues (see Hartmann, Kris, & Loewenstein, 1946) were, to a significant extent, cognitive psychologists, and they actively read and attempted to integrate into psychoanalytic theory the work of Piaget and Werner. Hartmann discussed means–end problem solving and the way thought processes can become automatic on cognitive development and adaptation in ways that would be familiar to contemporary cognitive psychologists.

Rapaport (1951) and his colleagues systematically observed and described the organization and pathology of thinking in patients with psychoses and serious personality disturbances in ways that have yet to be integrated into contemporary cognitive models. Contemporary research on subpsychotic cognitive disturbances in patients with schizotypal personality disorders and relatives of schizophrenia patients continues in this tradition, although not always explicitly (e.g., Coleman, Levy, Lenzenweger, & Holzman, 1996; Handest & Parnas, 2005; Perry, Minassian, Cadenhead, Sprock, & Braff, 2003). Shedler and Westen (2004) found, for example, that patients with scores in the upper fifth percentile on a schizotypal thinking scale, derived by factor analysis in a large clinical sample, were highly likely to have biological relatives with schizophrenia, whereas those with high scores below that threshold were distinguished by a psychosocial history of childhood attachment disruptions and sexual abuse. These data suggest that above a certain high threshold with a low base rate, schizotypal thinking is taxonic (i.e., genuinely categorical rather than continuous; see Meehl, 1995) and best understood as a schizophrenia spectrum phenomenon, whereas phenotypically similar but slightly lower levels of thinking disturbance can reflect a troubled developmental history. Research in progress using both genotyping and subtle measures of thinking disturbances may shed further light on the diverse etiologies of disordered thinking that does not rise to the level of psychosis.

Menninger, Mayman, and Pruyser (1963) made a seminal contribution to the understanding of adaptive functions and coping processes, elaborating the concept of levels of ego functioning and dyscontrol. In a work that has probably been equally underappreciated both within psychoanalysis and empirical psychology, Redl and Wineman (1951) distinguished a vast number of quasi-independent functions in their study of delinquent adolescents, who manifested deficits in many domains of ego control. Bellack, Hurvich, and Gediman (1973) developed a taxonomy of ego functions that they operationalized for systematic empirical investigation. Erikson's (1963, 1968) elaboration of stages of psychosocial/ego development parallel to Freud's psychosexual stages, his explication

of processes of identity crisis and formation, and his elucidation of interactions of personality development with historical and cultural forces fall within the broad tradition of ego psychology as well, and have led to a body of research explicitly testing his hypotheses (Marcia, 1994, 2006; McAdams, 2006; McAdams, Reynolds, Lewis, Patten, & Bowman, 2001).

Object Relations Theory, Self Psychology, and Relational Theories

Undoubtedly, the major development in psychoanalysis since Freud has been the emergence of object relations theories and related approaches to personality (see Greenberg & Mitchell, 1983; Guntrip, 1971; Mitchell, 1988; Person, Cooper, & Gabbard, 2005; Scharf & Scharf, 1998). "Object relations" refers to enduring patterns of interpersonal functioning in intimate relationships and the cognitive and emotional processes that mediate those patterns.

Clinical practice has always focused on interpersonal relationships, but object relations theories emerged in the 1930s and 1940s as clinicians began confronting patients with personality disorders who were unable to maintain satisfying relationships and who seemed to be haunted by fears and fantasies about the dangers of intimate relations with others and by unrealistic, often malevolent, representations of significant others (Fairbairn, 1952; Guntrip, 1971; M. Klein, 1948). In contrast to classical psychoanalytic theory, object relations theory stresses the impact of actual negative experiences in early childhood, the importance of self-representations and representations of others (called "object representations") in mediating interpersonal functioning, and the primary need for human relatedness that begins in infancy.

Psychoanalytic theory has seen a gradual shift from viewing objects as the repositories of drives (Freud, 1905/1953), to objects as fantasy figures (Fairbairn, 1952; M. Klein, 1948), to objects as mental representations of real people (Sandler & Rosenblatt, 1962). Alongside this shift has been a continuing debate about whether human social motivation is best conceived of as motivated by the desire for sexual/sensual pleasure or the desire for human contact and relatedness.

Fairbairn (1952) and Sullivan (1953) clearly specified interpersonal alternatives to Freud's theories of motivation and psychic structure, with Fairbairn asserting that libido is object seeking and not pleasure seeking, and Sullivan developing a comprehensive model of the structure and development of personality that emphasized the distortions in personality and self-concept necessitated by the avoidance of interpersonally generated anxiety.

Two major developments in object relations theory in the 1960s were Sandler and Rosenblatt's (1962) paper on the representational world and Bowlby's (1969) enunciation of the theory of attachment (see also Fraley & Shaver, Chapter 20, this volume). Following Jacobson (1954) and others, Sandler and Rosenblatt described the cognitive–affective structure of the "representational world"—that is, people's representations of the self and others—in ways that could still profitably be assimilated by researchers studying social cognition. In their 1962 paper, for example, they described the self-concept as a self-schema and elaborated the importance of distinguishing momentary from prototypic self-representations. Bowlby (1969, 1973, 1982) elaborated on Sandler and Rosenblatt's concept of "internal working models" of people and relationships but added a powerful reformulation of motivational constructs such as "instinct" by integrating psychoanalytic thinking with ethology. He argued that attachment is a primary motivational system in humans as in other species, and that its evolutionary significance is the provision of security to immature members of the species. He suggested, furthermore, that the expectations of relationships and the patterns of affective experience and regulation shaped in the first relationships are central determinants of later interpersonal functioning. As will be seen later, his theory has led to an enormous body of empirical research and a confirmation of many of these ideas.[3]

Although numerous theorists have proposed models of object relations, one of the major contemporary theories is Kernberg's (1975, 1984; Kernberg & Caligor, 2005) attempt to wed drive theory, ego psychology, and object relations theory. From the perspective of personality theory, one of Kernberg's (1975, 1984) central contributions has been his model of levels of personality orga-

nization. According to Kernberg, personality organization—that is, the enduring ways in which people perceive themselves and others, behave interpersonally, pursue their goals, and defend against unpleasant feelings—can be understood on a continuum of pathology. Individuals with a borderline level of personality organization have difficulty maintaining consistent views of themselves and others over time, and they are prone to severe distortions in the way they perceive reality—particularly, interpersonal reality—when the going gets rough. People at a neurotic to normal level of personality organization may have all kinds of conflicts, concerns, and problems (such as low self-esteem, anxiety, and so forth), but they are generally able to love and to work effectively.

Kernberg proposes a model of normal and pathological development that attempts to account for these different levels of personality organization. The basic logic of Kernberg's model is that development proceeds from a lack of awareness in infancy of the distinction between self and other (which he initially linked to psychotic levels of functioning), to a differentiation of representations based on affective valence (i.e., "good" vs. "bad" people and experiences) in the toddler years (related to borderline functioning), to an eventual construction of mature representations that integrate ambivalent feelings by age 5 or 6 (linked to the capacity for healthier functioning). Kernberg formulated his theory to account for phenomena observed in the treatment of severe personality disorders, notably the tendency of these patients toward "splitting" (the separation of good and bad representations, so that the person cannot see the self or others at a particular time with any richness or complexity). The preschooler scolded by his or her mother who yells, "Mommy, I hate you! You don't love me!" is evidencing this normal developmental incapacity to retrieve memories of interactions with the mother associated with a different affective tone. Later, according to Kernberg, splitting can be used defensively to maintain idealizations of the self or significant others, or to protect the other from the individual's own aggressive impulses. Kernberg's theory has proven useful in recent randomized clinical trials of treatment for borderline personality disorder (Levy et al., 2006).

Whereas Kernberg retains many elements of the classical theory of drive, conflict, and defense, self psychology, developed by Heinz Kohut (1966, 1971, 1977, 1984), represents a much more radical departure. (For a review of developments on the concept of the self since Kohut, see Pinel & Constantino, 2003.) Kohut originally developed his theory as an attempt to explain the phenomenology and symptomatology of patients with narcissistic personality disorders (Kohut, 1966). In his early work Kohut defined the "self" as other psychoanalysts since Hartmann (1950) had (and many contemporary social psychologists do), as a collection of self-representations. Later, however, Kohut (1971, 1977) came to view a psychology of the self as complementary to the classical theory of drive and defense. By the end of his life, Kohut (1984; Kohut & Wolf, 1978) argued that defects in the self, not the conflicts emphasized by classical psychoanalysis, are central to psychopathology more generally. "Self" in this later work refers to a psychic structure similar to Freud's id, ego, and superego. Kohut describes this structure as bipolar, with ambitions on one side, ideals on the other, and talents and skills driven by these two poles "arched" between them.

Although Kohut's terminology can be confusing, the thrust of his argument is that having a core of ambitions and ideals, the talents and skills with which to try to actualize them, and a cohesive and positive sense of self constitutes mental health. The extent to which children develop these characteristics reflects, according to Kohut, the extent to which their caretakers in the first years of life themselves are healthy along these dimensions and can thus respond empathically when their children need them, imparting their own sense of security and self-esteem to their children. For Kohut, ambitions, ideals, and the need for self-esteem are three primary motivational systems in humans.

Kohut's developmental theory, like that of most psychoanalytic theorists, proposes that the infant begins in a state of relatively poor differentiation of self and other, characterized by fragmented, unintegrated representations; he calls this the *stage of the fragmented self*. At some point in the second year a "nuclear self," or core sense of self, emerges, with the bipolar structure described above. In this stage the child is driven by a fantasized sense of the self as able to do anything, which Kohut calls the *grandiose self*, and identification with parents endowed by the child with a similar sense of greatness, which Kohut calls the *idealized parent imago*. If the child's primary caretakers are unempathic, chronically responding to their own needs instead of those of the infant, the child will develop defects in one or both poles of the self. This may lead to symptoms such as grandiosity, poor self-esteem, a desperate need to be attended to and admired, and severe problems in establishing a cohesive sense of identity. Kohut's self psychology remains influential in psychoanalysis, and some have attempted to investigate his theories and concepts and adapt them for empirical testing (see Banai, Mikulincer, & Shaver, 2005).

Perhaps the most important recent development in psychoanalysis is the emergence of *relational theories* (Aron, 1996; Aron & Harris, 2005; Mitchell, 1988, 1993, 1997; Mitchell & Aron, 1999), which in many respects are an outgrowth of both object relations theories within mainstream psychoanalysis and the interpersonal theory of Harry Stack Sullivan (1953) that was once on its fringes. Like both of these theoretical viewpoints, relational theories stress the importance of motives for relatedness and place less emphasis on the motivational significance of sex and aggression. They also emphasize the importance of the internalization of interpersonal interactions in the development of personality, arguing that the child's fundamental adaptations occur in response to the interpersonal world, and that the building blocks of personality are the ideas and images the child forms of the self and significant others.

For example, whereas Freud's model of intrapsychic conflict emphasized conflicts among drives, reality, and the dictates of conscience, Stephen Mitchell, the originator of the relational approach in psychoanalysis, viewed conflicts as relational configurations (1993, 1997). In other words, conflict is inherent in relationships, and these conflicted relationships are internalized from early in life and reexperienced in adulthood, as people seek interactions with others that actualize often competing and sometimes destructive prototypes from earlier in life. Mitchell's relational approach has roots in both traditional object relations theories as well as the work of Sullivan, who emphasized the role of actual relationships in shaping and maintaining personality processes.

Developments in Classical Psychoanalysis

Alongside these various developments have come changes in the classical model since Freud's time. Although these have been many, some of the major changes have come about through the systematizing and revisionist efforts of Charles Brenner (1982). Arlow and Brenner (1964) translated accounts of phenomena explained by Freud's topographic model, such as dreams, into the language of Freud's structural model. Since that time, Brenner, in particular, has reformulated many basic Freudian constructs while attempting to preserve what is most important in the classical theory. His attempts at reformulation are set forth most succinctly in *The Mind in Conflict* (1982), which expresses the classical theory, as revised by decades of psychoanalytic practice, probably as clearly and persuasively as it could be expressed. (For reviews of the development of Brenner's work, see also Brenner, 1991, 2002, 2003; Richards, 1986.)

Brenner's major contribution has been his elaboration of the concept of *compromise formation*, probably one of the most important constructs Freud ever developed. Freud proposed that neurotic symptoms represent compromises among competing forces in the mind, particularly impulses, superego prohibitions, and the constraints of reality. In *The Interpretation of Dreams* (1900/1953), Freud proposed that compromise is crucial in dream formation as well. Brenner's extension of Freud's theory suggests that all psychological events are compromise formations that include various elements of wishes, anxiety, depressive affect, defense, and superego prohibitions. For example, the academic who derives pleasure from his or her work may simultaneously (1) gratify wishes to be superior to competitors, which are satisfied by feelings of intellectual superiority; (2) gratify wishes to be admired, which are achieved by being surrounded by a cadre of graduate students (probably an illusory gratification); (3) allay anxiety by mastering intellectual domains of uncertainty and solving small problems in the discipline; (4) ward off depressive affect by bolstering self-esteem

through publishing papers, making presentations, and winning the esteem of colleagues; and (5) satisfy superego mandates by being disciplined in scientific method and seeking truth.

From the perspective of personality theory, Brenner's list of the ingredients involved in compromise formations probably requires some tinkering (Westen, 1985, 1998b, 2007; Westen, Weinberger, & Bradley, 2007). Notably absent is the need to see things as they really are, as well as cognitive processes leading to relatively veridical perception and cognition, which surely get expressed in beliefs along with more dynamic processes. Nevertheless, the basic point is that people are always synthesizing momentary compromises among multiple and competing mental processes. Some of these compromises are relatively stable and enduring, whereas others exist only briefly, because the "balance of forces" within the person is constantly changing in response to thoughts, feelings, fantasies, and environmental events.

CURRENT CONTROVERSIES IN PSYCHOANALYSIS

Currently psychoanalysis is in a state of flux, with no single theory in the ascendant. Indeed, in some ways, the last two decades have seen a flight from theory, as psychoanalysts have increasingly recognized the limitations of Freud's models of the mind but have not agreed upon any comprehensive alternative. The loss of consensus in Freud's models of the mind within psychoanalysis began to take shape in the 1970s with a growing disenchantment with drive theory, energy concepts, aspects of the structural model, the distance of concepts such as "libidinal cathexis" and "drive fusion" from observable psychological events, and the persistent tendency in psychoanalytic literature for Freud's structures to be reified (as if "the ego" feels or chooses something). An influential group of psychoanalytic theorists began to suggest abandoning much of Freud's theoretical superstructure, denoted his "metapsychology," in favor of the more experience-near concepts (e.g., defense, conflict) that constitute what has been called the "clinical theory" of psychoanalysis (G. S. Klein, 1976; Schafer, 1976). One of us (D. W.) and a colleague (see, e.g., Westen & Shedler, 2007) have gone a step further, attempting to operationalize, using plain clinical language, the psychoanalytic (and other) concepts about mental states and processes derived from personality, developmental, and clinical psychology that are relevant to personality pathology. Clinically skilled observers can apply the Q-sort instrument they developed with high reliability (e.g., "Appears unable to describe important others in a way that conveys a sense of who they are as people; descriptions of others come across as two-dimensional and lacking in richness").

Perhaps the most positive side of this "cultural revolution" within psychoanalysis is that it ultimately changed the nature of psychoanalytic discourse, which once required rigid adherence to particular dogmas and discouraged testing of specific hypotheses. The negative is that psychoanalytic practice is now guided less by an explicit set of theoretical propositions about personality and psychopathology than by an implicit one. Indeed, psychoanalytic theory today is less about personality and more about clinical technique and the nature of subjectivity. Nevertheless, a number of interrelated issues are at the forefront of thinking in contemporary psychoanalysis and have substantial relevance to personality psychology. Here we address two of these issues: the nature of motivation, and what it means to know a person.

The Nature of Motivation

Freud's theory of motivation has always been both the heart and the Achilles heel of psychoanalytic theory. Psychoanalysis is, above all else, a theory of the complexities of human motivation and the ways in which motives interact, conflict, and attain surreptitious expression. Despite multiple changes in his motivational theories throughout his career, Freud was unflagging in his view of sexuality as the primary instinct in humans that draws them to each other and motivates much of their behavior, and in his corresponding implication of sexuality in the etiology of neurosis. As an inveterate biologist who never entirely relinquished his wish to ground his theory in physiology (Sulloway, 1979), Freud maintained a theory of psychic energy in his latest models of the mind that was a clear descendent of a purely physiological theory he

had developed in 1895 but abandoned and chose never to publish (Freud, 1950/1966; see Pribram & Gill, 1976).

The Demise of the Classical Freudian Theory of Motivation

The libido theory was, as noted earlier, the point of contention that drove many of Freud's adherents from the fold in the early part of the 20th century. By the 1980s, fealty to Freud's theory of motivation was becoming "optional" for maintaining good standing in psychoanalytic circles, and by the 1990s, most psychoanalysts and psychoanalytic psychologists had abandoned much of Freud's theory of motivation, including his dual-instinct theory, his model of a displaceable psychic energy, his drive–discharge model of motivation, and the notion of a primary aggressive drive (see Gill, 1976; Holt, 1976; Rubenstein, 1976; Shevrin, 1984). The reasons are complex and many, but perhaps the most important were the recognition that not all motives can be reduced to sex and aggression; that motives for intimacy are not reducible to sexual desire; that not all motives (particularly aggressive motives) build up and require discharge; and that Freud's energy concepts (the notion of a displaceable psychic energy), though powerful metaphors, were too unwieldy and scientistic.

Even before Freud's death, Melanie Klein (1948) argued for the importance of motives such as envy. Fairbairn (1952) and other object relations theorists argued for the importance of relatedness to others, which Bowlby (1969) developed into a more systematic theory of attachment-related motivation years later, and which relational theorists (Mitchell, 1988) view as the primary motive in humans. Robert White (1959) emphasized the need to be effective or to attain mastery, and he reinterpreted Freud's psychosexual stages along these lines. Kohut (1971) emphasized the needs for self-esteem and for a sense of cohesion and described what could go wrong in development to lead some people to have difficulty regulating their self-esteem or to be vulnerable to feelings of fragmentation. Whereas many theorists have attempted to replace Freud's relatively simple two-motive theory with equally reductionist theories, others have offered more complex formulations. For example, Lichtenberg (1989) proposed that human motivation involves five motivational systems, including physiological regulation, attachment, exploration/assertion, withdrawal or antagonism in response to aversive events, and sensual/sexual pleasure.

Virtually all contemporary psychoanalytic approaches to motivation continue to retain some key features of Freud's theory, notably the recognition of the importance of unconscious motives, which has now been amply documented empirically (Ferguson & Bargh, 2004; McClelland, Koestner, & Weinberger, 1989). Nevertheless, the psychoanalytic theory of motivation would profit from greater acquaintance with both evolutionary theory and relevant psychological and neuroscientific research (Panksepp, 1998; Westen, 1997). For example, rather than speculating about how many motives human have, researchers might instead develop a relatively comprehensive list of motives as expressed in clinical sessions, everyday interactions, and ethnographies, and combine them with motives studied in over 70 years of psychological research, using factor analysis to identify common factors and see if motives have a hierarchical structure. Knowing something about the neural pathways that mediate different psychological motive systems and considering their possible evolutionary functions might also be useful in deciding to what extent various motives should be considered part of the same system or relatively independent. The notion that the desires for sex and for relatedness to others are transformations of the same underlying drive makes little sense in light of what we now know about the two motive systems from neuroimaging research (Adolphs, 2003; Hamann, 2006; Lieberman, 2007). For example, interpersonal thought, feeling, and motivation virtually always activate ventromedial prefrontal cortex, whereas sexual motivation may or may not do so.

Affect and Motivation

If any consensus is beginning to emerge in the psychoanalytic literature, it is probably a deceptively simple one that has always implicitly guided clinical practice and was anticipated in the psychological literature by Tomkins (1962) and others: that affect is a primary motivational mechanism in humans (Pervin, 1982; Sandler, 1987; Spez-

zano, 1993; Watson & Clark, 1984; Westen, 1985, 1997, 2007; Westen & Blagov, 2007). In other words, people are drawn to actions, objects, and representations associated with positive feelings or the anticipation of positive feelings and are repulsed by those associated with negative feelings or their likely activation.

This simple formula has a number of complications and ramifications, four of which are of particular significance. First, these affect-driven motivational pulls need not be conscious. As we predicted in this chapter two decades ago, experimental research increasingly supports the proposition that people often respond simultaneously to multiple such pulls in various directions (for models of how this happens, see Thagard, 2005; Westen, 2007; Westen et al., 2007).

Second, precisely how to integrate an affect theory of motivation with phenomena such as eating and sex, which have traditionally been understood in both psychology and psychoanalysis in terms of drives, is not yet entirely clear. One possibility is that drive states may take on motivational significance only to the extent that they lead to feeling-states such as sexual arousal or hunger, or to the extent that they become associatively linked with experiences of pleasure. Alternatively, they may be quasi-independent processes that evolved earlier and remain influenced by hypothalamic nuclei that may be activated or downregulated by cortical and subcortical circuits but can be activated independent of these later-evolved circuits and may provide both their own sources of "energy" for behavior and the direction of behavior (e.g., toward or away from same- vs. opposite-sex sexual partners).

Third, thinking of motives in terms of emotions and efforts at emotion regulation (see Gross, 2007)—that is, the selection of behaviors and mental processes based on their emotional consequences—allows one to avoid choosing among overly reductionistic single-motive or dual-motive systems that are unlikely to do justice to the complexity of human motivation. Fairbairn, for example, brought something very important into psychoanalysis by challenging the view that the desire for relationships is really just a derivative of the sexual drive. He argued, instead, that things are the other way around: that libido (desire) is object seeking (desirous of relationships), not pleasure seeking (desirous of sex).

Yet the antinomy between pleasure seeking and object seeking is only an antinomy in the context of Freud's specific meaning of libido, which confounds pleasure seeking with sexual pleasure seeking. People have a number of desires for connectedness with others, from wishes for physical proximity and security to desires for affiliation (J. D. Klein & Schnackenberg, 2000), intimacy (McAdams & Powers, 1981), and a sense of belongingness (Newman, Lohman, & Newman, 2007). These are clearly mediated by affective systems—that is, characterized by "pleasure seeking" (and pain avoidance)—just as surely as are sexual desires, although they may also combine with sexual desire, as in romantic love. In some ways, psychoanalysis and psychology may have simply rediscovered a thesis proposed by many of the ancient Greek philosophers and perhaps best articulated by the 16th-century philosopher Hobbes: namely, that much of motivation reflects the seeking of pleasure and avoidance of pain, whether physical or psychic—a postulate consistent with theory and research on the biologically based behavioral inhibition and activation systems (BIS/BAS, see Carver & White, 1994; Demaree, Robinson, & Everhart, 2005; J. A. Gray, 1990; Mathews, Yiend, & Lawrence, 2004). What psychoanalysis adds is the notion that many, if not most, of our behaviors are multiply influenced by competing and collaborating emotional pulls that reflect the range and strength of emotional associations we routinely form to anyone or anything we have encountered on multiple occasions.

As Bowlby (1969, 1973) elucidated, the child's attachment behavior is mediated by feelings such as separation distress, pleasure at being held in the mother's arms, and/or relief at reunion—and may be influenced, as well, by competing pulls to avoid close connection to the mother reflecting maternal insensitivity (Fonagy, Gergely, Jurist, & Target, 2002; van IJzendoorn et al., 2000). There is no a priori reason why a person cannot be motivated simultaneously by several motive systems, each mediated by pleasurable and unpleasurable feelings (Westen, 1985, 1997). This view is supported by findings that negative and positive affectivity are relatively independent dimensions (e.g., Clark, 2005;

Clark & Watson, 1991) and have overlapping but distinct neuroanatomy (Kim & Hamann, 2007). The interplay of these affective states and dispositions can help explain the complex motives behind seemingly irrational behavior (e.g., an abused spouse fleeing a shelter to return to an abusive partner, or an abused child clinging to a parent who is simultaneously abusing him or her).

A fourth ramification, implicit in the first three, is that a shift to an affect theory of motivation permits more coherent thinking about interactions of affect and cognition than has previously been the case, and is likely to allow much more (and more useful) contact between psychoanalysis and research on affect and cognition in empirical psychology (see Dalgleish & Power, 1999; Westen, 1999a). One example is the growing recognition that motives involve representations of desired, feared, or valued outcomes associatively linked with various feeling-states (see Manian, Papadakis, Strauman, & Essex, 2006; Oyserman & Fryberg, 2006; Shah, Higgins, & Friedman, 1998; Strauman, 1996). A prime example is the concept of *wish*, which has begun to replace the concept of drive in even classical analytic circles (Brenner, 1982; Dahl, 1983; Holt, 1976; Sandler & Sandler, 1978; Westen, 1985, 1997). "Wish" is an experience-near construct that does not rely on 19th-century energy concepts and is intuitively much more compelling.

Wishes may arise through the interaction of biological and environmental events, as affects become associated in preprogrammed and learned ways with various cognitive representations and structures. For example, in the second half of the first year, separation from a primary attachment figure (we will use the example of the mother) may trigger a distress response that is genetically programmed (given, of course, the proper environmental input, referred to in the psychoanalytic literature since Hartmann, 1939/1958, as an "average expectable environment"). When the return of the mother repeatedly quells this distress, the association of her representation with regulation of an aversive affective state creates an affect-laden representation of a desired state, which is then activated when the mother has been out of sight for a period of time, setting in motion a wish for proximity in the child.

Implications for Personality Theory

Although some of the links may not be readily apparent, these trends in psychoanalysis are of considerable relevance to personality psychology more broadly. They bear on questions about the role of affect and cognition in motivation, the extent to which motives endure over time, the circumstances under which motives and affects are chronically elicited in ways that bear the signature of an individual's personality, and the interaction of nature and nurture in generating the motives that underlie human behavior. Trait approaches to personality tend to remain silent on motivational issues. Social learning and social-cognitive approaches tend to emphasize conscious, cognitive, rational, and environmentally induced motivations, and to study them without reference to their developmental course. Each of these approaches could profitably wrestle with some of the issues psychoanalysis has been facing for decades in this respect.

From a psychoanalytic standpoint, what is crucial to any reconceptualization of the concept of motivation are several elements of classical Freudian theory that remain central, if implicit, in psychoanalytically oriented clinical thinking about motives and are too easily forgotten: that motives can (1) be conscious or unconscious; (2) combine and interact in complex ways; (3) conflict with equally compelling wishes, fears, or internal standards in which a person has invested emotionally; (4) be rooted in the biology of the organism and hence not readily "shut off"; and (5) feel "it-like" (Freud's clinical concept of the "id," or "it"), or like non-self, precisely because they are peremptory and cannot be readily eliminated. As we will see, many of these features of psychoanalytic approaches to motivation have considerable empirical support.[4]

What Does it Mean to Know a Person?

Alongside these theoretical issues is an epistemological question about what it means to know a person—and how we know when we know. To what extent are the narratives a patient tells in clinical hours best understand as (1) a record, albeit an imperfect one, offered from one point of view, of something usually interpersonally significant that occurred in the patient's life; (2) an index of the patient's ways of experiencing the self and others (a

central aspect of personality); or (3) an index of the efforts of two people to come to terms with the person's past and present in the context of a particular relationship that is inherently shaped by the psychology of both participants (a mixture of true variance and error variance)?

As we will see, these issues are—or should be—central to the study of personality in psychology as well. Clinicians since Freud have struggled with how much to accept at face value what their patients tell them about themselves and their lives. In contrast, researchers tend to accept respondents' self-reports on questionnaires as an index of who they are, rather than as compromise formations reflecting an amalgam of their efforts to perceive themselves accurately, regulate their self-esteem, manage guilt or shame, and so forth. Personality researchers only occasionally use scales designed to assess variables such as social desirability and inconsistent responding when studying normal populations, and they seldom attempt to parse variance attributable to the person, the way the person is being studied (via questionnaire), and the informant (typically self-report) (although see, e.g., Colvin, Block, & Funder, 1995; Shedler, Mayman, & Manis, 1993).

Capturing the Interactive Nature of Personality in Clinical Settings

Questions about the veracity of patients' self-report first came to the fore in psychoanalysis as theorists began to wrestle with the extent to which historical events in the life of a patient are psychoanalytically knowable or useful. Freud initially believed hysteria to result from sexual abuse, but the extremely high prevalence of reports of childhood seductions by his patients eventually led him to believe that many of these reports likely represented childhood fantasies. In so doing, Freud ultimately came to underestimate the prevalence of actual abuse (although he and clinicians following in his footsteps have somehow been blamed on both sides of the issue, for understating the occurrence of abuse and for implanting false memories). However, his gestalt switch also led him to think more deeply about "psychic reality" as opposed to "actual reality" (see Arlow, 1985). "Psychic reality" refers to the way in which a person experiences an event in light of his or her motives, fantasies, and affect-laden ideas about the self, others, and the world. In many ways, this shift in Freud's thinking foreshadowed a later shift from behaviorism to cognitive-behavioral theories in the 1950s through 1980s, as researchers recognized that behavior reflects not only contingencies of reinforcement but the way in which the person or animal construes those contingencies (i.e., the mediating role of expectancies and schemas).[5]

In psychoanalysis, Spence (1982) opened a Pandora's box by advancing the argument that what happens in psychoanalytic therapy is not an act of archeology, or recovering the past, but an act of mutual storymaking in which patient and analyst construct a compelling narrative that provides the patient with an integrated view of his of her history and helps explain seemingly inexplicable aspects of the patient's life. In so doing, Spence was describing, in part, an evolution in the practice of psychodynamic psychotherapy, reflecting a shift away from an archeological search for hidden memories—psychic boils in need of lancing—toward a more interactive therapeutic stance aimed at understanding the patient's inner world and its interactive effects on other people. The quest for understanding the patient's dynamics in light of his or her description of past experiences is an example of what the philosopher and cognitive scientist Paul Thagard (Thagard et al., 2006) calls *explanatory coherence*, that is, our brain's attempt to converge on cognitive solutions that have as good a fit as possible to the "facts on the ground" and help explain how they might occur together. This process in clinical work is, in principle, no different from the one scientists use when they synthesize a body of research or design their next study based on their best guesses about why their and other scientists' prior studies produced a particular pattern of results in need of better explanation.

The last two decades in psychoanalytic thinking have seen an increasing recognition of the extent to which psychoanalysis as a therapy is a "two-person psychology," an attempt by two people (the patient and the therapist), working collaboratively, to understand the subjectivity of one of them, with the goal of helping that person escape from repetitive cognitive, affective, and interpersonal patterns that compromise the patient's well-being (and often the well-being of oth-

ers). From this point of view, not only do clinicians influence what they observe in the patient in an ongoing way (a truism Freud understood from the start, which contributed to his therapeutic shift from hypnotic suggestion and related techniques to free association, which he did in part to try to minimize the role of suggestion), but patients are constantly exerting interpersonal influences on the clinician. By virtue of their personality dynamics, patients often re-create their characteristic modes of relatedness in their relationship with the clinician and elicit certain ways of reacting, feeling, and thinking from the clinician—which in turn affect the way the patient and therapist engage (Gabbard, 2005). Patients also elicit similar or complementary emotions in the therapist in ways long hypothesized by psychodynamic theorists but now better understood in light of neuroscientific research on phenomena such as mirror neurons, which literally lead one person to experience another person's emotions directly, if unconsciously (Iacoboni, 2008; Rizzolatti & Craighero, 2004). Hence therapists engage in introspection regarding their own internal experience of the patient and study their unconscious enactments with the patient carefully, knowing that their "countertransference" reactions are important, if imperfect, diagnostic tools in understanding the patient.

Freud initially introduced the concept of countertransference as something to be avoided (as an idiosyncratic personal reaction to the patient that led away from accurate understanding of the person). In contrast, contemporary theorists recognize that the way the clinician thinks, feels, and acts with a particular patient (the contemporary definition of countertransference—parallel to the definition of transference as the way the patient tends to respond cognitively, emotionally, and behaviorally to the therapist; see Bradley, Heim, & Westen, 2005)—is a joint function of what is unique to the therapist's personality and history (what Freud had in mind) and what is induced by the patient's affect and behavior (Gabbard, 1995; Westen & Gabbard, 2002b). By observing their own responses to a particular patient—what the patient seems to "pull"—in comparison to their typical responses to other patients, and integrating those observations with data from the narratives the patient has told about other relationships, clinicians attempt to understand better what their patients tend both to experience and to draw from others.

Recent research suggests that patients with particular personality disorders—and likely, by extension, less problematic personality styles as well (Blagov, Bradley, & Westen, 2007)—tend to elicit "average expectable countertransference" patterns across therapists that are not only clinically but diagnostically useful. Betan, Heim, Conklin, and Westen (2005) factor-analyzed data from a countertransference questionnaire completed by a large sample of psychiatrists and psychologists describing their work with a randomly selected patient. They identified eight conceptually and clinically coherent factors that were independent of the clinicians' theoretical orientation and varied in predictable ways with personality diagnosis. For example, a composite description of countertransference patterns in the treatment of patients who met diagnostic criteria for narcissistic personality disorder showed that therapists treating narcissistic patients tended to feel anger, resentment, and dread, and often felt criticized and devalued by these patients. They often felt distracted during their appointments with narcissistic patients and felt like they were "walking on eggshells" with them.

These data make considerable sense in light of what Paul Wachtel (1977, 1997) has called "cyclical psychodynamics"—the tendency of patients to draw from other people precisely what they worry about. In the social-psychological literature, Swann (1997; Bosson & Swann, 1999) has shown how these processes work with depressed people, who often draw critical responses from those around them, including well-trained clinicians. Downey (Downey, Freitas, Michaelis, & Khouri, 1998; London, Downey, Bonica, & Paltin, 2007) has similarly shown how people characterized by rejection sensitivity tend to draw precisely what they fear, for example, by pushing romantic partners away by prematurely requiring a level of commitment not commensurate with the history of the relationship.

Postmodern Views

The notion of psychoanalysis as a "two-person psychology" has gone a long way toward ending the caricature of the psychoanalytic relationship as one in which one person is on the couch while the other sits in a chair, trying to be a dispassionate observer who chimes in with an occasional "And what comes to mind about that?" or "How does that make you feel?" However, it has also led some theorists to embrace a radical relativism akin to an approach the cultural anthropologist Clifford Geertz (1973) once described, in the interpretation of cultural meanings, as suggesting that as long as we cannot create a completely antiseptic environment, we might as well perform surgery in the sewer. By the late 1980s and early 1990s, the increasing obsolescence of the view of the analyst as omniscient observer converged with postmodern approaches in the humanities that radically challenge the nature of knowledge and the scientific pursuit of it.

According to some postmodern psychoanalysts, Freud and the classical psychoanalysis that he developed are exemplars of the "modernist," positivist search for a single, objective truth (the dispassionate analyst seeking objective truth about the patient). A variety of contemporary schools of thought have challenged traditional views of the psychoanalytic enterprise, some of them under the banner of postmodernism and some of them simply reflecting greater humility than the psychoanalysis of old. These approaches go under a number of names, including mutuality, intersubjectivity, social constructivism, relativism, and perspectivism, all of which regard absolute objectivity as a myth (Aron, 1996; Gill, 1994; Greenberg, 1991; I. Z. Hoffman, 1991, 1998; Levine, 1994; Mitchell, 1993, 1997; Natterson, 1991; Ogden, 1994; Renik, 1993, 1998; Stolorow, Brandchaft, & Atwood, 1987).

A common theme in this literature is that the perceptions of the patient are inevitably colored by the subjectivity of the therapeutic interpreter, and that any efforts at theory are inherently flawed by the assumption of an objective reality "out there" (I. Z. Hoffman, 1998; Holland, 1993; Leary, 1994). Many of these critiques of "modernism" in psychoanalysis seem philosophically, historically, and empirically somewhat naive (Eagle, Wolitzky, & Wakefield, 2001; Westen, 2002). "Postmodern" concerns have been influential in the social sciences at least since the "premodern" writing of Karl Marx, who similarly viewed objectivity as a myth (and a motivated one at that), and there is something deeply ironic about postmodernists attacking the work of Sigmund Freud, who is so widely viewed in empirical psychology as anything but a positivist. Radical postmodern approaches are also vulnerable to precisely the same critiques that rendered "premodern" relativism (e.g., of early 20th-century anthropology) untenable. For example, if nothing is objectively true, then the statement that "nothing is true" is just one more assertion among competing assertions, all of which should ultimately be discarded because none is true.[6] Most psychoanalytic theorists and clinicians, however, approach the therapeutic situation with a more pragmatic combination of realism and perspectivism that acknowledges the presence of an external reality but recognizes that each participant in the therapeutic dyad brings his or her own perspective to bear on that reality (Gabbard, 1997c).

Science or Hermeneutics?

The question of the nature of truth in psychoanalysis dovetails with a broader question about what it means to know a person that is central to any understanding of personality. Freud believed (at least most of the time) that psychoanalysis should be a science just like any other (Freud, 1940/1964a), and many psychoanalysts and psychoanalytic psychologists remain committed to the view that psychoanalysis should identify regularities in nature and attempt to establish causal connections among events (e.g., thoughts, feelings, and behaviors; e.g., Holzman, 1985). On the other hand, others within psychoanalysis have suggested that psychoanalysis is instead a hermeneutic discipline, aimed at the *interpretive understanding* of human actions (Habermas, 1971; Ricoeur, 1971; Spence, 1982). In this view, the crucial difference between humans and the objects of natural science, such as planets or molecules, is that humans confer meanings to their experiences, and that these meanings in turn influence what they do. Thus, as a social scientist (or, in this case, a psychotherapist) the goal is not to attribute *causes* but to interpret behavior and understand people's *reasons* for doing what they are doing—that is, their intentions. In psychoanalysis, these reasons are presumed often to be unconscious.

Many psychoanalysts have argued against this approach (see, e.g., Edelson, 1985; Luyten, Blatt, & Corveleyn, 2006; Westen, 1998b, 2002), contending that it ignores many of its factual assertions about stages of development, psychological mechanisms, and the like, which can and should be tested just as the hypotheses of any approach to human mental life and behavior can and should be tested. As Holzman (1985) observes, psychoanalysis was, from the start, replete with causal theories (e.g., symptoms are caused by problematic compromise formations; attempting to defend against a wish can lead to its unconscious expression in some other form). Furthermore, reasons themselves have their causes (e.g., people have sexual fantasies because sexual motivation is rooted in their biology; narcissistic patients may consider a situation only in terms of its relevance to their own needs because they did not experience appropriate empathy as a child). Grunbaum (1984) offered a trenchant critique of the hermeneutic account of psychoanalysis, arguing, among other things, that reasons are simultaneously causes. Whether an event is physical or psychological makes no difference to an account of causality: To be causal, an event X must simply *make a difference* to the occurrence of another event Y, and intentions can do this as well as material causes (see also Edelson, 1984, 1985; Holt, 1981).

In some respects, we suspect the controversy over whether psychoanalysis should be a scientific or interpretative/hermeneutic enterprise reflects a failure to consider the sometimes distinct but often overlapping circumstances under which scientific and interpretive thinking are useful. There can be little doubt that one of the most important legacies of psychoanalysis for psychology is the recognition that meaning often does not lie on the surface of people's actions or communications and hence requires interpretation. To put it another way more congenial to contemporary thinking in cognitive neuroscience, the crux of psychoanalysis as an interpretive approach is in the exploration and mapping of a patient's associational networks, which are, by virtue of both mental architecture and efforts at affect regulation, not available to introspection (Westen, 1998b, 1999a, 1999b, 2007). What skilled clinicians do, and what skilled clinical supervisors teach, is a way of listening to the manifest content of a patient's communications and recognizing patterns of thought, feeling, motivation, and behavior that seem to co-occur and become activated under particular circumstances. This is one of the major reasons we believe that psychoanalysis has a great deal to offer personality psychology in terms of methods of inquiry, which aim less at asking people to *describe themselves* than to express themselves, and in so doing to reveal aspects of themselves.

On the other hand, the principles that underlie psychoanalytic interpretative efforts are empirical propositions, such as the view that people often reveal their characteristics ways of experiencing themselves and others in the therapeutic relationship, that their conscious beliefs can reflect transformations of unconscious beliefs distorted by their wishes, that their behaviors and beliefs can reflect compromises among multiple competing motives, and so forth. As we will see, many of these broad assumptions have received considerable empirical support. This support does not, however, absolve clinicians or theorists from the need to test the more specific theoretical assumptions that underlie their interpretations with their patients. These interpretations are frequently guided by theories of motivation, emotion, or development that lead particular clinicians to offer interpretations from a Freudian, object relational, interpersonal, self psychological, relational, or other point of view. Given the multitude of ways in which a clinician can interpret a particular piece of clinical data, it is surely not a matter of indifference whether some or all of the theoretical propositions underlying his or her preferred theoretical orientation are empirically inaccurate.

Implications for Personality Theory

The points of controversy currently enlivening the psychoanalytic scene point to several fundamental issues for personality theory more generally. From the perspective of personality psychology, one way to describe the changing psychoanalytic landscape is to suggest that psychoanalytic theory is increasingly catching up with its clinical practice in recognizing the extent to which personality lies in person-by-situation interactions. Personality is not something people carry with

them and express everywhere; rather, personality processes are essentially if–then contingencies (Kammrath, Mendoza-Denton, & Mischel, 2005; Mischel & Shoda, 1995), in which particular circumstances—including external situations as well as conscious and unconscious configurations of meaning—elicit particular ways of thinking, feeling, or behaving.

From a methodological standpoint, these issues have a number of implications for personality psychology as well. The increasing focus in psychoanalytic writing on countertransference and the role of the analyst's own history, feelings, beliefs, and subjectivity on the way he or she interprets data suggests that researchers' choice of theories, hypotheses, and methods are also unlikely independent of their own affective, motivational, and cognitive biases. (Some of the most virulent attacks on Freud would be difficult to understand—most dead people do not draw such passion—without considering such affective biases.) Similarly, the personal demands of handing subjects questionnaires versus engaging them in in-depth interviews about poignant personal experiences are very different, and it would be surprising if a preference for one or another were completely orthogonal to interpersonal needs, attachment styles, and so forth. Furthermore, just as psychoanalysts can no longer assume the objectivity of their interpretations and must pay more attention to the interpretive frames of their actively constructing subjects, so, too, personality psychologists need to think more carefully about the circumstances under which asking participants to describe themselves using statements constructed by the observer—that is, questionnaires—does justice to the subjectivity, and hence the personality, of the observed.

ENDURING CONTRIBUTIONS AND EMPIRICAL RESEARCH

Psychoanalysis has made a number of enduring contributions to psychology, and particularly to personality theory. Many of these take the form of testable propositions that have stood the test of time, whereas others are better conceived as guiding assumptions that are theoretically or methodologically useful. With respect to testable propositions, when one considers not only research generated by psychoanalytic researchers but also experimental findings from other research traditions that corroborate, dovetail with, or refine basic psychoanalytic hypotheses, one finds that the empirical basis of psychoanalytic concepts is far better documented, and that psychoanalytic thinking is far more widely applicable, than is typically assumed. Westen (1998b) has reviewed the empirical data on five basic postulates of contemporary psychodynamic thinking that have stood the test of time: (1) Much of mental life is unconscious, including thoughts, feelings, and motives. (2) Mental processes, including affective and motivational processes, operate in parallel, so that individuals can have conflicting feelings toward the same person or situation, which motivate them in opposing ways and often lead to compromise solutions. (3) Stable personality patterns begin to form in childhood, and childhood experiences play an important role in personality development, particularly in shaping the ways people form later social relationships. (4) Mental representations of the self, others, and relationships guide people's interactions with others and influence the ways in which they become psychologically symptomatic. (5) Personality development involves not only learning to regulate sexual and aggressive feelings but also moving from an immature, socially dependent state to a mature, interdependent one. We do not repeat that review here but instead briefly describe what we believe are a set of fundamental insights, concepts, and ways of orienting to the data of personality that psychoanalytic approaches continue to offer.

Unconscious Processes

The most fundamental assumption of psychoanalytic theory, which once provided the major distinction between it and every other approach to personality, is that much of mental life is unconscious, including thought, feeling, and motivation. Freud was not, of course, the first to recognize unconscious processes; he was, in many respects, the end of the line of a long tradition of German philosophy that focused on "the unconscious" (Ellenberger, 1970). Yet he was the first and only theorist to base an entire approach to personality on the notion that much of what

people consciously think and feel and most of their conscious choices are determined outside of awareness. He was also the first to try to explore the nature of unconscious processes systematically.

During the 1940s and 1950s, and into the 1960s, researchers associated with the "New Look" in perception (see Bruner, 1973; Erdelyi, 1974, 1985) studied the influence of motives, expectations, and defenses on perception. As early as 1917, Poetzl (1917/1960) had demonstrated that tachistoscopic presentation of stimuli could influence subsequent dread content. A basic idea behind New Look research was that considerable cognitive processing goes on before a stimulus is ever consciously perceived. These investigators argued, furthermore, that the emotional content of subliminally perceived stimuli can have an important impact on subsequent thought and behavior. The evidence is now clear that both of these suppositions are correct (Dixon, 1971, 1981; Weinberger, 2008).

The research of the New Look was, oddly, dismissed by most psychologists in the late 1950s just as the information-processing perspective, which could have assimilated its findings, began to emerge (see Erdelyi, 1974). Since then, this work has rarely been cited. However, in 1977, Nisbett and Wilson (1977) demonstrated that people have minimal access to their cognitive processes; that they often "tell more than they can know" about these psychological events; and that the explanations people typically offer about why they did or thought as they did involve application of general attributional knowledge rather than access to their own cognitive processes. One study reported by Nisbett and Wilson documented that subjects are unaware of the activation of associational networks. After learning the word pair *ocean–moon*, for example, participants were more likely to respond with "Tide" to a question about laundry detergents, even though they had no conscious idea that a network was active and had influenced their response.

In 1980, Shevrin and Dickman marshaled evidence form several fields of research—notably, work on selective attention, subliminal perception, and cortical evoked potentials—to argue that a concept of unconscious psychological processes is both necessary for, and implicit in, much psychological research and theory. Within 4 years, two prominent psychologists not identified with psychoanalysis (Bowers & Meichenbaum, 1984) edited a volume, *The Unconscious Reconsidered*, and stated unequivocally that unconscious processes pervasively influence thought, feeling, and behavior. Unconscious processes became a fully respectable area of research with the publication in *Science* of John Kihlstrom's (1987) article on the "cognitive unconscious."

By the 1990s, the notion that much of memory and cognition is unconscious was no longer a matter of much debate (Holyoak & Spellman, 1993; Roediger, 1990; Schacter, 1992, 1995; Squire, 1987). Two important forms of implicit memory—that is, memory expressed in behavior rather than in conscious recollection—are associative memory and procedural memory. Associative memory can be observed in priming experiments, as described above, in which prior exposure to the same or related information facilitates the processing of new information. Procedural memory, which refers to "how-to" knowledge of procedures or skills, can be seen in everyday activities, such as playing a complex piece of music on the piano, which requires the performer to move her fingers far faster than she can consciously remember how the piece goes or how to play it. Various literatures on thinking have similarly come to distinguish between implicit and explicit thought and learning processes (Gebauer & Mackintosh, 2007; Holyoak & Spellman, 1993; Jacoby & Kelly, 1992; Kahneman, 2003; Kihlstrom, Chapter 23, this volume; Lewicki, 1986; Reber, 1992; Seger, 1994). These literatures have demonstrated that people can learn to respond to regularities in the environment (e.g., the tendency of people in a culture to respond in certain ways to people of higher or lower status) without any awareness of these regularities, and that patients with damage to the neural systems involved in conscious recollection or manipulation of ideas can nevertheless respond to environmental contingencies (e.g., associations between stimuli with pleasure or pain) even without explicit knowledge of those contingencies. In general, for the past two decades, cognitive psychology has witnessed a radical shift from serial processing models to parallel processing models (e.g., Balleine & Killcross, 2006; Wagar & Thagard, 2004)

that share a central assumption with psychoanalytic theory: that most mental processes occur outside of awareness in parallel, rather than one at a time in consciousness.

As I argued in the first edition of this handbook (Westen, 1990a), if serial processing models are inadequate for describing cognitive processes, we have little reason to presume their adequacy for describing affective and motivational processes. At that time, researchers were limiting unconscious processes to unconscious cognition, but today the landscape has changed for motivation and is now doing so for emotion as well, just as it did 20 years ago for cognition. In fact, psychodynamically oriented researchers published the first systematic reviews of unconscious motivation (McClelland et al., 1989) and emotion (Westen, 1985) around the same time as cognitive scientists were establishing the existence of implicit memory.

Whereas unconscious motivation was once viewed by most empirical psychologists as on par with extrasensory perception, today the notion that behavior can be influenced by motives activated outside of awareness is widely accepted (Ferguson & Bargh, 2004). In a classic paper, McClelland and colleagues (1989) reviewed decades of research on self-report and Thematic Apperception Test (TAT) measures of motivation. They found that these two ways of measuring motives—one explicit and the other implicit—rarely correlate with one another, but each has predictable external correlates. For example, over the long run, motives assessed from TAT stories are highly predictive of entrepreneurial or managerial success, whereas self-report measures are not. On the other hand, self-report measures are highly predictive of achievement when people's conscious motives are aroused with instructions such as "You should work really hard on this and do the best you can." These and other data suggest that when conscious motives are activated, they guide behavior. When they are not, which is much of the time, unconscious motives guide behavior. More recently, Bargh and colleagues (Bargh & Barndollar, 1996; Chen & Bargh, 1999; Gillath et al., 2006) have conducted an extraordinary series of experiments over a decade, using priming procedures to prime implicit motives, just as cognitive psychologists have used these procedures to prime implicit memories.

With respect to unconscious affective processes, Broadbent (1977) found that neutral words were more easily perceived than unpleasant words, suggesting preconscious processing of the affective significance of stimuli. Moray (1969) found that words paired with electric shocks in a classical conditioning procedure altered galvanic skin response (suggesting an emotional reaction) when presented to the unattended ear in a dichotic listening task; although participants never consciously perceived the word that had been "tagged" with fear, presentation of the stimulus produced an emotional response that could be measured physiologically. Subsequent studies have shown that conditioned emotional responses can be both acquired and elicited outside of awareness (see, e.g., Ohman, 1994; Ohman, Carlsson, Lundqvist, & Ingvar, 2007; Wong, Shevrin, & Williams, 1994). Heinemann and Emrich (1971), studying cortical evoked potentials, found that emotion-laden words presented subliminally elicited significantly greater alpha rhythms than neutral words, even before subjects reported seeing anything, suggesting differential processing of emotional and neutral material outside of awareness.

Studies of amnesic patients demonstrate that these patients can retain affective associations without any conscious recollection of having seen the stimulus about which they nevertheless have retained feelings (e.g., Johnson, Kim, & Risse, 1985). Perhaps the most convincing evidence of unconscious affect comes from recent attitude research, which finds that people's implicit and explicit attitudes—including the emotional components of those attitudes—can be very different (e.g., Fazio, Jackson, Dunton, & Williams, 1995; Greenwald & Banaji, 1995; Greenwald et al., 2002). A particularly important area of research in this respect regards implicit racism. For example, Greenwald, McGhee, and Schwartz (1998) used the Implicit Association Test (IAT) to test the existence of unconscious negative attitudes toward African Americans by Caucasians who appeared nonprejudiced by self-report. The IAT is a response–competition task that uses reaction time to assess interference of one set of associations (e.g., emotionally positive words) with another (e.g., typically African American names). They found that although three-quarters of subjects reported no pref-

erence for European Americans over African Americans, all but one showed at least a slight preference for Caucasians as measured by the IAT. Although critics have raised several issues about potential confounds and the validity of the IAT (Blanton, Jaccard, Christie, & Gonzales, 2007; Blanton, Jaccard, Gonzales, & Christie, 2006), IAT data predict amygdala responses suggestive of fear or negative affect when white participants are presented with black faces (Cunningham et al., 2004), just as occurs with subliminal presentation of black faces among even explicitly nonprejudiced white respondents (Phelps et al., 2000). IAT data predict actual behavior above and beyond self-reported attitudes in other domains, such as drinking (Ostafin & Palfai, 2006) and self-concept (Steffens & König, 2006).

Although many of the studies described above have been conducted by researchers with little interest in psychodynamic ideas, the idea that affective processes activated outside of awareness can influence thought and behavior has been the basis of two major programs of psychoanalytically inspired research using subliminal activation for over two decades (see Klein Villa, Shevrin, Snodgrass, Bazan, & Brakel, 2006; Liddell, Williams, Rathjen, Shevrin, & Gordon, 2004; Shevrin, Bond, Brakel, Hertel, & Williams, 1996; Siegal & Weinberger, 1998; Silverman & Weinberger, 1985; Snodgrass & Shevrin, 2006; Weinberger & Silverman, 1988). Recently, Weinberger, Seifert, and Siegal (2008) have integrated psychodynamic and behavioral theory and therapy to see whether exposure procedures that can be extremely useful in the treatment of phobias can be conducted using subliminal stimulation. In a set of studies on unconscious flooding in people with self-reported spider phobias, Weinberger and colleagues found, and replicated the finding, that individuals with spider phobias who were repeatedly exposed to subliminal spider-related stimuli showed behavior change in their ability to approach spiders than phobic participants in control conditions. The theoretical and clinical implications of these findings are clearly important to future attempts at integrating psychodynamic approaches with both behavior therapy and cognitive neuroscience.

Work on effects of unconscious perception has also been applied to the political realm. In the 2000 presidential race, controversy arose when a Bush campaign commercial against Gore had what appeared to be the word *RATS* hidden within the ad. Intentional or not, some feared the subliminal presentation could have influenced voter attitudes toward Gore. To test whether this was possible, Weinberger and Westen (in press) recruited participants to complete a study online that presented the word *RATS* and other control words subliminally before presenting a picture of an unknown politician. As expected, ratings of the unknown politician were significantly more negative for the RATS condition than the others. In a follow-up study to address the concern that this effect would work only for unknown politicians, Weinberger and Westen found that whereas partisans' ratings were less affected by subliminal presentation (in this case, a picture of Bill Clinton) before a picture of then soon-to-be-recalled California Governor Gray Davis, independent voters' ratings of Davis switched from negative in the control condition to positive in the subliminal condition. With the empirical evidence now clear, we would argue that political campaigns should be discouraged, if not forbidden, from using even "unintentional" methods of subliminal priming in campaign ads.

These propositions about unconscious (implicit) cognitive, motivational, and emotional processes, many of them now buttressed by data collected by social and clinical psychologists and affective neuroscientists, have methodological implications that have not yet been fully appreciated in the personality literature. The methods used in most studies of personality, particularly in trait psychology, rely heavily on self-report data and were crafted long before the 1990s, when what could be called the "second cognitive revolution" ushered in this new wave of research on unconscious cognitive processes. Self-report methods implicitly presume that people are aware of most of what is important about their personalities—either that they have direct access to it or that they are likely to observe enough of their own behaviors to hold empirically viable views of themselves. If, as now appears to the be the case, psychoanalytic theory turns out to have been right that (1) much of what we think and do is determined unconsciously and (2) affective and motivational processes can be un-

conscious, this will likely require a paradigm shift in the way we measure personality.

In the last edition of this handbook, we argued, based on the emerging data, that we would likely see within the next 10 years personality researchers routinely including implicit and explicit measures of the same constructs because we would expect such measures to show moderate correlations with one another but independently predict relevant criterion variables. In retrospect, we were too sanguine about the pace of change in science. In the field of personality disorders, for example, the data are now clear that correlations between self-reports and aggregated peer reports hover in the range of $r = .25-.35$, and for some disorders (e.g., narcissistic), the correlation is essentially zero (Clifton, Turkheimer, & Oltmanns, 2005; Klonsky, Oltmanns, & Turkheimer, 2002). These findings suggest that much of the association between self-reported personality data and other self-reported variables, at least in clinical samples, largely reflects method variance. The implication is clear, especially since self- and peer reports show incremental validity in predicting different outcomes, that researchers should always supplement self-reported personality disorder data with diagnostic data from other informants, yet that is as rarely the case as in the field of normal personality. At some point, we hope, sound scientific procedures will prevail over tradition and expedience in leading researchers to use a mixture of methods of assessing both the implicit and explicit components of personality, given the overwhelming evidence that implicit and explicit measures of what appears to be the same construct (e.g., anxiety, avoidant attachment, power motivation) often measure different constructs (or the same construct at different levels of consciousness).

The Inner World

By 1914, Freud (1914/1957b) had begun to recognize the extent to which the people who inhabit our minds—ghosts from the past as well as goblins from the present—influence who we are and what we do. As described earlier, this emphasis on "internal objects"— mental representations of the self, others, and relationships—became the cornerstone of object relations theories.

As with unconscious processes, this view is no longer so distinctive of psychoanalytic theories. George Kelly's (1955) approach to personality had similar elements, as do contemporary social-cognitive and cognitive-behavioral approaches (Beck, Freeman, & Davis, 2004; Young, 1999). (Interestingly, so does every approach that clinicians find useful. Empirically, clinicians find trait approaches, which do not assess people's mental representations and expectations of others and relationships, relatively unhelpful in working with patients; Spitzer, First, Shedler, Westen, & Skodol, 2008.) One of the features that remains distinctive about object relations approaches, however, is the presumed complexity of these representations and the pervasiveness of the cognitive, affective, and behavioral precipitates of childhood attachment relationships in adult relationship patterns.

Empirical Studies of Object Relations

Object relations theory has served as the major impetus to psychoanalytically inspired research over the last 25 years, at first relying primarily on projective data and gradually expanding to including a range of data, from self-reports (M. D. Bell, Billington, Cicchetti, & Gibbons, 1988; M. D. Bell, Greig, Bryson, & Kaplan, 2001), to respondents' descriptions of significant others (Blatt & Auerbach, 2003; Harpaz-Rotem & Blatt, 2005), to narratives of interpersonally significant relationship episodes (e.g., Luborsky & Crits-Christoph, 1998), to psychotherapy hours (Peters, Hilsenroth, Eudell-Simmons, Blagys, & Handler, 2006).

These methods, particularly those that involve coding of some form of narrative data, have produced largely convergent findings. Although many personality and clinical researchers would be surprised that even well-conducted projective studies using stimuli such as the Rorschach and the TAT have produced solid findings in this area, social-cognitive research (Bargh, 1984; Cesario, Plaks, & Higgins, 2006; Higgins, King, & Mavin, 1982) suggests that chronically activated or accessible categories developed through experience are readily employed in the processing of social stimuli. Not surprisingly, the characters subjects see in the Rorschach or the TAT are likely to bear the imprint of enduring cognitive–affective processes and structures as long as the stimuli activate representations that resemble those activated interpersonally under other circumstances. Indeed, the recent explosion of research on implicit processes and the emergence of research on individual differences in implicit associations (e.g., Greenwald et al., 1998; Wittenbrink & Schwarz, 2007) suggest that measures applied to projective data may have considerably more validity than once presumed (Westen, Feit, & Zittel, 1999). Recent neuroimaging data, for example, has found that patients with borderline personality disorder (who are rejection sensitive, emotionally dysregulated, and often have a childhood history of interpersonal abuse, particularly sexual abuse) show amygdala activation when perceiving facial expressions designed to be neutral, to which normal controls do not have a similar neural response (Donegan et al., 2003). This finding would have been predicted from research a decade earlier using both TATs and early memories identifying a "malevolent attributional bias" in borderline patients (Nigg, Lohr, Westen, Gold, & Silk, 1992; Westen, 1991; Westen, Lohr, et al., 1990).

Mayman (1967, 1968) demonstrated 40 years ago for the potential utility of using projective tests to study the affective quality and cognitive structure of representations of self and others, hypothesizing that the extent to which individuals describe characters who are psychologically rich, differentiated, and interacting in benign ways should predict relative psychological health and capacity for intimacy. Research since Mayman's initial studies, primarily by Mayman and his students (e.g., Krohn & Mayman, 1974; Shedler et al., 1993; Urist, 1980) and by Blatt and his students and colleagues at Yale, has consistently confirmed this hypothesis (Huprich & Greenberg, 2003).

Blatt and his colleagues (Blatt, Brenneis, & Schimek, 1976; Blatt & Lerner, 1991; Diamond, Kaslow, Coonerty, & Blatt, 1990; Porcerelli, Hill, & Dauphin, 1995) have carried out an extensive program of research measuring several dimensions of object relations from Rorschach responses. They have found predicted differences among various clinical and normal populations, developmental changes through adolescence, and theoretically predicted patterns of change in patients receiving long-term psychodynamic treatments. Blatt has also developed a scale for assessing dimensions of object relations from free-response descriptions of significant others (Besser & Blatt, 2007; Blatt, Auerbach, & Levy, 1997; Blatt, Wein, Chevron, & Quinlan, 1979; Levy, Blatt, & Shaver, 1998), which assesses dimensions such as the cognitive or conceptual level of representations and the degrees of ambivalence and malevolence expressed toward the person. Blatt's methods reflect an attempt to integrate psychoanalytic object relations theories with Wernerian and Piagetian cognitive developmental theories. Blatt has also developed an approach to depression, grounded in object relations theory, which distinguishes self-critical and dependent styles and which he has extended to multiple forms of psychopathology (Blatt, Shahar, & Zuroff, 2001; Blatt & Zuroff, 1992).

Another program of research, initially developed by Westen and his colleagues, reflects an integration of object relations theory and research in social cognition (e.g., Westen, 1990a, 1991; Westen, Lohr, Silk, Gold, & Kerber, 1990). This research uses TAT stories and individuals' descriptions of salient interpersonal episodes from interviews and psychotherapy hours to assess momentarily active representations that shape thought and behavior, rather than the conscious, prototypical representations elicited by questions such as "Do you think people can usually be trusted?" Most research on the Social Cognition and Object Relations Scales (SCORS) has focused on five dimensions: (1) complexity of representations of people; (2) affective quality of relationship paradigms (the extent to which the person expects malevolence and pain or benevolence and pleasure in relationships); (3) capacity for emotional investment in relationships; (4) capacity for emotional investment in ideals and moral standards; and (5) understanding of social causality (the ability to tell logical and coherent narratives about interpersonal events, reflecting an understanding of why people do what they do). Later, Westen and colleagues added four additional variables: self-esteem, identity and coherence of sense of self, regulation of interpersonal aggression, and dominant interpersonal concerns (thematic content) (see Ackerman, Clemence, Weatherill, & Hilsenroth, 2001; Conklin & Westen, 2001; Eudell-Simmons, Stein, DeFife, & Hilsenroth, 2005; Pinsker-Aspen, Stein, & Hilsenroth, 2007).

A number of studies have found predicted differences among various patient groups (e.g., Fowler, Hilsenroth, & Handler, 1996; Hibbard, Hilsenroth, Hibbard, & Nash, 1995; Porcerelli et al., 1995; Westen, 1991; Westen, Lohr, et al., 1990), and developmental studies have documented developmental differences between second and fifth graders and between ninth and twelfth graders, as predicted (Westen et al., 1991). In addition, the SCORS has demonstrated interrater reliability, convergent validity, and utility in a variety of research and clinical contexts, including treatment outcome research (e.g., Ackerman, Clemence, Weatherill, & Hilsenroth, 1999; Eudell-Simmons et al., 2005; Porcerelli et al., 2006).

Attachment Research and Internal Working Models

A major development in the empirical study of object relations has come from attachment research based on Bowlby's (1969, 1973, 1982) integration of psychoanalysis, ethology, and systems theory. Ainsworth (1979; Ainsworth, Blehar, Waters, & Wall, 1978) developed a procedure for measuring different styles of secure and insecure attachment in infancy. Subsequent research has found these to be predictive of later adjustment and interpersonal styles in the school years (see Bretherton, 1985; Sroufe & Fleeson, 1986) and to be influenced substantially by the quality of the primary caretaker's relatedness to the child (see de Wolff & van IJzendoorn, 1997; Ricks, 1985; Steele, Steele, & Fonagy, 1996).

A quantum leap in our understanding of the ramifications of early attachment was made possible by the development of instruments for assessing adult attachment, particularly the Adult Attachment Interview (AAI), created by Main and her colleagues (Main & Goldwin, 1991). This interview elicits information about the way individuals recall separation and attachment experiences as they describe significant events with attachment figures. Transcripts are coded for the way respondents talk about their attachment relationships, yielding data analogous to infant attachment classifications: secure or autonomous; anxious or preoccupied with attachment; avoidant or dismissive of attachment; and an additional qualifier, unresolved with respect to loss or trauma, which maps roughly onto disorganized attachment status in infancy (Hesse & Main, 2006; Lyons-Ruth, Yellin, Melnick, & Atwood, 2005).[7] AAI attachment classification of parents (in relation to their own attachment figures) has proven highly predictive of the attachment status of their children, providing important data on the intergenerational transmission of attachment (Fonagy, Steele, & Steele, 1991; Hesse & Main, 1999; Main, 1990; Main, Kaplan, & Cassidy, 1985; Steele et al., 1996).

Self-report measures of adult attachment have also produced compelling findings in dozens of studies (e.g., Gillath et al., 2006; Mikulincer, 1998a, 1998b; Mickelson, Kessler, & Shaver, 1997; Stein et al., 2002; see also Fraley & Shaver, Chapter 20, this volume). However, narrative and self-report measures tend, as in other areas of research, not to be highly correlated (Calabrese, Farber, & Westen, 2005), and researchers are just beginning to tease apart what the two types of instruments may be measuring (see Brennan, Clark, & Shaver, 1998; Riggs et al., 2007; Westen, Nakash, Thomas, & Bradley, 2006). Research has also just begun to link some of these measures to distinct patterns of neural activity using functional magnetic resonance imaging (fMRI) (Buchheim et al., 2006; Lemche et al., 2006).

Attachment research is arguably the most "mainstream" research approach derived directly from psychoanalytic theory (see, e.g., Mikulincer, Shaver, Gillath, & Nitzberg, 2005), and reciprocally, the recent surge of empirical work on attachment is having a significant impact on psychoanalytic theories of development. Peter Fonagy and colleagues have recently focused both theoretical and empirical attention on what they call *mentalization*, the ability to take one's own and others' mental states as objects of thought (see Fonagy et al., 2002; Fonagy & Target, 2006). The concept of mentalization is closely tied to what developmental psychologists call theory of mind (see Gopnik & Wellman, 1992; Saxe, Carey, & Kanwisher, 2004), as well as to a number of related constructs, such as complexity of mental representations and understanding of social causality (Westen, 1991), psychological mindedness, perspective taking, empathy, and emotional intelligence (see Allen, 2006), although Fonagy emphasizes its emergence from childhood experiences with attachment figures.

The development of mentalization is associated with attachment figures' sensitiv-

ity to the child's internal states (Fonagy & Bateman, 2005). Conversely, Fonagy's work suggests a link between serious maltreatment in childhood and difficulties with mentalization, as seen, for example, in patients with borderline personality disorder. Abused children may learn to avoid thinking about their abusive caregivers' subjectivity so as not to have to consider why they would wish to harm them. As a result, these children grow up with an incapacity to understand mental states in themselves and others. Not surprisingly, the research literatures on unresolved and disorganized attachments and their antecedents have begun to dovetail with research on the attachment status and object relations of patients with borderline personality spectrum disorders (see Agrawal, Gunderson, Holmes, & Lyons-Ruth, 2004; Bradley & Westen, 2006).

Methodological Implications

Some of the central claims of psychoanalytic object relations theories—such as the theory that as adults we live with representations, motives, defenses, and interpersonal strategies forged in significant relationships from the past, and that many of these psychological processes emerge in our behavior without our knowledge of them—have substantial methodological implications. One of the most important is that people are likely to reveal important aspects of their inner worlds through their associations, ways of interacting with others (particularly with people who are emotionally significant), and narratives about themselves and significant interpersonal events. As we have seen, several bodies of research are now converging on the finding that what people reveal about their internal experience of the self and others explicitly through conscious self-reports, and what they reveal implicitly through narratives or other tasks that provide access to their associational networks, are often very different. Enduring object relational patterns can also be ascertained through the patterns of feeling and behavior people draw from others—for example, in the role relationships in which they manage to get others to engage (Sandler, 1976; Wachtel, 1997)—which is a central feature of contemporary views of countertransference (Tansey & Burke, 1989). What this convergence suggests is that we may need to broaden substantially the ways we assess personality, relying on multiple methods and measures rather than those that are relatively quick and easily administered, which may provide a window to only one aspect of people's experience of the self and others.

The Bodily, the Animal, and the Uncomfortable

Psychoanalysis repeatedly leads one to think about what one does not wish to think about. It is an approach to personality that one does not care to discuss with one's mother (or regrets once having done so). Motivation and fantasy are rich and sometimes aggressive, socially inappropriate, or perverse, and any theory that is entirely comfortable to discuss is probably missing something very important about what it means to be human.

A good example is social learning research on the influence of television aggression on children's behavior. This line of research, which has been productive for decades, is important and suggestive, but it fails to ask a crucial question: Why is it that aggressive television shows appeal to people so much? Would Freud be surprised to learn that the two variables that censors keep an eye on in television shows and movies are sex and aggression? One can read a thousand pages of the best social-cognitive work on personality and never know that people have genitals—or, for that matter, that they have bodies—let alone fantasies.

One of us (D. W.) once evaluated a patient who had been treated for his "poor social skills" and difficulties in his marriage for a year by a cognitive-behavioral therapist, who sent a glowing report of his progress in his treatment. Within the first session, however, the patient disclosed that he had had active fantasies of raping and murdering his therapist, which were clearly tied to a core sexual fantasy that was troubling him in his relationship with his wife. His therapist did not know about this fantasy because, the patient noted with a sly shrug, "She never asked." Psychoanalysis is the only theory of personality that suggests why one might want to ask.

Another example is Freud's psychosexual hypotheses. No doubt, many of his theories of development were off base, such as his view that penis envy is *the* central psychological event in a young girl's personality

development (see Fisher & Greenberg, 1985, 1996). On the other hand, Freudian psychosexual theory can often provide a compelling explanation of phenomena from everyday life about which competing theories can offer no rival explanations. For example, if readers try generating for themselves a list of all the profanities they can call a person, they will notice an overrepresentation of Freud's erogenous zones. Indeed, the worst epithet a person in our culture can hurl at another person has a distinctly Oedipal ring (Sophocles, circa 500 B.C.E.), and we doubt this term came to the United States via the Viennese doctor.

Defensive Processes

From the start, a central assumption of psychoanalytic theory and technique has focused on the pervasive nature of human self-deception. Whether this takes the form of turning feelings or beliefs into their opposite (e.g., persecution of homosexuals by politicians and preachers who turn out to have been struggling, at whatever level of consciousness, with homosexual desires; for relevant empirical work, see Adams, Wright, & Lohr, 1996), manipulating arguments or perceptions so that they point to the desired conclusion, or sundry other ways, from a psychodynamic point of view, every act of cognition is simultaneously an act of affect regulation (Westen & Blagov, 2007).

A wealth of research now provides incontrovertible evidence for the existence of defensive processes by which people adjust their conscious thoughts and feelings in an effort to maximize positive affect and minimize negative affect (see Campbell-Sills, Barlow, Brown, & Hofmann, 2006; Conte & Plutchik, 1995; N. Haan, 1977; Paulhus, Fridhandler, & Hayes, 1997; Perry & Cooper, 1987; Plutchik, 1998; Vaillant, 1992; Westen, 1998b).

The concept of hierarchical levels of defenses, originally developed by Anna Freud (1936), has been refined and studied empirically by Vaillant (1977, 2000), who has made major empirical contributions to the concept of defense. Theoretically, defenses involving rigidly held and gross distortions of reality are viewed as more pathological and hence are expected to be used with much greater frequency by individuals with severe character pathology or by relatively healthy people in times of severe stress (e.g., bereaved individuals who imagine the presence of recently deceased love ones). For example, individuals with narcissistic personality disorders may find even minor inadequacies so intolerable that they have to externalize the causes of any failure. Research supports such a view, linking particular defensive styles to particular types and levels of personality disturbance (Bond & Perry, 2004; Perry & Cooper, 1989; Vaillant & Drake, 1985; Westen, Mudderriso-glu, Fowler, Shedler, & Koren, 1997; Westen & Shedler, 1999a).

Other researchers studying defensive processes have converged on a defensive style that has adverse impact on physical health. Weinberger and colleagues (Weinberger, 1992; Weinberger, Schwartz, & Davidson, 1979) isolated individuals who simultaneously report a low level of distress on the Taylor Manifest Anxiety Scale and a high level of social desirability, defensiveness, or overcontrol as measured by the Marlowe–Crowne Scale (Crowne & Marlow, 1964). These "repressors" (low anxiety, high social desirability) are distinguished from other subjects by, among other things, greater reaction time when confronted with sexual and aggressive verbal stimuli; more difficulty retrieving unpleasant childhood memories; and health risks linked to hyperreactivity to potentially stressful events (e.g., Bonanno & Singer, 1995; L. L. Brown et al., 1996; Davis & Schwartz, 1987). Shedler and colleagues (1993) have isolated a related group of individuals who report minimal emotional disturbance on standard self-report measures such as Eysenck's neuroticism scale but whose narratives of early experience (early memories) manifest distress or a lack of narrative coherence. In a series of studies, Shedler and colleagues found that, when presented with a stressful or mildly threatening task (such as telling TAT stories), these individuals were hyperreactive on a combined index of heart rate and blood pressure used by cardiologists and empirically related to heart disease. Furthermore, although these individuals self-reported less subjective anxiety, their verbal productions revealed significantly more manifestations of anxiety (e.g., laughing, sighing, stuttering, blocking, avoiding the content of the stimulus) than individuals whose narratives and self-reports were concordant—that

is, who were either genuinely distressed or genuinely nondistressed.

Perhaps the most definitive study to date is one using neuroimaging to examine defensive or "motivated reasoning" among political partisans (Westen, Blagov, Haren-ski, Kilts, & Hamann, 2006). The investigators studied the neural responses of partisan Democrats and Republicans during the polarized 2004 presidential election between John Kerry and George W. Bush. The brains of Democrats and Republicans were mirror images, with Republicans responding to slides presenting threatening information about their candidate the same way Democrats did with theirs, and with each consciously denying the threat immediately afterward (i.e., having no trouble recognizing the duplicity, flip-flopping, or pandering of the opposition candidate). When presented with threatening information, partisan brains showed activation in multiple circuits indicating distress (e.g., right orbital frontal cortex, amygdala, insular gyrus), emotion regulation (medial orbital prefrontal cortex), and conflict (anterior cingulate, including the ventral or "emotional" regions). Immediately afterward, not only did these areas become relatively quiescent, but partisans showed activations in dopamine-rich regions associated with reward, suggesting the positive reinforcement of defensive bias.

Conflict and Ambivalence

Another enduring contribution of psychoanalysis is the concept of intrapsychic conflict. From the start, Freud emphasized that nothing about the mind requires that any given stimulus be associated exclusively or primarily with one feeling, and that our experiences with anyone of significance to us are likely to be mixed. What led Freud to this view was not only his clinical experience, in which he observed people who seemed to be in turmoil when their wishes and moral standards came into conflict, but a remarkably modern view of competing and conflicting psychological processes that operate in parallel outside of awareness.

A substantial body of research has begun to emerge across a number of areas of psychology, documenting the importance of conflict and ambivalence in human psychology (see Westen, 1998b). For example, many attitude researchers in social psychology now suggest that attitudes may be better conceived as including two distinct evaluative dimensions, positive and negative, than as bipolar (and hence measurable using Likert scales running from negative to positive) (Cacioppo, Gardner, & Berntson, 1997; de Liver, van der Pligt, & Wigboldus, 2007; Priester & Petty, 1996). The reason is that the same attitude object can engender both positive and negative feelings, which can be relatively independent and can vary in strength. Low positive–low negative attitudes tend to have minimal impact on behavior because they leave the person neutrally inclined toward a person, product, political issue, or other attitude object. Empirically, low positive–low negative attitudes are very different from high positive–high negative (ambivalent) attitudes, which nonetheless yield similar (moderate) scores on traditional bipolar attitude measures. For example, when people have fallen out of love and mourned the end of their relationship, their feelings toward each other may be relatively neutral. Months earlier, their feelings may have been intensely ambivalent, leading to the experience of tremendous conflict, psychosomatic symptoms, anxiety, and so forth. In both cases, the former partners' attitudes might be expressed as midway between positive and negative—but surely this assessment would mask the difference between being "over the relationship" and being in the midst of psychological turmoil about it.

The literature on ambivalence is consistent with research suggesting that positive and negative affect are only moderately negatively correlated—that is, that people who often feel good may also often feel bad—and are mediated by overlapping but largely distinct neural circuits (see, e.g., Barrett, Mesquita, Ochsner, & Gross, 2007; Davidson, 2003; J. A. Gray, 1990). Indeed, neuroimaging data indicate that the anterior cingulate is involved in dealing with both emotional and cognitive conflicts (e.g., Haas, Omura, Constable, & Canli, 2006). If the brain has evolved regions that deal with conflict, psychological theories should seriously consider the role of conflict in the development of personality and psychopathology.

Moreover, several literatures are independently converging on the notion that positive and negative interpersonal interactions, and their attendant feelings, are only moderately correlated and have distinct correlates. Developmental research suggests that supportive and harsh parenting, for example, do not appear to be opposite ends of a continuum. Rather, they correlate only imperfectly with each other, and each predicts unique components of the variance in children's adjustment (Pettit, Bates, & Dodge, 1997). Some parents are harsh but also loving; others, who might receive a similar rating on the overall affective quality of their parenting, are distant but not overtly punishing. These distinct parenting styles are likely to have very different consequences. Similarly, ingroup favoritism and outgroup denigration are not simply opposite sides of the same coin (Brewer, 2001; Brewer & Brown, 1998). In most situations, ingroup favoritism is more common than outgroup derogation. Indeed, a subtle form of racism or group antagonism may lie less in the presence of hostile feelings than in the absence of the positive feelings that normally bind people together (Pettigrew & Meertens, 1995).

The Concept of Personality Structure

Central to psychoanalytic approaches to personality is the concept of personality organization or structure. A search for simple behavioral regularities is likely to miss much about human beings that is important, because qualitatively different behaviors can stem from the same structure (see Sroufe & Waters, 1977). Several studies using Q-sort methods have attempted to operationalize this construct (Block, 1971; Block & Block, 1980; Westen & Shedler, 1999b, 2007). A study from Jack Block's longitudinal project is instructive in this respect. Shedler and Block (1990) found a systematic relationship between patterns of drug use at age 18, personality as assessed by Q-sort at age 18, personality as assessed in childhood, and quality of parenting as assessed at age 5. The investigators did not find a simple linear relation between drug use (from none to plenty), on the one hand, and personality characteristics or parenting styles, on the other. Participants who had experimented with marijuana were the *most* well-adjusted in the sample, compared with those who had never tried the drug (who were described by Q-sort as relatively anxious, emotionally constricted, and lacking in social skills) and those who abused marijuana (who were observed to be alienated and impulsive). Mothers of both the abstainers and the abusers had been previously rated as relatively cold and unresponsive.

As the authors point out, in the context of a relatively intact, flexible personality structure that permits experimentation and individuation in adolescence, drug use may be relatively healthy, depending on the historical and cultural moment. Educational or social learning approaches that focus on peer pressure as a primary cause of adolescent drug abuse and attempt to teach teenagers about the problems with drugs may be missing the point (and have proven, empirically, to be of little value in the long run; see Coggans, 2006; Klepp, Kelder, & Perry, 1995) because of their focus on discrete behaviors divorced from the personality structure in which they are embedded. The learning of behaviors occurs within the context of a personality structure, including characteristic ways of coping with, and defending against, impulses and affects; perceiving the self and others; obtaining satisfaction of one's wishes and desires; responding to environmental demands; and finding meaning in one's activities, values, and relationships (see Westen, Gabbard, & Blagov, 2006).

Viewing the Present in the Context of the Past

Axiomatic for psychoanalytic accounts of any mental or behavioral event is that current psychological processes must be viewed in the context of their development. Psychological experience is assumed to be so rich, and current thoughts, feelings, and actions are presumed to be so densely interconnected with networks of association at various levels of consciousness developed over time, that studying an adult form without its developmental antecedents is like trying to make sense of current politics without any knowledge of their history. This does not mean that psychoanalytic theory is wedded to a psychosocial determinism. Nothing about a psychodynamic theory of the development of any adult psychological tendency requires that temperamental factors play little or no role. Freud the neurologist would certainly never have taken such an antibiological stance; indeed, he was convinced that both schizophrenia and what we call today bipolar disorder (manic–depression) were brain diseases.

We suspect that Freud would have been as stunned and electrified as the rest of us by the research made possible only in the last few years by genetic and cross-fostering research in animals (particularly nonhuman primates) and the cracking of the human genome, and clearly psychoanalytic developmental theories will either grow with these advances or wither on the vine. As long hypothesized by psychodynamic clinicians, childhood maltreatment does substantially affect development, but its effects depend considerably on genetic liabilities to risk or resilience (e.g., Kim-Cohen et al., 2006; see Rutter, 2005). For example, in an already classic longitudinal study of a birth cohort of 1,037 New Zealand children, Caspi and colleagues (2002) found, as researchers are increasingly finding, that the main effects of genes and childhood experiences are often dwarfed by their interactions. In this study, the investigators defined childhood maltreatment as sexual abuse, physical abuse, maternal rejection, harsh discipline, or repeated loss of a primary caregiver. A functional polymorphism in the gene responsible for the neurotransmitter metabolizing enzyme monoamine oxidase A (MAO-A) moderated the effect of maltreatment, such that males with low MAO-A activity who were maltreated in childhood had elevated antisocial scores, whereas those with high MAO-A activity tended to be low on antisocial behavior, even if they had experienced childhood maltreatment. However, of males with both the low MAO-A activity genotype and severe maltreatment, 85% developed antisocial behavior. Foley and colleagues (2004) have replicated these findings.

On the other side of the coin, genetic predispositions to psychopathology may be short-circuited in the presence of a warm, nurturing environment. Animal research with rhesus monkeys and rats has used cross-fostering designs in which genetically anxious or aggressive infants are raised by normal mothers. Results indicate that adequate rearing (or rearing by "super-moms") can lead to normal outcomes, despite the presence of genes that create a liability for an anxious or aggressive temperament (e.g., Fish et al., 2004; Suomi, 2004, 2005).

What a psychodynamically informed account of development may have to add, however, is some complexity to our understanding of mind–brain–gene–environment relationships. For example, clinicians have long recognized, and research has subsequently documented, a link between early trauma (particularly sexual abuse and disrupted attachments) and a subsequent tendency to experience both depression and what is increasingly coming to be called emotional dysregulation, that is, a tendency for negative emotions to spiral out of control and lead to maladaptive efforts at coping, such as suicide attempts or self-injurious behavior (see J. D. Miller & Pilkonis, 2006; Shedler & Westen, 2004). Although it would be tempting to propose a simple hypothesis—that early trauma disrupts the capacity for self-regulation for strictly psychosocial reasons (e.g., lack of a nurturant caregiver who protects the child from abuse and who helps the child internalize the capacity for self-soothing)—we now know that early trauma also has long-lasting effects on neuroendocrine functioning, by setting off a cascade of processes that alters normal cortisol release and regulation, which in turn affects stress reactivity (Nemeroff, 2004; Nemeroff et al., 2006). Thus, trauma may not only create expectations of malevolence that lead a person later to avoid or seek relationships in dysfunctional ways or to have difficulty self-soothing in the face of readily perceived rejection or hostility, but the person's ability to cope may be further compromised by a dysregulated hypothalamic–pituitary axis, which makes more functional coping and defensive processes more difficult to muster. This, in turn, can lead to behaviors that drive others away, creating a vicious circle that is difficult to break. Add to that the influence of the multitude of genes that appear likely to moderate different aspects of stress reactivity and interpersonal functioning, and we have a portrait of development that is far more complex than anyone could have imagined even a decade ago.

Cognitive Science, Neuroscience, and Psychoanalysis

One of the most exciting developments in recent years in psychoanalysis has been its growing interface with neuroscience (e.g., Gabbard, 2006; Gabbard & Westen, 2003; Gordon, Panksepp, Dennis, & McSweeney, 2005; Hassin et al., 2005; Solms & Turnbull, 2002; Westen & Gabbard, 2002a, 2002b). Freud was himself a neurologist, and his theories were developed in the context of his understanding of the nervous system (Pribram & Gill, 1976; see also Kaplan-Solms & Solms, 2002).

Freud's "cognitive psychology" was extensive (see Erdelyi, 1985). His distinction between "primary-process" thought, which is organized by associations rather than by logic, and "secondary-process" thought, which is more rational and directed by conscious concerns, is similar in many respects to contemporary distinctions between controlled and automatic information processing and serial and parallel processing. However, an important difference between psychoanalytic and information-processing approaches to thought and memory is that the former were tied, from the start, to considerations of affect, cognitive–affective interaction, and consciousness. For psychoanalysis, it is axiomatic that cognition is largely, if not entirely, in the service of affective and motivational processes, and that needs, wishes, and conflicts are involved in categorizing and selecting information to be consciously perceived and processed. As we predicted in the last two editions of this handbook, the recent shift that has occurred in cognitive science, from a computer metaphor to a brain metaphor, has led to some rapprochement between psychoanalysis and cognitive neuroscience, as the latter has increasingly incorporated the view that brains, unlike computers, process fears, wishes, and other feelings.

A major impetus for psychoanalytic investigations of thinking in the middle of the last century was the attempt to understand disordered thought in patients with schizophrenia. Rapaport and his colleagues (see Allison, Blatt, & Zimet, 1968; Rapaport, 1951; Rapaport, Schafer, & Gill, 1945–1946) painstakingly analyzed the verbatim psychological testing protocols of hundreds of institutionalized patients, in an attempt to categorize the pathological processes characterizing schizophrenic thought. For example, they found, from examination of Rorschach responses, that psychotic patients frequently contaminated one percept with another; that is, they superimposed one perceptual response on another without recognizing the impossibility of the superimposition. Such patients were also found to make logical errors and category errors of various sorts and to suffer from associative intrusions (see Coleman et al., 1996; Johnson & Holtzman, 1979).

Subsequent research on thought disorder in patients with borderline personality disorder has found more attenuated forms of thought disturbance, such as egocentric or fanciful elaborations and intrusions of aggressive content into perceptions (see Gartner, Hurt, & Gartner, 1987). To our knowledge, no one has integrated these various observations with contemporary cognitive models, although they may provide insight into the nature of both well-ordered and disordered cognitive processes.

In a rarely cited but important book, Blum (1961) developed a model of cognitive–dynamic interactions based on systematic experimental research using hypnosis. Relying upon a computer model similar to the emerging models that guided the cognitive revolution in the 1960s, Blum described networks of association that he related to neural circuits; elaborated a theory of spreading activation (which he described as "reverberation" from an activated node in a network to related representations); described networks linking cognitive and affective representations; discussed cognitively controlled inhibitory mechanisms responsible for defenses such as repression; and used an experimental paradigm for exploring cognitive–affective interactions that predated similar work in cognitive psychology by 20 years.

Beginning in the 1960s, several theorists attempted to bring together psychodynamic concepts of motivation and affect with various mainstream approaches to cognition. Shared by all of these approaches was an attention to cognitive–affective interactions. For example, a number of theorists attempted to wed psychoanalytic and Piagetian notions, exploring the interaction of the child's developing understanding of the self, others, and the world with evolving wishes and fears (e.g., Basch, 1977; Fast, 1985; Greenspan, 1979; Wolff, 1960). Others offered potential integrations of psychoanalytic concepts of conflict, defense, and motivation with information-processing approaches to cognition, focusing on concepts such as networks of association and cognitive–affective schemas (Bucci, 1997; Erdelyi, 1985; M. J. Horowitz, 1987, 1988, 1998; Peterfreund, 1971; Shevrin et al., 1996; Singer & Salovey, 1991; Westen, 1985, 1994, 1999b).

Of particular importance for integrations of psychodynamic and cognitive approaches has been the emergence of connectionist and related models in cognitive science (Niedenthal, Barsalou, Winkielman, Krauth-Gruber, & Ric, 2005; Rumelhart, McClelland, & the PDP Research Group, 1986; Smith, 1998; Thagard, 2000). These models diverged, in multiple respects, from the information-processing models that dominated cognitive psychology for three decades: (1) they assume that most information processing occurs outside of awareness, in parallel; (2) they view representations as distributed throughout a network of neural units, each of which attends to some part of the representation; (3) they view knowledge as residing in associative links established through repeated coactivation, such that activation of one node in a network can either *facilitate* or *inhibit* nodes associatively linked to it; (4) they propose an equilibration model of cognition involving *parallel constraint satisfaction*, in which the brain simultaneously and unconsciously processes multiple features of a stimulus or situation; and (5) they rely on the metaphor of mind as brain, rather than mind as computer.

These models are of particular relevance because they suggest that conscious perception, memory, and thought occur through the collaboration and competition of multiple processes outside of awareness. Whereas connectionist models focus on parallel satisfaction of *cognitive* constraints—that is, "data" as represented by processing units within the brain—psychoanalytic theories of conflict and compromise focus on the way in which thoughts and behaviors reflect a similar equilibration process involving *feelings* and *motives* (see Westen, 1998b, 1999a, 2007; Westen & Blagov, 2007). An integrated model suggests that most of the time our beliefs and inferences reflect a process of parallel constraint satisfaction that includes both cognitive *and* emotional constraints, such that we tend to make judgments or inferences that best fit the data only to the extent that we are indifferent about the solutions to which our minds equilibrate. In everyday life, we are rarely so indifferent. Thus, our judgments and beliefs tend to reflect not only the activation and inhibition of neural networks by the data of observation but also by their hedonic significance—that is, based on how we would feel if we came to one conclusion or another. In other words, we see ourselves and others as accurately as we can within the constraints imposed by our wishes, fears, values, and efforts at self-esteem regulation.

As suggested earlier, another exciting area of convergence has emerged from the discovery of mirror neurons, which fire in the brain in response to the actions or affects of others (see Rizzolatti & Craighero, 2004). Mirror neurons form the basis for imitation and, according to some, provide building blocks for many aspects of communication and empathy (e.g., Iacoboni & Dapretto, 2006). Additionally, their existence has informed theories of embodied cognition, in which human thought is conceptualized in terms of bodily action and mental "simulations," a concept Freud himself, like both Piaget and Luria, used in thinking of thought as interiorized action (e.g., Garbarini & Adenzato, 2004; Niedenthal, Barsalou, Ric, & Krauth-Gruber, 2005). Mirror neurons provide one mechanism for helping us understand a range of phenomena, long described by psychoanalytic clinicians in a way that often had the feel of magic or voodoo, such as "transference," "countertransference," and "unconscious communication between patient and therapist." Not surprisingly, psychoanalysts have already begun to make connections between psychodynamic thinking and research on mirror neuron systems (e.g., Gallese, Eagle, & Migone, 2007; Wolf, Gales, Shane, & Shane, 2001).

Evolutionary Psychology and Psychoanalysis

One of the major developments today in contemporary psychology is the return of evolutionary thinking (Buss, 2005; Buss, Haselton, Shackelford, Bleske, & Wakefield, 1998; see also Buss, Chapter 2, this volume), which dominated functionalist approaches (such as Freud's) at the turn of the century and has now been invigorated by developments in Darwinian thinking since the rise of "sociobiology" in the 1960s (Williams, 1966) and 1970s (Trivers, 1971; E. O. Wilson, 1978). Freud was deeply influenced by Darwinian thinking, which was in the intellectual air he breathed in his youth. Freud's drive theory reflected his understanding of the importance of sexual motivation and intra-species competition, particularly for mates, but he never thought to evaluate his ideas systematically

in relation to Darwinian thinking. Thus, he proposed some concepts such as the "death instinct" that were evolutionarily untenable.

The first evolutionary approaches in psychoanalysis were arguably the writings of the ego psychologists, who emphasized the development of ego functions that foster adaptation to the natural and social environments (Hartmann, 1939/1958). For many years, however, the primary psychoanalytic voices heralding an integration of psychoanalysis and evolutionary thinking were those of Robert Plutchik (1980, 1998), John Bowlby (1973), and Robert LeVine (1982). Plutchik proposed an evolutionary theory of emotion and defense that stressed the adaptive nature of human emotions and the way in which individuals develop defenses to cope with particular emotions. Bowlby focused on attachment-related motives and emotions, drawing links between the primate literature on imprinting and the psychoanalytic literature on the effects of maternal deprivation and disturbances in the attachment relationship on subsequent development. Bowlby explicitly argued for the origin of object relational strivings in the infant's immaturity and need for security. LeVine, in work that has not yet been fully integrated into the mainstream, came at evolutionary theory from a different angle, focusing on the natural selection of cultural practices.

Since that time, evolutionary thinking has begun to creep into the psychoanalytic literature, though only slowly. One of the first thoroughgoing attempts to wed psychodynamic and evolutionary accounts was Westen's (1985) book on personality and culture, which drew on the work of Plutchik, Bowlby, and LeVine and explicitly addressed the implications of then-recent work in sociobiology for personality theory. Westen argued that emotions were naturally selected adaptations that themselves perform the function of "naturally selecting" thoughts, feelings, and actions that foster adaptation. In this view, emotions and sensory feeling-states evolved to lead people toward ways of thinking and behaving that maximize survival and reproduction and lead them away from pain-inducing acts that, in aggregate, tend to be maladaptive. From this point of view, pathology of affect regulation and motivation often involves the maladaptive use of mechanisms "designed" by nature to foster adaptation (e.g., avoidance of thoughts or stimuli associated with anxiety). Slavin and Kriegman (1992) and Badcock (1994) have both developed explicitly evolutionary approaches to psychoanalysis, although links between evolutionary psychology and psychoanalysis remain less developed than links with neuroscience (see Strenger, 2006).

So what might a psychodynamic account of personality look like 100 years after Freud began his inquiries and nearly 150 years after Darwin's *Origin of Species*? Here we briefly outline the directions an evolutionarily informed psychodynamic point of view might take. Humans are organisms endowed through natural selection with motives, feelings, cognitive processes, and behaviors— and the capacity to develop these processes through learning—that foster survival, adaptation, reproduction, and concern for the well-being of significant others. Biologically, we are all endowed with processes that serve self-preservative, sexual, and social functions that we cannot escape because they are built into our brains and our guts. We need to eat, to drink, to have sex, to form attachments and affiliative relationships with others, to nurture the next generation, and to experience ourselves and be viewed by others as important and worthwhile. Pursuit of these motives often entails expressing aggression or seeking dominance because status, sexual access to attractive others, and in some ecological circumstances, survival, necessarily engender clashes between relationship seeking, on the one hand, and self-interest or the interest of others in whose welfare we are emotionally invested, on the other (for views of empathy in other animals, particularly primates, see Preston & de Waal, 2002). To what extent aggression and sadism can be gratifying in and of themselves, and if so, why we evolved that way, remains unclear. The motives that drive people reflect universal biology, biologically and environmentally influenced gender differences, individual differences in genotype, culturally normative experiences, and idiosyncratic personal experience and associations. Thus, the strength of various motivations and the extent to which they are compatible with one another vary across individuals.

Conflict between motives is built into human life for at least three reasons. First, naturally selected motive systems at times inevitably come into conflict. Whether the conflict is a struggle between two good friends over the affection of a potential love object or the conflict between two siblings for their mother's attention, there is no innate requirement of human motives that they be harmonious. A second and related factor is our tendency to internalize the needs and motives of significant others as our own. We care about the welfare of people with whom we interact closely, particularly those to whom we are attached, so that their motives become, to a greater or lesser extent, our motives. Once inside us, either as wishes for their happiness and relief of their pain or as the set of moral standards Freud called the superego, these motives will inevitably conflict at times with our own personal desires (for the concept of morality in evolutionary theory, see M. Hauser, 2006). Third, one of the primary mechanisms that evolved in humans and other animals to register the effects of prior experience is associative learning. In the course of daily life, we associate any frequently encountered person or stimulus with whatever emotions the person or object engenders. Thus, over time, our representations of anything or anyone who is significant in our lives will be ambivalent, and different situations and associations will trigger different, and sometimes conflicting, affective reactions.

Organisms survived for millions of years without consciousness. Precisely when consciousness, as we think of it, arose evolutionarily is unknown and depends substantially on how one defines it. Yet millions of years before the evolution of consciousness, organisms learned to avoid aversive stimuli and seek rewarding ones that fostered survival and reproduction. With the development of limbic structures, most adaptively significant learning came to involve feeling-states of pleasure, pain, and more specific emotions. Nothing in the architecture of the human brain requires that these feeling-states be conscious in order for us to associate them with stimuli or to develop motives to avoid or approach stimuli associated with them. With the evolution of the neocortex, the capacity to form associations expanded dramatically, as did the ability to plan, remember, and make conscious choices and decisions. Yet most associations, cognitive patterns, decisions, and plans occur outside awareness; we simply could not attend to all the motives relevant to adaptation at any given moment because we have limited working memory capacity. The function of consciousness is to focus attention on stimuli that are potentially adaptively significant and require more processing than can be carried out unconsciously and automatically. Often this means that consciousness is drawn to anomalies, affectively significant stimuli, and stimuli that are salient because of their familiarity or unfamiliarity.

Consciousness of feeling-states is a useful guide to the potential significance of environmental events, internal processes, and possible courses of action. The downside of conscious emotion, however, is that we can experience emotional pain. When possible, people tend to respond at any given moment by trying to solve problems of adaptation directly. Under three circumstances, however, they tend, instead, to alter their conscious cognitive or affective states or keep certain mental contents out of awareness that are nonetheless adaptively significant. First, when circumstances do not allow control over painful events, people turn to coping and defensive strategies that protect them from the conscious experience of mental and physical pain, such as dissociation during sexual abuse or torture, or denial in the face of abandonment by a love object. Second, people routinize many affect-regulatory procedures, just as they routinize other forms of procedural knowledge (e.g., tying their shoes) during childhood. To the extent that childhood cognition places limits on the affect-regulatory procedures that become selected and routinized, and to the extent that these routinized procedures interfere with learning of more adaptive procedures, people will regulate their affects using unconscious procedures that prevent certain ideas, feelings, or motives from becoming conscious. Third, to the extent that consciousness of a thought, feeling, or desire conflicts with other powerful goals, such as moral standards or wishes, defensive distortion of conscious representations is likely to result.

Humans are not born as adults. They have a longer apprenticeship at the hands of parental figures than members of other species, and their experience in these hands influences their beliefs, expectations, feelings, motives, and behaviors. Their caretaking environment is not independent of their actions; what they experience involves a transaction between their own innate tendencies and the personalities and situational constraints of their caregivers. Cognitively and affectively, children reorganize continuously throughout development, as we do throughout our lives. Yet every decision that works—that solves a problem of adaptation, lends order where previously there was subjective disorder, or regulates an affect—becomes a conservative dynamic, a schema in the Piagetian sense. Often, however, cognitive, affective, and motivational "decisions" that resist accommodation prevent psychological development along different pathways. A child who learns to fear intimacy in his interactions with his avoidant/dismissing mother is likely to bring his characteristic working models of self and relationships, along with the motives and affect-regulatory strategies associated with them, into other relationships. In turn, this pattern constrains the reactions of others and the consequent feedback that might disconfirm expectations and challenge procedures that are maladaptive or at least nonoptimal.

Humans are also born into bodies. Our feelings, wishes, fears, and representations of self are, from the start, tied to our physical existence. And physical experiences are frequently linked to emotionally salient interpersonal encounters. The nurturant touch of a caretaker or the gleam in a proud parent's eyes is an intensely pleasurable experience. It is natural—and perhaps naturally selected—that children would at times want to be the *only* apple of their parents' eyes and would wish they could eliminate the competition—even though they may also be deeply attached to the competitors for their parents' love. Requirements to control one's body—to eat on schedule, to defecate in particular places at particular times, or to sit at a desk for hours at a day in school—begin early in life and cannot avoid creating conflicts of obedience versus disobedience or identification with respected others versus pursuit of one's own desires. And with the development of full-blown sexual wishes at puberty, children must negotiate a remarkably complex process of directing sexual and loving feelings toward particular others and avoiding sexual feelings toward some who are loved, with whom mating would be biologically disadvantageous—all without the aid of conscious attention. An affective aversion to incest is probably one more example of "prepared" emotional potentialities—in this case, a spontaneous feeling of disgust—that render certain associations between affects and representations more likely than others, just as humans and other animals are more likely to associate nausea with tastes than with sounds (on taste and nausea, see Garcia & Koelling, 1966).

Humans, like all other primates, are social animals for whom survival and reproduction require considerable good will from others, including caretakers, family, potential mates, and friends and coalition partners. Most of our wishes can only be attained interpersonally, which means that much of life involves an *external* negotiation with significant others to adjudicate and balance conflicting desires and an *internal* negotiation among competing feelings and motives associated with those we care about or need. From birth, our survival depends on the benevolence of others whose subjectivity and individuality we scarcely understand. For the young child, caretaking others are a given—ground, not figure—and their help, nurturance, and selflessness is expected and generally unacknowledged. At the same time, these important people in our lives invariably frustrate us, because they have competing needs and demands on their time and energy, because as young children we have only a limited understanding of their thoughts and motives, and because their own imperfections often lead them to respond in ways that are emotionally destructive. Thus, the fundamental templates for our later social representations are always ambivalent—associated with love and hate—which is why there is no one who can elicit our anger or aggression more than the ones we most love.

These templates—internal working models of the self, relationships, and others; wishes, fears, and emotions associated with them; and modes of relating and regulating affects—are by no means unalterable or monolithic. From early in life, children develop multiple working models even of the same caregiver, and they form significant relationships with siblings and others in their environment that establish templates for future relationships. Once again, however, it is important to bear in mind that routinized cognitive, affective, and affect-regulatory "decisions" can not only foster development,

by directing behavior in adaptive directions selected through learning, but also derail it, as they lock people into patterns maintained by avoidance of consciously or unconsciously feared alternatives, or lead them to behave in ways that result in confirmation of their beliefs and fears (Wachtel, 1997).

This is just an outline of what an evolutionarily influenced psychodynamic model of personality might look like, but we believe it is an important start. In any case, psychoanalytic theorists would do well in the future to weigh evolutionary considerations whenever they propose theories of motivation, development, or personality, because personality processes, like other psychological processes, likely bear the clear imprint of natural selection.

The Clinical Database

That psychoanalysts seriously shot themselves in the foot by never evolving from case study methods as their primary mode of hypothesis testing is beyond doubt. Over the last century, for example, psychoanalysts have offered a plethora of competing developmental theories, few of which have even been subjected to empirical scrutiny, and some of which are empirically unfalsifiable (or already falsified, such as most of Melanie Klein's speculations about infancy, which fly in the face of research on what infants are cognitively capable of doing at the ages she proposes them to engage in highly elaborate mental gymnastics). On the other hand, no other method allows the depth of observation of a single personality offered by the psychoanalytic method of intensive interviewing, observation, and interaction with a person, aimed at coming to understand the individual's associative networks, meaning structures, affective proclivities, ways of regulating affect, and so forth, over a period of years. With all its limitations and vulnerabilities for confirmation biases and other sources of contamination, the value of such observation cannot be overemphasized.

Clinical observation casts an extraordinary net for observing psychologically meaningful phenomena, particularly in the "context of discovery," where theories and hypotheses are spawned. The laboratory may be much more useful in the "context of justification," where hypotheses are tested, but in the context of discovery, it is much less valuable (see Westen & Weinberger, 2005). The reason for its relative lack of value in observing new phenomena and creating broader networks of ideas is precisely the reason for its strength in the context of justification: The experimenter exercises as much control as possible, limiting participants' responses to a small number in which the investigator is interested.

Indeed, one could make a strong case that the quest for relative certainty at the level of hypothesis testing in psychology (exemplified by decades of preoccupation with p-values) leads to the certainty of falsehood at the level of theory. If psychologists base their theoretical frameworks exclusively on well-replicated experiments, they create a collective "availability bias" that leads them to understate the importance of processes and variables that, for technological, practical, or ethical reasons, are relatively inaccessible to the scientific community. We need not, of course, choose between relatively rich theories containing numerous specific falsehoods or relatively impoverished theories containing numerous likely truths that, when aggregated, produce a narrow and distorted view. One way to avoid this is to consider psychological data as forming an evidentiary hierarchy, in which experimental demonstrations are especially convincing forms of evidence, and nonreplicable clinical observations are less compelling but important sources of data for theory building. This perspective is particularly important for the field of personality, which deals with phenomena of considerable complexity, many of which cannot be easily brought into a laboratory for systematic investigation.

The Interpretation of Meaning

Perhaps above all, psychoanalytic approaches offer an approach to interpreting what people mean by their communications and actions that allows the psychologist to understand human behavior in ways that may not seem intuitive or obvious to a layperson. This may well be the reason the vast majority of clinicians, whose work requires that they understand personal meanings, rely exclusively or in part on psychodynamic conceptualizations, whereas most experimentalists remain dubious of psychodynamic proposi-

tions. Learning to listen psychoanalytically and to interpret meanings in this manner requires years of experience and supervision, just as does learning to design and conduct valid experiments.

Of course, the "art" inherent in interpretation is precisely what has let the postmodern cat out of the bag in psychoanalysis. This does not mean, however, that meaning cannot be coded with some reliability, or that there are no principles that can be used to recognize salient themes (see Alexander, 1988; Westen & Muderrisoglu, 2006; Westen & Weinberger, 2004). In everyday life, we decode meaning all the time, and much of the time observers reach considerable consensus on what they have observed. The same is true when researchers apply coding systems to narratives in an effort to quantify either thematic content or structural aspects of the narrative that provide insight into what the person may be implicitly thinking or feeling—that is, meaning. From a methodological standpoint, the recognition that humans inherently attach meaning to their experiences, and that these meanings affect the way in which they behave, once again suggests limits to approaches that take people's responses—even their responses to highly structured stimuli, such as questionnaires—at face value.

DIRECTIONS FOR THE FUTURE

True to our psychodynamic stripes, we are probably better at interpreting the past than at predicting future behavior, so we describe only briefly here what we believe to be three directions that psychoanalysis, and psychoanalytic approaches to personality, in particular, will (and, we think, must) take in the future. Either our prognostic skills were uncharacteristically accurate or our schemas are rigid, because these are essentially the same as those we proposed in the last two editions of this handbook.

Psychoanalysis has already moved substantially in the first direction, namely, the attempt to upgrade its credentials as an empirical science. Barriers to a more thoroughgoing, mutually constructive dialogue between psychoanalysis and empirical psychology remain, however, from both sides. On the one hand, only a handful of psychoanalytic institutes are associated in any meaningful way with universities, and academic clinical psychology has, ironically, become more hostile to psychodynamic thinking as the field as a whole has moved progressively toward accepting many of its fundamental assumptions. Today, psychoanalytic thinking in universities is almost entirely confined to the humanities, where empiricism is taken as seriously as psychoanalysis is taken in academic psychology departments.

The second direction is enhanced attention to microprocesses and more precision in describing precisely how psychological events transpire. Perhaps the most important contribution of a mind such as Freud's or Piaget's is to pose big questions and big solutions. The historian H. R. Trevor-Roper once said something to the effect that the function of a genius is not to provide answers but to pose questions that time and mediocrity will resolve. Freud, like Piaget, drew the big picture and proposed broad stages and structures that could account for an astonishing array of observable phenomena.

Scientific progress seems to require a dialectic not only between theory and detailed observation but also between the holistic purview of thinkers such as Freud and the more atomistic view characteristic of most academic psychology, at least in North America. The time is overdue in psychoanalysis for a move toward exploration of microprocesses, as is beginning to occur, for example, with the recognition of the many types of unconscious processes—both functionally and neuroanatomically distinct (e.g., associative and procedural memory) that psychoanalysts all too frequently lump under the rubric of "the unconscious." Similarly, although psychoanalysis is, above all, a dynamic theory, which, at least clinically, seldom posits trait-like phenomena that express themselves across all or most situations, psychoanalytic theories need to pay closer attention to the activating conditions of various processes. We do not know, for example, whether borderline patients are uniformly unable to mentalize or form relatively rich, differentiated representations of people, or whether they use less mature representations and make illogical attributions under certain conditions, such as poorly modulated affect.

Finally, a shift that has been occurring over the last three decades appears to be continuing, namely, that psychoanalysis is becoming a theory about cognitive–affective interactions that has shown less of the need for 19th-century jargon as it has moved into the 21st century. In the first edition of this handbook, we suggested that someday the basic theoretical concepts in psychoanalysis would likely be denoted by terms such as "thoughts," "feelings," "wishes," "actions," and "compromises," rather than by more obscure terms lacking clear empirical referents, such as "countercathexis," "symbiotic fusion," "drive derivative," and the like. We hope that trend continues.

CONCLUSION

A story is told of a student who asked his mentor, "Professor, what is science?" The professor paused and finally answered, "Science is looking for a black cat in a dark room." Momentarily satisfied, the student began to turn away, but then another question came to him. "Professor," he asked, "what is philosophy?" The academic furrowed his brow and after some thought replied, "Philosophy is looking for a black cat in a dark room where there is no black cat." Once again the student, satisfied that his question was answered, took leave of his mentor, only to return to ask one further question: "Professor, what is psychoanalysis?" "Psychoanalysis," the professor responded after a moment of deep contemplation, "is looking for a black cat in a dark room where there is no black cat—and finding one anyway."

Although, as we have attempted to show, the cat has actually been there lurking in the dark more often than has been supposed, one can have little doubt that in the history of psychoanalysis, clinicians and theorists have mistaken more than one shadow for substance, and more than one of our own eyelashes for a feline whisker. The alternative, which personality psychologists who rely exclusively on more conservative methods have chosen, is to turn on the light, see what can be seen, and assume that what goes on in the dark is unknowable or unimportant. If psychoanalysis has, and will continue to have, anything to offer the psychology of personality, it is the insight that we need not be in the dark about processes that are not manifestly observable, and that in the shadows sometimes lies the substance.

NOTES

1. Given the roots of psychoanalysis in clinical practice, an ironic turn of events from the standpoint of intellectual history is that psychoanalytic thinking is finding its way back into personality and social psychology as its last vestiges are disappearing from clinical psychology, where the cognitive-behavioral revolution is all but complete.

2. Although, as we will see, Freud's theory of psychic energy has increasingly fallen into disrepute in psychoanalysis because of the many ways it is problematic (Holt, 1976), certain aspects of it are intuitively appealing and even have empirical support. One is the notion that actively keeping knowledge from oneself may require expenditure of considerable psychic energy, and that this may have a cost (Cousineau & Shedler, 2006; Shedler et al., 1993; Weinberger, 1995).

3. Also of considerable importance in the 1960s and 1970s was Mahler's research (Mahler et al., 1975) based on observation of infants and young children, in which she and her colleagues traced the development of separation–individuation—that is, of the child's struggle to develop a sense of autonomy and independent selfhood while maintaining an attachment to (or, in Mahler's theory, libidinal investment in) the primary caretaker.

4. On the other hand, one of the dangers inherent in a theory that begins with the assumption that everything is motivated is its potential to overestimate the role of motivation and underestimate the importance of expectations derived partly from social learning. The pervasive expectations of malevolence in borderline patients, which have been documented in several studies (e.g., Lerner & St. Peter, 1984; Nigg et al., 1992; Westen, Lohr, et al., 1990), were for years interpreted from within the classical framework as projections of aggression. Although this view is not wholly without merit, research over the last two decades has documented extremely high frequencies of childhood abuse, particularly sexual abuse, in the histories of patients with borderline personality disorder (Herman, Perry, & van der Kolk, 1989; Zanarini, 1997). The malevolent object world of the patient with borderline personality disorder is thus likely to reflect, in part, real experiences of abuse. Where dynamic explanations are essential, however, is in recognizing the extent to which such expectations can be perpetuated by the ways in which the person subsequently behaves, which themselves may reflect motives, affect-regulation strategies, and interpersonal patterns shaped in the context of abusive or neglectful childrearing experiences. These patterns (e.g., readily switching to a malevolent view of someone who is being momentarily frustrating, and hence behaving impulsively or responding angrily) can in turn elicit precisely what the person fears, leading to further confirmatory experiences of rejection or abuse (see Wachtel, 1997, on "cyclical psychodynamics"). Perhaps the take-home message is that a theory of personality must take seriously both cognition and conation. Any effort to reduce one consistently to the other is likely to oversimplify.

5. The concept of psychic reality is closely tied to another issue that has come to the fore in the last decade in psychoanalysis: namely, the role of actual events, particularly traumatic events, in shaping personality. Although Freud never entirely abandoned the idea that actual childhood seduction was a common and pathogenic phenomenon, he certainly emphasized the role of fantasy in his psychoanalytic writing. Simon (1990) noted that cases of actual incest were remarkably absent from much of the psychoanalytic literature until the decade of the 1980s. More recently, psychoanalytic thought has been heavily influenced by the rediscovery of the relatively high prevalence of incest and other forms of childhood abuse. A byproduct of the increased interest in traumatic experiences in childhood has been a widespread controversy about the veridicality of recovered memories in clinical practice. Critics of psychoanalysis (Crews, 1995, 1996) have tended to blame Freud for the so-called recovered memory therapists who supposedly encourage patients to believe in the absolute accuracy of false memories of childhood seductions. These attacks are based on the assumption that Freud's model of treatment in the 1890s was never superseded by advances in theory or technique. In fact, Freud abandoned the cathartic abreaction model of derepressing pathogenic memories before the turn of the century. Indeed, there is great irony in the linkage of recovered memory therapists to Freud, because in actuality he was the first to recognize the fallibility of recovered memories of childhood sexual abuse (Lear, 1998).

6. Furthermore, no analyst actually believes, or could believe, such a radically relativistic point of view and survive in the world (or make an honest living). If no knowledge is privileged, or at least probabilistically more likely than other points of view, then analysts should be just as happy to become behaviorists and tell a different set of stories to their patients. Or better yet, they should become barbers, because there is nothing about their training or knowledge that renders their potential co-constructions any more useful than those of the patient's

barber, as barber and patient chat away, co-constructing an intersubjective field.

7. Since Ainsworth's identification of three infant attachment statuses, researchers have identified an additional infant attachment style of particular relevance to psychopathology research because it is primarily characterized by disorganized behaviors of simultaneous approach and withdrawal from caregivers (see Cassidy & Mohr, 2001). In addition, Bartholomew and Horowitz (1991) proposed a revised model of attachment that partitions anxious-ambivalent attachment into preoccupied and fearful adult attachment styles (i.e., profoundly distrustful attachment, Holmes & Lyons-Ruth, 2006). These developments, and others, have added further complexity to contemporary attachment research.

REFERENCES

Ackerman, S. J., Clemence, A. J., Weatherill, R., & Hilsenroth, M. J. (1999). Use of the TAT in the assessment of DSM-IV Cluster B personality disorders. *Journal of Personality Assessment, 73,* 422–442.

Ackerman, S. J., Hilsenroth, M. J., Clemence, A. J., Weatherill, R., & Fowler, J. C. (2001). Convergent validity of Rorschach and TAT scales of object relations. *Journal of Personality Assessment, 77,* 295–306.

Adams, H. E., Wright, L. W., & Lohr, B. A. (1996). Is homophobia associated with homosexual arousal? *Journal of Abnormal Psychology, 105,* 440–445.

Adler, A. (1929). *The science of living.* Garden City, NY: Doubleday/Anchor.

Adler, A. (1939). *Social interest.* New York: Putnam.

Adolphs, R. (2003). Cognitive neuroscience of human social behavior. *Nature Reviews Neuroscience, 4,* 165–178.

Agrawal, H. R., Gunderson, J., Holmes, B. M., & Lyons-Ruth, K. (2004). Attachment studies with Borderline patients: A review. *Harvard Review of Psychiatry, 12,* 94–104.

Ainsworth, M. D. S. (1979). Attachment as related to mother–infant interaction. *Advances in the Study of Behavior, 9,* 2–52.

Ainsworth, M. D. S., Blehar, M. C., Waters, E., & Wall, S. (1978). *Patterns of attachment: A psychological study of the strange situation.* Hillsdale, NJ: Erlbaum.

Alexander, I. (1988). Personality, psychological assessment, and psychobiography. *Journal of Personality, 56,* 265–294.

Allen, J. G. (2006). Mentalizing in practice. In J. G. Allen & P. Fonagy (Eds.), *Handbook of mentalization-based treatment* (pp. 3–30). West Sussex, UK: Wiley.

Allison, J., Blatt, S. J., & Zimet, C.N. (1968). *The interpretation of psychological tests.* New York: Harper & Row.

Andersen, S., & Baum, A. (1994). Transference in interpersonal relations: Inferences and affect based on significant-other representations. *Journal of Personality, 62,* 460–497.

Arlow, J. (1985). The concept of psychic reality and related problems. *Journal of the American Psychoanalytic Association, 33,* 521–535.

Arlow, J., & Brenner, C. (1964). Psychoanalytic concepts and the structure model. *Journal of the American Psychoanalytic Association Monographs* (No. 3).

Aron, L., & Harris, A. (Eds.). (2005). *Relational psychoanalysis: Innovation and expansion* (Vol. 2). Mahwah, NJ: Analytic Press.

Badcock, C. (1994). *Psychodarwinism: The new synthesis of Darwin and Freud.* London: HarperCollins.

Balay, J., & Shevrin, H. (1988). The subliminal psychodynamic activation method: A critical review. *American Psychologist, 43,* 161–174.

Balleine, B. W., & Killcross, S. (2006). Parallel incentive processing: An integrated view of amygdala function. *Trends in Neurosciences, 29,* 272–279.

Banai, E., Mikulincer, M., & Shaver, P. R. (2005). "Selfobject" needs in Kohut's self psychology: Links with attachment, self-cohesion, affect regulation, and adjustment. *Psychoanalytic Psychology, 22,* 224–260.

Bargh, J. (1984). Automatic and conscious processing of social information. In R. S. Wyer & T. K. Srull (Eds.), *Handbook of social cognition* (Vol. 3, pp. 1–43). Hillsdale, NJ: Erlbaum.

Bargh, J., & Barndollar, K. (1996). Automaticity in action: The unconscious as repository of chronic goals and motives. In P. M. Gollwitzer & J. Bargh (Eds.), *The psychology of action: Linking cognition and motivation to behavior* (pp. 457–481). New York: Guilford Press.

Barrett, L. F., Mesquita, B., Ochsner, K. N., & Gross, J. J. (2007). The experience of emotion. *Annual Review of Psychology, 58,* 373–403.

Bartholomew, K., & Horowitz, L. M. (1991). Attachment styles among young adults: A test of a four-category model. *Journal of Personality and Social Psychology, 61,* 226–244.

Basch, F. M. (1977). Developmental psychology and explanatory theory in psychoanalysis. *Annual of Psychoanalysis, 5,* 229–263.

Beck, A. T., Freeman, A., Davis, D. D., & Associates. (2004). *Cognitive therapy of personality disorders* (2nd ed.). New York: Guilford Press.

Bell, M. D., Billington, R., Cicchetti, D., & Gibbons, J. (1988). Do object relations deficits distinguish BPD from other diagnostic groups? *Journal of Clinical Psychology, 44,* 511–516.

Bell, M. D., Greig, T. C., Bryson, G., & Kaplan, E. (2001). Patterns of object relations and reality testing deficits in schizophrenia: Clusters and their symptom and personality correlates. *Journal of Clinical Psychology, 57*, 1353–1367.

Bellack, L., Hurvich, M., & Gediman, H. K. (1973). *Ego functions in schizophrenics, neurotics, and normals.* New York: Wiley.

Besser, A., & Blatt, S. J. (2007). Identity consolidation and internalizing and externalizing problem behaviors in early adolescence. *Psychoanalytic Psychology, 24*, 126–149.

Betan, E., Heim, A. K., Conklin, C. Z., & Westen, D. (2005). Countertransference phenomena and personality pathology in clinical practice: An empirical investigation. *American Journal of Psychiatry, 162*, 890–898.

Bettelheim, B. (1983). *Freud and man's soul.* New York: Knopf.

Blagov, P. S., Bradley, R., & Westen, D. (2007). Under the Axis II radar: Clinically relevant personality constellations that escape DSM-IV diagnosis. *Journal of Nervous and Mental Disease, 195*, 477–483.

Blanck, G., & Blanck, R. (1974). *Ego psychology: Theory and practice.* New York: Columbia University Press.

Blanck, G., & Blanck, R. (1979). *Ego psychology: II. Psychoanalytic developmental psychology.* New York: Columbia University Press.

Blanton, H., Jaccard, J., Christie, C., & Gonzales, P. M. (2007). Plausible assumptions, questionable assumptions and post hoc rationalizations: Will the real IAT, please stand up? *Journal of Experimental Social Psychology, 43*, 399–409.

Blanton, H., Jaccard, J., Gonzales, P. M., & Christie, C. (2006). Decoding the Implicit Association Test: Implications for criterion prediction. *Journal of Experimental Social Psychology, 42*, 192–212.

Blatt, S. J., & Auerbach, J. S. (2003). Psychodynamic measures of therapeutic change. *Psychoanalytic Inquiry, 23*, 268–307.

Blatt, S. J., Auerbach, J., & Levy, K. (1997). Mental representations in personality development, psychopathology, and the therapeutic process. *Review of General Psychology, 1*, 351–374.

Blatt, S. J., Brenneis, C. B., & Schimek, J. G. (1976). Normal development and psychopathological impairment of the object on the Rorschach. *Journal of Abnormal Psychology, 85*, 364–373.

Blatt, S. J., & Lerner, H. (1991). Psychoanalytic perspectives on personality theory. In M. Hersen, A. Bellack, & J. A. E. Kazdin (Eds.), *Handbook of clinical psychology* (pp. 147–169). New York: Pergamon Press.

Blatt, S. J., Shahar, G., & Zuroff, D. C. (2001). Anaclitic (sociotropic) and introjective (autonomous) dimensions. *Psychotherapy: Theory, Research, Practice, Training, 38*, 449–454.

Blatt, S. J., Wein, S., Chevron, E. S., & Quinlan, D. M. (1979). Parental representations and depression in normal young adults. *Journal of Abnormal Psychology, 78*, 388–397.

Blatt, S. J., & Zuroff, D. (1992). Interpersonal relatedness and self-definition: Two prototypes for depression. *Clinical Psychology Review, 12*, 527–562.

Block, J. (1971). *Lives through time.* Berkeley, CA: Bancroft.

Block, J., & Block, J. (1980). The role of ego-control and ego-resiliency in the organization of behavior. In W. A. Collins (Ed.), *Minnesota Symposium on Child Development* (Vol. 13). Hillsdale, NJ: Erlbaum.

Blum, G. S. (1961). *A model of the mind.* New York: Wiley.

Bonanno, G., & Singer, J. L. (1995). Repressive personality style: Theoretical and methodological implications for health and pathology. In J. Singer (Ed.), *Repression and dissociation: Implications for personality theory, psychopathology, and health* (pp. 435–470). Chicago: University of Chicago Press.

Bond, M., & Perry, J. C. (2004). Long-term changes in defense styles with psychodynamic psychotherapy for depressive, anxiety, and personality disorders. *American Journal of Psychiatry, 161*, 1665–1671.

Bosson, J. K., & Swann, W. B., Jr. (1999). Self-liking, self-competence, and the quest for self-verification. *Personality and Social Psychology Bulletin, 25*, 1230–1241.

Bowers, K., & Meichenbaum, D. (Eds.). (1984). *The unconscious reconsidered.* New York: Wiley.

Bowlby, J. (1969). *Attachment and loss: Vol. 1. Attachment.* New York: Basic Books.

Bowlby, J. (1973). *Attachment and loss: Vol. 2. Separation.* New York: Basic Books.

Bowlby, J. (1982). Attachment and loss: Retrospective and prospect. *American Journal of Orthopsychiatry, 52*, 664–678.

Bradley, R., Heim, A. K., & Westen, D. (2005). Transference patterns in the psychotherapy of personality disorders: Empirical investigation. *British Journal of Psychiatry, 186*, 342–349.

Bradley, R., & Westen, D. (2006). The psychodynamics of borderline personality disorder: A view from developmental psychopathology. *Development and Psychopathology, 17*, 927–957.

Brennan, K., Clark, C. L., & Shaver, P. (1998). Self-report measurement of adult attachment: An integrative overview. In J. A. Simpson & W. S. Rholes (Eds.), *Attachment theory and close relationships* (pp. 46–76). New York: Guilford Press.

Brenner, C. (1982). *The mind in conflict*. New York: International Universities Press.

Brenner, C. (1991). A psychoanalytic theory of affects. *Journal of the American Psychoanalytic Association*, 39, 305–314.

Brenner, C. (2002). Conflict, compromise formation, and structural theory. *Psychoanalytic Quarterly*, 71, 397–417.

Brenner, C. (2003). Is the structural model still useful? *International Journal of Psychoanalysis*, 84, 1093–1103.

Bretherton, I. (1985). Attachment theory: Retrospect and prospect. In I. Bretherton & E. Waters (Eds.), Growing points of attachment theory and research. *Monographs of the Society for Research in Child Development*, 50(1–2, Serial No. 209), 3–35.

Breuer, J., & Freud, S. (1955). Studies on hysteria. In J. Strachey (Ed. & Trans.), *The standard edition of the complete psychological works of Sigmund Freud* (Vol. 2). London: Hogarth Press. (Original work published 1893–1895)

Brewer, M. B. (2001). Ingroup identification and intergroup conflict: When does ingroup love become outgroup hate? In R. D. Ashmore, L. Jussim, & D. Wilder (Eds.), *Social identity, intergroup conflict, and conflict reduction* (pp. 17–41). New York: Oxford University Press.

Brewer, M. B., & Brown, R. J. (1998). Intergroup relations. In D. T. Gilbert, S. T. Fiske, & G. Lindzey (Eds.), *Handbook of social psychology* (Vol. 2, pp. 554–594). New York: McGraw-Hill.

Broadbent, D. E. (1977). The hidden preattentive processes. *American Psychologist*, 32, 109–118.

Brown, L. L., Tomarken, A., Orth, D., Loosen, P., Kalin, N., & Davidson, R. (1996). Individual differences in repressive-defensiveness predict basal salivary cortisol levels. *Journal of Personality and Social Psychology*, 70, 362–371.

Bruner, J. S. (1973). *Beyond the information given: Studies in the psychology of knowing*. New York: Norton.

Bucci, W. (1997). *Psychoanalysis and cognitive science: A multiple code theory*. New York: Guilford Press.

Buchheim, A., Erk, S., George, C., Kachele, H., Ruchsow, M., Spitzer, M., et al. (2006). Measuring attachment representation in an fMRI environment: A pilot study. *Psychopathology*, 39, 144–152.

Busch, F. (1995). *The ego at the center of clinical technique*. Northvale, NJ: Aronson.

Buss, D. M. (2005). *The handbook of evolutionary psychology*. Hoboken, NJ: Wiley.

Buss, D. M., Haselton, M., Shackelford, T., Bleske, A., & Wakefield, J. (1998). Adaptations, exaptations, and spandrels. *American Psychologist*, 53, 533–548.

Cacioppo, J., Gardner, W., & Berntson, G. (1997). Beyond bipolar conceptualizations and measures: The case of attitudes and evaluative space. *Personality and Social Psychology Review*, 1, 3–25.

Calabrese, M. L., Farber, B. A., & Westen, D. (2005). The relationship of adult attachment constructs to object relational patterns of representing self and others. *Journal of the American Academy of Psychoanalysis and Dynamic Psychiatry*, 33, 513–530.

Campbell-Sills, L., Barlow, D. H., Brown, T. A., & Hofmann, S. G. (2006). Acceptability and suppression of negative emotion in anxiety and mood disorders. *Emotion*, 6, 587–595.

Carver, C. S., & White, T. L. (1994). Behavioral inhibition, behavioral activation, and affective responses to impending reward and punishment: The BIS/BAS scales. *Journal of Personality and Social Psychology*, 67, 319–333.

Caspi, A., McClay, J., Moffitt, T. E., Mill, J., Martin, J., Craig, I. W., et al. (2002). Role of genotype in the cycle of violence in maltreated children. *Science*, 297, 851–854.

Cassidy, J., & Mohr, J. J. (2001). Unsolvable fear, trauma, and psychopathology: Theory, research, and clinical considerations related to disorganized attachment across the life span. *Clinical Psychology: Science and Practice*, 8, 275–298.

Cesario, J., Plaks, J. E., & Higgins, E. T. (2006). Automatic social behavior as motivated preparation to interact. *Journal of Personality and Social Psychology*, 90, 893–910.

Chartrand, T. L., van Baaren, R. B., & Bargh, J. A. (2006). Linking automatic evaluation to mood and information processing style: Consequences for experienced affect, impression formation, and stereotyping. *Journal of Experimental Psychology: General*, 135, 70–77.

Chen, M., & Bargh, J. A. (1999). Consequences of automatic evaluation: Immediate behavioral predispositions to approach or avoid the stimulus. *Personality and Social Psychology Bulletin*, 25, 215–224.

Clark, L. A. (2005). Temperament as a unifying basis for personality and psychopathology. *Journal of Abnormal Psychology*, 114, 505–521.

Clark, L. A., & Watson, D. (1991). Tripartite model of anxiety and depression: Psychometric evidence and taxonomic implications. *Journal of Abnormal Psychology*, 100, 316–336.

Clifton, A., Turkheimer, E., & Oltmanns, T. F. (2005). Self- and peer perspectives on pathological personality traits and interpersonal problems. *Psychological Assessment*, 17, 123–131.

Coggans, N. (2006). Drug education and prevention: Has progress been made? *Drugs: Education, Prevention and Policy, 13,* 417–422.

Coleman, M. J., Levy, D. L., Lenzenweger, M. F., & Holzman, P. S. (1996). Thought disorder, perceptual aberrations, and schizotypy. *Journal of Abnormal Psychology, 105,* 469–473.

Colvin, R., Block, J., & Funder, D. C. (1995). Overly positive self-evaluations and personality: Negative implications for mental health. *Journal of Personality and Social Psychology, 68,* 1152–1162.

Conklin, A., & Westen, D. (2001). Thematic Apperception Test. In W. I. Dorfman & M. Hersen (Eds.), *Understanding psychological assessment* (pp. 107–133). Dordrecht, Netherlands: Kluwer.

Conte, H. R., & Plutchik, R. (Eds.). (1995). *Ego defenses: Theory and measurement.* New York: Wiley.

Cousineau, T. M., & Shedler, J. (2006). Predicting physical health: Implicit mental health measures versus self-report scales. *Journal of Nervous and Mental Disease, 194,* 427–432.

Crews, F. (1995). *The memory wars: Freud's legacy in dispute.* New York: New York Review of Books.

Crews, F. (1996). The verdict on Freud. *Psychological Science, 7,* 63–67.

Crowne, D. P., & Marlowe, D. (1964). *The approval motive: Studies in evaluative dependence.* New York: Wiley.

Cunningham, W. A., Johnson, M. K., Raye, C. L., Gatenby, J. C., Gore, J. C., & Banaji, M. R. (2004). Separable neural components in the processing of black and white faces. *Psychological Science, 15,* 806–813.

Dahl, H. (1983). On the definition and measurement of wishes. In J. Masling (Ed.), *Empirical studies of psychoanalytic theories* (Vol. 1, pp. 39–67). Hillsdale, NJ: Erlbaum.

Dalgleish, T., & Power, M. J. (Eds.). (1999). *Handbook of cognition and emotion.* New York: Wiley.

Davidson, R. (2003). Affective neuroscience and psychophysiology: Toward a synthesis. *Psychophysiology, 40,* 655–665.

Davis, P. J., & Schwartz, G. E. (1987). Repression and the inaccessibility of affective memories. *Journal of Personality and Social Psychology, 52,* 155–162.

de Liver, Y., van der Pligt, J., & Wigboldus, D. (2007). Positive and negative associations underlying ambivalent attitudes. *Journal of Experimental Social Psychology, 43,* 319–326.

Demaree, H. A., Robinson, J. L., & Everhart, D. E. (2005). Behavioral inhibition system (BIS) strength and trait dominance are associated with affective response and perspective taking when viewing dyadic interactions. *International Journal of Neuroscience, 115,* 1579–1593.

de Wolff, M., & van IJzendoorn, M. (1997). Sensitivity and attachment: A meta-analysis on parental antecedents of infant attachment. *Child Development, 68,* 571–591.

Diamond, D., Kaslow, N., Coonerty, S., & Blatt, S. J. (1990). Changes in separation–individuation and intersubjectivity in long-term treatment. *Psychoanalytic Psychology, 7,* 363–397.

Ditto, P. H., Munro, G. D., Apanovitch, A. M., Scepansky, J. A., & Lockhart, L. K. (2003). Spontaneous skepticism: The interplay of motivation and expectation in responses to favorable and unfavorable medical diagnoses. *Personality and Social Psychology Bulletin, 29,* 1120–1132.

Dixon, N. F. (1971). *Subliminal perception: The nature of controversy.* New York: McGraw-Hill.

Dixon, N. F. (1981). *Preconscious processing.* New York: Wiley.

Donegan, N. H., Sanislow, C. A., Blumberg H. P., Fulbright, R. K., Lacadie, C., Skudlarkis, P., et al. (2003). Amygdala hyperreactivity in borderline personality disorder: Implications for emotional dysregulation. *Biological Psychiatry, 54,* 1284–1293.

Downey, G., Freitas, A. L., Michaelis, B., & Khouri, H. (1998). The self-fulfilling prophecy in close relationships: Rejection sensitivity and rejection by romantic partners. *Journal of Personality and Social Psychology, 75,* 545–560.

Eagle, M., Wolitzky, D. L., & Wakefield, J. C. (2001). The analyst's knowledge and authority: A critique of the "new view" in psychoanalysis. *Journal of the American Psychoanalytic Association, 49,* 457–489.

Edelson, M. (1984). *Hypothesis and evidence in psychoanalysis.* Chicago: University of Chicago Press.

Edelson, M. (1985). The hermeneutic turn and the single case study in psychoanalysis. *Psychoanalysis and Contemporary Thought, 8,* 567–614.

Ellenberger, H. F. (1970). *The discovery of the unconscious: The history and evolution of dynamic psychiatry.* New York: Basic Books.

Erdelyi, M. (1974). A "new look" at the New Look in perception. *Psychological Review, 81,* 1–25.

Erdelyi, M. (1985). *Psychoanalysis: Freud's cognitive psychology.* San Francisco: Freeman.

Erikson, E. (1963). *Childhood and society* (rev. ed.). New York: Norton.

Erikson, E. (1968). *Identity: Youth and crises.* New York: Norton.

Eudell-Simmons, E. M., Stein, M. B., DeFife, J. A., & Hilsenroth, M. J. (2005). Reliability and validity of the Social Cognition and Object Relations Scale (SCORS) in the assessment of dream narratives. *Journal of Personality Assessment, 85*, 325–333.

Fairbairn, W. R. D. (1952). *Psychoanalytic studies of the personality*. London: Routledge & Kegan Paul.

Fast, I. (1985). *Event theory*. Hillsdale, NJ: Erlbaum.

Fazio, R., Jackson, J. R., Dunton, B., & Williams, C. J. (1995). Variability in automatic activation as an unobtrusive measure of racial attitudes: A bona fide pipeline? *Journal of Personality and Social Psychology, 69*, 1013–1027.

Ferguson, M. J., & Bargh, J. A. (2004). How social perception can automatically influence behavior. *Trends in Cognitive Sciences, 8*, 33–39.

Fish, E. W., Shahrokh, D., Bagot, R., Caldji, C., Bredy, T., Szyf, M., et al. (2004). Epigenetic programming of stress responses through variations in maternal care. In J. Devine, J. Gilligan, K. A. Miczek, R. Shaikh, & D. Pfaff (Eds.), *Youth violence: Scientific approaches to prevention* (pp. 167–186). New York: New York Academy of Sciences.

Fisher, S., & Greenberg, R. P. (1985). *The scientific credibility of Freud's theories and therapy*. New York: Columbia University Press.

Fisher, S., & Greenberg, R. P. (1996). *Freud scientifically reappraised: Testing the theories and therapy*. New York: Wiley.

Foley, D. L., Eaves, L. J., Wormley, D., Silberg, J. L., Maes, H. H., Kuhn, J., et al. (2004). Childhood adversity, monoamine oxidase A genotype, and risk for conduct disorder. *Archives of General Psychiatry, 61*, 738–744.

Fonagy, P., & Bateman, A. (2005). Attachment theory and mentalization-oriented model of borderline personality disorder. In J. M. Oldham, A. E. Skodol, & D. S. Bender (Eds.), *Textbook of personality disorders* (pp. 187–207). Washington, DC: American Psychiatric Association.

Fonagy, P., Gergely, G., Jurist, E., & Target, M. (2002). *Affect regulation, mentalization, and the development of the self*. New York: Other Press.

Fonagy, P., Moran, G. S., Steele, M., Steele, H., & Higgitt, A. C. (1991). The capacity for understanding mental states: The reflective self in parent and child and its significance for security of attachment. *Infant Mental Health Journal, 13*, 200–216.

Fonagy, P., Steele, M., & Steele, H. (1991). The capacity for understanding mental states: The reflective self in parent and child and its significance for security of attachment. *Infant Mental Health Journal, 12*, 201–218.

Fonagy, P., & Target, M. (2006). The mentalization-focused approach to self pathology. *Journal of Personality Disorders, 20*, 544–576.

Fowler, C., Hilsenroth, M., & Handler, L. (1996).

Two methods of early memories data collection: An empirical comparison of the projective yield. *Assessment, 3*, 63–71.

Freud, A. (1936). *The ego and the mechanisms of defense*. New York: International Universities Press.

Freud, S. (1953a). The interpretation of dreams. In J. Strachey (Ed. & Trans.), *The standard edition of the complete psychological works of Sigmund Freud* (Vol. 4, pp. 1–338; Vol. 5, pp. 339–621). London: Hogarth Press. (Original work published 1900)

Freud, S. (1953b). Three essays on the theory of sexuality. In J. Strachey (Ed. & Trans.), *The standard edition of the complete psychological works of Sigmund Freud* (Vol. 7, pp. 123–245). London: Hogarth Press. (Original work published 1905)

Freud, S. (1957). On narcissism. In J. Strachey (Ed. & Trans.), *The standard edition of the complete psychological works of Sigmund Freud* (Vol. 14, pp. 67–102). London: Hogarth Press. (Original work published 1914)

Freud, S. (1961). The ego and the id. In J. Strachey (Ed. & Trans.), *The standard edition of the complete psychological works of Sigmund Freud* (Vol. 19, pp. 1–66). London: Hogarth Press. (Original work published 1923)

Freud, S. (1964a). An outline of psycho-analysis. In J. Strachey (Ed. & Trans.), *The standard edition of the complete psychological works of Sigmund Freud* (Vol. 23, pp. 139–207). London: Hogarth Press. (Original work published 1940)

Freud, S. (1964b). New introductory lectures on psychoanalysis. In J. Strachey (Ed. & Trans.), *The standard edition of the complete psychological works of Sigmund Freud* (Vol. 22, pp. 1–182). London: Hogarth Press. (Original work published 1933)

Freud, S. (1966). Project for a scientific psychology. In J. Strachey (Ed. & Trans.), *The standard edition of the complete psychological works of Sigmund Freud* (Vol. 1, pp. 281–397). London: Hogarth Press. (Original work written in 1895, published 1950)

Fromm, E. (1947). *Man for himself: An inquiry into the psychology of ethics*. New York: Holt, Rinehart & Winston.

Fromm, E. (1962). *The sane society*. Greenwich, CT: Fawcett Books.

Gabbard, G. O. (1995). Countertransference: The emerging common ground. *International Journal of Psycho-Analysis, 76*, 475–485.

Gabbard, G. O. (1997). A reconsideration of objectivity in the analyst. *International Journal of Psycho-Analysis, 78*, 15–26.

Gabbard, G. O. (2005). Personality disorders come of age. *American Journal of Psychiatry, 162*, 833–835.

Gabbard, G. O. (2006). A neuroscience perspective on transference. *Psychiatric Annals, 36,* 283–288.

Gabbard, G. O., & Westen, D. (2003). On therapeutic action. *International Journal of Psycho-Analysis, 84,* 823–841.

Gallese, V., Eagle, M. N., & Migone, P. (2007). Intentional attunement: Mirror neurons and the neural underpinnings of interpersonal relations. *Journal of the American Psychoanalytic Association, 55,* 131–176.

Garbarini, F., & Adenzato, M. (2004). At the root of embodied cognition: Cognitive science meets neurophysiology. *Brain and Cognition, 56,* 100–106.

Garcia, J., & Koelling, R. (1966). Relation of cue to consequence in avoidance learning. *Psychonomic Science, 4,* 123–124.

Gartner, J., Hurt, S. W., & Gartner, A. (1987, September). *Psychological test signs of borderline personality disorder: A review of the empirical literature.* Paper presented at the annual convention of the American Psychological Association, New York.

Gebauer, G. F., & Mackintosh, N. J. (2007). Psychometric intelligence dissociates implicit and explicit learning. *Journal of Experimental Psychology: Learning, Memory, and Cognition, 33,* 34–54.

Geertz, C. (1973). *The interpretation of cultures.* New York: Basic Books.

Gill, M. M. (1976). Metapsychology is not psychology. In M. M. Gill & P. S. Holzman (Eds.), Psychology versus metapsychology: Psychoanalytic essays in memory of George S. Klein. *Psychological Issues, 9*(4, Monograph No. 36).

Gill, M. M. (1994). *Psychoanalysis in transition: A personal view.* Hillsdale, NJ: Analytic Press.

Gillath, O., Mikulincer, M., Fitzsimons, G. M., Shaver, P. R., Schachner, D. A., & Bargh, J. A. (2006). Automatic activations of attachment-related goals. *Personality and Social Psychology Bulletin, 32,* 1375–1388.

Gladwell, M. (2005). *Blink: The power of thinking without thinking.* New York: Little, Brown.

Gopnik, A., & Wellman, H. M. (1992). Why the child's theory of mind really is a theory. *Mind and Language, 7,* 145–171.

Gordon, N. S., Panksepp, J., Dennis, M., & McSweeny, J. (2005). The instinctual basis of human affect: Affective and fMRI imaging of laughter and crying. *Neuro-Psychoanalysis, 7,* 215–217.

Gray, J. A. (1990). Brain systems that mediate both emotion and cognition. *Cognition and Emotion, 4,* 269–288.

Gray, P. (1994). *The ego and the analysis of defense.* Northvale, NJ: Aronson.

Greenberg, J. R. (1991). *Oedipus and beyond: A clinical theory.* Cambridge, MA: Harvard University Press.

Greenberg, J. R., & Mitchell, S. A. (1983). *Object relations in psychoanalytic theory.* Cambridge, MA: Harvard University Press.

Greenspan, S. (1979). *Intelligence and adaptation.* New York: International Universities Press.

Greenwald, A. G., & Banaji, M. (1995). Implicit social cognition: Attitudes, self-esteem, and stereotypes. *Psychological Review, 102,* 4–27.

Greenwald, A. G., Banaji, M. R., Rudman, L. A., Farnham, S. D., Nosek, B. A., & Mellott, D. S. (2002). A unified theory of implicit attitudes, stereotypes, self-esteem, and self-concept. *Psychological Review, 109,* 3–25.

Greenwald, A. G., McGhee, D. E., & Schwartz, J. L. K. (1998). Measuring individual differences in implicit cognition: The Implicit Association Test. *Journal of Personality and Social Psychology, 74,* 1464–1480.

Gross, J. J. (Ed.). (2007). *Handbook of emotion regulation.* New York: Guilford Press.

Grunbaum, A. (1984). *The foundations of psychoanalysis: A philosophical critique.* Berkeley: University of California Press.

Guntrip, H. (1971). *Psychoanalytic theory, therapy, and the self.* New York: Basic Books.

Haan, N. (1977). *Coping and defending.* New York: Academic Press.

Haas, B. W., Omura, K., Constable, R. T., & Canli, T. (2006). Interference produced by emotional conflict associated with anterior cingulated activation. *Cognitive, Affective, and Behavioral Neuroscience, 6,* 152–156.

Habermas, J. (1971). *Knowledge and human interests* (J. J. Shapiro, Trans.) London: Heinemann.

Hamann, S. (2006). Sex differences in neural responses to sexual stimuli in humans. In T. Canli (Ed.), *Biology of personality and individual differences* (pp. 184–202). New York: Guilford Press.

Handest, P., & Parnas, J. (2005). Clinical characteristics of first-admitted patients with ICD-10 schizotypal disorder. *British Journal of Psychiatry, 187,* 49–54.

Harpaz-Rotem, I., & Blatt, S. J. (2005). Changes in representations of a self-designated significant other in long-term intensive inpatient treatment of seriously disturbed adolescents and young adults. *Psychiatry: Interpersonal and Biological Processes, 68,* 266–282.

Hartmann, H. (1958). *Ego psychology and the problem of adaptation.* New York: International Universities Press. (Original work published 1939)

Hartmann, H., Kris, E., & Loewenstein, R. (1946). Comments on the formation of psychic structure. *Psychoanalytic Study of the Child, 2,* 11–38.

Hassin, R. R., Uleman, J. S., & Bargh, J. A. (Eds.). (2005). *The new unconscious*. New York: Oxford University Press.

Hauser, M. (2006). Moral ingredients: How we evolved the capacity to do the right thing. In S. C. Levinson & J. Pierre (Eds.), *Evolution and culture: A Fyssen Foundation symposium* (pp. 219–245). Cambridge, MA: MIT Press.

Heinemann, L., & Emrich, H. (1971). Alpha activity during inhibitory brain processes. *Psychophysiology, 7*, 442–450.

Herman, J., Perry, J. C., & van der Kolk, B. A. (1989). Childhood trauma in borderline personality disorder. *American Journal of Psychiatry, 146*, 490–495.

Hesse, E., & Main, M. (1999). Second-generation effects of unresolved trauma in nonmaltreating parents: Dissociated, frightened, and threatening parental behavior. *Psychoanalytic Inquiry, 19*, 481–540.

Hesse, E., & Main, M. (2006). Frightened, threatening, and dissociative parental behavior in low-risk samples: Description, discussion, and interpretations. *Development and Psychopathology, 18*, 309–343.

Hibbard, S., Hilsenroth, M., Hibbard, J. K., & Nash, M. (1995). A validity study of two projective object representations measures. *Psychological Assessment, 7*, 432–439.

Higgins, E. T., & Bargh, J. A. (1987). Social cognition and social perception. *Annual Review of Psychology, 38*, 369–425.

Higgins, E. T., King, G. A., & Mavin, G. H. (1982). Individual construct accessibility and subjective impressions and recall. *Journal of Personality and Social Psychology, 43*, 35–47.

Hoffman, I. Z. (1991). Discussion: Toward a social constructivist view of the psychoanalytic situation. *Psychoanalytic Dialogues, 1*, 74–105.

Hoffman, I. Z. (1998). *Ritual and spontaneity in the psychoanalytic process: A dialectical–constructivist view*. Hillsdale, NJ: Analytic Press.

Holland, N. N. (1993). Post-modern psychoanalysis. In I. Hassan & S. Hassan (Eds.), *Innovation/renovation: New perspectives on the humanities* (pp. 291–309). Madison: University of Wisconsin Press.

Holmes, B. M., & Lyons-Ruth, K. (2006). The Relationship Questionnaire—Clinical Version (RQ-CV): Introducing a profoundly-distrustful attachment style. *Infant Mental Health Journal, 27*, 310–325.

Holt, R. R. (1976). Drive or wish? In M. M. Gill & P. S. Holzman (Eds.), Psychology versus metapsychology: Psychoanalytic essays in memory of George S. Klein. *Psychological Issues, 9*(4, Monograph No. 36).

Holt, R. R. (1981). The death and transfiguration of metapsychology. *International Review of Psycho-Analysis, 8*, 129–143.

Holyoak, K., & Spellman, B. (1993). Thinking. *Annual Review of Psychology, 44*, 265–315.

Holzman, P. (1985). Psychoanalysis: Is the therapy destroying the science? *Journal of the American Psychoanalytic Association, 33*, 725–770.

Horney, K. (1950). *Neurosis and human growth*. New York: Norton.

Horney, K. (1967). *Feminine psychology*. New York: Norton.

Horowitz, M. J. (1987). *States of mind: Configurational analysis of individual psychology* (2nd ed.). New York: Plenum Press.

Horowitz, M. J. (1988). *Introduction to psychodynamics: A synthesis*. New York: Basic Books.

Horowitz, M. J. (1998). *Cognitive psychodynamics: From conflict to character*. New York: Wiley.

Huprich, S. K., & Greenberg, R. P. (2003). Advances in the assessment of object relations in the 1990s. *Clinical Psychology Review, 23*, 665–698.

Iacoboni, M. (2008). *Mirroring people: The new science of how we connect with others*. New York: Farrar, Straus & Giroux.

Iacoboni, M., & Dapretto, M. (2006). The mirror neuron system and the consequences of its dysfunction. *Nature Reviews Neuroscience, 7*, 942–951.

Jacobson, E. (1954). The self and the object world. *Psychoanalytic Study of the Child, 9*, 75–127.

Jacoby, L., & Kelly, C. M. (1992). A process-dissociation framework for investigating unconscious influences: Freudian slips, projective tests, subliminal perception, and signal detection theory. *Current Directions in Psychological Science, 1*, 174–179.

Jahoda, M. (1977). *Freud and the dilemmas of psychology*. London: Hogarth Press.

Johnson, M. K., Kim, J. K., & Risse, G. (1985). Do alcoholic Korsakoff's syndrome patients acquire affective reactions? *Journal of Experimental Psychology: Learning, Memory, and Cognition, 11*, 22–36.

Johnston, M. H., & Holzman, P. S. (1979). *Assessing schizophrenic thinking*. San Francisco: Jossey-Bass.

Jost, J. T., Glaser, J., Kruglanski, A. W., & Sulloway, F. J. (2003). Political conservatism as motivated social cognition. *Psychological Bulletin, 129*, 339–375.

Jung, C. G. (1971). *The portable Jung* (J. Campbell, Ed.). New York: Viking.

Kahneman, D. (2003). A perspective on judgment and choice: Mapping bounded rationality. *American Psychologist, 58*, 697–720.

Kammrath, L. K., Mendoza-Denton, R., & Mischel, W. (2005). Incorporating if … then …

personality signatures in person perception: Beyond the person–situation dichotomy. *Journal of Personality and Social Psychology, 88,* 605–618.

Kaplan-Solms, K., & Solms, M. (2002). *Clinical studies in neuro-psychoanalysis: Introduction to a depth neuropsychology* (2nd ed.). London: Karnac Books.

Kelly, G. A. (1955). *Psychology of personal constructs.* New York: Norton.

Kernberg, O. (1975). *Borderline conditions and pathological narcissism.* New York: Aronson.

Kernberg, O. (1984). *Severe personality disorders: Psychotherapeutic strategies.* New Haven, CT: Yale University Press.

Kernberg, O. F., & Caligor, E. (2005). A psychoanalytic theory of personality disorders. In M. F. Lenzenweger & J. F. Clarkin (Eds.), *Major theories of personality disorder* (2nd ed., pp. 114–156). New York: Guilford Press.

Kihlstrom, J. F. (1987). The cognitive unconscious. *Science, 237,* 1445–1452.

Kim, S. H., & Hamann, S. (2007). Neural correlates of positive and negative emotion regulation. *Journal of Cognitive Neuroscience, 19,* 776–798.

Kim-Cohen, J., Caspi, A., Taylor, A., Williams, B., Newcombe, R., Craig, I. W., et al. (2006). MAO-A, maltreatment, and gene–environment interaction predicting children's mental health: New evidence and a meta-analysis. *Molecular Psychiatry, 11,* 903–913.

Klein, G. S. (1976). Freud's two theories of sexuality. In M. M. Gill & P. S. Holzman (Eds.), Psychology versus metapsychology: Psychoanalytic essays in memory of George S. Klein. *Psychological Issues, 9*(4, Monograph No. 36).

Klein, J. D., & Schnackenberg, H. L. (2000). Effects of informal cooperative learning and the affiliation motive on achievement, attitude, and student interactions. *Contemporary Educational Psychology, 25,* 332–341.

Klein, M. (1948). *Contributions to psychoanalysis,* 1921–1945. London: Hogarth Press.

Klein Villa, K., Shevrin, H., Snodgrass, M., Bazan, A., & Brakel, L. A. W. (2006). Testing Freud's hypothesis that word forms and word meaning are functionally distinct: Subliminal primary-process cognition and its link to personality. *Neuro-Psychoanalysis, 8,* 117–138.

Klepp, K. I., Kelder, S. H., & Perry, C. L. (1995). Alcohol and marijuana use among adolescents: Long-term outcomes of the class of 1989 study. *Annals of Behavioral Medicine, 17,* 19–24.

Klonsky, E. D., Oltmanns, T. F., & Turkheimer, E. (2002). Informant-reports of personality disorder: Relation to self-reports and future research directions. *Clinical Psychology: Science and Practice, 9,* 300–311.

Kohut, H. (1966). Forms and transformations of narcissism. *Journal of the American Psychoanalytic Association, 14,* 243–272.

Kohut, H. (1971). *The analysis of the self: A systematic psychoanalytic approach to the treatment of narcissistic personality disorders.* New York: International Universities Press.

Kohut, H. (1977). *The restoration of the self.* New York: International Universities Press.

Kohut, H. (1984). *How does analysis cure?* (A. Goldberg, Ed., with collaboration of P. E. Stepansky). Chicago: University of Chicago Press.

Kohut, H., & Wolf, E. (1978). The disorders of the self and their treatment: An outline. *International Journal of Psycho-Analysis, 59,* 413–425.

Krohn, A., & Mayman, M. (1974). Object representations in dreams and projective tests. *Bulletin of the Menninger Clinic, 38,* 445–466.

Lear, J. (1998). *Open minded: Working out the logic of the soul.* Cambridge, MA: Harvard University Press.

Leary, K. (1994). Psychoanalytic "problems" and postmodern "solutions." *Psychoanalytic Quarterly, 63,* 433–465.

Lemche, E., Giampietro, V. P., Surguladze, S. A., Amaro, E. J., Andrew, C. M., Williams, S. C. R., et al. (2006). Human attachment security is mediated by the amygdala: Evidence from combined fMRI and psychophysiological measures. *Human Brain Mapping, 27,* 623–635.

Lerner, H. D., & St. Peter, S. (1984). Patterns of object relations in neurotic, borderline, and schizophrenic patients. *Psychiatry, 47,* 77–92.

Levine, H. B. (1994). The analyst's participation in the analytic process. *International Journal of Psycho-Analysis, 75,* 665–676.

LeVine, R. (1982). *Culture, behavior, and personality* (2nd ed.). Chicago: Aldine.

Levy, K.N., Blatt, S., & Shaver, P. (1998). Attachment styles and parental representations. *Journal of Personality and Social Psychology, 74,* 407–419.

Levy, K. N., Meehan, K. B., Kelly, K. M., Reynoso, J. S., Weber, M., Clarkin, J. F., et al. (2006). Change in attachment patterns and reflective function in a randomized control trial of transference-focused psychotherapy for borderline personality disorder. *Journal of Consulting and Clinical Psychology, 74,* 1027–1040.

Lewicki, P. (1986). *Nonconscious social information processing.* New York: Academic Press.

Lichtenberg, J. (1989). *Psychoanalysis and motivation.* Hillsdale, NJ: Analytic Press.

Liddell, B. J., Williams, L. M., Rathjen, J., Shevrin, H., & Gordon, E. (2004). A temporal dissociation of subliminal versus supraliminal fear perception: An event-related potential study. *Journal of Cognitive Neuroscience, 16,* 479–486.

Lieberman, M. D. (2007). Social cognitive neuroscience: A review of core processes. *Annual Review of Psychology, 58,* 259–289.

London, B., Downey, G., Bonica, C., & Paltin, I. (2007). Social causes and consequences of rejection sensitivity. *Journal of Research on Adolescence, 17,* 481–506.

Luborsky, L., & Crits-Christoph, P. (1998). *Understanding transference: The Core Conflictual Relationship Theme method* (2nd ed.). Washington, DC: American Psychological Association.

Luyten, P., Blatt, S. J., & Corveleyn, J. (2006). Minding the gap between positivism and hermeneutics in psychoanalytic research. *Journal of the American Psychoanalytic Association, 54,* 571–610.

Lyons-Ruth, K., Yellin, C., Melnick, S., & Atwood, G. (2005). Expanding the concept of unresolved mental states: Hostile/helpless states of mind on the Adult Attachment Interview are associated with disrupted mother–infant communication and infant disorganization. *Development and Psychopathology, 17,* 1–23.

Mahler, M., Pine, F., & Bergman, A. (1975). *The psychological birth of the human infant: Symbiosis and individuation.* New York: Basic Books.

Main, M. (1990). Cross-cultural studies of attachment organization: Recent studies, changing methodologies, and the concept of conditional strategies. *Human Development, 33,* 48–61.

Main, M., & Goldwin, R. (1991). *Adult attachment classification system, version 5.* Unpublished manuscript, University of California, Berkeley.

Main, M., Kaplan, N., & Cassidy, J. (1985). Security in infancy, childhood, and adulthood: A move to the level of representation. In I. Bretherton & E. Waters (Eds.), Growing points of attachment theory and research. *Monographs of the Society for Research in Child Development, 50*(1–2, Serial No. 209), 67–104.

Manian, N., Papadakis, A. A., Strauman, T. J., & Essex, M. J. (2006). The development of children's ideal and ought self-guides: Parenting, temperament, and individual differences in guide strength. *Journal of Personality, 74,* 1619–1645.

Marcia, J. E. (1994). Ego identity and object relations. In J. M. Masling & R. E. Bornstein (Eds.), *Empirical perspectives on object relations theory* (pp. 59–103). Washington, DC: American Psychological Association.

Marcia, J. E. (2006). Ego identity and personality disorders. *Journal of Personality Disorders, 20,* 577–596.

Mathews, A., Yiend, J., & Lawrence, A. D. (2004). Individual differences in the modulation of fear-related brain activation by attentional control. *Journal of Cognitive Neuroscience, 16,* 1683–1694.

Mayman, M. (1967). Object-representation and object relationships in Rorschach responses. *Journal of Projective Techniques and Personality Assessment, 31,* 17–24.

Mayman, M. (1968). Early memories and character structure. *Journal of Projective Techniques and Personality Assessment, 32,* 303–316.

McAdams, D. P. (2006). The redemptive self: Generativity and the stories Americans live by. *Research in Human Development, 3,* 81–100.

McAdams, D. P., & Powers, J. (1981). Themes of intimacy in behavior and thought. *Journal of Personality and Social Psychology, 40,* 573–587.

McAdams, D. P., Reynolds, J., Lewis, M., Patten, A. H., & Bowman, P. J. (2001). When bad things turn good and good things turn bad: Sequences of redemption and contamination in life narratives and their relation to psychosocial adaptation in midlife adults and in students. *Personality and Social Psychology Bulletin, 27,* 474–485.

McClelland, D. C., Koestner, R., & Weinberger, J. (1989). How do self-attributed and implicit motives differ? *Psychological Review, 96,* 690–702.

Meehl, P. E. (1995). Bootstraps taxometrics: Solving the classification problem in psychopathology. *American Psychologist, 50,* 266–275.

Menninger, K., Mayman, M., & Pruyser, P. (1963). *The vital balance: The life process in mental health and illness.* New York: Viking.

Mickelson, K., Kessler, R. C., & Shaver, P. (1997). Adult attachment in a nationally representative sample. *Journal of Personality and Social Psychology, 73,* 1092–1106.

Mikulincer, M. (1998a). Adult attachment style and affect regulation: Strategic variations in self-appraisals. *Journal of Personality and Social Psychology, 75,* 420–435.

Mikulincer, M. (1998b). Adult attachment style and individual differences in functional versus dysfunctional experiences of anger. *Journal of Personality and Social Psychology, 74,* 513–524.

Mikulincer, M., Shaver, P., Gillath, O., & Nitzberg, R. (2005). Attachment, caregiving, and altruism: Boosting attachment security increases compassion and helping. *Journal of Personality and Social Psychology, 89,* 817–839.

Miller, J. D., & Pilkonis, P. A. (2006). Neuroticism and affective instability: The same or different? *American Journal of Psychiatry, 163,* 839–845.

Mischel, W., & Shoda, Y. (1995). A cognitive–affective system theory of personality: Reconceptualizing situations, dispositions, dynamics, and invariance in personality structure. *Psychological Review, 102,* 246–268.

Mitchell, S. A. (1988). *Relational concepts in psychoanalysis: An integration. Cambridge, MA: Harvard University Press.

Mitchell, S. A. (1993). Hope and dread in psychoanalysis. New York: Basic Books.

Mitchell, S. A. (1997). Autonomy and influence in psychoanalysis. Hillsdale, NJ: Analytic Press.

Mitchell, S. A., & Aron, L. (Eds.). (1999). Relational psychoanalysis: The emergence of a tradition. Mahwah, NJ: Analytic Press.

Moray, N. (1969). Attention: Selective processes in vision and hearing. London: Hutchinson.

Munro, G. D., Ditto, P. H., Lockhart, L. K., Fagerlin, A., Gready, M., & Peterson, E. (2002). Biased assimilation of sociopolitical arguments: Evaluating the 1996 U.S. presidential debate. Basic and Applied Social Psychology, 24, 15–26.

Natterson, J. (1991). Beyond countertransference: The therapist's subjectivity in the therapeutic process. Northvale, NJ: Aronson.

Nemeroff, C. B. (2004). Neurobiological consequences of childhood trauma. Journal of Clinical Psychiatry, 65, 18–28.

Nemeroff, C. B., Bremner, J. D., Foa, E. B., Mayberg, H. S., North, C. S., & Stein, M. B. (2006). Posttraumatic stress disorder: A state-of-the-science review. Journal of Psychiatric Research, 40, 1–21.

Newman, B. M., Lohman, B. J., & Newman, P. R. (2007). Peer group membership and a sense of belonging: Their relationship to adolescent behavior problems. Adolescence, 42, 241–263.

Niedenthal, P. M., Barsalou, L. W., Ric, F., & Krauth-Gruber, S. (2005). Embodiment in the acquisition and use of emotion knowledge. In L. F. Barrett, P. M. Niedenthal, & P. Winkielman (Eds.), Emotion and consciousness (pp. 21–50). New York: Guilford Press.

Niedenthal, P. M., Barsalou, L. W., Winkielman, P., Krauth-Gruber, S., & Ric, F. (2005). Embodiment in attitudes, social perception, and emotion. Personality and Social Psychology Review, 9, 184–211.

Nigg, J., Lohr, N. E., Westen, D., Gold, L., & Silk, K. R. (1992). Malevolent object representations in borderline personality disorder and major depression. Journal of Abnormal Psychology, 101, 61–67.

Nisbett, R. E., & Wilson, T. D. (1977). Telling more than we can know: Verbal reports on mental processes. Psychological Review, 84, 231–259.

Ogden, T. H. (1994). The analytic third: Working with intersubjective clinical facts. International Journal of Psycho-Analysis, 75, 3–19.

Ohman, A. (1994). "Unconscious anxiety": Phobic responses to masked stimuli. Journal of Abnormal Psychology, 103, 231–240.

Ohman, A., Carlsson, K., Lundqvist, D., & Ingvar, M. (2007). On the unconscious subcortical origin of human fear. Physiology and Behavior, 92, 180–185.

Ostafin, B. D., & Palfai, T. P. (2006). Compelled to consume: The Implicit Association Test and automatic alcohol motivation. Psychology of Addictive Behaviors, 20, 322–327.

Oyserman, D., & Fryberg, S. (2006). The possible selves of diverse adolescents: Content and function across gender, race and national origin. In C. Dunkel & J. Kerpelman (Eds.), Possible selves: Theory, research and applications (pp. 17–39). Hauppauge, NY: Nova Science.

Panksepp, J. (1998). Affective neuroscience: The foundations of human and animal emotions. New York: Oxford University Press.

Paulhus, D., Fridhandler, B., & Hayes, S. (1997). Psychological defense: Contemporary theory and research. In R. Hogan, J. Johnson, & S. R. Briggs (Eds.), Handbook of personality psychology (pp. 543–579). San Diego, CA: Academic Press.

Perry, J. C., & Cooper, S. H. (1987). Empirical studies of psychological defense mechanisms. In R. Michels & J. O. Cavenar (Eds.), Psychiatry (pp. 1–19). Philadelphia: Lippincott.

Perry, J. C., & Cooper, S. H. (1989). An empirical study of defense mechanisms: I. Clinical interview and life vignette ratings. Archives of General Psychiatry, 46, 444–460.

Perry, W., Minassian, A., Cadenhead, K., Sprock, J., & Braff, D. (2003). The use of the Ego Impairment Index across the schizophrenia spectrum. Journal of Personality Assessment, 80, 50–57.

Person, E., Cooper, A. M., & Gabbard, G. O. (Eds.). (2005). American Psychiatric Publishing textbook of psychoanalysis. Washington, DC: American Psychiatric Association.

Pervin, L. A. (1982). The stasis and flow of behavior: Toward a theory of goals. In M. M. Page (Ed.), Nebraska Symposium on Motivation (pp. 1–32). Lincoln: University of Nebraska Press.

Peterfreund, E. (1971). Information, systems, and psychoanalysis: An evolutionary biological approach to psychoanalytic theory. Psychological Issues, 7(1/2, Monograph No. 25/26).

Peters, E. J., Hilsenroth, M. J., Eudell-Simmons, E. M., Blagys, M. D., & Handler, L. (2006). Reliability and validity of the Social Cognition and Object Relations Scale in clinical use. Psychotherapy Research, 16, 606–614.

Pettigrew, T., & Meertens, R. (1995). Subtle and blatant prejudice in Western Europe. European Journal of Social Psychology, 25, 57–75.

Pettit, G., Bates, J., & Dodge, K. (1997). Supportive parenting, ecological context, and children's adjustment: A seven-year longitudinal study. Child Development, 68, 908–923.

Phelps, E. A., O'Connor, K. J., Cunningham, W. A., Funayama, E. S., Gatenby, J. C., Gore, J. C., et al. (2000). Performance on indirect measures of race evaluation predicts amygdala activation. *Journal of Cognitive Neuroscience, 12,* 729–738.

Pine, F. (1990). *Drive, ego, object, and self: A synthesis for clinical work.* New York: Basic Books.

Pinel, E. C., & Constantino, M. J. (2003). Putting self psychology to good use: When social and clinical psychologists unite. *Journal of Psychotherapy Integration, 13,* 9–32.

Pinsker-Aspen, J. H., Stein, M. B., & Hilsenroth, M. J. (2007). Clinical utility of early memories as a predictor of early therapeutic alliance. *Psychotherapy: Theory, Research, Practice, Training, 44,* 96–109.

Plutchik, R. (1980). A general psychoevolutionary theory of emotion. In R. Plutchik & H. Kellerman (Eds.), *Emotion: Vol. 1. Theories of emotion.* New York: Academic Press.

Plutchik, R. (1998). Emotions, diagnoses and ego defenses: A psychoevolutionary perspective. In W. Flack & J. D. Laird (Eds.), *Emotions in psychopathology: Theory and research* (pp. 367–379). New York: Oxford University Press.

Poetzl, O. (1960). The relationship between experimentally induced dream images and indirect vision. *Psychological Issues, 2*(Monograph No. 7), 41–120. (Original work published 1917)

Pope, K. S., Tabachnick, B. A., & Keith-Spiegel, P. (1987). Ethics of practice: The beliefs and behaviors of psychologists as therapists. *American Psychologist, 42,* 993–1006.

Porcerelli, J. H., Hill, K., & Dauphin, V. B. (1995). Need-gratifying object relations and psychopathology. *Bulletin of the Menninger Clinic, 59,* 99–104.

Porcerelli, J. H., Shahar, G., Blatt, S. J., Ford, R. Q., Mezza, J. A., & Greenlee, L. M. (2006). Social Cognition and Object Relations Scale: Convergent validity and changes following intensive inpatient treatment. *Personality and Individual Differences, 41,* 407–417.

Preston, S. D., & de Waal, F. B. M. (2002). Empathy: Its ultimate and proximate bases. *Behavioral and Brain Sciences, 25,* 1–72.

Pribram, K. H., & Gill, M. M. (1976). *Freud's "Project" re-assessed: Preface to contemporary cognitive theory and neuropsychology.* New York: Basic Books.

Priester, J. R., & Petty, R. E. (1996). The gradual negative threshold model of ambivalence: Relating positive and negative bases of attitudes to subjective ambivalence. *Journal of Personality and Social Psychology, 71,* 431–449.

Rapaport, D. (1951). *Organization and pathology of thought: Selected sources.* New York: Columbia University Press.

Rapaport, D. (1967). The scientific methodology of psychoanalysis. In M. Gill (Ed.), *The collected papers of David Rapaport* (pp. 165–220). New York: Basic Books. (Original work published 1944)

Rapaport, D., Schafer, R., & Gill, M. (1945–1946). *Diagnostic psychological testing* (2 vols.). Chicago: Year Book Medical.

Reber, A. (1992). The cognitive unconscious: An evolutionary perspective. *Consciousness and Cognition, 1,* 93–133.

Redl, R. A., & Wineman, D. (1951). *Children who hate.* New York: Collier.

Renik, O. (1993). Analytic interaction: Conceptualizing technique in light of the analyst's irreducible subjectivity. *Psychoanalytic Quarterly, 62,* 553–571.

Renik, O. (1998). The analyst's subjectivity and the analyst's objectivity. *International Journal of Psycho-Analysis, 79,* 487–497.

Richards, A. (1986). Introduction. In A. Richards & M. S. Willick (Eds.), *Psychoanalysis, the science of mental conflict: Essays in honor of Charles Brenner* (pp. 1–27). Hillsdale, NJ: Erlbaum.

Ricks, M. H. (1985). The social transmission of parental behavior: Attachment across generations. In I. Bretherton & E. Waters (Eds.), Growing points of attachment theory and research. *Monographs of the Society for Research in Child Development, 50,* (1–2, Serial No. 209), 211–227.

Ricoeur, P. (1971). *Freud and philosophy: An essay on interpretation* (D. Savage, Trans.). New Haven, CT: Yale University Press.

Riggs, S. A., Paulson, A., Tunnell, E., Sahl, G., Atkinson, H., & Ross, C. A. (2007). Attachment, personality, and psychopathology among adult inpatients: Self-reported romantic attachment style versus Adult Attachment Interview states of mind. *Development and Psychopathology, 19,* 263–291.

Rizzolatti, G., & Craighero, L. (2004). The mirror-neuron system. *Annual Review of Neuroscience, 27,* 169–192.

Roediger, H. L. (1990). Implicit memory: Retention without remembering. *American Psychologist, 45,* 1043–1056.

Rubenstein, B. (1976). On the possibility of a strictly clinical theory: An essay on the philosophy of psychoanalysis. In M. M. Gill & P. S. Holzman (Eds.), Psychology versus metapsychology: Psychoanalytic essays in memory of George S. Klein. *Psychological Issues, 9*(4, Monograph No. 36).

Rumelhart, D. E., McClelland, J. L., & the PDP Research Group. (1986). *Parallel distributed processing: Explanations in the microstructures of cognition* (2 vols.). Cambridge, MA: MIT Press.

Rutter, M. (2005). Environmentally mediated risks for psychopathology: Research strategies and findings. *Journal of the American Academy of Child and Adolescent Psychiatry, 44,* 3–18.

Sandler, J. (1976). Countertransference and role-responsiveness. *International Review of Psycho-Analysis, 3,* 43–47.

Sandler, J. (1991). Character traits and object relationships. *Psychoanalytic Quarterly, 50,* 694–708.

Sandler, J., & Rosenblatt, B. (1962). The concept of the representational world. *Psychoanalytic Study of the Child, 17,* 128–145.

Sandler, J., & Sandler, A. (1978). On the development of object relationships and affects. *International Journal of Psycho-Analysis, 59,* 285–296.

Saxe, R., Carey, S., & Kanwisher, N. (2004). Understanding other minds: Linking developmental psychology and functional neuroimaging. *Annual Review of Psychology, 55,* 87–124.

Schacter, D. L. (1992). Understanding implicit memory: A cognitive neuroscience approach. *American Psychologist, 47,* 559–569.

Schacter, D. L. (1995). Implicit memory: A new frontier for cognitive neuroscience. In M. Gazzaniga (Ed.), *The cognitive neurosciences* (pp. 815–824). Cambridge, MA: MIT Press.

Schacter, D. L. (1998). Memory and awareness. *Science, 280,* 59–60.

Schafer, R. (1976). *A new language for psychoanalysis.* New Haven, CT: Yale University Press.

Scharf, J. S., & Scharf, D. (1998). *Object relations individual therapy.* New York: Aronson.

Seger, C. A. (1994). Implicit learning. *Psychological Bulletin, 115,* 163–196.

Shah, J., Higgins, T., & Friedman, R. S. (1998). Performance incentives and means: How regulatory focus influences goal attainment. *Journal of Personality and Social Psychology, 174,* 285–293.

Shedler, J., & Block, J. (1990). Adolescent drug use and psychological health: A longitudinal inquiry. *American Psychologist, 45,* 612–630.

Shedler, J., Mayman, M., & Manis, M. (1988). *Defensive self-esteem: Overview of research to date.* Unpublished manuscript, University of California, Berkeley.

Shedler, J., Mayman, M., & Manis, M. (1993). The illusion of mental health. *American Psychologist, 48,* 1117–1131.

Shedler, J., & Westen, D. (2004). Dimensions of personality pathology: An alternative to the five-factor model. *American Journal of Psychiatry, 161,* 1743–1754.

Shevrin, H. (1984). The fate of the five metaphysical principles. *Psychoanalytic Inquiry, 4,* 33–58.

Shevrin, H., Bond, J. A., Brakel, L. A. W., Hertel, R. K., & Williams, W. J. (1996). *Conscious and unconscious processes: Psychodynamic, cognitive, and neurophysiological convergences.* New York: Guilford Press.

Shevrin, H., & Dickman, S. (1980). The psychological unconscious: A necessary assumption for all psychological theory? *American Psychologist, 35,* 421–434.

Siegel, P., & Weinberger, J. (1998). Capturing the "Mommy and I are one" merger fantasy: The oneness motive. In R. F. Bornstein & J. M. Masling (Eds.), *Empirical perspectives on the psychoanalytic unconscious* (pp. 71–97). Washington, DC: American Psychological Association.

Silverman, L. H., & Weinberger, J. (1985). Mommy and I are one: Implication for psychotherapy. *American Psychologist, 12,* 1296–1308.

Simon, H. (1990). Invariants of human behavior. *Annual Review of Psychology, 41,* 1–19.

Singer, J. L., & Salovey, P. (1991). Organized knowledge structures and personality: Person schemas, prototypes, and scripts. In M. J. Horowitz (Ed.), *Person schemas and maladaptive interpersonal patterns* (pp. 33–79). Chicago: University of Chicago Press.

Slavin, M. O., & Kriegman, D. (1992). *The adaptive design of the human psyche: Psychoanalysis, evolutionary biology, and the therapeutic process.* New York: Guilford Press.

Smith, E. R. (1998). Mental representation and memory. In D. T. Gilbert, S. T. Fiske, & G. Lindzey (Eds.), *Handbook of social psychology* (Vol. 1, pp. 391–445). New York: McGraw-Hill.

Snodgrass, M., & Shevrin, H. (2006). Unconscious inhibition and facilitation at the objective detection threshold: Replicable and qualitatively different unconscious perceptual effects. *Cognition, 101,* 43–79.

Solms, M., & Turnbull, O. (2002). *The brain and the inner world: An introduction to the neuroscience of subjective experience.* New York: Other Press.

Spence, D. P. (1982). *Narrative truth and historical truth: Meaning and interpretation in psychoanalysis.* New York: Norton.

Spezzano, C. (1993). *Affect in psychoanalysis: A clinical synthesis.* Hillsdale, NJ: Analytic Press.

Spitzer, R. L., First, M. B., Shedler, J., Westen, D., & Skodol, A. E. (2008). Clinical utility of five dimensional systems for personality diagnosis: A "consumer preference" study. *Journal of Nervous and Mental Disease, 196*(5), 356–374.

Squire, L. R. (1987). *Memory and brain.* New York: Oxford University Press.

Sroufe, L. A., & Fleeson, J. (1986). Attachment and the construction of relationships. In W. W. Hartup & Z. Rubin (Eds.), *Relationships and development.* Hillsdale, NJ: Erlbaum.

Sroufe, L. A., & Waters, E. (1977). Attachment as an organizational construct. *Child Development, 48*, 1184–1199.

Steele, H., Steele, M., & Fonagy, P. (1996). Associations among attachment classifications of mothers, fathers, and their infants. *Child Development, 67*, 541–555.

Steffens, M. C., & König, S. S. (2006). Predicting spontaneous Big Five behavior with Implicit Association Test. *European Journal of Psychological Assessment, 22*, 13–20.

Stein, H., Koontz, A. D., Fonagy, P., Allen, J. G., Fultz, J., Brethour, J. R., et al. (2002). Adult attachment: What are the underlying dimensions? *Psychology and Psychotherapy: Theory, Research and Practice, 75*, 77–91.

Stolorow, R., Brandchaft, B., & Atwood, G. (1987). *Psychoanalytic treatment: An intersubjective approach.* Hillsdale, NJ: Analytic Press.

Strauman, T. J. (1996). Stability within the self: A longitudinal study of the structural implications of self-discrepancy theory. *Journal of Personality and Social Psychology, 71*, 1142–1153.

Strenger, C. (2006). Freud's forgotten evolutionary project. *Psychoanalytic Psychology, 23*, 420–429.

Sullivan, H. S. (1953). *The interpersonal theory of psychiatry.* New York: Norton.

Sulloway, F. J. (1979). *Freud: Biologist of the mind.* New York: Basic Books.

Suomi, S. J. (2004). How gene–environment interactions influence mental development in rhesus monkeys. In C. G. Coll, E. L. Bearer, & R. M. Lerner (Eds.), *Nature and nurture: The complex interplay of genetic and environmental influences on human behavior and development* (pp. 35–51). Mahwah, NJ: Erlbaum.

Suomi, S. J. (2005). How gene–environment interactions shape the development of impulsive aggression in rhesus monkeys. In D. M. Stoff & E. J. Susman (Eds.), *Developmental psychobiology of aggression* (pp. 252–268). New York: Cambridge University Press.

Swann, W. B., Jr. (1997). The trouble with change: Self-verification and allegiance to the self. *Psychological Science, 8*, 177–180.

Tansey, M. J., & Burke, W. F. (1989). *Understanding countertransference: From projective identification to empathy.* Hillsdale, NJ: Analytic Press.

Thagard, P. (2000). *Coherence in thought and action.* Cambridge, MA: MIT Press.

Thagard, P. (2005). The emotional coherence of religion. *Journal of Cognition and Culture, 5*, 58–74.

Thagard, P., Kroon, F., Nerb, J., Sahdra, B., Shelley, C., & Wagar, B. (2006). *Hot thought: Mechanisms and applications of emotional cognition.* Cambridge, MA: MIT Press.

Tomkins, S. (1962). *Affect, imagery, consciousness* (Vol. 1). New York: Springer.

Trivers, R. (1971). The evolution of reciprocal altruism. *Quarterly Review of Biology, 46*, 35–57.

Urist, J. (1980). Object relations. In R. W. Woody (Ed.), *Encyclopedia of clinical assessment* (Vol. 2, pp. 821–833). San Francisco: Jossey-Bass.

Vaillant, G. E. (1977). *Adaptation to life.* Boston: Little, Brown.

Vaillant, G. E. (Ed.). (1992). *Ego mechanisms of defense: A guide for clinicians and researchers.* Washington, DC: American Psychiatric Association.

Vaillant, G. E. (2000). Adaptive mental mechanisms: Their role in a positive psychology. *American Psychologist, 55*, 89–98.

Vaillant, G. E., & Drake, R. E. (1985). Maturity of defenses in relation to DSM-III Axis II personality disorder. *Archives of General Psychiatry, 42*, 597–601.

van IJzendoorn, M. H., Moran, G., Belsky, J., Pederson, D., Bakermans-Kranenburg, M. J., & Kneppers, K. (2000). The similarity of siblings' attachments to their mother. *Child Development, 71*, 1086–1098.

Wachtel, P. L. (1977). *Psychoanalysis and behavior therapy.* New York: Basic Books.

Wachtel, P. L. (1987). *Action and insight.* New York: Guilford Press.

Wachtel, P. L. (1997). *Psychoanalysis, behavior therapy, and the relational world.* Washington, DC: American Psychological Association.

Wagar, B. M., & Thagard, P. (2004). Spiking Phineas Gage: A neurocomputational theory of cognitive–affective integration in decision making. *Psychological Review, 111*, 67–79.

Wallerstein, R. S. (1988). One psychoanalysis or many? *International Journal of Psycho-Analysis, 69*, 5–22.

Watson, D., & Clark, L. A. (1984). Negative affectivity: The disposition to experience aversive emotional states. *Psychological Bulletin, 96*, 465–490.

Weinberger, D. A. (1995). The construct validity of the repressive coping style. In J. L. Singer (Ed.), *Repression and dissociation: Implications for personality theory, psychopathology, and health* (pp. 337–386). Chicago: University of Chicago Press.

Weinberger, D. A., Schwartz, G. E., & Davidson, R. J. (1979). Low-anxious, high-anxious, and repressive coping styles: Psychometric patterns and behavioral and psychological responses to stress. *Journal of Abnormal Psychology, 88*, 369–380.

Weinberger, J. (2008). *The unconscious.* Unpublished manuscript, Adelphi University.

Weinberger, J., Seifert, C., & Siegal, P. (2008). *What you can't see can help you: The effects of subliminal exposure to spiders on approach behavior.* Unpublished manuscript.

Weinberger, J., & Silverman, L. (1988). *Testability and empirical verification of psychoanalytic dynamic propositions through subliminal psychodynamic activation.* Unpublished manuscript, H. A. Murray Center, Harvard University, Cambridge, MA.

Weinberger, J., & Westen, D. (in press). RATS, we should have used Clinton: Subliminal priming in political campaigns. *Political Psychology.*

Wenzlaff, R. M., & Wegner, D. M. (2000). Thought suppression. *Annual Review of Psychology, 51,* 59–91.

Westen, D. (1985). *Self and society: Narcissism, collectivism, and the development of morals.* New York: Cambridge University Press.

Westen, D. (1990a). Psychoanalytic approaches to personality. In L. Pervin (Ed.), *Handbook of personality: Theory and research* (pp. 21–65). New York: Guilford Press.

Westen, D. (1990b). Toward a revised theory of borderline object relations: Implications of empirical research. *International Journal of Psycho-Analysis, 71,* 661–693.

Westen, D. (1991). Social cognition and object relations. *Psychological Bulletin, 109,* 429–455.

Westen, D. (1994). Toward an integrative model of affect regulation: Applications to social-psychological research. *Journal of Personality, 62,* 641–647.

Westen, D. (1997). Toward an empirically and clinically sound theory of motivation. *International Journal of Psycho-Analysis, 78,* 521–548.

Westen, D. (1998a). Case formulation and personality diagnosis: Two processes or one? In James Barron (Ed.), *Making diagnosis meaningful* (pp. 111–138). Washington, DC: American Psychological Association.

Westen, D. (1998b). The scientific legacy of Sigmund Freud: Toward a psychodynamically informed psychological science. *Psychological Bulletin, 124,* 333–371.

Westen, D. (1999a). Psychodynamic theory and technique in relation to research on cognition and emotion: Mutual implications. In T. Dalgleish & M. J. Power (Eds.), *Handbook of cognition and emotion* (pp. 727–746). New York: Wiley.

Westen, D. (1999b). The scientific status of unconscious processes: Is Freud really dead? *Journal of the American Psychoanalytic Association, 47,* 1061–1106.

Westen, D. (2002). The language of psychoanalytic discourse. *Psychoanalytic Dialogues, 12,* 857–898.

Westen, D. (2007). *The political brain: The role of emotion in deciding the fate of the nation.* New York: Public Affairs Books.

Westen, D., & Blagov, P. (2007). A clinical–empirical model of emotion regulation: From defense and motivated reasoning to emotional constraint satisfaction. In J. J. Gross (Ed.), *Handbook of emotion regulation* (pp. 373–392). New York: Guilford Press.

Westen, D., Blagov, P. S., Harenski, K., Kilts, C., & Hamann, S. (2006). Neural bases of motivated reasoning: An fMRI study of emotional constraints on partisan political judgment in the 2004 U.S. presidential election. *Journal of Cognitive Neuroscience, 18,* 1947–1958.

Westen, D., Feit, A., & Zittel, C. (1999). Methodological issues in research using projective techniques. In P. C. Kendall, J. N. Butcher, & G. Holmbeck (Eds.), *Handbook of research methods in clinical psychology* (2nd ed., pp. 224–240). New York: Wiley.

Westen, D., & Gabbard, G. O. (2002a). Developments in cognitive neuroscience: 1. Conflict, compromise, and connectionism. *Journal of the American Psychoanalytic Association, 50,* 53–98.

Westen, D., & Gabbard, G. O. (2002b). Developments in cognitive neuroscience: 2. Implications for the concept of transference. *Journal of the American Psychoanalytic Association, 50,* 99–133.

Westen, D., Gabbard, G. O., & Blagov, P. (2006). Back to the future: Personality structure as a context for psychopathology. In R. F. Krueger & J. L. Tackett (Eds.), *Personality and psychopathology* (pp. 335–384). New York: Guilford Press.

Westen, D., Klepser, J., Ruffins, S., Silverman, M., Lifton, N., & Boekamp, J. (1991). Object relations in childhood and adolescence: The development of working representations. *Journal of Consulting and Clinical Psychology, 59,* 400–409.

Westen, D., Lohr, N., Silk, K., Gold, L., & Kerber, K. (1990). Object relations and social cognition in borderlines, major depressives, and normals: A TAT analysis. *Psychological Assessment: A Journal of Consulting and Clinical Psychology, 2,* 355–364.

Westen, D., & Muderrisoglu, S. (2006). Clinical assessment of pathological personality traits. *American Journal of Psychiatry, 163,* 1285–1297.

Westen, D., Muderrisoglu, S., Fowler, C., Shedler, J., & Koren, D. (1997). Affect regulation and affective experience: Individual differences, group differences, and measurement using a Q-sort procedure. *Journal of Consulting and Clinical Psychology, 65,* 429–439.

Westen, D., Nakash, O., Thomas, C., & Bradley,

R. (2006). Clinical assessment of attachment patterns and personality disorder in adolescents and adults. *Journal of Consulting and Clinical Psychology, 74,* 1065–1085.

Westen, D., & Shedler, J. (1999a). Revising and assessing Axis II: Part I. Developing a clinically and empirically valid assessment method. *American Journal of Psychiatry, 156,* 258–272.

Westen, D., & Shedler, J. (1999b). Revising and assessing Axis II: Part II. Toward an empirically based and clinically useful classification of personality disorders. *American Journal of Psychiatry, 156,* 273–285.

Westen, D., & Shedler, J. (2007). Personality diagnosis with the Shedler–Westen Assessment Procedure (SWAP): Integrating clinical and statistical measurement and prediction. *Journal of Abnormal Psychology, 116,* 810–822.

Westen, D., & Weinberger, J. (2004). When clinical description becomes statistical prediction. *American Psychologist, 59,* 595–613.

Westen, D., & Weinberger, J. (2005). In praise of clinical judgment: Meehl's forgotten legacy. *Journal of Clinical Psychology, 61,* 1257–1276.

Westen, D., Weinberger, J., & Bradley, R. (2007). Motivation, decision making, and consciousness: From psychodynamics to subliminal priming and emotional constraint satisfaction. In P. D. Zelazo, M. Moscovitch, & E. Thompson (Eds.), *The Cambridge handbook of consciousness* (pp. 673–702). New York: Cambridge University Press.

White, R. W. (1959). Motivation reconsidered: The concept of competence. *Psychological Review, 66,* 297–333.

Williams, G. C. (1966). *Adaptation and natural selection: A critique of some current evolutionary thought.* Princeton, NJ: Princeton University Press.

Wilson, E. O. (1978). *On human nature.* New York: Bantam.

Wilson, T. D. (2002). *Strangers to ourselves: Discovering the adaptive unconscious.* Cambridge, MA: Harvard University Press.

Wittenbrink, B., & Schwarz, N. (Eds.). (2007). *Implicit measures of attitudes.* New York: Guilford Press.

Wolf, N. S., Gales, M. E., Shane, E., & Shane, M. (2001). The developmental trajectory from amodal perception to empathy and communication: The role of mirror neurons in this process. *Psychoanalytic Inquiry, 21,* 94–112.

Wolff, P. H. (1960). The developmental psychologies of Jean Piaget and psychoanalysis. *Psychological Issues, 2* (Monograph 5).

Wong, P., Shevrin, H., & Williams, W. J. (1994). Conscious and nonconscious processes: An ERP index of an anticipatory response in a conditioning paradigm using visually masked stimuli. *Psychophysiology, 31,* 87–101.

Young, J. E. (1999). *Cognitive therapy for personality disorders: A schema-focused approach* (3rd ed.). Sarasota, FL: Professional Resource Press.

Zanarini, M. C. (1997). *Role of sexual abuse in the etiology of borderline personality disorder.* Washington, DC: American Psychiatric Association.

CHAPTER 4

Paradigm Shift
to the Integrative Big Five Trait Taxonomy
History, Measurement, and Conceptual Issues

Oliver P. John
Laura P. Naumann
Christopher J. Soto

Since the first version of this chapter (John, 1990) was completed in the late 1980s, the field of personality trait research has changed dramatically. At that time, the Big Five personality dimensions, now seemingly ubiquitous, were hardly known. Researchers, as well as practitioners in the field of personality assessment, were faced with a bewildering array of personality scales from which to choose, with little guidance and no organizing theory or framework at hand. What made matters worse was that scales with the same name might measure concepts that were quite different, and scales with different names might measure concepts that were quite similar. Although diversity and scientific pluralism can be useful, systematic accumulation of findings and communication among researchers had become almost impossible amidst the cacophony of competing concepts and scales.

At the University of California, Berkeley, for example, researchers studied personality with as few as two, and as many as 20 concepts, including the two dimensions of ego-resilience and ego-control that Block and Block (1980) measured with their California Q-sort; the four scales on the Myers–Briggs Type Indicator (MBTI; Myers & McCaulley, 1985) that measure extraversion, feeling, judging, and intuition; and the 20 scales on the California Psychological Inventory (CPI; Gough, 1987) measuring folk concepts such as capacity for status, self-control, well-being, tolerance, and achievement via independence (see Table 4.1). At the time, many personality researchers were hoping to be the one who would discover the right structure that all others would then adopt, thus transforming the fragmented field into a community speaking a common language. However, we now know that such an integration was not to be achieved by any one researcher or by any one theoretical perspective. As Allport once put it, "each assessor has his own pet units and uses a pet battery of diagnostic devices" (1958, p. 258).

What personality psychology lacked was a descriptive model, or taxonomy, of its subject matter. One of the central goals of scientific taxonomies is the definition of overarching domains within which large numbers of specific instances can be understood in a simplified way. Thus, in person-

TABLE 4.1. Personality Dimensions in Questionnaires and in Models of Personality and Interpersonal Behavior: Classified by Big Five Domain

Theorist	Extraversion I	Agreeableness II	Conscientiousness III	Neuroticism IV	Openness/Intellect V
Bales (1970)	Dominant–Initiative	Social–Emotional Orientation	Task Orientation[a]		—
Block & Block (1980)	Undercontrol	Overcontrol		Ego-Resiliency[b] (R)	
A. H. Buss & Plomin (1975)	Activity Sociability	—	Impulsivity (R)	Emotionality	—
Cattell (1943)	Exvia (vs. Invia)	Pathemia (vs. Cortertia)	Superego Strength	Adjustment (R) (vs. Anxiety)	Independence
Clark & Watson (1999)	Positive Emotionality	Constraint (vs. Disinhibition)[c]		Negative Emotionality	
Comrey (1970)	Extraversion, Activity	Femininity (vs. Masculinity)	Orderliness, Social Conformity	Emotional Stability (R)	Rebelliousness
Eysenck (1986)	Extraversion	Psychoticism[c] (R)		Neuroticism	—
Gough (1987) CPI Vectors	Externality		Norm-Favoring	Self-Realization[d] (R)	
CPI Scales	Sociability	Femininity	Achievement via Conformance	Well-Being (R)	Achievement via Independence
Guilford (1975)	Social Activity	Paranoid Disposition (R)	Thinking Introversion	Emotional Stability (R)	—
Hogan (1986)	Sociability	Likeability	Prudence (vs. Impulsivity)	Adjustment (R)	Intellectance
Jackson (1984)	Outgoing, Social Leadership	Self-Protective Orientation (R)	Work Orientation	Dependence (R)	Aesthetic–Intellectual
MMPI; Myers & McCauley (1985)	Extraversion (vs. Introversion)	Feeling (vs. Thinking)	Judging (vs. Perceiving)	—	Intuition (vs. Sensing)
MBTI; Tellegen (1982)	Positive Emotionality Agentive	Communal	Constraint	Negative Emotionality	Absorption
Tellegen et al. (2003)	Histrionic	Paranoid (R)	Compulsive	Borderline	Schizotypal
Wiggins[e] (1979)	Power/Dominance	Nurturance	(Conscientiousness)	(Neuroticism)	(Openness)

Note. Based on John (1990) and McCrae and John (1992). (R) indicates that the dimension was reverse-scored in the direction *opposite* to that of the Big Five label listed above. MBTI, Myers–Briggs Type Indicator; MMPI-2, Minnesota Multiphasic Personality Inventory—2.

[a] This dimension contrasts a work-directed, emotionally neutral orientation with an erratic, emotionally expressive orientation (Bales, 1970), and thus seems to combine elements of both Conscientiousness and Neuroticism.

[b] Ego-resiliency seems to subsume aspects of both Openness and low Neuroticism, because an ego-resilient individual is considered both intellectually resourceful and effective in controlling anxiety (Block & Block, 1980). However, Robins, John, and Caspi (1994) found that in adolescents, ego-resiliency is related to all of the Big Five dimensions in the well-adjusted direction. The ego-control construct was related to Extraversion, Conscientiousness, and Agreeableness, with the undercontrolled pole most similar to Extraversion and overcontrolled pole most similar to Conscientiousness and Agreeableness.

[c] High scores on the GTS Constraint scale are correlated with both Agreeableness and Conscientious (L. A. Clark & Watson, 1999; Markon et al., 2005). Conversely, the EPQ Psychoticism scale is associated with low scores on both Agreeableness and Conscientiousness (Goldberg & Rosolack, 1994; McCrae & Costa, 1985a).

[d] The third vector scale on the CPI (Gough, 1987) measures levels of psychological integration and realization and should reflect aspects of both low Neuroticism (e.g., Well-Being) and high Openness (e.g., Achievement via Independence).

[e] Wiggins (1979) originally focused on Dominance and Nurturance, which define the interpersonal circumplex. The dimensions in parentheses indicate that Trapnell and Wiggins (1990) added adjective scales for Conscientiousness, Neuroticism, and Openness after the emergence of the Big Five (see also Wiggins, 1995).

ality psychology, a taxonomy would permit researchers to study specified domains of related personality characteristics, rather than examining separately the thousands of particular attributes that make human beings individual and unique. Moreover, a generally accepted taxonomy would facilitate the accumulation and communication of empirical findings by offering a standard vocabulary, or nomenclature.

After decades of research, the field has now achieved an initial consensus on a general taxonomy of personality traits, the "Big Five" personality dimensions. These dimensions do not represent a particular theoretical perspective but were derived from analyses of the natural-language terms people use to describe themselves and others. Rather than replacing all previous systems, the Big Five taxonomy serves an integrative function because it can represent the various and diverse systems of personality description in a common framework, as shown by the columns organizing Table 4.1.

OUTLINE AND GOALS OF THIS CHAPTER

The first version of this chapter (John, 1990) offered a comprehensive and detailed review of most of the available research. This is no longer possible as we are writing this chapter in 2007. What has happened? Figure 4.1 uses publication trends over the past 25 years to illustrate how fundamentally the field has changed. Specifically, we show the number of publications related to the Big Five personality traits for each 5-year interval, beginning in the early 1980s, obtained from keyword searches of the PsycINFO database. To provide a comparison, we also show the publication trend for the influential models developed earlier by Cattell and by Eysenck. Although both were then close to retirement age, their influence had continued during the 1980s. In fact, both Cattell (1990) and Eysenck (1990) had written chapters on personality traits for the first edition of this handbook.

What did we expect to find? Our intuitions suggested that publications on the Big

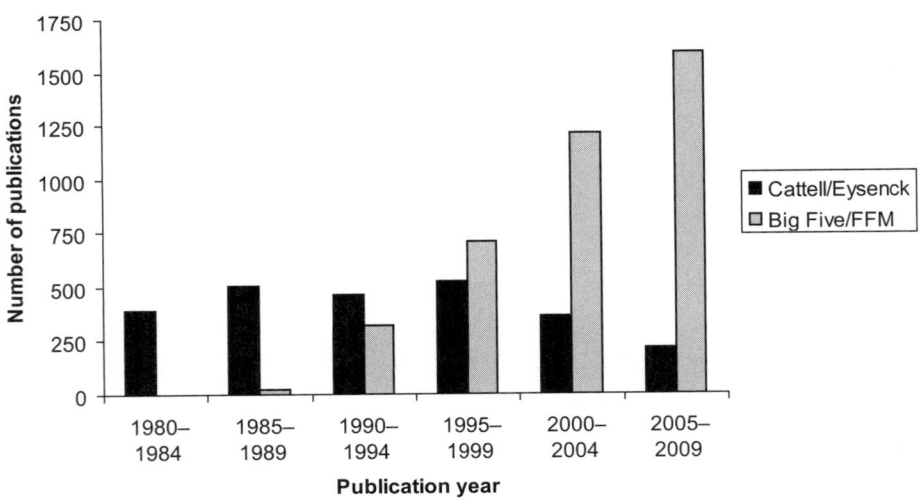

FIGURE 4.1. Number of publications related to either the Big Five personality traits or to the influential models developed earlier by Cattell and by Eysenck (in 5-year intervals), identified in keyword searches of the PsycINFO database. *Note*: The numbers identified in the figure as *Cattell/Eysenck* refer to the sum of all articles that used one of the measures developed by either Eysenck or Cattell as a keyword, such as "EPI," "EPQ," and "16PF"; those identified as *Big Five/FFM* are the sum of all articles that used as one of their keywords "Big Five," "Five Factor Model," "5 Factor Model," and "+ personality" (to rule out misidentifications of articles using these keywords in other literatures, such as the "big five game animals in Africa"). To estimate the projected publication trends for 2005–2009 (which were not yet available when this chapter was completed), we computed the sum of articles for 2005 and 2006 and multiplied that 2-year period by 2.5.

Five had increased substantially since the mid-1980s, with Cattell's and Eysenck's influence decreasing. But we were surprised by the data. First, the ascent of the Big Five happened much more gradually than we had expected, and Cattell's and Eysenck's influence held steady much longer. As Figure 4.1 shows, it took until the late 1990s for the number of Big Five publications to finally overtake the two older models. Second, whereas references to Cattell and Eysenck models have finally begun to decline in absolute numbers, their decline has been small compared to the amazing increase in research publications on the Big Five. By 2006, the last year for which we had figures available, the number of Big Five publications exceeded 300 per year, compared with less than 50 for the two older models.

In the 9 years since the previous version of this chapter (John & Srivastava, 1999) was completed, almost 2,000 new publications on the Big Five have appeared. As a result, we can now cover only a small fraction of all the relevant work in this chapter. Our main goal remains to provide a general overview and introduction to the field that focuses on the main issues and can serve as a useful reference resource. We therefore refer the reader to more specialized sources or reviews as needed. We begin our chapter with the history of the Big Five, including the discovery of the five dimensions, research replicating and extending the model, its convergence with research in the questionnaire tradition, and the development of several instruments to measure the Big Five. Then we compare three of the most frequently used instruments and discuss some new data regarding their reliability and validity. Finally, we address a number of conceptual issues, including how the Big Five taxonomy is structured hierarchically, how the five dimensions develop, whether they predict important life outcomes, and whether they are descriptive or explanatory concepts.

THE LEXICAL APPROACH AND DISCOVERY OF THE BIG FIVE

One starting place for a shared taxonomy is the natural language of personality description. Beginning with Klages (1932), Baumgarten (1933), and Allport and Odbert (1936), various psychologists have turned to the natural language as a source of attributes for a scientific taxonomy. This work, beginning with the extraction of all personality-relevant terms from the dictionary, has been guided by the lexical approach (see John et al., 1988; Saucier & Goldberg, 1996b). The *lexical hypothesis* posits that most of the socially relevant and salient personality characteristics have become encoded in the natural language (e.g., Allport, 1937). Thus, the personality vocabulary contained in the dictionaries of a natural language provides an extensive, yet finite, set of attributes that the people speaking that language have found important and useful in their daily interactions (Goldberg, 1981).

Allport and Odbert's Psycholexical Study: Traits, States, Activities, and Evaluations

Following Baumgarten's (1933) work in German, Allport and Odbert (1936) conducted a seminal lexical study of the personality terms in an unabridged English dictionary. They included all terms that could be used to "distinguish the behavior of one human being from that of another" (Allport & Odbert, 1936, p. 24) and identified almost 18,000 terms—"a semantic nightmare" (Allport, 1937, pp. 353–354) that would keep psychologists "at work for a life time" (Allport & Odbert, 1936, p. vi). Indeed, this task has preoccupied personality psychologists for more than 60 years (for details, see John et al., 1988; John, 1990).

What kinds of person descriptors are included in the dictionary? Allport and Odbert identified four major categories: (1) personality traits (e.g., *sociable*, *aggressive*, and *fearful*), defined as "generalized and personalized determining tendencies—consistent and stable modes of an individual's adjustment to his environment" (p. 26); (2) temporary states, moods, and activities, such as *afraid*, *rejoicing*, and *elated*; (3) highly evaluative judgments of personal conduct and reputation, such as *excellent*, *worthy*, *average*, and *irritating*—although these terms presuppose some traits within the individual, they do not indicate the specific attributes that gave rise to the individual's evaluation by others or by society in general; and (4) physical characteristics, capacities and talents, and other terms of doubtful relevance to personality. Norman

(1967) elaborated these classifications into seven content categories: Individuals can be described by their enduring *traits* (e.g., irrascible), by the *internal states* they typically experience (furious), by the *physical states* they endure (trembling), by the *activities* they engage in (screaming), by the *effects* they have on others (frightening), by the *roles* they play (murderer), and by social *evaluations* of their conduct (unacceptable, bad). Moreover, individuals differ in their anatomical and morphological characteristics (short) and in the personal and societal evaluations attached to these appearance characteristics (cute).

Both Allport and Odbert (1936) and Norman (1967) classified the terms culled from the dictionary into mutually exclusive categories. However, their categories clearly overlap and have fuzzy boundaries. Chaplin, John, and Goldberg (1988) proposed a prototype conception where each category is defined in terms of its clear cases rather than its boundaries. Chaplin and colleagues applied this prototype conception to traits, states, and activities. Prototypical *states* were seen as temporary, brief, and externally caused. Prototypical traits were seen as stable, longlasting, internally caused, and needed to be observed more frequently and across a wider range of situations than states before they were attributed to an individual. These findings replicated the earlier classifications and confirmed that the lay conceptions of traits and states are widely shared and understood.

Identifying the Major Dimensions of Personality Description: Cattell's Early Efforts

Allport and Odbert's (1936) classifications provided some initial structure for the personality lexicon. However, to be of practical value, a taxonomy must provide a systematic framework for distinguishing, ordering, and naming individual differences in people's behavior and experience (John, 1989). Aiming for such a taxonomy, Cattell (1943) used the Allport and Odbert list as a starting point. Because the size of that list was too overwhelming for research purposes, Cattell (1943, 1945a, 1945b) began with the subset of 4,500 trait terms. Indeed, most taxonomic research has focused on the trait category, although the other categories are no less important; the emotional-state and social-

evaluation categories have recently received more attention (Almagor, Tellegen, & Waller, 1995; Benet-Martínez & Waller, 1997).

Using both semantic and empirical clustering procedures as well as his own reviews of the literature available at the time (for reviews, see John, 1990; John et al., 1988), Cattell reduced the 4,500 trait terms to a mere 35 variables, eliminating more than 99% of the initial terms. This drastic reduction was dictated primarily by the data-analytic limitations of his time, which made factor analyses of large variable sets prohibitively costly and complex. Using this small set of 35 variables, Cattell conducted several oblique factor analyses (i.e., allowing for correlated factors) and concluded that he had identified 12 factors, which became part of his 16 Personality Factors (16PF) questionnaire (Cattell, Eber, & Tatsuoka, 1970).

Cattell also claimed that his factors showed excellent correspondence across methods, such as self-reports, ratings by others, and objective tests; however, these claims have not gone unquestioned (e.g., Becker, 1960; Nowakowska, 1973). Moreover, reanalyses of Cattell's own correlation matrices by others have not confirmed the number and nature of the factors he proposed (e.g., Tupes & Christal, 1961, 1992). Digman and Takemoto-Chock (1981) concluded that Cattell's "original model, based on the unfortunate clerical errors noted here, cannot have been correct" (p. 168), although the second-order factors of the 16PF show some correspondence between Cattell's system and the Big Five dimensions discovered later.

THE "BIG FIVE" FACTORS IN PERSONALITY TRAIT RATINGS

Initial Discovery of the Big Five in Cattell's Variable List

Cattell's pioneering work and the availability of a relatively short list of variables stimulated other researchers to examine the dimensional structure of trait ratings. Several investigators were involved in the initial discovery of the Big Five dimensions. First, Fiske (1949) constructed much simplified descriptions from 22 of Cattell's variables; the factor structures derived from self-ratings, ratings by peers, and ratings by psychological staff members were highly similar and resembled what would later become known as the Big Five. To clarify these factors, Tupes and Christal (1961) reanalyzed correlation matrices from eight samples and found "five relatively strong and recurrent factors and nothing more of any consequence" (1961, p. 14). This five-factor structure has been replicated by Norman (1963), Borgatta (1964), and Digman and Takemoto-Chock (1981) in lists derived from Cattell's 35 variables. Following Norman (1963), the factors were initially labeled (I) Extraversion or Surgency (talkative, assertive, energetic); (II) Agreeableness (good-natured, cooperative, trustful); (III) Conscientiousness (orderly, responsible, dependable); (IV) Emotional Stability (calm, not neurotic, not easily upset); and (V) Culture (intellectual, polished, independent-minded).

These factors (see Table 4.2 for more recent labels, definitions, and examples) eventually became known as the "Big Five"—a name Goldberg (1981) chose not to reflect their intrinsic greatness but to emphasize that each of these factors is extremely broad. Thus, the Big Five structure does not imply that personality differences can be reduced to only five traits. Rather, these five dimensions represent personality at a very broad level of abstraction; each dimension summarizes a large number of distinct, more specific personality characteristics.

Testing the Big Five in a Comprehensive Set of English Trait Terms

After a period of dormancy during the 1970s and early 1980s, research on personality structure increased dramatically during the mid-1980s. Factor structures resembling the Big Five were identified in numerous sets of variables (e.g., Botwin & Buss, 1989; Conley, 1985; De Raad, Mulder, Kloosterman, & Hofstee, 1988; Digman & Inouye, 1986; Goldberg, 1981, 1990; John, 1990; McCrae & Costa, 1985a, 1987; Peabody & Goldberg, 1989; Saucier & Goldberg, 1996a). Because a number of these studies were influenced by Cattell's selection of variables (Block, 1995), it was important to test the generality of the Big Five in more comprehensive variable sets. To update the Allport and Odbert list and rectify the problems with Cattell's reduction steps, Norman (1967) compiled an ex-

haustive list of personality descriptive terms, which he sorted into 75 semantic categories. Goldberg (1990; see also 1981, 1982) used this list to clarify the composition of the Big Five factors and to test their generalizability across methodological variations and data sources. Goldberg (1990) constructed an inventory of 1,710 trait adjectives and had participants rate their own personality. He then scored Norman's semantic categories as scales and factor-analyzed their intercorrelations in the self-rating data. The first five factors represented the expected Big Five, replicated across a variety of different methods of factor extraction and rotation, and remained virtually invariant even when more than five factors were rotated.

To ensure independence from any a priori classification, Goldberg (1990) conducted two additional studies using abbreviated sets of more common terms. In one study, Goldberg obtained self- and peer ratings on 475 very common trait adjectives, which he had grouped into 131 sets of "tight synonym" clusters. The five-factor self- and peer-report structures were very similar to each other and to the structure obtained in the more comprehensive list of 1,710 terms. Most important were the null results from the search for replicable additional factors. Saucier and Goldberg (1996a) selected 435 highly familiar trait adjectives; a factor analysis of these adjectives closely replicated the Big Five. Another thorough search for factors beyond the Big Five showed that these five were the only consistently replicable factors (Saucier, 1997).

Assessing the Big Five with Trait Descriptive Adjectives: Simple and Circumplex Approaches

Goldberg (1990, 1992) distilled his extensive taxonomic findings into several adjective lists. A 50-item instrument using the so-called "transparent format" (Goldberg, 1992) is not used much for research but is excellent for instructional purposes (Pervin, Cervone, & John, 2005): 10 bipolar adjective scales (e.g., quiet–talkative) are grouped together under the factor name, thus making the constructs being measured transparent to the subject. The list used more commonly in research is the set of 100 unipolar trait descriptive adjectives (TDA). Goldberg (1992) conducted a series of factor-analytic studies

TABLE 4.2. The OCEAN[a] of Personality: Definition and Explication of the Big Five Domains

Factor initial (number)	E (Factor I)	A (Factor II)	C (Factor III)	N (Factor IV)	O (Factor V)
Verbal labels	Extraversion Energy Enthusiasm	Agreeableness Altruism Affection	Conscientiousness Constraint Control of impulse	Neuroticism Negative Emotionality Nervousness	Openness Originality Open-Mindedness
Conceptual definition	Implies an *energetic approach* toward the social and material world and includes traits such as sociability, activity, assertiveness, and positive emotionality.	Contrasts a *prosocial and communal orientation* toward others with antagonism and includes traits such as altruism, tender-mindedness, trust, and modesty.	Describes *socially prescribed impulse control* that facilitates task- and goal-directed behavior, such as thinking before acting, delaying gratification, following norms and rules, and planning, organizing, and prioritizing tasks.	Contrasts emotional stability and even-temperedness with *negative emotionality*, such as feeling anxious, nervous, sad, and tense.	Describes the breadth, depth, originality, and complexity of an individual's *mental and experiential life.*
Behavioral examples	Approach strangers at a party and introduce myself; Take the lead in organizing a project; Keep quiet when I disagree with others (R)	Emphasize the good qualities of other people when I talk about them; Lend things to people I know (e.g., class notes, books, milk); Console a friend who is upset	Arrive early or on time for appointments; Study hard in order to get the highest grade in class; Double-check a term paper for typing and spelling errors; Let dirty dishes stack up for more than one day (R)	Accept the good and the bad in my life without complaining or bragging (R); Get upset when somebody is angry with me; Take it easy and relax (R)	Take the time to learn something simply for the joy of learning; Watch documentaries or educational TV; Come up with novel set-ups for my living space; Look for stimulating activities that break up my routine
Examples of external criteria predicted	*High pole:* Social status in groups and leadership positions; selection as jury foreperson; positive emotion expression; number of friends and sex partners *Low pole:* Poorer relationships with parents; rejection by peers	*High pole:* Better performance in work groups *Low pole:* Risk for cardiovascular disease, juvenile delinquency, interpersonal problems	*High pole:* Higher academic grade-point averages; better job performance; adherence to their treatment regimens; longer lives *Low pole:* Smoking, substance abuse, and poor diet and exercise habits; attention-deficit/hyperactivity disorder (ADHD)	*High pole:* Poorer coping and reactions to illness; experience of burnout or job changes *Low pole:* Feeling committed to work organizations; greater relationship satisfaction	*High pole:* Years of education completed; better performance on creativity tests; success in artistic jobs; create distinctive-looking work and home environments *Low pole:* Conservative attitudes and political party preferences

Note. Conceptual definitions are based on John and Srivastava (1999). Behavioral examples are based on significant correlations between Big Five Inventory scales and self-reported act frequencies in an undergraduate sample ($N = 375$; John & Naumann, 2007). (R) denotes that the act was a reverse-keyed item (i.e., correlated negatively with the Big Five domain). [a]The first letter of the Big Five dimensions form the anagram OCEAN. For more examples of predictive validity criteria and relevant references, see the text.

to develop and refine the TDA, selecting only adjectives that uniquely defined each factor. These scales have high internal consistency, and their factor structure is easily replicated.

Another adjectival measure of the Big Five was developed by Wiggins (1995; Trapnell & Wiggins, 1990), who used trait adjectives to elaborate the two major dimensions of interpersonal behavior: dominance (or agency) and nurturance (or communion). As shown in Table 4.1, the first dimension resembles Extraversion in the Big Five, and the second resembles Agreeableness. Wiggins thus extended his circumplex scales by adding simple adjective measures for the other three Big Five factors (Trapnell & Wiggins, 1990).

The circumplex approach has also been extended to a perennial problem in lexical research on personality factors: namely, to describe more clearly those characteristics that fall in the fuzzy regions between the factors. Using 10 two-dimensional circumplexes, Hofstee, De Raad, and Goldberg (1992) devised a novel empirical approach, called the Abbreviated Big Five Circumplex (AB5C), to represent the two-dimensional space formed by each pair of factors and define eight facets that reflect various combinations of the two factors. The facets differ in whether they are more closely related to one or the other factor. For example, there are two facets that reflect high Agreeableness and high Conscientiousness, but they differ in which of the two factors is given more prominence. The *responsibility* facet represents agreeable Conscientiousness, whereas the *cooperation* facet represents conscientious Agreeableness (Hofstee et al., 1997).

Cross-Language and Cross-Cultural Studies

The results reviewed so far suggest that the Big Five structure provides a replicable representation of the major dimensions of trait description in English—the five dimensions generalize across different types of samples, raters, and methodological variations when comprehensive sets of variables are factored. Generalizability across languages and cultures is another important criterion for evaluating personality taxonomies (John, Goldberg, & Angleitner, 1984). The existence of cultural universals (Goldberg, 1981) would be consistent with an evolutionary perspective: If

the tasks most central to human survival are universal, then the most important individual differences, and the terms people use to label these individual differences, should be universal as well (D. M. Buss, 1996; Hogan, 1983). Conversely, if cross-cultural research reveals a culturally specific dimension, variation on that dimension may be uniquely important within that culture's particular social context. Although central from the vantage point of the lexical approach, cross-language research is difficult and expensive to conduct, and until the 1990s it was quite rare. In the initial taxonomic studies, English was the language of choice, primarily because the researchers were American (see John et al., 1984; John, Angleitner, & Ostendorf, 1988).

Initial Studies in Dutch and German

The first two non-English taxonomy projects involved Dutch and German, both Germanic languages closely related to English. The Dutch projects, carried out by Hofstee, De Raad, and their colleagues at the University of Groningen (De Raad et al., 1988; Hofstee et al., 1997; see De Raad, Perugini, et al., 1998, for a review), yielded conclusions generally consistent with those from the American English research: Only five factors were replicable across different selections of trait adjectives and across different subject samples. Those five factors were similar to the English Big Five, although the fifth Dutch factor emphasized Unconventionality and Rebelliousness rather than Intellect and Imagination, as found in English.

The German taxonomy project, begun in Bielefeld, carried out a comprehensive "psycholexical" study of the German personality vocabulary (Angleitner, Ostendorf, & John, 1990). This study was explicitly based on the prototype conception and improved on earlier studies in several respects. In particular, 10 independent judges classified all the terms obtained from the dictionary as traits, states, social evaluations, etc., thus providing a continuous measure of the prototypicality of each term for each category and also a check on the reliability and validity of the judgments. The resulting German personality lexicon is more convenient to use than the unwieldy Allport and Odbert lists because prototypicality values are available for each term in 13 different content categories. Thus, it is easy to select subsets of prototypical traits, states, social evaluations, and so on, from the total pool for further studies. Angleitner and colleagues' (1990) research has served as a blueprint for subsequent taxonomic efforts in other languages.

To test the structure underlying the German trait terms, Ostendorf (1990) selected the most prototypical trait adjectives from the German taxonomy, and his factor analyses of about 450 traits yielded the clearest replication of the Big Five so far. In addition to the prototypical traits representing the distillation of the German trait lexicon, Ostendorf also included German translations of several English personality instruments—a combined emic–etic design that allows researchers to establish empirically the similarity of indigenous (emic) factors to the factors translated from other languages and cultures (etic). Using correlational analyses, Ostendorf conducted an a priori, quantitative evaluation of the fit between his emic German factors and the etic Big Five in the same sample of German subjects, and he found evidence for substantial cross-language convergence.

However, this combined emic–etic strategy is difficult to implement and, unfortunately, has not been used consistently in research. Thus, researchers often reach conclusions about factor similarity by "eyeballing" the item content of the factors in the indigenous language and comparing it to the typical factor definitions in English. That leaves much leeway to the investigators in finding (or not finding) a factor that another investigator might not have found. For example, a Hebrew factor defined primarily by traits such as sophisticated, sharp, knowledgeable, articulate, and impressive would lead some researchers to conclude that they had found a clear Intellect factor, whereas Almagor and colleagues (1995) interpreted it as Positive Valence.

Problems with Translations and Underestimating Cross-Language Congruence

Another methodological difficulty in cross-language research involves translations. Researchers working within their indigenous language have to translate their concepts into English to communicate their findings in

scientific journals, and much too often considerable slippage occurs in the translation process. For example, because "temperamental" was listed as a definer of Extraversion in German, one might hypothesize an important cultural difference here until one realizes that the German trait was probably *temperamentvoll*, which has nothing to do with temper but means "full of life and energy," as in *vivacious*. Similarly, the Italian trait term *frizzante* (translated as *sparkling*) was not found related to intellect, as one might expect, but to extraversion and probably means something close to *bubbly*.

An initial study of German–English bilinguals, which provided support for cross-language generalizability (John et al., 1984), directly addressed the issue of translation equivalence. The unique advantage of the bilingual design is that sample differences can be controlled and translation checks can be made at the level of individual items because the same subject provides descriptions in both languages (see also Benet-Martínez & John, 1998). Using a careful back-translation procedure, translation equivalence between English and German trait adjectives was acceptable, with a mean correlation of .52 across a 2-week interval between administrations (John et al., 1984). However, a few translations proved to be inadequate, with item-translation correlations approaching zero. These findings, obtained for closely related languages, suggest that mistranslations are even more likely to occur in monolingual investigations of personality structure and lead to severe underestimations of cross-language generality.

These difficulties are illustrated in a study by Hofstee and colleagues (1997) who used 126 words they felt could be translated and matched across previous lexical studies in English, Dutch, and German to assess factor congruence coefficients among all pairs of factors in the three languages. Their findings seemed to show considerable congruence; with one exception (the Openness factors in Dutch and English), the pairwise congruence coefficients all exceeded .70. Strangely, the authors interpreted these levels of cross-language congruence as "disappointing" (Hofstee et al., 1997, p. 27). We are more optimistic about these findings. The observed levels of factor congruence can be taken as absolute estimates only if one assumes that the translations are perfectly equivalent and that the factor structures in each language are perfectly stable. When the cross-language congruence coefficients were corrected for the imperfect reliabilities (replication) of the within-language factor structures, the corrected English–German congruence coefficients ranged from .84 to .93, impressive values given that they have not been corrected for the imperfect translations (John & Srivastava, 1999). Moreover, the correspondence for the fifth factor was .93, suggesting that the Intellect or Openness factor was defined almost identically in English and German. This reexamination suggests that translation-based comparisons across languages are heuristically useful but should not be interpreted in terms of absolute effect sizes. These results also suggest that the fifth factor in Dutch is defined differently than in the other two languages, and explanations for this finding need to be sought.

Rules for Including Trait Descriptors in Taxonomic Studies

In all likelihood, some of the differences observed among the factor structures in these three languages are due to the different inclusion rules adopted by the taxonomy teams. The selection criterion used by the Dutch researchers favored terms related to temperament, excluded terms related to intellect, talents, and capacities, and included a number of extremely negative evaluative terms, such as *perverse*, *sadistic*, and *criminal*. The German team explicitly included intellect and talent descriptors but omitted attitudes and evaluative terms, which were included as categories separate from traits. Finally, the American English taxonomy included attitudinal terms such as *liberal*, *progressive*, and *provincial*, along with a number of intellect terms. Given the diverse range of traits related to the fifth factor, it is less surprising that the German and English factors shared the intellect components, whereas the Dutch factor included some imagination-related traits (e.g., *inventive*, *original*, *imaginative*) but otherwise emphasized unconventionality and was thus interpreted initially as a "Rebelliousness" factor.

One Italian trait taxonomy (Caprara & Perugini, 1994) found a similar fifth factor interpreted as Unconventionality. Not surpris-

ingly, these Italian researchers had followed the Dutch selection procedures rather than the German procedures, which likely would have represented more Intellect terms in the initial item pool. A second (and independent) team of Italian taxonomers (Di Blas & Forzi, 1998) failed to find the same factors as the first (see also De Raad, Di Blas, & Perugini, 1998). Given that both teams started with the same lexical material (Italian personality descriptors), this notable lack of convergence within the same language is disconcerting and serves to illustrate the inherent difficulties in standardizing taxonomic procedures and factor-analytic decisions across cultures and languages. How can we expect the Big Five to generalize across languages when two studies of the same language fail to show factor generalizability?

Thus, apparent failures to replicate the Big Five structure can be hard to interpret. For example, Szirmak and De Raad (1994) examined Hungarian personality descriptors and found strong support for the first four of the Big Five but failed to obtain a factor resembling the fifth of the Big Five. Instead, when they forced a five-factor solution, the Agreeableness factor split into two factors. Should this finding be counted as failure to replicate the Big Five, suggesting that Hungarians do not differ systematically on traits related to imagination, creativity, and intellect? Probably not: When six factors were rotated, an Intellect/Openness factor did emerge in the Hungarian data. Again, we suspect that this finding may be due to differences in the way the initial item pool was selected. In their review of this literature, Saucier, Hampson, and Goldberg (2000) conclude that "Given these and other differences among studies, is it any wonder that investigators might disagree about the evidential basis for a particular structural representation?" (p. 23).

Evidence in Non-Germanic Languages

Lexical research has now been extended to a growing range of non-Germanic languages, such as Chinese (Yang & Bond, 1990), Czech (Hrebickova & Ostendorf, 1995), Greek (Saucier, Georgiades, Tsouasis, & Goldberg, 2005), Hebrew (Almagor et al., 1995), Hungarian (Szirmak & De Raad, 1994), Italian (e.g., De Raad et al., 1998),

Polish (Szarota, 1995), Russian (Shmelyov & Pokhil'ko, 1993), Spanish (Benet-Martínez & Waller, 1997), Tagalog in the Philipines (e.g., Church & Katigbak, 1989; Church, Reyes, Katigbak, & Grimm, 1997), Turkish (Somer & Goldberg, 1999), and others. This literature has now grown far beyond the scope of this chapter, and we thus refer the reader to several in-depths reviews (e.g., Ashton et al., 2004; De Raad & Perugini, 2002; De Raad et al., 1998; Saucier & Goldberg, 2001; Saucier et al., 2000).

Most generally, our reading of this literature is that factors similar to the Big Five have been found in many other languages, but often more than five factors needed to be rotated, and sometimes two indigenous factors corresponded to one of the Big Five. The Big Five have been well-replicated in Germanic languages, but the evidence for non-Western languages and cultures tends to be more complex. Overall, the evidence is least compelling for the fifth factor, which appears in various guises, ranging from pure Intellect (in German) to Unconventionality and Rebelliousness (in Dutch and Italian). Moreover, when we only consider which factors are the *most* replicable, then structures with fewer factors (such as two or three) are often even more robust than the more differentiated Big Five (e.g., Saucier et al., 2005). Finally, a number of studies have suggested more than five factors. For example, the seven-factor solutions in Spanish and English (see Benet-Martínez & Waller, 1997) suggested additional separate positive and negative self-evaluation factors. The more recent six-factor solutions, obtained in reanalyses of data from several different languages (Ashton et al., 2004), suggest an additional honesty–humility factor.

While it is too early to decide whether these additional factors hold sufficient promise, two conclusions are apparent now. First, note that these factors are indeed "additional"; that is, they provide evidence for the generalizability of the Big Five *plus* one or two further factors. Second, when more factors than the Big Five have been identified, the additional factors rarely replicate across multiple studies conducted by independent investigators. Thus, we agree with De Raad and colleagues (1998), who concluded that the findings show "the general contours of the Big Five model as the best working hy-

pothesis of an omnipresent trait structure" (p. 214). Although this cautious conclusion falls short of an unequivocal endorsement of the universality of the Big Five, it nonetheless offers a strong disconfirmation of the linguistic-relativism hypothesis that many of us had expected to hold true before the lexical data became available: There are no data to suggest that each culture and language has its own, unique set of personality dimensions; at least at the level of broad trait dimensions, cultures are more alike than we may have expected.

THE BIG FIVE IN PERSONALITY QUESTIONNAIRES

While researchers in the lexical tradition were accumulating evidence for the Big Five, the need for an integrative framework became more pressing among researchers who studied personality with questionnaire scales. Joint factor analyses of questionnaires developed by different investigators had shown that two broad dimensions, Extraversion and Neuroticism, appear in one form or another in most personality inventories. Beyond these "Big Two" (Wiggins, 1968), however, the various questionnaire-based models had shown few signs of convergence. For example, Eysenck (1991) observed that "Where we have literally hundreds of inventories incorporating thousands of traits, largely overlapping but also containing specific variance, each empirical finding is strictly speaking only relevant to a specific trait. ... This is not the way to build a unified scientific discipline" (p. 786).

Costa and McCrae's Research

The situation began to change in the early 1980s when Costa and McCrae were developing the NEO Personality Inventory (eventually published in 1985), labeled N-E-O because it was designed to measure the three dimensions of Neuroticism, Extraversion, and Openness to experience. Costa and McCrae (1976) had begun their work with cluster analyses of the 16PF (Cattell et al., 1970), which, as we described above, originated in Cattell's early lexical work. Their analyses again yielded the ubiquitous Extraversion and Neuroticism dimensions, but also convinced Costa and McCrae of the importance of Openness, which originated from several of Cattell's primary factors (e.g., imaginative; experimenting).

In 1983 Costa and McCrae realized that their NEO system closely resembled three of the Big Five factors but did not encompass traits in the Agreeableness and Conscientiousness domains. They therefore extended their model with preliminary scales measuring Agreeableness and Conscientiousness. In several studies, McCrae and Costa (1985a, 1985b, 1987) demonstrated that their five questionnaire scales converged with adjective-based measures of the Big Five, although their conception of Openness was considerably broader than the Intellect or Imagination factor emerging from the lexical analyses (Saucier & Goldberg, 1996a). A series of influential papers in the late 1980s and early 1990s showed that these five factors could also be recovered in various other personality questionnaires, as well as in self-ratings on the California Adult Q-sort (see Costa & McCrae, 1992; McCrae & Costa, 2003).

The Revised NEO Personality Inventory

The initial NEO Personality Inventory (Costa & McCrae, 1985) included scales to measure six conceptually derived facets each for Neuroticism, Extraversion, and Openness but did not include facet scales for the newly added Agreeableness and Conscientiousness. In 1992, Costa and McCrae published the 240-item NEO Personality Inventory—Revised (NEO-PI-R; Costa & McCrae, 1992), which permits differentiated measurement of each Big Five dimension in terms of six more specific facets per factor (Costa & McCrae, 1995). Table 4.3 shows the six facets defining each of the factors. In contrast to most of the lexical studies, which relied on college student samples, the NEO-PI-R was developed in samples of middle-age and older adults, using both factor-analytic and multimethod validational procedures of test construction. The scales have shown substantial internal consistency, temporal stability, and convergent and discriminant validity against spouse and peer ratings (Costa & McCrae, 1992; McCrae & Costa, 2003).

For many research applications, the NEO-PI-R is rather lengthy. To provide a shorter measure, Costa and McCrae (1989, 1992) developed the 60-item NEO-FFI, an abbreviated version based on an item-level factor analysis of the 1985 version of the NEO PI (Costa & McCrae, 1985). The 12-item scales of the FFI consist of items that loaded highly on one of the five factors. The item content of the scales was adjusted somewhat to ensure adequate content coverage of the facets; however, these scales represent the core elements of each Big Five factor as defined on the NEO PI and therefore do not represent equally each of the six facets defining each factor. For example, the Agreeableness scale includes five items from the Altruism facet, three from Compliance, two from Trust, one from Tender-Mindedness, one from Straightforwardness, and none from Modesty. The reliabilities (Costa & McCrae, 1992) are adequate, with a mean of .78, and the NEO-FFI scales are substantially correlated with the NEO-PI-R scales.

DEFINING THE BIG FIVE ACROSS STUDIES: A PROTOTYPE APPROACH

So far, we have reviewed both Goldberg's (1990) lexically based research and Costa and McCrae's (1992) questionnaire-based research on the Big Five. Despite this extensive research, the Big Five structure was initially not widely welcomed in the field and, in fact, explicitly rejected by some senior researchers (e.g., Block, 1995; Eysenck, 1992, 1997; McAdams, 1992; Pervin, 1994). One problem, it seems, was the perception that there is no *single* Big Five, in the same way as there was just one 16PF, namely Cattell's, because he owned it. In contrast, the Big Five emerged in multiple labs and studies and is therefore not owned by any one person in the field, which makes it possible to ask questions such as *"which* Big Five?" or *"whose* Big Five?" (John, 1989). For example, the first factor has been labeled as surgency, confident self-expression, assertiveness, social extraversion, and power (see John, 1990, Table 3.1), and the second factor as social adaptability, likability, friendly compliance, agreeableness, and love. Of course, some variation across studies is to be expected with dimensions as broad and inclusive as the Big Five because researchers differ in the variables they include, thus representing different parts of the factor's total range of meaning. Moreover, researchers dif-

TABLE 4.3. Defining Facets for the Big Five Trait Domains: Three Approaches

Lexical facets (18) (Saucier & Ostendorf, 1999)	NEO-PI-R facets (30) (Costa & McCrae, 1992)	CPI-Big Five facets (16) (Soto & John, 2008)
Extraversion (E) facets		
E Sociability	E Gregariousness	E Gregariousness
E Assertiveness	E Assertiveness	E Assertiveness/Leadership
	E Activity	
E Activity/Adventurousness	E Excitement-Seeking	[O Adventurousness]
		E Social Confidence vs. Anxiety
	E Positive emotions	
E Unrestraint		
[A Warmth/Affection]	E Warmth	
Agreeableness (A) facets		
A Warmth/Affection	[E Warmth]	
A Modesty/Humility	A Modesty	A Modesty vs. Narcissism
	A Trust	A Trust vs. Suspicion
	A Tender-Mindedness	A Empathy/Sympathy
A Generosity		A Altruism
A Gentleness	A Compliance	
	A Straightforwardness	
Conscientiousness (C) facets		
C Orderliness	C Order	C Orderliness
C Industriousness	C Achievement Striving	
C Reliability	C Dutifulness	C Industriousness
C Decisiveness		
	C Self-Discipline	C Self-Discipline
[O Perceptiveness]	C Competence	
	C Deliberation	
Neuroticism (N) facets		
N Insecurity	N Anxiety	N Anxiety
N Emotionality		
N Irritability	N Angry Hostility	N Irritability
	N Depression	N Depression
		N Rumination–Compulsiveness
	N Self-Consciousness	[E Social Confidence vs. Anxiety]
	N Vulnerability	
	N Impulsiveness	
Openness (O) facets		
O Intellect	O Ideas	O Intellectualism
	O Aesthetics	O Idealism
O Imagination/Creativity	O Fantasy	
		O Adventurousness
	O Actions	
	O Feelings	
	O Values	
O Perceptiveness		

Note. The NEO-PI-R facets are listed in the middle column because that instrument makes the largest number of distinctions below the Big Five (30 facets), as compared with the 18 lexical facets and the 16 CPI facets. CPI-Big Five facets are matched with NEO-PI-R facets on the basis of both rational judgments by the authors and correlations between the two sets of facets in a sample of 520 adults (see Soto & John, 2008). Lexical facets are matched with NEO-PI-R facets on the basis of rational judgments by the authors. Some facets (e.g., CPI Adventurousness) are listed once under their primary Big Five domain (e.g., Openness) and again in brackets under another Big Five domain if their best-matching facet appears there (e.g., next to NEO Excitement-Seeking, which is an Extraversion facet on the NEO-PI-R but also has a substantial secondary correlation with Openness). Note that the Warmth facet belongs to the Extraversion domain in the NEO-PI-R, whereas a very similar Warmth/Affection facet belongs to the Agreeableness domain in the lexical approach.

fer in their preferences for factor labels even when the factor content is quite similar. The fact that the labels differ does not necessarily mean that the factors are different, too. Thus, there may be more commonality than meets the eye.

A prototype approach may help identify these commonalities across studies (John, 1990). Natural categories such as the Big Five typically have fuzzy and partially overlapping definitions (Rosch, 1978), but they can still be extremely useful when defined in terms of prototypical exemplars. Similarly, the Big Five may be defined with prototypical traits that occur consistently across studies. One way to integrate the various interpretations of the factors is to conceptually map the five dimensions into a common language. Human judges were used to abstract the common elements in these findings (John, 1989, 1990), and the 300 terms included in the Adjective Check List (ACL; Gough & Heilbrun, 1983) served as the standard language.

Conceptually Derived Prototype Descriptions of the Big Five and Their Validation in Observer Data

A set of 10 judges first developed a detailed understanding of the Big Five by reviewing the factor solutions and interpretations of all major Big Five articles published by 1988. The judges then independently sorted each of the 300 items in the ACL into one of the Big-Five domains or into a sixth "other" category, with substantial interjudge agreement. In all, 112 of the 300 ACL terms were assigned to one of the Big Five with 90% or better agreement. These terms form a relatively narrow, or "core," definition of the five factors because they include only those traits that appeared consistently across studies. As with any rationally constructed measure, the validity of these categorizations was tested empirically in a factor analysis of the 112 terms. Whereas most Big Five research has been based on college students' self- and peer ratings, this study used observer data: psychologists rated 140 men and 140 women who had participated in groups of 10–15 in one of the assessment weekends at the Institute of Personality and Social Research (IPSR, formerly IPAR) at Berkeley (John, 1990). Because each subject had been described on the ACL by 10 staff members, a

factor analysis could be performed on more reliable, aggregated observer judgments. The varimax rotated factor loadings, shown in Table 4.4, provide a compelling confirmation of the initial prototypes. All but one item loaded on its hypothesized factor in the expected direction, and most of the loadings were substantial.

Note that the items defining each of the factors cover a broad range of content. For example, Factor I includes traits such as *active, adventurous, assertive, dominant, energetic, enthusiastic, outgoing, sociable,* and *show-off*. In light of this substantial bandwidth, the heterogeneity of the previous factor labels is understood more easily— different investigators have focused on different components, or facets, of the total range of meaning subsumed by each factor. In this study, the Extraversion factor includes at least five distinguishable components: activity level (active, energetic), dominance (assertive, forceful, bossy), sociability (outgoing, sociable, talkative), expressiveness (adventurous, outspoken, noisy, show-off), and positive emotionality (enthusiastic, spunky). Note that these five components are similar to five of the six facets Costa and McCrae (1992) included in their definition of the Extraversion domain: activity, assertiveness, gregariousness, excitement-seeking, and positive emotions (see Table 4.3)—and four of the five have been identified in a lexical study that empirically identified facets across two languages (Saucier & Ostendorf (1999), shown on the left-hand side of Table 4.3. Costa and McCrae's sixth Extraversion facet, warmth, is here considered a component of Factor II; all 10 judges interpreted past research to imply that warmth is part of Agreeableness, and the empirical loading of .82 confirmed this interpretation, just as the lexical facet of warmth/affection appears on Agreeableness. In addition to warmth (affectionate, gentle, warm), Factor II covers themes such as tender-mindedness (sensitive, kind, soft-hearted, sympathetic), altruism (generous, helping, praising), and trust (trusting, forgiving), as contrasted with hostility, criticality, and distrust; again, note the convergence with Costa and McCrae's facets. More generally, the adjectival definitions of the Big Five in Table 4.4 seem to capture the prototypical traits found in other studies and the facets shown in Table 4.3.

TABLE 4.4. Big Five Prototypes: Most Central Trait Adjectives Selected Consensually by Expert Judges and Their Factor Loadings in Personality Ratings by 10 Psychologists Serving as Observers

Extraversion		Agreeableness		Conscientiousness		Neuroticism		Openness	
Low	High	Low	High	Low	High	Low	High	Low	High
−.83 Quiet	.85 Talkative	−.52 Fault-finding	.87 Sympathetic	−.58 Careless	.80 Organized	−.39 Stable	.73 Tense	−.74 Commonplace	.76 Wide interests
−.80 Reserved	.83 Assertive	−.48 Cold	.85 Kind	−.53 Disorderly	.80 Thorough	−.35 Calm	.72 Anxious	−.73 Narrow interests	.76 Imaginative
−.75 Shy	.82 Active	−.45 Unfriendly	.85 Appreciative	−.50 Frivolous	.78 Planful	−.21 Contented	.72 Nervous	−.67 Simple	.72 Intelligent
−.71 Silent	.82 Energetic	−.45 Quarrelsome	.84 Affectionate	−.49 Irresponsible	.78 Efficient		.71 Moody	−.55 Shallow	.73 Original
−.67 Withdrawn	.82 Outgoing	−.45 Hard-hearted	.84 Soft-hearted	−.40 Slipshot	.73 Responsible		.71 Worrying	−.47 Unintelligent	.68 Insightful
−.66 Retiring	.80 Outspoken	−.38 Unkind	.82 Warm	−.39 Undependable	.72 Reliable		.68 Touchy		.64 Curious
	.79 Dominant	−.33 Cruel	.81 Generous	−.37 Forgetful	.70 Dependable		.64 Fearful		.59 Sophisticated
	.73 Forceful	−.31 Stern	.78 Trusting		.68 Conscientious		.63 High-strung		.59 Artistic
	.73 Enthusiastic	−.28 Thankless	.77 Helpful		.66 Precise		.63 Self-pitying		.59 Clever
	.68 Show-off	−.24 Stingy	.77 Forgiving		.66 Practical		.60 Temperamental		.58 Inventive
	.68 Sociable		.74 Pleasant		.65 Deliberate		.59 Unstable		.56 Sharp-witted
	.64 Spunky		.73 Good-natured		.46 Painstaking		.58 Self-punishing		.55 Ingenious
	.64 Adventurous		.73 Friendly		.26 Cautious		.54 Despondent		.45 Witty
	.62 Noisy		.72 Cooperative				.51 Emotional		.45 Resourceful
	.58 Bossy		.67 Gentle						.37 Wise
			.66 Unselfish						
			.56 Praising						
			.51 Sensitive						

Note. Based on John (1990). These items were assigned to one Big Five domain by at least 90% of the judges and thus capture the most prototypical (or central) content of each Big Five domain. The factor loadings, shown here only for the expected factor, were obtained in a sample of 140 males and 140 females, each of whom had been described by 10 psychologists serving as observers during an assessment weekend at the Institute of Personality and Social Research at the University of California at Berkeley (see also John, 1989).

The Prototypical Definition of Factor V: Culture, Intellect, or Openness?

The findings in Table 4.4 also address questions about the definition of the fifth factor. None of the items referring to aspects of "high" culture (e.g., civilized, polished, dignified, foresighted, logical) loaded substantially on Factor V (see John, 1990), and many loaded more highly on Factor III (Conscientiousness), thus discrediting an interpretation of Factor V as Culture. Apparently, the initial interpretation of Tupes and Christal's (1961) fifth factor as Culture was a historical accident (Peabody & Goldberg, 1989). The items that did load substantially on the fifth factor (see Table 4.4) include both the "open" characteristics (e.g., artistic, curious, original, wide interests) highlighted by McCrae and Costa (1985a, 1985b) and the "intellectual" characteristics (intelligent, insightful, sophisticated) emphasized by Digman and Inouye (1986), Peabody and Goldberg (1989), and Goldberg (1990).

These findings are also consistent with Goldberg's (1990) result that Factor V is defined as originality, wisdom, objectivity, knowledge, reflection, and art, thus involving facets of Openness related to ideas, fantasy, and aesthetics (Costa & McCrae, 1992). Similarly, Goldberg's analyses of the 133 synonym clusters showed intellectuality (intellectual, contemplative, meditative, philosophical, and introspective) and creativity (creative, imaginative, inventive, ingenious, innovative) with the highest loadings, only then followed by intelligence, versatility, wisdom, perceptiveness, art, logic, curiosity, and nonconformity (nonconforming, unconventional, rebellious), which loaded positively, and conventionality (traditional, conventional, unprogressive), which loaded negatively in all four samples. These and other lexical findings (see John & Srivastava, 1999) are inconsistent with both the Culture and a narrow Intellect interpretation and instead favor the broader Openness interpretation proposed by McCrae (1996); the inclusion of unconventionality and nonconformity also makes an important link to the definition of this lexical factor in Dutch and Italian (De Raad et al., 1998). Similarly, in a recent AB5C analysis designed to derive Big Five facets from the CPI item pool (summarized here in Table 4.3), we found three distinct Openness facets (being idealistic, adventurous, and intellectual) that were related both to adjective and NEO measures of the fifth factor (Soto & John, 2008). Moving away from a narrow Intellect interpretation, Saucier (1992, 1994) has suggested the label imagination, which is somewhat closer to Openness and emphasizes the emerging consensus that fantasy, ideas, and aesthetics, rather than intelligence, are most central to this factor. In this chapter, we therefore adopt the term *Openness*.

The Big Five Inventory: Measuring the Core Features of the Big Five with Short Phrases

To address the need for a short instrument measuring the prototypical components of the Big Five that are common across investigators, the Big Five Inventory (BFI) was constructed (John, Donahue, & Kentle, 1991; see also Benet-Martínez & John, 1998; John & Srivastava, 1999; Rammstedt & John, 2005, 2007). The 44-item BFI was developed to represent the Big Five prototype definitions described above (see Table 4.4)—a canonical representation of the factors intended to capture their core elements across the particulars of previous studies, samples, or instruments. The final items were selected on the basis of factor analyses in large samples of both junior college and public university students. Thus, Hampson and Goldberg (2006) were mistaken when they suggested that "John developed each of the five BFI scales to fall roughly between the lexical Big Five factors (Goldberg, 1992) and the five domain scores from the NEO PI-R" (p. 766), nor was this outcome either intended or entailed by the procedures used, as we will see below. The goal was to create a brief inventory that would allow efficient and flexible assessment of the five dimensions when there is no need for more differentiated measurement of individual facets. There is much to be said in favor of brevity: "Short scales not only save testing time, but also avoid subject boredom and fatigue. ... There are subjects ... from whom you won't get any response if the test looks too long" (Burisch, 1984, p. 219).

The BFI does not use single adjectives as items because such items are answered less consistently than when they are accompanied by definitions or elaborations (Goldberg & Kilkowski, 1985). Instead, the BFI uses short phrases based on the trait adjectives known to be prototypical markers of the Big Five (John, 1989, 1990). One or two prototypical trait adjectives served as the item core to which elaborative, clarifying, or contextual information was added. For example, the Openness adjective *original* became the BFI item "Is original, comes up with new ideas" and the Conscientiousness adjective *persevering* served as the basis for the item "Perseveres until the task is finished." Thus the BFI items (which are reprinted here in Appendix 4.1) retain the advantages of adjectival items (brevity and simplicity) while avoiding some of their pitfalls (ambiguous or multiple meanings and salient desirability). Indeed, DeYoung (2006, p. 1140) hypothesized that with their more contextualized trait content, the BFI items should elicit higher interrater agreement than single-adjective items, and found that pairwise interrater agreement was indeed somewhat higher for the BFI.

Although the BFI scales include only eight to ten items, they do not sacrifice either content coverage or good psychometric properties. For example, the nine-item Agreeableness scale includes items related to at least five of the six facets postulated by Costa and McCrae (1992)—namely, trust (trusting, forgiving), altruism (helpful and unselfish), compliance (not quarrelsome), modesty (not faultfinding with others), and tender-mindedness (considerate and kind). In U.S. and Canadian samples, the alpha reliabilities of the BFI scales range from .75 to .90 and average above .80. Three-month test–retest reliabilities range from .80 to .90, with a mean of .85 (Rammstedt & John, 2005; 2007). In a middle-age sample, Hampson and Goldberg (2006) found a mean test–retest stability of .74, with stability correlations of .79 for Extraversion and Openness and about .70 for Agreeableness, Conscientiousness, and Neuroticism. Validity evidence includes substantial convergent and divergent relations with other Big Five instruments as well as with peer ratings (Rammstedt & John, 2005, 2007). DeYoung (2006) analyzed a large community data set with BFI self-reports and BFI ratings by three peers; however, he did not report validity correlations between self-reports and the aggregated peer ratings. We therefore reanalyzed these data and found validity correlations of .67 for Extraversion, .60 for Openness, .52

for Neuroticism, .48 for Agreeableness, and .47 for Conscientiousness, averaging .55. The sizes of these convergent correlations are even more impressive given that the (absolute) hetero-trait, hetero-method discriminant correlations averaged .09, and 19 of the 20 correlations were below .20, with only one reaching –.21 (indicating that individuals who described themselves as high in neuroticism were rated by their peers as slightly more disagreeable).

MEASUREMENT: COMPARING THREE BIG FIVE INSTRUMENTS

So far, we have discussed Goldberg's (1992) TDA, Costa and McCrae's (1992) NEO questionnaires, and the BFI. In addition, a variety of other measures are available to assess the Big Five in English and other languages (see De Raad & Perugini, 2002). Many of them were developed for specific research applications. Digman (e.g., 1989) constructed several different adjective sets to study teacher ratings of personality in children and adolescents, and Wiggins's (1995) scales were described above. Big Five scales have also been constructed using items from existing instruments. For example, scales were developed to measure the Big Five in adolescents using personality ratings on the California Child Q-sort obtained from their mothers (John et al., 1994). Measelle, John, Ablow, Cowan, and Cowan (2005) developed scales to measure the Big Five with a puppet interview in children ages 4–7. In behavior genetic research, Loehlin, McCrae, Costa, and John (1998) used Big Five scales constructed from the ACL (Gough & Heilbrun, 1983) and the CPI (Gough, 1987); for the latter, we (Soto & John, 2008) recently developed new Big Five domain and facet scales. As shown in Table 4.1, another broadband personality inventory that provides scores for the Big Five is the Hogan Personality Inventory (Hogan, 1986). The availability of so many different instruments to measure the Big Five makes clear that there is no single instrument that represents *the* gold standard.

Comparing the TDA, NEO-FFI, and BFI

In general, the NEO questionnaires represent the best-validated Big Five measures in the questionnaire tradition. Goldberg's (1992) 100-item TDA and its abbreviated 40-item version (Saucier, 1994) are the most commonly used measures consisting of single adjectives. The BFI has been used frequently in research settings where subject time is at a premium, and its short-phrase item format provides more context than Goldberg's single-adjective items but less complexity than the sentence format used by the NEO questionnaires; the BFI items are also somewhat easier to understand (Benet-Martínez & John, 1998).

How well do these different Big Five measures converge? And are the five dimensions really independent? There has been concern that some of the Big Five dimensions are highly intercorrelated (Block, 1995; Eysenck, 1992). How high are these intercorrelations, and do they involve the same dimensions across instruments? A number of studies have reported on the psychometric characteristics of these instruments, and a few studies have compared two of them with each other (e.g., Benet-Martínez & John, 1998; DeYoung, 2006; Goldberg, 1992; McCrae & Costa, 1987). However, little is known about how all three compare to each other (see John & Srivastava, 1999, for an exception). To provide such a comparison, we summarize findings from a new large data set of self-reports on all three measures. The sample consisted of 829 undergraduates at the University of California, Berkeley (see John & Soto, 2007; Soto & John, 2008) who completed the BFI, Saucier's (1994) 40-item version of Goldberg's (1992) TDA, as well as Costa and McCrae's (1992) NEO-PI-R from which we scored both the 30 facets (see Table 4.3) and the NEO-FFI domain scores. The data thus represent a multitrait, multimethod (MTMM) design where the methods are the three Big Five self-report instruments (see John & Benet-Martínez, 2000).

Reliability of the Three Instruments

Overall, the coefficient alpha reliabilities, shown in Table 4.5, were impressive for these short scales, and relatively similar in size across instruments; the mean of the alphas was .84 for the TDA scales, .83 for the BFI, and .81 for the NEO-FFI, which had the longest scales (12 items compared to 8 for the TDA and about 9 for the BFI). Across

instruments, Extraversion, Neuroticism, and Conscientiousness were measured most reliably (all clearly above .80 on all instruments), whereas Agreeableness and Openness tended to be somewhat less reliable. The scales with the lowest reliabilities were the NEO-FFI Openness and Agreeableness scale, similar to the values reported in the NEO-PI-R manuals and also replicating two other college samples (e.g., Benet-Martínez & John, 1998). Several NEO-FFI Openness items did not correlate well with the total scale, and these less reliable items came from particular openness facets, namely from openness to action (e.g., trying new and foreign foods) and from openness to values (e.g., looking to religious authorities for decisions on moral issues, reverse scored) (John & Srivastava, 1999).

Convergent Validity across the Three Instruments

Overall, we expected the convergent validities across the three instruments to be substantial. However, we already noted some potential differences in the way the three instruments define Extraversion and Openness. The NEO Extraversion domain had already been defined in terms of six facets before Costa and McCrae added domain scales for Agreeableness and Conscientiousness in 1985 and facet scales for these two factors in 1992. Thus, the warmth facet scale, included in the NEO-PI-R Extraversion domain (see Table 4.3), also correlates substantially with their Agreeableness domain scale (Costa & McCrae, 1992). In contrast, different lexical researchers (e.g., Goldberg, 1992; John, 1990; Saucier & Ostendorf, 1999) all found, in independent analyses, that trait adjectives related to warmth correlate more highly with Agreeableness than with Extraversion (see Tables 4.3 and 4.4). Thus, the NEO-FFI Extraversion scale showed much less convergence with either the TDA or the BFI than those two instruments with each other (John & Srivastava, 1999).

The other potential difference involves the fifth factor. As described above, Goldberg (1992) prefers to interpret this factor as Intellect or Imagination (Saucier, 1992), thus emphasizing openness to ideas and to fantasy over the other four facets. Similarly, the BFI Openness scale does not include items conceptually related to Costa and McCrae's

TABLE 4.5. Reliability and Convergent Validity Coefficients for Three Short Big Five Measures: Big Five Inventory, NEO Five-Factor Inventory, and Trait Descriptive Adjectives

Measures	Extraversion	Agreeableness	Conscientiousness	Neuroticism	Openness	Mean
			Internal consistency			
BFI	.86	.79	.82	.87	.83	.83
NEO-FFI	.82	.75	.82	.87	.76	.81
TDA	.88	.84	.84	.83	.83	.84
Mean	.85	.80	.83	.85	.81	.83
			Uncorrected convergent validity correlations (across measures)			
BFI–TDA	.90	.75	.79	.70	.79	.80
BFI–NEO-FFI	.73	.76	.80	.81	.72	.77
TDA–NEO-FFI	.70	.66	.75	.64	.62	.68
Mean	.80	.73	.78	.73	.72	.75
			Corrected convergent validity correlations (across measures)			
BFI–TDA	.99	.93	.96	.82	.95	.95
BFI–NEO-FFI	.87	.99	.97	.94	.90	.95
TDA–NEO-FFI	.83	.83	.91	.76	.78	.83
Mean	.94	.95	.95	.86	.90	.93
			Standardized convergent validity coefficients from CFA (controlling for acquiescence factors)			
BFI–TDA	.99	.91	.91	.84	.97	.95
BFI–NEO-FFI	.83	.98	.95	.93	.90	.93
TDA–NEO-FFI	.76	.84	.87	.78	.74	.80
Mean	.92	.93	.92	.86	.91	.91

Note. N = 829 (see John & Soto, 2007). BFI, Big Five Inventory (John et al., 1991); TDA, Trait Descriptive Adjectives (Goldberg, 1992; 40-item mini-marker version, Saucier, 1994); NEO-FFI, NEO Five-Factor Inventory (Costa & McCrae, 1992); CFA, confirmatory factor analysis. Means are shown in **bold**. All means computed with Fisher *r*-to-Z transformations.

(1992) values and actions facets because preliminary BFI items, based on prototype items related to conventionality (i.e., relevant to the NEO-PI-R values facet) and behavioral flexibility (relevant to the action facet), failed to cohere with the other items on the BFI Openness scale (John et al., 1991). Thus, the NEO-FFI Openness scale showed less convergence with either the TDA or the BFI than those two instruments with each other (John & Srivastava, 1999).

As a first test of cross-instrument convergence, we examined the full 15 × 15 MTMM correlation matrix formed by the five factors crossed with the three instruments. The cross-instrument validity correlations, computed between pairs of instruments and shown in Table 4.5, were generally substantial in size. Across all five factors, the mean of the convergent validity correlations across instruments was .75, as compared with the much smaller discriminant correlations that averaged .19. As shown in Table 4.5, BFI

and TDA showed the strongest overall convergence (mean *r* = .80), followed closely by BFI and NEO-FFI (.77), and finally TDA and NEO-FFI (mean *r* = .68).

To determine the extent to which the validity correlations simply reflect the imperfect reliability of the scales rather than substantive differences among the instruments, we corrected for attenuation using alpha. As shown in Table 4.5, the corrected validity correlations averaged .93. However, this excellent overall result masks some important differences. Across instruments, the first three of the Big Five (Extraversion, Agreeableness, and Conscientiousness) showed mean validities of about .95, suggesting very high equivalence of the reliable variance of the three instruments. However, Neuroticism (.86) and Openness (.90) were notably lower. Focusing on the pairwise comparisons between instruments, the patterns were more differentiated. BFI and TDA (corrected mean *r* = .95) shared virtually all of their reliable variance, with the highest correlation for Extraversion; only the correlation for Neuroticism (.82) fell below .90. BFI and NEO-FFI showed the same substantial mean convergence (.95); here the highest correlation was for Agreeableness, and again only one correlation fell below .90 (for Extraversion). In contrast, TDA and NEO-FFI shared less in common (mean corrected $r = .83$); only one correlation (for Conscientiousness) exceeded .90, and those for Neuroticism and Openness did not even reach .80, suggesting that the conceptualization of four of the Big Five dimensions is not fully equivalent across these two instruments. On average, then, the BFI converged much better with both TDA and NEO-FFI than did TDA and NEO-FFI with each other. However, in contrast to Hampson and Goldberg's (2006) impression, the empirical findings show that the BFI does not simply occupy an intermediate position between the lexically derived TDA and the questionnaire-based NEO-FFI. Instead, the pattern of convergence correlations depends on the Big Five domain: The BFI achieved practical equivalence with the TDA for Extraversion (.99) but with the NEO-FFI for Agreeableness (.99), was much closer to the NEO-FFI than the TDA for Neuroticism (.94 vs. .82), a pattern that was reversed for Openness (.90 vs. .95), and finally converged equally well with both for Conscientiousness (.97 vs. .96).

Discriminant Correlations

Overall, discriminant correlations were low, with absolute values averaging .19 overall and .16 for the TDA and .20 for both the NEO-FFI and the BFI. Moreover, none of the discriminant correlations reached .35 on any of the instruments, and the largest correlations were .30 for the TDA, .34 for the NEO-FFI, and .31 for the BFI. Averaged across instruments, only four of the 10 discriminant correlations even exceeded .20: the mean correlation was .26 for Agreeableness and Conscientiousness, −.26 for Agreeableness and Neuroticism, −.26 for Conscientiousness and Neuroticism, and −.25 for Extraversion and Neuroticism. Thus, there was little support for Eysenck's (1992) contention that Agreeableness and Conscientiousness are highly correlated "primary" traits that should be combined into a broader dimen-

sion that contrasts Eysenck's Psychoticism with what might be called "good character." The size of these intercorrelations should also dampen some of the current enthusiasm (e.g., DeYoung, 2006; Markon, Krueger, & Watson, 2005) for higher-order factors above the Big Five (Digman, 1997). Yes, as has been noted repeatedly (e.g., John & Srivastava, 1999; Paulhus & John, 1998), the Big Five dimensions, as assessed by self and peer observers, are not strictly orthogonal, and scale intercorrelations of .26 are statistically significant. However, the size of these intercorrelations represents barely 10% shared variance—hardly enough, it would seem, to support the two substantively interpreted superordinate factors initially reported by Digman (1997). An alternative view showed that at least some of that covariance may be explained in terms of self-enhancing biases in self-reports (Paulhus & John, 1998).

Estimating Convergent and Discriminant Validity While Controlling Acquiescence

Finally, we tested whether individual differences in acquiescent response style (i.e., "yea-saying" vs. "nay-saying") might serve to influence cross-instrument validity estimates, such as inflating convergent validity correlations or depressing discriminant validity correlations (Soto, John, Gosling, & Potter, 2008). We found small but systematic acquiescence effects in the BFI; they appear as a small response-style factor in addition to the five substantive personality factors. We have therefore developed a new, content-balanced approach that controls acquiescence variance at the BFI item level and eliminates the response-style factor; this approach is described here in Appendix 4.2. For the present analyses, we used a bifactor approach to modeling an acquiescence factor, in addition to the five substantive personality factors, for each of the three instruments.

These structural equation models have a number of important properties. First, each instrument (BFI, TDA, NEO-FFI) has its own acquiescence factor, which was defined by setting the raw regression path from its acquiescence factor to each individual item equal to 1. By setting all of these loadings equally, we ensured that the acquiescence factor would represent *positive* covariance shared across all items on the instrument, rather than letting it estimate something else (e.g., social desirability). By setting all of the loadings equal to 1 (rather than setting the factor variance equal to 1), we allow the variance of the acquiescence factor to be estimated and can thus compare the amount of acquiescence variance across instruments.

Second, the 15 substantive personality factors (Big Five times three instruments) were allowed to correlate with each other freely, both within and across each instrument, thus allowing us to estimate latent convergent and discriminant validity correlations across pairs of instruments. Also, the three acquiescence factors were allowed to correlate with each other across instruments, thus allowing us to test whether individual differences in acquiescent responding generalize across the Big Five instruments. Third, the substantive factors were not allowed to correlate with the acquiescence factors—further ensuring that the acquiescence factors did not contain any substantive personality variance.

We tested two general predictions about acquiescent responding. First, does the single-adjective item format of the TDA and its longer nine-step response scale elicit more acquiescence variance than the more contextualized item formats of the BFI and NEO-FFI, with their shorter five-step response scales? Indeed, the estimated variance of the acquiescence factor was .106 for the TDA, compared with .033 for the BFI and .013 for the FFI. Constraining the acquiescence factor variances to be equal across instruments significantly reduced fit; $\Delta\chi^2(2) = 375$, $p < .001$. Second, is acquiescent responding instrument-specific or a broad response disposition that generalizes across these instruments? Our findings suggested considerable generalizability; the correlations between the acquiescence factors were all significant: .62 for BFI–TDA, .61 for BFI–NEO-FFI, and .43 for TDA–FFI.

Third, what are the effects of including the acquiescence factors on the estimates of the convergent and discriminant correlations? The results for the convergent correlations with the acquiescence factors included (thus controlling the effects of acquiescence) are shown in Table 4.5. They were virtually identical to those without the acquiescence factors and, most important, the pattern was very similar to that for the corrected convergent validity correlations in Table 4.5,

where acquiescence was not controlled. Including the acquiescence factors also did not change the mean estimated discriminant correlations, suggesting that at the scale level, the three Big Five instruments are not particularly susceptible to acquiescence effects. Together, the findings in this section show that the Big Five are fairly independent dimensions that can be measured by several instruments with impressive convergent and discriminant validity.

How Well Do BFI, TDA, and NEO-FFI Scales Represent the Six NEO-PI-R Facets?

The findings in Table 4.5 suggest that some pairs of scales define the intended Big Five domain in very similar ways (e.g., the BFI and TDA scales for Extraversion) whereas other pairs of scales do not (e.g., the TDA and NEO-FFI scales for Neuroticism). One way to explicate how the three Big Five instruments define each Big Five domain is to use the six facets included on the NEO-PI-R for each trait domain as a shared point of reference and correlate them, for each Big Five domain, with the scales on the three instruments. These correlations can then be graphed, yielding profiles that show how well each particular scale represents each of the six facets defined by the NEO-PI-R. The results are shown in Figure 4.2; we begin with Extraversion in the middle of the figure to illustrate how to read and interpret these profile graphs. In the Extraversion panel, it is immediately obvious that the profile curves for the BFI Extraversion scale and the TDA Extraversion scale are extremely similar. Both show correlations of about .55 with the four center facets (i.e., activity, gregariousness, warmth, and positive emotions), indicating that they weigh these facets all about equally. Both scales correlate most highly with assertiveness (about .70) and least highly with excitement-seeking (about .35), indicating that assertiveness is emphasized much more in their definition of Extraversion than is excitement-seeking, which is peripheral, at best. In contrast, the NEO-FFI Extraversion scale puts much more emphasis on positive emotions and warmth than do BFI and TDA, and less emphasis on assertiveness, as shown by the crossover pattern of their facet profiles. In other words, the NEO-FFI defines Extraversion as a somewhat different

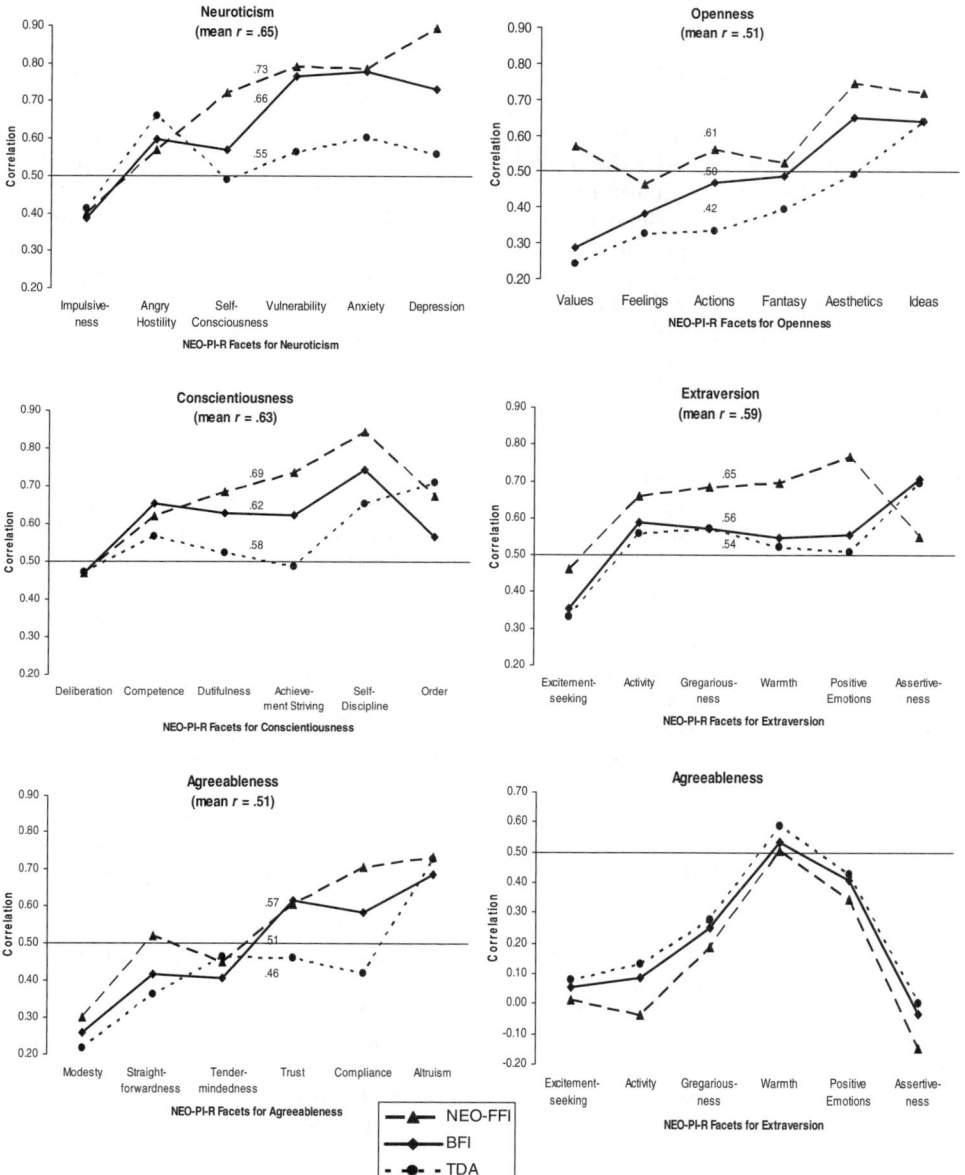

FIGURE 4.2. How do the three most commonly used, short Big Five instruments define each of the five broad trait domains? Profiles of the Big Five domains, as measured by the NEO Five-Factor Inventory (NEO-FFI), Big Five Inventory (BFI), and Trait Descriptive Adjectives (TDA) across the 30 facet traits defined by the NEO Personality Inventory—Revised (NEO-PI-R). *Note*: For each Big Five domain, the figure shows the convergent correlations of the scales of the three instruments, each shown as a profile curve, with the six NEO-PI-R facets for that domain. The average correlation between the domain scales from each Big Five instrument and the six NEO-PI-R facets is presented next to their respective profile curve. For the NEO-FFI (but not the other two instruments), these coefficients represent part–whole correlations; everything else being equal, the NEO-FFI profile curve should thus always be higher than the curves for the other two instruments (BFI and TDA). Therefore, the absolute elevation of the three profile curves is of less interest than their shape—that is, their relative similarity and differences. To illustrate that the interpersonal dimensions of Extraversion and Agreeableness show some overlap (see also Figure 4.3), the sixth panel (on the lower right) shows the discriminant validity correlations of the three Agreeableness domain scales with the Extraversion facets from the NEO-PI-R.

mixture of lower-level personality attributes than do the BFI and TDA.

We should comment on other features of these facet profiles. First, consider the overall elevation of these three Extraversion profiles, which is summarized by the mean correlation presented next to each profile line: .65 (highest overall) for the NEO-FFI, followed by .56 for the BFI and .54 for the TDA. The NEO-FFI's highest elevation here (and everywhere else in this figure) is due, in part, to partial item overlap and cannot be interpreted unambiguously—after all, the 60 items that make up the 12-item NEO-FFI scales are also included in the 30 facet scales that we used to generate the correlations for Figure 4.2. Thus, whereas the absolute elevation is informative for the BFI and TDA, it is less so for the NEO-FFI, and the shape of the profile is much more critical, like the crossover for assertiveness. Second, these graphs also tell us something about the facets that define the profiles. Note that all but one facet had correlations with all three Extraversion scales above the .50 line, suggesting that they are all substantially relevant to the way Extraversion is conceptualized on all three instruments. The finding that excitement-seeking had, by far, the lowest correlations with all three Extraversion scales suggests that it is a relatively peripheral facet within the Extraversion domain. Apparently, the NEO-PI-R facets are not all equal in their centrality to their Big Five domains.

This point is even more apparent in the Agreeableness panel on the lower left. The BFI, TDA, and NEO-FFI Agreeableness scales all correlate about .70 with the altruism facet, showing remarkable Agreement about the centrality of this facet to this domain. In contrast, all three correlated less than .30 with modesty, suggesting that this facet is peripheral to the Agreeableness domain. In terms of profile similarity, BFI and NEO-FFI are much closer to each other than either is to the TDA, especially for trust and compliance, which seem relatively underrepresented on the TDA. Finally, consider the sixth panel (on the lower right), which is the one panel that shows discriminant validity correlations, relating the three Agreeableness scales with the facets from the NEO-PI-R Extraversion domain. Here the Agreeableness scales show impressive profile similarity, indicating that all three correlate above .50 with warmth and about .40 with positive emotions.

This fuzzy boundary between the Extraversion and Agreeableness domain is also illustrated in Figure 4.3 which shows the Big Five trait version of the interpersonal circumplex (Wiggins, 1979). This figure shows factor loadings for the Extraversion and Agreeableness scales from the NEO-FFI, BFI, and TDA, which were factored along with the six NEO-PI-R facets defining Extraversion, the six defining Agreeableness, and the angry hostility facet from the Neuroticism domain, because it is also highly negatively related to Agreeableness (as indicated by its substantial negative loading on that factor). As we noted earlier, warmth and positive emotions are the Extraversion facets with the largest (positive) loadings on Agreeableness. The Agreeableness facets such as trust and altruism have positive loadings on Extraversion, whereas modesty and compliance have negative loadings. Finally, the locations of the TDA, BFI, and NEO-FFI scales are also compatible with our earlier observations. BFI and TDA Extraversion are almost in exactly the same spot in this two-dimensional space, and certainly closer to assertiveness than is NEO-FFI Extraversion, which is rotated to the right toward Agreeableness and thus closer to positive emotions and warmth. Both TDA and BFI Agreeableness are located very close to the altruism facet, which turned out to be so central to all three Agreeableness scales in Figure 4.2.

Although two-dimensional plots of factor loadings, such as those in Figure 4.3, have long been used in trait taxonomic and especially circumplex work, they seem to offer less specific information than the facet profiles in Figure 4.2. For Openness, for example, the biggest difference involves the value facet, which seems barely represented on either TDA or BFI. In contrast, for Neuroticism it is the underweighting of depression, anxiety, and vulnerability and the relative overweighting of hostility that make the TDA scale so different from both the BFI and NEO-FFI Neuroticism scales.

Big Five Measurement: Conclusions and Limitations

One of the limitations of the findings presented here is that we did not examine external (or predictive) validity. However, both the NEO questionnaires and the BFI have

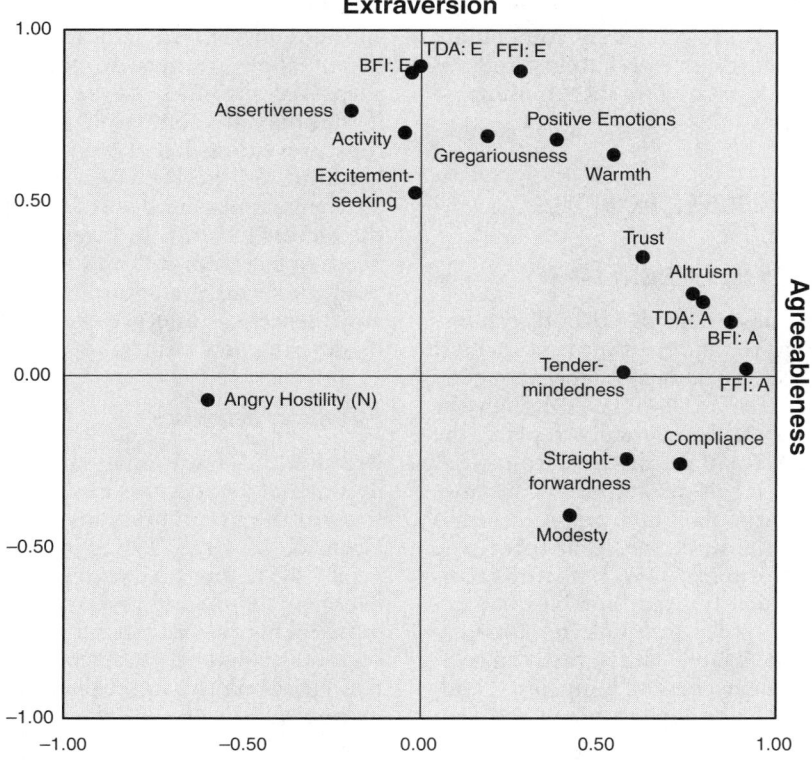

FIGURE 4.3. The interpersonal circumplex formed by the Big Five domains of Extraversion and Agreeableness. The Extraversion and Agreeableness domain scales from three Big Five instruments (NEO-FFI, BFI, and TDA) were factored along with the six NEO-PI-R facets defining Extraversion, the six defining Agreeableness, and the angry hostility facet from the Neuroticism domain (because it is also highly related to Agreeableness). FFI, NEO Five-Factor Inventory; BFI, Big Five Inventory; TDA, Trait Descriptive Adjectives; E, Extraversion; A, Agreeableness; N, Neuroticism.

been shown to predict peer ratings; and initial evidence is now available for the TDA scales (DeYoung, 2006). Future research needs to study the comparative validity of all three instruments using peer ratings and other external criteria. One of the advantages of the BFI is its efficiency, taking only about 5 minutes of administration time, compared with about 15 minutes for the NEO-FFI and the 100-item TDA. Moreover, the BFI items are shorter and easier to understand than the NEO-FFI items (Benet-Martínez & John, 1998; Soto et al., 2008). The 100 (or 40) adjectives on the TDA are even shorter; however, single-trait adjectives can be ambiguous in their meanings.

When should researchers use each of these instruments? When participant time is not at a premium, participants are well educated and test-savvy, and the research question calls for the assessment of multiple facets for the Big Five, then the full 240-item NEO-PI-R would be most useful. Otherwise, the 44-item BFI would seem to offer a measure of the core attributes of the Big Five that is at least as efficient and easily understood as the 60-item NEO-FFI and the 100-item TDA. At this point, we cannot recommend the use of even shorter instruments, with as few as 10 items (e.g., Gosling, Rentfrow, & Swann, 2003; Rammstedt & John, 2007), unless a researcher encounters truly exceptional circumstances, such as the need to measure the Big Five as part of a national phone survey. From our perspective, the gains in time achieved by moving from a measure such as the BFI (i.e., 5 minutes of subject time) to an even shorter measure can rarely compensate for the potential losses in reliability and validity one has to risk with such minimalist measurement.

FACTOR NAMES, NUMBERS, OR INITIALS: WHICH SHALL WE USE?

Problems with the English Factor Labels

Now that we have considered both the history of the Big Five and their measurement, it is time to revisit the names or labels assigned to the factors (see Table 4.2). Although the constructs that will eventually replace the current Big Five may be different from what we know now, labels are important because they imply particular interpretations and thus influence the directions that theorizing might take. Norman's (1963) factor labels have been frequently used, but Norman offered little theoretical rationale for their selection. Norman's labels differ vastly in their breadth or inclusiveness (Hampson, Goldberg, & John, 1987); in particular, Conscientiousness and Culture are much too narrow to capture the enormous breadth of these two dimensions. Moreover, researchers have abandoned Culture as a label for Factor V, in favor of Intellect or Imagination (Saucier & Goldberg, 1996a) or Openness to Experience (McCrae & Costa, 1985b). Neither label is truly satisfactory, however, because Intellect is too narrow and Openness, while broad enough, is somewhat vague.

Agreeableness is another problematic label. For one, it refers to the behavioral tendency to *agree* with others, thus incorrectly implying submissiveness, which is more closely related to the introverted pole of Factor I. Agreeableness is also too detached, too neutral a label for a factor supposed to capture intensely affective characteristics, such as love, compassion, and sympathy. Freud viewed love and work as central; following this lead, we could call Factor II simply *Love* (Peabody & Goldberg, 1989).

However, *Work* is too narrow a label for Factor III. Even Conscientiousness is too narrow because it omits a central component that Peabody and Goldberg (1989) called "favorable impulse control." Thus, Responsibility or even Degree of Socialization (see Gough, 1987) might be labels more appropriate for Factor III than Conscientiousness.

More could be said about the many shortcomings of the traditional labels, but better labels are hard to come by. The unsurpassed advantage of the traditional labels is that they are commonly known and used, thus preventing Babel from taking over the literature on the Big Five. Moreover, before any new names are devised, the definition of the factors in terms of facets or components needs to be elaborated and sharpened. At this point, it seems premature to settle the scope and theoretical interpretation of the factors by devising new names.

Preliminary Definitions

Because the traditional labels are so easily misunderstood, we provide short definitions of the five dimensions in Table 4.2 (cf., Costa & McCrae, 1992; John, 1990; Tellegen, 1985). Briefly, Extraversion implies an *energetic approach* toward the social and material world and includes traits such as sociability, activity, assertiveness, and positive emotionality. Agreeableness contrasts a *prosocial and communal orientation* toward others with antagonism and includes traits such as altruism, tender-mindedness, trust, and modesty. Conscientiousness describes *socially prescribed impulse control* that facilitates task- and goal-directed behavior, such as thinking before acting, delaying gratification, following norms and rules, and planning, organizing, and prioritizing tasks. Neuroticism contrasts emotional stability and even-temperedness with *negative emotionality*, such as feeling anxious, nervous, sad, and tense. Finally, Openness to Experience (vs. closed-mindedness) describes the breadth, depth, originality, and complexity of an individual's *mental and experiential life*.

The numbering convention from I to V, favored by Saucier and Goldberg (1996b) and Hofstee and colleagues (1997), is useful because it reflects the relative size of the factors in lexical studies. Factors I and II, which primarily summarize traits of an interpersonal nature, tend to account for the largest percentage of variance in personality ratings, followed by Factor III, whereas the last two factors are the smallest, by far, in lexical studies (De Raad et al., 1998). However, the Roman numerals are hard to remember, and the order of the factors is not invariant across studies. Thus, we favor the mnemonic convention suggested by the initials given in Table 4.2. These initials evoke multiple associations that represent more fully than a single word the broad range of meaning captured by each of the factors: *E* stands for Extraversion, Energy, or Enthusiasm; *A* for Agreeableness, Altruism, or Affection; *C* for Conscientiousness, Control, or Constraint; *N* for Neuroticism, Negative Affectivity, or Nervousness; and *O* for Openness, Originality, or Open-Mindedness. The reader intrigued by anagrams may have noticed that these letters form the OCEAN of personality dimensions.

CONVERGENCE BETWEEN THE BIG FIVE AND OTHER STRUCTURAL MODELS

McCrae and Costa's (1985a, 1985b, 1985c, 1987) findings, like the cross-instrument convergence described above, showed that the factor-analytic results from the lexical tradition converged surprisingly well with those from the questionnaire tradition. This convergence eventually led to a dramatic change in the acceptance of the five factors in the field. With regard to their empirical status, the findings accumulated since the mid-1980s show that the five factors replicate across different types of subjects, raters, and data sources, in both dictionary-based and questionnaire-based studies. Indeed, even more skeptical reviewers were led to conclude that "Agreement among these descriptive studies with respect to *what* are the appropriate dimensions is impressive" (Revelle, 1987, p. 437; see also McAdams, 1992). The finding that it doesn't matter whether Conscientiousness is measured with trait adjectives, short phrases, or questionnaire items suggests that the Big Five dimensions have the same conceptual status as other personality constructs. For example, Loehlin and colleagues (1998) found that all five factors show substantial and about equal heritabilities, regardless of whether they are measured with questionnaires or with adjective scales derived from the lexical approach.

One of the great strengths of the Big Five taxonomy is that it can capture, at a broad level of abstraction, the commonalities among most of the existing systems of personality traits, thus providing an integrative descriptive model for research. Table 4.1 summarizes the personality dimensions proposed by a broad range of personality theorists and researchers. These dimensions, although by no means a complete tabulation, emphasize the diversity of current conceptions of personality. However, they also point to some important convergences. First, almost every one of the theorists includes a dimension akin to Extraversion. Although the labels and exact definitions vary, nobody seems to doubt the fundamental importance of this dimension. The second almost universally accepted personality dimension is Emotional Stability, as contrasted with Neuroticism, Negative Emotionality, and Proneness to Anxiety. Interestingly, however, not all the researchers listed in Table 4.1 include a separate measure for this dimension. This is particularly true of the interpersonal approaches, such as Wiggins's and Bales's, as well as the questionnaires primarily aimed at the assessment of basically healthy, well-functioning adults, such as Gough's CPI, the MBTI, and even Jackson's Personality Research Form (PRF; 1984). In contrast, all of the temperament-based models include Neuroticism. There is less agreement on the third dimension, which appears in various guises, such as Control, Constraint, Super-Ego Strength, or Work Orientation, as contrasted with Impulsivity, Psychoticism, or Play Orientation. The theme underlying most of these concepts involves the control, or moderation, of impulses in a normatively and socially appropriate way (cf. Block & Block, 1980). However, Table 4.1 also points to the importance of Agreeableness and Openness, which are neglected by temperament-oriented theorists such as A. H. Buss and Plomin, Eysenck, and Zuckerman. In a comprehensive taxonomy, even at the broadest level, we need a "place" for an interpersonal dimension related to Communion, Feeling Orientation, Altruism, Nurturance, Love Styles, and Social Closeness, as contrasted with Hostility, Anger Proneness, and Narcissism. The existence of these questionnaire scales, and the cross-cultural work on the interpersonal origin and consequences of personality, stress the need for a broad domain akin to Agreeableness, Warmth, or Love.

Similar arguments apply to the fifth and last factor included in the Big Five. For one, there are the concepts of Creativity, Originality, and Cognitive Complexity, which are measured by numerous questionnaire scales (Gough, 1979; Helson, 1967, 1985). Although these concepts are cognitive, or, more appropriately, *mental* in nature, they are clearly different from IQ. Second, limited-domain scales measuring concepts such as Absorption, Fantasy Proneness, Need for Cognition, Private Self-Consciousness, Independence, and Autonomy would be difficult to subsume under Extraversion, Neuroticism, or Conscientiousness. Indeed, the fifth factor is necessary because individual differences in intellectual and creative functioning underlie artistic interests and performances, inventions and innovation, and even humor. Individual differences in these domains of human behavior and experience cannot be neglected by personality psychologists.

Finally, the matches between the Big Five and other constructs noted in Table 4.1 should be considered with a healthy dose of skepticism. Some of these correspondences are indeed based on solid research findings, but others are conceptually derived and await empirical confirmation. These matches reflect broad similarities, ignoring some important, implicative, and useful differences among the concepts proposed by different investigators. Nonetheless, at this stage in the field, we are more impressed by the newly apparent similarities than by the continuing differences among the various models. Indeed, the Big Five are useful primarily because of their integrative and heuristic value, a value that becomes apparent in Table 4.1. The availability of a taxonomy, even one that is as broad and incomplete as the Big Five, permits the comparison and potential integration of dimensions that, by their names alone, would seem entirely disparate.

CRITICAL ISSUES AND THEORETICAL PERSPECTIVES

Like any scientific model, the Big Five taxonomy has limitations. Critics have argued that the Big Five does not provide a complete theory of personality (e.g., Block, 1995; Eysenck, 1997; McAdams, 1992; Pervin, 1994), and we agree. In contrast to McCrae and Costa's (1996; see also McCrae & Costa, Chapter 5, this volume) five-factor theory, the Big Five taxonomy was never intended as a comprehensive personality theory; it was developed to account for the structural relations among personality traits (Goldberg,

1993). Thus, like most structural models it provides an account of personality that is primarily descriptive rather than explanatory, emphasizes regularities in behavior rather than inferred dynamic and developmental processes, and focuses on variables rather than on individuals or types of individuals (cf. John & Robins, 1993, 1998). Nonetheless, the Big Five taxonomy of trait terms provides a conceptual foundation that helps us examine these theoretical issues. In this section, we begin with the hierarchical structure defined by the Big Five and then review how the Big Five predict important life outcomes, how they develop, how they combine into personality types, and how different researchers view their conceptual status.

Hierarchy, Levels of Abstraction, and the Big Five

A frequent objection to the Big Five is that five dimensions cannot possibly capture all of the variation in human personality (e.g., Block, 1995; McAdams, 1992; Mershon & Gorsuch, 1988), and that they are much too broad. However, the objection that five dimensions are too few overlooks the fact that personality can be conceptualized at different levels of abstraction or breadth. Indeed, many trait domains are hierarchically structured (Hampson, John, & Goldberg, 1986).

The advantage of categories as broad as the Big Five is their enormous bandwidth. Their disadvantage, of course, is their low fidelity. In any hierarchical representation, one always loses information as one moves up the hierarchical levels. For example, categorizing something as a guppy is more informative than categorizing it as a fish, which in turn is more informative than categorizing it as a vertebrate. Or, in psychometric terms, one necessarily loses item information as one aggregates items into scales, and one loses scale information as one aggregates scales into factors (John, Hampson, & Goldberg, 1991).

The Big Five dimensions represent a rather broad level in the hierarchy of personality descriptors. In that sense, they are to personality what the categories "plant" and "animal" are to the world of biological objects—extremely useful for some initial rough distinctions but of less value for predicting specific behaviors of a particular individual. The hierarchical level a researcher selects depends on the descriptive and predictive tasks to be addressed (Hampson et al., 1986). In principle, the number of specific distinctions one can make in the description of an individual is infinite, limited only by one's objectives.

Norman, Goldberg, McCrae and Costa, and Hogan all recognized that there was a need in personality, just as in biology, "to have a system in which different levels of generality or inclusion are recognized" (Simpson, 1961, p. 12). A complete trait taxonomy must include middle-level categories, such as assertiveness, orderliness, and creativity, and even narrower descriptors, such as talkative, punctual, and musical (John et al., 1991). At this point, Costa and Mc-Crae's (1992) 30 facets, shown in Table 4.4, represent the most widely used and empirically validated model. Soto and John (2008) developed 16 facets (see Table 4.4) from the CPI item pool that tend to be broader than Costa and McCrae's facets. Hofstee and colleagues' (1992) circumplex-based AB5C approach defines 45 facets as unique, pairwise combinations or "blends" of the Big Five factors (e.g., Poise as a blend of high Extraversion and low Neuroticism); measures of these facets have now developed as part of Goldberg's collaborative and Web-based International Personality Item Pool (IPIP) project. Saucier and Ostendorf (1999) provide a thoughtful discussion of the fundamental issues in developing empirically based facets and present 18 facets (see Table 4.4) that show initial cross-language generalizability. Although Table 4.4 shows some promising convergences, the three approaches differ substantially in the number and nature of the facets they propose, indicating that further conceptual and empirical work is needed to achieve a consensual specification of the Big Five factors at lower level of abstraction.

Person–Environment Interactions: Do the Big Five Predict Important Life Outcomes?

Given that the Big Five dimensions were derived initially from analyses of the personality lexicon, one might wonder whether they merely represent linguistic artifacts. Do the Big Five actually predict important behavioral and life outcomes in people's lives? Initially, external validity and predictive utility did not receive much attention from researchers working in the Big Five tradition. Indeed,

Eysenck (1991) challenged the field, arguing that "Little is known about the social relevance and importance of openness, agreeableness, and conscientiousness. ... What is lacking is a series of large-scale studies which would flesh out such possibilities" (p. 785).

Over the past two decades, however, researchers have taken up the task of identifying the particular Big Five dimensions that predict particular life outcomes in such fundamental domains as physical and mental health, work, and relationships (see Table 4.2 for examples). This research is based on the assumption that personal factors (such as the individual's traits) and environmental factors (such as aspects of a job or a relationship partner) interact to jointly produce behavioral and experiential outcomes that accumulate over the individual's lifespan (e.g., Caspi & Bem, 1990; Scarr & McCartney, 1984). In other words, personality traits are important because they influence the way individuals interact with particular environments. As we review below, traits influence how individuals construe and interpret the personal meaning a particular environment or situation has for them (e.g., how they interpret a potential health risk), and to which aspects of the environment they attend (e.g., a doctor's prescribed treatment regimen). In addition to these cognitive processes of perceiving and attending to the environment, traits also influence the way individuals select both social and nonsocial environments (e.g., college classes, jobs, places to live, relationship partners, even music) and how they then modify those environments (e.g., their bedrooms). It is through their systematic interaction with environmental affordances and risks that traits are hypothesized to influence the behavioral, emotional, social, and material life outcomes of the individual.

Links to Health, Health Behaviors, and Longevity

Although research on personality and health has a long tradition in the field, the emergence of the Big Five taxonomy has greatly helped clarify and organize the links between personality, health behaviors, illness, and mortality across the lifespan. Multiple studies have provided converging evidence that Conscientiousness, for example, predicts good health habits, health outcomes, and longevity (for a review, see Hampson

& Friedman, Chapter 31, this volume). For example, low Conscientiousness predicts the likelihood of engaging in risky behaviors such as smoking, substance abuse, and poor diet and exercise habits (Bogg & Roberts, 2004; Hampson, Andrews, Barckley, Lichtenstein, & Lee, 2000; Trull & Sher, 1994). Moreover, highly conscientious individuals, when diagnosed with an illness, are more likely to adhere to their treatment regimens (Kenford et al., 2002) and have been shown to live longer lives (Danner, Snowden, & Friesen, 2001; Friedman, Hawley, & Tucker, 1994; Weiss & Costa, 2005). Other Big Five dimensions are also related to health-related risk factors. Low Agreeableness (especially hostility) predicts cardiovascular disease (Miller, Smith, Turner, Guijarro, & Hallet, 1996). High Neuroticism predicts less successful coping and poorer reactions to illness, in part because highly neurotic individuals are more likely to ruminate about their situation (David & Suls, 1999; Scheier & Carver, 1993). Individuals high in Extraversion, on the other hand, have available more social support and close relationships important for coping with illness (Berkman, Glass, Brissette, & Seeman, 2000).

Links to Psychopathology, Personality Disorders, and Adjustment Problems

The availability of the Big Five taxonomy has also renewed interest in the links between personality and psychopathology, especially personality disorders (e.g., Costa & Widiger, 2002; Wiggins & Pincus, 1989); findings from this burgeoning literature have been reviewed by Krueger and Tackett (2006) and Widiger and Smith (Chapter 30, this volume). From a developmental perspective, the Big Five dimensions may serve as risks or buffers for subsequent adjustment problems. In adolescents, for example, both low Agreeableness and low Conscientiousness predict delinquency and externalizing problems, whereas high Neuroticism and low Conscientiousness predict internalizing problems such as depression and anxiety (John et al., 1994; Measelle et al., 2005; Robins et al., 1994; 1996). Low Conscientiousness is also the personality trait most strongly linked to ADHD, at least when diagnosed in adulthood (Nigg et al., 2002); more specifically, low Conscientiousness predicts attentional

and organizational problems that can lead to broader adjustment problems in school settings and even relationships. Ultimately, findings linking Big Five profiles to developmental or adjustment problems may help us identify children at risk and design appropriate interventions, such as teaching children relevant behaviors and skills (e.g., strategies for delaying gratification).

Links to Academic and Work Outcomes

Industrial and organizational researchers have also rediscovered the importance of personality traits, and a growing body of research has linked the Big Five to academic and work achievement. Early studies showed that Conscientiousness as well as Openness predict school performance as measured with objective tests in early adolescence (John et al., 1994; Robins et al., 1994). In college, Conscientiousness predicts higher academic grade-point averages (Noftle & Robins, 2007; Paunonen, 2003), whereas Openness predicts the total years of education completed by middle adulthood (Goldberg, Sweeney, Merenda, & Hughes, 1998).

Beyond primary and secondary schooling, Conscientiousness has emerged also as a general predictor of job performance across a wide range of jobs (for reviews, see Barrick & Mount, 1991; Mount, Barrick, & Stewart, 1998). The other Big Five dimensions relate to more specific aspects of job performance, such as better performance or satisfaction in specific job types or positions. For example, Agreeableness and Neuroticism predict performance in jobs where employees work in groups, Extraversion predicts success in sales and management positions, Openness predicts success in artistic jobs, and Conscientiousness predicts success in conventional jobs (Barrick, Mount, & Gupta, 2003; Larson, Rottinghaus, & Borgen, 2002). Neuroticism is an important predictor of job satisfaction. Highly neurotic individuals are more likely to experience burnout and to change jobs, whereas more emotionally stable individuals feel satisfied and committed to their organizations (Thoresen, Kaplan, Barsky, Warren, & de Chermont, 2003). These trait-by-job interactions help researchers develop a more fine-grained understanding of how different traits are instrumental to performance and satisfaction in various job environments.

Links to Social Outcomes in Relationship and Group Contexts

The Big Five dimensions are also relevant for social behaviors and experiences, such as relationship maintenance and satisfaction, both in dyadic relationships and in groups. In terms of family relationships, adolescents high in Neuroticism, low in Conscientiousness, and low in Extraversion tend to have poorer relationships with parents (Belsky, Jaffee, Caspi, Moffitt, & Silva, 2003). Individuals low in Agreeableness and Extraversion are more likely to experience peer rejection (Newcomb, Bukowski, & Pattee, 1993). Extraversion, Conscientiousness, and low Neuroticism predict greater relationship satisfaction and less conflict, abuse, or dissolution (Karney & Bradbury, 1995; Robins, Caspi, & Moffitt, 2002; Watson, Hubbard, & Wiese, 2000). Because most social groups develop formal or informal status hierarchies, one important social goal is to attain status (respect, influence, and prominence) in one's social groups. Across several types of groups (Anderson, John, Keltner, & Kring, 2001), Extraversion substantially predicted higher status attainment for both sexes; high Neuroticism, incompatible with male gender norms, predicted lower status only in men. Consistent with these findings, extraverted individuals were more likely to be chosen as the jury foreperson (J. Clark, Boccaccini, Caillouet, & Chaplin, 2007) and more likely to have a firmer "power" handshake (Chaplin, Phillips, Brown, Clanton, & Stein, 2000).

Whereas status and leadership positions are not chosen by the individual but awarded by peers or coworkers, individuals do select or modify their environments. Individuals differ in their selection and modification efforts and successes, and these individual differences are related to personality traits. For example, several Big Five dimensions predict how and where people spend their time. In a study monitoring students' daily life (Mehl, Gosling, & Pennebaker, 2006), students high in Conscientiousness spent more time in the classroom or on campus; students high in Openness spent more time in coffee houses and restaurants; and students high in Extraversion engaged in more conversations and spent less time alone. In a series of studies relating independent assessments of bedrooms and offices to their inhabitants' personality traits (Gosling, Ko, Mannarelli, & Morris, 2002), the Big Five dimensions predicted how individuals shape and modify their physical environments: Highly open individuals tend to create distinctive-looking work and living spaces (with a large variety of different kinds of books), whereas highly conscientious individuals tend to keep their rooms well-organized and clutter-free. High Openness also predicts the expression of a wider variety of interests (e.g., complex music genres) and preferences in personal and social networking websites (Rentfrow & Gosling, 2006; Vazire & Gosling, 2004).

This brief review of Big Five research on person–environment interactions illustrates that the nomological network emerging for each of the Big Five domains now includes an ever-broadening range of life outcome variables. These findings have been summarized in greater detail in several reviews (e.g., Graziano & Eisenberg, 1997; Hogan & Ones, 1997; McCrae, 1996; Ozer & Benet-Martínez, 2006; Watson & Clark, 1997). In interpreting these findings, however, it is important to realize that although individual differences in personality traits are relatively stable over time (e.g., Roberts & DelVecchio, 2000), they are not fixed or "set like plaster" (e.g., Srivastava, John, Gosling, & Potter, 2003). Many people have the capacity to change their patterns of behavior, thought, and feeling, for example, as a result of therapy or intervention programs. Thus, the links between the Big Five and the life outcomes reviewed above are neither fixed nor inevitable for the individual. Instead, they point to critical domains of behavior and emotion that the individual may target for personal development and change. In the health domain, for example, people can improve how conscientiously they adhere to a diet, exercise regimen, or medical treatment plan (Friedman et al., 1994), thus greatly influencing their ultimate health outcomes and longevity.

The Big Five and Personality Development

Historically, personality psychology has concerned itself with a range of developmental issues that are relevant to the Big Five: the antecedents of adult personality traits, how traits develop, the timelines for the emergence and peak expression of traits, their stability or change throughout the lifespan, and the effects of traits on other aspects of personal development. Some critics have suggested that Big Five researchers have not paid enough attention to issues of personality development in childhood and adolescence (Pervin, 1994). This criticism has some merit: Although the Big Five taxonomy has influenced research on adult development and aging (e.g., Helson, Kwan, John, & Jones, 2002; McCrae & Costa, 2003; Roberts, Walton, & Viechtbauer, 2006; see also Roberts, Wood, & Caspi, Chapter 14, this volume), there has been much less research on personality structure in childhood. Developmental and temperament psychologists have studied a number of important traits (e.g., sociability, fearful distress, shyness, impulsivity), but many studies examine one trait at a time, in isolation from the others, and the available research has not been integrated in a coherent taxonomic framework. Until this work is done, however, research on personality development across the lifespan is likely to remain fragmented (Halverson, Kohnstamm, & Martin, 1994).

The adult personality taxonomy defined by the Big Five can offer some promising leads. In our view, the Big Five should be examined in developmental research for two reasons (John et al., 1994). Theoretically, it may be necessary to examine the developmental origins of the Big Five: Given that the Big Five emerge as basic dimensions of personality in adulthood, researchers need to explain how they develop. Practically, the Big Five have proven useful as a framework for organizing findings on adult personality in areas as diverse as behavior genetics and industrial psychology. Thus, extension of the Big Five into childhood and adolescence would facilitate comparisons across developmental periods.

Work on these issues has now begun, and researchers are drawing on existing models of infant and child temperament to make connections to the Big Five dimensions in adulthood (for reviews, see Caspi, Roberts, & Shiner, 2005; De Clerq, De Fruyt, Van Leeuwen, & Mervielde, 2006; Halverson et al., 1994; Shiner & Caspi, 2003). Some research suggests that the Big Five may provide a good approximation of personality structure in childhood and adolescence

(Digman, 1989; Graziano & Ward, 1992). Extending Digman's (1989) earlier work on Hawaiian children, Digman and Shmelyov (1996) examined both temperament dimensions and personality dimensions in a sample of Russian children. Based on analyses of teachers' ratings, they concluded that the Big Five offer a useful model for describing the structure of temperament. Studies using free-response techniques found that the Big Five can account for a substantial portion of children's descriptions of their own and others' personalities (Donahue, 1994), as well as teachers' and parents' descriptions of children's personality (Kohnstamm, Halverson, Mervielde, & Havill, 1998). In a large Internet sample providing self-reports on the BFI, we analyzed data from children and adolescents, ages 10–20, and found substantial changes in the coherence and differentiation of the Big Five domains, even though a variant of the adult Big Five factor structure was apparent as early as age 10 when individual differences in response acquiescence were controlled (see Appendix 4.2; Soto et al., 2008). In an even younger sample, Measelle and colleagues (2005) found that using an age-appropriate puppet interview task, children as young as ages 5–7 were able to self-report on their personality; by age 6, their self-reports were beginning to show evidence of coherence, longitudinal stability, and external validity (using ratings by adults) for the Big Five domains of Extraversion, Agreeableness, and Conscientiousness.

Two large-scale studies suggest that the picture may be more complicated. One study tested whether the adult Big Five structure would replicate in a large and ethnically diverse sample of adolescent boys (John et al., 1994). The California Child Q-sort provided a comprehensive item pool for the description of children and adolescents that was not derived from the adult Big Five and does not represent any particular theoretical orientation. Factor analyses identified five dimensions that corresponded closely with a priori scales representing the adult Big Five. However, two additional dimensions emerged. *Irritability* involved negative affect expressed in age-inappropriate behaviors, such as whining, crying, tantrums, and being overly sensitive to teasing. *Activity* was defined by items involving physical activity, energy, and high tempo, such as running, playing, and moving and reacting quickly. In several Dutch samples of boys and girls ages 3–16 years, van Lieshout and Haselager (1994) also found the Big Five plus two additional factors—one similar to Activity factor observed earlier in the United States (John et al., 1994), and a Dependency dimension defined primarily by eagerness to please and reliance on others. Although these findings need to be replicated and extended, they leave open the possibility that the structure of personality traits may be more differentiated in childhood than in adulthood. Specifically, the additional dimensions may originate in temperamental features of childhood personality (e.g., activity level) that become integrated into adult personality structure over the course of adolescence (John et al., 1994).

These studies illustrate how the Big Five can help stimulate research that connects and integrates findings across long-separate research traditions. They also provide initial insights about the way in which personality structure may develop toward its adult form. Yet a great deal of work still lies ahead. Studies need to examine the antecedents of the Big Five and their relations to other aspects of personality functioning in childhood and adolescence. In this way, the Big Five can help connect research on adult personality with the vast field of social development.

Theoretical Perspectives on the Big Five: Description and Explanation

Over the years, researchers have articulated a number of different perspectives on the conceptual status of the Big Five dimensions. Because of their lexical origin, the factors were initially interpreted as dimensions of trait description or attribution (John et al., 1988). Subsequent research, however, has shown that the lexical factors converge with dimensions derived in other personality research traditions, that they have external or predictive validity (as reviewed above), and that all five of them show about equal amounts of heritability (Loehlin et al., 1998). We thus need to ask how these differences should be conceptualized (e.g., Wiggins, 1996); below we briefly summarize some of the major theoretical perspectives.

Researchers in the lexical tradition tend to take an agnostic stance regarding the conceptual status of traits. For example, Saucier and Goldberg (1996b) argued that their studies of personality description do not address issues of causality or the mechanisms underlying behavior. Their interest is primarily in the language of personality. This level of self-restraint may seem dissatisfactory to psychologists who are more interested in personality itself. However, the findings from the lexical approach are informative because the lexical hypothesis is essentially a functionalist argument about the trait concepts in the natural language. These concepts are of interest because language encodes the characteristics that are central, for cultural, social, or biological reasons, to human life and experience. Thus, Saucier and Goldberg argue that lexical studies define an agenda for personality psychologists because they highlight the important and meaningful psychological phenomena (i.e., phenotypic characteristics) that personality psychologists should study and explain. Thus, issues such as the accuracy of self and peer descriptions and the causal origin of traits (i.e., genotypes) are left as open questions that need to be answered empirically. However, important characteristics may exist that people may not be able to observe and describe verbally; if so, the agenda specified by the lexical approach may be incomplete and would need to be supplemented by more theoretically driven approaches (Block, 1995; Tellegen, 1993).

Several theories conceptualize the Big Five as relational constructs. Interpersonal theory (Wiggins & Trapnell, 1996), emphasizes the individual in relationships. The Big Five are taken to describe "the relatively enduring pattern of recurrent interpersonal situations that characterize a human life" (Sullivan, 1953, pp. 110–111), thus conceptualizing the Big Five as descriptive concepts. Wiggins and Trapnell emphasize the interpersonal motives of agency and communion and interpret all of the Big Five dimensions in terms of their interpersonal implications. Because Extraversion and Agreeableness are the most clearly interpersonal dimensions in the Big Five, they receive conceptual priority in this model.

Socioanalytic theory (Hogan, 1996) focuses on the social functions of self- and other perceptions. According to Hogan, trait concepts serve as the "linguistic tools of observers" (1996, p. 172) used to encode and communicate reputations. This view implies that traits are socially constructed to serve interpersonal functions. Because trait terms fundamentally reflect reputation, individuals who self-report their traits engage in a symbolic–interactionist process of introspection (i.e., the individual considers how others view him or her). Hogan emphasizes that individuals may distort their self-reports with self-presentational strategies; another source of distortion are self-deceptive biases (cf. Paulhus & John, 1998), which do not reflect deliberate impression management but honestly held, though biased, beliefs about the self.

The evolutionary perspective on the Big Five holds that humans have evolved "difference-detecting mechanisms" to perceive individual differences that are relevant to survival and reproduction (D. M. Buss, 1996, p. 185; see also Botwin, Buss, & Shackelford, 1997). Buss views personality as an "adaptive landscape" where the Big Five traits represent the most salient and important dimensions of the individual's survival needs. The evolutionary perspective equally emphasizes person perception and individual differences: Because people vary systematically along certain trait dimensions, and because knowledge of others' traits has adaptive value, humans have evolved a capacity to perceive those individual differences that are central to adaptation to the social landscape. The Big Five summarize these centrally important individual differences.

McCrae and Costa (1996; see also Chapter 5, this volume) view the Big Five as causal personality dispositions. Their five-factor theory (FFT) is a general trait theory that provides an explanatory interpretation of the empirically derived Big Five taxonomy. One central tenet of the FFT is based on the finding that all of the Big Five dimensions have a substantial genetic basis (e.g., Loehlin et al., 1998; Plomin, DeFries, Craig, & McGuffin, 2003; see also Krueger & Johnson, Chapter 10, this volume) and must therefore derive, in part, from biological structures and processes, such as specific gene loci, brain regions (e.g., the amygdala), neurotransmitters (e.g., dopamine), hormones (e.g., testosterone), and so on (e.g., Canli, 2006; see also Canli, Chapter 11, this volume); it is in this sense that traits are assumed to have causal status. McCrae and Costa distinguish between "basic tendencies"

and "characteristic adaptations." Personality traits are basic tendencies that refer to the abstract underlying potentials of the individual, whereas attitudes, roles, relationships, and goals are characteristic adaptations that reflect the interactions between basic tendencies and environmental demands accumulated over time. According to McCrae and Costa, basic tendencies remain stable across the life course, whereas characteristic adaptations can undergo considerable change. From this perspective, then, a statement such as "Paul likes to go to parties because he is extraverted" is not circular, as it would be if *extraverted* were merely a description of typical behavior (Wiggins, 1997). Instead, the concept *extraverted* stands in for biological structures and processes that remain to be discovered. This view is similar to Allport's (1937) account of traits as neuropsychic structures and Eysenck's view of traits as biological mechanisms (Eysenck & Eysenck, 1985).

The idea that personality traits have a biological basis is also fundamental to Gosling's proposal that personality psychology must be broadened to include a comparative approach to study individual differences in both human and nonhuman animals (Gosling, 2001; Gosling, Kwan, & John, 2003). Although scientists are understandably reluctant to ascribe personality traits, emotions, and cognitions to animals, evolutionary theory predicts cross-species continuities not only for physical but also for behavioral traits; for example, Darwin (1872/1998) argued that emotions exist in both human and nonhuman animals. A review of 19 studies of personality factors in 12 nonhuman species showed substantial cross-species continuity (Gosling & John, 1999). Chimpanzees and other primates, dogs, cats, donkeys, pigs, guppies, and octopuses all showed reliable individual differences in Extraversion and Neuroticism, and all but guppies and octopuses varied in Agreeableness as well, suggesting that these three Big Five factors may capture fundamental dimensions of individual differences. Further evidence suggests that elements of Openness (such as curiosity and playfulness) are present in at least some nonhuman animals. In contrast, only humans and our closest relatives, chimpanzees, appear to show systematic individual differences in Conscientiousness. Given the relatively complex social-cognitive functions involved in this dimension (i.e., following norms and rules, thinking before acting, and controlling impulses), it makes sense that Conscientiousness may have appeared rather recently in our evolutionary history. The careful application of ethological and experimental methodology and the high interobserver reliability in these studies make it unlikely that these findings merely reflect anthropomorphic projections (c.f., Gosling et al., 2003; Kwan, Gosling, & John, 2008). Rather, these surprising cross-species commonalities suggest that personality traits reflect, at least in part, biological mechanisms that are shared by many mammalian species.

In summary, researchers subscribe to a diversity of perspectives on the conceptual status of the Big Five, ranging from purely descriptive concepts to biologically based causal concepts. This diversity might be taken to imply that researchers cannot agree about the definition of the trait concept and that the field is in disarray. It is important to recognize, however, that these perspectives are not mutually exclusive. For example, although Saucier and Goldberg (1996b) caution against drawing inferences about genotypes from lexical studies, the lexical hypothesis does not preclude the possibility that the Big Five are embodied in biological structures and processes. In our view, "what is a trait?" is fundamentally an empirical question. Research in diverse areas such as behavior and molecular genetics, personality stability and change, and accuracy and bias in self-reports and interpersonal perception will be instrumental in building and refining a comprehensive theoretical account of the Big Five.

CONCLUSIONS AND IMPLICATIONS

At the beginning of this chapter, we argued that a personality taxonomy should provide a systematic framework for distinguishing, ordering, and naming the behavioral, emotional, and experiential characteristics of individuals. Ideally, that taxonomy would be built around principles that are causal and dynamic, exist at multiple levels of abstraction or hierarchy, and offer a standard nomenclature for scientists working in the field of personality. The Big Five taxonomy does

not yet meet this high standard. It provides descriptive concepts that still need to be explicated theoretically, and a nomenclature that is still rooted in the "vernacular" English.

The Big Five structure has the advantage that everybody can understand the words that define the factors. Moreover, the natural language is not biased in favor of any existing scientific conceptions; although the atheoretical nature of the Big Five dimensions makes them less appealing to some psychologists, it also makes them more palatable to researchers who reject dimensions cast in a theoretical mold different from their own. Whatever the inadequacies of the natural language for scientific systematics, broad dimensions inferred from folk usage are *not* a bad place to start a taxonomy. Even in the biological taxonomy of animals, "the technical system evolved from the vernacular" (Simpson, 1961, pp. 12–13).

Obviously, a system that initially derives from the natural language does not need to reify such terms indefinitely. Indeed, several of the dimensions included among the Big Five, most notably Extraversion and Neuroticism, have been the target of various physiological and mechanistic explanations (e.g., Canli et al., 2001; see also L. A. Clark, 2005). In research on emotion regulatory processes, the links between the Big Five, the chronic use of particular regulatory strategies, and their emotional and social consequences are being articulated (John & Gross, 2007). Similarly, the conceptual explication of Extraversion and Neuroticism as persistent dispositions toward thinking and behaving in ways that foster, respectively, positive and negative affective experiences (e.g., Tellegen, 1985; see also Clark & Watson, Chapter 9, this volume) promises to connect the Big Five with individual differences in affective functioning, which, in turn, may be studied in more tightly controlled laboratory settings (see Gross, Chapter 28, this volume). At this point, the Big Five differentiate domains of individual differences that have similar surface manifestations—just like the early animal taxonomy that was transformed by better accounts of evolutionary processes and by the advent of new tools, such as molecular genetics. Likewise, the structures and processes underlying these personality trait domains are now beginning to be explicated. Explanatory and mechanistic terms will likely change the definition and assessment of the Big Five dimensions as we know them today.

As Gould (1981) observed, even in the biological and physical sciences, "taxonomy is always a contentious issue because the world does not come to us in neat little packages" (p. 158). Since the early 1980s when the Big Five barely registered a blip in the published personality literature (see Figure 4.1), we have come a long way in understanding the "messy packages" that are personality traits. Researchers have made enormous progress on the Big Five trait taxonomy, producing an initial consensus that we can differentiate five replicable domains of personality as summarized by the broad concepts of *Extraversion, Agreeableness, Conscientiousness, Neuroticism,* and *Openness to experience.* Viewed from a historical vantage point, the emergence of the Big Five structure, and the fact that multiple groups of researchers worked on it jointly, brought about a major change in the field of personality that is akin to a paradigm shift. Personality trait research has moved from a stage of early individualistic pioneers to a more mature stage of normal scientific inquiry: Researchers interested in studying the effects of personality traits on important theoretical or applied phenomena, such as emotion, social behavior and relationships, work and achievement, or physical and mental health, now use a commonly understood framework to conceptualize their research and choose from several well-validated instruments to operationalize these personality domains. Literature reviews and meta-analyses are commonly done to organize all the available empirical findings on a phenomenon, such as whether and how much personality traits change during particular periods of adulthood (e.g., Helson et al., 2002; Roberts et al., 2006), into one coherent set of hypotheses and findings. This is indeed a paradigm shift (or a seismic shift here in California) in a field dominated, until recently, by seemingly incompatible systems that caused fragmentation and competition, rather than fostering commonalities and convergences. As illustrated in Table 4.1, the Big Five structure captures, at a broad level of abstraction, the commonalities among the existing systems of personality description and thus provides an integrative descriptive taxonomy for personality research.

ACKNOWLEDGMENTS

This chapter summarizes and updates previous reviews by John (1990) and John and Srivastava (1999). The preparation of this chapter was supported in part by research grants from the Retirement Research Foundation and the Metanexus Foundation, and by National Science Foundation Predoctoral Fellowships to Laura Naumann and Christopher Soto. The support and resources provided by the Institute of Personality and Social Research are also gratefully acknowledged.

REFERENCES

Allport, G. W. (1937). *Personality: A psychological interpretation.* New York: Holt.

Allport, G. W. (1958). What units shall we employ? In G. Lindzey (Ed.), *Assessment of human motives* (pp. 238–260). New York: Rinehart.

Allport, G. W., & Odbert, H. S. (1936). Trait-names: A psycho-lexical study. *Psychological Monographs, 47,* No. 211.

Almagor, M., Tellegen, A., & Waller, N. G. (1995). The Big Seven model: A cross-cultural replication and further exploration of the basic dimensions of natural language trait descriptors. *Journal of Personality and Social Psychology, 69,* 300–307.

Anderson, C., John, O. P., Keltner, D., & Kring, A. (2001). Who attains social status? Effects of personality and physical attractiveness in social groups. *Journal of Personality and Social Psychology, 81,* 116–132.

Angleitner, A., Ostendorf, F., & John, O. P. (1990). Towards a taxonomy of personality descriptors in German: A psycho-lexical study. *European Journal of Personality, 4,* 89–118.

Ashton, M. C., Lee, K., Perugini, M., Szarota, P., de Vries, R. E., Di Blas, L., et al. (2004). A six-factor structure of personality-descriptive adjectives: Solutions from psycholexical studies in seven languages. *Journal of Personality and Social Psychology, 86,* 356–366.

Bales, R. F. (1970). *Personality and interpersonal behavior.* New York: Holt, Rinehart & Winston.

Barrick, M. R., & Mount, M. K. (1991). The Big Five personality dimensions and job performance: A meta-analysis. *Personnel Psychology, 44,* 1–26.

Barrick, M. R., Mount, M. K., & Gupta, R. (2003). Meta-analysis of the relationship between the five factor model of personality and Holland's occupational types. *Personnel Psychology, 56,* 45–74.

Baumgarten, F. (1933). *Die Charktereigenschaften* [The character traits]. In Beitraege zur Charakter- und Persoenlichkeitsforschung (Whole No. 1). Bern, Switzerland: A. Francke.

Becker, W. C. (1960). The matching of behavior rating and questionnaire personality factors. *Psychological Bulletin, 57,* 201–212.

Belsky, J., Jaffee, S. R., Caspi, A., Moffitt, T., & Silva, P. A. (2003). Intergenerational relationships in young adulthood and their life course, mental health, and personality correlates. *Journal of Family Psychology, 17,* 460–471.

Benet-Martínez, V., & John, O. P. (1998). Los Cinco Grandes across cultures and ethnic groups: Multitrait–multimethod analyses of the Big Five in Spanish and English. *Journal of Personality and Social Psychology, 75,* 729–750.

Benet-Martínez, V., & Waller, N. G. (1997). Further evidence for the cross-cultural generality of the Big Seven Factor model: Indigenous and imported Spanish personality constructs. *Journal of Personality, 65,* 567–598.

Berkman, L. F., Glass, T., Brissette, I., & Seeman, T. E. (2000). From social integration to health. *Social Science and Medicine, 51,* 843–857.

Block, J. (1995). A contrarian view of the five-factor approach to personality description. *Psychological Bulletin, 117,* 187–215.

Block, J. H., & Block, J. (1980). The role of ego-control and ego-resiliency in the organization of behavior. In W. A. Collins (Ed.), *Minnesota Symposia on Child Psychology* (Vol. 13, pp. 39–101). Hillsdale, NJ: Erlbaum.

Bogg, T., & Roberts, B. W. (2004). Conscientiousness and health behaviors: A meta-analysis. *Psychological Bulletin, 130,* 887–919.

Borgatta, E. F. (1964). The structure of personality characteristics. *Behavioral Science, 9,* 8–17.

Botwin, M. D., & Buss, D. M. (1989). Structure of act–report data: Is the five-factor model of personality recaptured? *Journal of Personality and Social Psychology, 56,* 988–1001.

Botwin, M. D., Buss, D. M., & Shackelford, T. K. (1997). Personality and mate preferences: Five factors in mate selection and marital satisfaction. *Journal of Personality, 65,* 107–136.

Burisch, M. (1984). Approaches to personality inventory construction. *American Psychologist, 39,* 214–227.

Buss, A. H., & Plomin, R. (1975). *A temperament theory of personality development.* New York: Wiley.

Buss, D. M. (1996). Social adaptation and five major factors of personality. In J. S. Wiggins (Ed.), *The five-factor model of personality: Theoretical perspectives* (pp. 180–207). New York: Guilford Press.

Canli, T. (Ed.). (2006). *Biology of personality and individual differences.* New York: Guilford Press.

Canli, T., Zhao, Z., Desmond, J. E., Kang, E., Gross, J., & Gabrieli, J. D. (2001). An fMRI study of personality influences on brain reactivity to emotional stimuli. *Behavioral Neuroscience, 115,* 33–42.

Caprara, G. V., & Perugini, M. (1994). Personality described by adjectives: The generalizability of the Big Five to the Italian lexical context. *European Journal of Personality, 8,* 357–369.

Caspi, A., & Bem, D. J. (1990). Personality continuity and change across the life course. In L. A. Pervin (Ed.), *Handbook of personality: Theory and research* (pp. 549–575). New York: Guilford Press.

Caspi, A., Roberts, B. W., & Shiner, R. L. (2005). Personality development: Stability and change. *Annual Review of Psychology, 56,* 453–484.

Cattell, R. B. (1943). The description of personality: Basic traits resolved into clusters. *Journal of Abnormal and Social Psychology, 38,* 476–506.

Cattell, R. B. (1945a). The description of personality: Principles and findings in a factor analysis. *American Journal of Psychology, 58,* 69–90.

Cattell, R. B. (1945b). The principal trait clusters for describing personality. *Psychological Bulletin, 42,* 129–161.

Cattell, R. B. (1990). Advances in Cattellian personality theory. In L. A. Pervin (Ed.), *Handbook of personality: Theory and research* (pp. 101–110). New York: Guilford Press.

Cattell, R. B., Eber, H. W., & Tatsuoka, M. M. (1970). *Handbook for the Sixteen Personality Factor Questionnaire (16PF).* Champaign, IL: IPAT.

Chaplin, W. F., John, O. P., & Goldberg, L. R. (1988). Conceptions of states and traits: Dimensional attributes with ideals as prototypes. *Journal of Personality and Social Psychology, 54,* 541–557.

Chaplin, W. F., Phillips, J. B., Brown, J. D., Clanton, N. R., & Stein, J. L. (2000). Handshaking, gender, personality, and first impressions. *Journal of Personality and Social Psychology, 79,* 110–117.

Church, A. T., & Katigbak, M. S. (1989). Internal, external, and self-report structure of personality in a non-Western culture: An investigation of cross-language and cross-cultural generalizability. *Journal of Personality and Social Psychology, 57,* 857–872.

Church, A. T., Reyes, J. A. S., Katigbak, M. S., & Grimm, S. D. (1997). Filipino personality structure and the Big Five model: A lexical approach. *Journal of Personality, 65,* 477–528.

Clark, J., Boccaccini, M. T., Caillouet, B., & Chaplin, W. F. (2007). Five factor model personality traits, jury selection, and case outcomes in criminal and civil cases. *Criminal Justice and Behavior, 34,* 641–660.

Clark, L. A. (2005). Temperament as a unifying basis for personality and psychopathology. *Journal of Abnormal Psychology, 114,* 505–521.

Clark, L. A., & Watson, D. (1999). Temperament: A new paradigm for trait psychology. In L. A. Pervin & O. P. John (Eds.), *Handbook of personality* (2nd ed., pp. 399–423). New York: Guilford Press.

Comrey, A. L. (1970). *Manual for the Comrey Personality Scales.* San Diego, CA: Educational and Industrial Testing Service.

Conley, J. J. (1985). Longitudinal stability of personality traits: A multitrait–multimethod–multioccasion analysis. *Journal of Personality and Social Psychology, 49,* 1266–1282.

Costa, P. T., Jr., & McCrae, R. R. (1976). Age differences in personality structure: A cluster analytic approach. *Journal of Gerontology, 31,* 564–570.

Costa, P. T., Jr., & McCrae, R. R. (1985). *The NEO Personality Inventory manual.* Odessa, FL: Psychological Assessment Resources.

Costa, P. T., Jr., & McCrae, R. R. (1989). *NEO PI/FFI manual supplement.* Odessa, FL: Psychological Assessment Resources.

Costa, P. T., Jr., & McCrae, R. R. (1992). *NEO PI-R professional manual.* Odessa, FL: Psychological Assessment Resources.

Costa, P. T., Jr., & McCrae, R. R. (1995). Domains and facets: Hierarchical personality assessment using the Revised NEO Personality Inventory. *Journal of Personality Assessment, 64,* 21–50.

Costa, P. T., Jr., & Widiger, T. A. (Eds.). (2002). *Personality disorders and the five factor model of personality* (pp. 203–214). Washington, DC: American Psychological Association.

Danner, D. D., Snowdon, D. A., & Friesen, W. V. (2001). Positive emotions in early life and longevity: Findings from the nun study. *Journal of Personality and Social Psychology, 80,* 804–813.

Darwin, C. (1998). *The expression of emotions in man and animals* (3rd ed.). New York: Oxford University Press. (Original work published 1872)

David, J., & Suls, J. (1999). Coping efforts in daily life: Role of Big Five traits and problem appraisal. *Journal of Personality, 67,* 119–140.

De Clercq, B., De Fruyt, F., Van Leeuwen, K., & Mervielde, I. (2006). The structure of maladaptive personality traits in childhood: A step toward an integrative developmental perspective for DSM-V. *Journal of Abnormal Psychology, 115,* 639–657.

De Raad, B., di Blas, L., & Perugini, M. (1998). Two independently constructed Italian trait taxonomies: Comparisons among Italian and between Italian and Germanic languages. *European Journal of Personality, 12,* 19–41.

De Raad, B., Mulder, E., Kloosterman, K., &

Hofstee, W. K. (1988). Personality-descriptive verbs. *European Journal of Personality, 2,* 81–96.

De Raad, B., & Perugini, M. (Eds.). (2002). *Big Five assessment.* Kirkland, WA: Hogrefe & Huber.

De Raad, B., Perugini, M., Hrebickova, M., & Szarota, P. (1998). *Lingua franca* of personality: Taxonomies and structures based on the psycholexical approach. *Journal of Cross-Cultural Psychology, 29,* 212–232.

DeYoung, C. G. (2006). Higher-order factors of the Big Five in a multi-informant sample. *Journal of Personality and Social Psychology, 91,* 1138–1151.

Di Blas, L., & Forzi, M. (1998). An alternative taxonomic study of personality-descriptive adjectives in the Italian language. *European Journal of Personality, 12,* 75–101.

Digman, J. M. (1989). Five robust trait dimensions: Development, stability, and utility. *Journal of Personality, 57,* 195–214.

Digman, J. M. (1997). Higher-order factors of the Big Five. *Journal of Personality and Social Psychology, 73,* 1246–1256.

Digman, J. M., & Inouye, J. (1986). Further specification of the five robust factors of personality. *Journal of Personality and Social Psychology, 50,* 116–123.

Digman, J. M., & Shmelyov, A. G. (1996). The structure of temperament and personality in Russian children. *Journal of Personality and Social Psychology, 71,* 341–351.

Digman, J. M., & Takemoto-Chock, N. K. (1981). Factors in the natural language of personality: Re-analysis and comparison of six major studies. *Multivariate Behavioral Research, 16,* 149–170.

Donahue, E. M. (1994). Do children use the Big Five, too?: Content and structural form in personality description. *Journal of Personality, 62,* 45–66.

Eysenck, H. J. (1986). Models and paradigms in personality research. In A. Angleitner, A. Furnham, & G. Van Heck (Eds.), *Personality psychology in Europe (Vol. 2): Current trends and controversies* (pp. 213–223). Lisse, The Netherlands: Swets & Zeitlinger.

Eysenck, H. J. (1990). Biological dimensions of personality. In L. A. Pervin (Ed.), *Handbook of personality: Theory and research* (pp. 244–276). New York: Guilford Press.

Eysenck, H. J. (1991). Dimensions of personality: 16, 5, or 3?—criteria for a taxonomic paradigm. *Personality and Individual Differences, 12,* 773–790.

Eysenck, H. J. (1992). Four ways five factors are not basic. *Personality and Individual Differences, 13,* 667–673.

Eysenck, H. J. (1997). Personality and experimental psychology: The unification of psychology and the possibility of a paradigm. *Journal of Personality and Social Psychology, 73,* 1224–1237.

Eysenck, H. J., & Eysenck, M. W. (1985). *Personality and individual differences: A natural science approach.* New York: Plenum Press.

Fiske, D. W. (1949). Consistency of the factorial structures of personality ratings from different sources. *Journal of Abnormal and Social Psychology, 44,* 329–344.

Friedman, H. S., Hawley, P. H., & Tucker, J. S. (1994). Personality, health, and longevity. *Current Directions in Psychological Science, 3,* 37–41.

Goldberg, L. R. (1981). Language and individual differences: The search for universals in personality lexicons. In L. Wheeler (Ed.), *Review of personality and social psychology* (Vol. 2, pp. 141–165). Beverly Hills: Sage.

Goldberg, L. R. (1982). From ace to zombie: Some explorations in the language of personality. In C. D. Spielberger & J. N. Butcher (Eds.), *Advances in personality assessment* (Vol. 1, pp. 203–234). Hillsdale, NJ: Erlbaum.

Goldberg, L. R. (1990). An alternative "description of personality": The Big-Five factor structure. *Journal of Personality and Social Psychology, 59,* 1216–1229.

Goldberg, L. R. (1992). The development of markers for the Big-Five factor structure. *Psychological Assessment, 4,* 26–42.

Goldberg, L. R. (1993). The structure of phenotypic personality traits. *American Psychologist, 48,* 26–34.

Goldberg, L. R., & Kilkowski, J. M. (1985). The prediction of semantic consistency in self-descriptions: Characteristics of persons and of terms that affect the consistency of responses to synonym and antonym pairs. *Journal of Personality and Social Psychology, 48,* 82–98.

Goldberg, L. R., & Rosolack, T. K. (1994). The Big Five factor structure as an integrative framework: An empirical comparison with Eysenck's P-E-N model. In C. F. Halverson, G. A. Kohnstamm, & R. P. Martin (Eds.), *The developing structure of temperament and personality from infancy to adulthood* (pp. 7–35). Hillsdale, NJ: Erlbaum.

Goldberg, L. R., Sweeney, D., Merenda, P. F., & Hughes, J.E. (1998). Demographic variables and personality: The effects of gender, age, education, and ethnic/racial status on self-descriptions of personality attributes. *Personality and Individual Differences, 24,* 393–403.

Gosling, S. D. (2001). From mice to men: What can we learn about personality from animal research? *Psychological Bulletin, 127,* 45–86.

Gosling, S. D., & John, O. P. (1999). Personality dimensions in nonhuman animals: A cross-species review. *Current Directions in Psychological Science, 8,* 69–75.

Gosling, S. D., Ko, S. J., Mannarelli, T., & Morris, M. E. (2002). A room with a cue: Personality judgments based on offices and bedrooms. *Journal of Personality and Social Psychology, 82,* 379–398.

Gosling, S. D., Kwan, V. S. Y., & John, O. P. (2003). A dog's got personality: A cross-species comparative approach to evaluating personality judgments. *Journal of Personality and Social Psychology, 85,* 1161–1169.

Gosling, S. D., Rentfrow, P. J., & Swann, W. B., Jr. (2003). A very brief measure of the Big Five personality domains. *Journal of Research in Personality, 37,* 504–528.

Gough, H. G. (1979). A creative personality scale for the Adjective Check List. *Journal of Personality and Social Psychology, 37,* 1938–1405.

Gough, H. G. (1987). *The California Psychological Inventory administrator's guide.* Palo Alto, CA: Consulting Psychologists Press.

Gough, H. G., & Heilbrun, A. B., Jr. (1983). *The Adjective Check List manual.* Palo Alto, CA: Consulting Psychologists Press.

Gould, S. J. (1981). *The mismeasure of man.* New York: Norton.

Graziano, W. G., & Eisenberg, N. (1997). Agreeableness: A dimension of personality. In R. Hogan, J. A. Johnson, & S. R. Briggs (Eds.), *Handbook of personality psychology* (pp. 795–824). San Diego, CA: Academic Press.

Graziano, W. G., & Ward, D. (1992). Probing the Big Five in adolescence: Personality and adjustment during a developmental transition. *Journal of Personality, 60,* 425–439.

Guilford, J. P. (1975). Factors and factors of personality. *Psychological Bulletin, 82,* 802–814.

Halverson, C. F., Kohnstamm, G. A., & Martin R. P. (1994). *The developing structure of temperament and personality from infancy to adulthood.* Hillsdale, NJ: Erlbaum.

Hampson, S. E., Andrews, J. A., Barckley, M., Lichtenstein, E., & Lee, M. E. (2000). Conscientiousness, perceived risk, and risk-reduction behaviors: A preliminary study. *Health Psychology, 19,* 247–252.

Hampson, S. E., & Goldberg, L. R. (2006). A first large cohort study of personality trait stability over the 40 years between elementary school and midlife. *Journal of Personality and Social Psychology, 91,* 763–779.

Hampson, S. E., Goldberg, L. R., & John, O. P. (1987). Category-breadth and social-desirability values for 573 personality terms. *European Journal of Personality, 1,* 241–258.

Hampson, S. E., John, O. P., & Goldberg, L. R. (1986). Category breadth and hierarchical structure in personality: Studies of asymmetries in judgments of trait implications. *Journal of Personality and Social Psychology, 51*, 37–54.

Helson, R. (1967). Personality characteristics and developmental history of creative college women. *Genetic Psychology Monographs, 76*, 205–256.

Helson, R. (1985). Which of those young women with creative potential became productive? Personality in college and characteristics of parents. In R. Hogan & W. H. Jones (Eds.), *Perspectives in personality theory, measurement, and interpersonal dynamics* (Vol. 1, pp. 49–80). Greenwich, CT: JAI Press.

Helson, R., Kwan, V. S. Y., John, O. P., & Jones, C. (2002). The growing evidence for personality change in adulthood: Findings from research with personality inventories. *Journal of Research in Personality, 36*, 287–306.

Hofstee, W. K. B., De Raad, B., & Goldberg, L. R. (1992). Integration of the Big Five and circumplex approaches to trait structure. *Journal of Personality and Social Psychology, 63*, 146–163.

Hofstee, W. K. B., Kiers, H. A., De Raad, B., & Goldberg, L. R. (1997). A comparison of Big-Five structures of personality traits in Dutch, English, and German. *European Journal of Personality, 11*, 15–31.

Hogan, R. (1983). A socioanalytic theory of personality. In M. Page (Ed.), *Nebraska Symposium on Motivation, 1982: Personality—current theory and research* (Vol. 29, pp. 55–89). Lincoln: University of Nebraska Press.

Hogan, R. (1986). *Hogan Personality Inventory manual*. Minneapolis, MN: National Computer Systems.

Hogan, R. (1996). A socioanalytic perspective on the five-factor model. In J. S. Wiggins (Ed.), *The five-factor model of personality: Theoretical perspectives* (pp. 180–207). New York: Guilford Press.

Hogan, R., & Ones, D. S. (1997). Conscientiousness and integrity at work. In R. Hogan, J. A. Johnson, & S. R. Briggs (Eds.), *Handbook of personality psychology* (pp. 849–870). San Diego, CA: Academic Press.

Hrebickova, M., & Ostendorf, F. (1995). *Lexikalni pristup k osobnosti. V: Klasifikace pridavnych jmen do kategorii osobnostni deskripce* [Lexical approach to personality: V. Classification of adjectives into categories of personality description]. *Ceskoslovenska Psychologie, 39*, 265–276.

Jackson, D. N. (1984). *Personality Research Form manual* (3rd ed.). Port Huron, MI: Research Psychologists Press.

John, O. P. (1989). Towards a taxonomy of personality descriptors. In D. M. Buss & N. Cantor (Eds.), *Personality psychology: Recent*

trends and emerging directions (pp. 261–271). New York: Springer-Verlag.

John, O. P. (1990). The "Big Five" factor taxonomy: Dimensions of personality in the natural language and questionnaires. In L. A. Pervin (Ed.), *Handbook of personality: Theory and research* (pp. 66–100). New York: Guilford Press.

John, O. P., Angleitner, A., & Ostendorf, F. (1988). The lexical approach to personality: A historical review of trait taxonomic research. *European Journal of Personality, 2*, 171–203.

John, O. P., & Benet-Martínez, V. (2000). Measurement, scale construction, and reliability. In H. T. Reis & C. M. Judd (Eds.), *Handbook of research methods in social and personality psychology* (pp. 339–369). New York: Cambridge University Press.

John, O. P., Caspi, A., Robins, R. W., Moffitt, T. E., & Stouthamer-Loeber, M. (1994). The "Little Five": Exploring the nomological network of the five-factor model of personality in adolescent boys. *Child Development, 65*, 160–178.

John, O. P., Donahue, E. M., & Kentle, R. L. (1991). *The Big Five Inventory—Versions 4a and 54*. Berkeley: University of California at Berkeley, Institute of Personality and Social Research.

John, O. P., Goldberg, L. R., & Angleitner, A. (1984). Better than the alphabet: Taxonomies of personality-descriptive terms in English, Dutch, and German. In H. Bonarius, G. van Heck, & N. Smid (Eds.), *Personality psychology in Europe: Theoretical and empirical developments* (pp. 83–100). Berwyn, PA: Swets North America.

John, O. P., & Gross, J. J. (2007). Individual differences in emotion regulation. In J. J. Gross (Ed.), *Handbook of emotion regulation* (pp. 351–372). New York: Guilford Press.

John, O. P., Hampson, S. E., & Goldberg, L. R. (1991). Is there a basic level of personality description? *Journal of Personality and Social Psychology, 60*, 348–361.

John, O. P., & Naumann, L. P. (2007). *Correlations of BFI scales and self-reported act frequencies in an undergraduate sample*. Unpublished data, Institute of Personality and Social Research, University of California at Berkeley.

John, O. P., & Robins, R. W. (1993). Gordon Allport: Father and critic of the five-factor model. In K. H. Craik, R. T. Hogan, & R. N. Wolfe (Eds.), *Fifty years of personality research* (pp. 215–236). New York: Plenum Press.

John, O. P., & Robins, R. W. (1998). Recent trends in Big Five research: Development, predictive validity, and personality types. In J. Bermudez et al. (Eds.), *Personality psychology in Europe*

(Vol. 6, pp. 6–16). Tilburg, The Netherlands: Tilburg University Press.

John, O. P., & Soto, C. J. (2007). The importance of being valid: Reliability and the process of construct validation. In R. W. Robins, R. C. Fraley, & R. F. Krueger (Eds.), *Handbook of research methods in personality psychology* (pp. 461–494). New York: Guilford Press.

John, O. P., & Srivastava, S. (1999). The Big Five trait taxonomy: History, measurement, and theoretical perspectives. In L. A. Pervin & O. P. John (Eds.), *Handbook of personality: Theory and research* (2nd ed., pp. 102–138). New York: Guilford Press.

Karney, B. R., & Bradbury, T. N. (1995). Assessing longitudinal change in marriage: An introduction to the analysis of growth curves. *Journal of Marriage and the Family*, 57, 1091–1108.

Kenford, S. L., Smith, S. S., Wetter, D. W., Jorenby, D. E., Fiore, M. C., & Baker, T. B. (2002). Predicting relapse back to smoking: Contrasting affective and physical models of dependence. *Journal of Consulting and Clinical Psychology*, 70, 216–227.

Klages, L. (1932). *The science of character*. London: Allen & Unwin.

Kohnstamm, G. A., Halverson, C. F., Mervielde, I., & Havill, V. L. (Eds.). (1998). *Parental descriptions of child personality: Developmental antecedents of the Big Five?* Mahwah, NJ: Erlbaum.

Krueger, R. F., & Tackett, J. L. (Eds.). (2006). *Personality and psychopathology*. New York: Guilford Press.

Kwan, V. S. Y., Gosling, S. D., & John, O. P. (2008). Anthropomorphism as a special case of social perception: A cross-species comparative approach and a new empirical paradigm. *Social Cognition*, 26, 129–142.

Larson, L. M., Rottinghaus, P. J., & Borgen, F. H. (2002). Meta-analyses of Big Six interests and Big Five personality factors. *Journal of Vocational Behavior*, 61, 217–239.

Loehlin, J. C., McCrae, R. R., Costa, P. T., Jr., & John, O. P. (1998). Heritabilities of common and measure-specific components of the Big Five personality factors. *Journal of Research in Personality*, 32, 431–453.

Markon, K. E, Krueger, R. F., & Watson, D. (2005). Delineating the structure of normal and abnormal personality: An integrative hierarchical approach. *Journal of Personality and Social Psychology*, 88, 139–157.

McAdams, D. P. (1992). The five-factor model in personality: A critical appraisal. *Journal of Personality*, 60, 329–361.

McCrae, R. R. (1996). Social consequences of experiential openness. *Psychological Bulletin*, 120, 323–337.

McCrae, R. R., & Costa, P. T., Jr. (1985a). Updating Norman's adequate taxonomy: Intelligence and personality dimensions in natural language and in questionnaires. *Journal of Personality and Social Psychology*, 49, 710–721.

McCrae, R. R., & Costa, P. T., Jr. (1985b). Openness to experience. In R. Hogan & W. H. Jones (Eds.), *Perspectives in personality* (Vol. 1, pp. 145–172). Greenwich, CT: JAI Press.

McCrae, R. R., & Costa, P. T., Jr. (1985c). Comparison of EPI and psychoticism scales with measures of the five-factor model of personality. *Personality and Individual Differences*, 6, 587–597.

McCrae, R. R., & Costa, P. T., Jr. (1987). Validation of the five-factor model of personality across instruments and observers. *Journal of Personality and Social Psychology*, 52, 81–90.

McCrae, R. R., & Costa, P. T., Jr. (1996). Toward a new generation of personality theories: Theoretical contexts for the five-factor model. In J. S. Wiggins (Ed.), *The five-factor model of personality: Theoretical perspectives* (pp. 51–87). New York: Guilford Press.

McCrae, R. R., & Costa, P. T., Jr. (2003). *Personality in adulthood: A five-factor theory perspective* (2nd ed.). New York: Guilford Press.

McCrae, R. R., & John, O. P. (1992). An introduction to the five-factor model and its applications. *Journal of Personality*, 60, 175–215.

Measelle, J. R., John, O. P., Ablow, J. C., Cowan, P. A., & Cowan, C. P (2005). Can children provide coherent, stable, and valid self-reports on the Big Five dimensions? A longitudinal study from ages 5 to 7. *Journal of Personality and Social Psychology*, 89, 90–106.

Mehl, M. R., Gosling, S. D., & Pennebaker, J. W. (2006). Personality in its natural habitat: Manifestations and implicit folk theories of personality in daily life. *Journal of Personality and Social Psychology*, 90, 862–877.

Mershon, B., & Gorsuch, R. L. (1988). Number of factors in the personality sphere: Does increase in factors increase predictability of real-life criteria? *Journal of Personality and Social Psychology*, 55, 675–680.

Miller, T. Q., Smith, T. W., Turner, C. W., Guijarro, M. L., & Hallet, A. J. (1996). A meta-analytic review of research on hostility and physical health. *Psychological Bulletin*, 119, 322–348.

Mount, M. K., Barrick, M. R., & Stewart, G. L. (1998). Five-factor model of personality and performance in jobs involving interpersonal interactions. *Human Performance*, 11, 145–165.

Myers, I. B., & McCaulley, M. H. (1985). *Manual: A guide to the development and use of the Myers–Briggs Type Indicator*. Palo Alto, CA: Consulting Psychologists Press.

Newcomb, A. F., Bukowski, W. M., & Pattee, L. (1993). Children's peer relations: A meta-analytic review of popular, rejected, neglected, controversial, and average sociometric status. *Psychological Bulletin, 113*, 99–128.

Nigg, J. T., John, O. P., Blaskey, L. G., Huang-Pollock, C. L., Willcutt, E. G., Hinshaw, S. P., et al. (2002). Big Five dimensions and ADHD symptoms: Link between personality traits and clinical syndromes. *Journal of Personality and Social Psychology, 83*, 451–469.

Noftle, E. E., & Robins, R. W. (2007). Personality predictors of Academic Outcomes: Big Five correlates of GPA and SAT scores. *Journal of Personality and Social Psychology, 93*, 116–130.

Norman, W. T. (1963). Toward an adequate taxonomy of personality attributes: Replicated factor structure in peer nomination personality ratings. *Journal of Abnormal and Social Psychology, 66*, 574–583.

Norman, W. T. (1967). *2,800 personality trait descriptors: Normative operating characteristics for a university population*. Unpublished paper, Department of Psychology, University of Michigan.

Nowakowska, M. (1973). The limitations of the factor-analytic approach to psychology with special application to Cattell's research strategy. *Theory and Decision, 4*, 109–139.

Ostendorf, F. (1990). *Sprache und Persoenlichkeitsstruktur: Zur Validitaet des Fuenf-Faktoren-Modells der Persoenlichkeit* [Language and personality structure: On the validity of the five factor model of personality]. Regensburg, Germany: S. Roderer Verlag.

Ozer, D. J., & Benet-Martínez, V. (2006). Personality and prediction of consequential outcomes. *Annual Review of Psychology, 57*, 401–421.

Paulhus, D. L., & John, O. P. (1998). Egoistic and moralistic biases in self-perception: The interplay of self-deceptive styles with basic traits and motives. *Journal of Personality, 66*, 1025–1060.

Paunonen, S. V. (2003). Big Five factors of personality and replicated prediction of behavior. *Journal of Personality and Social Psychology, 84*, 411–424.

Peabody, D., & Goldberg, L. R. (1989). Some determinants of factor structures from personality-trait descriptors. *Journal of Personality and Social Psychology, 57*, 552–567.

Pervin, L. A. (1994). A critical analysis of current trait theory. *Psychological Inquiry, 5*, 103–113.

Pervin, L. A., Cervone, D., & John, O. P. (2005). *Personality: Theory and research* (9th ed.). Hoboken, NJ: Wiley.

Plomin, R., DeFries, J. C., Craig, I. W., & McGuffin, P. (Eds.). (2003). *Behavioral genetics in the postgenomic era*. Washington, DC: American Psychological Association.

Rammstedt, B., & John, O. P. (2005). Short version of the Big Five Inventory (BFI-K): Development and validation of an economic inventory for assessment of the five factors of personality. *Diagnostica, 51*, 195–206.

Rammstedt, B., & John, O. P. (2007). Measuring personality in one minute or less: A 10-item short version of the Big Five Inventory in English and German. *Journal of Research in Personality, 41*, 203–212.

Rentfrow, P. J., & Gosling, S. D. (2006). Message in a ballad: The role of music preferences in interpersonal perception. *Psychological Science, 17*, 236–242.

Revelle, W. (1987). Personality and motivation: Sources of inefficiency in cognitive performance. *Journal of Research in Personality, 21*, 436–452.

Roberts, B. W., & DelVecchio, W. F. (2000). The rank-order consistency of personality traits from childhood to old age: A quantitative review of longitudinal studies. *Psychological Bulletin, 126*, 3–25.

Roberts, B. W., Walton, K. E., & Viechtbauer, W. (2006). Patterns of mean-level change in personality traits across the life course: A meta-analysis of longitudinal studies. *Psychological Bulletin, 132*, 1–25.

Robins, R. W., Caspi, A., & Moffitt, T. E. (2002). It's not just who you're with, it's who you are: Personality and relationship experiences across multiple relationships. *Journal of Personality, 70*, 925–964.

Robins, R. W., John, O. P., & Caspi, A. (1994). Major dimensions of personality in early adolescence: The Big Five and beyond. In C. F. Halverson, J. A. Kohnstamm, & R. P. Martin (Eds.), *The developing structure of temperament and personality from infancy to adulthood* (pp. 267–291). Hillsdale, NJ: Erlbaum.

Robins, R. W., John, O. P., Caspi, A., Moffitt, T. E., & Stouthamer-Loeber, M. (1996). Resilient, overcontrolled, and undercontrolled boys: Three replicable personality types? *Journal of Personality and Social Psychology, 70*, 157–171.

Rosch, E. (1978). Principles of categorization. In E. Rosch & B. B. Lloyd (Eds.), *Cognition and categorization* (pp. 27–48). Hillsdale, NJ: Erlbaum.

Rentfrow, P. J., & Gosling, S. D. (2006). Message in a ballad: The role of music preferences in interpersonal perception. *Psychological Science, 17*, 236–242.

Saucier, G. (1992). Openness versus Intellect: Much ado about nothing. *European Journal of Personality, 6*, 386–391.

Saucier, G. (1994). Mini-markers: A brief version

of Goldberg's unipolar Big-Five markers. *Journal of Personality Assessment, 63*, 506–516.

Saucier, G. (1997). Effects of variable selection on the factor structure of person descriptors. *Journal of Personality and Social Psychology, 73*, 1296–1312.

Saucier, G., Georgiades, S., Tsouasis, I., & Goldberg, L. R. (2005). Factor structure of Greek personality-descriptive adjectives. *Journal of Personality and Social Psychology, 88*, 856–875.

Saucier, G., & Goldberg, L. R. (199a). Evidence for the Big Five in analyses of familiar English personality adjectives. *European Journal of Personality, 10*, 61–77.

Saucier, G., & Goldberg, L. R. (1996b). The language of personality: Lexical perspectives on the five-factor model. In J. S. Wiggins (Ed.), *The five-factor model of personality: Theoretical perspectives* (pp. 21–50). New York: Guilford Press.

Saucier, G., & Goldberg, L. R. (2001). Lexical studies of indigenous personality factors: Premises, products, and prospects. *Journal of Personality, 69*, 847–879.

Saucier, G., Hampson, S. E., & Goldberg, L. R. (2000). Cross-language studies of lexical personality factors. In S. E. Hampson (Ed.), *Advances in personality psychology* (Vol. 1, pp. 1–36). London: Routledge.

Saucier, G., & Ostendorf, F. (1999). Hierarchical subcomponents of the Big Five personality factors: A cross-language replication. *Journal of Personality and Social Psychology, 76*, 613–627.

Scarr, S., & McCartney, K. (1984). How people make their own environments: A theory of genotype–environment effects. *Annual Progress in Child Psychiatry and Child Development*, 98–118.

Scheier, M. F., & Carver, C. S. (1993). On the power of positive thinking: The benefits of being optimistic. *Current Directions in Psychological Science, 2*, 26–30.

Shiner, R., & Caspi, A. (2003). Personality differences in childhood and adolescence: Measurement, development, and consequences. *Journal of Child Psychology and Psychiatry, 44*, 2–32.

Shmelyov, A. G., & Pokhil'ko, V. I. (1993). A taxonomy-oriented study of Russian personality-trait names. *European Journal of Personality, 7*, 1–17.

Simpson, G. G. (1961). *Principles of animal taxonomy*. New York: Columbia University Press.

Somer, O., & Goldberg, L. R. (1999). The structure of Turkish trait-descriptive adjectives. *Journal of Personality and Social Psychology, 76*, 431–450.

Soto, C. J., & John, O. P. (2008). *Measuring Big Five domains and 16 facets using the California Psychological Inventory*. Manuscript submitted for publication.

Soto, C. J., John, O. P., Gosling, S. D., & Potter, J. (2008). The developmental psychometrics of Big Five self-reports: Acquiescence, factor structure, coherence, and differentiation from ages 10 to 20. *Journal of Personality and Social Psychology, 94*, 718–737.

Srivastava, S., John, O. P., Gosling, S. D., & Potter, J. (2003). Development of personality in early and middle adulthood: Set like plaster or persistent change? *Journal of Personality and Social Psychology, 84*, 1041–1053.

Sullivan, H. S. (1953). *The interpersonal theory of psychiatry*. New York: Norton.

Szarota, P. (1995). *Polska Lista Przymiotnikowa (PLP): Narzedzie do diagnozy Pieciu Wielkich czynnikow osobowosci* [Polish Adjective List: An instrument to assess the five-factor model of personality]. *Studia Psychologiczne, 33*, 227–256.

Szirmak, Z., & De Raad, B. (1994). Taxonomy and structure of Hungarian personality traits. *European Journal of Personality, 8*, 95–117.

Tellegen, A. (1982). *Brief manual for the Differential Personality Questionnaire*. Unpublished manuscript, University of Minnesota, Minneapolis.

Tellegen, A. (1985). Structures of mood and personality and their relevance to assessing anxiety, with an emphasis on self-report. In A. H. Tuma & J. D. Maser (Eds.), *Anxiety and the anxiety disorders* (pp. 681–716). Hillsdale, NJ: Erlbaum.

Tellegen, A. (1993). Folk concepts and psychological concepts of personality and personality disorder. *Psychological Inquiry, 4*, 122–130.

Tellegen, A., Ben-Porath, Y. S., McNulty, J. L., Arbisi, P. A., Graham, J. R., & Kaemmer, B. (2003). *MMPI-2 Restructured Clinical (RC) Scales: Development, validation, and interpretation*. Minneapolis: University of Minnesota Press.

Thoresen, C. J., Kaplan, S. A., Barsky, A. P., Warren, C. R., & de Chermont, K. (2003). The affective underpinnings of job perceptions and attitudes: A meta-analytic review and integration. *Psychological Bulletin, 129*, 914–945.

Trapnell, P. D., & Wiggins, J. S. (1990). Extension of the Interpersonal Adjective Scales to include the Big Five dimensions of personality. *Journal of Personality and Social Psychology, 59*, 781–790.

Trull, T. J., & Sher, K. J. (1994). Relationship between the five-factor model of personality and Axis I disorders in a nonclinical sample. *Journal of Abnormal Psychology, 103*, 350–360.

Tupes, E. C., & Christal, R. C. (1961). *Recur-

rent personality factors based on trait ratings. Technical Report, U.S. Air Force, Lackland Air Force Base, TX.

Tupes, E. C., & Christal, R. C. (1992). Recurrent personality factors based on trait ratings. *Journal of Personality, 60,* 225–251.

van Lieshout, C. F. M., & Haselager, G. J. T. (1994). The Big Five personality factors in Q-sort descriptions of children and adolescents. In C. F. Halverson, G. A. Kohnstamm, & R. P. Martin (Eds.), *The developing structure of temperament and personality from infancy to adulthood* (pp. 293–318). Hillsdale, NJ: Erlbaum.

Vazire, S., & Gosling, S. D. (2004). e-Perceptions: Personality impressions based on personal websites. *Journal of Personality and Social Psychology, 87,* 123–132.

Watson, D., & Clark, L. A. (1997). Extraversion and its positive emotional core. In R. Hogan, J. A. Johnson, & S. R. Briggs (Eds.), *Handbook of personality psychology* (pp. 767–793). San Diego, CA: Academic Press.

Watson, D., Hubbard, B., & Wiese, D. (2000). General traits of personality and affectivity as predictors of satisfaction in intimate relationships: Evidence from self- and partner-ratings. *Journal of Personality, 68,* 413–449.

Weiss, A., & Costa, P. T., Jr. (2005). Domain and facet personality predictors of all-cause mortality among Medicare patients aged 65–100. *Psychosomatic Medicine, 67,* 724–733.

Wiggins, J. S. (1968). Personality structure. In P. R. Farnsworth (Ed.), *Annual review of psychology* (Vol. 19, pp. 320–322). Palo Alto, CA: Annual Reviews.

Wiggins, J. S. (1979). A psychological taxonomy of trait-descriptive terms: The interpersonal domain. *Journal of Personality and Social Psychology, 37,* 395–412.

Wiggins, J. S. (1995). *Interpersonal Adjective Scales: Professional manual.* Odessa, FL: Psychological Assessment Resources.

Wiggins, J. S. (Ed.). (1996). *The five-factor model of personality: Theoretical perspectives.* New York: Guilford Press.

Wiggins, J. S. (1997). In defense of traits. In R. Hogan, J. A. Johnson, & S. R. Briggs (Ed.), *Handbook of personality psychology* (pp. 649–679). San Diego, CA: Academic Press.

Wiggins, J. S., & Pincus, A. L. (1989). Conceptions of personality disorders and dimensions of personality. *Psychological Assessment, 1,* 305–316.

Wiggins, J. S., & Trapnell, P. D. (1996). A dyadic–interactional perspective on the five-factor model. In J. S. Wiggins (Ed.), *The five-factor model of personality: Theoretical perspectives* (pp. 180–207). New York: Guilford Press.

Yang, K. S., & Bond, M. H. (1990). Exploring implicit personality theories with indigenous or imported constructs: The Chinese case. *Journal of Personality and Social Psychology, 58,* 1087–1095.

APPENDIX 4.1. BIG FIVE INVENTORY RESPONSE FORM AND INSTRUCTIONS TO PARTICIPANTS

Instructions: Here are a number of characteristics that may or may not apply to you. For example, do you agree that you are someone who *likes to spend time with others*? Please write a number next to each statement to indicate the extent to which you agree or disagree with that statement.

1 Disagree strongly	2 Disagree a little	3 Neither agree nor disagree	4 Agree a little	5 Agree strongly

I see myself as someone who ..

1. ____ Is talkative
2. ____ Tends to find fault with others
3. ____ Does a thorough job
4. ____ Is depressed, blue
5. ____ Is original, comes up with new ideas
6. ____ Is reserved
7. ____ Is helpful and unselfish with others
8. ____ Can be somewhat careless
9. ____ Is relaxed, handles stress well
10. ____ Is curious about many different things
11. ____ Is full of energy
12. ____ Starts quarrels with others
13. ____ Is a reliable worker
14. ____ Can be tense
15. ____ Is ingenious, a deep thinker
16. ____ Generates a lot of enthusiasm
17. ____ Has a forgiving nature
18. ____ Tends to be disorganized
19. ____ Worries a lot
20. ____ Has an active imagination
21. ____ Tends to be quiet
22. ____ Is generally trusting
23. ____ Tends to be lazy

24. ____ Is emotionally stable, not easily upset
25. ____ Is inventive
26. ____ Has an assertive personality
27. ____ Can be cold and aloof
28. ____ Perseveres until the task is finished
29. ____ Can be moody
30. ____ Values artistic, aesthetic experiences
31. ____ Is sometimes shy, inhibited
32. ____ Is considerate and kind to almost everyone
33. ____ Does things efficiently
34. ____ Remains calm in tense situations
35. ____ Prefers work that is routine
36. ____ Is outgoing, sociable
37. ____ Is sometimes rude to others
38. ____ Makes plans and follows through with them
39. ____ Gets nervous easily
40. ____ Likes to reflect, play with ideas
41. ____ Has few artistic interests
42. ____ Likes to cooperate with others
43. ____ Is easily distracted
44. ____ Is sophisticated in art, music, or literature

Please check: Did you write a number in front of each statement?

Note. From John, Donahue, and Kentle (1991). Copyright 1991 by Oliver P. John. Reprinted by permission.

APPENDIX 4.2. SCORING THE BFI SCALES AND ACQUIESCENCE INDEX, AND IPSATIZING THE BFI ITEMS

Computing Simple BFI Scale Scores

BFI scale scoring: Reverse score the items labeled "R" and compute scale scores as the mean of the following items:

> Extraversion (8 items): 1, 6R, 11, 16, 21R, 26, 31R, 36
> Agreeableness (9 items): 2R, 7, 12R, 17, 22, 27R, 32, 37R, 42
> Conscientiousness (9 items): 3, 8R, 13, 18R, 23R, 28, 33, 38, 43R
> Neuroticism (8 items): 4, 9R, 14, 19, 24R, 29, 34R, 39
> Openness (10 items): 5, 10, 15, 20, 25, 30, 35R, 40, 41R, 44

Computing the Content-Balanced Acquiescence Index and Ipsatizing the BFI Items

To index individuals' acquiescent response style (where high scores mean "yea-saying" and low scores mean "nay-saying"), we compute their acquiescence score as their mean response across 32 BFI items that form 16 pairs of items with opposite implications for personality (e.g., item 1 "Is talkative" and item 21 "Tends to be quiet"). As described in Soto, John, Gosling, and Potter (2008), we devised these 16 pairs of opposite items on the basis of item content and the size of their (negative) interitem correlations. Using the standard BFI item numbers (see Appendix A; see also Benet-Martínez & John, 1998; John & Srivastava, 1999), these item pairs are 1 and 21, 6 and 16, 31 and 36, 2 and 17, 7 and 12, 27 and 42, 32 and 37, 3 and 43, 8 and 13, 18 and 33, 23 and 28, 9 and 19, 24 and 29, 34 and 39, 5 and 35, 30 and 41.

The Statistical Package for the Social Sciences (SPSS) syntax given below first computes each person's acquiescence score ("bfiave"; the average of his or her 16 × 2 = 32 item responses) and response extremeness ("bfistd"; the standard deviation of that person's 32 item responses). Both of these individual-difference scores may be retained and used in research on individual or group differences in response-scale use (e.g., comparing Asian Americans and European Americans). The syntax below shows how these two scores can be used to ipsatize the full set of 44 BFI items, by removing from each item score the individual's acquiescence score (i.e., content-balanced response mean) and then adjusting the resulting deviation scores by dividing them by the individual's standard deviation, resulting in person-centered standard (or Z) scores. The syntax below assumes that the variables for the 44 BFI items are named bfi1 to bfi44 in standard order.

SPSS Syntax to Ipsatize the 44 BFI Items before Scoring the Scales

```
* Compute within-person response means (bfiave) and standard deviations
(bfistd).

COMPUTE bfiave = mean(bfi1, bfi6, bfi16, bfi21, bfi31, bfi36, bfi2, bfi7, bfi12,
bfi17, bfi27, bfi32, bfi37, bfi42, bfi3, bfi8, bfi13, bfi18, bfi23, bfi28, bfi33,
bfi43, bfi9, bfi19, bfi24, bfi29, bfi34, bfi39, bfi5, bfi30, bfi35, bfi41).

COMPUTE bfistd = sd(bfi1, bfi6, bfi16, bfi21, bfi31, bfi36, bfi2, bfi7, bfi12, bfi17,
bfi27, bfi32, bfi37, bfi42, bfi3, bfi8, bfi13, bfi18, bfi23, bfi28, bfi33, bfi43, bfi9,
bfi19, bfi24, bfi29, bfi34, bfi39, bfi5, bfi30, bfi35, bfi41).
EXECUTE.

* Compute ipsatized BFI items (zbfi).

COMPUTE zbfi1 = (bfi1 - bfiave)/bfistd.
COMPUTE zbfi2 = (bfi2 - bfiave)/bfistd.
COMPUTE zbfi3 = (bfi3 - bfiave)/bfistd.
                     .
                     .
                     .
COMPUTE zbfi44 = (bfi44 - bfiave)/bfistd.
EXECUTE.
```

Then use the ipsatized item scores to compute scale scores as mean item responses, as described above.

CHAPTER 5

The Five-Factor Theory of Personality

Robert R. McCrae
Paul T. Costa, Jr.

EMPIRICAL AND CONCEPTUAL BASES OF A PERSONALITY THEORY

In a narrow sense, the five-factor model (FFM) of personality is an empirical generalization about the covariation of personality traits. As Digman and Inouye (1986) put it, "if a large number of rating scales is used and if the scope of the scales is very broad, the domain of personality descriptors is almost completely accounted for by five robust factors" (p. 116). The five factors, frequently labeled Neuroticism (N), Extraversion (E), Openness (O), Agreeableness (A), and Conscientiousness (C), have been found not only in the peer rating scales in which they were originally discovered (Tupes & Christal, 1961/1992), but also in self-reports on trait descriptive adjectives (Saucier, 1997), in questionnaire measures of needs and motives (Costa & McCrae, 1988), in expert ratings on the California Q-Set (Lanning, 1994), and in personality disorder symptom clusters (Clark & Livesley, 2002). Much of what psychologists mean by the term "personality" is summarized by the FFM, and the model has been of great utility to the field by integrating and systematizing diverse conceptions and measures.

In a broader sense, the FFM refers to the entire body of research that it has inspired, amounting to a reinvigoration of trait psychology itself. Research associated with the FFM has (1) included studies of diverse populations (McCrae, Terracciano, et al., 2005a), often followed over decades of the lifespan (Terracciano, Costa, & McCrae, 2006); (2) employed multiple methods of assessment (Funder, Kolar, & Blackman, 1995); and (3) even featured case studies (Costa & McCrae, 1998a; McCrae, 1993–1994). As Carlson (1984) might have predicted, these research strategies have paid off handsomely in substantive findings: The FFM "is the Christmas tree on which findings of stability, heritability, consensual validation, cross-cultural invariance, and predictive utility are hung like ornaments" (Costa & McCrae, 1993, p. 302). After decades of floundering, personality psychology has begun to make steady progress, accumulating a store of replicable findings about the origins, development, and functioning of personality traits (McCrae, 2002a).

But neither the model itself nor the body of research findings with which it is associated constitutes a theory of personality. A theory organizes findings to tell a coherent story, to bring into focus those issues and phenomena that can and should be explained. As Mayer (1998) argued, personality may be viewed as a system, and an adequate theory of personality must provide a definition of the system, a specification of its components, a model of their organization and interaction, and an account of the system's development. Five-factor theory (FFT; McCrae & Costa, 1996) represents an effort to construct such a theory that is consistent with current knowledge about personality. In this chapter we summarize and elaborate it.

The FFM and Trait Theory

Although the FFM is not a theory of personality, McCrae and John (1992) argued that it implicitly adopts the basic tenets of *trait theory*: that individuals can be characterized in terms of relatively enduring patterns of thoughts, feelings, and actions; that traits can be quantitatively assessed; that they show some degree of cross-situational consistency; and so on. The hundreds of studies of personality correlates that employ measures of the FFM both presume and confirm that personality traits exist.

It is therefore somewhat surprising that, in a volume on its theoretical basis (Wiggins, 1996), some of the psychologists most closely associated with the FFM explicitly disavowed a trait perspective. Saucier and Goldberg (1996) stated that their "lexical perspective is not an instance of 'trait theory,'" which they described as "a rubric that may have no meaning outside introductory personality texts" (p. 25). They are concerned only with the phenotypic level of personality and do not even presume that trait descriptive adjectives refer to temporally stable attributes. Hogan (1996), who advocates a socioanalytic perspective, argued that personality attributes are not neuropsychic structures within the individual, but "categories that people use to evaluate one another" that "reveal the amount of status and acceptance that a person has been granted" (p. 173). Responses to personality questionnaires, according to Hogan, are not veridical self-descriptions but strategic self-presentations; socioanalytic theory does not presume that there is any "link between item endorsements and other behavior" (p. 176). Wiggins and Trapnell (1996) follow Sullivan in seeing the locus of personality not within the individual but in patterns of interpersonal relationships; their major conceptual orientation is guided by the metatheoretical concepts of agency and communion.

Perhaps these positions can be understood historically as reactions to the disrepute into which traits had fallen in the 1970s. Today, however, they seem needlessly modest: Why restrict theoretical ambitions to the phenotypic level, especially in light of the accelerating advances in behavior genetics? Why not postulate temporal stability for traits, when stability is already well documented? Why doubt neuropsychic structures exist when many neuroscientists are explicating the biological bases of personality (Canli, 2006)? Why locate personality only in interpersonal space, as Wiggins and Trapnell did, when we can understand interpersonal behavior as a result of characteristics within the individual (Côté & Moskowitz, 1998)? FFT is unabashedly a trait theory, making full use of the empirical results of the last two decades that constitute the FFM in the broader sense.

Personality traits are recognized by laypersons, who have a rich vocabulary for describing themselves and others (e.g., *anxious, bold, curious, docile, efficient*), and traits have been studied formally by psychologists from Francis Galton to Gordon Allport to Hans Eysenck. Despite theoretical distinctions, on an empirical level other individual-difference variables (including needs, types, and folk concepts) appear to be closely related to traits (Costa & McCrae, 1988; McCrae & Costa, 1989; McCrae, Costa, & Piedmont, 1993). In fact, most psychological questionnaires measure some form of personality trait, broadly construed.

Traits (under one name or another) have proven so very interesting to personality psychologists because they explain much of what defines the individual person—the chosen focus of personologists. Universal characteristics—such as the need for oxygen or the capacity for language—tell us much about the species but nothing about the individual. Conversely, specific behaviors, transient moods, and biographical details tell us about the individual-in-context but may not permit generalizable insights. From the perspective of trait theory, these two levels appear to yield only truisms and trivia. By contrast, traits point to more-or-less consistent and recurrent patterns of acting and reacting that simultaneously characterize individuals and differentiate them from others, and they allow the discovery of empirical generalizations about how others with similar traits are likely to act and react.

As a practical matter, trait psychologists do routinely ignore the universal and the particular in their research. Except when dealing with very unusual populations, trait researchers do not bother to remind readers that their subjects could understand the questionnaires, had self-concepts on which to base their self-reports, and continued to breathe normally for the duration of the testing session. Nor, except in the occasional case study, do they give concrete instances of how traits are expressed in specific times and circumstances.

But a theory of personality cannot afford to ignore these two levels of explanation. Part of making sense of trait findings requires putting them into a broader context and showing how they, in turn, form the context for specific behaviors and individual lives. In Mayer's (1998) terminology, the trait system must be identified in terms of its boundaries with other systems, higher and lower. These links form a recurrent theme in this chapter.

Assumptions about Human Nature

The trait perspective, like every personality theory, is based on a set of assumptions about what people are like and what a theory of personality ought to do. Most of these assumptions—for example, that explanations for behavior are to be sought in the circumstances of this life, not karma from a previous one—are implicit. FFT explicitly acknowledges four assumptions about human nature (cf. Hjelle & Siegler, 1976)—its *knowability*, *rationality*, *variability*, and *proactivity;* all of these appear to be implicit in the standard enterprise of trait research.

Knowability is the assumption that personality is a proper object of scientific study. In contrast to some humanistic and existential theories that celebrate human freedom and the irreducible uniqueness of the individual, FFT assumes that there is much to be gained from the scientific study of personality in individuals and groups.

Scientific study does not necessarily imply experimentation, nor do we agree with Eysenck (1997) that a persuasive paradigm for personality psychology must involve a unification of correlational and experimental methods. Science proceeds by many methods and works best when the method is dictated by the nature of the problem rather than academic fashion and prestige. In particular, correlational methods can capitalize on natural experiments, especially in longitudinal, twin, and cross-cultural studies. Yang,

McCrae, and Costa (1998), for example, explored the impact of China's Cultural Revolution on personality development—a quasi-experimental manipulation whose scope, intensity, and duration could never be matched in the laboratory.

Rationality is the assumption that people are generally capable of understanding themselves and others (cf. Funder, 1995). This is an unpopular view. Psychoanalysts hold that people are driven by unconscious forces; their self-understanding is fundamentally self-deception. Contemporary social psychologists (and personologists; see Robins & John, 1997) document cognitive biases and errors, and Jussim (2005) noted that reading social psychology convinces most of his students that "people are fundamentally irrational" (p. 7). That perspective in social psychology can perhaps be traced back to Simon (1957), who responded to simplistic models of economic behavior that assumed pure rationality on the part of consumers by proposing the concept of *bounded rationality*—rationality limited by the imperfections of human thought processes. Perhaps it is time for the pendulum to swing back, and to describe human thought and behavior in terms of *bounded irrationality*, for if our perceptions and judgments were wholly out of touch with reality, we would not have survived as a species. Jussim cites reviews of scientific evidence of accuracy in a wide range of human judgments, and studies of cross-observer agreement (e.g., McCrae et al., 2004) show that this accuracy applies also to judgments about personality traits.

In this respect, trait psychology is an unusual science. As Kagan (2005) noted, "No biologist would use the reports of informants to decide on the basic human diseases" (p. 7). But trait psychologists routinely—and properly—ask people how sociable or competitive or irritable they are, and interpret the answers (suitably aggregated and normed) as meaning what they say. Psychologists are able to do this because with respect to personality traits, laypersons are extraordinarily sophisticated judges who employ a trait language evolved over centuries to express important social judgments (cf. Saucier & Goldberg, 1996). Kagan's objection is a reasonable basis for requiring evidence of the validity of self-reports, but he failed to point out that such evidence is abundant: The dimensions of personality revealed by analyses of lay self-reports are confirmed in the ratings of expert observers (Lanning, 1994), reflected in behavior counts (Funder & Sneed, 1993), based on the structure of the genotype (Yamagata et al., 2006), and so on.

The assumption of rationality does not mean that FFT is merely folk psychology. Lay understanding is largely limited to a superficial level, whereas FFT attempts to account for the underlying structure and its operations. People understand whether someone is arrogant or modest, but they do not intuitively know the heritability of modesty, or its lifespan developmental course, or its evolutionary significance. To laypeople, trait psychology is thus like representational art: Viewers recognize the face or flower, although they may know nothing about the laws of perspective or the techniques of overpainting.

Variability asserts that people differ from each other in psychologically significant ways—an obvious premise for differential psychology. Note, however, that this position sets trait theories apart from all those views of human nature, philosophical and psychological, that seek a single answer to what human nature is really like. Are people basically selfish or altruistic? Creative or conventional? Purposeful or lazy? Within FFT, those are all meaningless questions; terms such as "creative" and "conventional" define opposite poles of dimensions along which people vary.

Proactivity refers to the assumption that the locus of causation of human action is to be sought in the person. It goes without saying that people are not absolute masters of their destinies, and that (consistent with the premise of variability) people differ in the extent to which they control their lives. But trait theory holds that it is worthwhile to seek the origins of behavior in characteristics of the person. People are not passive victims of their life circumstances, nor are they empty organisms programmed by histories of reinforcements. Personality is actively—and interactively—involved in shaping people's lives (Soldz & Vaillant, 1999).

It is important to recognize that proactivity of personality is not equivalent to proactivity of the person; an individual's proactive traits are not necessarily the same as his or her conscious goals. Failure to adhere to a diet may be as much an expression of an individual's personality as success in dieting;

anxiety and depression may be a person's own natural, albeit noxious, way of life.

A UNIVERSAL PERSONALITY SYSTEM

Personality traits are individual-difference variables; to understand them and how they operate, it is necessary to describe personality itself, the dynamic psychological organization that coordinates experience and action. Previously we described our account of this as a "model of the person," but to distinguish it from the FFM, it would perhaps be better to call it the FFT *personality system* (Costa & McCrae, 1994; McCrae & Costa, 1996). This system is represented schematically in Figure 5.1.

Components of the Personality System

The personality system consists of *components* that correspond to the definitions of FFT and *dynamic processes* that indicate how these components are interrelated—the basic postulates of FFT. The definitions would probably seem reasonable to personologists from many different theoretical backgrounds; the postulates distinguish FFT from most other theories of personality and reflect interpretations of empirical data.

The core components of the personality system, indicated in rectangles in Figure 5.1, are designated as *basic tendencies*, *characteristic adaptations*, and the *self-concept*—which is actually a subcomponent of characteristic adaptations, but one of sufficient interest to warrant its own box. The elliptical peripheral components, which represent the interfaces of personality with adjoining systems, are labeled *biological bases*, *external influences*, and the *objective biography*. Figure 5.1 can be interpreted cross-sectionally as a diagram of how personality operates at any given time; in that case the external influences constitute the situation or context, and the objective biography is a specific instance of behavior, the output of the system. Figure 5.1 can also be interpreted longitudinally to indicate personality development (in basic tendencies and characteristic adaptations) and the evolution of the life course (objective biography).

It may be helpful to consider some of the substance of personality to flesh out the abstractions in Figure 5.1. Table 5.1 presents

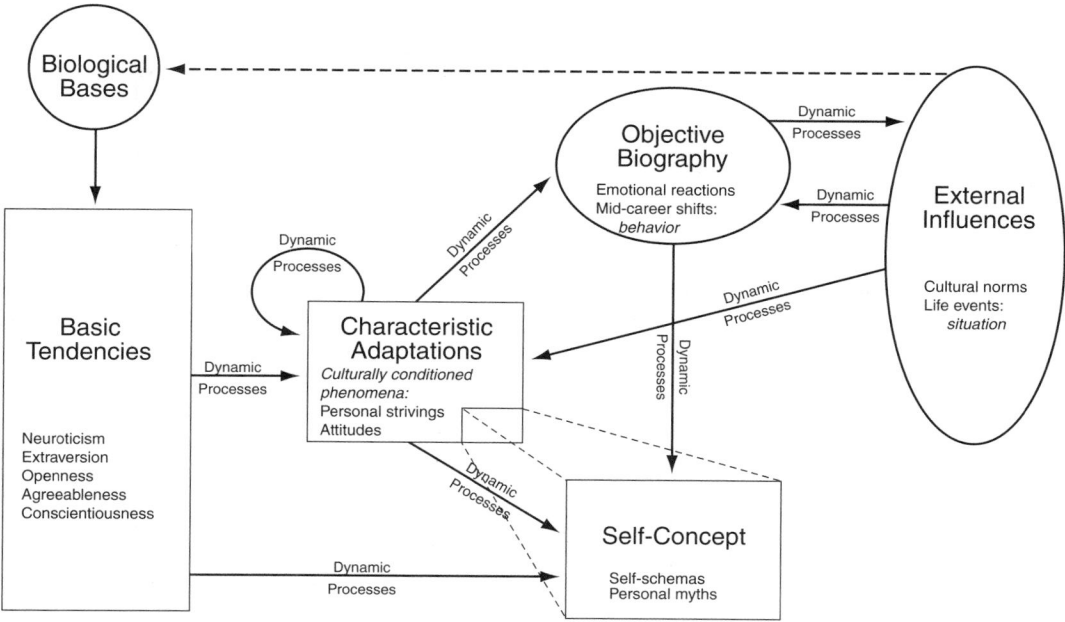

FIGURE 5.1. A representation of the five-factor theory personality system. Core components are in rectangles; interfacing components are in ellipses. From McCrae and Costa (1996).

some examples. For each of the five factors, a single facet (one of the specific traits that define the factor) is identified as a basic tendency in the first column of the table. The intrapsychic and interpersonal features that develop over time as expressions of these facet traits are illustrated as characteristic adaptations in the second column, and the third column mentions an instance of behavior—a datum from the objective biography—of an individual characterized by the high or low pole of the facet.

At present, FFT has relatively little to say about the peripheral components of the personality system. Biological bases certainly include genes and brain structures, but the precise mechanisms—developmental, neuroanatomical, or psychophysiological—are not yet specified. Similarly, FFT does not detail types of external influences or aspects of the objective biography. Like most theories of personality, FFT presumes that "situation" and "behavior" are more or less self-evident.

What FFT does focus attention on is the distinction between *basic tendencies* (abstract psychological potentials) and *characteristic adaptations* (their concrete manifestations in the personality system). Some-

what similar distinctions have been made by others—for example, in the familiar contrast of genotypic and phenotypic traits (Wiggins, 1973/1997), and in McAdams's (1996) distinction between Level 1 and Level 2 personality variables. FFT, however, insists on a distinction that other theories usually make only in passing, and it assigns traits exclusively to the category of basic tendencies. In FFT, traits are not patterns of behavior (Buss & Craik, 1983), nor are they the plans, skills, and desires that lead to patterns of behavior (Johnson, 1997). They are directly accessible neither to public observation nor to private introspection. Instead, they are deeper psychological entities that can only be *inferred* from behavior and experience. Self-reports of personality traits are based on such inferences, just as observer ratings are.

Although it seems to smack of obfuscation, there are good reasons to uncouple personality traits from the more observable components of personality. Characteristic adaptations—habits, attitudes, skills, roles, relationships—are influenced both by basic tendencies and by external influences. They are *characteristic* because they reflect the enduring psychological core of the individual, and they are *adaptations* because they help

TABLE 5.1. Some Examples of FFT Personality System Components

Basic tendencies	Characteristic adaptations	Objective biography
Neuroticism N3: Depression (a tendency to experience dysphoric affect—sadness, hopelessness, guilt)	Low self-esteem, irrational perfectionistic beliefs, pessimistic attitudes	"Betty" (very high N3) feels guilty about her low-prestige job (Bruehl, 2002)
Extraversion E2: Gregariousness (a preference for companionship and social stimulation)	Social skills, numerous friendships, enterprising vocational interests, participation in team sports, club memberships	J.-J. Rousseau (very low E2) leaves Paris for the countryside (McCrae, 1996)
Openness to Experience O4: Actions (a need for variety, novelty, and change)	Interest in travel, many different hobbies, knowledge of foreign cuisine, diverse vocational interests, friends who share tastes	Diane Ackerman (high O4) cruises the Antarctic (McCrae, 1993–1994)
Agreeableness A4: Compliance (a willingness to defer to others during interpersonal conflict)	Forgiving attitudes, belief in cooperation, inoffensive language, reputation as a pushover	Case 3 (very low A4) throws things at her husband during a fight (Costa & McCrae, 1992a)
Conscientiousness C4: Achievement Striving (strong sense of purpose and high aspiration levels)	Leadership skills, long-term plans, organized support network, technical expertise	Richard Nixon (very high C4) runs for president (Costa & McCrae, 2005)

the individual fit into the ever-changing social environment. Characteristic adaptations and their configurations inevitably vary tremendously across cultures, families, and portions of the lifespan. *But personality traits do not*: The same five factors are found in all cultures studied so far (McCrae & Costa, 1997b; McCrae, Terracciano, et al., 2005a); parent–child relations have little lasting effect on personality traits (Rowe, 1994); and traits are generally stable across the vicissitudes of the adult lifespan (McCrae & Costa, 2003). These well-replicated empirical generalizations make sense only if personality traits are insulated from the direct effects of the environment. Human nature is proactive because personality traits are endogenous basic tendencies (McCrae et al., 2000).

Operation of the System

The welter of arrows in Figure 5.1 indicate some of the most important paths by which personality components interact. The plural *processes* is used because many quite distinct processes may be involved in each pathway. For example, the arrow from *objective biography* to *self-concept* implies that we learn who we are, in part, from observing what we

do. But interpreting what we have done may involve social comparison, selective attention, defensive denial, implicit learning, or any number of other cognitive–affective processes. (Evolutionary psychologists such as Buss [1991; see also Chapter 2, this volume] have also emphasized that there are likely to be a very large number of evolved psychological mechanisms for specific problems in adaptation.)

One implication is that personality theories that posit a small handful of key dynamic processes (e.g., repression, learning, self-actualization, getting ahead and getting along) are unlikely to prove adequate. Another is that psychologists who prefer to study processes instead of traits—"doing" instead of "having" (Cantor, 1990)—face the challenging prospect of identifying the most important of these many processes to study. There is as yet nothing like an adequate taxonomy of processes, and creating such a taxonomy should become a priority for personality theorists. FFT acknowledges the issue of multiple dynamic processes and specifies important categories of processes that share a common function in the organization of the personality system. It does not, however, detail the specifics. A complete theory of personality will ultimately include subtheories that elaborate on such specific topics.

Table 5.2 lists 16 postulates intended to specify how the personality system operates (McCrae & Costa, 1996, 2006b). Postulates 1b through 2b spell out the ways in which traits develop from biological bases and interact with the environment to create characteristic adaptations (or maladaptations). Postulate 5a says that behavior is a function of the interaction of characteristic adaptations and external influences. An example of the operation of the system is provided by the need for closure (Kruglanski & Webster, 1996). This tendency to "seize" the first credible answer and to "freeze" on one's initial decisions was shown to be strongly inversely related to Openness to Experience. It is easy to imagine the paths by which such habits of thought might develop:

TABLE 5.2. FFT Postulates

1. Basic tendencies

1a. Individuality. All adults can be characterized by their differential standing on a series of personality traits that influence patterns of thoughts, feelings, and actions.

1b. Origin. Personality traits are endogenous basic tendencies that can be altered by exogenous interventions, processes, or events that affect their biological bases.

1c. Development. The development of personality traits occurs through intrinsic maturation, mostly in the first third of life but continuing across the lifespan; and through other biological processes that alter the basis of traits.

1d. Structure. Traits are organized hierarchically from narrow and specific to broad and general dispositions; Neuroticism, Extraversion, Openness to Experience, Agreeableness, and Conscientiousness constitute the highest level of the hierarchy.

2. Characteristic adaptations

2a. Adaptation. Over time, individuals react to their environments by evolving patterns of thoughts, feelings, and behaviors that are consistent with their personality traits and earlier adaptations.

2b. Maladjustment. At any one time, adaptations may not be optimal with respect to cultural values or personal goals.

2c. Plasticity. Characteristic adaptations change over time in response to biological maturation, social roles and/or expectations, and changes in the environment or deliberate interventions.

3. Objective biography

3a. Multiple determination. Action and experience at any given moment are complex functions of all those characteristic adaptations that are evoked by the situation.

3b. Life course. Individuals have plans, schedules, and goals that allow action to be organized over long time intervals in ways that are consistent with their personality traits.

4. Self-concept

4a. Self-schema. Individuals maintain a cognitive–affective view of themselves that is accessible to consciousness.

4b. Selective perception. Information is selectively represented in the self-concept in ways that (i) are consistent with personality traits; and (ii) give a sense of coherence to the individual.

5. External influences

5a. Interaction. The social and physical environment interacts with personality dispositions to shape characteristic adaptations, and with characteristic adaptations to regulate the flow of behavior.

5b. Apperception. Individuals attend to and construe the environment in ways that are consistent with their personality traits.

5c. Reciprocity. Individuals selectively influence the environment to which they respond.

6. Dynamic processes

6a. Universal dynamics. The ongoing functioning of the individual in creating adaptations and expressing them in thoughts, feelings, and behaviors is regulated in part by universal cognitive, affective, and volitional mechanisms.

6b. Differential dynamics. Some dynamic processes are differentially affected by basic tendencies of the individual, including personality traits.

Note. Adapted from McCrae and Costa (1996, 2006b).

Lacking a need for change and uncertainty, closed people come to prefer a simple, structured, familiar world. Through experience they discover that tradition, conventionality, and stereotypes offer tried-and-true answers that they can adopt without much thought. They begin to think of themselves as conservative, down-to-earth people, and they seek out like-minded friends and spouses who will not challenge their beliefs. Thus, Basic Tendencies of closedness develop into preferences, ideologies, self-construals, and social roles; these Characteristic Adaptations habitualize, legitimatize, and socially support a way of thinking that expresses a high need for closure. (Costa & McCrae, 1998b, p. 117)

Revisions to FFT

The postulates in Table 5.2 are empirically testable, and in fact most of them are based on a body of empirical literature. In a few cases, recent data have suggested the need for revision or clarification of some of the original postulates, and we have proposed new versions (McCrae & Costa, 2006b).

Most of the 16 postulates are apparently not controversial. No one seems to dispute that people have a self-concept (4a) or that some characteristic adaptations may be maladaptive (2b). In fact, much research has tied maladaptive *DSM-IV* personality disorders to personality traits, consistent with FFT (Costa & Widiger, 2002). Although they did not couch it as a test of FFT, McAdams and his colleagues (2004) recently published data that support Postulate 4b, *selective perception*. McAdams believes that people come to understand themselves not by amassing a catalogue of relevant descriptors but by constructing a coherent life narrative (McAdams, 1996; see also Chapter 8, this volume). Given that interpretation of the self-concept, Postulate 4b implies that life narratives should be consistent with personality traits, and this is precisely what McAdams and colleagues found. Stories with themes of sadness and distress were associated with Neuroticism; themes of love and friendship were associated with Agreeableness; and the complexity of the narratives was strongly related to Openness to Experience.

There are, however, three postulates that have been challenged by recent literature and should be reconsidered.

Issues of Structure

Postulate 1d, *Structure*, claims that the five factors "constitute the highest level of the hierarchy." In a major article on personality structure, Markon, Krueger, and Watson (2005) suggested that, although the five factors are most fundamental, there are even broader higher-order factors: At the higher levels, Extraversion and Openness combine to form Digman's (1997) Personal Growth factor, β; Agreeableness and Conscientiousness combine to form (low) Disinhibition; and Disinhibition and Neuroticism merge into Digman's (low) Socialization factor, α. Markon and colleagues argued that each of these levels corresponds to a major model in the literature, and that all of them are useful for some purposes. Should we revise Postulate 1d?

Not yet. In 1999 we argued that Digman's factors might well be artifacts of evaluation, specifically, that Socialization corresponded to (low) negative valence, and Personal Growth to positive valence (McCrae & Costa, 1995a). Paulhus and John (1998) argued similarly that factors such as α and β arise from moralistic and egoistic self-enhancing biases. Strong evidence in favor of an artifactual interpretation was offered by Biesanz and West (2004), who reported multitrait, multimethod confirmatory factor analyses of self-reports and peer and parent ratings. Within informant type (e.g., self-reports), where evaluative biases are shared, the five factors were intercorrelated as Digman predicted. Across informant types, however, the five factors were orthogonal. This study raises the question of whether the higher-order factor structure reported by Markon and colleagues (2005) is a product of monomethod assessment: "Theoretical frameworks that integrate [FFM factors] as facets of a broader construct may need to be reexamined" (Biesanz & West, 2004, p. 871). A lexical study that examined a two-factor solution also failed to replicate Digman's factors (Ashton, Lee, & Goldberg, 2004). However, recent unpublished analyses suggest that the Digman structure may be the result of both within-method bias and substantive higher-order associations; if such findings are replicated, some modification of Postulate 1d would be warranted.

Other researchers dispute the claim that personality is well described by only five factors. Ashton, in particular, has energetically pushed the case for a six-factor, HEXACO, model (Ashton & Lee, 2005; Ashton, Lee, Perugini, et al., 2004). He has argued that in lexical studies, a sixth factor of Honesty-Humility is identified, and that some of the other factors are reoriented. But honesty and humility correspond conceptually and empirically to the Straightforwardness and Modesty facets of Agreeableness (Ashton & Lee, 2005), as assessed by the Revised NEO Personality Inventory (NEO-PI-R; Costa & McCrae, 1992a). In natural languages there are likely to be many terms related to Agreeableness/Honesty, because these traits are so central to social interactions. In this large collection of variables, relatively subtle distinctions may be sufficient to define different factors, and in this case it appears that the more introverted aspects of Agreeableness (Honesty and Humility) are distinguished from the more extraverted aspects. Both, however, can be subsumed by the broader Agreeableness factor found in the NEO-PI-R.

Cheung has also advocated a sixth factor, which was defined by scales from the Chinese Personality Assessment Inventory (CPAI) such as Face, *Ah-Q* Mentality (Defensiveness), and Thrift vs. Extravagance, representing indigenous Chinese personality constructs. The sixth factor was initially called Chinese Tradition (Cheung & Leung, 1998). Subsequent research in non-Chinese samples showed a similar factor and led to a broader label, Interpersonal Relatedness (Cheung, Cheung, Leung, Ward, & Leong, 2003). In a joint factor analysis of the CPAI and item parcels from the NEO Five-Factor Inventory (NEO-FFI; Costa & McCrae, 1992a), a six-factor solution showed an Interpersonal Relatedness factor defined solely by scales from the CPAI. But a five-factor solution simply redistributed the Interpersonal Relatedness scales among the usual FFM factors. For example, Face loaded on the N factor, *Ah-Q* Mentality on the (low) A factor, and Thrift on the C factor. The FFM is sufficiently comprehensive to include all these indigenous Chinese constructs.

Issues of Development

The original statement of the development postulate (1c in Table 5.2) asserted that traits "reach mature form in adulthood; thereafter they are stable." This statement was perhaps misleading; it has apparently been interpreted to mean that traits are absolutely immutable after full adulthood is reached (Roberts, Walton, & Viechtbauer, 2006; Srivastava, John, Gosling, & Potter, 2003), which was not our intended meaning. At the time that we formulated this postulate, we did not have good evidence of normative mean-level change after age 30, but we already knew that individual differences were not perfectly stable. In 1992 we had estimated that only "about three-fifths of the variance in personality traits is stable across the full adult age range. Is there change as well as stability in individual differences?" we asked. "Yes, of course" (Costa & McCrae, 1992b, p. 182). Perhaps our postulate should have read "*relatively* stable."

Curiously, new analyses spanning over 40 years suggest that our earlier assessment actually underestimated the long-term stability of individual differences, because the decay of stability reaches a non-zero asymptote after about 20 years (Jones, Livson, & Peskin, 2006; Terracciano et al., 2006). Perhaps four-fifths of the true-score variance is stable across the adult lifespan. But even that estimate is inconsistent with the "immutability" interpretation of Postulate 1c.

Furthermore, we now know that there are continuing mean-level changes after age 30 in all five factors (Roberts et al., 2006; Terracciano, McCrae, Brant, & Costa, 2005), although they are very gradual. The 30-year-old extravert is still likely to be an extravert at age 70, though not quite as active or keen on excitement. Finally, there appear to be a few individuals who change substantially (although such changes have not been demonstrated across methods; see McCrae, 1993; Watson & Humrichouse, 2006). We could revise Postulate 1c to say "relatively stable for most people," or we could specify more concretely what we now think we know (e.g., "with an accelerating decline in activity and a small increase in warmth"), but the major postulates of a theory are not meant to be repositories of technical information that may need to be updated with each new study. The real point of our development postulate is that the course of personality development is determined by biological maturation, not by life experience, and the statement in Table 5.2 now reflects that view.

But personality development is a broader topic than the development of traits. Postulate 2a acknowledges that characteristic adaptations also evolve over time, and Postulate 3b notes that the life course unfolds under the enduring influence of traits. But characteristic adaptations and the life course are also determined by the environment, in part by shared age norms and expectations (cf. Roberts, Wood, & Smith, 2005), although the influence of age norms appears to have declined in modern societies (Neugarten, 1982). The developmental psychology of characteristic adaptations is a fertile field for future research and theorizing.

Issues of Origin

Postulate 1b is even more controversial, because it denies any role to the environment in determining trait levels. Decades of personality theorizing on the role of childrearing in shaping adult personality are supported by almost no empirical data, except perhaps in extreme cases (Caspi et al., 2002). The debate on the role of adult experience in shaping personality continues. As the next section shows, the evidence for Postulate 1b is stronger now than it was in 1996. Most behavior genetic studies have continued to show little or no role for the shared environment (Bouchard & Loehlin, 2001), and ambitious attempts to pin down substantive contributions of the non-shared environment have largely failed (Reiss, Neiderhiser, Hetherington, & Plomin, 2000). However, a number of studies have reported findings that seem to imply some role for the environment:

- Living in Canada increased Openness and Agreeableness among Chinese undergraduates (McCrae, Yik, Trapnell, Bond, & Paulhus, 1998).
- Work experiences were associated with personality changes in young adults (Roberts, Caspi, & Moffit, 2003).
- Physical demands and hazardous work conditions were associated with a decline in trust over a 10-year interval (Sutin & Costa, 2008).
- General cultural changes led to changes in personality traits (Roberts & Helson, 1997).
- Large cohort differences were found in Extraversion in successive generations of college students (Twenge, 2001).

- In women, the experience of divorce was related to decreased dominance (Roberts, Helson, & Klohnen, 2002).
- In women, the experience of divorce was related to increased Extraversion (Costa, Herbst, McCrae, & Siegler, 2000).

Readers sympathetic to the environmental causation hypothesis may take this list as powerful evidence that FFT is flawed, and that there are indeed environmental influences on basic tendencies. But in fact the data do not bear close scrutiny. Dominance is strongly related to Extraversion, so why do the Roberts and colleagues' (2002) and Costa and colleagues' (2000) studies reach opposite conclusions on the effect of divorce? Twenge's (2001) dramatic cohort effects were not replicated in a study of nearly 2,000 adults assessed repeatedly over 15 years (Terracciano et al., 2005). The analyses in Roberts, Caspi, and Moffit are causally ambiguous: They showed that personality changes between ages 18 and 26 were associated with work variables at age 26, but it was not clear whether the changes preceded or followed the work experience. Finally, with the exception of McCrae and colleagues (1998), these studies relied exclusively on self-report data, so we do not know whether they reflected changes in personality or merely changes in the self-concept or reporting biases. Under certain conditions the environment may directly affect traits, but that effect has not yet been reliably or pervasively demonstrated.

However, there is one undeniable way in which the environment can affect personality traits, and that is through the mediation of biological bases. A metal rod through the brain of 19th-century railroad worker Phineas Gage created dramatic changes in his personality. More benignly, psychotropic medications can affect personality traits (Bagby, Levitan, Kennedy, Levitt, & Joffe, 1999). Psychotherapy, a nonbiological intervention, can cure depression (a brain disease; Mayberg et al., 2000) and thus lead to changes in personality trait levels (Costa, Bagby, Herbst, & McCrae, 2005). These findings suggest the rephrasing of Postulate 1b in Table 5.2 and lead to the introduction of a new arrow in Figure 5.1, dashed to indicate that it occurs outside the confines of personality proper.

New Cross-Cultural Evidence for FFT

FFT was formulated to organize and explain a body of findings; in particular, it was intended to provide an explanation for the remarkable stability of personality that longitudinal studies had revealed. How was it possible that years of experience, marriage, divorce, career changes, chronic and acute illnesses, wars and depressions, and countless hours of television viewing could have so little impact on personality traits? Combined with emerging findings on the heritability of personality traits and the general lack of evidence for common environmental influences on personality (Plomin & Daniels, 1987), these findings suggested to us that traits are categorically distinct from learned behaviors and beliefs, which certainly do change with age and which certainly are shaped by childhood experiences. FFT is really an elaboration of this basic insight, formulated in the early 1990s.

Ideally, theories go beyond a post hoc interpretation of observations and lead to testable hypotheses. Perhaps the most compelling tests of FFT have been the cross-cultural studies on the FFM that have been conducted in the past decade. Researchers around the world began to translate the NEO-PI-R (to date, into more than 40 languages) and conduct research in their own cultures. There was, of course, no guarantee that the instrument would be translatable or that the intended factors would be replicated in different cultures. Indeed, one skeptic wrote that "different cultures and different languages should give rise to other models that have little chance of being five in number nor of having any of the factors resemble those derived from the linguistic/social network of middle-class Americans" (Juni, 1996, p. 864).

That was a reasonable view if one assumed that culture dictates personality, as generations of anthropologists and personality psychologists had done. But the implications of FFT are clear: Personality traits are a function of biology, and all human being share a common genome. Therefore, the structure of personality ought to be universal.

Lexical studies, in which the personality traits encoded in natural languages are analyzed, have now been conducted in a number of cultures. Many of them do show the FFM seen in American lexical studies (e.g., Somer & Goldberg, 1999), but the case is less clear in other cultures (Saucier, Hampson, & Goldberg, 2000), and some researchers, as noted earlier, discern a common six-factor model (Ashton, Lee, Perugini, et al., 2004). Historically, lexical studies played a crucial role in the identification of the FFM, but it must be recalled that they are studies of personality *language* and only indirectly of personality itself. The lexical hypothesis asserts that all socially significant traits will be encoded in language, but that hypothesis may be too strong. There are, after all, languages in which the only color words are *dark* and *light* (see Kay, Berlin, Maffi, & Merrifield, 1997), but this does not mean that the speakers are color-blind.

An appropriate test of the universality of structure would need to use the same variables in each culture, and translations of a standard personality inventory provide such variables. Evidence for the universality of the FFM is clear across different instruments (McCrae & Costa, 1997b; Paunonen et al., 1996) and different methods of measurement. A large-scale observer rating study showed factor replications in 50 different cultures (McCrae, Terracciano, et al., 2005a). The traits of the FFM exist and are similarly related in all cultures so far studied. This does not preclude the possibility that there are other, indigenous personality factors unique to particular cultures, although such factors would probably be interpretable as characteristic adaptations within FFT.

Postulate 1c claims that the development of traits is guided by intrinsic maturation, and thus development too should be species-wide. There are few longitudinal studies outside Western cultures, and normally cross-sectional studies are difficult to interpret, because age differences at any given time may reflect cohort effects—that is, influences of the particular time and place in which people's personalities developed. Education levels, for example, decline cross-sectionally, not because people become less educated with age, but because education has become more widespread in more recent times.

But according to FFT, early life experience should not matter, because experience does not shape personality traits. Trait development in the People's Republic of China should parallel development in the United States, despite the different experiences posed by the Cultural Revolution and the subsequent rise of capitalism. And, in fact, cross-sectional age differences in personality are very similar in these two countries (Yang et al., 1998) and in such diverse cultures as Zimbabwe and Estonia (McCrae & Costa, 2006a). Similar age trends were found in 50 cultures when observer ratings were analyzed (McCrae, Terracciano, et al., 2005a), with a reduced rate of (cross-sectional) change after age 40.

Much the same story can be told for sex differences, which are also universal (Costa, Terracciano, & McCrae, 2001; McCrae, Terracciano, et al., 2005a), despite large differences in gender roles and expectations across cultures. A curious twist, however, is that the magnitude of sex differences varies across cultures in a surprising fashion: The largest differences are found in modern, progressive nations that ostensibly emphasize equality of the sexes. Those differences are probably artifacts; for example, women in traditional cultures may assess their personality relative to other women, thus norming away gender differences. Whatever the explanation, the phenomenon is not consistent with the naive environmentalism that would expect greater sex differences in traditional cultures.

McCrae and colleagues (2004) reported cross-cultural analyses of self–other agreement on personality ratings. Some cultural psychologists (see Church, 2000) have suggested that traits are Western, individualistic phenomena, and that even if they existed in collectivistic cultures, they were likely to go unnoticed. Instead, roles and social relationships are more important in collectivistic cultures. However, Buss (1991, p. 471) used evolutionary reasoning to argue that "perceiving, attending to, and acting upon differences in others is crucial" for survival and reproduction, and thus should be built in, species-wide. In their review, McCrae and colleagues found almost identical levels of self–other agreement in North American and cross-cultural studies. These data suggest that both personality traits and the mechanisms for their perception are rooted in evolved human biology.

The fact that the same traits and the same structure are found everywhere does not mean that average trait levels need be universal. People everywhere have hair, but there are more blonds in Europe than in Asia. Comparisons of mean levels across cul-

tures is a demanding task, because apparent differences may be due to translation of the instrument, or to cultural differences in response sets, or to different sampling biases in different cultures. However, a series of studies addressing these concerns led to the conclusion that there are reliable differences in the mean levels of traits across cultures (McCrae, 2002b; McCrae, Terracciano, et al., 2005b). The clearest finding was that cultures of European descent scored higher in Extraversion than Asian and African cultures. It is not clear at this point whether that finding is attributable to shared culture or shared ancestry (or both), but in itself it is not inconsistent with FFT. A century ago, geographers subscribed to the doctrine of environmental determinism, which held that culture and character were formed by the soil, climate, and landscape in which a people lived (Mitchell, 2000). Yet generations of life in South Africa created little resemblance between blacks and whites. In personality profiles, black South Africans resembled other black Africans; white South Africans resembled Europeans.

The effects of culture and ethnicity are most easily distinguished in acculturation studies. If the personality profile of an immigrant group comes to resemble that of the host culture, then cultural influences are indicated; if not, the profile may reflect the enduring influence of the immigrants' gene pool. Europeans living in South Africa do not offer a clear test of this hypothesis, because they did not acculturate to the indigenous culture; instead, they transported their language and culture with them. McCrae and colleagues (1998), however, examined personality profiles of Chinese undergraduates in Hong Kong and in Canada. Recent immigrants to Canada showed profiles very similar to Hong Kong undergraduates, but ethnic Chinese students born in Canada more closely resembled European Canadian students, especially with respect to levels of O and A. This is an important piece of evidence against FFT; if it is a replicable finding, some modification of the proscription of environmental influences on trait levels would be needed.

Evolutionary Explanations of the Factors

As noted in Table 5.2, Postulate 1d of FFT states that "traits are organized hierarchically from narrow and specific to broad and general dispositions; Neuroticism, Extraversion, Openness to Experience, Agreeableness, and Conscientiousness constitute the highest level of the hierarchy." This is the only postulate in which the FFM is even mentioned; otherwise the theory could just as well be adopted by proponents of a three- or seven- or N-factor model.

And Postulate 1d does not offer to explain the FFM, it merely asserts it. Shouldn't a five-factor theory explain why there are five factors and not six? And why these factors and not others? That would be an impressive feat, but it is not essential to scientific understanding. The speed of light is crucial to the theory of special relativity, but that theory gives no clue as to why $c \approx 300,000$ km/sec.

Postulate 1d reflects the position of McCrae and John (1992), who explained the recurrent finding of five robust factors by saying "we believe it is an empirical fact, like the fact that there are seven continents or eight American presidents from Virginia" (p. 194). McCrae and John were not trying to make a dogmatic pronouncement about the true number of factors (although the quote seems sometimes to have been interpreted that way; see, e.g., Block, 1995). Instead, they hoped to offer an alternative to the seductive but ultimately unpersuasive notion that the number somehow reflected the information-processing capacities of human raters (Goldberg, 1983; Miller, 1956). There is nothing magic about the number 5; it is simply what the data seem to show.

Without further rationale, Postulate 1d is vulnerable to empirical falsification. The continent of Atlantis may rise again from the sea, a ninth Virginian may be elected president, and trait researchers may discover another factor or factors of personality of comparable scope to N, E, O, A, and C. At that point it will be time to modify FFT. Although they could not explain the number 8, historians could certainly give some reasons why natives of Virginia were disproportionately chosen as U.S. presidents, and could give very specific reasons for the selection of Washington, Jefferson, and Madison. Can personality psychologists explain why people differ in levels of N, E, O, A, or C?

Given that personality traits have a biological basis and that human beings are the products of evolution, it is natural to seek answers in evolutionary psychology. Buss (1996; see also Chapter 2, this volume) made a strong case for the relevance of personality traits to social adaptation. People with different personality traits go about the tasks of survival and reproduction in different ways. For example, to retain their mates, extraverts show off, agreeable men express affection, and men low in C try to make their mates jealous. Personality traits influence the ability to make strategic alliances and to compete with others for resources. Personality traits, and specifically the five major factors, are of central relevance to the tasks people have evolved to solve. Because of this, people have learned to attend to individual differences in personality, and to base their choices of leaders, friends, and mates partly on inferred personality characteristics.

This perspective does not, in itself, explain the evolution of the FFM, however. Normally natural and sexual selection are invoked to explain a species-wide characteristic, not variation within the species. A number of evolutionary approaches have been taken to explain individual differences, and Figueredo and colleagues (2005) review them and the slim evidence that currently can be used to evaluate them.

Tooby and Cosmides (1990) offered what must be considered the null position: Traits exist because they are adaptively neutral; they are perpetuated as genetic noise. This is a valuable fall-back position for traits such as Openness to Aesthetics that are of dubious adaptive value (see also Buss, Haselton, Shackelford, Bleske, & Wakefield, 1998). A step higher are models that claim that traits are the result of stabilizing selection (Bouchard & Loehlin, 2001)—that is, that extreme values may have been selected out. (This position is consistent with views of personality disorder that identify pathology with extreme scores.) Individuals who were too introverted to find a mate or too extraverted to conceal themselves from an enemy may not have survived and reproduced. But variation within the normal range may be of no evolutionary consequence.

MacDonald (1998) takes a more substantive position, arguing that the five factors represent evolved mechanisms for solving social and nonsocial problems. For example, he links Extraversion to a behavioral approach system "designed to motivate organisms to approach sources of reward" (p. 125). Individual differences in such adaptive traits are incidental and explainable by noting that there are alternative viable strategies associated with different levels of traits. Agreeableness makes it easier to acquire allies, but antagonism sharpens one's ability to compete with enemies; open exploration leads to new resources, but closed conventionality exploits the tried-and-true.

Figueredo and King (2001) offer a more formal explanation for individual differences. They agree that traits are adaptive but invoke the notion of frequency-dependent selection to account for individual differences. Agreeableness is usually adaptive, leading to cooperation and shared resources. But if a group consists chiefly of highly agreeable individuals, the occasional antagonist can prosper by taking advantage of them. If antagonists proliferate, however, their competition will lower the adaptive value of being antagonistic. Individual differences in an evolving population thus sustain a dynamic equilibrium.

Such theorizing illustrates the ways in which evolutionary thinking might account for the factors of the FFM, but no compelling case has yet been made. Ideally, we would begin with basic principles of evolution, such as parental investment, reciprocal altruism, and deception strategies (see Hendrick, 2005), and deduce the existence and nature of the five factors—but that seems unlikely to happen. As Buss (1991) acknowledged, "general evolutionary theory broadly outlines what is *unlikely* to have evolved ... [but] it can rarely specify what must have evolved" (p. 465).

One complication in formulating evolutionary hypotheses is that we do not yet know to which evolutionary era they must be pegged. Buss (1991) sought to analyze personality by identifying *"adaptive problems confronted by ancestral human populations"* (p. 476; original emphasis), but evidence shows that the FFM can also be glimpsed in chimpanzees (King, Weiss, & Farmer, 2005). This finding suggests that precursors of these personality factors may have evolved in ancestors common to some or all primates. Indeed, for all we know, Extraversion evolved when fish first formed schools. Identifying the relevant adaptive problems may require much more data from comparative personality psychology.

Another problem concerns the adaptive core of each factor. MacDonald (1998) identifies Extraversion with excitement seek-

ing and reward sensitivity; Ashton and Lee (2001) more narrowly focus on "behaviours that tend to attract social attention" (p. 342). Other theorists might emphasize the element of dominance in Extraversion and seek an explanation based on adaptive variations in dominance versus submission. MacDonald cautions that "there is no reason to suppose that the dimensions revealed by factor analysis map in a 1:1 manner with biological adaptations" (p. 127), which, if true, effectively undermines the search for evolutionary explanations for the factors in the FFM.

Nevertheless, Figueredo and colleagues (2005) concluded that there is "a modicum of evidence supporting each of the major evolutionary theories explaining ... individual differences" (p. 873). The problem of defining the adaptive core of each factor might be obviated by proposing theories on the evolution of facet-level traits, which are more narrowly defined. And it must be recalled that different evolutionary explanations may apply to different traits. Openness to Aesthetics may be a matter of genetic noise; Depression may reflect stabilizing selection; Compliance may result from frequency-dependent selection. Evolutionary explanation, like evolution itself, may be a convoluted process.

Subtheories of the Five Factors

The postulates of FFT deal uniformly with all five factors and thus must offer quite general propositions. It would be entirely possible to construct more specific subtheories to deal with each of the five factors separately. Conceptual analyses of the individual factors have been offered in several articles (Costa & McCrae, 1998a; Costa, McCrae, & Dembroski, 1989; McCrae & Costa, 1997a; Watson & Clark, 1997); formal theorizing could be guided by Figure 5.1. The agenda might be as follows:

1. Define the basic tendencies involved for the factor and its defining facet traits.
2. Identify specific biological bases, from genes to brain structures and functions.
3. Identify dynamic processes, such as defenses, cognitive styles, or planning and scheduling, that are differentially affected by the factor (see Postulate 6b).
4. Catalogue the characteristic adaptations—interests, roles, skills, self-image, psychiatric symptoms—associated with the fac-

tor and explain how they reflect common basic tendencies.

5. Account for the lifespan development of the factor, its objective reflection in the life course, and its subjective representation in life narratives.

Different parts of this agenda appeal to different psychologists. Factor analysts are concerned with identifying the facet traits and interpreting the resulting factors (Hofstee, Kiers, De Raad, Goldberg, & Ostendorf, 1997). Psychobiologists emphasize the identification of underlying biological mechanisms (Eysenck, 1967). Clinicians might be most concerned with problematic characteristic adaptations (see Postulate 2b), which they might be able to modify (Harkness & Lilienfeld, 1997).

Perhaps because they ground psychology in a more basic science, theories that offer biological explanations for traits seem particularly desirable, and we encourage research on which such theories could be based. In our present state of relative ignorance, however, theories of biological mechanisms may be premature. For example, Cloninger's neurohormonal theory of personality, which staked so much on the initial findings in the molecular genetics of personality (Cloninger, Adolfsson, & Svrakic, 1996), was surely shaken by subsequent failures to replicate (Herbst, Zonderman, McCrae, & Costa, 2000; Malhotra et al., 1996).

Steps 1 through 3 of the above agenda are presumably universal to all human beings. Steps 4 and 5, however, deal with the interaction of the person and the environment and speak only to particular contexts. How Conscientiousness is expressed in Italy is likely to be very different from how it is expressed in Iran. Ethnographic methods might be needed to identify the culturally prescribed forms in which personality factors are manifested, and comparative cross-cultural studies could illuminate links between personality and culture (McCrae, 2000).

Alternatives to FFT

In our first full statement of FFT we suggested that it was likely to be only one of a new generation of personality theories informed by research findings (McCrae & Costa, 1996). Alternative theories have, in fact, been proposed, and some comparisons to FFT seem warranted.

Roberts and colleagues (e.g., Roberts, Wood, & Smith, 2005) have offered a midlevel theory concerned with trait development. Their social investment perspective offers a reinterpretation of the cross-cultural consistency of age differences and changes. Specifically, they propose that life tasks such as finding a mate and raising children are universal, and that cultures everywhere promote traits, such as increased A and C, that assist in these tasks. The mechanism for these changes is the individual's internalized investment in social roles such as work or parenting. Actually occupying the role does not matter; this explains (within social investment theory) why people who become parents do not become more conscientious than those who remain childless (Neyer & Asdendorpf, 2001)—although one might have guessed that, on average, people who have children would be more invested in the parenting role.

FFT does not dispute that the maturational changes typically seen between adolescence and adulthood are useful for perpetuating the next generation, or that societies generally reward such changes. But the rewards cannot (according to FFT) be the cause of the changes. Instead, one might argue that they have evolved biologically because individuals whose A and C levels increased after adolescence successfully raised more children. Perhaps the most informative tests of these competing theories will come from longitudinal studies in developing countries: Is psychological maturity hastened by the earlier life responsibilities often found there?

On a larger scale, the most extensive theoretical work has been done by McAdams and his colleagues. In 1992 (in the same symposium in which we introduced FFT) McAdams proposed that personality might be conceived as occupying three levels: Level 1 consisted of relatively stable traits, Level 2 of personal concerns, and Level 3 of life stories. Levels 2 and 3 were more plastic than Level 1 and should show change across the lifespan (see McAdams, Chapter 8, this volume). There are obvious parallels between this model and FFT: Basic tendencies, characteristic adaptations, and the self-concept are clearly related to the Levels 1, 2, and 3, respectively. In next few years, the chief difference between the two theories was McAdams' (1996) insistence that the three levels were essentially independent, requiring their own methods of investigation and their own explanations. This stance was apparently motivated by the fear that higher levels of personality might be reduced to mere expressions of traits.

In 2002, Hooker began to link McAdams's levels to each other and to dynamic processes, and soon McAdams had endorsed this revision (Hooker & McAdams, 2003). The major innovation was the pairing of levels with processes: For example, traits were paired with states (phenomena that FFT would class not as processes but as outcomes—the subjective side of the objective biography). Most recently, McAdams and Pals (2006) have offered a new formulation, based not on components of a personality system, but on five principles that relate and set in context the three Levels, now called "dispositional traits," "characteristic adaptations," and "integrative life narratives." In place of biological bases, McAdams and Pals put "evolved human nature," and in place of external influences they specify "culture," plus a residual box of the "social ecology of everyday life." The objective biography is what is to be explained, so it is not identified as a separate principle, but the arrow joining *characteristic adaptations* and *social ecology* is labeled "most daily behavior."

Perhaps the most important difference between McAdams and Pals's (2006) model and that in Figure 5.1 is that most of their arrows are two-headed, suggesting reciprocal influence. Even that aspect is not quite as different as it appears. They acknowledge that culture's effects on traits may be limited, but argue that "culture does provide demand characteristics and display rules for the behavioral expression of traits" (p. 211), and it is this feature that accounts for the arrow from *culture* to *dispositional traits*. Yet that interpretation is entirely consistent with FFT, which regards trait expression as a function of culturally conditioned characteristic adaptations.

Sheldon (2004) offered an ambitious synthesis of contemporary research in the social and biological sciences, combined with prescriptions for optimizing human functioning. At the level of personality, situated between the brain and culture, four levels are identified: organismic characteristics, personality traits, goals and intentions, and selves and life stories. Sheldon's chief criticism of FFT is that it is reductionistic, apparently granting primacy to basic tendencies instead of postu-

lating the reciprocal influences among levels that Sheldon favors.

FFT acknowledges that some characteristic adaptations are maladaptive but says nothing about why; it is a very meager theory of psychopathology and says nothing about positive mental health (but see McCrae, Löckenhoff, & Costa, 2005, for an elaboration of personality psychopathology based on FFT). By contrast, Sheldon hopes to offer a comprehensive theory of optimal human being. His intention is to articulate general principles that reflect what is known about human nature, such as "Satisfy your basic bodily needs," "Try to develop more positive personality traits," "Set and pursue goals, as effectively as possible," and "Adapt to one's culture's norms and prescriptions" (pp. 184–185). Stated so baldly, these may seem mere platitudes, but they do offer a systematic survey of what may be considered desirable at many of the levels identified in this new generation of personality theories, and they are worth serious consideration by anyone concerned with positive psychology.

FFT AND THE INDIVIDUAL

Although it is doubtless true that every person is, in some respects, like no other person (Kluckhohn & Murray, 1953), FFT (like most personality theories) has nothing to say about this aspect of the person. It is, from a trait perspective, error variance. However, this most emphatically does not mean that personality is irrelevant to understanding the individual.

In the typical application in clinical or personnel psychology, the individual case is understood by inferring personality traits from one set of indicators and using the resulting personality profile to interpret a life history or predict future adjustment. This is not circular reasoning, because if valid personality measures are used, the traits identified carry surplus meaning that allows the interpreter to go beyond the information given (McCrae & Costa, 1995b). If respondents tell us that they are cheerful and high-spirited, we detect Extraversion and can guess with better-than-chance accuracy that they will be interested in managerial and sales positions. However, it would be much harder to predict their current occupation: Just as the theory of evolution is better at explaining how existing species function than it is at predicting which species will evolve, so personality profiles are more useful in understanding a life than in making specific predictions about what a person will do. This is not a limitation of FFT; it is an intrinsic feature of complex and chaotic systems.

Postulate 3a, multiple determination, points out that there is rarely a one-to-one correspondence between characteristic adaptations and behaviors; the same is, of course, equally true for the traits that underlie characteristic adaptations. Consequently, interpreting individual behaviors even when the personality profile is well known is a somewhat speculative art. Consider the case of Horatio, Lord Nelson (Costa & McCrae, 1998a; Southey, 1813/1922). In the course of his campaigns against Napoleon's France, he spent many months defending the woefully corrupt court of Naples against a democratic insurrection that had been encouraged by the French. Why would so heroic a figure take on so shabby a task?

We know from a lifetime of instances that Nelson was a paragon of dutifulness, and we might suspect that he was simply following orders—certainly he would have rationalized his conduct as devotion to the war against France. But we also know that Nelson was fiercely independent in his views of what constituted his duty: "I always act as I feel right, without regard to custom" (Southey, 1813/1922, p. 94). He might equally well have supported the insurrection and won its allegiance to the English cause.

We should also consider another trait Nelson possessed: He was excessively low in modesty. Great as his naval achievements were, he never failed to remind people of them. His sympathies were thus with the aristocracy, and he was flattered by the court of Naples, which ultimately named him Duke Di Bronte. Together, diligence (C), independence (O), and vanity (low A) go far to explain this episode of behavior.

To be sure, there are other factors, including Nelson's relationship to the English ambassador's wife, Lady Hamilton (Simpson, 1983). That notorious affair itself reflects Nelson's independence and vanity but seems strikingly incongruent with his dutifulness. At the level of the individual, the operations of personality traits are complex and often inconsistent (a phenomenon Mischel & Shoda, 1995, have tried to explain).

The Subjective Experience of Personality

A number of writers (e.g., Hogan, 1996) have suggested that the FFM does not accurately represent personality as it is subjectively experienced by the individual. Daniel Levinson dismissed the whole enterprise of trait psychology as a concern for trivial and peripheral aspects of the person (Rubin, 1981). McAdams (1996) has referred to it as the "psychology of the stranger," because standing on the five factors is the sort of thing one would want to know about a stranger to whom one has just been introduced. Ozer (1996) claimed that traits are personality as seen from the standpoint of the other, not the self.

We believe this last position represents a slight confusion. Individuals, who have access to their own private thoughts, feelings, and desires, and who generally have a more extensive knowledge of their own history of behavior, have a quite different perspective on their own traits than do external observers. What they nonetheless share with others is the need to infer the nature of their own traits and to express their inference in the comparative language of traits. We have no direct intuition of our trait profile; we can only guess at it from its manifestations in our actions and experience. (One possible reason for the increasing stability of personality as assessed by self-reports from ages 12 to 30—see McCrae et al., 2002; Siegler et al., 1990—is that we continue to learn about ourselves in this time period.)

The fact that traits must be inferred does not, however, mean that they are or seem foreign. When adults were asked to give 20 different answers to the question "Who am I?", about a quarter of the responses were worded as personality traits, and many others combined trait and role characteristics (e.g., "a loving mother"). Traits seem to form an important component of the spontaneous self-concept (McCrae & Costa, 1988); even children use trait terms to describe themselves (Donahue, 1994).

Sheldon, Ryan, Rawsthorne, and Ilardi (1997) brought a humanistic perspective to this issue by assessing sense of authenticity in individuals as they occupied different social roles. They also asked for context-specific self-reports of personality (e.g., how extraverted respondents were as students and as romantic partners). They found that individuals who described themselves most consistently across roles also claimed the highest feelings of authenticity. They concluded that "more often than not, one's true self and one's trait self are one and the same" (p. 1392).

CONCLUSION

FFT is an attempt to make sense of the explosion of findings that researchers have reported in the wake of the FFM. FFT is a contemporary version of trait theory, based on the assumptions that people are knowable, rational, variable, and proactive. FFT explains personality functioning as the operation of a universal personality system, with defined categories of variables and classes of dynamic processes that indicate the main causal pathways. The five personality factors—Neuroticism, Extraversion, Openness, Agreeableness, and Conscientiousness—form the substantive nucleus of the system; FFT traces their ramifications throughout the personality system. FFT provides a framework in which to understand the development and operation of psychological mechanisms (such as need for closure) and the behavior and experience of individual men and women.

FFT is a Grand Theory in the sense that it attempts to provide an overview of the functioning of the whole person across the complete lifespan. To do so it necessarily omits many specifics that a complete theory of personality would include. We have described in some detail the need for, and possible form of, subtheories of each of the individual factors. Also needed are subtheories that catalogue the contents of characteristic adaptations and systematize dynamic processes; more formal treatment of the self-concept; theories of psychopathology and psychotherapy (see Widiger, Costa, & McCrae, 2002); theories of personality perception and assessment; and an account of the basic executive mechanism—the operating system—that coordinates the ongoing flow of behavior and experience. Much is already known about all these topics; the theorist's task is to organize the information and integrate it into the overall scheme of FFT.

Historically, personality psychology has been characterized by elaborate and ambitious theories with only the most tenuous links to empirical findings, and theorists have often been considered profound to the extent that their visions of human nature departed from common sense. Freud's glorification of the taboo, Jung's obscure mysticism, Skinner's denial of that most basic experience of having a mind—such esoteric ideas set personality theorists apart from normal human beings and suggested that they were privy to secret knowledge. By contrast, FFT is closely and strongly tied to the empirical findings it summarizes, and its vision of human nature, at least at the phenotypic level, is not far removed from folk psychology. If that makes it a rather prosaic Grand Theory, so be it. What matters is how far it takes us in understanding that endlessly fascinating phenomenon, personality.

ACKNOWLEDGMENTS

Preparation of this chapter was supported by the Intramural Research Program, National Institutes of Health, National Institute on Aging. Thanks to Aurelio Jose Figueredo for comments on our discussion of evolutionary psychology. Portions of the chapter appear (in French) in McCrae and Costa (2006b).

REFERENCES

Ashton, M. C., & Lee, K. (2001). A theoretical basis for the major dimensions of personality. *European Journal of Personality*, 15, 327–353.

Ashton, M. C., & Lee, K. (2005). Honesty–humility, the Big Five, and the five-factor model. *Journal of Personality*, 73, 1321–1353.

Ashton, M. C., Lee, K., & Goldberg, L. R. (2004). A hierarchical analysis of 1,710 English personality-descriptive adjectives. *Journal of Personality and Social Psychology*, 87, 707–721.

Ashton, M. C., Lee, K., Perugini, M., Szarota, P., De Vries, R. E., Di Blass, L., et al. (2004). A six-factor structure of personality descriptive adjectives: Solutions from psycholexical studies in seven languages. *Journal of Personality and Social Psychology*, 86, 356–366.

Bagby, R. M., Levitan, R. D., Kennedy, S. H., Levitt, A. J., & Joffe, R. T. (1999). Selective alteration of personality in response to noradrenergic and serotonergic antidepressant medication in depressed sample: Evidence of non-specificity. *Psychiatry Research*, 86, 211–216.

Biesanz, J. C., & West, S. G. (2004). Towards

understanding assessments of the Big Five: Multitrait–multimethod analyses of convergent and discriminant validity across measurement occasion and type of observer. *Journal of Personality, 72,* 845–876.

Block, J. (1995). A contrarian view of the five-factor approach to personality description. *Psychological Bulletin, 117,* 187–215.

Bouchard, T. J., & Loehlin, J. C. (2001). Genes, evolution, and personality. *Behavior Genetics, 31,* 243–273.

Bruehl, S. (2002). A case of borderline personality disorder. In P. T. Costa & T. A. Widiger (Eds.), *Personality disorders and the five-factor model of personality* (2nd ed., pp. 283–291). Washington, DC: American Psychological Association.

Buss, D. M. (1991). Evolutionary personality psychology. *Annual Review of Psychology, 42,* 459–491.

Buss, D. M. (1996). Social adaptation and the five major factors of personality. In J. S. Wiggins (Ed.), *The five-factor model of personality* (pp. 180–207). New York: Guilford Press.

Buss, D. M., & Craik, K. H. (1983). The act frequency approach to personality. *Psychological Review, 90,* 105–126.

Buss, D. M., Haselton, M. G., Shackelford, T. K., Bleske, A. L., & Wakefield, J. C. (1998). Adaptations, exaptations, and spandrels. *American Psychologist, 53,* 533–548.

Canli, T. (Ed.). (2006). *Biology of personality and individual differences.* New York: Guilford Press.

Cantor, N. (1990). From thought to behavior: "Having" and "doing" in the study of personality and cognition. *American Psychologist, 45,* 735–750.

Carlson, R. (1984). What's social about social psychology? Where's the person in personality research? *Journal of Personality and Social Psychology, 47,* 1304–1309.

Caspi, A., McClay, J., Moffitt, T. E., Mill, J., Martin, J., Craig, I. W., et al. (2002). Role of genotype in the cycle of violence in maltreated children. *Science, 297,* 851–853.

Cheung, F. M., Cheung, S. F., Leung, K., Ward, C., & Leong, F. (2003). The English version of the Chinese Personality Assessment Inventory. *Journal of Cross-Cultural Psychology, 34,* 433–452.

Cheung, F. M., & Leung, K. (1998). Indigenous personality measures: Chinese examples. *Journal of Cross-Cultural Psychology, 29,* 233–248.

Church, A. T. (2000). Culture and personality: Toward an integrated cultural trait psychology. *Journal of Personality, 68,* 651–703.

Clark, L. A., & Livesley, W. J. (2002). Two approaches to identifying dimensions of personality disorder: Convergence on the five-factor model. In P. T. Costa & T. A. Widiger (Eds.), *Personality disorders and the five-factor model of personality* (2nd ed., pp. 161–176). Washington, DC: American Psychological Association.

Cloninger, C. R., Adolfsson, R., & Svrakic, N. M. (1996). Mapping genes for human personality. *Nature Genetics, 12,* 3–4.

Costa, P. T., Jr., Bagby, R. M., Herbst, J. H., & McCrae, R. R. (2005). Personality self-reports are concurrently reliable and valid during acute depressive episodes. *Journal of Affective Disorders, 89,* 45–55.

Costa, P. T., Jr., Herbst, J. H., McCrae, R. R., & Siegler, I. C. (2000). Personality at midlife: Stability, intrinsic maturation, and response to life events. *Assessment, 7,* 365–378.

Costa, P. T., Jr., & McCrae, R. R. (1988). From catalog to classification: Murray's needs and the five-factor model. *Journal of Personality and Social Psychology, 55,* 258–265.

Costa, P. T., Jr., & McCrae, R. R. (1992a). *Revised NEO Personality Inventory (NEO-PI-R) and NEO Five-Factor Inventory (NEO-FFI) professional manual.* Odessa, FL: Psychological Assessment Resources.

Costa, P. T., Jr., & McCrae, R. R. (1992b). Trait psychology comes of age. In T. B. Sonderegger (Ed.), *Nebraska Symposium on Motivation: Psychology and aging* (pp. 169–204). Lincoln: University of Nebraska Press.

Costa, P. T., Jr., & McCrae, R. R. (1993). Bullish on personality psychology. *The Psychologist, 6,* 302–303.

Costa, P. T., Jr., & McCrae, R. R. (1994). "Set like plaster"? Evidence for the stability of adult personality. In T. Heatherton & J. Weinberger (Eds.), *Can personality change?* (pp. 21–40). Washington, DC: American Psychological Association.

Costa, P. T., Jr., & McCrae, R. R. (1998a). Six approaches to the explication of facet-level traits: Examples from Conscientiousness. *European Journal of Personality, 12,* 117–134.

Costa, P. T., Jr., & McCrae, R. R. (1998b). Trait theories of personality. In D. F. Barone, M. Hersen, & V. B. Van Hasselt (Eds.), *Advanced personality* (pp. 103–121). New York: Plenum Press.

Costa, P. T., Jr., & McCrae, R. R. (2005). Theories of personality and psychopathology: Approaches derived from philosophy and psychology. In B. J. Sadock & V. A. Sadock (Eds.), *Kaplan and Sadock's comprehensive textbook of psychiatry* (Vol. 1, pp. 778–793). Philadelphia: Lippincott, Williams & Wilkins.

Costa, P. T., Jr., McCrae, R. R., & Dembroski, T. M. (1989). Agreeableness vs. antagonism: Explication of a potential risk factor for CHD.

In A. Siegman & T. M. Dembroski (Eds.), *In search of coronary-prone behavior: Beyond Type A* (pp. 41–63). Hillsdale, NJ: Erlbaum.

Costa, P. T., Jr., Terracciano, A., & McCrae, R. R. (2001). Gender differences in personality traits across cultures: Robust and surprising findings. *Journal of Personality and Social Psychology*, *81*, 322–331.

Costa, P. T., Jr., & Widiger, T. A. (Eds.). (2002). *Personality disorders and the five-factor model of personality* (2nd ed.). Washington, DC: American Psychological Association.

Côté, S., & Moskowitz, D. S. (1998). On the dynamic covariation between interpersonal behavior and affect: Prediction from Neuroticism, Extraversion, and Agreeableness. *Journal of Personality and Social Psychology*, *75*, 1032–1046.

Digman, J. M. (1997). Higher-order factors of the Big Five. *Journal of Personality and Social Psychology*, *73*, 1246–1256.

Digman, J. M., & Inouye, J. (1986). Further specification of the five robust factors of personality. *Journal of Personality and Social Psychology*, *50*, 116–123.

Donahue, E. M. (1994). Do children use the Big Five, too? Content and structural form in personality description. *Journal of Personality*, *62*, 45–66.

Eysenck, H. J. (1967). *The biological basis of personality*. Springfield, IL: Thomas.

Eysenck, H. J. (1997). Personality and experimental psychology: The unification of psychology and the possibility of a paradigm. *Journal of Personality and Social Psychology*, *73*, 1224–1237.

Figueredo, A. J., & King, J. E. (2001, June). The evolution of individual differences. In S. D. Gosling & A. Weiss (Chairs), *Evolution and individual differences*. Symposium presented at the annual meeting of the Human Behavior and Evolution Society, London.

Figueredo, A. J., Sefcek, J. A., Vasquez, G., Brumbach, B. H., King, J. E., & Jacobs, W. J. (2005). Evolutionary personality psychology. In D. M. Buss (Ed.), *Handbook of evolutionary psychology* (pp. 851–877). Hoboken, NJ: Wiley.

Funder, D. C. (1995). On the accuracy of personality judgment: A realistic approach. *Psychological Review*, *102*, 652–670.

Funder, D. C., Kolar, D. C., & Blackman, M. C. (1995). Agreement among judges of personality: Interpersonal relations, similarity, and acquaintanceship. *Journal of Personality and Social Psychology*, *69*, 656–672.

Funder, D. C., & Sneed, C. D. (1993). Behavioral manifestations of personality: An ecological approach to judgmental accuracy. *Journal of Personality and Social Psychology*, *64*, 479–490.

Goldberg, L. R. (1983, June). *The magical number five, plus or minus two: Some considerations on the dimensionality of personality descriptors*. Paper presented at a research seminar, Gerontology Research Center, Baltimore.

Harkness, A. R., & Lilienfeld, S. O. (1997). Individual differences science for treatment planning: Personality traits. *Psychological Assessment*, *9*, 349–360.

Hendrick, C. (2005). Evolution as a foundation for psychological theories. In S. Strack (Ed.), *Handbook of personology and psychopathology* (pp. 3–23). Hoboken, NJ: Wiley.

Herbst, J. H., Zonderman, A. B., McCrae, R. R., & Costa, P. T., Jr. (2000). Do the dimensions of the Temperament and Character Inventory map a simple genetic architecture? Evidence from molecular genetics and factor analysis. *American Journal of Psychiatry*, *157*, 1285–1290.

Hjelle, L. A., & Siegler, D. J. (1976). *Personality: Theories, basic assumptions, research and applications*. New York: McGraw-Hill.

Hofstee, W. K. B., Kiers, H. A. L., De Raad, B., Goldberg, L. R., & Ostendorf, F. (1997). A comparison of Big Five structures of personality traits in Dutch, English, and German. *European Journal of Personality*, *11*, 15–31.

Hogan, R. (1996). A socioanalytic perspective on the five-factor model. In J. S. Wiggins (Ed.), *The five-factor model of personality* (pp. 163–179). New York: Guilford Press.

Hooker, K. (2002). New directions for research in personality and aging: A comprehensive model linking levels, structures, and processes. *Journal of Research in Personality*, *36*, 318–334.

Hooker, K., & McAdams, D. P. (2003). Personality reconsidered: A new agenda for aging research. *Journal of Gerontology: Psychological Sciences*, *58B*, P296–P304.

Johnson, J. A. (1997). Units of analysis for the description and explanation of personality. In R. Hogan, J. A. Johnson, & S. R. Briggs (Eds.), *Handbook of personality psychology* (pp. 73–93). New York: Academic Press.

Jones, C. J., Livson, N., & Peskin, H. (2006). Paths of psychological health: Examination of 40-year trajectories from the Intergenerational Studies. *Journal of Research in Personality*, *40*, 56–72.

Juni, S. (1996). Review of the Revised NEO Personality Inventory. In J. C. Conoley & J. C. Impara (Eds.), *12th Mental Measurements Yearbook* (pp. 863–868). Lincoln: University of Nebraska Press.

Jussim, L. (2005). Accuracy in social perception: Criticisms, controversies, criteria, components, and cognitive processes. *Advances in Experimental Social Psychology*, *37*, 1–93.

Kagan, J. (2005). Personality and temperament: Historical perspectives. In M. Rosenbluth, S. H. Kennedy, & R. M. Bagby (Eds.), *Depression and personality: Conceptual and clinical chal-*

lenges (pp. 3–18). Washington, DC: American Psychiatric Publishing.

Kay, P., Berlin, P., Maffi, L., & Merrifield, W. (1997). Color naming across languages. In C. L. Hardin & L. Maffi (Eds.), *Color categories in thought and language* (pp. 21–56). New York: Cambridge University Press.

King, J. E., Weiss, A., & Farmer, K. H. (2005). A chimpanzee (*Pan troglodytes*) analogue of cross-national generalization of personality structure: Zoological parks and an African sanctuary. *Journal of Personality, 73,* 389–410.

Kluckhohn, C., & Murray, H. A. (1953). Personality formation: The determinants. In C. Kluckhohn, H. A. Murray, & D. M. Schneider (Eds.), *Personality in nature, society, and culture* (pp. 53–67). New York: Knopf.

Kruglanski, A. W., & Webster, D. M. (1996). Motivated closing of the mind: "Seizing" and "freezing." *Psychological Review, 103,* 263–283.

Lanning, K. (1994). Dimensionality of observer ratings on the California Adult Q-Set. *Journal of Personality and Social Psychology, 67,* 151–160.

MacDonald, K. (1998). Evolution, culture, and the five-factor model. *Journal of Cross-Cultural Psychology, 29,* 119–149.

Malhotra, A. K., Virkkunen, M., Rooney, W., Eggert, M., Linnoila, M., & Goldman, D. (1996). The association between the dopamine D4 receptor (D4DR) 16 amino acid repeat polymorphism and Novelty Seeking. *Molecular Psychiatry, 1,* 388–391.

Markon, K. E., Krueger, R. F., & Watson, D. (2005). Delineating the structure of normal and abnormal personality: An integrative hierarchical approach. *Journal of Personality and Social Psychology, 88,* 139–157.

Mayberg, H. S., Brannan, S. K., Tekell, J. L., Silva, J. A., Mahurin, R. K., McGinnis, S., et al. (2000). Regional metabolic effects of fluoxetine in major depression: Serial changes and relationship to clinical response. *Biological Psychiatry, 48,* 830–843.

Mayer, J. D. (1998). A systems framework for the field of personality. *Psychological Inquiry, 9,* 118–144.

McAdams, D. P. (1992, August). Levels of stability and growth in personality across the lifespan. In J. Weinberger (Chair), *Personality in the life course.* Symposium presented at the American Psychological Association Convention, Washington, DC.

McAdams, D. P. (1996). Personality, modernity, and the storied self: A contemporary framework for studying persons. *Psychological Inquiry, 7,* 295–321.

McAdams, D. P., Anyidoho, N. A., Brown, C., Huang, Y. T., Kaplan, B., & Machado, M. A.

(2004). Traits and stories: Links between dispositional and narrative features of personality. *Journal of Personality, 72,* 761–784.

McAdams, D. P., & Pals, J. L. (2006). A new Big Five: Fundamental principles for an integrative science of personality. *American Psychologist, 61,* 204–217.

McCrae, R. R. (1992). The five-factor model: Issues and applications [Special issue]. *Journal of Personality, 60*(2).

McCrae, R. R. (1993). Moderated analyses of longitudinal personality stability. *Journal of Personality and Social Psychology, 65,* 577–585.

McCrae, R. R. (1993–1994). Openness to Experience as a basic dimension of personality. *Imagination, Cognition, and Personality, 13,* 39–55.

McCrae, R. R. (1996). Social consequences of experiential openness. *Psychological Bulletin, 120,* 323–337.

McCrae, R. R. (2000). Trait psychology and the revival of personality and culture studies. *American Behavioral Scientist, 44,* 10–31.

McCrae, R. R. (2002a). The maturation of personality psychology: Adult personality development and psychological well-being. *Journal of Research in Personality, 36,* 307–317.

McCrae, R. R. (2002b). NEO-PI-R data from 36 cultures: Further intercultural comparisons. In R. R. McCrae & J. Allik (Eds.), *The five-factor model of personality across cultures* (pp. 105–125). New York: Kluwer Academic/ Plenum.

McCrae, R. R., & Costa, P. T., Jr. (1988). Age, personality, and the spontaneous self-concept. *Journal of Gerontology: Social Sciences, 43,* S–77–S185.

McCrae, R. R., & Costa, P. T., Jr. (1989). Reinterpreting the Myers–Briggs Type Indicator from the perspective of the five-factor model of personality. *Journal of Personality, 57,* 17–40.

McCrae, R. R., & Costa, P. T., Jr. (1995a). Positive and negative valence within the five-factor model. *Journal of Research in Personality, 29,* 443–460.

McCrae, R. R., & Costa, P. T., Jr. (1995b). Trait explanations in personality psychology. *European Journal of Personality, 9,* 231–252.

McCrae, R. R., & Costa, P. T., Jr. (1996). Toward a new generation of personality theories: Theoretical contexts for the five-factor model. In J. S. Wiggins (Ed.), *The five-factor model of personality* (pp. 51–87). New York: Guilford Press.

McCrae, R. R., & Costa, P. T., Jr. (1997a). Conceptions and correlates of Openness to Experience. In R. Hogan, J. A. Johnson, & S. R. Briggs (Eds.), *Handbook of personality psychology* (pp. 269–290). Orlando, FL: Academic Press.

McCrae, R. R., & Costa, P. T., Jr. (1997b). Personality trait structure as a human universal. *American Psychologist, 52,* 509–516.

McCrae, R. R., & Costa, P. T., Jr. (2003). *Personality in adulthood: A five-factor theory perspective* (2nd ed.). New York: Guilford Press.

McCrae, R. R., & Costa, P. T., Jr. (2006a). Cross-cultural perspectives on adult personality trait development. In D. Mroczek & T. Little (Eds.), *Handbook of personality development* (pp. 129–145). Hillsdale, NJ: Erlbaum.

McCrae, R. R., & Costa, P. T., Jr. (2006b). *Perspectives de la théorie des cinq facteurs (TCF): Traits et culture* [A five-factor theory perspective on traits and culture]. *Psychologie Française, 51,* 227–244.

McCrae, R. R., Costa, P. T., Jr., Martin, T. A., Oryol, V. E., Rukavishnikov, A. A., Senin, I. G., et al. (2004). Consensual validation of personality traits across cultures. *Journal of Research in Personality, 38,* 179–201.

McCrae, R. R., Costa, P. T., Jr., Ostendorf, F., Angleitner, A., Hrebícková, M., Avia, M. D., et. al. (2000). Nature over nurture: Temperament, personality, and lifespan development. *Journal of Personality and Social Psychology, 78,* 173–186.

McCrae, R. R., Costa, P. T., Jr., & Piedmont, R. L. (1993). Folk concepts, natural language, and psychological constructs: The California Psychological Inventory and the five-factor model. *Journal of Personality, 61,* 1–26.

McCrae, R. R., Costa, P. T., Jr., Terracciano, A., Parker, W. D., Mills, C. J., De Fruyt, F., et al. (2002). Personality trait development from 12 to 18: Longitudinal, cross-sectional, and cross-cultural analyses. *Journal of Personality and Social Psychology, 83,* 1456–1468.

McCrae, R. R., & John, O. P. (1992). An introduction to the five-factor model and its applications. *Journal of Personality, 60,* 175–215.

McCrae, R. R., Löckenhoff, C. E., & Costa, P. T., Jr. (2005). A step towards *DSM-V*: Cataloging personality-related problems in living. *European Journal of Personality, 19,* 269–270.

McCrae, R. R., Terracciano, A., & 78 Members of the Personality Profiles of Cultures Project. (2005a). Universal features of personality traits from the observer's perspective: Data from 50 cultures. *Journal of Personality and Social Psychology, 88,* 547–561.

McCrae, R. R., Terracciano, A., & 79 Members of the Personality Profiles of Cultures Project. (2005b). Personality profiles of cultures: Aggregate personality traits. *Journal of Personality and Social Psychology, 89,* 407–425.

McCrae, R. R., Yik, M. S. M., Trapnell, P. D., Bond, M. H., & Paulhus, D. L. (1998). Interpreting personality profiles across cultures: Bilingual, acculturation, and peer rating studies of Chinese undergraduates. *Journal of Personality and Social Psychology, 74,* 1041–1058.

Miller, G. E. (1956). The magical number seven, plus-or-minus two: Some limits on our capacity for processing information. *Psychological Review, 63,* 81–97.

Mischel, W., & Shoda, Y. (1995). A cognitive–affective system theory of personality: Reconceptualizing situations, dispositions, dynamics, and invariance in personality structure. *Psychological Review, 102,* 246–268.

Mitchell, D. (2000). *Cultural geography: A critical introduction.* Oxford, UK: Blackwell.

Neugarten, B. (1982). *Age or need?* Beverly Hills: Sage.

Neyer, F. J., & Asendorpf, J. B. (2001). Personality–relationship transaction in young adulthood. *Journal of Personality and Social Psychology, 81,* 1190–1204.

Ozer, D. J. (1996). The units we should employ. *Psychological Inquiry, 7,* 360–363.

Paulhus, D. L., & John, O. P. (1998). Egoistic and moralistic biases in self-perception: The interplay of self-deceptive styles with basic traits and motives. *Journal of Personality, 66,* 1025–1060.

Paunonen, S. V., Keinonen, M., Trzebinski, J., Forsterling, F., Grishenko-Roze, N., Kouznetsova, L., et al. (1996). The structure of personality in six cultures. *Journal of Cross-Cultural Psychology, 27,* 339–353.

Plomin, R., & Daniels, D. (1987). Why are children in the same family so different from one another? *Behavioral and Brain Sciences, 10,* 1–16.

Reiss, D., Neiderhiser, J. M., Hetherington, E. M., & Plomin, R. (2000). *The relationship code: Deciphering genetic and social influences on adolescent development.* Cambridge, MA: Harvard University Press.

Roberts, B. W., Caspi, A., & Moffitt, T. E. (2003). Work experiences and personality development in young adulthood. *Journal of Personality and Social Psychology, 84,* 582–593.

Roberts, B. W., & Helson, R. (1997). Changes in culture, changes in personality: The influence of individualism in a longitudinal study of women. *Journal of Personality and Social Psychology, 72,* 641–651.

Roberts, B. W., Helson, R., & Klohnen, E. C. (2002). Personality development and growth in women across 30 years: Three perspectives. *Journal of Personality, 70,* 79–102.

Roberts, B. W., Walton, K. E., & Viechtbauer, W. (2006). Patterns of mean-level change in personality traits across the life course: A meta-analysis of longitudinal studies. *Psychological Bulletin, 132,* 3–25.

Roberts, B. W., Wood, D., & Smith, J. L. (2005). Evaluating five-factor theory and social investment perspectives on personality trait development. *Journal of Research in Personality, 39,* 166–184.

Robins, R. W., & John, O. P. (1997). Effects of visual perspective and narcissism on self-perceptions: Is seeing believing? *Psychological Science, 8,* 37–42.

Rowe, D. C. (1994). *The limits of family influence: Genes, experience, and behavior.* New York: Guilford Press.

Rubin, Z. (1981). Does personality really change after 20? *Psychology Today, 15,* 18–27.

Saucier, G. (1997). Effects of variable selection on the factor structure of person descriptors. *Journal of Personality and Social Psychology, 73,* 1296–1312.

Saucier, G., & Goldberg, L. R. (1996). The language of personality: Lexical perspectives on the five-factor model. In J. S. Wiggins (Ed.), *The five-factor model of personality* (pp. 21–50). New York: Guilford Press.

Saucier, G., Hampson, S. E., & Goldberg, L. R. (2000). Cross-language studies of lexical personality factors. In S. E. Hampson (Ed.), *Advances in personality psychology* (Vol. 1, pp. 1–36). Philadelphia: Taylor & Francis.

Sheldon, K. M. (2004). *Optimal human being: An integrated multi-level perspective.* Mahwah, NJ: Erlbaum.

Sheldon, K. M., Ryan, R. M., Rawsthrone, L. J., & Ilardi, B. (1997). Trait self and true self: Cross-role variation in the Big-Five personality traits and its relations with psychological authenticity and subjective well-being. *Journal of Personality and Social Psychology, 73,* 1380–1393.

Siegler, I. C., Zonderman, A. B., Barefoot, J. C., Williams, R. B., Jr., Costa, P. T., Jr., & McCrae, R. R. (1990). Predicting personality in adulthood from college MMPI scores: Implications for follow-up studies in psychosomatic medicine. *Psychosomatic Medicine, 52,* 644–652.

Simon, H. A. (1957). *Models of man: Social and rational.* Oxford, UK: Wiley.

Simpson, C. (1983). *Emma: The life of Lady Hamilton.* London: Bodley Head.

Soldz, S., & Vaillant, G. E. (1999). The Big Five personality traits and the life course: A 45-year longitudinal study. *Journal of Research in Personality, 33,* 208–232.

Somer, O., & Goldberg, L. R. (1999). The structure of Turkish trait-descriptive adjectives. *Journal of Personality and Social Psychology, 76,* 431–450.

Southey, R. (1922). *Life of Nelson.* New York: Dutton. (Original work published 1813)

Srivastava, S., John, O. P., Gosling, S. D., & Potter, J. (2003). Development of personality in early and middle age: Set like plaster or persistent change? *Journal of Personality and Social Psychology, 84,* 1041–1053.

Sutin, A. R., & Costa, P. T., Jr. (2008). *Reciprocal influences of personality and job characteristics across middle adulthood.* Manuscript submitted for publication.

Terracciano, A., Costa, P. T., Jr., & McCrae, R. R. (2006). Personality plasticity after age 30. *Personality and Social Psychology Bulletin, 32,* 999–1009.

Terracciano, A., McCrae, R. R., Brant, L. J., & Costa, P. T., Jr. (2005). Hierarchical linear modeling analyses of NEO-PI-R scales in the Baltimore Longitudinal Study of Aging. *Psychology and Aging, 20,* 493–506.

Tooby, J., & Cosmides, L. (1990). On the universality of human nature and the uniqueness of the individual: The role of genetics and adaptation. *Journal of Personality, 58,* 17–68.

Tupes, E. C., & Christal, R. E. (1992). Recurrent personality factors based on trait ratings. *Journal of Personality, 60,* 225–251. (Original work published 1961)

Twenge, J. M. (2001). Birth cohort changes in extraversion: A cross-temporal meta-analysis, 1966–1993. *Personality and Individual Differences, 30,* 735–748.

Watson, D., & Clark, L. A. (1997). Extraversion and its positive emotional core. In R. Hogan, J. A. Johnson, & S. R. Briggs (Eds.), *Handbook of personality psychology* (pp. 767–793). New York: Academic Press.

Watson, D., & Humrichouse, J. (2006). Personality development in emerging adulthood: Integrating evidence from self-ratings and spouse ratings. *Journal of Personality and Social Psychology, 91,* 959–974.

Widiger, T. A., Costa, P. T., Jr., & McCrae, R. R. (2002). A proposal for Axis II: Diagnosing personality disorders using the five-factor model. In P. T. Costa & T. A. Widiger (Eds.), *Personality disorders and the five-factor model of personality* (2nd ed., pp. 431–456). Washington, DC: American Psychological Association.

Wiggins, J. S. (Ed.). (1996). *The five-factor model of personality.* New York: Guilford Press.

Wiggins, J. S. (1997). In defense of traits. In R. Hogan, J. A. Johnson, & S. R. Briggs (Eds.), *Handbook of personality psychology* (pp. 97–115). San Diego, CA: Academic Press. (Original work presented 1973)

Wiggins, J. S., & Trapnell, P. D. (1996). A dyadic interactional perspective on the five-factor model. In J. S. Wiggins (Ed.), *The five-factor model of personality* (pp. 88–162). New York: Guilford Press.

Yamagata, S., Suzuki, A., Ando, J., Ono, Y., Kijima, N., Yoshimura, K., et al. (2006). Is the genetic structure of human personality universal? A cross-cultural twin study from North America, Europe, and Asia. *Journal of Personality and Social Psychology, 90,* 987–998.

Yang, J., McCrae, R. R., & Costa, P. T., Jr. (1998). Adult age differences in personality traits in the United States and the People's Republic of China. *Journal of Gerontology: Psychological Sciences, 53B,* P375–P383.

CHAPTER 6

When Is Personality Revealed?

A Motivated Cognition Approach

E. Tory Higgins
Abigail A. Scholer

What defines who someone *really* is? When is personality revealed? Many of us have an intuitive sense that some behaviors and situations unmask aspects of our underlying personality more than others. How high we sing, how far we jump, or how fast we walk are typically not accepted as evidence of our personality. On the other hand, individuals' ability to resist eating a tempting marshmallow (Mischel & Ebbesen, 1970), their responses to failure (Dweck, 1999) or rejection (Downey & Feldman, 1996), and their interpretation of splotches of ink (Exner, 1993; Rorschach, 1921/1951) or ambiguous pictures (Murray, 1938) have been accepted as revealing of personality.

This question of who someone *really* is, of course, essentially characterizes the debate about how best to define personality. This is no easy task, as others have noted (e.g., Allport & Vernon, 1930; Pervin, 1990). And while in the past some have argued that "it is in individual differences that we find the logical key to personality" (Guilford, 1959, p. 5) or even that "all individual differences in the behavioral realm may be regarded as the subject matter of personality research" (Jensen, 1958, p. 302), it is clear that some

individual differences are considered personality and others, such as walking speed, are not. So what is it that differentiates walking speed from the ability to resist a tempting marshmallow?

Exploring the nature of this difference, we argue, elucidates the conditions that must be present in order for personality to be revealed. It is true that there must be individual differences within a species to even consider that personality might exist. If we don't detect individual differences in how earthworms approach the task of living, we are unlikely to say that different earthworms have different personalities. But imagine that some earthworms burrow through soil quickly whereas others tunnel at a slow and jerky pace. Would those individual differences constitute personality? Or would those individual differences alone not be enough?

We believe that all variability is not created equal; it is simply *not* enough to have just individual differences. Individual differences are a necessary but not sufficient condition. Even among humans, for whom the contention that individual differences exist is not controversial, one can question whether personality is revealed through individual differences such as hair color and musical ability or through individual differences such as conscientiousness and sensitivity to rejection. And regardless of whether one attributes the source of variability to global dispositions or to complex interactions of cognitive–affective processing units (e.g., Mischel & Shoda, 1995), variability is only a *prerequisite* for personality.

The individual differences that reveal *personality*, we argue, are those that reflect *motivated* preferences and biases (cf. H. Grant & Dweck, 1999). More precisely, we suggest that *personality is revealed through motivated preferences and biases in the ways that people see the world and cope in the world*. The notion that motivation is key to personality is not new; many theories of personality have given a primary role to the motivations, intentions, and goals of an individual, from early psychodynamic theories (e.g., S. Freud, 1914/1955) to more recent social-cognitive approaches (e.g., Bandura, 1986; Cantor & Kihlstrom, 1987; Dweck & Leggett, 1988; Higgins, 1997; Mischel & Shoda, 1995; Molden & Dweck, 2006). Indeed, Gordon Allport (1937), in his classic book on personality, defined personality traits not in terms of a tendency to behave the same way across situations but, rather, as an individual characteristic that "renders many stimuli functionally equivalent" (p. 295) and, given this rendering, initiates and guides equivalent responses to these stimuli. The former feature relates to biases and preferences in the ways that an individual sees the world, and the latter feature relates to preferences and biases in the ways that an individual copes in the world. As we discuss later, an individual bias in the chronic accessibility of a specific construct can create functional equivalence across vague and ambiguous stimuli (i.e., high accessibility will produce an equivalent stimulus identification), and an individual preference for a specific strategic response to a particular type of demanding situation can create equivalent responses to this type of situation. Building on such past approaches and perspectives on personality, we place motivated cognition at the center of understanding personality.

These motivations may consciously or unconsciously determine preferences and biases as revealed in response choices, yet they can only emerge when there is a range of possible responses over which an individual has some control (including nonconscious control). In other words, motivated preferences and biases (and thus personality) can be inferred only when we know that an individual *could have responded in a different way*. Thus, personality is not just any individual difference. Personality is about individual differences that reflect the preferences and biases of an underlying motivational system. Along any dimension or within any dynamic that we would call personality, individuals have motivated preferences and biases for what they see or believe, what they want to have, how they want to get these desired states of being, and how they want to deal with failures to get them.

Although we highlight a motivated cognition perspective, our approach grows out of a broader social-cognitive framework of conceptualizing personality. A defining characteristic of social-cognitive theories of personality is that they take a person-in-context approach to understanding the individual (Bandura, 1986; Cantor & Kihlstrom, 1987; Dweck & Leggett, 1988; Higgins, 1997; Kelly, 1955; Mischel & Shoda, 1995; see also Caprara & Cervone, 2000). Personality is seen to emerge from interactions among cognitive and affective processes enacted in the social world (Cervone & Shoda, 1999). These interactions underscore the importance of jointly considering the content, organization, and structure of an individual's goals, strategies, and mental representations that include expectancies and beliefs (Bandura, 1986; Cantor & Kihlstrom, 1987; Dweck & Leggett, 1988; Higgins, 1997; Kelly, 1955; Mischel & Shoda, 1995). A critical factor in how these interactions play out in a given context is how an individual interprets the situation—"idiosyncratic histories produce idiosyncratic stimulus meanings" (Mischel, 1973, p. 259; see also Kelly, 1955). And differences in interpretations (i.e., psychological situations) will vary according to motivated preferences and biases that arise from either chronic or temporary sources (Higgins, 1990, 1996).

We suggested earlier that these motivated preferences and biases are revealed in both individuals' "ways of seeing" and "ways of coping" in the world—two different kinds of *sensitivities* that can define personality. We further suggest that there are particular situations that are most likely to reveal these ways of seeing and ways of coping. On the one hand, low-demand situations, where input is minimal or ambiguous, provide opportunities to observe how individuals' perceptions, judgments, and evaluations are shaped by their ways-of-seeing sensitivities (e.g., their chronically accessible constructs). On the other hand, high-demand situations, where individuals' self-regulatory systems are taxed or stressed, provide opportunities to observe how their handling of personal problems and pressures are shaped by their ways-of-coping sensitivities (see also Caspi & Moffitt, 1993; Wright & Mischel 1987). Thus, our chapter considers the special role of low- and high-demand situations while we explore *ways of seeing* and *ways of coping* as windows into understanding personality from a motivated cognition perspective.

WAYS OF SEEING

In the 1940s, when the "New Look" in perception emerged, the notion that differences in ways of seeing could reveal personality gained credence. Expectancies, needs, and beliefs influence perception (Bruner, 1957a, 1957b); knowledge structures derived from past experiences affect the perception of objects, events, and other individuals in the world (e.g., Bartlett, 1932; Bruner, 1957a, 1957b; Hebb, 1949; Kelly, 1955; Wertheimer, 1923). Furthermore, the way in which an individual "sees" an object, event, or person determines its significance, thereby affecting evaluations, preferences, and decisions regarding that stimulus. As envisioned in Kelly's (1955) personal constructs theory, individuals scan the perceptual field to "pick up blips of meaning" (p. 145) that relate to individuals' chronically accessible constructs (see Higgins, King, & Mavin, 1982; Robinson, 2004).

Indeed, some of the earliest research in personality took advantage of differences in ways of seeing to explore differences in personality (McClelland & Atkinson, 1948; McClelland, Atkinson, Clark, & Lowell, 1953; Murray, 1938). Although the terminology differed from what we use here, early work by McClelland and Atkinson (e.g., McClelland & Atkinson, 1948; McClelland et al., 1953) emphasized that differences in percep-

tion were driven by differences in an individual's highly accessible constructs, including motives. Projective tests of personality such as the Thematic Apperception Test (Murray, 1938) or the Rorschach inkblot test (Exner, 1993; Rorschach, 1921/1951) rely on the assumption that the meaning an individual imposes on ambiguous or vague stimuli reveals highly accessible motives (see Sorrentino & Higgins, 1986). Although much of the initial work was focused on chronically accessible motives, even early work demonstrated that motives could become temporarily accessible through the priming of a motivational construct such as achievement (McClelland et al., 1953) or affiliation (Atkinson, Heyns, & Veroff, 1954). As such, it is not surprising that individual differences in construct accessibility play a critical role in many social-cognitive theories of personality (e.g., Higgins, 1990, 1997; Mischel & Shoda, 1995).

The idea that differences in ways of seeing the world reflect differences in personality was also the core assumption in the cognitive styles approach to personality, which is a precursor to many social-cognitive theories of personality (Kagan & Kogan, 1970; for a review, see Cantor & Kihlstrom, 1987). Perhaps best known is the distinction between field-dependent versus field-independent individuals, or the extent to which individuals rely on either the context or the self as a reference point for judgments (Witkin, Dyk, Faterson, Goodenough, & Karp, 1962). Differences in reliance on the self versus the context for physical perception (e.g., the rod and frame test) were believed to reflect global perceptual styles that would also be observed in processes of social perception. In certain situations, cognitive styles such as field dependence did predict quite a number of behaviors in the social realm (Witkin & Goodenough, 1977). Interestingly, in terms of predicting the extent of reliance on the context in social situations, differences between these two cognitive styles tended to emerge primarily when situations were ambiguous. Field-dependent individuals were not more likely to seek information from others *in general* when making decisions, but were more likely to do so when there was *ambiguity* about the best possible decision (Witkin & Goodenough, 1977). These findings exemplify how personality differences in ways of seeing can be revealed especially in low-demand situations.

Low-Demand Situations

Although ways-of-seeing sensitivities can be revealed in almost any context, the evidence suggests that ambiguous or vague situations (i.e., low demand) afford particularly clear opportunities to observe biased motives. "To the degree that the situation is 'unstructured,' the subject will expect that virtually *any* response from him is equally likely to be equally appropriate ... and variance from individual differences will be the greatest" (Mischel, 1973, p. 276). Projective tests of personality thus take advantage not only of the supposition that an individual's motives will be reflected in what he or she sees, but also that this will be more clearly revealed when the stimuli are vague or ambiguous. There is greater potential for chronically accessible motives to influence behavior in such situations, given that the expression of people's motives, particularly for preferred outcomes, is bounded by reality constraints (Kruglanski, 1996; Kunda, 1990; see also Dunning, Meyerowitz, & Holtzberg, 1989).

These unstructured situations may take various forms. Following distinctions in the knowledge accessibility literature (Higgins, 1996), we describe low-demand situations as those that are either vague or ambiguous. Vague situations are those in which no particular response or behavior has objectively high applicability. Ambiguous situations, on the other hand, are those in which at least two alternative responses or behaviors have high applicability and are equally possible. These alternatives may arise either because both interpretations of a particular behavior are plausible, given the situation as a whole (e.g., your boss's behavior suggests either confidence or arrogance), or because different aspects of the situation, over time, suggest different interpretations (e.g., some of your boss's behaviors suggest confidence whereas other behaviors suggest arrogance).

Antecedents of Motivated Biases and Preferences in Ways of Seeing

Low-demand situations, because they provide relatively few reality constraints, may more clearly reveal an individual's ways of seeing. These ways of seeing, however, may arise from either person-related or situational factors and may reflect differences in the availability, accessibility, or judged usability of knowledge (Higgins, 1990, 1996, 1999a). In this section, we explore the implications of taking a "general principles" approach to personality and what it means for understanding ways of seeing.

The general principles perspective on personality proposes that "person" and "situation" variables are simply different sources of the same general underlying principles or mechanisms (Higgins, 1990, 1999a). Rather than distinguishing between person-related explanatory principles and situational explanatory principles, this approach argues that the same psychological principles underlie both person and situation explanations. In contrast, the personality "traits" perspective on personality has typically removed the influence of situations in order to study personality (see Epstein, 1979; John, 1990). Whereas the "interactionist" perspectives (see Endler, 1982; Magnusson, 1990; Magnusson & Endler, 1977) do not remove situational influences, they have tended to examine person and situation variables as distinct sources that reciprocally determine one another (Magnusson, 1990). More recent developments in the interactionist approach incorporate situational variability as a part of personality rather than separate from it, relating personality to individual differences in psychological processes rather than to differences in traits (Mischel & Shoda, 1995). Nonetheless, even the social-cognitive learning approach retains the distinction between person-related and situational sources of variability.

Though we generally embrace the social-cognitive learning emphasis on underlying psychological processes, we advocate for *one set* of general principles for which *both* person and situation are different sources of variability. As argued elsewhere (e.g., Higgins, 1999a), doing so not only provides a common language for personality and social psychologists but also offers a richer understanding of how a given principle plays out in a number of conditions. By taking a general principles perspective on personality, we thus entertain evidence from both person and situation sources of variability in understanding the nature of personality.

Principles Underlying Biased Ways of Seeing

As an illustration of the general principles perspective, the synapse model of knowledge activation and use outlines how chronic individual differences in construct accessibility function in the same way as temporary individual differences in construct accessibility from situational priming (Bargh, Lombardi, & Higgins, 1988; Higgins, 1996; Higgins, Bargh, & Lombardi, 1985). Temporary sources of accessibility include momentary contextual priming, situationally induced expectancies, and goals related to the immediate tasks or interaction at hand. Chronic sources include chronic contextual activation (e.g., institutionalized situations) and long-term expectancies, beliefs, standards, and goals (Higgins, 1989, 1990). Chronic and temporary sources of accessibility combine additively to increase the excitation level, but these different sources are not distinguishable experientially from each other (Higgins, 1989). In other words, people do not know the extent to which the activated subjective meanings they apply to objects, situations, and other individuals arise from the momentary context; their past experiences, expectancies, and goals; or features of the stimulus. In short, they don't know what the accessibility is "about" (Higgins, 1998). Rather, the chronic and temporary sources of a construct's accessibility, as well as its applicability to a stimulus, combine to produce knowledge activation that is simply experienced as an outcome (for similar effects, see Nisbett & Wilson, 1977; Schachter & Singer, 1962; Zillman, 1978).

The synapse model of knowledge activation and use also distinguishes accessibility from two other principles of knowledge activation: the availability of knowledge and the judged usability of knowledge (Higgins, 1996). "Availability" refers to whether or not knowledge is actually present in memory. Availability is a necessary condition for accessibility; if knowledge is not available, it has zero accessibility (Higgins & King, 1981). Once knowledge is available, it can be distinguished in terms of its "accessibility," or the activation potential of available knowledge (Higgins, 1996). We define accessibility as the potential for knowledge activation rather than the potential for knowledge use. Though knowledge might be accessible,

it may not be used. For instance, if an individual is aware that activated knowledge is inappropriate or irrelevant to the task at hand, he or she may try to minimize or correct its impact on his or her behavior (see Higgins, 1996; Martin, 1986). Thus, it is useful to distinguish between the activation of knowledge and its actual use.

Two critical factors influence the probability that some stored knowledge will be activated: (1) the accessibility of the knowledge prior to the presentation of some stimulus; and (2) the applicability of the knowledge; that is, the overlap of features between the individual's stored knowledge and the stimulus (Bruner, 1957b). As accessibility and applicability increase, the chances that the knowledge will be activated also increase (Higgins, 1996). Conversely, as applicability decreases, accessibility must be greater in order for knowledge activation to occur. For instance, Higgins and Brendl (1995) found that even when a description of a target was extremely vague, perceivers for whom the construct "conceited" was highly accessible (high chronic accessibility plus priming of the construct "conceited") were likely to have spontaneous conceited-related impressions of the target.

Even if the activated knowledge is applicable to the stimulus, it may not be judged relevant or appropriate, as noted earlier. "Judged usability" of knowledge is the judged appropriateness or relevance of applying that knowledge to a particular stimulus or situation (Higgins, 1996). Perceivers may not use information if they judge it to be irrelevant or inappropriate (Higgins & Bargh, 1987). If perceivers are aware that information is activated and feel that it is not appropriate or relevant, they may try to suppress its use in their judgments, and this suppression can lead to contrast rather than assimilation effects (Martin, 1986). Importantly, the judged usability of knowledge may itself be influenced by motivational factors. For example, whereas the fact that a job candidate graduated from the same high school as the employer is not actually relevant to a hiring decision, the increased motivation to hire this individual with a common social identity—a positive outcome—may lead an employer to construct a reason to make it relevant. What information is deemed appropriate or relevant to use depends on a person's mental model of the appropriateness and relevance of information use under different conditions, and mental models themselves can reflect motivated preferences and biases. Thus, motivations can influence both the accessibility and the judged usability of knowledge.

Given that activation is likely to come from both chronic (person-related) and temporary (situational) sources, low-demand situations that contribute a minimal amount of excitation from either contextual priming or applicability may be particularly likely to produce judgment effects that reflect chronic accessibilities. When the stimuli are ambiguous and could be characterized by more than one construct, the construct that receives additional excitation from greater chronic accessibility will be more likely to be used if judged relevant. When the stimuli are vague, chronic accessibility of a construct may compensate for the low contribution of the situation to activation (e.g., Higgins & Brendl, 1995). Thus, both ambiguous and vague situations increase the potential to observe the contributions of chronically accessible constructs.

So far, we have outlined the idea that the chronic accessibility of underlying constructs will influence how an individual sees the world, revealing motivated biases indicative of personality. A given individual's past experiences (e.g., socialization) can make different types of knowledge more chronically accessible and thus influence how likely it is that a construct (e.g., "conceitedness") will be used by that individual to characterize the social world (see Higgins & Brendl, 1995). For instance, Robinson, Vargas, Tamir, and Solberg (2004) have found a relationship between the speed with which participants classify words as negative or neutral and the intensity of daily negative affect. In other words, the extent to which making negative evaluations has become habitual influences the ease with individuals can "see" negativity in the world. These types of influence involve differences in the accessibility of different kinds of knowledge content that can be used to make judgments and decisions.

Personality differences in underlying goals and self-regulatory concerns can also influence ways of seeing by influencing preferences for particular outcomes and/or strategies when forming judgments and making decisions (for a review, see Molden & Higgins, 2005). Motivations to achieve particular outcomes influence information processing (e.g., how people search for, evaluate, and organize information) to make it more likely that individuals will reach their desired outcomes. Even if individuals are not biased toward a specific kind of outcome, preferences for the use of a particular strategy may influence what kind of information is deemed important and relevant, profoundly impacting judgments and behavior.

Consequences of Motivated Biases and Preferences in Ways of Seeing

The previous section described three types of principles that can produce motivated biases and preferences in ways of seeing: (1) principles of knowledge activation and use; (2) principles of preferences for outcomes that could be produced by making particular judgments and decisions; and (3) principles of preferences for using specific strategies in the process of forming judgments and decisions. This section reviews evidence of the consequences for individuals' decisions and social lives of these motivated biases and preferences in ways of seeing.

Consequences of Knowledge Activation and Use on Ways of Seeing

Differences in chronic accessibility influence social perception and social behavior (e.g., Bargh & Pratto, 1986; Bargh & Thein, 1985; Higgins et al., 1982; King & Sorrentino, 1988; Lau, 1989; Strauman & Higgins, 1987). When encountering ambiguous or vague social information, which is common when encountering new people, an individual's chronic accessibilities may be especially likely to affect how an individual perceives and responds to others. Given the primary role of social relationships to healthy human functioning (Baumeister & Leary, 1995; Fiske, 2003), such mechanisms are an essential part of understanding personality. Chronically accessible constructs shape social interaction by affecting how individuals judge and remember others. In one study, for instance, participants' chronically accessible constructs were measured by asking them to list the traits of the type of person they liked, disliked, sought out, avoided, and frequently encountered, and then identifying which traits were listed first in response to these questions (Higgins et al., 1982). About a week later, participants read an essay containing descriptions of a target person that related to either their own chronically accessible constructs or others' chronically accessible constructs (i.e., a yoked design). The information that was related to the participants' own chronically accessible constructs was reflected more in their subsequent impressions and memory of the target.

The work of Andersen and her colleagues on the accessibility of significant-other representations (see Andersen & Chen, 2002) provides a striking example of how chronically accessible constructs can shape behavior in interpersonal contexts. The relational-self model is grounded in the principles of knowledge accessibility (Higgins, 1996). It proposes that individuals have multiple selves that are experienced in relationship with significant others, and which can be situationally activated (Chen, Andersen, & Hinkley, 1999). Representations of significant others include not only representations of their characteristics and motives, but also the habitual ways of being with them (Andersen & Chen, 2002; Andersen, Reznik, & Chen, 1997; Hinkley & Andersen, 1996). The relational-self model is concerned with how *specific* representations of significant others, rather than general relational schemas, affect cognition and behavior. Consequently, the typical paradigm used to explore these effects involves an idiographic approach (see Andersen & Chen, 2002; Andersen & Saribay, 2005). Participants first provide an idiosyncratic description of a significant other before the experiment. After some delay, the effects of the accessibility of this significant-other information are assessed, such as the effects on impressions or recall of a fictional person who happens to resemble the significant other in some way.

These studies suggest that individuals are ready to use accessible significant-other representations to make sense of new individuals and social interactions (Andersen, Reznik, & Glassman, 2005, p. 432). Participants report greater confidence that they saw information—information that was *not* actually presented—when it was related to characteristics of their significant other (Andersen & Cole, 1990; Andersen, Glassman, Chen, & Cole, 1995; Glassman & Andersen,

1999). They also express more positive affect when they engage in an interaction with a target who happens to share some similarities with a liked, rather than a disliked, significant other (Berk & Andersen, 2000). Participants are also more likely to behave with the "similar" target in the way they would with their significant other (Andersen & Baum, 1994; Hinkley & Andersen, 1996). Even when the applicability of the target to the significant-other representation was minimal, the significant-other representation was used to derive meaning in new contexts, suggesting that such representations are highly accessible (Chen, Andersen, & Hinkley, 1999).

Activating *general* self–other representations can also affect an individual's ways of seeing. Baldwin and Holmes (1987), for example, asked participants to vividly imagine being with their parents or with two campus friends. Later they were asked to rate how much they enjoyed a number of written passages, including a critical passage that described a woman contemplating having sex with a man she did not know well. Participants rated the passage as more enjoyable and exciting after imagining being with their friends than their parents, presumably because activation of the "friend" relational schema was associated with more permissive standards than the "parent" relational schema.

Consequences of the Influence of Preferred Outcomes on Ways of Seeing

Two general classes of preferred outcomes have been studied: directional and nondirectional outcomes (Kruglanski, 1996; Kunda, 1990; Molden & Higgins, 2005). Motivation for directional outcomes reflect desires to reach particular conclusions (e.g., "I am an intelligent and kind person"; "My spouse is generous and attractive"). Motivations for nondirectional outcomes are about more general concerns. "Need for closure," for example, is the desire for any answer as long as it is definite (Kruglanski & Webster, 1996). Need for closure tends to bias judgments and decisions toward attaining closure quickly and permanently—"seizing" and "freezing."

Need for closure is often contrasted with need for accuracy (Fiske & Neuberg, 1990). Individuals with high (versus low) accuracy motivation consider detailed individuating information about a target (Kruglanski & Freund, 1983; Neuberg & Fiske, 1987), whereas people who have a high (versus low) need for closure rely instead on more categorical information during impression formation (Dijksterhuis, van Knippenberg, Kruglanski, & Schaper, 1996; Kruglanski & Freund, 1983; see also Moskowitz, 1993). Individuals high (versus low) in need for closure are more influenced by constructs made more accessible by priming, whereas those high in need for accuracy tend to be less influenced by primed constructs (Ford & Kruglanski, 1995; Thompson et al., 1994). The strength of correspondent inferences—that is, inferring that the cause of a person's "X" action is his or her "X" trait or attitude—also varies as a function of need for closure and need for accuracy. In a study by Tetlock (1985), for example, participants read an essay written by another participant who had been assigned by the experimenter to take a favorable or unfavorable position on affirmative action. Participants motivated to make accurate judgments took the experimenter's coercion into account and were less likely to make a correspondent inference. In contrast, Webster (1993) found that correspondent inferences were stronger for participants' high in need for closure.

Consequences of the Influence of Preferred Strategies on Ways of Seeing

Individuals not only differ in the outcomes that they prefer; they can also be motivated to prefer a particular *strategy* for reaching a decision, independent of any motivation to achieve a specific outcome (Higgins & Molden, 2003). Certain strategies may be more suitable—a better fit (Higgins, 2000b)—for a given motivational orientation. Such regulatory fit strengthens engagement in an activity, which in turn intensifies value experiences (Higgins, 2006).

To illustrate, consider the difference in strategic preferences between individuals who have a predominant promotion focus and individuals who have a predominant prevention focus. Regulatory focus theory posits the coexistence of two distinct motivational systems—the promotion system and the prevention system—that each serves fundamentally important but different survival needs (Higgins, 1997). Specifically, the promotion system is characterized by a sensitivity to the presence or absence of positive outcomes and concerns with ideals (hopes and aspirations), advancement, and accomplishment. Suitable to these concerns, promotion-focused individuals have been shown to prefer using eagerness-related means rather than vigilance-related means. In contrast, the prevention system is characterized by a sensitivity to the absence or presence of negative outcomes and concerns with "oughts" (duties and responsibilities), safety, and security. Suitable to these concerns, prevention-focused individuals have been shown to prefer using vigilance-related means rather than eagerness-related means (Crowe & Higgins, 1997; Higgins & Molden, 2003; Liberman, Molden, Idson, & Higgins, 2001).

Higgins, Roney, Crowe, and Hymes (1994) reasoned that if individuals with a promotion orientation have a stronger preference for using eager rather than vigilant means, they should be more sensitive to eager-related input than vigilant-related input, whereas the reverse should be true for individuals with a prevention orientation. Higgins and colleagues asked participants to report either on how their hopes and aspirations had changed over time (priming a promotion focus) or on how their sense of duty and obligation had changed over time (priming a prevention focus). They then read about the life of another student. In one set of episodes, the target used eager means to attain a goal, such as the target person waking up early to get to an exciting (of course!) psychology class that began at 8:30 A.M. In another set, the target used vigilant means to attain a goal, such as not registering for a Spanish class that was scheduled at the same time as a photography class the target person wanted to take. Promotion-focused participants showed better memory for the eager-related episodes than the vigilant-related episodes, whereas the opposite was true for prevention-focused participants.

Liberman and colleagues (2001) found that when participants were asked to identify vague stimulus objects depicted in photos, promotion-focused participants generated more alternatives for the identity of the objects than did those in a prevention focus (see also Crowe & Higgins, 1997). This was found both when regulatory focus was measured as a chronic individual difference and when focus was temporarily induced through priming. Participants in a promotion focus also generated more possible explanations for why a target person behaved in a helpful way, which in turned influenced their predictions about how the target would behave in the future. Specifically, because promotion participants had considered alternatives for the helpful behavior other than dispositional ones, they were less likely to endorse the idea that the helpful behavior would generalize in the future (Liberman et al., 2001).

Strategic preferences also influence how people evaluate their past decisions in life. Counterfactual thinking involves imagining what might have happened "if only" one had done things differently (Roese, 1997). Counterfactuals either take the form of reversing a previous inaction (e.g., "If only I *had done* X, then Y") or of reversing a previous action (e.g., "If only I *hadn't done* X, then Y"). Counterfactuals that reverse a previous inaction that missed an opportunity for a gain, known as additive counterfactuals, reflect an eager strategy of imagining moving from what was a "0" to a "+1" instead. In contrast, counterfactuals that reverse a previous action that produced a loss, known as subtractive counterfactuals, reflect a vigilant strategy of imagining moving from what was a "–1" to a "0" instead. Roese, Hur, and Pennington (1999) found that participants who considered promotion-related setbacks (their own or fictional examples) generated more additive counterfactuals, whereas participants who considered prevention-related setbacks generated more subtractive counterfactuals (see also Oishi, Schimmack, & Colcombe, 2003).

WAYS OF COPING

Whereas low-demand situations provide the clearest opportunities for revealing motivated preferences or biases in "ways of seeing," high-demand situations that tax or stress individuals provide the clearest opportunities for revealing the motivations and strategies underlying individual ways of coping (Cox & Ferguson, 1991; Wright & Mischel, 1987). Differences in coping have been identified as particularly important in explaining vari-

ability in how people function under stress (Folkman & Moskowitz, 2004). The coping literature suggests that it is differences in the ways people cope with stressful situations, rather than the nature of the stress itself, that is the best predictor of psychological and physical outcomes (see Zeidner & Endler, 1996). Individuals often have preferred coping strategies that they use to deal with stress (e.g., Carver, Scheier, & Weintraub, 1989; Endler & Parker, 1990; S. M. Miller, 1980; S. M. Miller & Mangan, 1983), suggesting that ways of coping can provide a meaningful insight into personality.

Early psychoanalytic approaches emphasized the importance of exploring differences in ways of coping in order to understand personality, with special emphasis on the defenses that individuals use to deal with conflict and frustration (Breuer & Freud, 1893/1956). When unwanted or disturbing thoughts become conscious, an individual had to find some way to cope, particularly because such thoughts and impulses could not be gratified acceptably. Following on Sigmund Freud's pioneer work (S. Freud, 1914/1955), Anna Freud advanced psychoanalytic ideas about the core defense mechanisms (A. Freud, 1936/1946). In addition to identifying several new defense mechanisms, she observed that individuals differ in their preferences for using some defense mechanisms more than others. Moreover, she argued that some coping defenses were more adaptive than others, and that particular defense "styles" could be associated with particular pathologies. Though current conceptions tend to identify coping in terms of strategies rather than defenses, many of these core ideas remain (e.g., Cantor & Kihlstrom, 1987).

There is increased attention to the importance of understanding self-control and self-regulatory mechanisms in human functioning (Baumeister, Schmeichel, & Vohs, 2007). In large part, coping is about self-regulation, "the self altering its own responses or inner states" (Baumeister et al., p. 5). Self-regulation has received substantial attention as a topic not because we excel at it, but because we so often fail. People sometimes lack the skills for successful regulation (H. N. Mischel & W. Mischel, 1983; Salovey, Hsee, & Mayer, 1993), lack a sense of efficacy that they can achieve their goals (Bandura, 1977, 1997), believe it's not possible (Martijn, Tenbult, Merckelbach, Dreezens, & de Vries, 2002), or are insufficiently motivated by the current goal or manner of goal pursuit (e.g., Higgins, 2000b). To understand failures of self-regulation, we must consider when they are most likely to occur and how they occur (i.e., the underlying processes).

Differences in coping strategies and abilities to self-regulate emerge most clearly when individuals are placed in stressful situations. The competency-demand hypothesis (Wright & Mischel, 1987) contends that psychologically demanding situations reveal certain aspects of an individual's characteristics with particular clarity (see also Caspi & Moffitt, 1993). Wright and Mischel (1987) provide an apt metaphor: "An attribution of brittleness is not a summary statement about a generalized tendency to shatter or break; rather, it expresses a set of subjunctive if–then propositions about how the object would respond to certain situations (e.g., cracking or shattering when physically stressed)" (p. 1161). For example, the difference between repressors (who prefer avoidant strategies such as denial) and sensitizers (who prefer approach strategies such as rumination) in attending to information about their personal liabilities is greatest following failure and least following success (Mischel, Ebbesen, & Zeiss, 1973). Though individuals with Type A personalities are not more hostile than individuals with Type B personalities, in general, they are more hostile following frustration (Strube, Turner, Cerro, Stephens, & Hinchey, 1984). In other words, differences in strategic coping observed in high-demand situations reveal motivated biases in personality. In order to explore how ways of coping reveal personality, we identify here only a handful of high-demand situations, with special attention to those studied by social-cognitive researchers. These situations include dealing with (1) failure or anticipated failure, (2) interpersonal rejection, and (3) conditions that tax self-regulatory capacity (e.g., delay of gratification or resisting temptation).

Ways of Coping with Failure

In this section we consider differences in individuals' behavioral, cognitive, and emotional responses to failure as differences in ways of coping. Before beginning our review, we need to state two caveats. Our first caveat is that we are treating emotions in this section as ways of coping in the world. However, emotions can also be considered as ways of seeing the world. Different emotions reflect different psychological situations or different meanings assigned to events in the world, such as the psychological situation of sadness being the absence of positive outcomes (see Higgins, 1987; Roseman, 1984). Indeed, it has been argued that cognitive appraisals are always involved in emotions (e.g., Lazarus, 1982). There are also chronic motivated preferences and biases in emotional appraisal. Shah and Higgins (2001), for example, found that individuals with stronger promotion concerns were faster in appraising how cheerful or dejected everyday objects made them feel, whereas individuals with stronger prevention concerns were faster in appraising how quiescent or agitated the same objects made them feel. In sum, we agree that emotions reflect both ways of seeing and ways of coping with the world. To avoid redundancy and save space, however, we have chosen to emphasize the coping nature of emotions in this chapter.

Our second caveat is that our discussion of ways of coping in this section emphasizes coping with failure and problems. This emphasis is consistent with the emphasis in the literature on coping and defense mechanisms—it concerns dealing with failure and how to respond when things are going wrong. However, people do manage and control success as well, and there are individual differences in preferences and biases for how to respond when things are going well. Again, because of space constraints, as well as the fact that most of the literature has examined how people deal with problems, this section emphasizes ways of coping with failure.

Individual Differences in Implicit Theories

As mentioned earlier with respect to judged usability, individuals' mental models or implicit theories about the world can create biases and preferences. These implicit theories can be conceptualized as meaning systems that contain core assumptions about the self that shape individuals' goals, beliefs, and motivations (Molden & Dweck, 2006). In particular, Dweck and her colleagues have studied two different implicit theories that individuals hold about the nature of intelligence (e.g., Dweck, 1999): the *entity* view that intelligence is fixed and stable, and the *incremental* view that intelligence is malleable and can change through effort over time. These different theories can be held chronically or induced experimentally (e.g., Dweck, Chiu, & Hong, 1995). Whereas holding an incremental theory is associated with having learning goals (i.e., goals about developing one's intelligence), holding an entity theory is associated with having performance goals (i.e., goals about validating one's intelligence). Incremental theorists tend to have more positive beliefs about effort and to display "mastery-oriented" strategies when they face failure, in contrast to the "helpless-oriented" strategies exhibited by entity theorists (Dweck, 1999).

A field study by Blackwell, Trzesniewski, and Dweck, described in Molden and Dweck (2006), explored how the effects of these implicit theories are especially likely to emerge in challenging situations that increase the threat of failure. Students were followed across the transition to junior high school. This life transition was selected because students are more likely to encounter greater challenges (and potential failures) in junior high courses than they had in elementary school. At the beginning of seventh grade, there was no difference in math achievement between students who held an entity versus incremental view of intelligence. However, subsequently the math grades of incremental theorists steadily increased whereas those of entity theorists decreased. Furthermore, path analyses showed that incremental theories had this effect on math grades through the adoption of positive beliefs about effort and mastery-oriented strategies (Blackwell et al., 2005; see also Dweck & Sorich, 1999; Henderson & Dweck, 1990). A study by Nussbaum and Dweck, described in Molden and Dweck (2006), found that, following failure, participants who had been induced to adopt an entity theory wanted to see the work of others who had done very poorly on the task, supposedly to protect their self-esteem (see Tesser, 2000), whereas incremental theorists wanted to see the work of those who had done better on the task, supposed-ly to learn more effective strategies. Recent work examining differences in attention deployment in learning tasks also found that, following a challenging task, incremental theorists orient more to learning feedback than do entity theorists (Dweck, Mangels, & Good, 2004).

Individual Differences in Self-Efficacy Beliefs

An individual's sense of personal efficacy—the belief that he or she can produce desired results by his or her actions—is also critical for understanding responses to potential failures and challenges (Bandura, 1977, 1997; Cervone, 2000; Cervone & Scott, 1995). Self-efficacy beliefs can arise from a number of different sources. Bandura (1997, 1999), for example, discusses four potential sources of self-efficacy: (1) experiences of overcoming obstacles oneself, (2) experiences of observing others overcome obstacles, (3) social situations that increase the likelihood of success, and (4) physical or emotional states that signal high (e.g., feeling energetic) or low (e.g., feeling exhausted) self-efficacy. Individual differences arise not only in whether a given individual has high or low self-efficacy, but also in how an individual integrates information about self-efficacy from different sources (see Bandura, 1999). As discussed earlier in the section on knowledge accessibility principles, underlying motivations influence perceived self-efficacy in how individuals attend to these different sources and in how different sources are judged applicable and/or relevant.

Although self-efficacy beliefs can be influenced by both chronic and temporary factors, most empirical approaches define self-efficacy in relation to particular contexts. Individuals may have high perceived self-efficacy in some domains but low perceived self-efficacy in others (Bandura, 1977; Cervone, 1997, 2000; Cervone, Shadel, & Jencius, 2001; Cervone & Williams, 1992). For instance, Artistico, Cervone, and Pezzuti (2003) found that older adults had higher self-efficacy (and performed better) on problems that were more ecologically relevant to the challenges they confronted in their daily lives (e.g., for grandparents dealing with grown-up sons, "dealing with excessive demands by one's sons to baby-sit their children"), whereas younger adults had higher self-efficacy (and performed better) on problems more relevant to their lives (e.g., "coping with loss of motivation to finish a degree").

Not surprisingly, differences between individuals with high and low self-efficacy often emerge in high-demand situations. Degree of self-efficacy predicts how much effort people will invest in a goal and how long they'll persist in attempting to attain it, particularly when challenges arise (Bandura, 1977; Bandura & Cervone, 1983, 1986; Cervone & Peake, 1986; Peake & Cervone, 1989; Schunk, 1981; Stock & Cervone, 1990). Individuals with low self-efficacy tend to see more risks, ruminate about dangers and their own inadequacies, and have greater anxiety when facing stressful situations (Sanderson, Rapee, & Barlow, 1989). Those with high self-efficacy are able to transform stressful situations into ones that are more controllable (Williams, 1992). Research has shown that efficacy beliefs about resisting peer pressure in a time of heightened demand and potential failure—the period of adolescence—predict academic achievement and decreases in antisocial conduct among adolescents. A 2-year longitudinal study (Caprara, Barbaranelli, Pastorelli, & Cervone, 2004; see also Caprara, Regalia, & Bandura, 2002) found that students who had high self-efficacy in the domain of peer pressure had better grades, less problem behavior, and were more popular among peers over time. Furthermore, efficacy beliefs predicted outcomes above and beyond ratings of the Big Five dimensions (see, e.g., McCrae & Costa, 1999).

Defensive Pessimism

Research on defensive pessimism also highlights individual differences in coping with the *potential* for failure. Cantor and colleagues (Norem & Cantor, 1986a, 1986b; Showers, 1992) identified different strategies that people use to cope with task pursuit when the possibility of failure exists. This work highlights not just differences in *how* people cope, but also *when* people cope. Work on defensive pessimism suggests that some individuals actually have better outcomes when they adopt a negative, rather than positive, outlook for anticipated events (Norem & Cantor, 1986a, 1986b; Showers, 1992). Defensive pessimists "expect the worst" when

entering a new situation, despite the fact that they generally don't perform differently than those with a more optimistic outlook (Cantor & Norem, 1989; Cantor, Norem, Niedenthal, Langston, & Brower, 1987). Defensive pessimism serves two goals: (1) a self-protective goal of preparation for possible failure in the future and (2) a motivational goal of increasing effort in the present to prevent negative possibilities. In support of this idea, Norem and Cantor (1986b) found that when the strategic coping mechanisms of defensive pessimists' were disrupted, they performed more poorly. It appeared that simply pointing out the inconsistency between their current expectations and past performance disrupted their ability to harness vigilance in their preferred way.

In another research program, Showers (1992) demonstrated that it is not only anticipated performance failure but more general anticipation of negative outcomes that appears to be important to defensive pessimists' strategic response to an upcoming task. For these studies, participants were selected based on chronic defensive pessimism or optimism scores in social situations. When participants arrived for the study, they were told that they would be having a "get acquainted" conversation with another participant—a social situation that has the potential to go badly. Prior to the conversation, some participants filled out a questionnaire that highlighted the possibilities for positive outcomes in the upcoming discussion, and other participants filled out a questionnaire highlighting negative outcome possibilities. Showers found that defensive pessimists in the "negative possibilities" condition exhibited more positive behaviors during the social interaction than did defensive pessimists in the "positive possibilities" condition—they talked more, exerted more effort, and the conversations were rated more positively by the confederates with whom they were interacting. Another study found that defensive pessimists in the negative (versus positive) possibilities condition reported feeling more prepared for the interaction. It appears that the act of reflecting on possible negative outcomes is a critical component of the defensive pessimists' way of coping with possible failure. In contrast, such negative reflection can interfere with the performance of optimists (see Norem & Illingworth, 1993).

Discrepancies from Own and Others' Standards for Oneself

When failure occurs, the discrepancy from one's expected or desired behavior or performance may be judged against a number of different standards. Self-discrepancy theory (Higgins, 1987) posits two dimensions as being critical for such evaluations: *domains of the self* (ideal self, ought self) and *standpoints on the self* (own, other). Self-guides or standards are represented by the ideal or ought selves that involve either the own or other standpoint (i.e., ideal–own, ideal–other; ought–own, ought–other). The self-concept is represented by the actual self-state and can be discrepant from any of the four types of self-guides.

Self-discrepancy theory proposes that individuals are motivated to maintain matches between their self-concept and their self-guides because discrepancies between these two produce negative psychological states. The consequences of the discrepancy, however, differ depending on the self-guide involved. Regarding domains of the self, for instance, when an actual–ideal discrepancy is present, the actual state does not match the ideal state that the individual (or other) hopes for and aspires to. This *absence of a positive outcome* produces a vulnerability to dejection-related emotions, such as feeling sad or discouraged. In contrast, when an actual–ought discrepancy is present, the actual state does not match the state that the individual (or other) believes is a duty or obligation to fulfill. This *presence of a negative outcome* produces a vulnerability to agitation-related emotions, such as feeling nervous or worried. Indeed, studies have found that actual–ideal discrepancies predict suffering from dejection-related emotions, whereas actual–ought discrepancies predict suffering from agitation-related emotions (e.g., Higgins, Bond, Klein, & Strauman, 1986; Strauman & Higgins, 1988). In addition, factors that moderate these two distinct relations, such as self-guide accessibility and self-guide strength or importance, have been identified (e.g., Boldero & Francis, 2000; Higgins, 1999b; Higgins, Shah, & Friedman, 1997).

Strauman and Higgins (1987) tested the idea that even when individuals are unobtrusively primed with self-discrepancies in a neutral context, the activation of the mismatch will still have a significant impact. In a first session, discrepancy scores were calculated for each participant based on the Selves Questionnaire (Higgins et al., 1985), and participants were classified as predominant ideal discrepant (high-ideal discrepancy with low-ought discrepancy) or predominant ought discrepant (high-ought discrepancy with low-ideal discrepancy). When participants returned for an experimental session about a month later, they were unobtrusively primed with self-relevant attributes that were taken from each subject's self-guides (ideal or ought) or from another participant's self-guides (in a yoked design). For self-relevant primes, participants were exposed either to ideal-discrepant attributes, ought-discrepant attributes, or nondiscrepant attributes. Critically, the attributes were presented in a neutral context: Each trial consisted of having participants complete sentences that began "A _____ person ... " with a different attribute inserted for each incomplete sentence. A subset of the sentences contained the critical attributes. The study found that for predominant ideal-discrepant participants, dejection-related emotions and symptoms (motor retardation, decreased arousal) increased when they were primed with ideal-discrepant attributes. For predominant ought-self discrepant participants, agitation-related emotions and symptoms (motor agitation, heightened arousal) increased when participants were primed with ought-discrepant attributes. Thus, even when chronic self-discrepancies are made momentarily more accessible in an indirect way, they can produce emotional and behavioral consequences.

Reznick and Andersen (2003; cited in Andersen & Saribay, 2005) found that similar effects extend to the interpersonal realm. When participants expected to interact with a target individual who resembled a significant other who held a self-guide for them from which they were discrepant, their emotional reactions to the target could be predicted based on which type of discrepancy was involved (ideal vs. ought). Ideal discrepancies produced increased dejection, whereas ought discrepancies produced increased agitation. Furthermore, participants for whom the target resembled an ideal-discrepant significant other were still eager to interact with the target, perhaps as a way to address the discrepancy. In contrast, participants for whom the target resembled an ought-discrepant significant other were more likely to want to avoid the anticipated interaction.

Alexander and Higgins (1993) found that actual–ought versus actual–ideal discrepancies predicted the emotional responses of mothers after giving birth to their first child. In addition to the new responsibilities and many life changes that accompany the birth of a child, it is also an event that can shift experienced discrepancies. For women who had high actual–ought discrepancies prior to the birth of their child, agitation *decreased* from pre- to postpartum. However, for women who had high actual–ideal discrepancies prior to the birth, dejection *increased* from pre- to postpartum. These results suggest that for women high in actual–ought discrepancies, fulfilling the stereotypical role duties of being a mother and a "good wife" may reduce their previous actual–ought discrepancies, thereby reducing their anxiety. For women high in actual–ideal discrepancies, however, the period immediately following childbirth may be especially distressing because they have fewer resources to devote to the pursuit of their ideals (e.g., professional accomplishments), thereby accentuating ideal discrepancies (failures) that produce depression.

It is not only self-guide domains that matter. Self-guide *standpoints* also matter. Using the Selves Questionnaire, Moretti, Higgins, Woody, and Leung (1998) distinguished between individuals who were "own standpoint regulators" (high actual–own self-discrepancies) and individuals who were "other standpoint regulators" (high actual–other self-discrepancies). In a subsequent experimental session, participants believed they were being socially evaluated and were given social feedback on their personality. They received negative feedback that targeted a self-discrepancy (or yoked negative feedback that targeted a self-discrepancy of another participant). Affect was measured immediately after feedback and a day later. Moretti and colleagues predicted that although all participants would feel badly immediately after the negative social feedback, it would be the "other standpoint regulators" who would be most likely to continue to feel negatively a day later. Indeed, only the "other standpoint regulators" reported negative af-

fect a day later that was comparable to the levels reported immediately after feedback. The impact of negative social feedback was determined by both the self-relevance of the feedback and how sensitive participants were to the standpoint of another (see Moretti & Higgins, 1999, for a review of self-vs. other standpoints in self-regulation).

Ways of Coping with Rejection

One form of failure that has special psychological significance for people is the failure of a social relationship. Indeed, the need or desire for belonging is often considered to be one of the core social motives (Baumeister & Leary, 1995; Fiske, 2003). Classic psychodynamic models of personality highlight the importance of problems in early relationships with significant others for the development of strategic biases and preferences in adults' current relationships (e.g., Adler, 1954; Sullivan, 1953). More recent social-cognitive models of personality have also addressed how people cope with interpersonal rejection and the threat of rejection. A prime example is the rejection sensitivity model of Downey and her colleagues (e.g., Downey & Feldman, 1996; Downey, Freitas, Michaelis, & Khouri, 1998). The model posits that those high in rejection sensitivity anxiously expect rejection, readily perceive rejection, and tend to overreact with hostility to rejection, often leading to the very rejection they most want to avoid (a form of the self-fulfilling prophecy). A social-cognitive model, it focuses on how individuals process cognitive and affective information within specific interpersonal situations (Pietrzak, Downey, & Ayduk, 2005). Individuals high in rejection sensitivity exhibit strategic biases in the ways they interpret and cope with social situations in which rejection might occur.

Ayduk, Downey, Testa, Yen, and Shoda (1999) demonstrated that women high in rejection sensitivity show an automatic association between rejection and hostility. Following a rejection prime, high-rejection-sensitive women pronounced hostility-related words more quickly. Low-rejection-sensitive women did not show this readiness to identify hostility following the rejection prime. Furthermore, no difference was found between high-rejection-sensitive and low-rejection-sensitive women in the chronic accessibility of hostile thoughts, demonstrating that it was the "rejection–hostility" link, not simply the hostility construct itself, that was highly accessible for high-rejection-sensitive women. Evidence from a diary study (Ayduk et al., 1999) also provides support for the link between rejection and hostility for high-rejection-sensitive individuals. High-rejection-sensitive women were more hostile toward their partner on days following rejection, but this relation was not observed for low-rejection-sensitive women (see also Downey et al., 1998). Importantly, there was no difference in the probability of conflicts on days not following rejection for high- versus low-rejection-sensitive women (Ayduk et al., 1999). Reflecting activation of the defensive motivational system (see Lang, Bradley, & Cuthbert, 1998), high-rejection-sensitive individuals are highly motivated to detect threat-congruent cues when in a state of threat (Downey, Mougios, Ayduk, London, & Shoda, 2004), showing, for example, a higher startle response to rejection-themed art, but not to other images, than low-rejection-sensitive individuals.

There is also evidence that people high in rejection sensitivity may respond differently depending on whether they think that ultimate rejection is preventable or not. When rejection is perceived as possible but not irrevocable, people high in rejection sensitivity can take extreme measures to adapt the self to the relationship in an attempt to prevent rejection. Romero-Canyas and Downey (2005) found, for example, that males who were high in rejection sensitivity were willing to engage in ingratiating behaviors (doing menial tasks for a group) and move their attitudes toward a group if they received moderately cold rather than clearly rejecting e-mail messages. It is perhaps because high-rejection-sensitive individuals are willing to align their beliefs and goals with others if doing so will prevent rejection that rejection sensitivity is associated with an unstable sense of self (Ayduk, Mischel, & Downey, 2002; see also Purdie & Downey, 2000). Thus, depending on how a particular interpersonal context is interpreted, the motivation to prevent rejection can either produce behaviors that actually increase the likelihood of rejection (e.g., Downey et al., 1998) when rejection is seen as inevitable, or it can produce ingratiation (Romero & Downey, 2005) or

self-silencing behaviors (Purdie & Downey, 2000) that increase acceptance when rejection is seen as preventable.

Ways of Coping with Taxing Self-Regulatory Demands

Yet another window on personality that was highlighted in the classic psychodynamic perspective was differences in how people dealt with the conflict between their immediate wishes and desires (e.g., id impulses) and their beliefs about what they should do in the long run (e.g., ego plans and super-ego demands). This conflict has often been characterized in terms of people's strategies for delaying gratification or resisting temptation. Social-cognitive models have also been concerned with this issue. In particular, Mischel and his colleagues have an extensive research program examining the person and situation factors that influence the ability to delay gratification (see Mischel & Ayduk, 2004; Mischel, Cantor, & Feldman, 1996).

A now classic paradigm has been used by Mischel and colleagues to explore children's ability to delay gratification (e.g., Mischel & Baker, 1975; Mischel & Ebbesen, 1970; Moore, Mischel, & Zeiss, 1976). Children are presented with two potential rewards, a smaller reward available immediately (e.g., one marshmallow) and a larger, more desirable reward (e.g., two marshmallows) that they will receive if they can wait until the experimenter returns to the room after some delay. The children do not know how long they might have to wait for the larger reward, but they know that they can claim the smaller reward at any time if they ring a bell to summon the experimenter. For young children, this delay period is difficult and frustrating; when both rewards are present, children on average wait only about 3 minutes before summoning the experimenter (Mischel & Ebbeson, 1970). Research has shown (Mischel et al., 1996) that the ability to wait for the deferred reward depends both on self-regulatory motivation (involving expectancies and values) and self-regulatory competencies (involving the cognitive and attentional strategies used for coping). In particular, differences in the way in which attention is deployed and differences in the ways in which rewards are mentally represented appear to be crucially important in determining a child's ability to wait (e.g., Mischel & Baker, 1975; Moore et al., 1976).

It is the way in which the reward is mentally represented, rather the presence of the reward itself, that is critical for children's ability to delay reward. In particular, whether the children in these studies represented the reward in terms of its hot or cool properties (Metcalfe & Mischel, 1999) turns out to be one of the most critical factors in the ability to delay gratification. Children can wait longer under three conditions: (1) when exposed to a symbolically presented reward (picture) rather than the actual reward (Mischel & Moore, 1973), (2) when they themselves mentally transform actual rewards into mental pictures (Moore et al., 1976), or (3) when they focus on the reward's abstract and cool properties (e.g., thinking of marshmallows as "white, fluffy clouds") rather than the reward's consummatory and hot properties (e.g., thinking of marshmallows as "sweet and sticky") (Mischel & Baker, 1975). Some of the children who delay best are able to flexibly shift their attention between the hot and cool features, reducing frustration while maintaining the motivation to delay (Peake, Hebl, & Michel, 2002). Although young children are better able to delay when provided with such strategies, there are significant individual differences in their ability to delay rewards. Long-term follow-ups (Mischel, Shoda, & Peake, 1988; Shoda, Mischel, & Peake, 1990) show that seconds of preschool delay time predict Scholastic Aptitude Tests (SAT) scores, parental ratings of reasoning ability, planfulness, and self-control years later in high school (see also Mischel & Ayduk, 2004). In accordance with the hypothesis proposed here, it is behavior in the most demanding situation (reward present, no strategies provided) that is predictive of these long-term outcomes (for a review, see Mischel et al., 1996).

Beyond the mental transformations that can be used to increase control in difficult self-regulatory situations, the types of strategies that individuals use may also be more or less effective, given their fit with those individuals' motivational orientations. Freitas, Liberman, and Higgins (2002) examined participants' evaluations of a task that involved resisting tempting diversions from task completion. Because avoiding obstacles to goal attainment is a preferred means of prevention-focused self-regulation, they predicted that this kind of task would better fit a prevention focus than a promotion focus. They indeed found that, whether deciphering encrypted messages or solving math problems, prevention-focused participants later reported *greater* enjoyment when the task required vigilantly ignoring attractive, distracting video clips, whereas promotion-focused participants later reported less enjoyment when the clips were presented.

The importance of regulatory fit in individuals' control of demanding situations is also illustrated in a study by S. J. Grant and Park (2003). They gave American students (typically more promotion focused) or Korean students (typically more prevention focused) two tasks, either framed in promotion- or prevention-focused ways. They predicted that individuals would be better able to perform consecutive tasks that involved the same regulatory focus and that fit their predominant focus than tasks that were not a fit. They also predicted that when participants' were given two consecutive tasks that fit their orientation, they would subsequently persist longer on an anagram task (a measure of self-control). American students persisted longer on the anagram task when it was preceded by two promotion tasks rather than two prevention tasks or the mixed set. In contrast, Korean students showed the worst performance on the anagram task after doing two promotion tasks.

Regulatory fit is one kind of regulatory compatibility. Another type of compatibility that may be important is that between the strategies employed and the type of stressor (Cantor, 1994; Carver & Scheier, 1994; Taylor & Aspinwall, 1996). For example, problem-solving strategies have been found to be a more effective response to controllable versus uncontrollable stressors. Indeed, Compas, Malcarne, and Fondacaro (1988) found that better adjustment was associated with coping strategies that matched the controllability of the stressor. Children who generated problem-focused strategies in response to controllable stressors did better in terms of emotional and behavioral adjustment than those who generated problem-focused strategies in response to uncontrollable stressors.

Goals can also buffer the demanding effects of self-regulation. Webb and Sheeran

(2002) took advantage of the demanding effects of the Stroop color interference task to explore how differences in intentions can influence self-regulatory processes. Because participants have to inhibit the automatic tendency to read the words in the task, it is used as a way to create demands on self-regulatory strength. Participants who had completed the Stroop task persisted less on a subsequent self-regulation task *unless* they had formed explicit implementation intentions (Gollwitzer, 1996) about the task. Although the process of forming implementation intentions was imposed by the experimental task in this case, it suggests that individuals who are motivated to form specific plans may be buffered from some of the depleting effects of high-demand situations. Weiland, Lassiter, Daniels, and Fisher (2004) also explored the effects of nonconsciously priming participants with achievement words before they engaged in a demanding editing task. Afterwards, participants who had not received the achievement-related primes persisted less on unsolvable puzzles than participants who had received these primes. The motivation to achieve, made more accessible by the prime, affected how participants coped in this demanding situation.

In sum, as illustrated in the evidence we have reviewed, individuals differ in the ways in which they cope and in the extent to which different coping strategies are effective for them. These differences emerge in situations as diverse as failing a challenging math test to being rejected by a lover, yet all consume self-regulatory energy and challenge the self-regulatory system. Personality is revealed through the characteristic ways in which individuals' underlying self-regulatory biases and preferences shape their responses to these challenges.

CONCLUDING REMARKS

In our review we have proposed that *personality is revealed through motivated preferences and biases in the ways that people see the world and cope in the world*. These preferences and biases, driven by an underlying motivational system, influence what individuals see or believe, what they want to have, how they want to get those desired states of being, and how they deal with failures to

get them. Regulatory focus theory (Higgins, 1997) provides a clear example of how an underlying motivational system influences both ways of seeing and ways of coping.

Whereas prevention-focused individuals are more likely to encode and remember loss-relevant information, promotion-focused individuals are more likely to encode and remember gain-relevant information (Higgins & Tykocinski, 1992). Such differences are particularly likely to emerge in low-demand situations, where input is minimal or ambiguous. In such situations, chronically accessible constructs have a greater influence in what draws attention, what meanings are assigned, and what judgments are deemed appropriate and relevant. Promotion- and prevention-focused individuals also have different ways of coping in the world. Differences in coping are particularly pronounced in high-demand situations, where an individual's self-regulatory system is taxed or stressed. As discussed earlier, failure to meet the standards and expectations of self or others is one such situation. For promotion-focused individuals, failure represents the loss of a hoped-for ideal or aspiration, producing dejection and depression; for prevention individuals, failure represents the presence of negativity and the failure to uphold a duty, producing agitation and anxiety (e.g., Strauman & Higgins, 1987).

Given such an approach to defining personality, one might ask: If personality is revealed in underlying biases and preferences in ways of seeing and ways of coping, at what level should we expect to find coherence in the system? The question of finding coherence in personality is an important one that has concerned researchers for years, including those who have taken a social-cognitive approach to personality (see Cervone & Shoda, 1999). It is fitting, perhaps, that we began our review by stating that *variability* in behavior across situations is a prerequisite for a consideration of personality; we end with a discussion of the *invariances* in personality.

We propose that coherence will not be found in specific behaviors across situations but in the underlying motivations, goals, or strategies that produce behavior (see also H. Grant & Dweck, 1999; Pervin, 1983; Showers & Cantor, 1985). A number of different approaches have emphasized the different levels at which personality, and self-regulation or goal pursuit in particular, can be represented. Different approaches have emphasized the importance of different kinds of distinctions—between goals and subgoals (G. A. Miller, Galanter, & Pribram, 1960); between principles, programs, and sequences of movement (Carver & Scheier, 1998); between life-task goals, strategies, and plans or tactics (Cantor & Kihlstrom, 1987); between goals and plans (Pervin, 1983, 1989); between self-regulatory systems and strategies (Higgins, 1997; Higgins et al., 1994); and between global motivational dispositions, goals, and behaviors (Elliot, 2006; Elliot & Church, 1997). Although these approaches differ somewhat in the preferred terminology and number of levels, a common thread runs throughout: At any lower level in the hierarchy, there are multiple means (e.g., tactics or behaviors) that can serve a higher level. Within such a framework, we suggest that the coherence of personality is most often reflected in the types of goals that individuals pursue and their strategic ways of pursuing them (also referred to as plans; Pervin, 1983) rather than at the level of behavior.

As has been noted by others (e.g., Cantor & Kihlstrom, 1987; McClelland, 1951; Murray, 1938; Pervin, 2001), the same motivation can produce opposing behaviors in different contexts, given that a variety of behaviors may be enacted to pursue a given strategy. As just one illustration of this principle of equipotentiality (Pervin, 2001), consider the classic example of the authoritarian personality (Adorno, Frenkel-Brunswik, Levinson, & Sanford, 1950). Individuals with an authoritarian personality perceive the world in terms of high- and low-status people, and the motivation to cope with the maintenance of power is central. However, this motivation produces opposing behaviors in situations involving superiors versus subordinates. When high authoritarians face a higher-status person, they are more submissive than low authoritarians (Wells, Weinert, & Rubel, 1956); however, when high authoritarians face a lower-status person, they are more dominant and punitive than low authoritarians (Dustin & Davis, 1967). It is also true that the same behavior can reflect different underlying motives; the submissiveness of a high authoritarian is likely to reflect a different underlying motive

than the submissiveness of a highly agreeable individual—an example of the principle of equifinality (Pervin, 2001). The importance of distinguishing between these levels is that we can predict coherence while accounting for dynamic and changing behaviors (see also Mischel & Shoda, 1995).

In our own work we have explored how coherence can be found at the strategic level within the promotion and prevention systems (Higgins, 1997). For instance, whereas prevention-focused individuals have been shown to have a conservative bias in a classic signal detection paradigm when the stimuli are neutral (Crowe & Higgins, 1997), this bias shifts when the context is negative (Scholer, Stroessner, & Higgins, 2008). In other words, when confronted with negative stimuli, prevention-focused individuals exhibit a risky bias. How is this shift in behavior accounted for by the same underlying motivation? A prevention-focused individual, concerned with the possibility of negativity and making a mistake, prefers vigilant strategies. When the context is neutral, cautious and conservative behaviors serve that strategy well. However, negative information poses a direct challenge to the primary concerns of an individual under prevention focus: maintaining safety and security. Thus, prevention-focused individuals should be especially motivated not to "miss" this negative information—to do anything necessary to return from this negative state back to the status quo. Consequently, when negative information is involved, individuals in a prevention focus modify their typical behaviors (i.e., the conservative tactic of attaining correct rejections while minimizing false alarms) and show a willingness to incur false alarms to ensure that negative information is not ignored (i.e., a risky tactic).

This finding suggests that invariance in personality will not be found at the level of tactics or behaviors but at the level of *underlying strategic biases and preferences*. The motivation for need for closure also produces opposing behaviors, depending on whether one has the information needed to form a judgment (see Kruglanski & Webster, 1996). When individuals high in need for closure have the information to form a judgment readily available, they "freeze" on a particular judgment. However, when the same individuals do not have the information they need, they may actually increase information search to "seize" upon additional information (Kruglanski, Webster, & Klem, 1993). Also, as reviewed earlier, rejection sensitivity may lead either to hostility (Downey et al, 1998) or ingratiation (Romero-Canyas & Downey, 2005), depending on whether rejection is perceived as preventable or not. Across these examples, it is clear that, in both how people see the world and how they cope in the world, the coherence of underlying biases and preferences is revealed at the strategic rather than the behavioral level.

If it is at the strategic level that coherence will be found, the challenge going forward will be to continue to find ways to identify the motivational biases and preferences that capture the essence of personality. In particular, if the same underlying motivation can produce opposing behaviors in different contexts, the links between the interpretations of situations and the behaviors enacted in them must be identified. In seeking such strategic equivalences across situations, the additional study of how multiple and interacting motivations underlie such strategies would also be fruitful (see also Molden & Higgins, 2005; Pervin, 2001). There is much yet to be revealed.

REFERENCES

Adler, A. (1954). *Understanding human nature.* New York: Fawcett.

Adorno, T. W., Frenkel-Brunswik, E., Levinson, D. J., & Sanford, R. N. (1950). *The authoritarian personality.* Oxford, UK: Harpers.

Alexander, M. J., & Higgins, E. T. (1993). Emotional trade-offs of becoming a parent: How social roles influence self-discrepancy effects. *Journal of Personality and Social Psychology, 65,* 1259–1269.

Allport, G. W. (1937). *Personality: A psychological interpretation.* New York: Holt.

Allport, G. W., & Vernon, P. E. (1930). The field of personality. *Psychological Bulletin, 27,* 677–730.

Andersen, S., & Saribay, S. A. (2005). The relational self and transference: Evoking motives, self-regulation, and emotions through activation of mental representations of significant others. In M. W. Baldwin (Ed.), *Interpersonal cognition* (pp. 1–32). New York: Guilford Press.

Andersen, S. M., & Baum, A. (1994). Transference in interpersonal relations: Inferences and affect based on significant-other representations. *Journal of Personality* [Special issue: Psychodynamics and social cognition: Perspectives on the representation and processing of emotionally significant information], *62,* 459–497.

Andersen, S. M., & Chen, S. (2002). The relational self: An interpersonal social-cognitive theory. *Psychological Review, 109,* 619–645.

Andersen, S. M., & Cole, S. W. (1990). "Do I know you?": The role of significant others in general social perception. *Journal of Personality and Social Psychology, 59,* 384–399.

Andersen, S. M., Glassman, N. S., Chen, S., & Cole, S. W. (1995). Transference in social perception: The role of chronic accessibility in significant-other representations. *Journal of Personality and Social Psychology, 69,* 41–57.

Andersen, S. M., Reznik, I., & Chen, S. (1997). The self in relation to others: Motivational and cognitive underpinnings. In J. G. Snodgrass & R. L. Thompson (Eds.), *The self across psychology: Self-recognition, self-awareness, and the self concept* (Vol. 818, pp. 233–275). New York: New York Academy of Sciences.

Andersen, S. M., Reznik, I., & Glassman, N. S. (2005). The unconscious relational self. In R. R. Hassin, J. S. Uleman, & J. A. Bargh (Eds.), *The new unconscious* (pp. 421–481). New York: Oxford University Press.

Artistico, D., Cervone, D., & Pezzuti, L. (2003). Perceived self-efficacy and everyday problem solving among young and older adults. *Psychology and Aging, 18,* 68–79.

Atkinson, J. W., Heyns, R. W., & Veroff, J. (1954). The effect of experimental arousal of the affiliation motive on thematic apperception. *Journal of Abnormal and Social Psychology, 49,* 405–410.

Ayduk, O., Downey, G., Testa, A., Yen, Y., & Shoda, Y. (1999). Does rejection elicit hostility in rejection sensitive women? *Social Cognition* [Special issue: Social cognition and relationships], *17,* 245–271.

Ayduk, O., Mischel, W., & Downey, G. (2002). Attentional mechanisms linking rejection to hostile reactivity: The role of "hot" versus "cool" focus. *Psychological Science, 13,* 443–448.

Baldwin, M. W., & Holmes, J. G. (1987). Salient private audiences and awareness of the self. *Journal of Personality and Social Psychology, 52,* 1087–1098.

Bandura, A. (1977). Self-efficacy: Toward a unifying theory of behavioral change. *Psychological Review, 84,* 191–215.

Bandura, A. (1986). *Social foundations of thought and action: A social cognitive theory.* Upper Saddle River, NJ: Prentice Hall.

Bandura, A. (1997). *Self-efficacy: The exercise of control.* New York: Freeman.

Bandura, A. (1999). Social cognitive theory of

personality. In D. Cervone & Y. Shoda (Eds.), *The coherence of personality: Social-cognitive bases of consistency, variability, and organization* (pp. 185–241). New York: Guilford Press.

Bandura, A., & Cervone, D. (1983). Self-evaluative and self-efficacy mechanisms governing the motivational effects of goal systems. *Journal of Personality and Social Psychology, 45*, 1017–1028.

Bandura, A., & Cervone, D. (1986). Differential engagement of self-reactive influences in cognitive motivation. *Organizational Behavior and Human Decision Processes, 38*, 92–113.

Bargh, J. A., Lombardi, W. J., & Higgins, E. T. (1988). Automaticity of chronically accessible constructs in person × situation effects on person perception: It's just a matter of time. *Journal of Personality and Social Psychology, 55*, 599–605.

Bargh, J. A., & Pratto, F. (1986). Individual construct accessibility and perceptual selection. *Journal of Experimental Social Psychology, 22*, 293–311.

Bargh, J. A., & Thein, R. D. (1985). Individual construct accessibility, person memory, and the recall-judgment link: The case of information overload. *Journal of Personality and Social Psychology, 49*, 1129–1146.

Bartlett, F. C. (1932). *Remembering.* Oxford, UK: University Press.

Baumeister, R. F., & Leary, M. R. (1995). The need to belong: Desire for interpersonal attachments as a fundamental human motivation. *Psychological Bulletin, 117*, 497–529.

Baumeister, R. F., Schmeichel, B. J., & Vohs, K. D. (2007). Self-regulation and the executive function: The self as controlling agent. In A. W. Kruglanski & E. T. Higgins (Eds.), *Social psychology: Handbook of basic principles* (2nd ed., pp. 516–539). New York: Guilford Press.

Berk, M. S., & Andersen, S. M. (2000). The impact of past relationships on interpersonal behavior: Behavioral confirmation in the social-cognitive process of transference. *Journal of Personality and Social Psychology, 79*, 546–562.

Boldero, J., & Francis, J. (2000). The relation of self-discrepancies and emotions: The moderating roles of self-guide achievement importance, location relevance, and social self-domain importance. *Journal of Personality and Social Psychology, 78*, 38–52.

Breuer, J., & Freud, S. (1956). On the psychical mechanism of hysterical phenomena (1893). *International Journal of Psycho Analysis, 37*, 8–13. (Original work published 1893)

Bruner, J. S. (1957a). Going beyond the information given. In J. S. Bruner, E. Brunswik, L. Festinger, F. Heider, K. F. Muenzinger, C. E. Osgood, et al. (Eds.). *Contemporary approaches to cognition* (pp. 41–69). Cambridge, MA: Harvard University Press.

Bruner, J. S. (1957b). On perceptual readiness. *Psychological Review, 64*, 123–152.

Cantor, N. (1994). Life task problem solving: Situational affordances and personal needs. *Personality and Social Psychology Bulletin, 20*, 235–243.

Cantor, N., & Kihlstrom, J. F. (1987). *Personality and social intelligence.* Englewood Cliffs, NJ: Prentice Hall.

Cantor, N., & Norem, J. K. (1989). Defensive pessimism and stress and coping. *Social Cognition* [Special issue: Stress, coping, and social cognition], *7*, 92–112.

Cantor, N., Norem, J. K., Niedenthal, P. M., Langston, C. A., & Brower, A. M. (1987). Life tasks, self-concept ideals, and cognitive strategies in a life transition. *Journal of Personality and Social Psychology, 53*, 1178–1191.

Caprara, G. V., Barbaranelli, C., Pastorelli, C., & Cervone, D. (2004). The contribution of self-efficacy beliefs to psychosocial outcomes in adolescence: Predicting beyond global dispositional tendencies. *Personality and Individual Differences, 37*, 751–763.

Caprara, G. V., & Cervone, D. (2000). *Personality: Determinants, dynamics, and potentials.* New York: Cambridge University Press.

Caprara, G.V., Regalia, C., & Bandura, A. (2002). Longitudinal impact of perceived self-regulatory efficacy on violent conduct. *European Psychologist, 7*, 63–69.

Carver, C. S., & Scheier, M. F. (1994). Situational coping and coping dispositions in a stressful transaction. *Journal of Personality and Social Psychology, 66*, 184–195.

Carver, C. S., & Scheier, M. F. (1998). On the self-regulation of behavior. Cambridge, UK: Cambridge University Press.

Carver, C. S., Scheier, M. F., & Weintraub, J. K. (1989). Assessing coping strategies: A theoretically based approach. *Journal of Personality and Social Psychology, 56*, 267–283.

Caspi, A., & Moffitt, T. E. (1993). When do individual differences matter?: A paradoxical theory of personality coherence. *Psychological Inquiry, 4*, 247–271.

Cervone, D. (1997). Social-cognitive mechanisms and personality coherence: Self-knowledge, situational beliefs, and cross-situational coherence in perceived self-efficacy. *Psychological Science, 8*, 43–50.

Cervone, D. (2000). Thinking about self-efficacy. *Behavior Modification, 24*, 30–56.

Cervone, D., & Peake, P. K. (1986). Anchoring, efficacy, and action: The influence of judgmental heuristics on self-efficacy judgments and behavior. *Journal of Personality and Social Psychology, 50*, 492–501.

Cervone, D., & Scott, W. D. (1995). Self-efficacy theory of behavioral change: Foundations, conceptual issues, and therapeutic implications. In W. T. O'Donohue & L. Krasner (Eds.), *Theories of behavior therapy: Exploring behavior change* (pp. 349–383). Washington, DC: American Psychological Association.

Cervone, D., Shadel, W. G., & Jencius, S. (2001). Social-cognitive theory of personality assessment. *Personality and Social Psychology Review, 5,* 33–51.

Cervone, D., & Shoda, Y. (1999). *The coherence of personality: Social-cognitive bases of consistency, variability, and organization.* New York: Guilford Press.

Cervone, D., & Williams, S. L. (1992). Social cognitive theory and personality. In G. V. Caprara & G. L. Van Heck (Eds.), *Modern personality psychology: Critical reviews and new direction.* New York: Harvester Wheatsheaf.

Chen, S., Andersen, S. M., & Hinkley, K. (1999). Triggering transference: Examining the role of applicability in the activation and use of significant-other representations in social perception. *Social Cognition, 17,* 332–365.

Compas, B. E., Malcarne, V. L., & Fondacaro, K. M. (1988). Coping with stressful events in older children and young adolescents. *Journal of Consulting and Clinical Psychology, 56,* 405–411.

Cox, T., & Ferguson, E. (1991). Individual differences, stress and coping. In C. L. Cooper & R. Payne (Eds.), *Personality and stress: Individual differences in the stress process* (pp. 7–30). Oxford, UK: Wiley.

Crowe, E., & Higgins, E. T. (1997). Regulatory focus and strategic inclinations: Promotion and prevention in decision-making. *Organizational Behavior and Human Decision Processes, 69,* 117–132.

Dijksterhuis, A., van Knippenberg, A., Kruglanski, A. W., & Schaper, C. (1996). Motivated social cognition: Need for closure effects on memory and judgment. *Journal of Experimental Social Psychology, 32,* 254–270.

Downey, G., & Feldman, S. I. (1996). Implications of rejection sensitivity for intimate relationships. *Journal of Personality and Social Psychology, 70,* 1327–1343.

Downey, G., Freitas, A. L., Michaelis, B., & Khouri, H. (1998). The self-fulfilling prophecy in close relationships: Rejection sensitivity and rejection by romantic partners. *Journal of Personality and Social Psychology, 75,* 545–560.

Downey, G., Mougios, V., Ayduk, O., London, B. E., & Shoda, Y. (2004). Rejection sensitivity and the defensive motivational system: Insights from the startle response to rejection cues. *Psychological Science, 15,* 668–673.

Dunning, D., Meyerowitz, J. A., & Holzberg, A. D. (1989). Ambiguity and self-evaluation: The role of idiosyncratic trait definitions in self-serving assessments of ability. *Journal of Personality and Social Psychology, 57,* 1082–1090.

Dustin, D. S., & Davis, H. P. (1967). Authoritarianism and sanctioning behavior. *Journal of Personality and Social Psychology, 6,* 222–224.

Dweck, C. S. (1999). *Self-theories: Their role in motivation, personality, and development.* New York: Psychology Press.

Dweck, C. S., Chiu, C.-Y., & Hong, Y.-Y. (1995). Implicit theories and their role in judgments and reactions: A world from two perspectives. *Psychological Inquiry, 6,* 267–285.

Dweck, C. S., & Leggett, E. L. (1988). A social-cognitive approach to motivation and personality. *Psychological Review, 95,* 256–273.

Dweck, C. S., Mangels, J. A., & Good, C. (2004). Motivational effects on attention, cognition, and performance. In D. Y. Dai & R. J. Sternberg (Eds.), *Motivation, emotion, and cognition: Integrative perspectives on intellectual functioning and development* (pp. 41–55). Mahwah, NJ: Erlbaum.

Dweck, C. S., & Sorich, L. (1999). Mastery-oriented thinking. In C. R. Snyder (Ed.), *Coping* (pp. 232–251). New York: Oxford University Press.

Elliot, A. J. (2006). The hierarchical model of approach–avoidance motivation. *Motivation and Emotion, 30,* 111–116.

Elliot, A. J., & Church, M. A. (1997). A hierarchical model of approach and avoidance achievement motivation. *Journal of Personality and Social Psychology, 72,* 218–232.

Endler, N. S. (1982). Interactionism comes of age. In M. P. Zanna, E. T. Higgins, & C. P. Herman (Eds.), *Consistency in social behavior: The Ontario Symposium* (Vol. 2, pp. 209–249). Hillsdale, NJ: Erlbaum.

Endler, N. S., & Magnusson, D. (1977). The interaction model of anxiety: An empirical test in an examination situation. *Canadian Journal of Behavioural Science, 9,* 101–107.

Endler, N. S., & Parker, J. D. (1990). Multidimensional assessment of coping: A critical evaluation. *Journal of Personality and Social Psychology, 58,* 844–854.

Epstein, S. (1979). The stability of behavior: I. On predicting most of the people much of the time. *Journal of Personality and Social Psychology, 37,* 1097–1126.

Exner, J. E., Jr. (1993). *The Rorschach: A comprehensive system. Vol. 1. Basic foundations* (3rd ed.). Oxford, UK: Wiley.

Fiske, S. T. (2003). Five core social motives, plus or minus five. In S. J. Spencer, S. Fein, M. P. Zanna, & J. M. Olson (Eds.), *Motivated social* perception: The Ontario Symposium (Vol. 9, pp. 233–246). Mahwah, NJ: Erlbaum.

Fiske, S. T., & Neuberg, S. L. (1990). A continuum of impression formation, from category-based to individuating processes: Influences of impression formation and motivation on attention and interpretation. In M. P. Zanna (Ed.), Advances in experimental social psychology (Vol. 23, pp. 1–74). New York: Academic Press.

Folkman, S., & Moskowitz, J. T. (2004). Coping: Pitfalls and promise. Annual Review of Psychology, 55, 745–774.

Ford, T. E., & Kruglanski, A. W. (1995). Effects of epistemic motivations on the use of accessible constructs in social judgment. Personality and Social Psychology Bulletin, 21, 950–962.

Freitas, A. L., Liberman, N., & Higgins, E. T. (2002). Regulatory fit and resisting temptation during goal pursuit. Journal of Experimental Social Psychology, 38, 291–298.

Freud, A. (1946). The ego and the mechanisms of defense. London: Hogarth Press. (Original work published 1936)

Freud, S. (1955). Further remarks on the neuro-psychoses of defence. In J. Strachey (Ed. & Trans.), The standard edition of the complete psychological works of Sigmund Freud (Vol. 3). London: Hogarth Press. (Original work published 1896)

Freud, S. (1955). History of the psychoanalytic movement. In J. Strachey (Ed. & Trans.), The standard edition of the complete psychological works of Sigmund Freud (Vol. 14). London: Hogarth Press. (Original work published 1914)

Glassman, N. S., & Andersen, S. M. (1999). Activating transference without consciousness: Using significant-other representations to go beyond what is subliminally given. Journal of Personality and Social Psychology, 77, 1146–1162.

Gollwitzer, P. M. (1996). The volitional benefits of planning. In P. M. Gollwitzer & J. A. Bargh (Eds.), The psychology of action: Linking cognition and motivation to behavior (pp. 287–312). New York: Guilford Press.

Grant, H., & Dweck, C. S. (1999). A goal analysis of personality and personality coherence. In D. Cervone & Y. Shoda (Eds.), The coherence of personality: Social-cognitive bases of consistency, variability, and organization (pp. 345–371). New York: Guilford Press.

Grant, S. J., & Park, J. W. (2003, October). The effect of goal orientation on self-regulatory depletion. Paper presented at the annual meeting of the Association for Consumer Research, Toronto.

Guilford, J. P. (1959). Personality. New York: McGraw-Hill.

Hebb, D. O. (1949). The organization of behavior: A neuropsychological theory. Oxford, UK: Wiley.

Henderson, V., & Dweck, C. S. (1990). Achievement and motivation in adolescence: A new model and data. In S. Feldman & G. Elliot (Eds.), At the threshold: The developing adolescent (pp. 308–329). Cambridge, MA: Harvard University Press.

Higgins, E. T. (1987). Self-discrepancy: A theory relating self and affect. Psychological Review, 94, 319–340.

Higgins, E. T. (1989). Knowledge accessibility and activation: Subjectivity and suffering from unconscious sources. In J. S. Uleman & J. A. Bargh (Eds.), Unintended thought (pp. 75–123). New York: Guilford Press.

Higgins, E. T. (1990). Personality, social psychology, and person–situation relations: Standards and knowledge activation as a common language. In L. A. Pervin (Ed.), Handbook of personality: Theory and research (pp. 301–338). New York: Guilford Press.

Higgins, E. T. (1996). Knowledge activation: Accessibility, applicability, and salience. In E. T. Higgins & A. W. Kruglanski (Eds.), Social psychology: Handbook of basic principles (pp. 133–168). New York: Guilford Press.

Higgins, E. T. (1997). Beyond pleasure and pain. American Psychologist, 52, 1280–1300.

Higgins, E. T. (1998). The aboutness principle: A pervasive influence on human inference. Social Cognition, 16, 173–198.

Higgins, E. T. (1999a). Persons and situations: Unique explanatory principles or variability in general principles? In D. Cervone & Y. Shoda (Eds.), The coherence of personality: Social-cognitive bases of consistency, variability, and organization (pp. 61–93). New York: Guilford Press.

Higgins, E. T. (1999b). When do self-discrepancies have specific relations to emotions?: The second-generation question of Tangney, Niedenthal, Covert, and Barlow (1998). Journal of Personality and Social Psychology, 77, 1313–1317.

Higgins, E. T. (2000a). Does personality provide unique explanations for behaviour?: Personality as cross-person variability in general principles. European Journal of Personality. Special Issue: Personality and Cognition, 14, 391–406.

Higgins, E. T. (2000b). Making a good decision: Value from fit. American Psychologist, 55, 1217–1230.

Higgins, E. T. (2006). Value from hedonic experience and engagement. Psychological Review, 13, 439–460.

Higgins, E. T., & Bargh, J. A. (1987). Social cognition and social perception. Annual Review of Psychology, 38, 369–425.

Higgins, E. T., Bargh, J. A., & Lombardi, W. J. (1985). Nature of priming effects on categorization. *Journal of Experimental Psychology: Learning, Memory, and Cognition, 11*, 59–69.

Higgins, E. T., Bond, R. N., Klein, R., & Strauman, T. (1986). Self-discrepancies and emotional vulnerability: How magnitude, accessibility, and type of discrepancy influence affect. *Journal of Personality and Social Psychology, 51*, 5–15.

Higgins, E. T., & Brendl, C. M. (1995). Accessibility and applicability: Some "activation rules" influencing judgment. *Journal of Experimental Social Psychology, 31*, 218–243.

Higgins, E. T., & King, G. A. (1981). Accessibility of social constructs: Information processing consequences of individual and contextual variability. In N. Cantor & J. Kihlstrom (Eds.), *Personality, cognition, and social interaction* (pp. 69–121). Hillsdale, NJ: Erlbaum.

Higgins, E. T., King, G. A., & Mavin, G. H. (1982). Individual construct accessibility and subjective impressions and recall. *Journal of Personality and Social Psychology, 43*, 35–47.

Higgins, E. T., Klein, R., & Strauman, T. (1985). Self-concept discrepancy theory: A psychological model for distinguishing among different aspects of depression and anxiety. *Social Cognition* [Special issue: Depression], *3*, 51–76.

Higgins, E. T., & Molden, D. C. (2003). How strategies for making judgments and decisions affect cognition: Motivated cognition revisited. In G. V. Bodenhausen & A. J. Lambert (Eds.), *Foundations of social cognition: A festschrift in honor of Robert S. Wyer, Jr.* (pp. 211–235). Mahwah, NJ: Erlbaum.

Higgins, E. T., Roney, C. J. R., Crowe, E., & Hymes, C. (1994). Ideal versus ought predilections for approach and avoidance distinct self-regulatory systems. *Journal of Personality and Social Psychology, 66*, 276–286.

Higgins, E. T., Shah, J., & Friedman, R. (1997). Emotional responses to goal attainment: Strength of regulatory focus as moderator. *Journal of Personality and Social Psychology, 72*, 515–525.

Higgins, E. T., & Tykocinski, O. (1992). Self-discrepancies and biographical memory: Personality and cognition at the level of psychological situation. *Personality and Social Psychology Bulletin, 18*, 527–535.

Hinkley, K., & Andersen, S. M. (1996). The working self-concept in transference: Significant-other activation and self change. *Journal of Personality and Social Psychology, 71*, 1279–1295.

Jensen, A. R. (1958). Personality. *Annual Review of Psychology, 9*, 295–322.

John, O. P. (1990). The "Big Five" factor taxonomy: Dimensions of personality in the natural language and in questionnaires. In L. A. Pervin (Ed.), *Handbook of personality: Theory and research* (pp. 66–100). New York: Guilford Press.

Kagan, J., & Kogan, N. (1970). Individual variation in cognitive processes. In P. Mussen (Ed.), *Carmichael's manual of child psychology* (Vol. 1, pp. 1273–1365). New York: Wiley.

Kelly, G. A. (1955). *The psychology of personal constructs: I. A theory of personality: Clinical diagnosis and psychotherapy.* Oxford, UK: Norton.

King, G. A., & Sorrentino, R. M. (1988). Uncertainty orientation and the relation between individual accessible constructs and person memory. *Social Cognition, 6*, 128–149.

Kruglanski, A. W. (1996). Motivated social cognition: Principles of the interface. In E. T. Higgins & A. W. Kruglanski (Eds.), *Social psychology: Handbook of basic principles* (pp. 493–520). New York: Guilford Press.

Kruglanski, A. W., & Freund, T. (1983). The freezing and unfreezing of lay inferences: Effects on impressional primacy, ethnic stereotyping, and numerical anchoring. *Journal of Experimental Social Psychology, 19*, 448–468.

Kruglanski, A. W., & Webster, D. M. (1996). Motivated closing of the mind: "Seizing" and "freezing." *Psychological Review, 103*, 263–283.

Kruglanski, A. W., Webster, D. M., & Klem, A. (1993). Motivated resistance and openness to persuasion in the presence or absence of prior information. *Journal of Personality and Social Psychology, 65*, 861–876.

Kunda, Z. (1990). The case for motivated reasoning. *Psychological Bulletin, 108*, 480–498.

Lang, P. J., Bradley, M. M., & Cuthbert, B. N. (1998). Emotion, motivation, and anxiety: Brain mechanisms and psychophysiology. *Biological Psychiatry, 44*, 1248–1263.

Lau, R. R. (1989). Construct accessibility and political choice. *Political Behavior, 11*, 5–32.

Lazarus, R. S. (1982). Thoughts on the relations between emotion and cognition. *American Psychologist, 37*, 1019–1024.

Liberman, N., Molden, D. C., Idson, L. C., & Higgins, E. T. (2001). Promotion and prevention focus on alternative hypotheses: Implications for attributional functions. *Journal of Personality and Social Psychology, 80*, 5–18.

Magnusson, D. (1990). Personality development from an interactional perspective. In L. A. Pervin (Ed.), *Handbook of personality: Theory and research* (pp. 193–222). New York: Guilford Press.

Magnusson, D., & Endler, N. S. (1977). *Personality at the crossroads: Current issues in interactional psychology.* Hillsdale, NJ: Erlbaum.

Martijn, C., Tenbult, P., Merckelbach, H.,

Dreezens, E., & de Vries, N. K. (2002). Getting a grip on ourselves: Challenging expectancies about loss of energy after self-control. *Social Cognition, 20*, 441–460.

Martin, L. L. (1986). Set/reset: Use and disuse of concepts in impression formation. *Journal of Personality and Social Psychology, 51*, 493–504.

McClelland, D. C. (1951). *Personality*. New York: Sloane.

McClelland, D. C., & Atkinson, J. W. (1948). The projective expression of needs: I. The effect of different intensities of the hunger drive on perception. *Journal of Psychology: Interdisciplinary and Applied, 25*, 205–222.

McClelland, D. C., Atkinson, J. W., Clark, R. A., & Lowell, E. L. (1953). *The achievement motive*. East Norwalk, CT: Appleton-Century-Crofts.

McCrae, R. R., & Costa, P. T., Jr. (1999). A five-factor theory of personality. In L. Pervin & O. P. John (Eds.), *Handbook of personality: Theory and research* (2nd ed., pp. 139–153). New York: Guilford Press.

Metcalfe, J., & Mischel, W. (1999). A hot/cool-system analysis of delay of gratification: Dynamics of willpower. *Psychological Review, 106*, 3–19.

Miller, G. A., Galanter, E., & Pribram, K. H. (1960). *Plans and the structure of behavior*. New York: Holt.

Miller, S. M. (1980). When is a little information a dangerous thing?: Coping with stressful life-events by monitoring vs. blunting. In S. Levine & H. Ursin (Eds.), *Coping and health* (pp. 145–169). New York: Plenum Press.

Miller, S. M., & Mangan, C. E. (1983). Interacting effects of information and coping style in adapting to gynaecologic stress: Should the doctor tell all? *Journal of Personality and Social Psychology, 45*, 223–236.

Mischel, H. N., & Mischel, W. (1983). The development of children's knowledge of self-control strategies. *Child Development, 54*, 603–619.

Mischel, W. (1973). Toward a cognitive social learning reconceptualization of personality. *Psychological Review, 80*, 252–283.

Mischel, W. (1974). Processes in delay of gratification. *Advances in Experimental Social Psychology, 7*, 249–292.

Mischel, W., & Ayduk, O. (2004). Willpower in a cognitive–affective processing system: The dynamics of delay of gratification. In R. F. Baumeister & K. D. Vohs (Eds.), *Handbook of self-regulation: Research, theory, and applications* (pp. 99–129). New York: Guilford Press.

Mischel, W., & Baker, N. (1975). Cognitive appraisals and transformations in delay behavior. *Journal of Personality and Social Psychology, 31*, 254–261.

Mischel, W., Cantor, N., & Feldman, S. (1996). Principles of self-regulation: The nature of willpower and self-control. In E. T. Higgins & A. W. Kruglanski (Eds.), *Social psychology: Handbook of basic principles* (pp. 329–360). New York: Guilford Press.

Mischel, W., & Ebbesen, E. B. (1970). Attention in delay of gratification. *Journal of Personality and Social Psychology, 16*, 329–337.

Mischel, W., Ebbesen, E. B., & Zeiss, A. R. (1973). Selective attention to the self: Situational and dispositional determinants. *Journal of Personality and Social Psychology, 27*, 129–142.

Mischel, W., & Moore, B. (1973). Effects of attention to symbolically presented rewards on self-control. *Journal of Personality and Social Psychology, 28*, 172–179.

Mischel, W., & Shoda, Y. (1995). A cognitive–affective system theory of personality: Reconceptualizing situations, dispositions, dynamics, and invariance in personality structure. *Psychological Review, 102*, 246–268.

Mischel, W., Shoda, Y., & Peake, P. K. (1988). The nature of adolescent competencies predicted by preschool delay of gratification. *Journal of Personality and Social Psychology, 54*, 687–696.

Molden, D. C., & Dweck, C. S. (2006). Finding "meaning" in psychology: A lay theories approach to self-regulation, social perception, and social development. *American Psychologist, 61*, 192–203.

Molden, D. C., & Higgins, E. T. (2005). Motivated thinking. In K. J. Holyoak & R. G. Morrison (Eds.), *The Cambridge handbook of thinking and reasoning* (pp. 295–317). New York: Cambridge University Press.

Moore, B., Mischel, W., & Zeiss, A. (1976). Comparative effects of the reward stimulus and its cognitive representation in voluntary delay. *Journal of Personality and Social Psychology, 34*, 419–424.

Moretti, M. M., & Higgins, E. T. (1999). Own versus other standpoints in self-regulation: Developmental antecedents and functional consequences. *Review of General Psychology, 3*, 188–223.

Moretti, M. M., Higgins, E. T., Woody, E., & Leung, D. (1998). *Predicting individual differences in response to negative feedback: "Own" versus "other" regulatory style*. Unpublished manuscript, Simon Fraser University, Burnaby, British Columbia, Canada.

Moskowitz, G. B. (1993). Individual differences in social categorization: The influence of personal need for structure on spontaneous trait inferences. *Journal of Personality and Social Psychology, 65*, 132–142.

Murray, H. A. (1938). *Explorations in personality*. Oxford, UK: Oxford University Press.

Neuberg, S. L., & Fiske, S. T. (1987). Motivational

influences on impression formation: Outcome dependency, accuracy-driven attention, and individuating processes. *Journal of Personality and Social Psychology, 53,* 431–444.

Nisbett, R., & Wilson, T. (1977). Telling more than we can know: Verbal reports on mental processes. *Psychological Review, 84,* 231–259.

Norem, J. K., & Cantor, N. (1986a). Anticipatory and post hoc cushioning strategies: Optimism and defensive pessimism in "risky" situations. *Cognitive Therapy and Research, 10,* 347–362.

Norem, J. K., & Cantor, N. (1986b). Defensive pessimism: Harnessing anxiety as motivation. *Journal of Personality and Social Psychology, 51,* 1208–1217.

Norem, J. K., & Illingworth, K. S. S. (1993). Strategy-dependent effects of reflecting on self and tasks: Some implications of optimism and defensive pessimism. *Journal of Personality and Social Psychology, 65,* 822–835.

Oishi, S., Schimmack, U., & Colcombe, S. J. (2003). The contextual and systematic nature of life satisfaction judgments. *Journal of Experimental Social Psychology, 39,* 232–247.

Peake, P. K., & Cervone, D. (1989). Sequence anchoring and self-efficacy: Primacy effects in the consideration of possibilities. *Social Cognition, 7,* 31–50.

Peake, P. K., Hebl, M., & Mischel, W. (2002). Strategic attention deployment for delay of gratification in working and waiting situations. *Developmental Psychology, 38,* 313–326.

Pervin, L. A. (1983). The stasis and flow of behavior: Toward a theory of goals. In M. M. Page (Ed.), *Personality: Current theory and research* (pp. 1–53). Lincoln: University of Nebraska Press.

Pervin, L. A. (1989). Goal concepts in personality and social psychology: A historical introduction. In L. A. Pervin (Ed.), *Goal concepts in personality and social psychology* (pp. 1–17). Hillsdale, NJ: Erlbaum.

Pervin, L. A. (1990). A brief history of modern personality theory. In L. A. Pervin (Ed.), *Handbook of personality: Theory and research* (pp. 3–18). New York: Guilford Press.

Pervin, L. A. (2001). A dynamic systems approach to personality. *European Psychologist, 6,* 172–176.

Pietrzak, J., Downey, G., & Ayduk, O. (2005). Rejection sensitivity as an interpersonal vulnerability. In M. W. Baldwin (Ed.), *Interpersonal cognition* (pp. 62–84). New York: Guilford Press.

Purdie, V., & Downey, G. (2000). Rejection sensitivity and adolescent girls' vulnerability to relationship-centered difficulties. *Child Maltreatment: Journal of the American Professional Society on the Abuse of Children, 5,* 338–349.

Robinson, M. D. (2004). Personality as performance: Categorization tendencies and their correlates. *Current Directions in Psychological Science, 13,* 127–129.

Robinson, M. D., Vargas, P. T., Tamir, M., & Solberg, E. C. (2004). Using and being used by categories: The case of negative evaluations and daily well-being. *Psychological Science, 15,* 521–526.

Roese, N. J. (1997). Counterfactual thinking. *Psychological Bulletin, 121,* 133–148.

Roese, N. J., Hur, T., & Pennington, G. L. (1999). Counterfactual thinking and regulatory focus: Implications for action versus inaction and sufficiency versus necessity. *Journal of Personality and Social Psychology, 77,* 1109–1120.

Romero-Canyas, R., & Downey, G. (2005). Rejection sensitivity as a predictor of affective and behavioral responses to interpersonal stress: A defensive motivational system. In K. D. Williams, J. P. Forgas, & W. von Hippel (Eds.), *The social outcast: Ostracism, social exclusion, rejection, and bullying* (pp. 131–154). New York: Psychology Press.

Rorschach, H. (1951). *Psychodiagnostics: A diagnostic test based on perception* (5th ed.). Oxford, UK: Grune & Stratton. (Original work published 1921)

Roseman, I. J. (1984). Cognitive determinants of emotion: A structural theory. *Review of Personality and Social Psychology, 5,* 11–36.

Salovey, P., Hsee, C. K., & Mayer, J. D. (1993). Emotional intelligence and the self-regulation of affect. In D. M. Wegner & J. W. Pennebaker (Eds.), *Handbook of mental control* (pp. 258–277). Upper Saddle River, NJ: Prentice-Hall.

Sanderson, W. C., Rapee, R. M., & Barlow, D. H. (1989). The influence of an illusion of control on panic attacks induced via inhalation of 5.5% carbon-dioxide-enriched air. *Archives of General Psychiatry, 46,* 157–162.

Schachter, S., & Singer, J. E. (1962). Cognitive, social and physiological determinants of emotional state. *Psychological Review, 69,* 379–399.

Scholer, A. A., Stroessner, S. J., & Higgins, E. T. (2008). Responding to negativity: How a risky tactic can serve a vigilant strategy. *Journal of Experimental Social Psychology, 44*(3), 767–774.

Schunk, D. H. (1981). Modeling and attributional effects on children's achievement: A self-efficacy analysis. *Journal of Educational Psychology, 73,* 93–105.

Shah, J., & Higgins, E. T. (2001). Regulatory concerns and appraisal efficiency: The general impact of promotion and prevention. *Journal of Personality and Social Psychology, 80,* 693–705.

Shoda, Y., Mischel, W., & Peake, P. K. (1990). Predicting adolescent cognitive and self-regulatory competencies from preschool delay of gratification: Identifying diagnostic conditions. *Developmental Psychology, 26,* 978–986.

Showers, C. (1992). The motivational and emotional consequences of considering positive or negative possibilities for an upcoming event. *Journal of Personality and Social Psychology, 63,* 474–484.

Showers, C., & Cantor, N. (1985). Social cognition: A look at motivated strategies. *Annual Review of Psychology, 36,* 275–305.

Sorrentino, R. M., & Higgins, E. T. (1986). Motivation and cognition: Warming up to synergism. In R. M. Sorrentino & E. T. Higgins (Eds.), *Handbook of motivation and cognition: Foundations of social behavior* (pp. 3–19). New York: Guilford Press.

Stock, J., & Cervone, D. (1990). Proximal goal-setting and self-regulatory processes. *Cognitive Therapy and Research, 14,* 483–498.

Strauman, T. J., & Higgins, E. T. (1987). Automatic activation of self-discrepancies and emotional syndromes: When cognitive structures influence affect. *Journal of Personality and Social Psychology* [Special issue: Integrating personality and social psychology], *53,* 1004–1014.

Strauman, T. J., & Higgins, E. T. (1988). Self-discrepancies as predictors of vulnerability to distinct syndromes of chronic emotional distress. *Journal of Personality, 56,* 685–707.

Strube, M. J., Turner, C. W., Cerro, D., Stephens, J., & Hinchey, F. (1984). Interpersonal aggression and the Type A coronary-prone behavior pattern: A theoretical distinction and practical implications. *Journal of Personality and Social Psychology, 47,* 839–847.

Sullivan, H. S. (1953). *The collected works of Harry Stack Sullivan: Vol. 1. The interpersonal theory of psychiatry* (H. S. Perry & M. L. Gawel, Eds.). New York: Norton.

Taylor, S. E., & Aspinwall, L. G. (1996). Mediating and moderating processes in psychosocial stress: Appraisal, coping, resistance, and vulnerability. In H. B. Kaplan (Ed.), *Psychosocial stress: Perspectives on structure, theory, life-course, and methods* (pp. 71–110). San Diego, CA: Academic Press.

Tesser, A. (2000). On the confluence of self-esteem maintenance mechanisms. *Personality and Social Psychology Review, 4,* 290–299.

Tetlock, P. E. (1985). Accountability: A social check on the fundamental attribution error. *Social Psychology Quarterly, 48,* 227–236.

Thompson, E. P., Roman, R. J., Moskowitz, G. B., Chaiken, S., & Bargh, J. A. (1994). Accuracy motivation attenuates covert priming: The systematic reprocessing of social information. *Journal of Personality and Social Psychology, 66,* 474–489.

Webb, T. L., & Sheeran, P. (2002). Can implementation intentions help to overcome ego-depletion? *Journal of Experimental Social Psychology, 39,* 279–286.

Webster, D. M. (1993). Motivated augmentation and reduction of the overattribution bias. *Journal of Personality and Social Psychology, 65,* 261–271.

Weiland, P. E., Lassiter, G. D., Daniels, L., & Fisher, A. (2004, January). *Can nonconscious goals moderate self-regulatory failure?* Paper presented at the annual meeting of the Society for Personality and Social Psychology, Austin, TX.

Wells, W. D., Weinert, G., & Rubel, M. (1956). Conformity pressure and authoritarian personality. *Journal of Psychology: Interdisciplinary and Applied, 42,* 133–136.

Wertheimer, M. (1923). Untersuchunger zur Lehre van der Gestalt: II. *Psychologische Forschung, 4,* 301–350.

Williams, S. L. (1992). Perceived self-efficacy and phobic disability. In R. Schwarzer (Ed.), *Self-efficacy: Thought control of action* (pp. 149–176). Washington, DC: Hemisphere.

Witkin, H. A., Dyk, R. B., Faterson, H. F., Goodenough, D. R., & Karp, S. A. (1962). *Psychological differentiation.* Potomac, MD: Erlbaum.

Witkin, H. A., & Goodenough, D. R. (1977). Field dependence and interpersonal behavior. *Psychological Bulletin, 84,* 661–689.

Wright, J. C., & Mischel, W. (1987). A conditional approach to dispositional constructs: The local predictability of social behavior. *Journal of Personality and Social Psychology* [Special issue: Integrating personality and social psychology], *53,* 1159–1177.

Zeidner, M., & Endler, N. S. (Eds.). (1996). *Handbook of coping: Theory, research, applications.* Oxford, UK: Wiley.

Zillman, D. (1978). Attribution and misattribution of excitatory reactions. In J. H. Harvey, W. J. Ickes, & R. F. Kidd (Eds.), *New directions in attribution research* (Vol. 2, pp. 335–368). Hillsdale, NJ: Erlbaum.

CHAPTER 7

Toward a Unified Theory of Personality

Integrating Dispositions and Processing Dynamics within the Cognitive–Affective Processing System

Walter Mischel
Yuichi Shoda

Psychologists and nonpsychologists alike assume that people have distinct, enduring personalities. Ample evidence exists that individuals do differ reliably in what they do and think and feel in any given situation (e.g., Mischel, Shoda, & Ayduk, 2008). But, historically, it has remained surprisingly difficult to demonstrate the *consistency* of such individual differences from one situation to another. Study after study has found that such consistency, although not zero, was only slightly above chance, rarely accounting for more than 5 of the variance when behavior is directly observed (Mischel, 1968; Mischel & Peake, 1982a, 1982b; Peterson, 1968; Shoda, Mischel, & Wright, 1994; Vernon, 1964). This finding has led many to ask: Which is correct, our intuitive belief in the existence of stable personality differences, or the repeated research findings of behavioral *in*consistency across situations (Bem & Allen, 1974)? This classic "personality paradox" challenged the basic premise of personality psychology and generated a sense of paradigm crisis, creating a deep split between those who study individual differences ("personality" psychologists) and those who study the effect of situations ("social" psychologists), even though the behavioral phenomena they study overlap considerably (reviewed in Mischel, 2004).

Findings to date show that neither the research nor the intuition was wrong about the nature of individual differences in social behavior, although each had given an incomplete picture. It turned out that hidden in the seemingly random variation of individuals' behavior across situations is a pattern that *is* stable and distinctive for every individual (e.g., Shoda & LeeTiernan, 2002). The behavior itself varies, but there is stability in how each individual's behavior varies from one situation to another. These stable and distinctive *if ... then ...* situation–behavior patterns form *behavioral signatures of personality* (Shoda, Mischel, & Wright, 1994) and suggest the existence of a higher-order consistency on which the intuitive belief in personality may be based (Mischel & Shoda, 1995). To understand these stable intraindividual patterns of variability requires a theory and research paradigm that goes beyond the traditional investigation of personality and social situations. The findings yield both new answers and new questions about the nature of personality and the interactions of persons and situations.

Happily, passionate debates in the search for the nature of personality are being replaced by findings and reconceptualizations that promise to resolve paradoxes and to overcome problems that have frustrated and divided the study of personality almost since its inception. This chapter focuses on the key implications of these developments in recent decades for building a unifying, cumulative personality theory and science, based on the findings from a century of theory-making and research in psychology and related fields. The question is: In light of advances in our science, is it possible to integrate, within a unitary framework, the dispositional (trait) and processing (social-cognitive–affective–dynamic) approaches that have so long been split virtually into two separate fields (e.g., Mischel & Shoda, 1994, 1998)?

PERSONALITY DISPOSITIONS AND PROCESSING DYNAMICS: COMPETING APPROACHES OR TWO SIDES OF ONE SYSTEM?

The first or *dispositional approach* and trait theory in recent years, led by the five-factor model (e.g., McCrae & Costa, 1996), identifies a few broad stable traits, factors, or behavioral dispositions to be the basic units for characterizing and understanding individuals and the differences among them. The fundamental goal is to characterize all people in terms of a comprehensive but small set of such stable *behavioral dispositions* or factors on which they differ. These factors are assumed to remain invariant across situations and to determine a broad range of important behaviors (e.g., Allport, 1937; Funder, 1991; Goldberg, 1993; Wiggins & Pincus, 1992). In this vein, empirical research has examined the breadth and durability of these differences across diverse situations, and their predictive utility (e.g., Hogan, Johnson, & Briggs, 1997; Roberts, Kuncel, Shiner, Caspi, & Goldberg, 2007).

The second or *processing approach* construes personality as an organized system of mediating units (e.g., encodings, expectancies, goals, motives) and psychological processes or cognitive–affective dynamics, conscious and unconscious, that interact with the situation the individual experiences (e.g., Cervone & Shoda, 1999; Mischel, 1973, 1990). In this view, in the last 30 years, the basic con-

cern has been to discover general principles about how the mind operates and influences social behavior as the person interacts with social situations, conceptualized within a broadly social-cognitive theoretical framework (e.g., Bandura, 1986; Cantor, 1994, Cantor & Kihlstrom, 1987; Higgins, 1990, 1996b, 1996c; Mischel, 1973, 1990; Mischel & Shoda, 1995; Pervin, 1990, 1994).

Each approach has its strengths and its distinctive vulnerabilities (Mischel, 1998a; Mischel et al., 2008). As trait psychologists are quick to note, while the general principles that emerge from research on social cognition and social learning are valuable, one can challenge their relevance for understanding some of the most essential aspects of personality. Perhaps the most common critique by traditional personality psychologists of social-cognitive processing approaches is that they contain lists of seemingly disconnected personality processes and they simply do not explain (or often do not even address) the coherent functioning of the whole person (Mischel, 1999). Thus although these principles, both singly and collectively, advance our understanding of basic social-cognitive–motivational processes, they must be applied in concert to understand the individual as an organized, coherent, functioning system—the fundamental unit of analysis to which personality psychology has been committed from its start (Allport, 1937). In addition, processing approaches also have been criticized for ignoring "what people are like" in general terms, neglecting the stable dispositional differences between individuals and thus missing the essence of the personality construct. In this vein, Funder (1994), for example, urges a return to a neo-Allportian global dispositional approach in which people are characterized in broad dispositional terms with the language of traits.

On the other side, however, trait-dispositional approaches are vulnerable to the criticism that they do not adequately consider, or even address, the psychological processes and dynamics that underlie behavioral dispositions and are of little utility for facilitating behavioral change, for example, in psychotherapy (e.g., Block, 1995; Mischel, 1968; Pervin, 1994). To make this point, Epstein drew a vivid analogy with the assessment of automobiles (Epstein, 1994). Like people, automobiles are readily characterized according to certain dimensions: Are they gas guzzlers or economical? Are they clunky or speedy? Silent or noisy? Sexy and sporty or staid, quiet, and conservative? Such generalizations are, of course, useful in orienting buyers toward a particular brand or type, but only provide distal cues about the mechanisms that lead to these differences—about what is going on under the hood (Cervone, 2005). As a result, characterization of an automobile as sporty and economical does not help much when your car breaks down in the middle of nowhere, and you try to repair it (Epstein, 1994).

It is obviously essential for personality psychology to take serious account of important, stable differences between people. The question is not the existence of such differences but rather how to capture (1) the nature of the stability and consistency that exists in the behavioral expressions of individual differences relevant to personality, and (2) the psychological processes and structures that underlie those expressions and that function in a coherent fashion. The stable differences between people in their behavioral tendencies and qualities of temperament or other social-cognitive–affective characteristics and behavior patterns need to be captured. But they also need to be understood and explained in terms of the psychological processes that characterize the intra-individual dynamics of persons and not just described in trait terms.

Advances in theory and research in the last few decades have led to the development of at least the framework for such a unifying theory of personality (Cervone & Shoda, 1999; Mischel & Shoda, 1995, 1998; Shoda & Mischel, 1998), which is the focus of the present chapter. We hope to show that personality dispositions and the psychological processes that underlie them are two aspects of the same personality system. They therefore need to be integrated within a unifying theory rather than split into alternative or even competing fields. That goal is now becoming feasible in light of rapidly accumulating findings on the nature of the consistencies and coherence that characterizes individuals (e.g., Borkenau, Riemann, Spinath, & Angleitner, 2006; Fournier, Moskowitz, & Zuroff, 2008; Mischel & Shoda, 1995; Shoda et al., 1994). A comprehensive, unifying theory of personality also needs to build on, and incorporate, the enduring contributions that have come from a century of psychological work directly relevant to developing a science of personality (see Mischel et al., 2008, for a review). In this chapter, we also indicate how these contributions are integrated within the type of unifying meta-theory represented by the Cognitive–Affective Processing System (CAPS) framework.

A COGNITIVE–AFFECTIVE PROCESSING SYSTEM

A theoretical integration that reconciles dispositions and the psychological processes that underlie them within a comprehensive theory of personality needs at its foundation a processing model of the personality system at the level of the individual (Mischel & Shoda, 1995). In such a model, person variables are important, and it is valuable to understand the basic psychological processes underlying, for example, how people construe or encode situations and themselves, their self-efficacy expectations and beliefs, their goals, and so on, as has long been recognized (e.g., Mischel, 1973). But these variables do not function singly and in isolation; rather, they are components that are dynamically interconnected within an organized system of relationships, a unique network that functions as a whole, and that interacts with the social–psychological situations in which the system is activated and contextualized (e.g., Shoda & Mischel, 1998).

An adequate personality system also must account for intra-individual coherence and stability within the person as well as for plasticity and discriminativeness in adaptive behavior across situations. It must encompass the individual's characteristic dispositions as well as the dynamic mediating processes that underlie them. Moreover, it needs to incorporate not only social-cognitive–motivational and affective determinants but also biological and genetic antecedents. And this system must be able to deal with the complexity of human personality and the cognitive–affective dynamics, conscious and unconscious—both "cool" and "hot," cognitive and emotional, rational and impulsive—that underlie the individual's distinctive, characteristic internal states and external behavioral expressions (see Metcalfe & Jacobs, 1998; Metcalfe & Mischel, 1999). In such a system the individual is not conceptualized as a bundle of mediating variables and procedural decision rules or as fixed points on dimensions. Instead, in this view the individual is a complex, multi-level, parallel and distributed (rather than serial, centralized) social information processing system (e.g., Kunda & Thagard, 1996; Read & Miller, 1998; Shultz & Lepper, 1996) that operates cognitively and emotionally at various levels of awareness (e.g., Westen, 1990). The Cognitive–Affective Processing System, or CAPS theory (Mischel & Shoda, 1995, 1998; Shoda & Mischel, 1998), was developed in part to move personality psychology in this direction, connecting it to advances in related fields as well as within personality and social psychology.

TWO BASIC ASSUMPTIONS

With the above ambitious goals, but also with a commitment to parsimony, CAPS theory makes two fundamental assumptions. Namely:

Individual Differences in Chronic Accessibility

CAPS theory assumes, first, that people differ in the *chronic accessibility*, that is, the ease, with which particular cognitive and affective mental representations or units, called CAUs, become activated. These CAUs refer to the cognitions and affects or feelings that are available to the person. Such mediating units were conceptualized initially in terms of five relatively stable person variables on which individuals differ in processing self-relevant information, such as individuals' encodings or construal (of self, other people, situations) and expectancies (Mischel, 1973). In the years since that formulation, research developments (reviewed in Mischel & Shoda, 1995) have suggested a set of CAUs, largely based on the person variables previously proposed, that are represented in the personality system, as summarized in Table 7.1. Namely, encodings or construals, efficacy and outcome expectancies, beliefs, goals and values, affects and feeling states, as well as competencies and self-regulatory plans and

strategies, exemplify the types of units in the system that interact as the individual selects, interprets, and generates situations.

The cognitive–affective units in the system are not conceptualized as isolated, static components. They are organized, for example, into subjective equivalence classes, as illustrated in theory and research on encoding, person prototypes, and personal constructs, (e.g., Cantor & Mischel, 1977, 1979; Cantor, Mischel, & Schwartz, 1982; Higgins, King, Mavin, 1982; Forgas, 1983a, 1983b; Kelly, 1955; Linville & Clark, 1989; Vallacher & Wegner, 1987). Some aspects of the organization of relations among the cognitions and affects, such as evaluative-affective associations, and inter-concept relations (e.g., Cantor & Kihlstrom, 1987; Mendoza-Denton & Mischel, 2007; Murphy & Medin, 1985), are common among members of a culture, whereas others may be unique for an individual (e.g., Rosenberg & Jones, 1972). But whether common or unique, cognitive–affective representations are not unconnected units that are simply elicited as discrete "responses" in isolation; rather, these cognitive representations and affective states interact dynamically and influence each other reciprocally. It is the organization of the relationships among them that forms the core of the personality structure and that guides and constrains their effects.

TABLE 7.1. Types of Cognitive–Affective Units in the Personality Mediating System

1. *Encodings*: Categories (constructs) for the self, people, events, and situations (external and internal).
2. *Expectancies and beliefs*: About the social world, about outcomes for behavior in particular situations, about self-efficacy.
3. *Affects*: Feelings, emotions, and affective responses (including physiological reactions).
4. *Goals and values*: Desirable outcomes and affective states; aversive outcomes and affective states; goals, values, and life projects.
5. *Competencies and self-regulatory plans*: Potential behaviors and scripts, and plans and strategies for organizing action and for affecting outcomes and one's own behavior and internal states.

Note. From Mischel (1973, p. 275). Copyright 1973 by the American Psychological Association. Adapted by permission.

Individual Differences in the Stable Organization of Interconnections among Units

Thus the CAPS model makes a second assumption: Individual differences reflect not only the accessibility of particular cognitions and affects but also the distinctive *organization of relationships* among them (see Figure 7.1, which shows a schematic, greatly simplified CAPS system). This organization constitutes the basic, stable *structure of the personality system* and underlies the behavioral expressions that characterize the individual. It is this organization that guides and constrains the activation of the particular cognitions, affects, and actions that are available within the system.

As Figure 7.1 illustrates, when the individual perceives certain features of a situation, a characteristic pattern of cognitions and affects (shown schematically as circles) becomes activated through this distinctive network of connections. Mediating units in the system become activated in relation to some situation features (positive connections) but are deactivated or inhibited in relation to others (negative connections, shown as broken lines). The CAPS system interacts continuously and dynamically with the social world in which it is contextualized. The interactions with the external word involve a two-way reciprocal interaction: The behaviors that the personality system generates influence the interpersonal situations the person subsequently faces and that, in turn, influence the person (e.g., Bandura, 1986; Buss, 1987; Mischel, 1973).

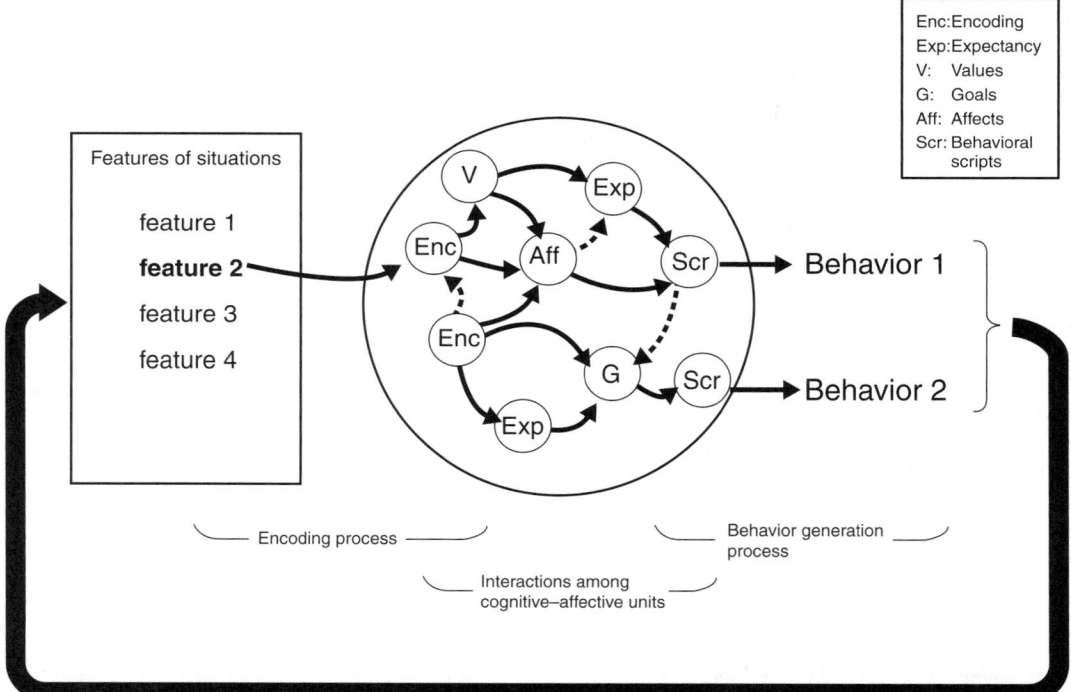

FIGURE 7.1. The Cognitive–Affective Processing System (CAPS). Situational features activate a given mediating unit, which activates specific subsets of other mediating units through a stable network of relations that characterizes an individual, generating a characteristic pattern of behavior in response to different situations. The relation may be positive (solid line), which increases the activation, or negative (dashed line), which decreases the activation. From Mischel and Shoda (1995, p. 254). Copyright 1995 by the American Psychological Association. Adapted by permission.

APPLYING THE CAPS FRAMEWORK

CAPS is a meta-theory. A meta-theory provides the building blocks and "the requirements for a more specific theoretical model of intra-individual personality structure" (Cervone, Shadel, Smith, & Fiori, 2006, p. 19). In biology, a fundamental metatheory is that DNA contains genetic information. It tells us where to look for genetic information and spells out the rule with which information is coded and decoded. Based on this, a biologist constructs a specific theory of how a given organism functions.

Similarly, in the CAPS model each individual is characterized by a distinctive pattern and strength of associations among mental representations. Based on this, if one is interested in why one individual succeeds in his or her effort to quit smoking whereas another individual fails to do so, one asks questions such as, how strongly is the concept of smoking associated with that of *relaxing* or *socializing*? This then allows one to understand why seemingly the same social contexts lead one person to smoke, whereas another person successfully resists the urge to smoke.

CAPS as a Guide for Constructing Content-Full, Domain-Specific Theories

To illustrate the basic principles of the CAPS model, Figure 7.1 is necessarily oversimplified and generic. For example, some of the small circles refer to mental representations. But representations of what? And just how many such representations are there? An individual's mind contains an immense number of mental representations. But not all of them are equally important in any given situation or sets of situations. The particular mental representations that are important depend on the individual, the behavior one wants to predict, and the situations in which these behaviors are expected to occur. Therefore the small circles in Figure 7.1 are deliberately left unfilled. The potential power, as well as the challenge, of the CAPS model comes from its ability to generate a locally optimized, specific theory—a theory that is guided by general principles but that is targeted to the specific problem and goals of interest.

Historically, nomothetic theories of personality, starting with the humors of the ancient Greeks, sought generalizability by proposing that the same handful of qualities, such as conscientiousness and open-mindedness, accounted for most behaviors of most people in most situations. Similarly, biology's meta-theory that a DNA sequence contains genetic information is generalizable precisely because it leaves up to the researchers the identification of a particular gene and its function. A meta-theoretical framework such as the CAPS model approaches the same goals in a very different fashion. It seeks generalizability by providing the conceptual and methodological tools in the form of simple and generalizable components and principles, but it leaves the task of identifying the qualities up to empirical investigation and the investigator. The meta-theory thus provides general principles and conceptualizations for building a theory about a particular behavior and the dynamics that underlie it, such as the dynamics of rejection sensitivity under conditions of relationship threat (e.g., Ayduk, Downey, Testa, Yen, & Shoda, 1999; Ayduk et al., 2000), or about the struggles of the narcissist to maintain a grandiose self-concept when faced with evidence of personal failure (e.g., Morf, 2006). To illustrate these points, we consider an example of how the general CAPS network has been used to construct models of domain-specific behavior, namely reactions to the verdict in the highly controversial O. J. Simpson criminal trial (for another example, see Miller, Shoda, & Hurley, 1996).

CAPS Analysis of Reactions to the O. J. Simpson Trial Verdict

In this study, the CAPS meta-theory was used to generate a specific theory of the passionately diverse emotional reactions aroused by the O. J. Simpson murder trial verdict. Mendoza-Denton, Ayduk, Shoda, and Mischel (1997) did an empirical investigation of the thoughts and feelings that become activated when people were reminded of various aspects of the trial. Figures 7.2 and 7.3 illustrate the processing dynamics that mediate between situational features in the environment and people's responses to them. For example, the researchers traced the thought patterns within two groups: the *dismayed* and the *elated*. The statements in quotations are verbatim quotes from respondents; the numbers in parentheses show corresponding arrow numbers within the maps being discussed.[1]

The Dismayed

Figure 7.2 indicates that Simpson's escape in the Bronco, the physical evidence, and his past history of spousal abuse all positively activated thoughts that he was guilty (1–4). These cognitions inhibited recognition of the argument that the evidence may have been questionable (5–7). Information related to police detective Mark Fuhrman led to thoughts that "the trial should not have been turned into a debate on racism" (8), which

further strengthened the idea that the evidence was solid (9), while inhibiting the idea that the evidence may have been tainted (10). Thoughts that "the fact that he was famous in America exonerated him from wrongdoing" (21), and thoughts about his domestic abuse (22) further strengthened the idea that the "not guilty" verdict was wrong (23) and led to dismay over it (24).

The Elated

Figure 7.3 represents a prototypical cognitive–affective dynamic that led to elation in reaction to the verdict. Some respondents noted that Nicole Brown Simpson "had always been using drugs, borrowing money, and

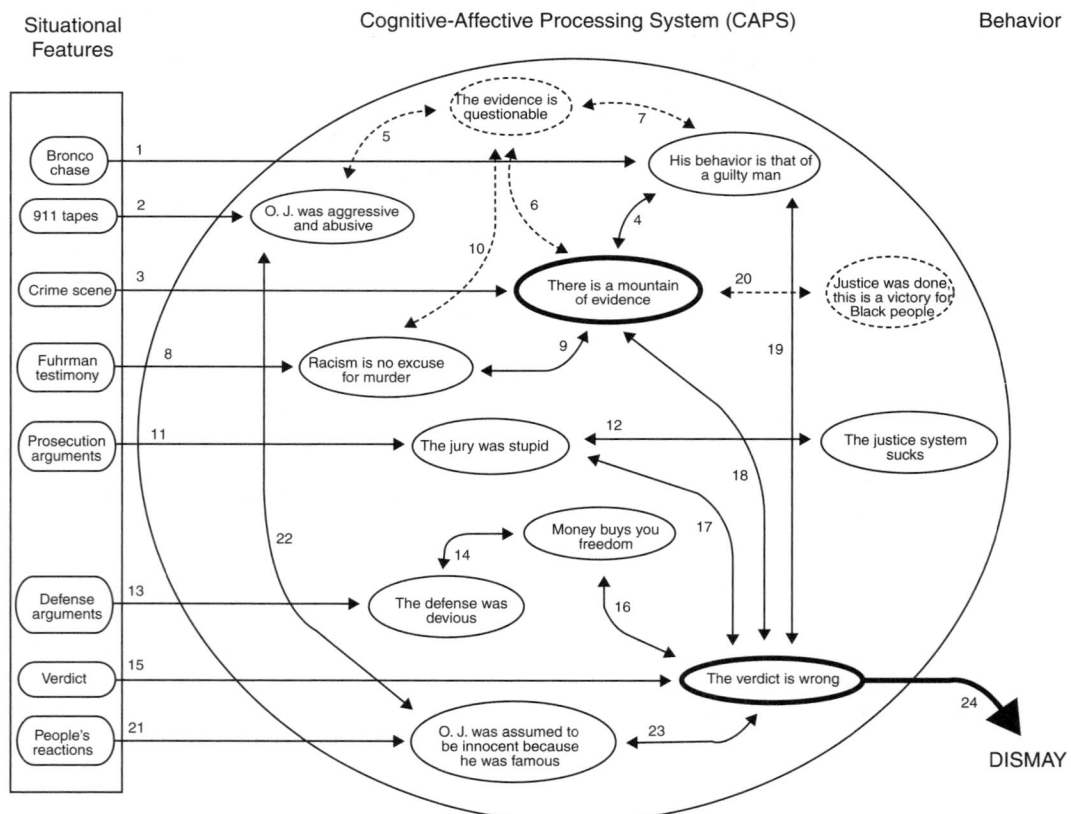

FIGURE 7.2. CAPS network typical of those who were dismayed by the Simpson criminal trial verdict. Solid lines indicate positive (activating) relations among units; broken lines indicate negative (deactivating) relations. The darkness of a thought unit corresponds to its accessibility. Dashed units indicate inhibited thoughts in the system. From Mendoza-Denton, Ayduk, Shoda, and Mischel (1997, p. 575). Copyright 1997 by Blackwell Publishing. Adapted by permission.

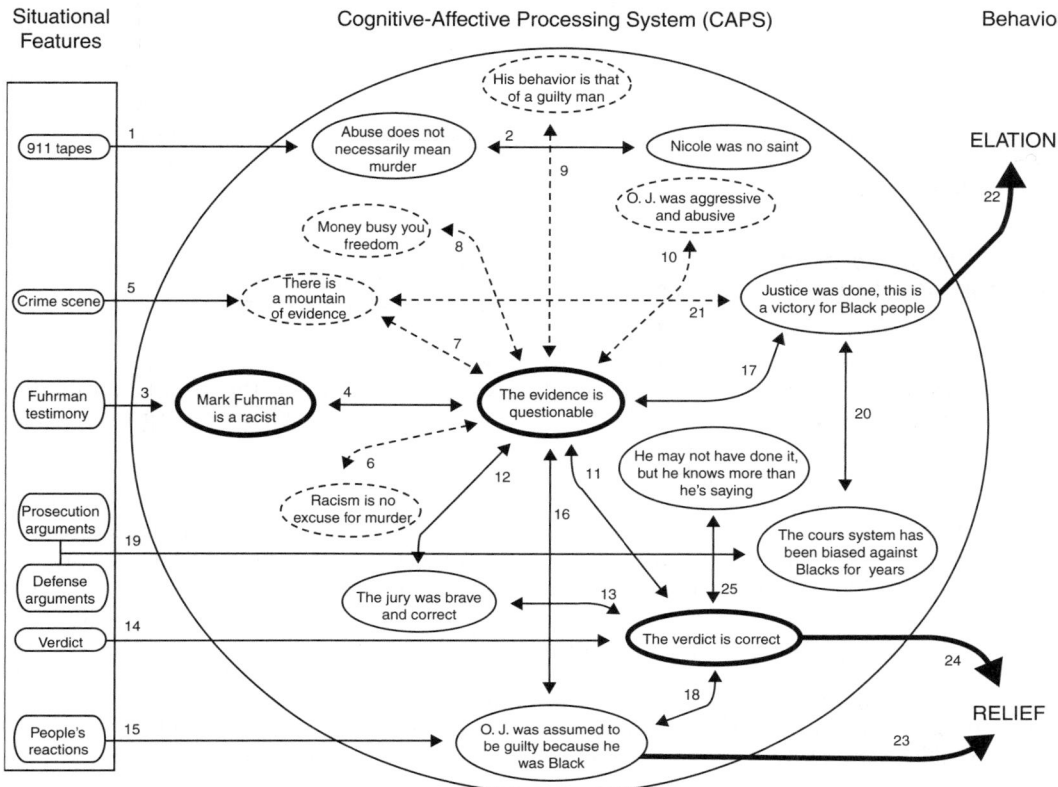

FIGURE 7.3. CAPS network typical of those who were elated by the Simpson criminal trial verdict. Solid lines indicate positive (activating) relations among units; broken lines indicate negative (deactivating) relations. The darkness of a thought unit corresponds to its accessibility. Dashed units indicate inhibited thoughts in the system. From Mendoza-Denton, Ayduk, Shoda, and Mischel (1997, p. 577). Copyright 1997 by Blackwell Publishing. Adapted by permission.

drinking and sleeping around" (2), that "Mark Fuhrman is a racist cop" (3), and that "the evidence is questionable" (4). The idea that the evidence was questionable in turn inhibited many of the thoughts that were highly accessible to the dismayed (6–10). To the elated, the evidence seemed dubious, the verdict was just (11), the jury "made a brave decision" (12, 13), and these thoughts further increased their skepticism about the evidence (14–18).

In sum, the figures illustrate qualitatively different dynamics that underlie different emotional reactions to the verdict. Describing the two types merely by the reaction (e.g., "dismayed" vs. "elated") would obscure the important differences in the underlying dynamics. Indeed, the main prediction

from these figures is not that a person whose cognitive–affective dynamics resemble Figure 7.2 is more likely to be in a bad mood more than a person who resembles Figure 7.3. In fact, it probably is not true that those who were elated upon hearing the "not guilty" Simpson verdict were generally less distressed than those who were dismayed on the same occasion.

Instead, the figures predict that *when* a person whose system resembles Figure 7.2 activates a certain thought (e.g., "O. J. was aggressive and abusive"), *then* he or she is likely to be thinking "O. J. was assumed to be innocent because he was famous." That is, the behavioral manifestation of the domain-specific theory depicted in Figure 7.2 is an intra-individual *if … then …* pattern, or "behavioral signature." This point is also supported by computer simulations showing that network models of the type depicted in the figure generally lead to distinct patterns of *if … then …* behavioral signatures, characterizing how behavior varies within a given person (Shoda, 2007).

A Person-Centered Approach to the Individual as a Dynamic Cognitive–Affective System

The previous example illustrates how the specific applications of the meta-theory to particular domains of behavior begin to reveal the unique configuration of individuals' cognitive–affective networks. It also underlines the fundamental difference in approach with the meta-theory that guides traditional personality psychology. In the CAPS approach, generalizability comes from the broad applicability of its basic principles for building domain-specific theories, while the predictive power comes from its domain specificity.

Biology again offers an analogy here. Biologists try to understand the functioning of each species separately first, before seeking cross-species generalization. They do not try to build a model of "plants in general" or "mammals in general" or view species as a cluster of variables, such as "bird-ness," "mammal-ness," or size, shape, number of limbs, presence of feathers, and so on, examining the "effects" of each of these characteristics in a regression equation. Rather, they take each species one at a time and study the functions of its structure, as encoded by the unique DNA sequence that defines that species. Yet in developing an understanding of specific species, they apply their meta-theory: the fundamental principles by which the DNA sequence affects the development and functioning of all species. And they also utilize a general set of conceptual and analytical tools, in order to discover the species-specific mechanisms.

CAPS is a meta-theory for building theories to account for individuals' characteristic intra-individual dynamics. The principles basic to the CAPS meta-theory suggest a view of people not as an operationalization of variables, but rather as a distinctive social–cognitive–affective system. It is a system that dynamically interacts with situations and generates contextualized thoughts, feelings, and behaviors. In this framework, one route for pursuing generalizable knowledge is by enabling domain-specific theories that can identify types of individuals who are similar in their cognitive–affective social information processing system.

MULTIPLE LEVELS IN THE EXPRESSIONS AND ANALYSIS OF PERSONALITY

CAPS expands the conception of personality to contextualize the individual within the social world. This view of the person within a person–environment system allows us to examine the reciprocal interaction. The person's behavior affects how the environment responds, which in turn generates the situation the person faces. These continuous person–situation interactions raise further questions about the dynamics of development and change in personality over the life trajectory. The outlines for a view of the person–environmental system and its developmental origin are shown in Figure 7.4.

At a first level is the psychological processing system of personality with its structures and the *processing dynamics* in the cognitive–affective system that become activated within it. Second, the expressions and manifestations of the system are visible at the level of the individual's characteristic *behaviors* (including *thoughts and feelings*) as they unfold *in vivo* across situations and over time (shown in the situation–behavior, *if … then …* profile data in the figure). At a third level are the *perceptions* of personality and of the person's behavior, including the individual's self-perceptions (as indicated by the eye shown in Figure 7.4). A fourth level consists of the stable personal environment of situations that come to characterize the individual's life space (depicted as the inputs into the system). Finally, at the fifth level are the *pre*-dispositions, consisting of genetic-biochemical, somatic structures and states, as well as the cumulative social learning and sociocultural influences that constitute the person's total history and current endowment. All of these levels, and the interactions among them, are relevant to personality; each is discussed from the CAPS framework in the remainder of this chapter.

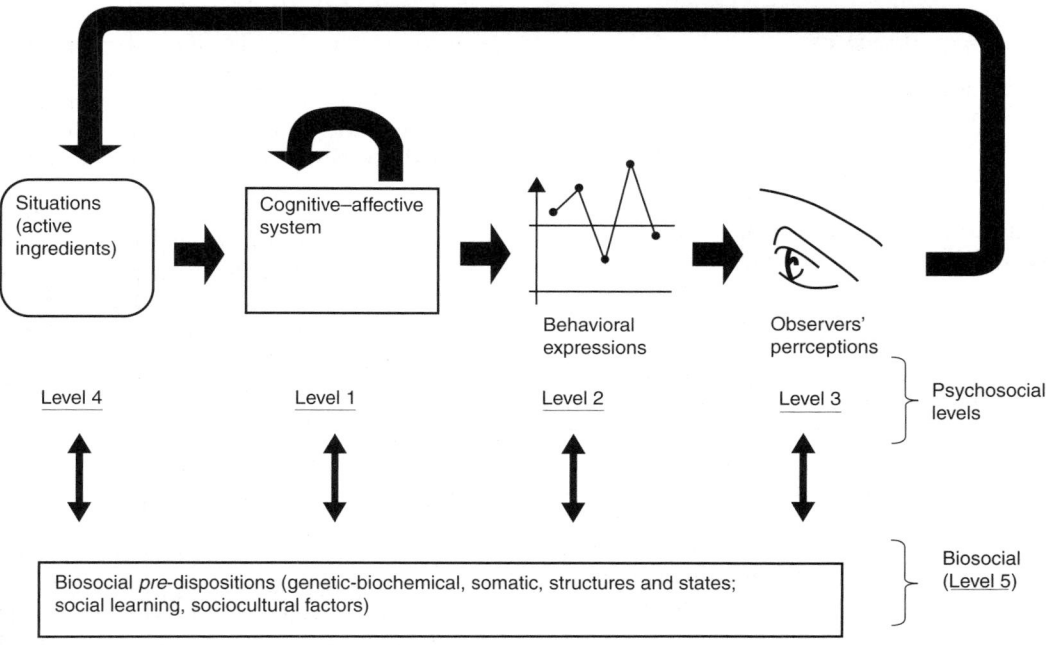

FIGURE 7.4. Personality stability and invariance: Five levels of analysis. From Mischel and Shoda (1995, p. 262). Copyright 1995 by the American Psychological Association. Adapted by permission.

Level 1: Processing Dynamics of Personality

At the processing system level, CAPS theory conceptualizes dispositions as having distinctive cognitive–affective processing structures that underlie and generate characteristic processing dynamics (Mischel & Shoda, 1995). In this section we define and illustrate these dynamics and discuss how they operate.

Processing Dynamics Defined

The *processing dynamics* of a disposition consist of an organized pattern and sequence of activation among cognitive–affective mediating units in CAPS that are generated when persons with this disposition experience situations with relevant features (e.g., rejection cues, failure cues, achievement cues). As an example (in highly simplified form) of the processing dynamics for a disposition or personality prototype (Cantor & Mischel, 1979), consider the construct of "rejection sensitivity" (e.g., Downey, Freitas, Michaelis, & Khouri, 1998; Feldman & Downey, 1994). Many rejection-sensitive

persons have had histories of exposure to family violence and rejection. Later in life, when they encounter what could be perceived as uncaring behavior from a romantic partner (e.g., he or she is attentive to someone else), they easily experience thoughts such as "She doesn't love me," which in turn trigger expectations of rejection, abandonment, and associated emotions. These expectations and affects interact and combine to lead the person to readily perceive rejection even in ambiguous situations. In turn, perceived rejection tends to activate behavioral scripts for hostility (Ayduk et al., 1999). A wide range of controlling and coercive behaviors may be enacted and often are blamed on the behavior of the partner rather than seen as self-generated. These behaviors in turn tend to elicit the partner rejection that is most feared. Over time this process increasingly erodes the relationship in a self-defeating pattern that ultimately confirms and maintains rejection expectations and strengthens the vicious cycle (Downey et al., 1998).

Incorporating the Psychological Situation into Personality Dynamics

As the rejection-sensitivity example indicates, CAPS theory incorporates the situation into the conception of the personality processing dynamics that characterize the individual and the type: The situation activates the processing dynamics and in part defines them. But although the situation plays an important role in this model, it is not conceptualized as a simple external stimulus, unlike how situations were conceptualized in early behaviorism as mechanically evoking responses from an organism's repertoire. In CAPS theory it is the person, or more precisely, the *personality system*, that is sensitized to particular features of situations and ready to scan for, and potentially over-react to, them in an organized, predictable pattern. In the example of rejection-sensitive persons, this is seen in their tendency to scan for and find potential rejection cues even in ambiguous situations, which then triggers their vulnerable, characteristic pattern of reactions.

Most important, CAPS theory (Shoda et al., 1994) distinguishes between *nominal situations* (e.g., meeting in the dean's office) and the *active ingredients* or *psychological features* of situations (e.g., having your ideas rejected). "Nominal situations" refer to the particular places and activities in the particular setting, for example, woodworking activities in a summer camp, or arithmetic tests and dining halls, or playgrounds in a school setting (e.g., Hartshorne & May, 1928; Newcomb, 1929). Individual differences in relation to such specific nominal situations, even if highly stable, would be of limited generalizability. These are valid and reliable definitions, but they don't tell us what aspects of each situation are responsible for the observed pattern of behavior variation. If Mary is usually relaxed in the nominal situation "meeting with Jane" but often tense in the situation "having lunch with Joe," will she be anxious when picking up a job candidate at the airport? It is this lack of generalizability that made demonstrations of situation specificity a threat to the fundamental goal of personality psychology. It is therefore important to try to characterize "situations" in terms of their common psychological features (Shoda & LeeTiernan, 2002). Once the

feature of the situation to which the individual is responding is identified (e.g., having one's ideas rejected by an authority), predictive generalization to other situations that contain known features becomes possible, even if those situations are nominally quite different.

There has been an increasing call for a systematic analysis of the "stimulus field" (e.g., Kelley, 1997). Such top-down approaches to this challenge (e.g., Kelley et al., 2003) can also be complemented by seeking to develop a comprehensive, ground-up methodology (e.g., Zayas, Whitsett, Lee, Wilson, & Shoda, in press). Ultimately, identifying the psychological features of situations may provide a language to understand the meaning of various social situations for the individuals who experience them.

This challenge is analogous to one faced by an allergy specialist. Suppose a patient has reliably identified that he has an allergic reaction every time he eats breakfast cereal brands A and E, but he can eat brands B, C, and D without problems. Note that the "situations"—the brands of cereal—are defined nominally. The pattern of variation in the patient's reactions across the situations (brands of cereal) is reliable and reflects some stable characteristics of his immune system. But to go further and predict whether or not he can safely eat brand X, a new brand he has not tried before, it would first be necessary to identify just what it is about brands A and E that causes the allergic reaction.

If social situations are analyzed to capture their basic psychological features (i.e., the active ingredients that impact on the person's behavior), it becomes possible to predict behavior across a broad range of contexts that contain the same psychological features (Shoda et al., 1994). People differ characteristically in the particular situational features (e.g., being teased, being frustrated, being approached socially, feeling rejected) that are the salient active ingredients for them and that thus activate their characteristic and relatively predictable patterns of cognitions and affects in those situations—that is, their distinctive processing dynamics (Mischel & Shoda, 1995).

Equally important, there also are internal feedback loops within the system through which self-generated stimuli (e.g., thinking, fantasy, daydreaming) serve as "internal situations." They also activate the individual's personality dynamics, triggering characteristic cognitive–affective–behavioral reaction patterns (e.g., Shoda & Mischel, 1998). The features of situations that activate the person's processing dynamics are generated internally within the personality system through thought, planning, fantasy, and imagination (e.g., Antrobus, 1991; Gollwitzer, 1996; Klinger, 1996; Mischel, Shoda, & Rodriguez, 1989; Nolen-Hoeksema, Parker, & Larson, 1994). And they encompass not just social and interpersonal situations (as when lovers "reject" or peers "tease and provoke") but also internal situations, as in mood states (e.g., Isen, Niedenthal, & Cantor, 1992; Schwarz, 1990) as well as in the everyday stream of experience and feeling (e.g., Bolger & Eckenrode, 1991; Emmons, 1991; C. A. Smith & Lazarus, 1990; Wright & Mischel, 1988).

Personality States

The pattern of activation among cognitions and affects that exists at a given time in this system is the *personality state*, and it depends on the particular context and the psychological situations experienced by the individual at that moment. Whereas the personality system and its structure or organization can remain stable across diverse situations, the personality state can change easily when the situational features that are active change (e.g., Mischel & Shoda, 1995). But the change is not random. It is guided by the personality system, which mediates the *relationships* between the types of situations encountered and the cognitive, affective, and behavioral reaction patterns—the dynamics—that become activated. Thus, if the situations change, so do the reactions patterns to them, but the *relationship* between the situations and the reaction patterns is stable as long as the personality system remains unchanged. This assumption leads CAPS theory to predict characteristic, predictable patterns of *variation* in the individual's behavior across situations—that is, the sorts of stable situation–behavior, *if ... then ...* profiles that are found in empirical studies of the structure of social behavior in relation to situations and over time (Mischel

& Shoda, 1995; Shoda et al., 1994). These patterns are discussed further in a later section on the behavioral expressions of the personality system.

Identifying features of situations is only half the challenge. The other half is an assessment of the CAPS network, describing how, within a given individual, a particular situational feature (e.g., Joe's facial features that remind Mary of her father) activates cognitive (e.g., a memory of the father's disdain for mediocrity) and emotional (e.g., Mary's anxiety) reactions. Combining this CAPS network assessment with assessments of situations in relation to their psychological characteristics should facilitate more specific predictions of a given individual's reaction to particular types of psychological situations. This goal is a formidable challenge, particularly because individuals are often not aware of the associations among their thoughts. Thus it becomes important to develop empirical methodologies for the assessment of automatic (i.e., not consciously controlled) associations among personally significant cognitions and affects.

Probing the Associations in the Network

In recent years, research has demonstrated the value and feasibility of assessing links between specific cognitive, affective, and behavioral reactions. For example, links between situation features and cognitive and emotional reactions have repeatedly been shown to underlie the phenomenon of "transference" (Andersen & Chen, 2002; English & Chen, 2007). Another approach for assessing strengths of automatic associations within each individual's CAPS network utilizes implicit measures, such as the Implicit Association Test (Greenwald, McGhee, & Schwartz, 1998). For example, people with secure attachment styles, compared to those with insecure styles, were shown to have stronger automatic associations between the concept of their current romantic partner and positive reactions (Zayas & Shoda, 2005). For these individuals, thoughts about their partner more strongly (compared to insecure individuals) activated positive reactions. Furthermore, the strength of such associations was found to be meaningfully related to relationship outcomes, such as greater satisfaction and emotional commitment.

Basic findings in research on brain activities also are leading to promising new methods for personality researchers to probe more deeply into the internal processes of the personality system. Specifically, a particular component of electroencephalogram (EEG) waves in response to an event, called N400, has been shown to be magnified when participants analyze the semantic meaning of words. Applying this finding and methodology to the social and personality domain, greater N400 reactions are observed when women encounter a negative interpersonal outcome (e.g., partner's inattention) in response to a bid for a partner's support, compared to encountering the same situation in more neutral contexts (Zayas et al., 2008). Furthermore, women who were anxiously attached and low in attachment avoidance (also referred to as preoccupied with attachment) showed the greatest reaction to rejection words, as assessed by the N400.

The focus on the analysis of psychological features of situations, and identifying individuals' behavioral signatures with regard to such features, also requires expanding the general paradigms used for social and personality psychology research. Specifically, traditional research designs examine individuals' reactions to a single situation, their reaction to an unspecified situation, or an average of their reactions to multiple situations. Such designs have intrinsic limitations for discovering patterns of psychological regularities within each person. To address this problem, one may adopt an alternative approach, which might be called a "highly repeated within subject design" (Shoda, 2003). Application of this method (Shoda & LeeTiernan, 2002; Zayas & Shoda, 2007) allows a systematic and quantitative characterization of individual-level situation–behavior relations by within-subject regression analyses. These individual-level characterizations can in turn be predicted from individual-difference variables, using a multilevel modeling approach (e.g., hierarchical linear modeling [HLM]), as discussed by Zayas and colleagues (in press).

Hot and Cool Processing Subsystems and Their Dynamic Interactions

The characteristic reactions of the personality system to situations often are immediate, automatic, emotional, and virtually reflexive. But just as often they are highly mediated and reflective, involving higher-order cognitive processes, as when the individual exerts effortful control strategies to prevent impulsive responses to "hot" trigger stimuli. To deal with these phenomena within a CAPS framework, and to incorporate the long-neglected but crucial role of emotion into the personality system, a distinction has been made between two subsystems, one a "hot" emotional "go" system, and one a "cool" cognitive "know" system, which closely interact (Metcalfe & Mischel, 1999).

The *hot system* is specialized for quick emotional processing and responding based on unconditional or conditional trigger features, as when rejection-sensitive people become abusive to their partners as automatic reactions to perceived rejection cues. Conceptualized as the basis of emotionality, fears, as well as passions—impulsive and reflexive— initially controlled by innate releasing stimuli (and thus literally under "stimulus control"), it is fundamental for emotional (classical) conditioning, and it undermines efforts at self-control, reflective thought, and planfulness (Metcalfe & Mischel, 1999). In contrast, the *cool cognitive system* is specialized for complex spatio-temporal and episodic representation and thought. Because it is cognitive, it is emotionally neutral, contemplative, flexible, integrated, coherent, spatio-temporal, slow, episodic, strategic—the seat of self-regulation and self-control.

The balance between the hot and cool systems is determined by stress, developmental level, and the individual's self-regulatory dynamics. Whereas stress—both chronic and situational—enhances the hot system and attenuates the cool system, with increasing development and maturation, the cool system becomes more developed and active, and the impact of the hot system becomes attenuated. The interactions between these systems allow prediction and explanation of findings on diverse phenomena involving the interplay of emotion and cognition, including goal-directed delay of gratification and the operation of "willpower" and self-directed change. Thus strategic interventions may be used to influence the interaction of the hot and cool systems to overcome the power of stimulus control, as people attempt to purposefully prevent powerful stimuli from eliciting their impulsive, immediate responses and dispositional vulnerabilities.

Purposeful Change

CAPS theory also suggests ways in which individuals may be able to facilitate goal-directed change. For example, if they understand their processing dynamics, people may become able to anticipate the events and conditions that will activate certain cognitions and affects in them. Such meta-cognitive knowledge may help them to recognize some of the key internal or external stimuli that activate or deactivate their problematic emotional, cognitive, and behavioral dynamics, and to modify them if they prove to be maladaptive or dysfunctional. Such knowledge—a goal to which therapy might be directed—could help them influence their personality states and behaviors (e.g., Mischel & Mischel, 1983; Rodriguez, Mischel, & Shoda, 1989), for example, by avoiding some situations and selecting or generating others, to the degree that they know their own processing dynamics and the features of situations that activate them.

People can powerfully change the impact of situations by reconstruing or reframing them with alternative encodings, and by altering their own thoughts and feelings in relation to particular problem-producing situations that cannot themselves be changed. For example, self-generated changes in the mental representations of a stimulus by cognitively focusing on its potentially affect-arousing "hot," consummatory features, versus on its more abstract, "cool" or informative features "in imagination" may dramatically influence self-regulatory behaviors of considerable long-term personal significance (Mischel et al., 1989). This is seen experimentally when four-year-olds are primed to focus on "hot" consummatory features of rewards—such as a pretzel's crunchy, salty taste; they want them immediately and further delay to obtain them becomes extremely difficult. In contrast, a focus on the abstract features (e.g., how the pretzels are "like little logs") makes it easy for them to continue to wait in order to get them. By influencing the stimuli-as-encoded, or by focusing attention on selected mental representations, individuals can exert some control over their own cognitions and affects. They can select,

structure, influence, and reinterpret or cognitively and emotionally transform situations to which they are exposed, and thus are not merely passive victims of the situations or stimuli that are imposed on them (e.g., Eigsti et al., 2006; Kross, Ayduk, & Mischel, 2005; Mischel, 1996; Mischel, Cantor, & Feldman, 1996). They also can enhance their control over the environment through *if ... then ...* implementation planning strategies for achieving even highly difficult and distal goals, as elaborated in the work of Gollwitzer and colleagues (e.g., Gollwitzer, 1996; Gollwitzer & Bargh, 1996).

Research also shows how such mental operations can be harnessed as effective interventions to deal with intense negative feelings and experiences. An example of such intervention possibilities comes from research examining the common belief that in order to "get over" intense negative emotional experiences such as rejection by significant others, one needs to work through and understand those negative feelings. However, people's attempts to do this are often counterproductive, leading to rumination that increases distress (Nolen-Hoeksema, 1991; Teasdale, 1988). Kross and colleagues (2005), guided by CAPS and the hot–cool system model, facilitated "emotional cooling" by instructing participants to adopt a *psychologically distanced* perspective (i.e., take a step back and watch the conflict happening to them from a distance) immediately after cueing them to recall an intense anger-arousing experience. Such distancing helped people to cognitively re-represent their experiences and the emotions they elicited in relatively cool, cognitive terms, making sense of them and working through them without becoming overwhelmed by them or engulfed in rumination and depression. The overall findings help to explain when people's attempts to understand their negative feelings are likely to be adaptive and when they are likely to trigger rumination instead.

Level 2: Behavioral Expressions of Personality

CAPS theory suggests that the second level of personality can be seen in the behavioral expressions of the processing system. The nature of the consistencies or coherences in these behavioral expressions of personality has been the focus of concern and intense debate in personality psychology for decades. This "consistency controversy" historically underlies much of the divisiveness between the two main approaches to personality that may still persist. The resolution of these issues is therefore a prerequisite for development of the integrative, unifying approach addressed in the present chapter, and is discussed next.

The Classic Consistency Problem

The belief that people are characterized by pervasive cross-situational consistencies in their behavior has been perhaps the most basic and intensely disputed assumption of personality psychology for most of the past century, defining much of the field's agenda (e.g., Mischel, 1968; Mischel & Shoda, 1995, 1998; Pervin, 1994). On the one hand, a belief in the consistency of personality is intuitively evident, captured as a fundamental principle in theories of impression formation: Perceivers expect consistency in the traits and behaviors of the perceived (e.g., Hamilton & Sherman, 1996). It is also the case, however, that the history of research in the pursuit of consistency at the behavioral level has long yielded perplexing results, marked by years of continuing disputes about the extent and nature of consistency and predictability in the individual's behavior across situations. The classic "personality paradox" has shown that such consistency is much less than our intuitions predict, and that the situation or context plays a crucial role in the regulation and structure of behavioral consistency (e.g., Bem & Allen, 1974; Krahe, 1990; Mischel, 1968; Mischel & Peake, 1982a, 1982b; Mischel & Shoda, 1998; Nisbett, 1980; Nisbett & Ross, 1980; Pervin, 1994; Ross & Nisbett, 1991; Shweder, 1975; Shweder & D'Andrade, 1980).

The Consistency Controversy Briefly Revisited

Throughout this consistency controversy, which arose early in the 20th century (e.g., Hartshorne & May, 1928) and continued over the years (e.g., Cervone & Shoda, 1999; Mischel, 2004; Pervin, 1994; Ross & Nisbett, 1991), the virtually unquestioned basic assumption was that personality consists of broad traits, expressed across many different situations as generalized, global

behavior tendencies. Given this assumption, the failure to find strong support for cross-situational consistency at the behavioral level, especially when juxtaposed with evidence for the importance of the situation (e.g., Ross & Nisbett, 1991), was often read as a basic threat to the construct of personality itself. The result was an unfortunate and prolonged "person versus situation" debate and a paradigm crisis in the field (e.g., Bem & Allen, 1974; Krahe, 1990; Magnusson & Endler, 1977; Mischel, 1968, 1984, 2007; Pervin, 1990, 1994).

After years of debate, culminating in the Carleton College study (Mischel & Peake, 1982a), consensus was reached about the state of the data: The average cross-situational consistency coefficient is nonzero, but not by much (Bem, 1983; Epstein, 1983; Funder, 1983). But there was, and remains, disagreement about how to interpret the data and proceed in the study of personality (e.g., as discussed in Mischel & Shoda, 1994, 1998; Pervin, 1994). The classic dispositional or trait approach generally has focused on the broad stable characteristics that differentiate individuals consistently on the whole, seeking evidence for the breadth and durability of these differences across diverse situations. Its most widely accepted strategy acknowledges the low cross-situational consistency in behavior found from situation to situation: It then systematically removes the situation by aggregating the individual's behavior on a given dimension (e.g., "conscientiousness") over many different situations (e.g., home, school, work) to estimate an overall "true score" (as discussed in Epstein, 1979, 1980; Mischel & Peake, 1982a), treating the variability across situations as "error."

Alternative Conception of Stability: Stable Situation–Behavior Relations

CAPS theory proposes a fundamentally different conception of personality invariance. Personality is construed as a relatively stable system of social-cognitive–affective mediating processes whose expressions are manifested in predictable patterns of situation–behavior relations; they therefore cannot be properly assessed unless the situation is incorporated into the conception and analysis of personality coherence (e.g., Mischel, 1973; Mischel & Shoda, 1995, 1998). In the analysis of the nature of personality invariance and its behavioral expressions, process models in general, and CAPS theory specifically, suggest that clues about the person's underlying qualities—the construals and goals, the motives and passions, that drive the individual—may be seen in *when* and *where* a type of behavior is manifested, not only in its overall frequency (Mischel, 1973; Mischel & Shoda, 1995, 1998).

Consider the differences between two people, A and B, whose behavior in a particular domain, for example, their helping behavior across situations, is shown on the horizontal axis of Figure 7.5.

In the traditional approach to behavioral dispositions, the observed variability within each person on a dimension is seen as "error" and averaged out to get the best approximation of the underlying stable "true score," so the question simply becomes: Is person A different overall in the level of helping behavior than person B? This question is important, and perhaps the best first question to ask in the analysis of personality invariance. But it may also be its premature end if we ignore the profile information about *when* and *where* A and B differ in their unique pattern with regard to the particular dimension of behavior. These differences in their pattern of variability in relation to situations may be a possible key to understanding individuality and personality coherence and their underlying motivations and personality systems. In that case, these patterns are potential signatures that need to be identified and harnessed rather than deliberately removed.

Empirical Evidence

As noted in the discussion of the assumptions of the CAPS model and its processing operations, in this theory, variation in the person's behavior in relation to changing situations in part constitutes a potentially meaningful reflection of the personality system itself. Empirical evidence to support this expectation came initially from a series of studies of social behavior as it unfolds *in vivo* in relation to situations. In these studies, the social behavior (e.g., "verbal aggression," "compliance") of children was systematically observed in relation to the inter-personal situations in which the behavior occurred in a residential summer camp setting. The results provided powerful evidence for behavioral signatures (e.g., Mischel & Shoda, 1995; Shoda, Mischel, & Wright, 1993b, 1994). Some children were found to be consistently more verbally aggressive than others when warned by an adult, for example, but were much less aggressive than most peers when peers approached them positively. In contrast, another group of children with a similar overall average level of aggression was distinguished by a striking and opposite pattern: They were more aggressive than any other children when peers approached them positively, but were exceptionally unaggressive when warned by an adult.

It is noteworthy that in classic trait approaches to behavioral dispositions, such intra-individual variations in a type of behavior across situations (after the effects of situations are removed by standardization) is

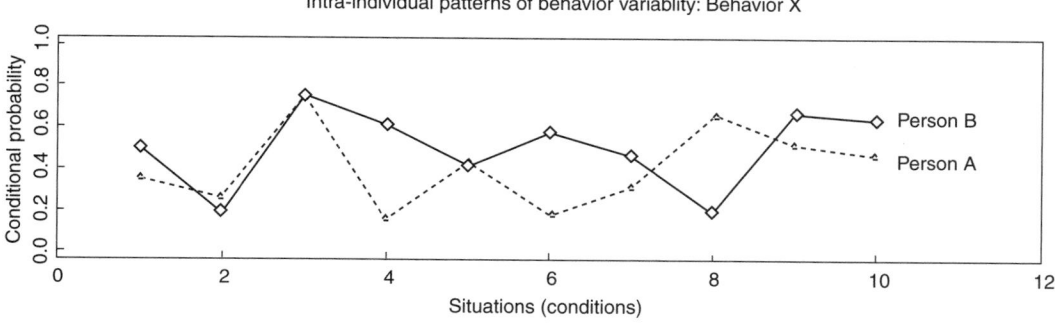

FIGURE 7.5. Typical individual differences in the conditional probability of a type of behavior in different situations. From Mischel and Shoda (1995, p. 247). Copyright 1995 by the American Psychological Association. Reprinted by permission.

assumed to reflect only intrinsic unpredictability or measurement error. Thus, from that perspective, the stability of the intra-individual pattern of variation should, on average, be zero. The obtained findings, yielding highly significant intra-individual stability coefficients for these profiles, obviously contradict this expectation. They reveal that meaningfully patterned behavioral expressions of personality, contextualized within particular situations, characterize individuals. They yield distinctive profiles of variability for particular types of behavior that form behavioral signatures of personality that have a meaningful shape as well as elevation or overall mean level, as illustrated in Figure 7.6.

These profiles characterize an individual by the situations in which he or she becomes particularly angry or depressed, anxious or relieved, revealing a stable pattern, such as: He *A* when *X*, but *B* when *Y*, and does *A* most when *Z*. When properly analyzed and assessed, these patterns of intra-individual variation of behavior across situations seem to reflect the structure and organization of the underlying personality system, such as how the situations are encoded and the expectations, affects, and goals that become activated within them (Mischel & Shoda, 1995). Although it had long been assumed that a focus on the role of the situation un-

dermined the search for personality consistency, in fact, by focusing on the effects of the situation on the organization of behavior in depth and detail, it became possible to find this second type of personality stability, enriching rather than undermining the personality construct and the conception of consistency. Researchers have replicated the existence of meaningful behavioral signatures in diverse domains, measured in a variety of ways (e.g., Andersen & Chen, 2002; Borkenau et al., 2006; Cervone & Shoda, 1999; English & Chen, 2007; Fournier et al., 2008; Shoda & LeeTiernan, 2002; Vansteelandt & Van Mechelen, 1998). Reliable patterns of behavior variability, or of *if … then …* behavioral signatures, seem to characterize individuals distinctively as a rule rather than an exception. The surprise is not simply that this type of behavioral signature of personality exists and is robust, but that it has so long been treated as error and deliberately removed by averaging behavior over diverse situations. Ironically, although such aggregation was intended to capture personality, it actually can delete information that reflects the individual's most distinctive qualities and unique intra-individual patterning, throwing out some of the essence of personality and individuality along with the error term.

Furthermore, the CAPS analysis shows that it is not necessary to have separate units

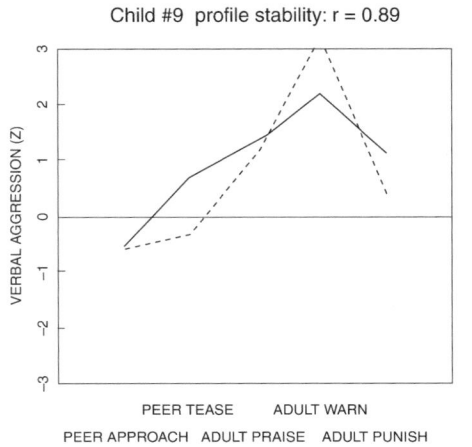

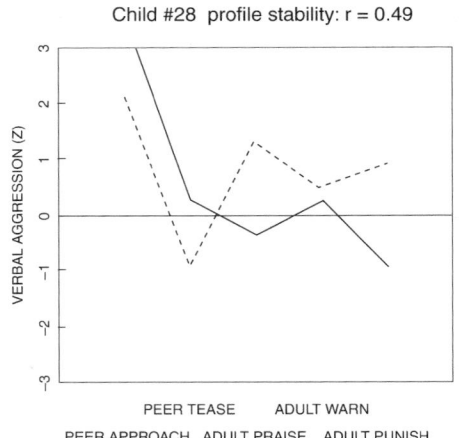

FIGURE 7.6. Illustrative intra-individual, situation–behavior profiles for verbal aggression in relation to five situations in two time samples (*solid* and *dotted lines*). Data are shown in standardized scores (*z*) relative to the normative levels of verbal aggression in each situation. From Shoda, Mischel, and Wright (1994, p. 678). Copyright 1994 by the American Psychological Association. Reprinted by permission.

or constructs to represent overall levels of behavior; the CAPS system can account for stable mean-level differences in particular types of behavior, as well as stable patterns of variability in that behavior across situations. This was seen, for example, in computer simulation of person–situation interactions within the CAPS model, in which individual differences were represented only in terms of the connections among the internal representations that were common to all individuals (patterns of activation pathways determining the links between features of situations and the outcomes generated by the system).

As predicted, an individual's unique configuration in the personality system was manifested in the uniqueness of the *if ... then ...* profiles that unfolded as the individual interacted with situations containing different psychologically active features. Interestingly, however, some individuals in this simulation consistently produced higher levels of the behavior in question, whereas the predicted behavior profiles of others were consistently low in elevation (Mischel & Shoda, 1995; Shoda & LeeTiernan, 2002; Shoda & Mischel, 1998). What is noteworthy is that such stable differences in global behavior tendencies—usually interpreted as directly reflecting the underlying disposition—were predicted and obtained even though the CAPS representation of personality did not contain any unit that directly represented chronic individual differences in generalized behavioral dispositions independent of situation features. This simulation thus showed that to account for stable differences in the overall levels of behavior observed does not require positing mediating units that correspond directly to behavioral dispositions. Individual differences in global behavioral tendencies, or traits as traditionally defined, and processing dynamics within an interactive model such as CAPS are not intrinsically incompatible: The CAPS system yields both types of behavioral expressions without additional assumptions.

To recapitulate, the personality system is expressed at the level of behavior in the pattern with which a type of behavior varies over a set of situations, as well as in the average level of the behavior aggregated across situations (i.e., its overall "act frequency"). Predictable patterns of variability in relation to context in CAPS theory is a potential key

to the individual's stability and coherence, a sign of the underlying system that generates it. Personality assessment needs to move beyond characterization of the person's overall average types of behavior to a more precise level of contextualized specific prediction of who is likely to do what when, that is, in relation to particular types of diagnostic situations (Shoda et al., 1994).

To illustrate, the rejection-sensitive person may be more prone than others to anger, disapproval, and coercive behaviors in certain types of situations in intimate relationships, and at the same time be more supportive, caring, and romantic than most people, for example, in initial encounters with potential partners who are not yet committed to them, or later in the relationship when they are about to lose the partner (Downey et al., 1998). The same rejection-sensitive man who coerces and abuses his partner also can behave in exceedingly tender and loving ways (e.g., Walker, 1979) in seemingly similar situations that have different "active ingredients" or psychological trigger features (e.g., Mischel & Shoda, 1995). In semantic terms, he is both hurtful and kind, caring and uncaring, violent and gentle.

Traditional analyses of such "inconsistencies" in personality lead to the question "which one of these two people is the real one? What is simply the effect of the situation?" In contrast, CAPS theory allows the same person to have contradictory facets that are equally genuine. The surface contradictions become comprehensible when one analyzes the network of relations among cognitions and affects and how they interact with situations. The research problem is to understand when and why different cognitions and affects become activated predictably in relation to different features of situations, external and internal. The theory views the individual's distinctive patterns of variability not necessarily as internal contradictions but as the potentially predictable expressions of a stable underlying system that itself may remain quite unchanged in its organization. The challenge is to discriminate, understand, and predict when each aspect will be activated, and the dynamics that underlie the pattern. For example, are the caring and uncaring behaviors two scripts in the service of the same goal? If so, how are they connected to, and guided by, the person's self-conceptions and belief system in relation to the psychological features of situations that activate them?

Identifying Common Dispositions, Types, and Dynamics: Shared Personality Signatures

The stable situation–behavior profiles generated by CAPS lend themselves not only to the idiographic study of persons in their life contexts, but also provide a nomothetic route to characterize groups or types of persons. Such a personality type consists of people who share a common organization of relations among mediating units in the processing of certain situation features (e.g., Shoda et al., 1994). One can identify these individuals by finding their shared *if ... then ...* patterns of behavior variation. Conversely, identifying similarities among people in their underlying dynamics should allow prediction of the common *if ... then ...* patterns they are likely to manifest behaviorally, and of the underlying dynamics that generate them. Examples of research to identify such personality types and to discover their distinctive behavioral signatures and dynamics, in a framework consistent with the CAPS approach, are seen in research on rejection sensitivity and borderline personality (e.g., Ayduk et al., 1999, 2000, 2008; Pietrzak, Downey, & Ayduk, 2005), narcissistic personality types (Morf, 2006; Morf & Rhodewalt, 2001), as well as on "relational selves" that play out in the individual's characteristic relationships with different types of significant others (e.g., Andersen & Chen, 2002; English & Chen, 2007).

Level 3: The Perception of Personality

The behavioral manifestations of a disposition may be easily and reliably encoded by observers as indicators of person prototypes or exemplars (e.g., Cantor et al., 1982; Wright & Mischel, 1987, 1988), and of traits and types in everyday psycholexical terms, both by lay perceivers (e.g., Jones, 1990) and psychologists (e.g., Goldberg, 1993; John, 1990; McCrae & Costa, 1996). What do the observers' reports of someone's personality tell us? On what aspects of behaviors of the observed are they based? One possibility is that such reports refer to the same kind of generalized behavioral tendency focused on by traditional trait personality psycholo-

gists. However, equating personality with behavioral dispositions easily leads one to construe personality and situation as mutually exclusive and even opposing influences (discussed in Shoda & Mischel, 1993; Shoda et al., 1989; Wright & Mischel, 1987). If one relies on such an equation, it makes sense to assume that perceivers dichotomize observed behavior into its situational versus dispositional components with the goal of partialing out the effect of the situation in order to discover the "true" score of the perceived (e.g., Kelley, 1973). But perceivers may, at least under some circumstances, base their perception on the behavioral variability and *if ... then ...* situation–behavior profiles of the observed. Then their perceptions depend not just on the average levels of different types of behavior displayed by a person, but also on the situations in which those behaviors are contextualized, that is, on the *if ... then ...* situation–behavior patterns of the person's variability across situations, e.g., "She *A* when *X* but *B* when *Y*."

The Intuitive Perceiver Can Be a Sophisticated Personality Theorist

In fact, judgments by observers of how well individuals fit particular dispositional prototypes (e.g., the "friendly" child, the "withdrawn" child, the "aggressive" child) are related clearly to the shape of the observed situation–behavior pattern or signature, as well as to the individuals' average level of prototype-relevant behaviors (Shoda et al., 1993b, 1994). If the pattern of variability is changed, so are the personality judgments (Shoda et al., 1989). Furthermore, by observing these *if ... then ...* patterns, perceivers—whether laypersons or professional observers—can more accurately predict the behaviors of the perceived, presumably because context allows the underlying meanings and motivation to be inferred (Shoda et al., 1989).

Extensive research now shows that intuitive perceivers are more sophisticated personality theorists than most experiments in person perception have allowed them to be. People spontaneously use contextual information in subtle ways (Trope, 1986), and their impressions of others are linked to the *if ... then ...* behavioral signatures of the perceived, which are interpreted as signs of their underlying motivations and intentions (e.g., Kammrath, Mendoza-Denton, & Mischel, 2005; Shoda et al., 1993b). To make sense of the behavior of significant others in their lives, peoples' intuitive lay theories include beliefs about their *if ... then ...* psychological states—"*If* Jack wants to create a good impression, *then* he acts friendly" (Chen, 2003). They try to infer the underlying stable personality system that generates and explains observed behavioral signatures when they are given the information to do so, and the motivation for expending the effort. Research has found that people do so, for example, when they are dealing with people who are important to them and not just with the strangers typically used in person perception experiments (Chen-Idson & Mischel, 2001; Shoda et al., 1989). Increasingly it seems that *if ... then ...* relations are basic units in lay conceptions of personality (Chen, 2003), and perceivers use them to infer the underlying mental states and personality characteristics that account for them.

To reveal these lay theories of personality, however, researchers have to give perceivers the opportunity to observe the behaviors of the perceived across diverse situations. Such information is absent in most studies of person perception. But when people can observe behavioral signatures, rather than discounting the situation, as classic attribution theory expects, they use the signatures instead to infer the underlying motivations and characteristics of the perceived (e.g., Cantor et al., 1982; Chen-Idson & Mischel, 2001; Vonk, 1998; Wright & Mischel, 1988). Moreover, stable patterns of variations lead to a greater, rather than diminished, sense of personality coherence (Plaks, Shafer, & Shoda, 2003).

In sum, the processing dynamics and structure of personality are inferred (regardless of accuracy) not only by professional psychologists but also by lay perceivers in their intuitive theories of personality: At least some of the time, some perceivers try to infer the beliefs, goals, and affects of the people they want to understand to see how these qualities underlie their behavior (Shoda & Mischel, 1993). Given that the expressions of the personality system are reflected in the shape as well as in the elevation of the *if ... then ...* situation–behavior profiles generated by the system, the perceiver (whether layperson or psychologist) needs such information

to infer the underlying structure and dynamics and generate a theory about the person (Plaks et al., 2003). In the studies in which such data are made available to lay perceivers, they seem to be linked to the social perceptions and inferences that are formed and suggest that the perceivers may be intuitive interactionists at least some of the time (e.g., Chiu, 1994; Dweck, Hong, & Chiu, 1993; Kruglanski, 1989, 1990; Read & Miller, 1993; Shoda, Mischel, & Wright, 1993a, 1993b; Wright & Mischel, 1987, 1988). Thus, even if traits appear to be the preferred language for the psychology of the stranger (McAdams, 1994), perceivers do make inferences about the goals and motivations of the perceived (Plaks et al., 2003) when necessary contextual information is available. This is true particularly when they try to understand themselves and their intimates or to take an empathic orientation (e.g., Chen-Idson & Mischel, 2001; Hoffman, Mischel, & Mazze, 1981; Kammrath et al., 2005; Vonk, 1998; Wright & Mischel, 1988).

Perceived Consistencies and Their Behavioral Roots: The Locus of Self-Perceived Consistency and Dispositional Judgments

The profiles of situation–behavior relations that characterize persons—their behavioral signatures of personality—also appear to be an important locus of self-perception regarding consistency and coherence. This was found in a reanalysis by Mischel and Shoda (1995) of the Carleton College field study (Mischel & Peake, 1982a). In that study college students were observed on campus in various situations relevant to their conscientiousness in the college setting (e.g., in the classroom, in the dormitory, in the library) and assessed over repeated occasions in the semester. Students who perceived themselves as consistent did not show greater overall cross-situational consistency than those who did not. But for individuals who perceived themselves as consistent, the average situation–behavior profile stability correlation was near .5, whereas it was trivial for those who viewed themselves as inconsistent. So it may be the stability in the situation–behavior profiles (e.g., conscientious about homework but not about punctuality), not the cross-situational consistency of behavior, that underlies the perception of consistency with regard to a type of behavior or disposition.

The Personality Paradox Demystified

The types of *if . . . then . . .* situation–behavior relations that a dynamic personality system such as CAPS necessarily generates has important implications for rethinking the classic personality paradox (Bem & Allen, 1974). As Bem and Allen noted two decades ago, on the one hand, the person's behavior across situations yields only modest cross-situational consistency coefficients (Hartshorne & May, 1928; Newcomb, 1929), but on the other hand, personality theory's fundamental assumption, and our intuition, insist that personality surely is stable (e.g., Bem & Allen, 1974; Heatherton & Weinberger, 1994; Krahe, 1990; Mischel, 1968; Moskowitz, 1982, 1994). Indeed such discriminative facility is an index of adaptive behavior and constructive functioning, whereas consistency regardless of subtle contextual cues can be a sign of rigidity (Chiu, Hong, Mischel, & Shoda, 1995).

This paradox dissolves, however, by recognizing that the variability of behaviors within individuals across situations is neither all "error" nor "due to the situation rather than to the person." Instead it is at least partly an essential expression of the enduring but dynamic personality system itself and its stable underlying organization. Thus the person's behaviors in a domain will necessarily change from one type of situation to another because when the *if* changes, so will the *then*, even when the personality structure remains entirely unchanged. How the individual's behavior and experience change across situations is part of the essential expression of personality (Mischel & Shoda, 1995) and becomes a key focus for personality assessment. From this perspective, the person's ability to make subtle discriminations among situations and to take these cues into account in the self-regulation of behavior in order to adapt it to changing situational requirements, is a basic aspect of social competence, not a reflection of inconsistency (Chiu et al., 1995; Shoda et al., 1993b). This type of discriminative facility seems to be a component of social intelligence, a sensitivity to the subtle cues in the situation that influence behavior. Such discriminative facility, for example, by encoding spontaneous social information in conditional versus global dispositional terms, was found to predict the quality of the person's social interaction (Chiu et al., 1995).

In sum, relatively stable situation–behavior profiles reflect characteristic intraindividual patterns in how the person relates to different psychological conditions or features of situations, forming a sort of behavioral signature of personality (Shoda et al., 1994). The stability of these situation–behavior profiles in turn predicts the self-perception of consistency as well as being linked to the dispositional judgments made about the person by others (Shoda et al., 1993b, 1994). These expectations and findings are congruent with classic processing theories, most notably Freud's conception of psychodynamics. In that view, peoples' underlying processing dynamics and qualities—the construals and goals, the motives and passions, that drive them—may be reflected not only in how often they display particular types of behavior but also in when and where, and thus also—and most importantly—*why* that behavior occurs. In short, the CAPS model expects that the stable patterns of situation–behavior relationships that characterize persons provide potential keys to their dynamics. They are informative roads to the underlying system that produces them, not sources of error to be eliminated systematically by aggregating out the situation.

Level 4: The Stable Interpersonal Space: Situational Signatures of Personality

Although different models of personality hypothesize different mediating processes, there is wide agreement among researchers, ranging from behavior geneticists (e.g., Plomin, DeFries, McClearn, & Rutter, 1997) to social-cognitive interactionists (e.g., Bandura, 1986; Mischel & Shoda, 1995), that individuals' characteristics and behaviors influence the environments or situations that they subsequently experience. As discussed above, these characteristics and behaviors are perceived and encoded by people who observe them, as well as by the people who enact them, and have important consequences for the stable psychological world that comes to characterize each person's life. For example, the dispositional inferences observers make about an individual in turn may influence their reactions (e.g., by avoiding contact), and thereby influence that individual's future interpersonal space. Thus people select, influence, and even generate their own interpersonal situations as well as being influenced by them in an interactive process (e.g., Bolger, DeLongis, Kessler, & Schilling, 1989; Bolger & Schilling, 1991; Buss, 1987; Ross & Nisbett, 1991; T. W. Smith & Rhodewalt, 1986; Snyder, 1983; Snyder & Gangestad, 1982).

Ultimately this process results in a degree of stability or equilibrium in the situations the person characteristically experiences in the psychological life space. Such stability "belongs" neither to the person nor to the situation in isolation, but is a reflection of the enduring pattern of reciprocal interactions between the individual and his or her distinctive interpersonal world as they dynamically influence each other, each impacting on the other.

To illustrate, Figures 7.7, 7.8, and 7.9 show the frequency (in z-scores) with which three children from the Wediko summer camp (Shoda, 1990) experienced the five types of situations measured repeatedly over the course of 6 weeks. For child #6 (Figure 7.7), everything happened often; he was positively approached by peers, teased by them, praised by adults, and also warned and given time out by them. In stark contrast, for child #20 (Figure 7.8) we see an empty summer, with far fewer experiences, either positive or

negative, than the average camper. It is a portrait of an isolated child, avoided or ignored by the social world around him. Child #78 (Figure 7.9) experienced a world in which the outstanding feature was the exceptional amount of teasing (and threatening/provoking) he endured from peers. If such different patterns of interpersonal encounters are characteristic and stable for each individual across different activities and contexts—and they often are—then they constitute an aspect of behavioral coherence that needs to be incorporated into the conception and assessment of personality consistency (Mischel & Shoda, 1995).

The features of situations that activate the person's processing dynamics are not just triggered by external situations encountered in the social world. They also are generated internally, within the personality system, through thought, planning, fantasy, and imagination (e.g., Antrobus, 1991; Gollwitzer, 1996; Klinger, 1996; Mischel et al., 1989; Nolen-Hoeksema et al., 1994). And they encompass not just social and interpersonal situations (e.g., when lovers "reject" or peers "tease and provoke") but also internal situations, as in mood states (e.g., Isen et al., 1992; Schwarz, 1990) as well as in the everyday stream of experience and feeling (e.g., Bolger & Eckenrode, 1991; Emmons, 1991; C. A. Smith & Lazarus, 1990; Wright & Mischel, 1988).

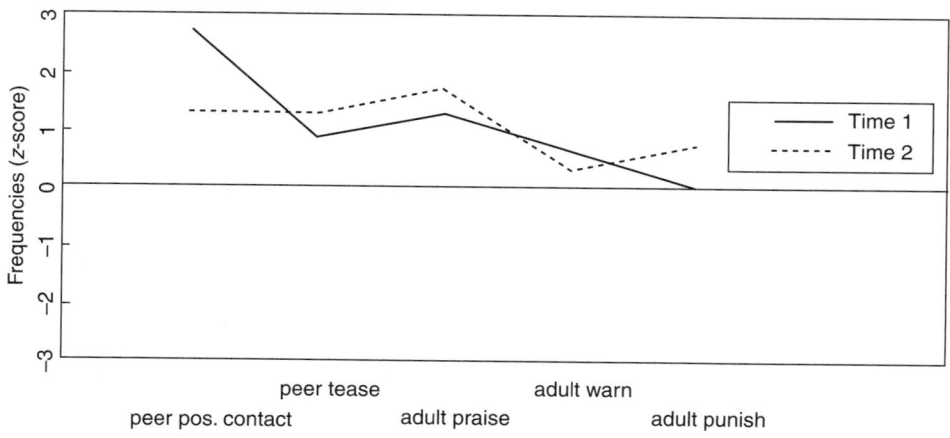

FIGURE 7.7. Frequencies of encountering psychological situations: Child #6, profile stability: $r = .53$. From Shoda (1990). Reprinted with permission from the author.

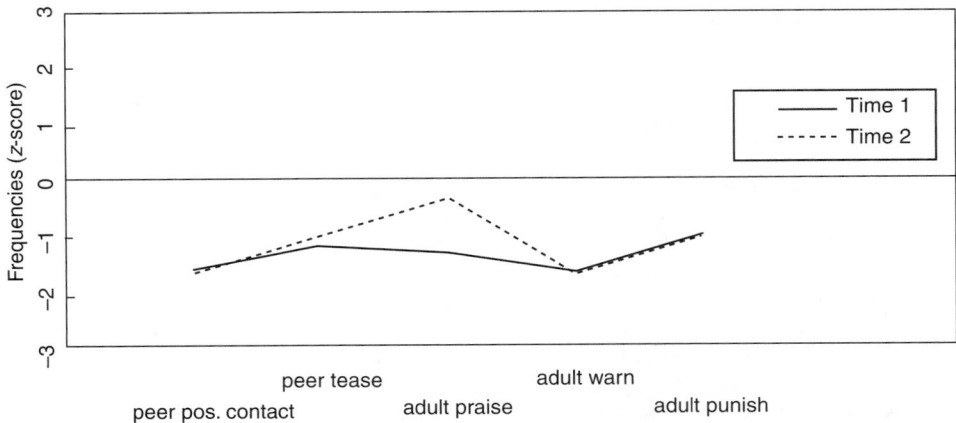

FIGURE 7.8. Frequencies of encountering psychological situations: Child #20, profile stability: $r = .63$. From Shoda (1990). Reprinted with permission from the author.

Level 5: Pre-Dispositions at the Biological–Genetic and Social History Substrate: Interactions among Levels

Together, Levels 1–4 form a person–environment system that guides the intra- and inter-personal dynamics that generate the individual's flow of cognition, affects, and behaviors. Thus, a person does X, the environment does Y in response, which activates the person's CAPS and produces Z. Levels 1–4 describe the functioning of the person within this person–environment system. The system produces large variations in

behavior, but the components of the system, for example, the person's CAPS network itself, may be largely stable during these interactions. The question we next consider is how the diverse individual differences in the person–environment system (i.e., those that underlie individual differences in Levels 1–4) develop in response to the individual's biological–genetic and learning level.

People differ importantly in diverse biochemical–genetic–somatic factors, which may be conceptualized as *pre*-dispositions. We emphasize the *pre* to underline that they are biological precursors that may manifest

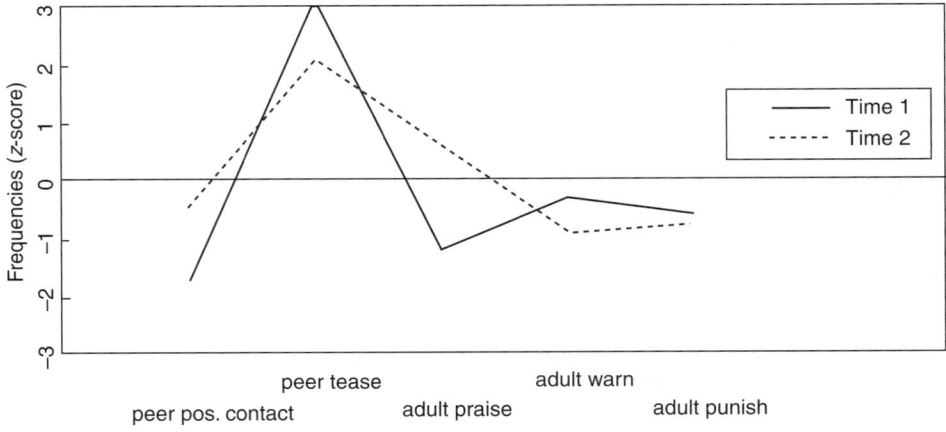

FIGURE 7.9. Frequencies of encountering psychological situations: Child #78, profile stability: $r = .77$. From Shoda (1990). Reprinted with permission from the author.

indirectly as well as directly, in diverse and complex forms, at the other levels of analysis. These *pre*-dispositions ultimately influence such personality-relevant qualities as sensory and psychomotor sensitivities and vulnerabilities, skills and competencies (including those essential for self-regulation and goal-directed delay of gratification), temperament (including activity level and emotionality), and chronic mood and affective states. These in turn interact with social-cognitive, social learning and cultural–societal influences, mediated by, and conjointly further influencing, the system—and the person—that emerges.

Individuals differ with regard to virtually every aspect of the biological human repertoire and genetic heritage, as well as in their social learning and emotional histories, and these differences can have profound predisposing implications for the personality processing system and its behavioral expressions that ultimately develop (e.g., Mischel et al., 2008; Plomin et al., 1997). Such differences may occur, for instance, in sensory, perceptual, cognitive, and affective systems, in metabolic clocks and hormones, in neurotransmitters—in short, in the person's total biochemical–genetic–somatic heritage. These *pre*-dispositions interact with conditions throughout development and play out in ways that influence what the person thinks, feels, and does and the processing dynamics and behavioral signatures that come to characterize the individual. Even small differences between persons at the biochemical–somatic level (e.g., in sensory–perceptual sensitivity, in allergy and disease proneness, in energy levels) may manifest ultimately as considerable differences in their experiences and behavior and in what comes to be perceived as their personalities.

Consequently, a comprehensive approach to personality has to address not only the structure and organization of the cognitive–affective–behavioral processing system at the psychological level at any one point in time but also its biochemical–genetic predisposing foundations (e.g., Plomin et al., 1997; Saudino & Plomin, 1996) and their interactions with social learning and cultural–societal sources of influence (Mischel, 1998b). Genetically influenced individual differences presumably affect, at least indirectly, how people construe or encode—and shape—their environments, which in turn

produce important person–context interactions throughout the life course (e.g., Kagan, 2006; Plomin, 1994; Rothbart, Derryberry, & Posner, 1994; Saudino & Plomin, 1996; Schmidt & Fox, 1999).

Given these considerations, in CAPS theory, both biochemical and social-cognitive influences, heritable and learned, are expected to affect the availability of cognitive–affective units and their organization that is the personality system. For example, variables of temperament or reactivity visible early in life, such as activity, irritability, tension, distress, and emotional lability visible early in life (Bates & Wachs, 1994), have important, albeit complexly interactive, links to emotional and attentional processing and self-regulation (e.g., Rothbart et al., 1994), and thus should influence the organization of relations among the mediating units in the system. Because this system, in turn, generates the specific *if ... then ...* situation–behavior relations manifested, the theory predicts that individual differences in genes and early social learning history will be seen not only in the mean level of behaviors, but in the behavioral signatures of personality—that is, the stable configuration of *if ... then ...* situation–behavior relations. When the system changes, either due to modification in the biological substrates or due to developmental changes and significant life events, the effects will also be manifested at the behavioral level, visible as a change in the relationships between the "ifs" and the "thens" in the person's characteristic situation–behavior profiles.

ENDURING CONTRIBUTIONS OF THE FIELD INCORPORATED INTO CAPS

As a glance at any textbook on personality theory quickly makes clear, the field has had a long and rich tradition in which each new theorist puts forth a particular view of personality that tries to be entirely original and to stand sharply distinguished from all that came before it, usually cast to conflict with its many predecessors. As a result, rather than a cumulative theory rooted in, building on, and integrating scientifically the best and most viable views that came before it, personality psychologists have been faced with a virtual mall of alternative theories. In it they shop for and select the one more for the mix they want (unless their mentors do it for them), from psychodynamic to behavioristic, from phenomenological–humanistic to social learning and social cognitive, from evolutionary and biological to a wide array of trait models and the Big Five. In contrast, CAPS from the start (Mischel & Shoda, 1995) was intended to be a meta-theory that explicitly builds on, and tries to incorporate, whatever scientific contributions of earlier theories proved to be enduring, while also leaving itself open to change that is certain to come as our science develops. We next point to some of these features, both to make clear CAPS's debt to the field's enduring heritage, and our commitment to try to help develop an increasingly cumulative and comprehensive approach to the rigorous study of individuals within their social worlds:

• CAPS predicts and generates both the type of overall average individual differences identified in trait approaches and the *if ... then ...* signatures originally proposed within a social-cognitive framework (discussed in Level 1 above).

• The contributions from biological and genetic work relevant to personality are fundamental in CAPS (Level 5). The biological substrate constrains and guides our model of mind–brain connections and ultimately links to the genetic endowment, as in studies of self-control that relate how people think and appraise situations to their brain activity (e.g., Metcalfe & Mischel, 1999).

• Consistent with the discovery initially within the psychodynamic–motivational tradition that much if not most of the mind operates at levels outside awareness and plays out in automatic ways, CAPS is conceptualized as a network that operates rapidly and functions at multiple levels, often outside conscious awareness (Kihlstrom, 1999, 2003). Such automatic processing (e.g., Bargh, 1997; Bargh & Ferguson, 2000; Bargh & Williams, 2006) relies on preexisting schemas and is usually involuntary and unconscious. There is a great deal of such automatic, uncontrolled processing in CAPS. But as the ego psychologists and social-cognitive theorists long recognized, much that is important in personality and adaptive functioning also requires cognition and thinking and plays out in controlled processing and conscious thought, as in planning, problem solving, future-oriented decision making, and self-control. This level requires motivation, effort, and self-regulatory competencies, and often is essential for overcoming impulsive responding that could lead to unfortunate future consequences. When one first begins to drive an automobile, it is a controlled process, but it soon becomes an automatic process that runs more or less on its own much of the time. The same is true for self-control patterns, as in control efforts to overcome eating or drug abuse problems: At first much effortful control may be required, but ultimately it can become mostly automatic.

• Drawing on discoveries from psychodynamic theorizing as well as current social-cognitive neuroscience research, CAPS encompasses a "hot" emotion-driven, reflexive affective personality system, just as much as it also contains a cool, more reflective, cognitive system. Behavior is seen as reflecting the continuous interaction of both systems, experienced at varying levels of awareness.

• The focus on both the situation and on behavior—on what the person does—was a core contribution originally rooted in contributions from the *behavioral conditioning theories* as well as from later work in a social learning and social-cognitive framework, and it is an integral part of CAPS. The connections activated in the personality system at any time depend on the particular situation with which the individual is interacting. Thus the CAPS personality structure continuously interacts with the situations experienced, and the processing of this information is played out at the behavioral level.

• Likewise, key findings from social-cognitive theories are integrated into CAPS by incorporating such person variables as expectancies, goals, values, and self-regulatory competencies. All of these schemas are represented in the CAUs that are interconnected within the personality system. They play out in the personality signatures activated in different psychological situations, which in turn account for the two types of consistency identified at the trait-dispositional level.

• The contributions of phenomenological–humanistic theories to CAPS are evident in the emphasis on the psychological situation, that is, the situation as perceived and appraised or construed by the individual, not just on the objective stimulus. The influence of such theorists as George Kelly as well as Carl Rogers is seen in the CAPS focus on the importance of construal (appraisal, encoding) from the perceiver's perspective as determining the psychological impact of situations on the individual. Likewise, in CAPS situations are not just external; they also are self-generated and internal, experienced in such processes as planning, thinking, remembering, daydreaming, and exercising effortful control in long-term goal pursuit, and so on, and even created by one's own mood and affective states.

• The dynamic processes within CAPS integrate the phenomenological focus on the self and the ability of individuals to be agentic and proactive in influencing their own futures with the information processing focus of social-cognitive models, while also drawing on neural network models from cognitive and social-cognitive neuroscience. At the same time it views the system as self-generating and emergent in continuous transaction with the social environment.

• CAPS theory emphasizes that the personality system is not simply a passive responder to the psychological situations encountered; it also generates and creates its own situations. Moreover, at least within its cool sub-system, CAPS is an active and indeed proactive, as well as reactive, system. It thus sees people as anticipating, interpreting, rearranging, and changing situations as well as reacting to them, not only responding to the environment but also generating, selecting, and modifying situations in reciprocal transactions.

• The proactive rather than merely reactive operations of the system take many forms. These include self-induced motivational changes by means of (1) various mental framing operations (e.g., a "promotion vs. prevention" focus; Higgins, 1996a, 1997, 1998); or (2) by the operation of different types of goals and the person's own theories (e.g., Grant & Dweck, in press); or (3) by cognitive transformations and reappraisals of the situation itself to reframe it strategically. The proactive operations can do so, for example, by focusing on different features within the system (e.g., Metcalfe & Mischel, 1999; Mischel, 1974, 1996) and through self-regulatory and control processes that function in the service of long-term goals and life projects (e.g., as reviewed in Mischel & Ayduk, 2004; Mischel et al., 1996).

Summary

Although we proposed the CAPS model, it was built on contributions from all sides of our science. Its over-arching goal is to provide a unifying, cumulative meta-theory and framework in which what we have learned about personality dispositions and processes are both incorporated, as seamlessly—we hope—and as presently possible, so that researchers can take both fully into account.

It has been widely assumed and asserted that process-oriented approaches to personality ignore or deny stable personality dispositions (e.g., Funder, 1991; Goldberg, 1993), but in fact, in CAPS theory they have a significant role in the personality system itself. As was seen, dispositions are defined by a characteristic cognitive–affective processing structure that underlies, and generates, distinctive processing dynamics. The processing structure of the disposition consists of a characteristic set of cognitions, affects, and behavioral strategies in an organization of inter-relations that guides and constrains their activation.

The behavioral manifestations of a disposition and its processing dynamics are seen in the elevations and shapes of the situation–behavior profiles—the dispositional signature—that distinguishes its exemplars, as well as in the overall level of different types of behaviors or act frequencies generated over time. Individuals who have similar organizations of relations among cognitions and affects that become activated in relation to a distinctive set of situational features may be said to have a particular processing disposition. Distinctive dispositions are characterized by distinctive processing dynamics that become activated and, over time and contexts, generate the situation–behavior profiles that have the characteristic elevations and shapes that identify the dispositional exemplars.

TOWARD A UNIFIED FIELD AND FRAMEWORK

This chapter posed the question: Can the two approaches to personality—dispositional (trait) and processing (social-cognitive–

affective–dynamic)—be reconciled and integrated within a unifying framework? Our analysis proposes that they can be, and probably should be, if personality psychology is to develop into a cumulative science. The CAPS model is an attempt toward such a unifying integration.

At present, however, we believe that barriers to such an integration remain, more because of the field's history and traditions and sociology than for scientific reasons. Thus to make this integration possible, many old "hot" reflexes as well as treasured assumptions will have to be overcome. One of the most pernicious of these is the preemptive definition of personality psychology as a science of personality "traits," conceptualized as causal, genotypic, entities that correspond to phenotypic behavioral dispositions. That view automatically makes narrowly defined "traits" *the* target of investigation—as well as the bases for explanations. If personality psychology is to become a cumulative science, researchers need to address the phenomena that demand explanation, rather than be governed by any set of preemptive explanatory constructs. These phenomena can be analyzed at each of the complementary levels outlined above, allowing an ultimately more comprehensive and cumulative science conception of personality and its diverse manifestations and antecedents. Seen that way, many of the differences between the two current major approaches of the field may reflect different goals and preferences in the level of analysis pursued more than fundamental incompatibilities.

There are some indications that significant moves toward an integration may be under way (Mischel, 2004, 2005; Mischel & Shoda, 1998). As we have emphasized, CAPS theory attempts to take account of overall important differences between people in qualities such as temperament, chronic mood and affective states, and skills and is compatible with data pointing to the substantial genetic contributions to personality, as noted above. Far from denying the importance of individual differences in personality and behavior, researchers within the CAPS framework, and in related processing approaches, have been identifying diagnostic situations in which such differences, for example, with regard to aggressive tendencies or self-control abilities, and cultural differences, may be-

come particularly visible (e.g., Ayduk et al., 2000; Baumeister, Heatherton, & Tice, 1993; Downey et al., 1998; Fleeson, 2001; Fournier et al., 2008; Mendoza-Denton & Mischel, 2007; Mischel et al., 1989, 1996; Shoda, Mischel, & Peake, 1990; Vansteelandt & Van Mechelen, 1998; Wright & Mischel, 1987, 1988). Furthermore, the stable correlates and consequences of individual differences in such social-cognitive person variables as (1) the goals and personal projects pursued over time (e.g., Cantor, 1994; Cantor & Fleeson, 1994), (2) the person's beliefs and goal structures (Weary & Edwards, 1994), (3) the person's own implicit theories about personality (e.g., Dweck & Leggett, 1988; Grant & Dweck, 1999), and (4) the type of focus primed in goal pursuit (e.g., gain-oriented vs. loss-avoidant; Higgins, 1996a, 1996b) are central to the agenda of current processing approaches.

In the same vein, analyses of cognitive–attentional processes during self-control efforts in young children in the last decade also have identified dramatic threads of long-term continuity and stability in the course of development (e.g., Ayduk et al., 2000; Eigsti et al., 2006; Mischel et al., 1989; Sethi, Mischel, Aber, Shoda, & Rodriguez, 2000). For example, significant and substantial links have been found between seconds of delay of gratification in certain diagnostic laboratory situations in preschool and behavioral outcomes years later in adolescence and early adulthood, showing levels of stability and meaningful networks of associated developmental outcomes that are clearly indicative of long-term personality coherence (e.g., Mischel & Ayduk, 2004; Mischel et al., 1989; Shoda et al., 1990).

It is also noteworthy that at least some dispositional theorists increasingly seem to take account of the contextualized, situation-bound expressions of traits, and try to include motivational and dynamic processing concepts in their models (e.g., Revelle, 1995). Such research is helping to identify the specific boundary conditions within which traits become activated (e.g., Stemmler, 1997). For many researchers, a quiet but dramatic transformation may be occurring in how personality dispositions are defined. That move seems to be away from the global and situation-free trait construct, criticized 30 years earlier for its empirically unviable assumption of cross-situational consistency (Mischel, 1968), to "likelihood and rates of change in behavior in response to particular situational cues" (Revelle, 1995, p. 315)—a definition free of the cross-situational consistency requirement, and acceptable to any processing theorist interested in individual differences. This trend is exemplified in research on such dispositions as anxious rejection expectations (e.g., Ayduk et al., 1999, 2000; Pietrzak et al., 2005), attachment types and interpersonal signatures (Andersen & Chen, 2002; Zayas et al., 2008), narcissistic personality types (e.g., Morf, 2006), and expressions of the self (e.g., Mischel & Morf, 2003).

In this chapter we have tried to show that personality psychologists do not have to choose between the study of dispositions or processes, but can analyze both the distinctive behavior patterns that characterize the exemplars of a disposition (defined in terms of characteristic behavior patterns) and the psychological processes and mediating units that underlie those. A theoretical integration and the building of a cumulative science of personality seem achievable, at least in the abstract, along the lines we have sketched in this chapter. If the field can embrace, but also move beyond, its history, the realization of that prospect promises to become an exciting time for the field and for the growth of personality psychology as a vibrant science of the individual at the hub of the behavioral sciences.

NOTE

1. On October 3, 1995, Simpson was acquitted of the murders of Nicole Brown Simpson and Ronald Goldman. Images of cheering faces of African Americans were juxtaposed with those of dismayed European Americans across front pages of newspapers and magazine covers, providing a reminder that Blacks and Whites in America live in different worlds, understanding and experiencing the same publicity about the trial differently. As easy as it may be to classify agreement and elation as the "Black" response and disagreement and dismay as the "White" response (as the media did), such generalizations are unlikely to be useful in understanding people's reactions. A CAPS model was generated to understand the process that brought about people's reactions to the verdict.

REFERENCES

Allport, G. (1937). *Personality: A psychological interpretation.* New York: Holt.

Andersen, S. M., & Chen, S. (2002). The relational self: An interpersonal social-cognitive theory. *Psychological Review, 109,* 619–645.

Antrobus, J. (1991). Dreaming: Cognitive processes during critical activation and high afferent thresholds. *Psychology Review, 98,* 96–121.

Ayduk, O., Downey, G., Testa, A., Yen, Y., & Shoda, Y. (1999). Does rejection elicit hostility in rejection sensitive women? *Social Cognition, 17,* 245–271.

Ayduk, O., Mendoza-Denton, R., Mischel, W., Downey, G., Peake, P. K., & Rodriguez, M. (2000). Regulating the interpersonal self: Strategic self-regulation for coping with rejection sensitivity. *Journal of Personality and Social Psychology, 79,* 776–792.

Ayduk, O., Zayas, V., Downey, G., Cole, A. B., Shoda, Y., & Mischel, W. (2008). Rejection sensitivity and executive control: Joint predictors of borderline personality features. *Journal of Research in Personality, 42,* 151–168.

Bandura, A. (1986). *Social foundations of thought and action: A social cognitive theory.* Englewood Cliffs, NJ: Prentice-Hall.

Bargh, J. A. (1997). The automaticity of everyday life. In R. S. Wyer (Ed.), *The automaticity of everyday life: Advances in social cognition* (Vol. 10, pp. 1–61). Mahwah, NJ: Erlbaum.

Bargh, J. A., & Ferguson, M. J. (2000). Beyond behaviorism: On the automaticity of higher mental processes. *Psychological Bulletin, 126,* 925–945.

Bargh, J. A., & Williams, E. L. (2006) The automaticity of social life. *Current Directions in Psychological Science, 15,* 1–4.

Bates, J. E., & Wachs, T. D. (1994). *Temperament: Individual differences at the interface of biology and behavior.* Washington, DC: American Psychological Association.

Baumeister, R. F., Heatherton, T. F., & Tice, D. M. (1993). When ego threats lead to self-regulation failure: Negative consequences of high self-esteem. *Journal of Personality and Social Psychology, 64,* 141–156.

Bem, D. J. (1983). Further déjà vu in the search for cross-situational consistency: A response to Mischel and Peake. *Psychological Review, 90,* 390–393.

Bem, D. J., & Allen, A. (1974). On predicting some of the people some of the time: The search for cross-situational consistencies in behavior. *Psychological Review, 81,* 506–520.

Block, J. (1995). A contrarian view of the five-factor approach to personality description. *Psychological Bulletin, 117,* 187–215.

Bolger, N., DeLongis, A., Kessler, R. C., & Schilling, E. A. (1989). Effects of daily stress on negative mood. *Journal of Personality and Social Psychology, 57,* 808–818.

Bolger, N., & Eckenrode, J. (1991). Social relationships, personality, and anxiety during a major stressful event. *Journal of Personality and Social Psychology, 61,* 440–449.

Bolger, N., & Schilling, E. A. (1991). Personality and the problems of everyday life: The role of neuroticism in exposure and reactivity to daily stressors. *Journal of Personality, 59,* 355–386.

Borkenau, P., Riemann, R., Spinath, F. M., & Angleitner, A. (2006). Genetic and environmental influences on person × situation profiles. *Journal of Personality, 74,* 1451–1479.

Buss, D. M. (1987). Selection, evocation, and manipulation. *Journal of Personality and Social Psychology, 53,* 1214–1221.

Cantor, N. (1994). Life task problem-solving: Situational affordances and personal needs. *Personality and Social Psychology Bulletin, 20,* 235–243.

Cantor, N., & Fleeson, W. (1994). Social intelligence and intelligent goal pursuit: A cognitive slice of motivation. In W. Spaulding (Ed.), *Integrative views of motivation, cognition, and emotion: Nebraska Symposium on Motivation* (Vol. 41, pp. 125–179). Lincoln: University of Nebraska Press.

Cantor, N., & Kihlstrom, J. F. (1987). *Personality and social intelligence.* Englewood Cliffs, NJ: Prentice Hall.

Cantor, N., & Mischel, W. (1977). Traits as prototypes: Effects on recognition memory. *Journal of Personality and Social Psychology, 35,* 38–48.

Cantor, N., & Mischel, W. (1979). Prototypes in person perception. In L. Berkowitz (Ed.), *Advances in experimental social psychology* (Vol. 12, pp. 3–52). New York: Academic Press.

Cantor, N., Mischel, W., & Schwartz, J. (1982). A prototype analysis of psychological situations. *Cognitive Psychology, 14,* 45–77.

Cervone, D. (2005). Personality architecture: Within-person structures and processes. *Annual Review of Psychology, 56,* 423–452.

Cervone, D., Shadel, W. G., Smith, R. E., & Fiori, M. (2006). Self-regulation: Reminders and suggestions from personality science. *Applied Psychology: An International Review, 55,* 333–385.

Cervone, D., & Shoda, Y. (1999). Social-cognitive theories and the coherence of personality. In D. Cervone & Y. Shoda (Eds.), *The coherence of personality: Social-cognitive bases of consistency, variability, and organization* (pp. 3–33). New York: Guilford Press.

Chen, S. (2003). Psychological state theories about significant others: Implications for the content and structure of significant-other representations. *Personality and Social Psychology Bulletin, 29,* 1285–1302.

Chen-Idson, L., & Mischel, W. (2001). The personality of familiar and significant people: The lay perceiver as a social cognitive theorist. *Journal of Personality and Social Psychology, 80,* 585–596.

Chiu, C. (1994). *Bases of categorization and person cognition.* Unpublished doctoral dissertation, Columbia University, New York.

Chiu, C., Hong, Y., Mischel, W., & Shoda, Y. (1995). Discriminative facility in social competence: Conditional versus dispositional encoding and monitoring–blunting of information. *Social Cognition, 13,* 49–70.

Downey, G., Freitas, A., Michaelis, B., & Khouri, H. (1998). The self-fulfilling prophecy in close relationships: Rejection sensitivity and rejection by romantic partners. *Journal of Personality and Social Psychology, 75,* 545–560.

Dweck, C. S., Hong, Y., Chiu, C. (1993). Implicit theories: Individual differences in the likelihood and meaning of dispositional inference. *Personality and Social Psychology Bulletin, 19,* 644–656.

Dweck, C. S., & Leggett, E. L. (1988). A social-cognitive approach to motivation and personality. *Psychological Review, 95,* 256–273.

Eigsti, I., Zayas, V., Mischel, W., Shoda, Y., Ayduk, O., Dadlani, M. B., et al. (2006). Predicting cognitive control from preschool to late adolescence and young adulthood. *Psychological Science, 17,* 478–484.

Emmons, R. A. (1991). Personal strivings, daily life events, and psychological and physical well-being. *Journal of Personality, 59,* 453–472.

English, T., & Chen, S. (2007). Culture and self-concept stability: Consistency across and within contexts among Asian Americans and European Americans. *Journal of Personality and Social Psychology, 93,* 478–490.

Epstein, S. (1979). The stability of behavior: On predicting most of the people much of the time. *Journal of Personality and Social Psychology, 37,* 1097–1126.

Epstein, S. (1980). The stability of behavior: II. Implications for psychological research. *American Psychologist, 35,* 790–806.

Epstein, S. (1983). Aggregation and beyond: Some basic issues on the prediction of behavior. *Journal of Personality, 51,* 360–392.

Epstein, S. (1994). Integration of the cognitive and the psychodynamic unconscious. *American Psychologist, 49,* 709–724.

Feldman, S., & Downey, G. (1994). Rejection sensitivity as a mediator of the impact of childhood exposure to family violence on adult attachment behavior. *Development and Psychopathology, 6,* 231–247.

Fleeson, W. (2001). Toward a structure- and

process-integrated view of personality: Traits as density distributions of states. *Journal of Personality and Social Psychology, 80,* 1011–1027.

Forgas, J. P. (1983a). Episode cognition and personality: A multidimensional analysis. *Journal of Personality, 51,* 34–48.

Forgas, J. P. (1983b). Social skills and the perception of interaction episodes. *British Journal of Clinical Psychology, 22,* 195–207.

Fournier, M. A., Moskowitz, D. S., & Zuroff, D. C. (2008). Integrating dispositions, signatures, and the interpersonal domain. *Journal of Personality and Social Psychology, 90,* 283–289.

Funder, D. C. (1983). Three issues in predicting more of the people: A reply to Mischel and Peake. *Psychological Review, 90,* 283–289.

Funder, D. C. (1991). Global traits: A neo-Allportian approach to personality. *Psychological Science, 2,* 31–39.

Funder, D. C. (1994). Explaining traits. *Psychological Inquiry, 5,* 125–127.

Goldberg, L. R. (1993). The structure of phenotypic personality traits. *American Psychologist, 48,* 26–34.

Gollwitzer, P. M. (1996). The volitional benefits of planning. In P. M. Gollwitzer & J. A. Bargh (Eds.), *The psychology of action: Linking cognition and motivation to behavior* (pp. 297–312). New York: Guilford Press.

Gollwitzer, P. M., & Bargh, J. A. (Eds.). (1996). *The psychology of action: Linking cognition and motivation to behavior.* New York: Guilford Press.

Grant, H., & Dweck, C. (1999). A goal analysis of personality and personality coherence. In D. Cervone & Y. Shoda (Eds.), *The coherence of personality: Social-cognitive bases of personality consistency, variability, and organization* (pp. 345–371). New York: Guilford Press.

Greenwald, A. G., McGhee, D. E., & Schwartz, J. L. K. (1998). Measuring individual differences in implicit cognition: The Implicit Association Test. *Journal of Personality and Social Psychology, 74,* 1464–1480.

Hamilton, D. L., & Sherman, S. J. (1996). Perceiving persons and groups. *Psychological Review, 103,* 336–355.

Hartshorne, H., & May, M. A. (1928). *Studies in the nature of character: Vol. 1. Studies in deceit.* New York: Macmillan.

Heatherton, T. F., & Weinberger, J. L. (Eds.). (1994). *Can personality change?* Washington, DC: American Psychological Association.

Higgins, E. T. (1990). Personality, social psychology, and person–situation relations: Standards and knowledge activation as a common language. In L. A. Pervin (Ed.), *Handbook of personality: Theory and research* (pp. 301–338). New York: Guilford Press.

Higgins, E. T. (1996a). Emotional experiences: The pains and pleasures of distinct regulatory systems. In R. D. Kavanaugh, B. Zimmerberg, & S. Fein (Eds.), *Emotion: Interdisciplinary perspectives* (pp. 203–241). Mahwah, NJ: Erlbaum.

Higgins, E. T. (1996b). Ideals, oughts, and regulatory focus: Relating affect and motivation from distinct pains and pleasures. In P. M. Gollwitzer & J. A. Bargh (Eds.), *The psychology of action: Linking cognition and motivation to behavior* (pp. 91–114). New York: Guilford Press.

Higgins, E. T. (1996c). Knowledge activation: Accessibility, applicability, and salience. In E. T. Higgins & A. W. Kruglanski (Eds.), *Social psychology: Handbook of basic principles* (pp. 133–168). New York: Guilford Press.

Higgins, E. T. (1997). Beyond pleasure and pain. *American Psychologist, 52,* 1280–1300.

Higgins, E. T. (1998). Promotion and prevention: Regulatory focus as a motivational principle. In M. P. Zanna (Ed.), *Advances in experimental social psychology* (Vol. 30, pp. 1–46). New York: Academic Press.

Higgins, E. T., King, G. A., & Mavin, G. H. (1982). Individual construct accessibility and subjective impressions and recall. *Journal of Personality and Social Psychology, 43,* 35–47.

Hoffman, C., Mischel, W., & Mazze, K. (1981). The role of purpose in the organization of information about behavior: Trait-based versus goal-based categories in person cognition. *Journal of Personality and Social Psychology, 40,* 211–225.

Hogan, R., Johnson, J., & Briggs, S. (1997). *Handbook of personality psychology.* New York: Academic Press.

Isen, A. M., Niedenthal, P. M., & Cantor, N. (1992). An influence of positive affect on social categorization. *Motivation and Emotion, 16,* 65–78.

John, O. P. (1990). The "Big Five" factor taxonomy: Dimensions of personality in the natural language and in questions. In L. A. Pervin (Ed.), *Handbook of personality: Theory and research* (pp. 66–100). New York: Guilford Press.

Jones, E. E. (1990). *Interpersonal perception.* New York: Macmillan.

Kagan, J. (2006). *An argument for mind.* New Haven, CT: Yale University Press.

Kammrath, L. K., Mendoza-Denton, R., & Mischel, W. (2005). Incorporating if … then … personality signatures in person perception: Beyond the person–situation dichotomy. *Journal of Personality and Social Psychology, 88,* 605–618.

Kelley, H. H. (1973). The processes of casual attribution. *American Psychologist, 28,* 107–128.

Kelley, H. H., Holmes, J. G., Kerr, N., Reis, H. T.,

Rusbult, C. E., & Van Lange, P. A. M. (2003). *An atlas of interpersonal situations*. New York: Cambridge University Press.

Kihlstrom, J. F. (1999). The psychological unconscious. In L. A. Pervin & O. P. John (Eds.), *Handbook of personality: Theory and research* (2nd ed., pp. 424–442). New York: Guilford Press.

Kihlstrom, J. F. (2004). Implicit methods in social psychology. In C. Sansone, C. C. Morf, & A. Panter (Eds.), *Handbook of methods in social psychology* (pp. 195–212). Thousand Oaks, CA: Sage.

Klinger, E. (1996). Emotional influences on cognitive processing, with implications for theories of both. In P. M. Gollwitzer & J. A. Bargh (Eds.), *The psychology of action: Linking cognition and motivation to action* (pp. 168–189). New York: Guilford Press.

Krahe, B. (1990). *Situation cognition and coherence in personality: An individual-centered approach*. Cambridge, UK: Cambridge University Press.

Kross, E., Ayduk, O., & Mischel, W. (2005). When asking *"why"* doesn't hurt: Distinguishing rumination from reflective processing of negative emotions. *Psychological Science*, *16*, 709–715.

Kruglanski, A. W. (1989). *Lay epistemics and human knowledge: Cognitive and motivational bases*. New York: Plenum Press.

Kruglanski, A. W. (1990). Lay epistemic theory in social-cognitive psychology. *Psychological Inquiry*, *1*, 181–197.

Kunda, Z., & Thagard, P. (1996). Forming impressions from stereotypes, traits, and behaviors: A parallel-constraint satisfaction theory. *Psychological Review*, *103*, 284–308.

Linville, P. W., & Clark, L. F. (1989). Can production systems cope with coping? *Social Cognition*, *7*, 195–236.

Magnusson, D., & Endler, N. S. (Eds.). (1977). *Personality at the crossroads: Current issues in interactional psychology*. Hillsdale, NJ: Erlbaum.

McAdams, D. P. (1994). A psychology of the stranger. *Psychological Inquiry*, *5*, 145–148.

McCrae, R. R., & Costa, P. T., Jr. (1996). Toward a new generation of personality theories: Theoretical contexts for the five-factor model. In J. S. Wiggins (Ed.), *The five-factor model of personality* (pp. 51–87). New York: Guilford Press.

Mendoza-Denton, R., Ayduk, O., Shoda, Y., & Mischel, W. (1997). A cognitive–affective processing system analysis of reactions to the O. J. Simpson verdict. *Journal of Social Issues*, *53*, 565–583.

Mendoza-Denton, R., & Mischel, W. (2007). Integrating system approaches to culture and personality: The cultural Cognitive–Affective Pro-

cessing System. In S. Kitayama & D. Cohen (Eds.), *Handbook of cultural psychology* (pp. 175–195). New York: Guilford Press.

Metcalfe, J., & Jacobs W. J. (1998). Emotional memory: The effects of stress on "cool" and "hot" memory systems. In D. L. Medin (Ed.), *The psychology of learning and motivation: Vol. 38. Advances in research and theory* (pp. 187–222). San Diego, CA: Academic Press.

Metcalfe, J., & Mischel, W. (1999). A hot/cool system analysis of delay of gratification: Dynamics of willpower. *Psychological Review*, *106*, 3–19.

Miller, S. M., Shoda, Y., & Hurley, K. (1996). Applying cognitive-social theory to health-protective behavior: Breast self-examination in cancer screening. *Psychological Bulletin*, *119*, 70–94.

Mischel, W. (1968). *Personality and assessment*. New York: Wiley.

Mischel, W. (1973). Toward a cognitive social learning reconceptualization of personality. *Psychological Review*, *80*, 252–283.

Mischel, W. (1974). Processes in delay of gratification. In L. Berkowitz (Ed.), *Advances in experimental social psychology* (Vol. 7, pp. 249–292). New York: Academic Press.

Mischel, W. (1984). Convergences and challenges in the search for consistency. *American Psychologist*, *39*, 351–364.

Mischel, W. (1990). Personality dispositions revisited and revised: A view after three decades. In L. A. Pervin (Ed.), *Handbook of personality: Theory and research* (pp. 111–134). New York: Guilford Press.

Mischel, W. (1996). From good intentions to willpower. In P. M. Gollwitzer & J. A. Bargh (Eds.), *The psychology of action: Linking cognition and motivation to action* (pp. 197–218). New York: Guilford Press.

Mischel, W. (1998a). *Introduction to personality* (6th ed.). Fort Worth, TX: Harcourt, Brace.

Mischel, W. (1998b). Metacognition at the hyphen of social-cognitive psychology. *Personality and Social Psychology Review*, *2*, 84–86.

Mischel, W. (1999). Personality coherence and dispositions in a cognitive–affective processing system (CAPS) approach. In D. Cervone & Y. Shoda (Eds.), *The coherence of personality: Social-cognitive bases of personality consistency, variability, and organization* (pp. 37–60). New York: Guilford Press.

Mischel, W. (2004). Toward an integrative science of the person. *Annual Review of Psychology*, *55*, 1–22.

Mischel, W. (2005). Alternative futures for our science. *American Psychological Society Observer*, *18*, 15–19.

Mischel, W. (2007). Walter Mischel. In G. Lindzay

& W. M. Runyan (Eds.), *A history of psychology in autobiography* (Vol. 9, pp. 229–267). Washington, DC: American Psychological Association.

Mischel, W., & Ayduk, O. (2004). Willpower in a cognitive–affective processing system: The dynamics of delay of gratification. In R. F. Baumeister & K. D. Vohs (Eds.), *Handbook of self-regulation: Research, theory, and applications* (pp. 99–129). New York: Guilford Press.

Mischel, W., Cantor, N., & Feldman, S. (1996). Principles of self-regulation: The nature of willpower and self-control. In E. T. Higgins & A. W. Kruglanski (Eds.), *Social psychology: Handbook of basic principles* (pp. 329–360). New York: Guilford Press.

Mischel, W., & Mischel, H. N. (1983). The development of children's knowledge of self-control strategies. *Child Development, 54,* 603–619.

Mischel, W., & Morf, C. C. (2003). The self as a psycho-social dynamic processing system: A meta-perspective on a century of the self in psychology. In M. R. Leary & J. P. Tangney (Eds.), *Handbook of self and identity* (pp. 15–43). New York: Guilford Press.

Mischel, W., & Peake, P. K. (1982a). Beyond déjà vu in the search for cross-situational consistency. *Psychological Review, 89,* 730–755.

Mischel, W., & Peake, P. (1982b). In search of consistency: Measure for measure. In M. P. Zanna, E. T. Higgins, & C. P. Herman (Eds.), *Consistency in social behavior: The Ontario Symposium* (Vol. 2, pp. 187–207). Hillsdale, NJ: Erlbaum.

Mischel, W., & Shoda, Y. (1994). Personality psychology has two goals: Must it be two fields? *Psychological Inquiry, 5,* 156–158.

Mischel, W., & Shoda, Y. (1995). A cognitive–affective system theory of personality: Reconceptualizing situations, dispositions, dynamics, and invariance in personality structure. *Psychological Review, 102,* 246–268.

Mischel, W., & Shoda, Y. (1998). Reconciling processing dynamics and personality dispositions. *Annual Review of Psychology, 49,* 229–258.

Mischel, W., Shoda, Y., & Ayduk, O. (2008). *Introduction to personality: Toward an integrative science of the person* (8th ed.). New York: Wiley.

Mischel, W., Shoda, Y., & Rodriguez, M. L. (1989). Delay of gratification in children. *Science, 244,* 933–938.

Morf, C. C. (2006). Personality reflected in a coherent idiosyncratic interplay of intra-and interpersonal self-regulatory processes. *Journal of Personality, 74,* 1527–1556.

Morf, C. C., & Rhodewalt, F. (2001). Expanding the dynamic self-regulatory processing model of narcissism: Research directions for the future. *Psychological Inquiry, 12,* 243–251.

Moskowitz, D. S. (1982). Coherence and cross-situational generality in personality: A new analysis of old problems. *Journal of Personality and Social Psychology, 43,* 754–768.

Moskowitz, D. S. (1994). Cross-situational generality and the interpersonal circumplex. *Journal of Personality and Social Psychology, 66,* 921–933.

Murphy, G. L., & Medin, D. L. (1985). The role of theories in conceptual coherence. *Psychological Review, 92,* 289–316.

Newcomb, T. M. (1929). *Consistency of certain extrovert–introvert behavior patterns in 51 problem boys.* New York: Columbia University, Teachers College, Bureau of Publications.

Nisbett, R. E. (1980). Evolutionary psychology, biology, and cultural evolution. *Motivation and Emotion, 14,* 255–263.

Nisbett, R. E., & Ross, L. D. (1980). *Human inference: Strategies and shortcomings of social judgment.* Englewood Cliffs, NJ: Prentice Hall.

Nolen-Hoeksema, S. (1991). Responses to depression and their effects on the duration of depressive episodes. *Journal of Abnormal Psychology, 100,* 569–582.

Nolen-Hoeksema, S., Parker, L. E., & Larson, J. (1994). Ruminative coping with depressed mood following loss. *Journal of Personality and Social Psychology, 67,* 92–104.

Pervin, L. A. (Ed.). (1990). *Handbook of personality: Theory and research.* New York: Guilford Press.

Pervin, L. A. (1994). A critical analysis of trait theory. *Psychological Inquiry, 5,* 103–113.

Peterson, D. R. (1968). *The clinical study of social behavior.* New York: Appleton-Century-Crofts.

Pietrzak, J., Downey, G., & Ayduk, O. (2005). Rejection sensitivity as an interpersonal vulnerability. In M. W. Baldwin (Ed.), *Interpersonal cognition* (pp. 62–84). New York: Guilford Press.

Plaks, J. E., Shafer, J. L., & Shoda, Y. (2003). Perceiving individuals and groups as coherent: How do perceivers make sense of variable behavior? *Social Cognition, 21,* 26–60.

Plomin, R. (1994). *Genetics and experience: The developmental interplay between nature and nurture.* Newbury Park, CA: Sage.

Plomin, R., DeFries, J. C., McClearn, G. E., & Rutter, M. (1997). *Behavioral genetics* (3rd ed.). New York: Freeman.

Read, S. J., & Miller, L. C. (1993). Rapist or "regular guy": Explanatory coherence in the construction of mental models of others. *Personality and Social Psychology Bulletin, 19,* 526–540.

Read, S. J., & Miller, L. C. (Eds.). (1998). *Connectionist models of social reasoning and social behavior.* Mahwah, NJ: Erlbaum.

Revelle, W. (1995). Personality processes. *Annual Review of Psychology*, 46, 295–328.

Roberts, B. W., Kuncel, N. R., Shiner, R., Caspi, A., & Goldberg, L. R. (2007). The power of personality: The comparative validity of personality traits, socio-economic status, and cognitive ability for predicting important life outcomes. *Perspectives on Psychological Science*, 2, 313–345.

Rodriguez, M., Mischel, W., & Shoda, Y. (1989). Cognitive person variables in the delay of gratification of older children at-risk. *Journal of Personality and Social Psychology*, 57, 358–367.

Rosenberg, S., & Jones, R. (1972). A method for investigating and representing a person's implicit theory of personality. *Journal of Personality and Social Psychology*, 22, 372–386.

Ross, L., & Nisbett, R. E. (1991). *The person and the situation: Perspectives of social psychology.* New York: McGraw-Hill.

Rothbart, M. K., Derryberry, D., & Posner, M. I. (1994). A psychobiological approach to the development of temperament. In J. E. Bates & T. D. Wachs (Eds.), *Temperament: Individual differences at the interface of biology and behavior* (pp. 83–116). Washington, DC: American Psychological Association.

Saudino, K. J., & Plomin, R. (1996). Personality and behavioral genetics: Where have we been and where are we going? *Journal of Research in Personality*, 30, 335–347.

Schmidt, L. A., & Fox, N. A. (1999). Conceptual, biological, and behavioral distinctions among different categories of shy children. In L. A. Schmidt & J. Schulkin (Eds.), *Extreme fear, shyness, and social phobia: Origins, biological mechanisms, and clinical outcomes* (pp. 47–66). New York: Oxford University Press.

Schwarz, N. (1990). Feelings and information: Informational and motivational functions of affective states. In R. M. Sorrentino & E. T. Higgins (Eds.), *Handbook of motivation and cognition: Foundations of social behavior* (Vol. 2, pp. 527–561). New York: Guilford Press.

Sethi, A., Mischel, W., Aber, L., Shoda, Y., & Rodriguez, M. (2000). The role of strategic attention deployment of self-regulation: Prediction of preschoolers' delay of gratification from mother–toddler interactions. *Developmental Psychology*, 36, 767–777.

Shoda, Y. (1990). *Conditional analyses of personality coherence and dispositions.* Unpublished doctoral dissertation, Columbia University, New York.

Shoda, Y. (2003). Individual differences in social psychology: Understanding situations to understand people, understanding people to understand situations. In C. Sansone, C. Morf,

& A. Panter (Eds.), *Handbook of methods in social psychology* (pp. 117–141). Thousand Oaks, CA: Sage.

Shoda, Y. (2007). Computational modeling of personality as a dynamical system. In R. W. Robins, R. C. Fraley, & R. F. Krueger (Eds.), *Handbook of research methods in personality psychology* (pp. 633–651). New York: Guilford Press.

Shoda, Y., & LeeTiernan, S. (2002). What remains invariant?: Finding order within a person's thoughts, feelings, and behaviors across situations. In D. Cervone & W. Mischel (Eds.), *Advances in personality science* (pp. 241–270). New York: Guilford Press.

Shoda, Y., & Mischel, W. (1993). Cognitive social approach to dispositional inferences: What if the perceiver is a cognitive–social theorist? *Personality and Social Psychology Bulletin*, 19, 574–585.

Shoda, Y., & Mischel, W. (1998). Personality as a stable cognitive–affective activation network: Characteristic patterns of behavior variation emerge from a stable personality structure. In S. Read & L. C. Miller (Eds.), *Connectionist models of social reasoning and social behavior* (pp. 175–208). Mahwah, NJ: Erlbaum.

Shoda, Y., Mischel, W., & Peake, P. K. (1990). Predicting adolescent cognitive and self-regulatory competencies from preschool delay of gratification: Identifying diagnostic conditions. *Developmental Psychology*, 26, 978–986.

Shoda, Y., Mischel, W., & Wright, J. C. (1989). Intuitive interactionism in person perception: Effects of situation–behavior relations on dispositional judgments. *Journal of Personality and Social Psychology*, 56, 41–53.

Shoda, Y., Mischel, W., & Wright, J. C. (1993a). Links between personality judgments and contextualized behavior patterns: Situation-behavior profiles of personality prototypes. *Social Cognition*, 4, 399–429.

Shoda, Y., Mischel, W., & Wright, J. C. (1993b). The role of situational demands and cognitive competencies in behavior organization and personality coherence. *Journal of Personality and Social Psychology*, 65, 1023–1035.

Shoda, Y., Mischel, W., & Wright, J. C. (1994). Intra-individual stability in the organization and patterning of behavior: Incorporating psychological situations into the idiographic analysis of personality. *Journal of Personality and Social Psychology*, 67, 674–687.

Shultz, T. R., & Lepper, M. R. (1996). Cognitive dissonance reduction as constraint satisfaction. *Psychological Review*, 103, 219–240.

Shweder, R. A. (1975). How relevant is an individual difference theory of personality? *Journal of Personality*, 43, 455–485.

Shweder, R. A., & D'Antrade, R. G. (1980). The systematic distortion hypothesis. In R. A. Shweder (Ed.), *Fallible judgment in behavioral research: New directions for methodology of behavioral science* (pp. 37–58). San Francisco: Jossey-Bass.

Smith, C. A., & Lazarus, R. S. (1990). Emotion and adaptation. In L. A. Pervin (Ed.), *Handbook of personality: Theory and research* (pp. 609–637). New York: Guilford Press.

Smith, T. W., & Rhodewalt, F. (1986). On states, traits, and processes: A transactional alternative to the individual difference assumptions in Type A behavior and physiological reactivity. *Journal of Research in Personality, 20,* 229–251.

Snyder, M. (1983). The influence of individuals on situations: Implications for understanding the links between personality and social behavior. *Journal of Personality, 51,* 497–516.

Snyder, M., & Gangestad, S. (1982). Choosing social situations: Two investigations of self-monitoring processes. *Journal of Personality and Social Psychology, 43,* 123–135.

Stemmler, G. (1997). Selective activation of traits: Boundary conditions for the activation of anger. *Personality and Individual Differences, 22,* 213–233.

Teasdale, J. D. (1988). Cognitive vulnerability to persistent depression. *Cognition and Emotion, 2,* 247–274.

Trope, Y. (1986). Identification and inferential processes in dispositional attribution. *Psychological Review, 93,* 239–257.

Vallacher, R. R., & Wegner, D. M. (1987). What do people think they're doing?: Action identification and human behavior. *Psychological Review, 94,* 3–15.

Vansteelandt, K., & Van Mechelen, I. (1998). Individual differences in situation–behavior profiles: A triple typology model. *Journal of Personality and Social Psychology, 75,* 751–765.

Vernon, P. E. (1964). *Personality assessment: A critical survey.* New York: Wiley.

Vonk, R. (1998). The slime effect: Suspicion and dislike of likeable behavior toward superiors. *Journal of Personality and Social Psychology, 74,* 849–864.

Walker, L. E. (1979). *The battered women.* New York: Harper & Row.

Weary, G., & Edwards, J. A. (1994). Individual differences in causal uncertainty. *Journal of Personality and Social Psychology, 67,* 308–318.

Westen, D. (1990). Psychoanalytic approaches to personality. In L. A. Pervin (Ed.), *Handbook of personality: Theory and research* (pp. 21–65). New York: Guilford Press.

Wiggins, J. S., & Pincus, A. L. (1992). Personality: Structure and assessment. *Annual Review of Psychology, 43,* 473–504.

Wright, J. C., & Mischel, W. (1987). A conditional analysis of dispositional constructs: The local predictability of social behavior. *Journal of Personality and Social Psychology, 53,* 1159–1177.

Wright, J. C., & Mischel, W. (1988). Conditional hedges and the intuitive psychology of traits. *Journal of Personality and Social Psychology, 3,* 454–469.

Zayas, V., & Shoda, Y. (2005). Do automatic reactions elicited by thoughts of romantic partner, mother, and self relate to adult romantic attachment? *Personality and Social Psychology Bulletin, 31,* 1011–1025.

Zayas, V., & Shoda, Y. (2007). Predicting preferences for dating partners from past experiences of psychological abuse: Identifying the "psychological ingredients" of situations. *Personality and Social Psychology Bulletin, 33,* 123–138.

Zayas, V., Shoda, Y., Osterhout, L., Takahashi, M. M., & Mischel, W. (2008). *ERP evidence of greater processing cost for negative partner behaviors in attachment-related situations.* Manuscript submitted for publication.

Zayas, V., Whitsett, D., Lee, J. J. Y., Wilson, N., & Shoda, Y. (in press). From situation assessment to personality: Building a social-cognitive model of a person. In G. Boyle, G. Matthews, & D. Saklofske (Eds.), *Handbook of personality theory and testing.* Newbury Park, CA: Sage.

CHAPTER 8

Personal Narratives and the Life Story

Dan P. McAdams

The study of stories people tell about their lives is no longer a promising new direction for the *future* of personality psychology. Instead, personal narratives and the life story *have arrived*. In the first decade of the 21st century, narrative approaches to personality have moved to the center of the discipline. Building on broadly based narrative theories of personality and identity (e.g., McAdams, 1985; Singer & Salovey, 1993; Tomkins, 1979) and incorporating insights regarding life stories and autobiographical memory to be found in cognitive science, developmental and clinical psychology, life-course sociology, anthropology, communications studies, and education, a new generation of personality psychologists has established psychological laboratories and research programs dedicated to the empirical study of personal narratives (see Singer, 2004). Hypothesis-testing studies of the structure, content, and dynamics of life stories now regularly appear in mainstream psychological journals. Moreover, narrative approaches to the study of individual lives are reviving personality psychology's historical commitment to idiographic research (Nasby & Read, 1997). Narrative theories and concepts offer a strong alternative to the tired dogmas of psychoanalysis for the interpretation of case studies, biographies, and

the intensive study of the single life over time and in society (Josselson, 2004; McAdams, 2005; Wiggins, 2003).

This chapter brings together the best research being done in personality psychology today on personal narratives and the life story. A key concept in much of this work is *narrative identity*, which refers to an individual's internalized, evolving, and integrative story of the self. A growing number of theorists and researchers agree that people begin to construct narrative identities in adolescence and young adulthood and continue to work on these stories across the adult life course (Birren, Kenyon, Ruth, Shroots, & Svendson, 1996; Cohler, 1982; Habermas & Bluck, 2000; McAdams, 1985). The stories people fashion to make meaning out of their lives serve to situate them within the complex social ecology of modern adulthood. It is within the realm of narrative identity, therefore, that personality shows its most important and intricate relations to culture and society (McAdams, 2006; Rosenwald, 1992). Put differently, the stories we construct to make sense of our lives are fundamentally about our struggle to reconcile who we imagine we were, are, and might be in our heads and bodies with who we were, are, and might be in the social contexts of family, community, the workplace, ethnicity, religion, gender, social class, and culture writ large. *The self comes to terms with society through narrative identity.*

THE NARRATIVE STUDY OF LIVES: SIX COMMON PRINCIPLES

Freud (1900/1953) wrote about dream narratives; Jung (1936/1969) explored universal life myths; A. Adler (1927) examined narrative accounts of earliest memories; Murray (1938) identified recurrent themes in the Thematic Apperception Test (TAT) stories and autobiographical accounts. But none of these classic personality theories from the first half of the 20th century explicitly imagined human beings as storytellers and human lives as stories to be told. The first *narrative* theories of personality emerged in the late 1970s and early 1980s. Tomkins (1979) proposed a *script theory* of personality that conceived of the developing individual as akin to a playwright who organizes emotional life in terms of salient scenes and recurrent scripts. In Tomkins's view, the most important individual differences in psychological life had little to do with basic traits or needs but instead referred to the particular kinds of affect-laden scenes and rule-generating scripts that individuals construct from their experiences as they move through life. In a somewhat similar vein, I (McAdams, 1985) formulated a *a life-story model of identity*, contending that people living in modern societies begin, in late adolescence and young adulthood, to construe their lives as evolving stories that integrate the reconstructed past and the anticipated future in order to provide life with some semblance of unity and purpose (see also Cohler, 1982). Among the most important individual differences between people are structural and content differences in their narrative identities, I argued, apparent in the story's settings, plots, characters, scenes, images, and themes. Singer and Salovey (1993) identified *self-defining memories* as representations of vivid and emotionally intense events in one's life that reflect recurrent life concerns. They asserted that self-defining memories are key components of narrative identity.

The original formulations of Tomkins, McAdams, and Singer viewed life stories as *autobiographical projects* (Thorne, 2006). Much like playwrights or novelists, people work on their stories in an effort to construct an integrative and meaningful product. As psycholiterary achievements, life stories function to make lives make sense by helping to organize the many different roles and features of the individual life into a synthetic whole and by offering causal explanations for how people believe they have come to be who they are (Habermas & Bluck, 2000). A rival perspective in life narrative studies emerged in the 1990s with the postmodern and social-constructionist approaches offered by Gergen (1991) and others (e.g., Bamberg, 1997; Shotter & Gergen, 1989). Developing out of communications studies and literary theory, these perspectives tended to view personal narratives and life stories as *situated performances* (Thorne, 2006). According to Gergen, for example, people tell and enact as many different kinds of stories in social life as there are social situations within which to tell and enact them. Each performance may be imagined as a text to be deconstructed so as to reveal the shifting dynamics involved, but no larger life patterns or meanings are likely to be found. Personal narratives reveal multiple and conflicting self-expressions, a point emphasized, as well, in Hermans's (1996) influential theory of the *dialogical self*. In Hermans's view, narrative identity is akin to a polyphonic novel that is authored by many different voices within the person, all of whom engage in dialogue with each other and with flesh-and-blood characters in the external world.

In recent years, theories of life narrative have tried to steer a middle course between the personal and the social, viewing narrative identity as both an autobiographical project and a situated performance (see McAdams, Josselson, & Lieblich, 2006, for a range of current views). Nonetheless, psychologists who study life stories represent a wide range of theoretical perspectives and corresponding methodological preferences. No single theory or research paradigm integrates all the work being done. Still, certain broad themes emerge again and again in the scholarly literature on the narrative study of lives. Across the many different approaches, there would appear to be general agreement on the validity of the following six common principles.

Principle 1: The Self Is Storied

The neuroscientist Antonio Damasio (1999) wrote: "Consciousness begins when brains acquire the power, the simple power I must add, of telling a story" (p. 10). This simple power may reflect a human universal: Human beings are storytellers by nature (Bruner, 1986). In a multitude of guises—as folktale, legend, myth, history, epic, opera, motion picture, novel, biography, joke, personal anecdote, and reality television—the story appears in every human culture. Stories are the best vehicles known to human beings for conveying how (and why) a human agent, endowed with consciousness and motivated by intention, enacts desires and strives for goals over time (Ricoeur, 1984). Invoking William James's (1892/1963) famous distinction, the self encompasses a subjective storytelling "I" whose stories about personal experience become part and parcel of a storied "me." The self is both the storyteller and the stories that are told.

From an early age, children tell stories about life, casting their personal experiences into the structure of setting, character, scene, and plot. As they move into adolescence and adulthood, they collect together remembered episodes from the past into an autobiographical storehouse that may be organized in terms of lifetime periods (e.g., "when I was in grade school," "before my father left my mother"), general events ("high school football games I enjoyed," "job interviews"), and event-specific knowledge ("my 7th birthday," "senior prom") (Conway & Pleydell-Pearce, 2000). Rather than representing a veridical recording of life as lived, autobiographical memories are highly selective and strategic. Although they may convey certain objective facts about a life, storied recollections of the past are more noteworthy for their expression of personal meaning (Schacter, 1996). Autobiographical memories, furthermore, are encoded and later retrieved in ways that serve the person's goals. As such, life strivings and ongoing projects influence how personal narratives about the past are organized in the first place, and goals for the future generate retrieval models to guide the search for memories later on (Conway & Pleydell-Pearce, 2000; Singer & Salovey, 1993). Life stories, therefore, are always about both the reconstructed past and the imagined future.

Principle 2: Stories Integrate Lives

Stories do many things: They entertain, educate, inspire, motivate, conceal and reveal, organize and disrupt. Among their most important functions, however, is *integration* (Habermas & Bluck, 2000; McAdams, 2001). Stories often bring together into an understandable frame disparate ideas, characters, happenings, and other elements of life that were previously set apart. Psychologically speaking, life stories may provide integration in two ways (McAdams, 1985). First, people's stories about themselves may bring together different self-ascribed tendencies, roles, goals, and remembered events into a *synchronic* pattern that expresses how the individual person, who seems to encompass so many different things in a complex social world, is, at the same time, one (complex and even contradictory) thing as well. A life story may explain, for example, how a person who describes herself as "gentle" and "caring" and who claims to avoid conflict in her personal life manages still to be a successful litigator for her law firm. Second, people's stories provide *diachronic* integration, that is, in time. They provide causal accounts regarding how a person moved from A to B to C in life, showing, for example, how a rebellious teenager at age 20 became a respectable stakeholder in society by the time he was 35; or how a successful 60-year-old entrepreneur believes he evolved, step by step, from an impoverished childhood to his current state of affluence.

The formulation of an integrative narrative identity is an especially salient challenge for individuals living in modern societies, who seek personal integration within an every-changing, contradictory, and multifaceted social world that offers no clear guidelines, no consensus on how to live and what life means (Giddens, 1991). Whereas some approaches to narrative identity examine integration at the broad level of one's life as a whole (McAdams, 1985), others focus on particular scenes and settings in everyday life (Pasupathi, 2001; Thorne, 2000). Whether talking about the full life story or a personal narrative of a single event, nonetheless, people typically engage in a process of *autobiographical reasoning*, wherein they seek to derive general/semantic meanings from particular/episodic experiences in life (Habermas & Bluck, 2000; McLean, 2005; Pals, 2006b). People may conclude, for instance, that a particular event in their lives (episodic knowledge) illustrates something general about themselves (semantic knowledge) or that a particular sequence of events helps to explain how they came to be who they are today. Whether aimed at finding meaning in yesterday's conversation around the water cooler or in a 15-year marriage that ended two decades ago, autobiographical reasoning is an exercise in personal integration— putting things together into a narrative pattern that affirms life meaning and purpose.

Principle 3: Stories Are Told in Social Relationships

A simple but profound truth about stories is that people *tell them*. People tell stories to other people. As such, stories are social phenomena, told in accord with societal expectations and norms. Underscoring the discursive and performative aspects of life storytelling, many investigators argue that any narrative expression of the self cannot be understood outside the context of its assumed listener or audience, with respect to which the story is designed to make a point or produce a desired effect (Pasupathi, 2001). Autobiographical narrators anticipate what their audiences want to hear, and these anticipations influence what they tell and how they tell it (Wortham, 2001).

Research suggests that people frequently share their most memorable events with others soon after the event occurs and on multiple occasions (Rime, Mesquita, Philippot, & Boca, 1991). Telling the story of the event again and again may help the teller to clarify the event's emotional meaning. Thorne and McLean (2003) suggest that the clarification may occur because audiences push storytellers to tell what the story means. "Interlocuters often demand meanings; sooner or later, they insist on knowing why the speaker is telling them the story" (Thorne & McLean, 2003, p. 170). Meaning is expressed not only in what the storyteller says but also in the way he or she says it. Storytellers adopt particular emotional and social *positions* vis-à-vis their audience, and as protagonists in their own personal narratives, they position themselves vis-à-vis other characters in the story (Bamberg, 1997). Thorne and McLean found that

students who told stories of traumatic events in their lives typically positioned themselves, as both narrators and protagonists, in one of three different ways: as brave and courageous (John Wayne), caring and concerned (Florence Nightingale), or weak and vulnerable. Because audiences responded more positively to the John Wayne and the Florence Nightingale stances, and because these two stances were so common, Thorne and McLean depict these as examples of *master narrative positioning* in personal storytelling, at least among young American people.

Pasupathi and colleagues have conducted a number of studies examining how the different conditions under which personal stories are told influence how storytellers feel about themselves and how they recall those stories later (Pasupathi, 2001, 2006; Pasupathi & Rich, 2005). In one experiment, Pasupathi and Rich (2005) asked participants to tell a good friend the story of a positive autobiographical event. In each case, the close friend (listener) was assigned to either an attentive role ("We'd like you to listen to your friend the way you typically do when you're being a good listener") or a distracted role. For the distracted role, the listener was asked to keep track (surreptitiously) of how many times the storyteller used a word beginning with "*th*." Storytellers reacted to the distracted role by providing accounts that were only half as long as those given in the attentive condition. Furthermore, they tended to rate the typicality of the event they described as significantly lower than did the storytellers in the attentive condition. Pasupathi and Rich concluded that distracted listeners tend to undermine the storyteller's confidence that what he or she is describing represents a true expression of the self. In a second experiment, Pasupathi and Rich showed that inattentiveness has more deleterious effects on experience sharing than even disagreeableness. When people are talking about important events in their lives, any kind of reaction—even a hostile one—is preferable to no reaction at all.

People narrate personal events in different ways for different listeners, and they may switch back and forth between different modes of telling. McLean (2005) showed that younger adolescents tend to tell self-defining memories to their parents, but as they get older they prefer peers as audiences for self-telling. Adolescents and young adults often tell personal stories in a humorous mode, aiming to entertain as much as explain (McLean & Thorne, 2006). They may switch back and forth between what Pasupathi (2006) calls *dramatic* and *reflective* modes of storytelling. In the dramatic mode, the storyteller makes frequent use of nonverbal signals, employs vivid quotes and dialogue, and attempts to reenact the original event in the telling. In the reflective mode, the storyteller spends relatively little time describing what happened in the event and focuses instead on what the event may mean or how the event made the person feel. Reflective modes more efficiently communicate information, especially interpretive information. Dramatic modes make for vivid and entertaining stories.

Principle 4: Stories Change over Time

Autobiographical memory is notoriously unstable. Although people typically remember well the *gist* of an important life event as time passes, they often misremember the details (Schacter, 1996). Factual errors in autobiographical recollection increase substantially as the temporal distance from the to-be-remembered event increases. For example, Talarico and Rubin (2003) found that accuracy in recollections of how people heard the news of the September 11, 2001, terrorist attacks in New York City decreased substantially over an 8-month period. Research on *flashbulb memories*—personal recollections of dramatic historical events—suggests that, despite people's beliefs to the contrary, accuracy for memories of the John F. Kennedy assassination (November 22, 1963) or the 9/11 attacks may be no greater than for memories of any other events in life.

The temporal instability of autobiographical memory, therefore, contributes to change in the life story over time. But many other processes are also at play, and many of these reflect changes in how the person comes to terms with the social world. Most obviously, people accumulate new experiences over time, some of which may prove to be so important as to make their way into narrative identity. As people's motivations, goals, personal concerns, and social positions change, furthermore, their memories of important events in their lives and the meanings they

attribute to those events may also change (Conway & Pleydell-Pearce, 2000; Singer & Salovey, 1993). People's autobiographical priorities change as well. Some events may increase in personal salience over time whereas others fade into the background. In a 3-year longitudinal study that asked college students to recall and describe 10 key scenes in their life stories on three different occasions, I and my colleagues (2006) found that only 28% of the memories described at Time 1 were repeated 3 months later (Time 2), and 22% of the original (Time 1) memories were chosen and described again 3 years after the original assessment (Time 3). (Despite change in manifest content of stories, however, we also documented noteworthy longitudinal consistencies in certain emotional and motivational qualities in the stories and in the level of narrative complexity.) Over the 3 years, students' life story accounts became more complex, and they incorporated a greater number of themes suggestive of personal growth and integration (McAdams, Bauer, et al., 2006). Consistent with the general idea that life stories change with personality development, a number of studies have documented significant associations between age, on the one hand, and various structural and content dimensions of personal narratives, on the other (e.g., Bauer, McAdams, & Sakaeda, 2005b; Pratt & Fiese, 2004).

Principle 5: Stories Are Cultural Texts

Life stories mirror the culture wherein the story is created and told (McAdams, 2006). Stories live in culture. They are born, they grow, they proliferate, and they eventually die according to the norms, rules, and traditions that prevail in a given society, according to a society's implicit understanding of what counts as a tellable life (Rosenwald, 1992). Habermas and Bluck (2000) contend that before a person can formulate a convincing life story, he or she must become acquainted with the culture's concept of biography. Indeed, Rubin (2005) argues that much of what people "remember" as part of their life story is really shared cultural knowledge about the life course. Denzin (1989) and I (McAdams, 1996) suggest that narrative accounts of the life course in modern Western cultures are expected to begin in the family, to involve growth and expansion in the early years, to trace later problems back to earlier conflicts, to incorporate epiphanies and turning points that mark changes in the protagonist's quest, and to be couched in the discourse of progress versus decline. But other societies tell lives in different ways and have different views regarding how a person should come to terms with the social world through narrative (Gregg, 1991).

In recent years, psychologists have noted strong differences in autobiographical memory and self-construction between East Asian and North American societies. For example, North American adults typically have an earlier age of first memory and have longer and more detailed memories of childhood than do Chinese, Japanese, and Korean adults (Leichtman, Wang, & Pillemer, 2003). In addition, several studies have noted that North Americans' personal memories tend to be more self-focused than are the memories of East Asians (e.g., Wang, 2001). The differences are consistent with the well-known argument that certain Eastern societies tend to emphasize interdependent construals of the self, whereas Western societies emphasize independent self-conceptions (e.g., Markus & Kitayama, 1991). From an early age, Westerners are encouraged to think about their own individual exploits and to tell stories about them. In a more collectivist culture that inculcates interdependent self-construals, by contrast, children may be encouraged to cultivate a listening role over a telling role and to construct narratives of the self that prioritize other people and social contexts.

Wang and Conway (2004) asked European American and Chinese midlife adults to recall 20 autobiographical memories. Americans provided more memories of individual experiences and one-time events, and they focused their attention on their own roles and emotions in the events. In contrast, Chinese adults were more inclined to recall memories of social and historical events, and they placed a greater emphasis on social interactions and significant others in their stories. The Chinese subjects also more frequently drew upon past events to convey moral messages than did Americans. Wang and Conway suggested that personal narratives and life stories fulfill both self-expressive and self-directive functions. European Americans may prioritize self-expressive functions, viewing personal narratives as vehicles for articulating the breadth, depth, and uniqueness of the inner self. By contrast, Chinese people may prioritize the self-directive function, viewing personal narratives as guides for good social conduct. Confucian traditions and values place a great deal of emphasis on history and respect for the past. Individuals are encouraged to learn from their own past experiences and from the experiences of others, including their ancestors. From a Confucian perspective, the highest purpose in life is *ren*—a blending of benevolence, moral vitality, and sensitive concern for others. One method for promoting *ren* is to scrutinize one's autobiographical past for mistakes in social conduct. Another method is to reflect upon historical events in order to understand one's appropriate position in the social world. It should not be surprising, then, that personal narratives imbued with a Confucian ethic should draw upon both individual and historical events in order to derive directions for life.

Within any society, different stories compete for dominance and acceptance. Feminists such as Heilbrun (1988) argue that, in Western societies, many women "have been deprived of the narratives, or the texts, plots, or examples, by which they might assume power over—take control over—their lives" (p. 17). It is painfully clear that life stories echo gender and class constructions in society and reflect, in one way or another, prevailing patterns of hegemony in the economic, political, and cultural contexts wherein human lives are situated. Power elites privilege certain life stories over others. At the same time, people may resist dominant cultural narratives, give voice to suppressed discourses, and struggle to bring marginalized ways of imagining and telling lives to the cultural fore (Gjerde, 2004). Bamberg and Andrews (2004) describe the effort to make sense of lives outside of, and in opposition to, dominant cultural modes as the construction of *counter-narratives*. Counter-narratives can be found in many different cultural venues and are especially salient among minorities, the economically disadvantaged, and other marginalized groups in society.

Principle 6: Some Stories Are Better Than Others

A life story always suggests a moral perspective, in that human characters are intentional, moral agents whose actions can always be construed from the standpoint of what is "good" and what is "bad" in a given society (MacIntyre, 1981). Furthermore, stories themselves can be evaluated as relatively good or bad from a psychological standpoint, though these evaluations also suggest moral perspectives and reflect the values and norms of the society within which a story is evaluated. The past decade has witnessed an upsurge of interest among narrative researchers in what exactly constitutes a *good life story* (e.g., King, 2001). Researchers have examined narrative coherence and complexity, as well as the extent to which certain features of life stories are associated with psychological maturity, mental health, and professional and marital satisfaction (e.g., J. Adler, Kissel, & McAdams, 2006; Bauer, McAdams, & Sakaeda, 2005a).

A growing number of clinical and counseling psychologists are beginning to see psychotherapy as fundamentally a process of story reformulation and repair (Angus & McLeod, 2004; Lieblich, McAdams, & Josselson, 2004; Singer, 2005). From the view of *narrative therapy*, clients often present disrupted and disorganized life stories that contribute to their symptoms and underlie poor mental health (Dimaggio & Semerari, 2004; Neimeyer & Tschudi, 2003). Narrative therapists help clients transform their faulty life narratives into new stories that affirm growth, health, and adaptation. Narrative interventions have also been developed for the penal system, wherein counselors work to rehabilitate offenders through the development of life stories that acknowledge wrongdoing, manage shame, and point the way to a reformed life (Maruna & Ramsden, 2004).

NARRATIVE IN PERSONALITY: TRAITS, ADAPTATIONS, AND STORIES

Where does narrative identity fit within the big picture of personality? Drawing on narrative studies, the Big Five traits, and other recent trends in the field, we (McAdams & Pals, 2006) proposed an integrative conceptual framework for personality psychology that views the big picture in terms of five broad and interrelated concepts (see also Hooker & McAdams, 2003; Sheldon, 2004; Singer, 2005). The five concepts are evolution,

traits, adaptations, life narratives, and culture. We (McAdams & Pals, 2006) conceive of personality as (1) an individual's unique variation on the general evolutionary design for human nature, expressed as a developing pattern of (2) dispositional traits, (3) characteristic adaptations, and (4) self-defining life narratives, complexly and differentially situated in (5) culture and social contexts. Figure 8.1 illustrates these five concepts and shows their relations to each other.

Evolution provides the general design for psychological individuality against which socially consequential variations in human lives can be conceived. Human beings have evolved, furthermore, to take note of those variations that were most important for group life in the environment of evolutionary adaptedness, many of which continue to play an important role in social life today. Among the most notable psychological variations are a small set of broad dispositional traits, such as extraversion, neuroticism, and other general dimensions to be found within the Big Five and related trait taxonomies. Beyond dispositional traits, human lives vary with respect to a wide range of motivational, social-cognitive, and developmental adaptations, contextualized in time, place, and/or social role. Characteristic adaptations include motives, goals, plans, strivings, strategies, values, self-schemas, mental representations of significant others, developmental tasks, and many other aspects of psychological individuality that speak to motivational, social-cognitive, and developmental concerns. If traits sketch the outline, characteristic adaptations fill in many of the details of personality.

Beyond dispositional traits and characteristic adaptations, human lives vary with respect to the integrative life stories and personal narratives that individuals construct to make meaning and identity in the modern world. Life stories draw from, and are layered upon, dispositional traits and characteristic adaptations, but they cannot be reduced to traits and adaptations. If traits sketch the outline and adaptations fill in details, then stories give individual lives their unique and culturally anchored meanings. Culture exerts different effects on different levels of personality. It exerts modest effects on dispositional traits by setting ground rules and demand characteristics for phenotypic trait expres-

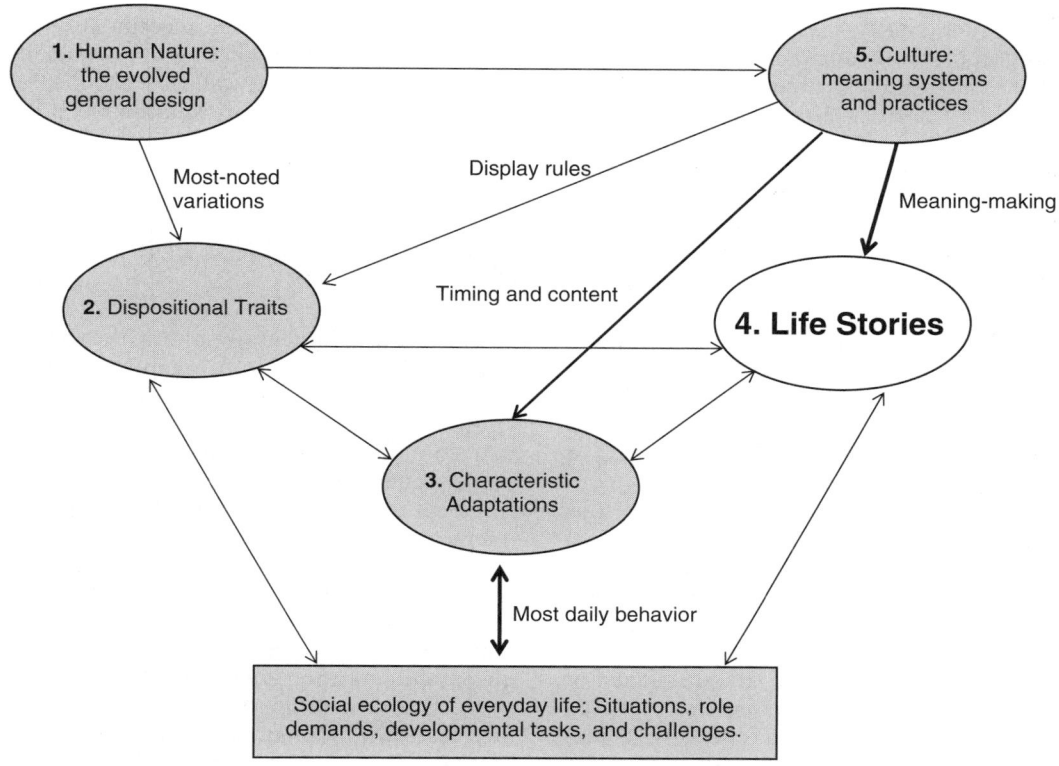

FIGURE 8.1. A framework for personality. From McAdams and Pals (2006, p. 213). Copyright 2006 by the American Psychological Association. Adapted by permission.

sion. It exerts moderately strong effects on characteristic adaptations by influencing the timing and content of goals, motives, values, and the like. Culture exerts its strongest effects, however, on life stories by providing the canonical narrative forms—a menu of life narrative choices—out of which people make meaning in, and out of, their lives (McAdams, 2006). Culture and personality interact in their most intricate and profound ways in the fashioning of narrative identity.

Personality researchers have conducted many studies examining linkages between life narratives and characteristic adaptations. For example, studies have shown that social motives concerning power and intimacy (viewed as characteristic adaptations in Figure 8.1) are systematically related to recurrent narrative themes in life stories (e.g., McAdams, 1982; McAdams, Hoffman, Mansfield, & Day, 1996; Woike, 1995; Woike, Gershkovich, Piorkowski, & Polo, 1999). People with strong power motives

tend to construct personal narratives and life stories that feature such agentic life themes as self-mastery, status and victory, achievement and responsibility, and empowerment; those high in intimacy motivation tend to construct more communal life narratives, emphasizing love and friendship, dialogue, caring for others, and belongingness. People with strong power motivation also tend to use an analytic and differentiated narrative style when describing agentic events, perceiving more differences, separations, and oppositions, compared to people lower in power motivation. By contrast, people with high intimacy motivation tend to use a synthetic style when describing communal events, detecting similarities, connections, and congruence among different elements in significant life story scenes.

Erikson's (1963) theory of psychosocial stages has framed inquiries into the relations between developmental adaptations and life stories. Conway and Holmes (2004) asked older adults to recall important autobiographical memories from each decade of life. They found that the content of these important life-story scenes tends to reflect stage-related themes corresponding to the age at which the scene was encoded. For example, themes of identity (vs. role confusion) tend to predominate in memories from the teenage and emerging adult years, themes of intimacy (vs. isolation) are highest in the 20s, and themes of generativity (vs. stagnation) tend to show up in the midlife decades. Young, Stewart, and Miner-Rubino (2001) found that divorced women tend to frame the stories of their failed marriages in terms of the Eriksonian stages that were relevant at the time of the divorce

Research has also examined relations between life narratives and dispositional traits. Sutin and Robins (2005) documented relations between content themes in self-defining memories and self-report measures of narcissism and self-esteem. Blagov and Singer (2004) found that the specificity of self-defining memories was inversely related to self-report measures of repressive defensiveness. Studies examining life narratives and the Big Five traits have found significant, though statistically modest, relations between the two (McAdams et al., 2004; Raggatt, 2006). Individuals high in neuroticism tend to construct stories with more negative emotional tones; agreeableness tends to be associated with communal themes (e.g., nurturing and caring for others) in life narratives; and people high in openness to experience tend to tell structurally complex stories about themselves that emphasize their creative and artistic tendencies.

Although some predictable relations between the content and structure of life stories, on the one hand, and measures of characteristic adaptations and dispositional traits, on the other, have been documented, the correlations are not so strong as to suggest that these are all interchangeable constructs. Narrative accounts are not merely methodological alternatives for getting at the same dimensions of personality that can be accessed through self-report scales. We (McAdams & Pals, 2006) conceive of traits, adaptations, and stories as three separate domains of personality—three separate categories of self-knowledge, three separate discourses for making sense of self. Assess-

ments of each of the three account for substantial variance in predicting important life outcomes (Bauer et al., 2005b; Pals, 2006c) and contribute unique information to understanding the person as a complex and developing whole (Wiggins, 2003).

THE EMERGENCE AND DEVELOPMENT OF NARRATIVE IDENTITY

Stories are fundamentally about the vicissitudes of human *intention* organized in time (Bruner, 1986). In virtually all intelligible stories, humans or humanlike characters act to accomplish intentions upon a social landscape, generating a sequence of actions and reactions extended as a plot in time. Human intentionality is at the heart of narrative, and therefore the development of intentionality is of prime importance in establishing the mental conditions necessary for storytelling and story comprehension. Research on imitation and attention suggests that by the end of the first year of life, human infants recognize that other human beings are intentional agents who act in a goal-directed manner (Kuhlmeier, Wynn, & Bloom, 2003). They implicitly understand that a story's characters act in accord with goals.

The second year of life marks the emergence of a storytelling, autobiographical self. By 24 months of age, toddlers have consolidated a sense of themselves as agentic and appropriating subjects in the social world who are, at the same time, the objects of others' observations (as well as their own). The 2-year-old self is a reflexive, duplex, I–me configuration: a subjective *I* that observes (and begins to construct) an objective *me*. Among those elements of experience that the *I* begins to attribute to the *me* are autobiographical events. Howe and Courage (1997) argue that children begin to encode, collect, and narrate autobiographical memories around the age of 2—*my* little stories about what happened to *me*—stories the *I* constructs and remembers about *me*.

With development and experience in the preschool years, the storytelling, autobiographical self becomes more sophisticated and effective. The burgeoning research literature on children's *theory of mind* shows that in the 3rd and 4th years of life most children come to understand that intentional human behavior is motivated by internal desires and beliefs. Interpreting the actions of others (and oneself) in terms of their predisposing desires and beliefs is a form of mind reading, according to Baron-Cohen (1995), a competency that is critical for effective social interaction. By the time children enter kindergarten, mind reading seems natural and easy. To most schoolchildren, it makes intuitive sense that a girl should eat an ice-cream cone because "she wants to" (desire) or that a boy should look for a cookie in the cookie jar because "he believes the cookies are there." But autistic children often find mind reading to be extraordinarily difficult, as if they never developed this intuitive sense about what aspects of mind are involved in the making of motivated human behavior. Characterized by what Baron-Cohen calls *mindblindness*, children with autism do not understand people as intentional characters, or do so only to a limited degree. Their lack of understanding applies to the self as well, suggesting that at the heart of severe autism may reside a disturbing dysfunction in "I-ness" and a corresponding inability to formulate and convey sensible narratives of the self (Bruner, 1994).

Autobiographical memory and self-storytelling develop in a social context. Parents typically encourage children to talk about their personal experiences as soon as children are verbally able to do so (Fivush & Nelson, 2004). Early on, parents may take the lead in stimulating the child's recollection and telling of the past by reminding the child of recent events, such as this morning's breakfast or yesterday's visit to the doctor. Taking advantage of this initial conversational scaffolding provided by adults, the young child soon begins to take more initiative in sharing personal events. By the age of 3 years, children are actively engaged in co-constructing their past experience in conversations with adults. By the end of the preschool years, they are able to give a relatively coherent account of their past experiences, independent of adult guidance. Yet individual differences in how parents converse with their children appear to have strong impacts on the development of the storytelling self. For example, when mothers consistently engage their children in an elaborative conversational pattern, asking children to reflect and elaborate upon their personal experiences, children develop richer autobiographical memories and tell more de-

tailed stories about themselves. Conversely, a more constricted style of conversation on the part of mothers is associated with less articulated personal narratives in children (Reese & Farrant, 2003).

By the time children are able to generate their own narrative accounts of personal memories, they also exhibit a good understanding of the canonical features of stories themselves. Five-year-olds typically know that stories are set in a particular time and place and involve characters that act upon their desires and beliefs over time. They expect stories to evoke suspense and curiosity and will dismiss as "boring" a narrative that fails to live up to these emotional conventions (Brewer & Lichtenstein, 1982). They expect stories to conform to a conventional *story grammar* (Mandler, 1984) or generic script concerning what kinds of events can occur and in what order. Stories are expected to have definite beginnings, middles, and endings. The ending is supposed to provide a resolution to the plot complications that developed over the course of the story. If a story does not conform to conventions such as these, children may find it confusing and difficult to remember, or they may recall it later with a more canonical structure than it originally had.

As children move through the elementary school years, they come to narrate their personal experiences in ways that conform to their implicit understandings of how good stories should be structured and what they should include. Importantly, they begin to internalize their culture's norms and expectations concerning what the story of an *entire human life* should contain. As they learn that a telling of a single life typically begins, say, with an account of birth and typically includes, say, early experiences in the family, eventual moves out of the family, getting a job, getting married, and so on, they acquire what Habermas and Bluck (2000) term a *cultural concept of biography*. Cultural norms define conventional phases of the life course and suggest what kinds of causal explanations make sense in telling a life story. As children learn the culture's biographical conventions, they begin to see how single events in their own lives—remembered from the past and imagined for the future—might be sequenced and linked together to create their own life story.

Still, it is not until adolescence, according to Habermas and Bluck (2000), that individuals craft causal narratives to explain how different events are linked together in the context of a biography. What Habermas and Bluck call *causal coherence* in life narratives is exhibited in the increasing effort across the adolescent years to provide narrative accounts of one's life that explain how one event caused, led up to, transformed, or in some way was/is meaningfully related to other events in one's life. An adolescent girl may explain, for example, why she rejects her parents' liberal political values, or why she feels shy around boys, or how it came to be that her junior year in high school represented a turning point in her understanding of herself in terms of personal experiences from the past that she has selected and reconstrued to make a coherent personal narrative. Furthermore, she may now identify an overarching theme, value, or principle that integrates many different episodes in her life and conveys the gist of who she is and what her biography is all about—a cognitive operation that Habermas and Bluck call *thematic coherence*. Studies reported in Habermas and Bluck suggest that causal and thematic coherence are relatively rare in autobiographical accounts in early adolescence but increase substantially through the teenage years and into early adulthood (see also Habermas & Paha, 2001).

The formulation of a narrative identity is the central psychosocial challenge of emerging adults in modern societies. Equipped now with the cognitive software to construct causally and thematically coherent narratives of the self, and motivated to do so by cultural demands, ranging from parental pressure to economic necessity, that proclaim the time "to get a life" is now (Habermas & Bluck, 2000; McAdams, 1985), young men and women begin to put their lives together into full life stories that make sense of the reconstructed past and position them to move forward with purpose into an unknown future. It is time to make some decisions about the future, about school, the armed services, work, and (for some) marriage and family. In general, modern societies "expect" adolescents and young adults to begin to examine the occupational, interpersonal, and ideological offerings of society and, eventually, to make commitments, even if only temporar-

ily, to personalized niches in the adult world. This is to say that both the society and the emerging adult are ready for the individual's experiments in narrative identity by the time he or she has, in fact, become an emerging adult.

If the formation of a narrative identity, then, emerges as a psychosocial problem in late adolescence and young adulthood, it should not be expected to fade away quickly once the individual resolves an identity "stage." The common reading of Erikson's (1963) theory to suggest that identity is a well-demarcated stage to be explored and resolved in adolescence and early adulthood is, from the standpoint of narrative theory and recent life-course research in psychology and sociology (e.g., Arnett, 2000), an increasingly misleading reading of how modern people live and think about their lives. More accurate, it now appears, is this view: *Once narrative identity enters the developmental scene, it remains a project to be worked on for much of the rest of the life course.* Into and through the midlife years, adults continue to refashion their narrative understandings of themselves, incorporating into their ongoing, self-defining life stories developmentally on-time and off-time events, expected and unexpected life transitions, gains and losses, and their changing perspectives on who they were, are, and may be (Birren et al., 1996; Cohler, 1982). Adults continue to come to terms with society and social life through narrative. The autobiographical storytelling self continues to make narrative sense of life, and its efforts may even improve with age. Recent empirical evidence suggests that as they move from adolescence up through midlife, adults use increasingly sophisticated forms of autobiographical reasoning and produce increasingly coherent narrative accounts of their personal experiences (Bluck & Gluck, 2004; Pasupathi & Mansour, 2006).

NARRATING SUFFERING, GROWTH, AND SELF-TRANSFORMATION

Life stories contain accounts of high points, low points, turning points, and other emotionally charged events (Singer & Salovey, 1993; Tomkins, 1979). Positive events involve emotions such as joy, excitement, and love; negative events are about experiences of distress, sadness, fear, anxiety, anger, guilt, shame, and the like. In his script theory of personality, Tomkins (1979) suggested that people tend to organize emotionally positive and negative scenes in their life stories in correspondingly different ways. Scenes built around the positive affects of joy and excitement tend to be construed and organized as *variants*, Tomkins argued. People accentuate variation in their positive scenes, and, in so doing, their stories affirm the notion that people can be happy in many different ways. By contrast, scenes built around negative affects tend to be construed and organized as *analogs*. People accentuate the similarities among their negative events, perceiving common patterns and repetitive sequences, as if to suggest that unhappiness tends to happen in the same old way, over and over again. Positive scenes in narrative identity feel like this: "Wow! This is cool!" For negative scenes, it is more like, "Oh no! Here we go again."

There are many reasons to believe that emotionally positive and negative events present correspondingly different challenges and fulfill different functions in life stories (Pals, 2006a). At a general level, many theories in psychological science link positive emotions to a behavioral approach system (BAS) in the brain, designed to regulate reward-seeking activities. By contrast, negative emotions may signal avoidance behaviors in response to threat or uncertainty, regulated by a behavioral inhibition system (BIS). In her mobilization–minimization theory, Taylor (1991) underscored the asymmetrical effects of positive and negative events. Negative (adverse or threatening) events evoke strong and rapid physiological, cognitive, emotional, and social responses, Taylor argued. The organism mobilizes resources in order to cope with, and ultimately minimize, the adverse effect of a negative event. Negative events produce more cognitive activity in general and more efforts to engage in causal reasoning, compared to positive events. At the level of the life story, negative events seem to *demand an explanation*. They challenge the storyteller to make narrative sense of the bad thing that happened—to explain why it happened and perhaps why it may not happen again, to explore the consequences of the negative event for later development in the story.

Many researchers and clinicians believe that the cognitive processing of negative events leads to insight and positive consequences for psychological well-being and health. Pennebaker's (1997) landmark studies show that writing about (and presumably working through) negative events in life produces positive effects on health and well-being. Whether reviewing and analyzing positive life events produce the same kinds of effects remains an open question (Burton & King, 2004), but at least one study suggests that extensively processing positive events may lead to *reduced* well-being (Lyubomirsky, Sousa, & Dickerhoff, 2006). It may be better simply to *savor* positive life-story scenes, to reexperience the positive emotions involved rather than trying to make cognitive sense of them (Burton & King, 2004). Negative scenes, however, seem to demand more storytelling work. In recent years, narrative research has examined the nature of that work: How do people process negative events in their life stories? And what are the psychological consequences of telling different kinds of stories about personal suffering and adversity?

When it comes to life storytelling, there are many ways to narrate negative events. Perhaps the most common response is to *discount* the event in some way. The most extreme examples of discounting fall under the rubrics of repression, denial, and dissociation. Some stories are so bad that they simply cannot be told—cannot be told to others and, in many cases, cannot really be told to the self. Freeman (1993) argued that some traumatic and especially shameful experiences in life cannot be incorporated into narrative identity because the narrator (and perhaps the narrator's audience as well) lacks the world assumptions, cognitive constructs, or experiential categories needed to make the story make sense. Less extreme are examples of what Taylor (1983) called *positive illusions*. People may simply overlook the negative aspects of life events and exaggerate the potentially positive meanings. "I may be sick, but I am not nearly as sick as my good friend's wife" or "God is testing my resolve, and I will rise to the challenge." Bonanno (2004) showed that many people experience surprisingly little angst and turmoil when stricken with harsh misfortunes in life. People often show *resilience* in the face of adversity, Bonanno argued. Rather than ruminate over the bad things that happen in their lives, they put it all behind them and move forward.

In many situations, however, people cannot or choose not to discount negative life events. Instead, they try to make meaning out the suffering they are currently experiencing, or experienced once upon a time. For example, McLean and Thorne (2003) showed that adolescents often find it necessary to discern lessons learned or insights gained in self-defining memories that involve conflict with others. Pals (2006a) argued that autobiographical reasoning about negative events ideally involves a two-step process. In the first step, the narrator explores the negative experience in depth, thinking long and hard about what the experience feels or felt like, how it came to be, what it may lead to, and what role the negative event may play in his or her overall understanding of self. In the second step, the narrator articulates and commits the self to a positive resolution of the event. Pals warned that one should not pass lightly over the first step. When it comes to narrative identity, Pals suggested, the unexamined life lacks depth and meaning.

Consistent with Pals (2006a), a number of studies have shown that exploring negative life events in detail is associated with psychological maturity. For example, King and her colleagues have conducted a series of intriguing studies wherein they ask people who have faced daunting life challenges to tell stories about "what might have been" had their lives developed in either a more positive or more expected direction (see King & Hicks, 2006, for an overview). In one study, mothers of infants with Down syndrome reflected upon what their lives might have been like had they given birth to babies not afflicted with the syndrome. Those mothers who were able to articulate detailed and thoughtful accounts, suggesting a great deal of exploration and meaning making in their processing of this negative life event, tended to score higher on Loevinger's (1976) measure of ego development than did mothers who discounted what might have been (King, Scollon, Ramsey, & Williams, 2000).

In a study of how midlife women respond to divorce, the elaboration of loss in narrative accounts interacted with time since divorce to predict ego development (King & Raspin, 2004). Among women who had

been divorced for an extended period of time, vivid and highly elaborate accounts of the married life they had lost were associated with higher ego development at the time of their life telling, and narrative elaboration predicted increases in ego development measured 2 years later. In a methodologically similar study, King and Smith (2004) found that the extent to which gay and lesbian individuals explored what might have been had their lives followed a more conventional (heterosexual) course predicted high levels of ego development at the time of their life-narrative accounts and increases in ego development 2 years later.

Narrative studies of life transitions have also shown that self-exploration and elaboration are associated with higher levels of ego development. Bauer and McAdams (2004b) examined narrative accounts from people who had undergone major life changes in either work or religion. People high in ego development tended to construct accounts of these difficult transitions that emphasized learning, growth, and positive personal transformation. The extent to which personal narratives emphasizing self-exploration, transformation, and integration are positively correlated with ego development has also been documented in studies of life goals (Bauer & McAdams, 2004a) and narrative accounts of life's high points, low points, and turning points (Bauer et al., 2005b). In another study linking development to narrative processing, McLean and Pratt (2006) found that young adults who used more elaborated and sophisticated forms of meaning making in narrating turning points in their lives tended also to score higher on an overall identity maturity index. Analyzing data from the Mills Longitudinal Study, Pals (2006c) found that the extent to which women at age 52 explored the ramifications of negative life events mediated the relationship between age 21 coping style and age 61 psychosocial maturity. Women who in early adulthood scored high on self-report scales assessing an open and nondefensive coping style constructed more elaborate and exploratory narrative accounts of difficult life events at age 52, and narrative exploration at age 52 predicted (and accounted for the relationship of coping openness to) clinical ratings of maturity at age 61.

If the first step in making narrative sense of negative life events is exploring and elaborating upon their nature and impact, the second step involves constructing a positive meaning or resolution (Pals, 2006a). Numerous studies have shown that deriving positive meanings from negative events is associated with indicators of life satisfaction and emotional well-being. In their studies of mothers of children with Down syndrome, divorced women, and gay and lesbian adults who reflected on what might have been in life, King and colleagues demonstrated that attaining a sense of closure regarding negative experiences from the past and/or lost possible selves predicts self-reported psychological well-being (see King & Hicks, 2006, for an overview). In her analysis of longitudinal data from the Mills study, Pals (2006c) found that coherent positive resolutions of difficult life events at age 51 predicted life satisfaction at age 61 and were associated with increasing ego resiliency between young adulthood and midlife.

Finding positive meanings in negative events is the central theme that runs through my (McAdams, 2006) conception of the *redemptive self*. In a series of nomothetic and idiographic studies conducted over the past 15 years, I and my colleagues have consistently found that midlife American adults who score especially high on self-report measures of generativity—suggesting a strong commitment to promoting the well-being of future generations and improving the world in which they live (Erikson, 1963)—tend to see their own lives as narratives of redemption (Mansfield & McAdams, 1996; McAdams & Bowman, 2001; McAdams, Diamond, de St. Aubin, & Mansfield, 1997; McAdams, Reynolds, Lewis, Patten, & Bowman, 2001). Compared to their less generative American counterparts, highly generative adults tend to construct life stories that feature redemption sequences, in which the protagonist is delivered from suffering to an enhanced status or state. In addition, highly generative American adults are more likely than their less generative peers to construct life stories in which the protagonist (1) enjoys a special advantage or blessing early in life; (2) expresses sensitivity to the suffering of others or societal injustice as a child; (3) establishes a clear and strong value system in adolescence that remains a source of unwavering conviction through the adult years; (4) experiences significant conflicts between desires for agency/power and desires for com-

munion/love; and (5) looks to achieve goals to benefit society in the future. Taken together, these themes articulate a general script or narrative prototype that many highly generative American adults employ to make sense of their own lives. For highly productive and caring midlife American adults, the redemptive self is a narrative model of *the good life*.

The redemptive self is a life-story prototype that serves to support the generative efforts of midlife men and women. Their redemptive life narratives tell how generative adults seek to give back to society in gratitude for the early advantages and blessings they feel they have received. In every life, generativity is tough and frustrating work, as every parent or community volunteer knows. But if an adult constructs a narrative identity in which the protagonist's suffering in the short run often gives way to reward later on, he or she may be better able to sustain the conviction that seemingly thankless investments today will pay off for future generations. Redemptive life stories support the kind of life strivings that a highly generative man or woman is likely to set forth.

At the same time, the redemptive self may say as much about American culture and tradition as it does about the highly generative American adults who tend to tell this kind of story about their lives. I (McAdams, 2006) argued that the life-story themes expressed by highly generative American adults recapture and couch in a psychological language especially cherished, as well as hotly contested, ideas in American cultural history—ideas that appear prominently in (1) spiritual accounts of 17th-century Puritans, (2) Benjamin Franklin's 18th-century autobiography, (3) slave narratives and Horatio Alger stories from the 19th century, and (4) the literature of self-help and American entrepreneurship from more recent times. Evolving from the Puritans to Emerson to Oprah, the redemptive self has morphed into many different storied forms in the past 300 years as Americans have sought to narrate their lives as redemptive tales of atonement, emancipation, recovery, self-fulfillment, and upward social mobility. The stories speak of heroic individual protagonists—the *chosen people*—whose *manifest destiny* is to make a positive difference in a dangerous world, even when the world does not wish to be redeemed. The stories translate a deep and abiding script of American exceptionalism into the many contemporary narratives of success, recovery, development, liberation, and self-actualization that so pervade American talk, talk shows, therapy sessions, sermons, and commencement speeches. It is as if especially generative American adults, whose lives are dedicated to making the world a better place for future generations, are, for better and sometimes for worse, the most ardent narrators of a general life-story format as American as apple pie and the Super Bowl.

NOMOTHETIC AND IDIOGRAPHIC RESEARCH

When some psychological scientists see the word "narrative," they immediately think: "qualitative methods and case studies." However, most of the narrative-based research published in personality journals (and nearly all of the research reviewed above) consists of *quantitative* studies designed to test hypotheses. Over the past two decades, researchers have developed structured protocols for obtaining life-narrative data and have validated a large number of procedures for coding psychological dimensions of life stories. For example, I and my colleagues have designed a variety of life-story interview protocols and a guided autobiography questionnaire, and we have developed objective coding systems for assessing narrative tone, themes of agency and communion in life-narrative accounts, redemption and contamination sequences, and goal articulation (see *www.sesp.northwestern.edu/foley/*). Singer and colleagues have developed quantitative procedures for assessing the specificity, meaning, content, and affective quality of self-defining memories (Blagov & Singer, 2004; Singer, 2005). Pennebaker and colleagues have employed computer-based word-count systems to assess many different features of narrative text (e.g., Pennebaker, Mayne, & Francis, 1997). Although no single compendium or clearing house has yet been established to organize and disseminate all of the many different coding schemes that narrative researchers use, Smith (2000) and King (2003) have written useful review chapters that lay out basic procedures for designing nomothetic studies of life narratives.

Following Allport (1937) and Murray (1938), a small but vocal contingent of personality psychologists has always argued strenuously for the idiographic approach, wherein subtle and complex patterns of human individuality can be exposed (e.g., Elms, 2007; Runyan, 1990; White, 1952). Case studies and other idiographic approaches are invaluable in the derivation of hypotheses, the construction of new theories, and the illustration of complex patterns of psychological individuality. In recent years, narrative theories, concepts, and methods have provided new tools for the psychological study of the single case. What Josselson and Lieblich (1993) first called the *narrative study of lives* has begun to revitalize personality psychology's historical, if hesitant, commitment to idiographic, case-based research.

When personality psychologists and the public at large thought about psychological case studies in the 20th century, they typically thought about Freud. Psychoanalytic theories—from Freud and Jung to Kohut and the object-relations theorists—provided compelling frameworks for making psychological sense of the individual human life, especially when the life presented interesting conflicts or mysteries to be resolved. As psychoanalytic theory has lost favor in scientific circles, however, personality psychologists have begun to turn to narrative theories for guidance in understanding the single case. For example, Nasby and Read (1997) applied my life-story theory of identity (and the five-factor model of traits) in an in-depth, *in vivo* case study of Dodge Morgan, a middle-age man who circumnavigated the globe in a small boat. Wiggins (2003) compared life-narrative approaches to other assessment strategies in the case study of "Madeline G.," a flamboyant young lawyer who volunteered to be the subject of an in-depth assessment protocol. Singer (1997, 2005) has employed narrative theories in elegant case studies of alcoholics and other patients in psychotherapy. De St. Aubin (1998) drew upon narrative theories, including Tomkins's (1979) script theory, in his psychobiography of the architect Frank Lloyd Wright. I (McAdams, 2005) developed a new set of guidelines for psychobiography, drawn from narrative theories of personality and from contemporary personality research.

Over the past 15 years, the narrative study of lives has inspired a wealth of case-based, idiographic research that continues to provide personality psychology with some of its freshest new ideas. For example, Schultz (2003) developed the concept of the *prototypical scene* in life stories, in order to illustrate a new method for deriving psychobiographical hypotheses. Landman (2001) and Maruna (2001) examined the dynamics of shame, confession, and rehabilitation in narrative studies of reformed criminals. Cohler and Hammack (2006) explored how gay men have struggled to construct coherent narrative identities at different points in American history, teasing out the intricate interrelationships of historical events, social movements, birth cohorts, and individual biographies. Halbertal and Koren (2006) showed how highly religious (Jewish) gays and lesbians construct multiple and contradictory life stories that run along parallel narrative tracks. In a line-by-line exegesis of interview transcripts, Gregg (2006) showed how multiple images of the self are related to each other in terms of structural oppositonality, like *thesis* and *antithesis* in a dialectic. Based on a reading of selected case studies, we (McAdams & Logan, 2006) derived a new theory of how certain creative adults, such as academic researchers in the arts and sciences, narrate the development of their passion for work, and how their narratives of creative work may relate to the stories of their personal lives. J. Adler and I (2007) analyzed autobiographical memories from former psychotherapy patients to derive an initial conception of "the good therapy story." In another study of psychotherapy narratives, Alon and Omer (2004) called into question the idea that progressive and redemptive life stories are always "good" psychological stories and made a compelling argument for the value of tragedy in narrative identity. All of these idiographic efforts put the complex relation between self and society at the center of the inquiry.

Idiographic, case-based studies of life narratives have proven to be especially valuable in generating new methods, concepts, and hypotheses for personality research. Examinations of the single case have also illustrated the sweep and power of narrative theories of personality. As documented in the current chapter as well, nomothetic research on personal narratives and life stories has begun to build up an impressive corpus of empirical findings on the relations between life narratives and other dimensions of personality, the development of narrative identity, the construction of meaning in the face of adversity, and the interpersonal and cultural shaping of the self. More than is true for any other realm of personality psychology today, narrative studies show how idiographic and nomothetic approaches to personality research can complement and enrich each other.

CONCLUSION

Once upon a time, personality psychologists viewed life stories as little different from fairy tales: charming, even enchanting on occasion, but fundamentally children's play, of little scientific value for understanding human behavior and experience. Today, the empirical study of personal narratives and the life story has moved to the center of personality psychology. Building on broad theories of narrative identity developed in the 1980s and 1990s, researchers have set up laboratories and developed ambitious programs to study the expression, development, function, and meaning of the stories people tell about their lives. Internalized and evolving narratives of the self provide people's lives with some measure of integration and purpose. Life stories speak directly to how people come to terms with their interpersonal worlds, with society, and with history and culture. As such, life stories make up a domain of personality structure and functioning that is separate from, though related to, the well-established domains of dispositional traits and characteristic adaptations. Empirical studies have begun to chart relations between stories, traits, and adaptations in human personality, and they have shown how measures of all three domains are needed if the personality psychologist is to provide a full and dynamic account of psychological individuality, an account that pays special attention to the ways in which lives and their social contexts make each other up.

A large and growing body of research traces the development of narrative identity from the infant's first glimmerings of human intentionality to the reworking of life stories in late middle age. Many studies address how people construct stories to make sense of suffering and setbacks in life, and how these redemptive narratives of the self contribute to psychological health, well-being, and maturity. Coming out of social psychology and communication studies, a parallel literature examines the co-construction of personal narratives and life stories in social interaction, in personal relationships, and in the complex cultural and societal contexts wherein narrative identity finds its ultimate meanings. Furthermore, narrative theories and methods have inspired new approaches to psychological case studies and revitalized personality psychology's efforts to build theory and derive new hypotheses through idiographic studies. No realm of personality psychology today so effectively blends the idiographic and the nomothetic as does the narrative study of lives.

In the year 1900, Sigmund Freud published what is arguably the most famous book ever written on the interpretation of personal narratives. In *The Interpretation of Dreams*, Freud argued that dream stories are the "royal road to the unconscious." Freud surely promised too much, and he placed too much faith in but one kind of story that people tell. But he had it right when he surmised that stories hold psychological truth. Over 100 years later, personality psychologists have finally taken on the task of exploring systematically the wide range of stories that people create, tell, and enact about their lives, from childhood through old age, in social interactions and in culture. The study of personal narratives and life stories may not be the *only* royal road to understanding psychological individuality. But until recent years it was the road less traveled. As more and more personality psychologists and other social, behavioral, and cognitive scientists are drawn down the narrative path, researchers will continue to develop new insights and build up systematic bodies of knowledge on how people make sense of their lives in society and culture and how the stories they tell largely determine who they are and affect what they do.

REFERENCES

Adler, A. (1927). *The practice and theory of individual psychology.* New York: Harcourt, Brace World.

Adler, J., Kissel, E., & McAdams, D. P. (2006). Emerging from the CAVE: Attributional style and the narrative study of identity in midlife adults. *Cognitive Therapy and Research, 30,* 39–51.

Adler, J., & McAdams, D. P. (2007). Telling stories about therapy: Ego development, well-being, and the healing relationship. In R. Josselson, A. Lieblich, & D. P. McAdams (Eds.), *The meaning of others: Narrative studies of relationships* (pp. 213–236). Washington, DC: American Psychological Association.

Allport, G. W. (1937). *Personality: A psychological interpretation.* New York: Holt, Rinehart & Winston.

Alon, N., & Omer, H. (2004). Demonic and tragic narratives in psychotherapy. In A. Lieblich, D. P. McAdams, & R. Josselson (Eds.), *Healing plots: The narrative basis of psychotherapy* (pp. 29–48). Washington, DC: American Psychological Association.

Angus, L. E., & McLeod, J. (Eds.). (2004). *The handbook of narrative and psychotherapy: Practice, theory, and research.* London: Sage.

Arnett, J. J. (2000). Emerging adulthood: A theory of development from the late teens through the twenties. *American Psychologist, 55,* 469–480.

Bamberg, M. G. W. (1997). Positioning between structure and performance. *Journal of Narrative and Life History, 7,* 335–342.

Bamberg, M. G. W., & Andrews, M. (Eds.). (2004). *Considering counter-narratives: Narrating, resisting, making sense.* Amsterdam: Benjamins.

Baron-Cohen, S. (1995). *Mindblindness: An essay on autism and theory of mind.* Cambridge, MA: MIT Press.

Bauer, J. J., & McAdams, D. P. (2004a). Growth goals, maturity, and well-being. *Developmental Psychology, 40,* 114–127.

Bauer, J. J., & McAdams, D. P. (2004b). Personal growth in adults' stories of life transitions. *Journal of Personality, 72,* 573–602.

Bauer, J. J., McAdams, D. P., & Sakaeda, A. R. (2005a). Crystallization of desire and crystallization of discontent in narratives of life-changing decisions. *Journal of Personality, 73,* 1181–1213.

Bauer, J. J., McAdams, D. P., & Sakaeda, A. R. (2005b). Interpreting the good life: Growth memories in the lives of mature, happy people. *Journal of Personality and Social Psychology, 88,* 203–217.

Birren, J., Kenyon, G., Ruth, J. E., Shroots, J. J. F., & Svendson, J. (Eds.). (1996). *Aging and biography: Explorations in adult development.* New York: Springer.

Blagov, P. S., & Singer, J. A. (2004). Four dimensions of self-defining memories (specificity, meaning, content, and affect) and their relationship to self-restraint, distress, and repressive defensiveness. *Journal of Personality, 72,* 481–511.

Bluck, S., & Gluck, J. (2004). Making things better and learning a lesson: Experiencing wisdom across the lifespan. *Journal of Personality, 72,* 543–572.

Bonanno, G. A. (2004). Loss, trauma, and human resilience: Have we underestimated the human capacity to thrive after extremely aversive events? *American Psychologist, 59,* 20–28.

Brewer, W. F., & Lichtenstein, E. H. (1982). Stories are to entertain: A structural–affect theory of stories. *Journal of Pragmatics, 6,* 473–486.

Bruner, J. S. (1986). *Actual minds, possible worlds.* Cambridge, MA: Harvard University Press.

Bruner, J. S. (1994). The "remembered" self. In U. Neisser & R. Fivush (Eds.), *The remembering self* (pp. 41–54). New York: Cambridge University Press.

Burton, C. M., & King, L. A. (2004). The health benefits of writing about intensely positive experiences. *Journal of Research in Personality, 38,* 150–163.

Cohler, B. J. (1982). Personal narrative and the life course. In P. Baltes & O. G. Brim, Jr. (Eds.), *Lifespan development and behavior* (Vol. 4, pp. 205–241). New York: Academic Press.

Cohler, B. J., & Hammack, P. L. (2006). Making a gay identity: Life story and the construction of a coherent self. In D. P. McAdams, R. Josselson, & A. Lieblich (Eds.), *Identity and story: Creating self in narrative* (pp. 151–172). Washington DC: American Psychological Association.

Conway, M. A., & Holmes, A. (2004). Psychosocial stages and the accessibility of autobiographical memories across the life cycle. *Journal of Personality, 72,* 461–480.

Conway, M. A., & Pleydell-Pearce, C. W. (2000). The construction of autobiographical memories in the self-memory system. *Psychological Review, 107,* 261–288.

Damasio, A. (1999). *The feeling of what happens: Body and emotion in the making of consciousness.* New York: Harcourt, Brace.

de St. Aubin, E. (1998). Truth against the world: A psychobiographical exploration of generativity in the life of Frank Lloyd Wright. In D. P. McAdams & E. de St. Aubin (Eds.), *Generativity and adult development: How and why we care for the next generation* (pp. 391–428). Washington, DC: American Psychological Association.

Denzin, N. (1989). *Interpretive biography.* Newbury Park, CA: Sage.

Dimaggio, G., & Semerari, A. (2004). Disorganized narratives: The psychological condition and its treatment. In L. E. Angus & J. McLeod (Eds.), *Handbook of narrative and psychotherapy: Practice, theory, and research* (pp. 263–282). London: Sage.

Elms, A. C. (2007). Psychobiography and case study methods. In R. W. Robins, R. C. Fraley, & R. F. Krueger (Eds.), *Handbook of research methods in personality psychology* (pp. 97–113). New York: Guilford Press.

Erikson, E. H. (1963). *Childhood and society* (2nd ed.). New York: Norton.

Fivush, R., & Nelson, K. (2004). Culture and language in the emergence of autobiographical memory. *Psychological Science, 15,* 573–577.

Freeman, M. (1993). *Rewriting the self: History, memory, narrative.* London: Routledge.

Freud, S. (1953). *The interpretation of dreams.* In J. Strachey (Ed.), *The standard edition of the complete psychological works of Sigmund Freud* (Vols. 4 and 5). London: Hogarth Press. (Original work published 1900)

Gergen, K. (1991). *The saturated self: Dilemmas of identity in contemporary life.* New York: Basic Books.

Giddens, A. (1991). *Modernity and self-identity: Self and society in the late modern age.* Stanford, CA: Stanford University Press.

Gjerde, P. (2004). Culture, power, and experience: Toward a person-centered cultural psychology. *Human Development, 47,* 138–157.

Gregg, G. (1991). *Self-representation: Life-narrative studies of identity and ideology.* New York: Greenwood Press.

Gregg, G. (2006). The raw and the bland: A structural model of narrative identity. In D. P. McAdams, R. Josselson, & A. Lieblich (Eds.), *Identity and story: Creating self in narrative* (pp. 63–87). Washington, DC: American Psychological Association.

Habermas, T., & Bluck, S. (2000). Getting a life: The emergence of the life story in adolescence. *Psychological Bulletin, 126,* 748–769.

Habermas, T., & Paha, C. (2001). The development of coherence in adolescents' life narratives. *Narrative Inquiry, 11,* 35–54.

Halbertal, T. H., & Koren, I. (2006). Between "being" and "doing": Conflict and coherence in the identity formation of gay and lesbian orthodox Jews. In D. P. McAdams, R. Josselson, & A. Lieblich (Eds.), *Identity and story: Creating self in narrative* (pp. 37–61). Washington, DC: American Psychological Association.

Heilbrun, C. (1988). *Writing a woman's life.* New York: Norton.

Hermans, H. J. M. (1996). Voicing the self: From information processing to dialogical interchange. *Psychological Bulletin, 119,* 31–50.

Hooker, K., & McAdams, D. P. (2003). Personality reconsidered: A new agenda for aging research. *Journal of Gerontology: Psychological Sciences, 58B,* P296–P304.

Howe, M. L., & Courage, M. L. (1997). The emergence and early development of autobiographical memory. *Psychological Review*, *104*, 499–523.

James, W. (1963). *Psychology*. Greenwich, CT: Fawcett. (Original work published 1892)

Josselson, R. (2004). The hermeneutics of faith and the hermeneutics of suspicion. *Narrative Inquiry*, *14*, 1–28.

Josselson, R., & Lieblich, A. (Eds.). (1993). *The narrative study of lives*. Thousand Oaks, CA: Sage.

Jung, C. G. (1969). *The archetypes and the collective unconscious: Vol. 9. The collected works of C. G. Jung*. Princeton, NJ: Princeton University Press. (Original work published 1936)

King, L. A. (2001). The hard road to the good life: The happy, mature person. *Journal of Humanistic Psychology*, *41*, 51–72.

King, L. A. (2003). Measures and meanings: The use of qualitative data in social and personality psychology. In C. Sansone, C. C. Morf, & A. T. Panter (Eds.), *Sage handbook of methods in social psychology* (pp. 173–194). Thousand Oaks, CA: Sage.

King, L. A., & Hicks, J. A. (2006). Narrating the self in the past and future: Implications for maturity. *Research in Human Development*, *3*, 121–138.

King, L. A., & Raspin, C. (2004). Lost and found possible selves, subjective well-being, and ego development in divorced women. *Journal of Personality*, *72*, 602–632.

King, L. A., Scollon, C. K., Ramsey, C., & Williams, T. (2000). Stories of life transition: Subjective well-being and ego development in parents of children with Down syndrome. *Journal of Research in Personality*, *34*, 509–536.

King, L. A., & Smith, N. G. (2004). Gay and straight possible selves: Goals, identity, subjective well-being, and personality development. *Journal of Personality*, *72*, 967–994.

Kuhlmeier, V., Wynn, K., & Bloom, P. (2003). Attribution of dispositional states by 12-month-olds. *Psychological Science*, *14*, 402–408.

Landman, J. (2001). The crime, punishment, and ethical transformation of two radicals: Or how Katherine Power improves on Dostoevsky. In D. P. McAdams, R. Josselson, & A. Lieblich (Eds.), *Turns in the road: Narrative studies of lives in transition* (pp. 35–66). Washington, DC: American Psychological Association.

Leichtman, M. D., Wang, Q., & Pillemer, D. B. (2003). Cultural variations in interdependence: Lessons from Korea, China, India, and the United States. In R. Fivush & C. A. Haden (Eds.), *Autobiographical memory and the construction of a narrative self* (pp. 73–97). Mahwah, NJ: Erlbaum.

Lieblich, A., McAdams, D. P., & Josselson, R. (Eds.). (2004). *Healing plots: The narrative basis of psychotherapy*. Washington, DC: American Psychological Association.

Loevinger, J. (1976). *Ego development*. San Francisco: Jossey-Bass.

Lyubomirsky, S., Sousa, L., & Dickerhoff, R. (2006). The costs and benefits of writing, talking, and thinking about life's triumphs and defeats. *Journal of Personality and Social Psychology*, *90*, 692–708.

MacIntyre, A. (1981). *After virtue*. Notre Dame, IN: University of Notre Dame Press.

Mandler, J. M. (1984). *Stories, scripts, and scenes: Aspects of schema theory*. Hillsdale, NJ: Erlbaum.

Mansfield, E. D., & McAdams, D. P. (1996). Generativity and themes of agency and communion in adult autobiography. *Personality and Social Psychology Bulletin*, *22*, 721–731.

Markus, H., & Kitayama, S. (1991). Culture and the self: Implications for cognition, emotion, and motivation. *Psychological Review*, *98*, 224–253.

Maruna, S. (2001). *Making good: How ex-convicts reform and rebuild their lives*. Washington, DC: American Psychological Association.

Maruna, S., & Ramsden, D. (2004). Living to tell the tale: Redemption narratives, shame management, and offender rehabilitation. In A. Lieblich, D. P. McAdams, & R. Josselson (Eds.), *Healing plots: The narrative basis of psychotherapy* (pp. 129–149). Washington, DC: American Psychological Association.

McAdams, D. P. (1982). Experiences of intimacy and power: Relationships between social motives and autobiographical memory. *Journal of Personality and Social Psychology*, *42*, 292–302.

McAdams, D. P. (1985). *Power, intimacy, and the life story: Personological inquiries into identity*. New York: Guilford Press.

McAdams, D. P. (1996). Personality, modernity, and the storied self: A contemporary framework for studying persons. *Psychological Inquiry*, *7*, 295–321.

McAdams, D. P. (2001). The psychology of life stories. *Review of General Psychology*, *5*, 100–122.

McAdams, D. P. (2005). What psychobiographers might learn from personality psychology. In W. T. Schultz (Ed.), *Handbook of psychobiography* (pp. 64–83). New York: Oxford University Press.

McAdams, D. P. (2006). *The redemptive self: Stories Americans live by*. New York: Oxford University Press.

McAdams, D. P., Anyidoho, N. A., Brown, C., Huang, Y. T., Kaplan, B., & Machado, M. A. (2004). Traits and stories: Links between dispositional and narrative features of personality. *Journal of Personality*, *72*, 761–783.

McAdams, D. P., Bauer, J. J., Sakaeda, A. R., Anyidoho, N. A., Machado, M. A., Magrino-Failla, K., et al. (2006). Continuity and change in the life story: A longitudinal study of autobiographical memories in emerging adulthood. *Journal of Personality, 74*, 1371–1400.

McAdams, D. P., & Bowman, P. (2001). Turning points in life: Redemption and contamination. In D. P. McAdams, R. Josselson, & A. Lieblich (Eds.), *Turns in the road: Narrative studies of lives in transition* (pp. 3–34). Washington, DC: American Psychological Association.

McAdams, D. P., Diamond, A., de St. Aubin, E., & Mansfield, E. D. (1997). Stories of commitment: The psychosocial construction of generative lives. *Journal of Personality and Social Psychology, 72*, 678–694.

McAdams, D. P., Hoffman, B. J., Mansfield, E., & Day, R. (1996). Themes of agency and communion in significant autobiographical scenes. *Journal of Personality, 64*, 339–378.

McAdams, D. P., Josselson, R., & Lieblich, A. (Eds.). (2006). *Identity and story: Creating self in narrative*. Washington, DC: American Psychological Association.

McAdams, D. P., & Logan, R. L. (2006). Creative work, love, and the dialectic in selected life stories of academics. In D. P. McAdams, R. Josselson, & A. Lieblich (Eds.), *Identity and story: Creating self in narrative* (pp. 89–108). Washington, DC: American Psychological Association.

McAdams, D. P., & Pals, J. L. (2006). A new Big Five: Fundamental principles for an integrative science of personality. *American Psychologist, 61*, 204–217.

McAdams, D. P., Reynolds, J., Lewis, M., Patten, A., & Bowman, P. J. (2001). When bad things turn good and good things turn bad: Sequences of redemption and contamination in life narrative, and their relation to psychosocial adaptation in midlife adults and in students. *Personality and Social Psychology Bulletin, 27*, 472–483.

McLean, K. C. (2005). Late adolescent identity development: Narrative meaning making and memory telling. *Developmental Psychology, 41*, 683–691.

McLean, K. C., & Pratt, M. W. (2006). Life's little (and big) lessons: Identity statuses and meaning-making in the turning point narratives of emerging adults. *Developmental Psychology, 42*, 714–722.

McLean, K. C., & Thorne, A. (2003). Late adolescents' self-defining memories about relationships. *Developmental Psychology, 39*, 635–645.

McLean, K. C., & Thorne, A. (2006). Identity light: Entertainment stories as a vehicle for self-development. In D. P. McAdams, R. Josselson, & A. Lieblich (Eds.), *Identity and story: Creating self in narrative* (pp. 111–127).

Murray, H. A. (1938). *Explorations in personality*. New York: Oxford University Press.

Nasby, W., & Read, N. (1997). The life voyage of a solo circumnavigator: Integrating theoretical and methodological perspectives. Introduction. *Journal of Personality, 65*, 787–794.

Neimeyer, R. A., & Tschudi, F. (2003). Community and coherence: Narrative contributions to the psychology of conflict and loss. In G. D. Fireman, T. E. McVay, Jr., & O. J. Flanagan (Eds.), *Narrative and consciousness: Literature, psychology, and the brain* (pp. 166–191). New York: Oxford University Press.

Pals, J. L. (2006a). Authoring a second chance in life: Emotion and transformational processing within narrative identity. *Research in Human Development, 3*, 101–120.

Pals, J. L. (2006b). Constructing the "springboard effect": Causal connections, self-making, and growth within the life story. In D. P. McAdams, R. Josselson, & A. Lieblch (Eds.), *Identity and story: Creating self in narrative* (pp. 175–199). Washington, DC: American Psychological Association.

Pals, J. L. (2006c). Narrative identity processing of difficult life events: Pathways of personality development and positive self-transformation in adulthood. *Journal of Personality, 74*, 1079–1109.

Pasupathi, M. (2001). The social construction of the personal past and its implications for adult development. *Psychological Bulletin, 127*, 651–672.

Pasupathi, M. (2006). Silk from sows' ears: Collaborative construction of everyday selves in everyday stories. In D. P. McAdams, R. Josselson, & A. Lieblich (Eds.), *Identity and story: Creating self in narrative* (pp. 129–150). Washington, DC: American Psychological Association.

Pasupathi, M., & Mansour, E. (2006). Adult age differences in autobiographical reasoning in narratives. *Developmental Psychology, 42*, 798–808.

Pasupathi, M., & Rich, B. (2005). Inattentive listening undermines self-verification in personal storytelling. *Journal of Personality, 73*, 1051–1085.

Pennebaker, J. (1997). Writing about emotional experiences as a therapeutic process. *Psychological Science, 8*, 162–166.

Pennebaker, J., Mayne, T. J., & Francis, M. E. (1997). Linguistic predictors of adaptive bereavement. *Journal of Personality and Social Psychology, 72*, 863–871.

Pratt, M. W., & Fiese, B. (Eds.). (2004). *Family stories and the life course: Across time and generations*. Mahwah, NJ: Erlbaum.

Raggatt, P. (2006). Putting the five-factor model in context: Evidence linking Big Five traits to narrative identity. *Journal of Personality, 74*, 1321–1347.

Reese, E., & Farrant, K. (2003). Social origins

of reminiscing. In R. Fivush & C. A. Haden (Eds.), *Autobiographical memory and the construction of a narrative self* (pp. 29–48). Mahwah, NJ: Erlbaum.

Ricoeur, P. (1984). *Time and narrative*. Chicago: University of Chicago Press.

Rime, B., Mesquita, B., Philippot, P., & Boca, S. (1991). Beyond the emotional event: Six studies on the social sharing of emotion. *Cognition and Emotion, 5*, 435–465.

Rosenwald, G. C. (1992). Conclusion: Reflections on narrative self-understanding. In G. C. Rosenwald & R. L. Ochberg (Eds.), *Storied lives: The cultural politics of self-understanding* (pp. 265–289). New Haven, CT: Yale University Press.

Rubin, D. C. (2005). A basic-systems approach to autobiographical memory. *Current Directions in Psychological Science, 14*, 79–83.

Runyan, W. M. (1990). Individual lives and the structure of personality psychology. In A. I. Rabin, R. A. Zucker, R. A. Emmons, & S. Frank (Eds.), *Studying persons and lives* (pp. 10–40). New York: Springer.

Schacter, D. L. (1996). *Searching for memory: The brain, the mind, and the past*. New York: Basic Books.

Schultz, W. T. (2003). The prototypical scene: A method for generating psychobiographical hypotheses. In R. Josselson, A. Lieblich, & D. P. McAdams (Eds.), *Up close and personal: The teaching and learning of narrative research* (pp. 151–175). Washington, DC: American Psychological Association.

Sheldon, K. M. (2004). *The psychology of optimal being: An integrated, multi-level perspective*. Mahwah, NJ: Erlbaum.

Shotter, J., & Gergen, K. (Eds.). (1989). *Texts of identity*. London: Sage.

Singer, J. A. (1997). *Message in a bottle: Stories of men and addiction*. New York: Free Press.

Singer, J. A. (2004). Narrative identity and meaning making across the adult lifespan: An introduction. *Journal of Personality, 72*, 437–459.

Singer, J. A. (2005). *Personality and psychotherapy: Treating the whole person*. New York: Guilford Press.

Singer, J. A., & Salovey, P. (1993). *The remembered self: Emotion and memory in personality*. New York: Free Press.

Smith, C. E. (2000). Content analysis and narrative analysis. In H. Reis & P. Shaver (Eds.), *Handbook of research methods in social and personality psychology* (pp. 313–335). New York: Academic Press.

Sutin, A. R., & Robins, R. W. (2005). Continuity and correlates of emotions and motives in self-defining memories. *Journal of Personality, 73*, 793–824.

Talarico, J. M., & Rubin, D. C. (2003). Confidence, not consistency, characterizes flashbulb memories. *Psychological Science, 14*, 455–461.

Taylor, S. E. (1983). Adjustment to threatening events: A theory of cognitive adaptation. *American Psychologist, 38*, 624–630.

Taylor, S. E. (1991). Asymmetrical effects of positive and negative events: The mobilization–minimization hypothesis. *Psychological Bulletin, 110*, 67–85.

Thorne, A. (2000). Personal memory telling and personality development. *Personality and Social Psychology Review, 4*, 45–56.

Thorne, A. (2006). Putting the person into social identity. *Human Development, 47*, 1–5.

Thorne, A., & McLean, K. C. (2003). Telling traumatic events in adolescence: A study of master narrative positioning. In R. Fivush & C. A. Haden (Eds.), *Autobiographical memory and the construction of a narrative self* (pp. 169–185). Mahwah, NJ: Erlbaum.

Tomkins, S. S. (1979). Script theory. In H. E. Howe & R. A. Dienstbier (Eds.), *Nebraska Symposium on Motivation* (Vol. 26, pp. 201–236). Lincoln: University of Nebraska Press.

Wang, Q. (2001). Culture effects on adults' earliest recollection and self-descriptions: Implications for the relation between memory and the self. *Journal of Personality and Social Psychology, 81*, 220–233.

Wang, Q., & Conway, M. A. (2004). The stories we keep: Autobiographical memory in American and Chinese middle-aged adults. *Journal of Personality, 72*, 911–938.

White, R. W. (1952). *Lives in progress*. New York: Holt, Rinehart & Winston.

Wiggins, J. S. (2003). *Paradigms of personality assessment*. New York: Guilford Press.

Woike, B. A. (1995). Most-memorable experiences: Evidence for a link between implicit and explicit motives and social cognitive processes in everyday life. *Journal of Personality and Social Psychology, 68*, 1081–1091.

Woike, B. A., Gershkovich, I., Piorkowski, R., & Polo, M. (1999). The role of motives in the content and structure of autobiographical memory. *Journal of Personality and Social Psychology, 76*, 600–612.

Wortham, S. (2001). *Narratives in action: A strategy for research and analysis*. New York: Teachers College Press.

Young, A. M., Stewart, A. J., & Miner-Rubino, K. (2001). Women's understandings of their own divorces: A developmental perspective. In D. P. McAdams, R. Josselson, & A. Lieblich (Eds.), *Turns in the road: Narrative studies of lives in transition* (pp. 203–226). Washington, DC: American Psychological Association.

PART III

Biological Bases

Temperament

An Organizing Paradigm for Trait Psychology

Lee Anna Clark
David Watson

ANCIENT HISTORY

Temperament is an ancient concept. As early as the fifth century B.C., Greek physicians believed that health depended on a harmonious blend of the four "humors." Extending this view, Galen later proposed that predominance of one or another humor resulted in a characteristic emotional style or temperament, which formed the core of one of four basic personality types (indeed, the word *temperament* derives from the Latin "to blend," so that differences in the blend of humors were equated with differences in temperament; Digman, 1994). The *sanguine* or cheerful, active temperament reflected an excess of blood; the *melancholic* or gloomy temperament reflected an excess of black bile; *choleric* or angry, violent types had an excess of yellow bile; and an excess of phlegm was associated with the *phlegmatic* or calm, passive temperament.

Two aspects of this ancient formulation remain alive in current theories of temperament: (1) Biological factors are seen to underlie observable characteristics, and (2) emotions are seen as core and defining features of temperament. As is so often the case with personality-related constructs, Allport

(1937) provided a definition that captures the essential features:

> Temperament refers to the characteristic phenomena of an individual's emotional nature, including his susceptibility to emotional stimulation, his customary strength and speed of response, the quality of his prevailing mood, and all peculiarities of fluctuation and intensity of mood; these phenomena being regarded as dependent on constitutional makeup and therefore largely hereditary in origin. (p. 54)

Researchers today investigate serotonin deficits, the noradrenergic system, and mesolimbic dopaminergic pathways rather than imbalances among the humors, but the recognition that behavior is partly a function of physical characteristics was a remarkable insight. Moreover, although debates on a precise definition of temperament and its distinction from personality remain (and we do not resolve them in this chapter), there is now widespread agreement (following Allport) that emotional experience and emotional regulation are intrinsic to these concepts (see Digman, 1994, for a brief history of the concept of temperament and further discussion of definitions).

A third aspect of the Greek model is humbling to admit. The Greek observation that there were four main temperaments maps remarkably well onto the four quadrants that emerge from crossing the two primary personality dimensions of the modern theorist Hans Eysenck, neuroticism (or emotional stability) and extraversion, which are found in all major models of temperament and personality. Thus, the stable extravert is sanguine, the unstable extravert is choleric, the unstable introvert is melancholic, and the stable introvert is phlegmatic (Eysenck & Eysenck, 1975).

A BRIEF MODERN HISTORY OF TEMPERAMENT RESEARCH

In addition to the notion that temperament reflects biologically based individual differences in emotional responding, modern temperament theories also have incorporated Allport's idea that these biological differences are innate and form the foundation upon which mature personality develops. Seminal in childhood temperament research, Thomas, Chess, and Birch's (1968; Thomas & Chess, 1977) nine-dimensional structure promoted the view that childhood behavior was structured, measurable, and systematically related to later personality development. Numerous spin-off measures spanned the developmental range from birth through adolescence. Most notably, Eysenck (1967) and Strelau (1983) offered early models of adult temperament derived from Pavlov's theory of central nervous system (CNS) properties. Not widely known in the United States, Strelau's work (Oniszcenko et al., 2003; Strelau & Zawadzki, 1995) has been quite influential among European temperament researchers, and both models spawned numerous learning-based experimental studies.

J. A. Gray (1982, 1987b) also offered a biological model of temperament that overlapped notably with Eysenck's work. Based largely on pharmacological studies with animals, Gray's work strongly influenced theorizing about adult personality or temperament dimensions, particularly among psychopathy researchers. J. A. Gray (Wilson, Barrett, & Gray, 1989) and others (most notably Carver & White, 1994) developed self-report questionnaires to assess Gray's hypothesized dimensions, but the former's measures "bore only a partial resemblance" to the constructs they were designed to measure (p. 1037; Wilson, Gray, & Barrett, 1990), and the latter's scales align closely with Eysenck's Neuroticism and Extraversion (e.g., Jorm et al., 1999), rather than with Gray's dimensions, which Gray viewed as 45 degrees rotated from Eysenck's (e.g., J. A. Gray, 1987a). Thus, relatively little direct testing of Gray's model has been conducted in people, due largely to these difficulties in assessing the hypothesized neuropsychological systems. By contrast, Buss and Plomin (1975) articulated a temperament model that had relatively little theoretical impact, but was widely used in research, because of the instrument they developed to measure their four proposed dimensions of emotionality, activity, sociability, and impulsivity (EASI Temperament Survey).

In various ways, these early efforts were instrumental in beginning to link biological variables with temperament dimensions and their adult personality outgrowths, and they now are starting to bear fruit in the form of (1) better measurement models (e.g., Rothbart & Ahadi, 1994), (2) a major revision of Gray's theory that is "biologically more accurate" (Revelle, 2008), and (3) more sophisticated and complex theoretical models emerging in the newly developing fields of cognitive and affective neuroscience (e.g., Corr, 2004). Indeed, the original edition of this chapter (Clark & Watson, 1999) contained a substantial section on biological models of temperament. However, because the literature on this topic has exploded in the relatively brief intervening period, we no longer can even pretend to do justice to it in the limited space allotted. We do offer interested readers an Appendix with a limited set of relevant references and also direct them to two relevant chapters in this volume: Krueger and Johnson, Chapter 10, on behavioral and molecular genetics and personality, and Canli, Chapter 11, on the neurobiological basis of personality.

THE STRUCTURAL "TRAIT" APPROACH

In contrast to developmentalists and European temperament researchers, American personologists showed relatively little interest in studying temperament as a biologically based concept through much of the 20th century. Rather, trait psychologists focused their attention on structural analyses, with the goal of creating comprehensive descriptive trait taxonomies, and tended to ignore the etiology of the identified dimensions. This structural emphasis led to the criticism that trait psychology offered only a sterile, static *description* of behavior, not a true *explanation* for it.

Mischel (1968) fanned the fires of criticism by suggesting that trait concepts accounted for relatively little variance in—and failed to provide even useful summary descriptions of—behavior, which ignited the longstanding "person–situation debate" (Epstein & O'Brien, 1985; Mischel & Peake, 1982) that still is reverberating (Funder, 2006; see also Funder, Chapter 22, this volume). Although diverse issues eventually were incorporated into this debate, the core controversy revolved around two central questions: (1) Are traits "real" in a basic psychological sense, or do they simply reflect cognitive constructions that people impose on reality to increase predictability and control? (2) Are trait concepts useful predictors of important real-world criteria? After nearly 20 years of theoretical and empirical debate, sufficient evidence accrued to satisfy most researchers that the answer to both questions was "yes": Traits represent real entities and predict important real-world phenomena.

CONVERGENCE OF TEMPERAMENT AND STRUCTURAL APPROACHES

A key element in resolving the debate was the recognition that the major personality traits represent basic *psychobiological* dimensions of temperament (e.g., Eysenck, 1992, 1997; Tellegen, 1985; Watson & Clark, 1993). The emergence of this recognition undoubtedly reflects several factors, three of which we highlight here. First, an explosion of research demonstrated that most personality traits have a substantial genetic component (e.g., Bouchard & Loehlin, 2001; Eysenck, 1990; Loehlin, McCrae, Costa, & John, 1998; McCartney, Harris, & Bernieri, 1990; Oniszczenko et al., 2003; Plomin & Daniels, 1987; Tellegen et al., 1988), indicating that more satisfying genotypic explanations of behavior underlie phenotypic descriptions of traits; we summarize these data in a later section.

Second, rapidly accumulating evidence in the 1980s and early 1990s established that major dimensions of personality—especially neuroticism and extraversion—are strongly associated with individual differences in affective experience (e.g., Meyer & Shack, 1989; Tellegen, 1985; Watson & Clark, 1984, 1992b, 1997). These data provided systematic links to the rich literature on the neurobiological basis of mood and emotion and to temperament research, because temperament had long been considered to have an emotional basis. This development thus held promise for integrating research in the three fields of personality: mood, emotion, and temperament. It was in part the extensive data regarding the genetic and biological etiology of individual differences that helped to establish that traits are real and represent true causes of behavior, rather than mere descriptive summaries.

Third, after decades of seemingly indifferent progress, structural research finally began to bear fruit, converging on a consensual phenotypic taxonomy of personality traits, which we describe subsequently (see also Markon, Krueger, & Watson, 2005). This development enabled more intensive focus on a relatively small number of consensually recognized traits, incorporating them into more complex and sophisticated conceptual schemes and generating more detailed, systematic hypotheses, which helped to clarify the real-world correlates of these traits (e.g., Watson & Clark, 1984, 1993, 1997). Thus, the emergence of a temperament-based paradigm elevated trait psychology to the status of a more mature science that—for the first time—promises a comprehensive explanation of human individual differences in personality.

A STRUCTURAL MODEL FOR STUDYING TEMPERAMENT

The "Big Three" as a Structural Framework

One factor that facilitated the convergence of personologists on a consensual, phenotypic taxonomy was the recognition that personality traits are ordered hierarchically, so that there is no fundamental incompatibility between models emphasizing a few general "superfactors" and those that include a much larger number of narrower traits (see Digman, 1997; Jang, Livesley, Angleitner, Riemann, & Vernon, 2002; Jang, McCrae, Angleitner, Riemann, & Livesley, 1998; Markon et al., 2005). At the apex of this hierarchy are the "big" traits—such as neuroticism and extraversion—that comprise the superfactor models. At the next lower level of the hierarchy, these very broad dispositions divide into several distinct yet empirically correlated traits. For instance, the general trait of extraversion can be subdivided into the more specific facets of assertiveness, gregariousness, cheerfulness, and energy (Depue & Collins, 1999; Watson & Clark, 1997). These facets, in turn, break down into even more specific constructs, including very narrow traits (e.g., talkativeness) and behavioral habits (Digman, 1997).

Of course, all of these levels need to be considered in a comprehensive assessment of personality. We focus primarily on the broad, higher order superfactors for two reasons. First, the available data are most extensive at this level of the hierarchy. For instance, there is much more evidence regarding the genetic basis (Bouchard & Loehlin, 2001; Viken, Rose, Kaprio, & Koskenvuo, 1994) and biological substrates (e.g., Depue & Collins, 1999; Eysenck, 1997; Tellegen, 1985) of extraversion and neuroticism than of other traits (although data on the three other traits comprising the "Big Five" is increasing; see Loehlin et al., 1998) or lower order facets. Second, there currently is much better consensus regarding these superfactors than there is for the traits comprising lower levels of the hierarchy (see Markon et al., 2005). Consequently, we use these superfactors as our basic organizing framework; nonetheless, we consider data related to the lower order facets when relevant.

What are the basic superfactors that form the apex of this hierarchy? Markon and colleagues (2005) recently clarified this issue by reporting a series of factor analyses on a rich collection of trait measures in two studies. Their results were highly consistent across the studies and established an integrative, multilevel hierarchical structure. At its most basic level, personality can be reduced to two superfactors, alpha and beta, originally proposed by Digman (1997). At the next level of the hierarchy, alpha decomposes into distinc-

tive negative emotionality and disinhibition factors, thereby reflecting the well-known Big Three model of personality (e.g., Eysenck & Eysenck, 1975; Gough, 1987; Tellegen, 1985; Watson & Clark, 1993). Disinhibition then splits into two dimensions: disagreeable disinhibition (i.e., low agreeableness [A] of the five-factor model [FFM]) and unconscientious disinhibition (i.e., low conscientiousness [C]). Finally, at the five-factor level, beta splits to form separate extraversion and openness factors, which yields the familiar FFM (e.g., Digman, 1990; McCrae & Costa, 1987, 1997). Thus, the major higher order traditions within personality—including the Big Two, Big Three, and Big Five—all can be organized neatly into a common multilevel structure.

We center our discussion around the Big Three model for two related reasons. First, this model long has guided our thinking and led us to develop our own Big Three instrument, the General Temperament Survey (GTS; Clark & Watson, 1990). Second, researchers within this tradition have placed greater value on explicating the underlying neurobiological substrates of the superfactors (e.g., Eysenck, 1992, 1997; Tellegen, 1985). In contrast, proponents of the Big Five have focused more on the phenotypic description of personality. It must be acknowledged, however, that this gap has narrowed substantially in recent years, as Big Five researchers recently have shown greater interest in the biological etiology of these dimensions (e.g., Jang et al., 2002; McCrae & Costa, 1996; Riemann, Angleitner, & Strelau, 1997).

As per its name, the Big Three model emphasizes the importance of three broad superfactors—which we call "neuroticism/ negative emotionality" (N/NE), "extraversion/positive emotionality" (E/PE), and "disinhibition versus constraint" (DvC). Briefly, N/NE reflects individual differences in the extent to which a person perceives the world as threatening, problematic, and distressing. High scorers experience elevated levels of negative emotions and report a broad array of problems, whereas those low on the trait are calm, emotionally stable, and self-satisfied. E/PE involves an individual's willingness to engage the environment. High scorers (i.e., extraverts) approach life actively, with energy, enthusiasm, cheerfulness, and confidence; as part of this general approach tendency, they seek out and enjoy the company of others and are facile and persuasive in interpersonal settings; in contrast, those low on the dimension (i.e., introverts) tend to be reserved and socially aloof, and they report lower levels of energy and confidence. Finally, DvC reflects individual differences in the tendency to behave in an undercontrolled versus overcontrolled manner. Disinhibited individuals are impulsive and somewhat reckless, and are oriented primarily toward the feelings and sensations of the immediate moment; in contrast, constrained individuals plan carefully, avoid risk and danger, and are controlled more strongly by the longer term implications of their behavior (see Watson & Clark, 1993).[1]

This model arose from the pioneering work of Eysenck and colleagues (e.g., Eysenck, 1967, 1992, 1997; Eysenck & Eysenck, 1975). As noted earlier, Eysenck originally created a widely influential two-factor model consisting of the broad traits of *neuroticism* (vs. emotional stability) and *extraversion* (vs. introversion) which, when crossed, yielded the four Greek temperaments, as noted. Subsequent analyses of expanded pools of questionnaire items led to the identification of a third broad dimension, labeled *psychoticism* (which, despite its name, is better viewed as a measure of psychopathy or disinhibition; see Digman, 1990; Watson & Clark, 1993). A scale assessing this third superfactor was included in the Eysenck Personality Questionnaire (EPQ; Eysenck & Eysenck, 1975).

Other theorists since have postulated very similar three-factor models. Tellegen (1985) proposed a scheme consisting of *negative emotionality* (cf. neuroticism), *positive emotionality* (cf. extraversion), and *constraint* (which has a strong negative correlation with psychoticism). We (Watson & Clark, 1993) subsequently articulated a highly similar model, with factors named *negative temperament*, *positive temperament*, and *disinhibition* (vs. constraint), respectively. Furthermore, in his reformulation of the California Psychological Inventory (CPI), Gough (1987) introduced three higher order "vectors" of *self-realization*, *internality*, and *norm-favoring*, which reflect the low ends of neuroticism, extraversion, and psychoticism, respectively.

These models define a single common structure. For example, Tellegen (1985) demonstrated a high degree of convergence between his factors and those of both Eysenck and Gough. Similarly, we have obtained strong correlations between our factors and those of Eysenck and Tellegen (Watson & Clark, 1993, 1997). Finally, Gough (1987) reported substantial correlations between his higher order vectors and Eysenck's scales. To document this important point further, we administered three purported Big Three instruments—the EPQ, the CPI, and our own GTS—to a sample of 250 University of Iowa undergraduates. We then subjected the nine higher order scales from these instruments—three for each superfactor—to a principal factor analysis (squared multiple correlations in the diagonal). As expected, three factors clearly emerged and were rotated using varimax.

The resulting factor loadings (see Table 9.1) clearly establish that these instruments define a common three-dimensional structure. The three factors—each of which is strongly defined by a scale from all three instruments—are identifiable easily as E/PE, N/NE, and DvC. It should be noted, however, that consistent with earlier studies in this area (e.g., Watson & Clark, 1993), the markers of the DvC dimension generally show the weakest level of convergence. In addition, the GTS and EPQ scales show the strongest convergence and consistently emerge as the best markers of the underlying dimensions.

Relating the Big Three and Big Five

As noted earlier, the Big Three and Big Five models define nested trait structures. Although we use the Big Three as our primary structural framework, we also can take advantage of the enormous amounts of available data using various Big Five measures. To integrate these findings into our framework, we need to expand upon our earlier discussion of Markon and colleagues' (2005) integrative hierarchical model and consider briefly how these two taxonomies relate.

The Big Five model developed originally out of attempts to understand the natural language of trait descriptors (see Digman, 1990; John & Srivastava, 1999; John, Naumann, & Soto, Chapter 4, this volume). Extensive structural analyses of these descriptors consistently revealed five broad factors: neuroticism (vs. emotional stability), extraversion (or surgency), conscientiousness (or dependability), agreeableness (vs. antagonism), and openness to experience (or imagi-

TABLE 9.1. Varimax-Rotated Factor Loadings of the Higher Order Scales from the EPQ, CPI, and GTS

Scale	Factor 1	Factor 2	Factor 3
EPQ Extraversion	**.84**	−.09	−.06
GTS Positive Temperament	**.71**	−.13	−.25
CPI Internality	**−.73**	.06	−.13
GTS Negative Temperament	−.09	**.84**	.09
EPQ Neuroticism	−.16	**.81**	.07
CPI Self-Realization	.02	**−.66**	−.16
GTS Disinhibition	.19	.20	**.73**
EPQ Psychoticism	−.05	.09	**.64**
CPI Norm-Favoring	.29	−.05	**−.61**

Note. N = 250. Loadings of |.40| or greater are shown in **boldface**. EPQ, Eysenck Personality Questionnaire; CPI, California Psychological Inventory; GTS, General Temperament Survey.

nation, intellect, or culture). This structure has proven to be remarkably robust, with the same five factors emerging in both self- and peer ratings (e.g., McCrae & Costa, 1987), children and adults (Digman, 1990, 1994), and across a wide range of languages and cultures (e.g., Ahadi, Rothbart, & Ye, 1993; De Clercq, De Fruyt, Van Leeuwen, & Mervielde, 2006; Jang et al., 1998; McCrae & Costa, 1997).

In addition to the Markon and colleagues (2005) results, other data also indicate that these five factors represent an expanded and more differentiated version of the Big Three. Most notably, it is clear that the neuroticism and extraversion factors of the Big Five essentially are equivalent to the N/NE and E/PE dimensions, respectively, of the Big Three (e.g., Watson & Clark, 1992b, 1993; Watson, Kotov, & Gamez, 2006). Thus, these taxonomic schemes share a common "Big Two" of N/NE and E/PE.

Furthermore, the DvC dimension of the Big Three has been shown to be a complex combination of (low) conscientiousness and agreeableness; that is, disinhibited individuals tend to be impulsive, carefree, reckless (low conscientiousness), uncooperative, deceitful, and manipulative (low agreeableness) (e.g., Digman, 1997; Eysenck, 1997; Markon et al., 2005). In this regard, as we document subsequently, our GTS Disinhibition scale contains both Carefree Orientation and Antisocial Behavior subscales that correlate differentially with (low) conscientiousness and

agreeableness, respectively. Finally, openness appears to be largely unrelated to the Big Three dimensions (Markon et al., 2005). Taken together, these data indicate that one can transform the Big Three into the Big Five by (1) decomposing the DvC dimension into component traits of conscientiousness and agreeableness and (2) including the additional dimension of openness.

BEYOND STRUCTURAL VALIDITY

Development of a clear structural model is an important first step in the articulation of scientific concepts, but we argued earlier that trait models have transcended structuralism to provide authentic explanations for human behavior. In the following sections, we present a portion of these data as illustrative offerings. The first section draws largely from our own research and presents, in overview, a systematic array of correlates for each of the Big Three. We first document relations between mood and temperament; thereafter, we avoid data on variables whose correlations with temperament can be explained, directly or in large part, by a shared mood component (e.g., the voluminous literature on life and job satisfaction). Subsequent sections summarize (1) accumulated genetic evidence that supports the existence of these traits, (2) factors that affect trait stability and change, and (3) relations with psychopathology.

Correlates of the Big Three Traits

Mood

As mentioned earlier, a great deal of evidence links N/NE and E/PE with individual differences in affective experience, to the point that affectivity may be viewed as a core—if not *the* core—of these two dimensions. More specifically, mood also has been shown to have two major dimensions, commonly labeled negative affect (or negative activation) and positive affect (or positive activation) (see Watson, 2000; Watson & Tellegen, 1985; Watson, Wiese, Vaidya, & Tellegen, 1999). Negative Affect (NA) is a general dimension of subjective distress, encompassing a number of specific negative emotional states, including fear, sadness, anger, guilt, contempt, and disgust. Positive Affect (PA), by contrast, reflects the co-occurrence among a wide variety of positive mood states, including joy, interest, attentiveness, excitement, enthusiasm, and pride.

Despite the conceptual distinctiveness of these various specific negative (or positive) mood states, it is quite well-established that they substantially co-occur both within and across individuals to form general (i.e., higher order) affect dimensions (Diener, Smith, & Fujita, 1995; Watson, 2000; Watson & Clark, 1992a, 1992b; Watson et al., 1999). These two highly robust mood dimensions have been recovered from mood ratings of widely ranging terms, formats, and time frames (e.g., from momentary mood to average mood over the past year) (Watson, 1988), as well as in diverse cultures and languages (e.g., Balatsky & Diener, 1993; Watson, Clark, & Tellegen, 1984). It is important to stress that, despite their opposite-sounding labels, these dimensions are largely orthogonal. That is, they represent independent biopsychosocial dimensions that are influenced by different external variables (Clark & Watson, 1988, 1991) and distinct internal biological systems (Clark, Watson, & Leeka, 1989; Watson et al., 1999).

Individuals high in N/NE report higher levels of NA in virtually any situation, from baseline conditions to highly stressful circumstances (e.g., Watson & Clark, 1984). Conversely, high E/PE individuals are more likely to report higher PA levels across a wide range of situations (Watson & Clark, 1992b, 1997). Indeed, as stated earlier, the propensity to experience NA/PA more frequently and intensely are core features of the N/NE and E/PE dimensions, respectively (Tellegen, 1985; Watson & Clark, 1984, 1992b). Although these relations have been well established in various ways by the studies cited (and many others, as well), we cannot resist the temptation to present additional data to document the point using yet another method.

The data in Table 9.2 are from four longitudinal studies of college students who completed mood and activity forms repeatedly over varying lengths of time. Mood ratings were obtained using the 20-item Positive and Negative Affect Schedule (PANAS; Watson, Clark, & Tellegen, 1988). Respondents rated the extent to which they had experienced each mood term (10 each for NA and PA) on a 5-point scale (*very slightly or not at all* to *very much*). The mood ratings in Table 9.2 represent respondents' mood "today" (Samples 1 and 2), "over the past few days" (Sample 3), or "over the past week" (Sample 4). In each sample, the data for each participant were averaged across the entire rating period to yield overall mean NA and PA scores. The

TABLE 9.2. Correlations between the Big Three and Aggregated Mood Ratings in Four Studies

Sample	N/NE	E/PE	DvC
Negative affect			
1	.41	−.02	.19
2	.41	.05	.23
3	.60	−.26	.18
4	.54	−.10	.29
Positive affect			
1	−.14	.35	−.03
2	−.12	.44	−.09
3	−.24	.49	−.06
4	.01	.44	.12

Note. Correlations of |.30| or greater are shown in **boldface**. N/NE, Neuroticism/Negative Emotionality; E/PE, Extraversion/Positive Emotionality; DvC, Disinhibition versus Constraint. Sample 1 *N* = 379; mood measured daily for an average of 44 days (range = 30–55). Sample 2 *N* = 136; mood measured daily for an average of 48 days (range = 21–54). Sample 3 *N* = 61; mood measured over a minimum of 42, 2-day periods (range = 39–45). Sample 4 *N* = 115; mood measured over an average of 13 weekly periods (range = 7–14). Temperament was measured using the GTS (Studies 1 and 3) or factor scores computed from the GTS, EPQ, and CPI (Studies 2 and 4).

TABLE 9.3. Correlations of Disinhibition and Its Subscales with Substance Use

Sample	DvC	CO	AB
Alcohol			
1	.46	**.44**	.35
2	.44	.40	.33
3	.43	**.41**	.29
4	.35	**.40**	.13
Cigarettes			
1	.25	.24	.21
2	.30	.26	.25
Marijuana			
1	.40	.34	.34
2	.36	.26	**.38**
Psychedelics			
1	.32	.24	.31
2	.25	.18	.27
Any nonalcohol substance			
3	.24	.19	.27
Substance-use-related problems			
1	.36	.31	.35
2	.38	.27	.34

Note. DvC, Disinhibition versus Constraint; CO, Carefree Orientation; AB, antisocial behavior. Sample 1 *N* = 638. Sample 2 *N* = 827. Sample 3 *N* = 197. See Watson and Clark (1993) for details regarding method, which were identical for Studies 1 and 2 and slightly modified for Sample 3. Sample 4 *N* = 115; see text for details. The larger of the two subscale correlations is in **boldface**; if the difference between them is significant, it is also underlined.

Big Three scores are from the GTS (Studies 1 and 3) or represent factor scores calculated from the GTS and EPQ combined (Sample 2) or from the GTS, EPQ, and CPI (Sample 4). The data in Table 9.2 demonstrate that, regardless of the time frame over which it is measured or the manner in which the Big Three scores are derived, NA is strongly and consistently related to N/NE, largely unrelated to E/PE, and slightly related to DvC. Conversely, PA is strongly and consistently related to E/PE and largely unrelated to either N/NE or DvC. Clearly and simply, N/NE and E/PE define the prototype for dimensions of temperament as individual differences in affectivity.

Social Behavior

Social engagement is a primary defining characteristic of the E/PE dimension. Indeed, it seems tautological to present data demonstrating that extraverts have a higher level of social involvement than introverts. Rather, it is important to establish that social activity is associated with the Positive Emotionality component of E/PE. We have written extensively on this topic elsewhere (e.g., Watson & Clark, 1997) and so only summarize these data here. First, in a series of studies, indices of social behavior were shown first to be correlated with measures of state positive affect (e.g., Clark & Watson, 1988). Second, social behavior was shown to be as highly correlated with measures of trait positive affect (e.g., the PANAS PA scale) as with "purer" measures of Extraversion (e.g., EPQ-E). For example, number of hours spent with friends (measured daily for approximately 6 weeks) was equally correlated (~.30) with measures of positive temperament and social dominance. Similarly, a 15-item scale of social activity, completed weekly for 13 weeks, correlated equally (again, ~.30) with the PANAS PA scale and with EPQ-E. In both cases, social activity was unrelated to either N/NE or DvC. More specific measures of social behavior, such as number of leadership roles, number of close friends or dating partners, and frequency of partying versus percent of weekend nights spent alone, showed similar patterns (see Watson & Clark, 1997). Although these nonaggregated indices of social behavior showed somewhat lower correlations with both types of E/PE measures (approximately .20), they again were virtually uncorrelated with the other two Big Three dimensions. These types of data demonstrate that positive emotionality and social engagement are specific to, and integral parts of, the E/PE dimension.

DAILY RHYTHMS AND SLEEP

Biologically based diurnal and seasonal rhythms are observed in many important behaviors of plants and animals; human behavior is no exception. For example, there is strong and consistent diurnal variation in mood: PA—but not NA—shows a roughly sinusoidal curve that tracks with other bodily cycles, such as body temperature (Clark et al., 1989; Thayer, 1989; Watson, 2000; Watson et al., 1999). Given that mood is a core feature of temperament, it is plausible that individual differences in daily behavior might reflect underlying variations in temperament. Research examining variation in diurnal mood cycles due to temperament, however, has been quite inconsistent, suggesting that there is no simple relation between temperament and daily mood rhythms (e.g., Clark et al., 1989). However, to investigate whether temperament might influence other aspects of daily behavior, we had students in Sample 2 record the number of hours they slept each day, whereas students in Sample 4 kept a daily log of their rising and retiring times, from which we computed total hours of sleep. The Sample 4 students also completed a revised version (Smith, Reily, & Midkiff, 1989) of the Horne and Ostberg (1977) Morningness–Eveningness Questionnaire (MEQ).

There was no relation between hours of sleep and either N/NE or E/PE in either study; this "non-finding" is consistent with the prior literature, which has found few simple or straightforward relations between diurnal rhythms and general affective temperament (E. K. Gray & Watson, 2002). In Sample 2, amount of sleep correlated modestly with DvC ($r = .27$, $p < .01$), with those high in disinhibition sleeping longer. In Sample 4, however, when actual rising and retiring times were recorded, so that we calculated the students' sleep time rather than having them estimate it themselves, this relation disappeared.

It is noteworthy, however, that although there was no clear relation with total sleep amount, there were significant associations between temperament and *when* students slept. First, disinhibited individuals both retired and arose later ($rs = .33$ and .36, respectively; $p < .001$). Moreover, this effect related significantly more to the DvC Carefree Orientation (low C) subscale ($rs = .39$ and .43, respectively) than to Antisocial Behavior (low A; $rs = .19$, $p < .05$ and .14, ns). Similarly, disinhibited individuals displayed a more characteristic "night owl" orientation on the MEQ than did those low in disinhibition ($r = -.27$), with a much stronger relation observed for Carefree Orientation ($r = -.34$) than Antisocial Behavior ($r = -.08$). Similarly, E. K. Gray and Watson (2002) found that DvC was associated significantly

with later rising and retiring times in a 7-day sleep log, with a particularly strong effect for the Carefree Orientation subscale (see their Table 5).

Conversely, individuals high in E/PE were more likely to be "morning larks" (MEQ $r = .34$, $p < .01$) and to record both earlier rising ($r = -.17$, $p < .07$) and retiring times ($r = -.21$, $p < .03$, respectively). Further analysis using the two GTS Positive Temperament subscales yielded interesting results. The 12-item Energy subscale reflects the more purely physical aspects of the dimension that likely are tied more directly to biological parameters (e.g., "Most days I have a lot of 'pep' or vigor" and "I can work hard, and for a long time, without feeling tired"). The Positive Affectivity subscale items, by contrast, are more laden with cognitive content (e.g., "I lead a very interesting life" and "I can make a game out of some things that others consider work"). The subscales are substantially related ($r = .57$), so strongly differential correlates are relatively rare; nevertheless, both earlier rising time ($rs = -.19$ vs. $-.06$) and MEQ scores ($rs = .33$ vs. .23) related significantly more to the Energy than to the Positive Affectivity subscale. (Curiously, however, retiring time was equally related to Energy and Positive Affectivity.) Although these relations are not strong nor the differences large, they clearly suggest that sleep behavior is tied more closely to the physical and biological (vs. social) aspects of positive temperament.

SUBSTANCE USE, SEXUALITY, AND SPIRITUALITY

We and others have documented the strong relation between DvC and substance use, as well as the striking *lack* of relation of substance use with both N/NE and E/PE. For example, in a large ($N = 901$) college student sample, alcohol use correlated .44 with DvC, $-.04$ with N/NE, and .05 with E/PE (Watson & Clark, 1993, Table 23.4). Correlations with use of marijuana, cigarettes, psychedelics, and caffeine pills ranged from .23 to .33 for DvC, but were all less than |.10| for N/NE and E/PE.

Two additional large-sample replications of these data are reported in Table 9.3, along with data from two other samples. Samples 1 and 2 used a slightly modified version of the inventory we described (Watson & Clark,

1993); the substance-use variables from this inventory are aggregations of multiple items that assess both frequency and quantity of use. Sample 3 participants completed an abbreviated version of the survey in which all substances other than alcohol were assessed with single items. Sample 4 is the same Sample 4 whose prospective, longitudinal data are presented in Table 9.2. The alcohol use variable is the percentage of days on which students reported drinking alcohol. Only correlations with DvC and its subscales, Carefree Orientation and Antisocial Behavior, are shown in Table 9.3, because all correlations with N/NE and E/PE hover around zero.

In the college student population, it appears that use of alcohol—which is quite widespread despite its general illegality in this age group (Wechsler, Davenport, Dowdall, Moeykens, & Castilllo, 1994)—is associated more strongly with a carefree than an antisocial lifestyle (in FFM terms, with low C more than low A). This relation emerges most clearly when the usage variable represents pure frequency of use (Sample 4). College students who "just want to have fun" turn to drink on many occasions. Similarly, cigarette use (which itself is correlated with alcohol use) is nonsignificantly more related to a carefree than an antisocial lifestyle. By contrast, use of substances that are illegal regardless of age (e.g., marijuana, psychedelics, or "any non-alcohol substance" [Sample 3]), as well as substance-use-related problems, are somewhat more indicative of an antisocial lifestyle. Although few of these differences were statistically significant, the consistency of the pattern is noteworthy. However, it is unclear whether this pattern will generalize to samples that include a significant proportion of individuals with serious, chronic alcohol use, in which case stronger correlations with antisocial behavior might be expected.

Promiscuous sexual behavior also has been shown to be related to DvC (e.g., Watson & Clark, 1993; Zuckerman, Tushup, & Finner, 1976). For example, in our (Watson & Clark, 1993) data set, sexual behavior (e.g., number of sex partners in past year) was correlated with DvC ($r = .37$) but not with either N/NE or E/PE ($r = -.02$ and $-.01$, respectively). Additional data—again, only for DvC and its subscales—are reported in Table 9.4. Samples 1–3 are the same as those

TABLE 9.4. Correlations of Disinhibition and Its Subscales with Sexual Behavior

Item/sample	DvC	CO	AB
Number of sexual partners in the past year			
1	.30	.19	**.34**
2	.30	.19	**.31**
4	.22	.14	**.20**
Positive attitudes toward casual sex[a]			
3	**.45**	.28	**.45**
4	**.43**	.26	**.45**
Variety of sexual partners (seven-item scale)			
3	.32	.20	**.33**
Risky sexual behavior (four-item scale)			
3	.32	.22	**.33**

Note. DvC, Disinhibition versus Constraint; CO, Carefree Orientation; AB, Antisocial Behavior. Sample 1 $N = 638$. Sample 2 $N = 827$. Sample 3 $N = 197$. See Watson and Clark (1993) for details regarding method, which were identical for Studies 1 and 2 and slightly modified for Sample 3. Sample 4 (Haig, 1997) $N = 408$; see text for details. The larger of the two subscale correlations is in **boldface**; if the difference between them is significant, it is also underlined. [a]Eight-item scale in Sample 3; three-item scale in Sample 4.

reported in Table 9.3; Sample 4 (Haig, 1997) is another large ($N = 408$) college sample that completed a modified version of the behavioral inventory we used previously (Watson & Clark, 1993). Once again, the pattern is clear: Disinhibited individuals have more positive attitudes toward casual sex and, concomitantly, engage more freely in a variety of sexual behaviors, including those associated with some risk. Moreover, this finding appears to reflect an antisocial more than simply a carefree lifestyle, which is consistent with the inclusion of "promiscuous sexual behavior" among the criteria for psychopathy (Cleckley, 1964; Hare, 1991).

We (Watson & Clark, 1993) also reported that "perceived spirituality" was related positively to E/PE and negatively to DvC. To examine this relation further, Samples 3 and 4 were asked to provide additional data on religious beliefs and behaviors, shown in Table 9.5. Scores from all Big Three factors are shown, because of the established relations of these behaviors to E/PE as well as DvC. Replicating our (Watson & Clark,

1993) findings, all measures relating to religious behaviors or beliefs were related to both E/PE and DvC, with some mild indication that nonreligiosity reflects a more antisocial than simply a carefree lifestyle. That religious people should be more behaviorally constrained comes as no great surprise, although it might be interesting to test the generalizability of these relations in cultures with a less puritanical streak than the United States. The extent to which the relation with E/PE may be due to the social aspects of religious behavior is unknown, and is an issue worth further investigation.

Work and Achievement

At the other end of the spectrum, a number of work- and achievement-related behaviors also have been shown to have associations with temperament (e.g., Barrick & Mount, 1991; Lodi-Smith & Roberts, 2007). For example, in Barrick and Mount's (1991) meta-analysis, Conscientiousness emerged as a significant predictor of all job performance criteria for all occupational groups, whereas E/PE was a valid predictor for two occupations involving substantial social interaction. We (Watson & Clark, 1993) reported that DvC scores were a stronger predictor of first-

year college grades than were Scholastic Aptitude Test (SAT) scores, even after controlling for the latter or for high school grades (the best overall predictor). To determine whether academic performance related differentially to the DvC subscales, we replicated this study in two large samples. The results, presented at the bottom of Table 9.5, indicate that college performance is unrelated to either N/NE or E/PE, but is predicted well by DvC, especially by Carefree Orientation. Thus, again not surprisingly, poor grades early in college are more likely to be obtained by those who lack discipline and prefer to live day-to-day rather than planning carefully for the future. The lower relation with antisocial behavior suggests that some students high on this dimension actually may succeed in "beating the system," whereas others do not.

Putting all of these data together creates a picture that is consistent with theoretical models positing that the DvC dimension is related more to the style of affective regulation than to the overall affective level (which is more the case with N/NE and E/PE). Disinhibited individuals experience greater reinforcement from positive stimuli and simultaneously are capable of diverting attention away from negative stimuli. This combination leads them to focus more strongly on the

TABLE 9.5. Correlations of the Big Three and DvC Subscales with Selected Lifestyle Variables

Variable (No. of items)	Big Three			DvC	
	N/NE	E/PE	DvC	CO	AB
Sample 3					
Religious behavior (10)	−.03	.14	−.32	−.28	−.27
Conservative religious beliefs (11)	−.01	.23	−.15	−.12	−.13
Sample 4					
Religious service attendance (1)	.06	.15	−.19	−.12	−.22
Importance of religion (1)	.02	.17	−.23	−.15	−.25
Reckless driving (4)	−.02	.01	.40	.26	.36
Thrill-seeking behaviors (17)	−.14	.24	.24	.15	.17
Sample 5					
High school GPA	.01	.03	−.22	−.25	−.13
College GPA	.06	−.02	−.27	−.30	−.17
Sample 6					
High school GPA	.02	.01	−.24	−.27	−.10
College GPA	.03	.04	−.42	−.41	−.30

Note. DvC, Disinhibition versus Constraint; CO, Carefree Orientation; AB, Antisocial Behavior; GPA, grade-point average. Sample 3 $N = 197$. See Watson and Clark (1993) for details regarding method, which were slightly modified for this study. Correlations $\geq |.15|$, $p < .05$; $r \geq |.19|$, $p < .01$. Sample 4 (Haig, 1997) $N = 408$; see text for details. Correlations $\geq |.10|$, $p < .05$; $r \geq |.13|$, $p < .01$. Sample 5 $N = 716$ for HS-GPA; $N = 831$ for college GPA. Sample 6 (E. K. Gray & Watson, 2002) $N = 300$. The larger of the two DvC subscale correlations is in **boldface**; if the difference between them is significant, it is also <u>underlined</u>.

rewards than the risks of behavior and thus to engage in a wide range of pleasurable behaviors. Nonetheless, they are not immune to the negative consequences of these behaviors, and so also report a greater number of behavior-related problems. The end result is a zero balance in terms of overall affective level (i.e., no strong correlation of either DvC or these various behaviors with N/NE or E/PE), but a broader range of affective experience.

Genetic and Environmental Contributions to the Big Three Traits

We have postulated that the major traits of personality represent basic biobehavioral dimensions of temperament. We now consider data supporting this assertion. That temperament is biologically based implies that observed individual differences are substantially heritable and that they are—at least in latent form—present at birth (e.g., Buss & Plomin, 1975; Digman, 1994). That is, although biological parameters may be changed by life experiences (cf. stress reactions), our basic biological makeup is innate. Therefore, one crucial line of evidence concerns the possible hereditary basis of these traits.

After decades of neglect, researchers began systematically exploring the genetic basis of personality approximately 30 years ago, starting with the seminal contribution of Loehlin and Nichols (1976). Interest in this topic accelerated in the latter half of the 1980s (e.g., Plomin & Daniels, 1987; Tellegen et al., 1988) and has continued unabated ever since. Consequently, we now have sufficient data to permit several basic conclusions. First, it is quite clear that all of the major dimensions—and, indeed, virtually every trait that has ever been examined—has a substantial genetic component. Heritability estimates based on twin studies generally fall in the .40–.60 range, with a median value of approximately .50 (e.g., Bouchard & Loehlin, 2001; Eid, Reimann, Angleitner, & Borkenau, 2003; Eysenck, 1990; Finkel & McGue, 1997; Jang et al., 2002; Loehlin et al., 1998; Luciano, Wainwright, Wright, & Martin, 2006; Plomin & Daniels, 1987). Adoption studies tend to yield somewhat lower heritability estimates, because they are not well suited to modeling nonadditive genetic variance (Bouchard & Loehlin, 2001;

Plomin, Corley, Caspi, Fulker, & DeFries, 1998; see Krueger & Johnson, Chapter 10, this volume, for a fuller discussion of this issue).

As stated earlier, the data are particularly extensive for N/NE and E/PE, and it is noteworthy that virtually identical findings have emerged across a wide variety of instruments, including the EPQ (e.g., Eysenck, 1990; Viken et al., 1994), CPI (Loehlin & Gough, 1990), Multidimensional Personality Questionnaire (MPQ; Bouchard & Loehlin, 2001; Finkel & McGue, 1997; McGue, Bacon & Lykken, 1993; Tellegen et al., 1988), Minnesota Multiphasic Personality Inventory (MMPI; Beer, Arnold, & Loehlin, 1998), NEO Personality Inventory—Revised (NEO-PI-R; Bouchard & Loehlin, 2001; Jang et al., 1998, 2002; Luciano et al., 2006), and Cloninger's Temperament and Character Inventory (Keller, Coventry, Heath, & Martin, 2005); see also Loehlin and colleagues (1998) for a study examining multiple measures in the same sample. The data for DvC also have been quite consistent, with the exception of one unusually low heritability estimate (.18), for the CPI Norm-Favoring vector scale (Loehlin & Gough, 1990). However, the data are inconsistent regarding the extent to which the genetic variance is additive versus nonadditive (see Keller et al., 2005). Nevertheless, it is noteworthy that nonadditive dominance effects are found much more frequently for E/PE than for the other superfactors (Eysenck, 1990; McGue et al., 1993; but see Loehlin et al., 1998, who also found them for N/NE). Finally, it is interesting to note that—paralleling the structure of phenotypic personality traits—the factor structure that emerges from genetic studies is hierarchical (Krueger & Johnson, Chapter 10, this volume).

Second, the data overwhelmingly suggest that a common rearing environment (i.e., the effects of living together in the same household) exerts virtually no effect on personality (e.g., Beer et al., 1998; Bouchard & Loehlin, 2001; Eid et al., 2003; Eysenck, 1990; Goldsmith, Buss, & Lemery, 1997; Jang et al., 2002; Loehlin et al., 1998; Plomin & Daniels, 1987; Tellegen et al., 1988). This finding was unanticipated and initially was met with some skepticism, but it has emerged so consistently that it now must be acknowledged as a necessary component in any model of personality development. Indeed, virtually the only supportive evidence comes from analyses of the E/PE factor: Three studies have reported significant shared environment effects (Beer et al., 1998; Goldsmith et al., 1997; Tellegen et al., 1988; see also Loehlin et al., 1998, who found shared environment effects for A and C on personality inventories but not trait or adjective rating scales). However, this positive evidence must be weighed against a much larger number of studies that have found no effects due to the common rearing environment (e.g., Eysenck, 1990; Finkel & McGue, 1997; Jang et al., 1998). Thus, we largely concur with Beer and colleagues' (1998) conclusion that "shared familial environmental variation is an unimportant source of individual differences in personality and interests" (p. 818).

In contrast, researchers consistently have reported substantial effects due to the unshared environment (i.e., idiosyncratic environmental stimuli experienced by a single individual but not by his or her biological relatives). A commonplace finding is that roughly half the variance is attributable to genes, with the other half attributable to unique aspects of the environment (see Bouchard & Loehlin, 2001; Loehlin et al., 1998; Plomin & Daniels, 1987; Tellegen et al., 1988). However, this neat symmetry almost certainly represents a substantial overestimate of the unshared environmental variance. The problem—frequently noted by investigators (e.g., Bouchard & Loehlin, 2001; Eysenck, 1990; Riemann et al., 1997; Tellegen et al., 1988)—is that the traditional method of estimating the unshared environment actually confounds (1) true environmental variance, (2) gene–environment interactions, and (3) measurement error. In this regard, it is noteworthy that Riemann and colleagues (1997) were able to separate out the first two effects from the last by conducting combined analyses of self- and peer ratings. Using this expanded approach, they found that nearly 70% of the systematic variance in both N/NE and E/PE was due to genetic factors, with only roughly 30% attributable to the unshared environment and gene–environment interactions. The latter takes on particular importance in the case of temperament, when conceptualized as a set of biologically based propensities to respond to the environment in certain ways. That is,

it is largely through gene–environment interactions that each individual's unique personality develops.

Researchers also have begun to examine how genetic and environmental influences may vary as a function of demographic variables such as sex and age. The data regarding sex have been markedly inconsistent, although several investigators have reported higher heritabilities for women than for men (for a review, see Finkel & McGue, 1997). The evidence regarding age is much more systematic, as several studies now have found that heritability estimates for both N/NE and E/PE are significantly lower in older respondents (McCartney et al., 1990; McGue et al., 1993; Pedersen, 1993; Viken et al., 1994). The causes of these age-related declines have not yet been clearly established, but it appears that they may differ across these two dimensions. Specifically, McGue and colleagues (1993) found that the lower value for N/NE was due to a true decline in heritability, whereas that for E/PE was attributable to the increased influence of the unshared environment (coupled with a stable genetic component).

Finally, the recent explosion of genetics research has yielded valuable data regarding the interesting issue of assortative mating, that is, whether or not people partner with individuals who are phenotypically (and, therefore, genotypically) similar to themselves. In other words, do "Birds of a feather flock together" or do "Opposites attract"? Assortative mating is of keen interest to behavior geneticists because if it occurs, people actually will be more genetically similar to their first-degree relatives than the 50% that traditionally is assumed in the classic models. Generally speaking, however, there appears to be little or no assortative mating on the Big Three superfactors (e.g., Beer et al., 1998; Eysenck, 1990; Finkel & McGue, 1997; Watson et al., 2004). Based on a review of earlier literature, Eysenck (1990) concluded that "mating is essentially random for personality differences" (p. 252), and more recent data support this conclusion. It is unclear, however, whether this is because temperament is irrelevant in mating or because both axioms are true to some extent and their effects cancel out. In contrast to the temperament data, there is evidence supporting assortative mating for more attitudinal aspects of personality (Watson et al., 2004), but this topic is beyond our scope.

The Temporal Stability of Personality

The Genetic and Environmental Basis of Stability

A discussion of the stability of personality over time may seem superfluous in light of our earlier review of heritability data. Indeed, a popular misconception is that because we are born with a full complement of genes, their influence necessarily must be stable and invariant throughout the lifespan, which, in turn, implies that there should be a direct, positive correlation between the heritability of a trait and its temporal stability (for discussions, see Pedersen, 1993; Viken et al., 1994). In actuality, however, genes can be a source of both stability and change in personality. Indeed, age-specific genes (e.g., a gene that influences temperament during adolescence but is quiescent during adulthood) generally can be expected to lead to instability in individual differences over time (McGue et al., 1993; Pedersen, 1993). Conversely, unchanging aspects of the environment (e.g., a long-term career or marriage) may well play an important role in maintaining the stability of temperament. Consequently, there is no necessary correlation between stability and heritability.

That said, however, we also must acknowledge that available data suggest that the popular view is reasonably accurate after all: Genes do appear to be the major source of observed stability in temperament, whereas environmental factors are primarily responsible for change (McGue et al., 1993; Pedersen, 1993; Viken et al., 1994). For instance, McGue and colleagues (1993) estimated the heritability of the stable component to be .71, .89, and .89 for N/NE, E/PE, and DvC, respectively. Note that although these values demonstrate that genetic factors are overwhelmingly responsible for phenotypic stability, they also indicate that the unshared environment has a nontrivial influence on the observed continuity of temperament. Conversely, McGue and colleagues found that although the unshared environment was primarily responsible for observed changes on these traits, genetic factors also played a moderate role in the instability of N/NE and DvC, and a more modest role in produc-

ing changes on E/PE. McGue and colleagues suggested these genetic sources of instability may be linked to the observed declines in heritability that were discussed earlier. For example, age-specific genes may exert a significant influence on N/NE in adolescence, but then decline in importance during adulthood, leading to both lower heritabilities and phenotypic instability in N/NE over time.

These data establish that genes are primarily responsible for stability, but they do not address the issue of stability itself. How stable are the major dimensions of temperament over time? In discussing this issue, it is useful to distinguish three different types of stability: *mean-level stability, rank-order stability*, and *structural stability* (see Pedersen, 1993).

Mean-Level Stability

Mean-level stability concerns whether average levels of a trait change systematically with age. For example, do people generally become more cautious and constrained as they grow older? Recent reviews of these data have yielded several clear conclusions (Caspi, Roberts, & Shiner, 2005; Roberts, Walton, & Viechtbauer, 2006; Vaidya, Gray, Haig, & Watson, 2002; Watson & Humrichouse, 2006).

First, trait levels of N/NE show a significant decline with age, the bulk of which occurs in adolescence and early adulthood; nevertheless, decreases continue to be seen later in life (Roberts et al., 2006). Similarly, DvC scores also decline with age, decreasing during both young adulthood and middle age (Roberts et al., 2006). In addition, Roberts and colleagues' (2006) recent meta-analysis indicated that the A- and C-related aspects of the trait show differential patterns over time. Specifically, C increased substantially between the ages of 22 and 40, and showed much more change overall; in contrast, A exhibited less overall change and displayed the largest increases later in life (Roberts et al., 2006, Tables 6 and 7).

Finally, the findings regarding E/PE have been much more inconsistent (Roberts et al., 2006; Vaidya et al., 2002). However, Roberts, Robins, Trzesniewski, and Caspi (2003) found that the data were more consistent at the specific trait level: Measures of dominance tended to increase from adolescence through early middle age, whereas levels of sociability increased during adolescence but then declined starting in young adulthood. In a related vein, Roberts and colleagues (2006) found that social dominance scores increased consistently throughout young adulthood and stabilized thereafter. In contrast, social vitality levels tended to be highly stable throughout most of the lifespan before showing a modest decline late in life.

Taken together, the available data indicate that mean-level changes are both meaningful and highly systematic across the lifespan. Indeed, Caspi and colleagues (2005) concluded that they reflect a *maturity principle*, arguing that these mean-level shifts "point to increasing psychological maturity over development, from adolescence to middle age" (p. 468). We must note, however, that virtually all of the relevant longitudinal evidence comes from participant self-ratings. Moreover, in an analysis of a relatively large newlywed sample, Watson and Humrichouse (2006) found that spouse-rated personality displayed a very different pattern over a 2-year interval, showing significant decreases in C, A, O, and E/PE over time. Interestingly, spouse ratings also showed evidence of a "honeymoon halo effect," such that they tended to be more positive than self-ratings at Time 1, but 2 years later tended to be more negative. These results highlight the value of collecting multimethod data in adult personality development studies.

Rank-Order Stability

Data on the extent to which individuals maintain their relative position on trait continua over time are quite consistent and yield several clear conclusions. First, stability correlations for personality traits are moderate to strong in magnitude, even when assessed in childhood and adolescence (Caspi et al., 2005; Roberts & DelVecchio, 2000). Thus, the stability of personality is not simply a characteristic of adulthood, but emerges early in life.

Second, stability correlations decline in magnitude as the time interval increases (Caspi et al., 2005; Roberts & DelVecchio, 2000; Watson, 2004). This consistent pattern has helped to establish the existence of true change in personality, given that change is more and more likely to occur with in-creasing retest intervals (Watson, 2004). It must be emphasized, however, that stability correlations never approach .00 and remain at least moderate in magnitude, even across several decades (Fraley & Roberts, 2004).

Third, stability correlations for personality increase systematically with age (Caspi et al., 2005; Roberts & DelVecchio, 2000). Older models of trait development assumed that most personality change occurred prior to the age of 30, after which stability correlations should be uniformly high (for a discussion, see Roberts & DelVecchio, 2000). However, the meta-analytic findings of Roberts and DelVecchio (2000) revealed that stability coefficients for personality continue to increase well into middle age.

Fourth, the available evidence indicates that rank-order stability coefficients essentially are invariant across methods (Caspi et al., 2005; Roberts & DelVecchio, 2000; Watson & Humrichouse, 2006). Most notably, in their meta-analytic review of the literature, Roberts and DelVecchio obtained virtually identical population estimates of overall trait stability across self-report (ρ = .52) and observer-rated (ρ = .48) data (see their Table 4).

Structural Stability

This type of stability reflects the extent to which correlations among phenotypic dimensions of temperament are invariant across the lifespan. An extensive body of evidence—based on measures of both the Big Three and the Big Five—has established that essentially identical structures can be identified in child, high school student, college student, normal adult, and older adult samples (e.g., Costa & McCrae, 1992; Digman, 1990; Eysenck & Eysenck, 1975; Kohnstamm, Halverson, Mervielde, & Avila, 1998; Mackinnon et al., 1995; Measelle, John, Ablow, Cowan, & Cowan, 2005). Thus, personality structure shows impressive stability from adolescence through old age.

Fewer data exist for pre-high-school ages, but the available evidence indicates that structures closely paralleling the Big Three and Big Five emerge at an early age. For instance, Digman and associates replicated the Big Five structure in a series of studies in which teachers rated the characteristics of elementary school children (Digman, 1997).

Similarly, analyses of the Children's Behavior Questionnaire (CBQ; Rothbart & Ahadi, 1994; Rothbart, Ahadi, & Hershey, 1994), a parent-report instrument that assesses temperament in children ages 3–8 years, consistently have identified three higher order factors that closely resemble the Big Three (Ahadi et al., 1993; Goldsmith et al., 1997; Rothbart & Ahadi, 1994; Rothbart et al., 1994). Shiner and Caspi's (2003) review of the childhood/adolescent personality literature identified four robust higher order factors (N/NE, E/PE, A, and C). Coupled with data demonstrating the broad cross-cultural robustness of these models (e.g., Ahadi et al., 1993; De Clercq et al., 2006; Jang et al., 1998), the evidence supports McCrae and Costa's (1997) claim that "personality structure is a human universal" (p. 514).

Temperament and Psychopathology

A prominent theme of this chapter is that the emergence of a theoretical model of temperament has led to widespread progress in the field. Like any good theory, this model not only explains a range of existing data but also suggests avenues for further exploration; moreover, it has the power to change in fundamental ways how certain phenomena are conceptualized. Psychopathology is one domain that the emerging temperamental paradigm has the potential to transform. For decades, research in personality and psychopathology developed independently, with little cross-fertilization. Eventually, however, investigators in each of these fields began to take notice of the work in the other, to note parallelisms between findings, and to ask how personality and psychopathology might be interrelated: Does personality act as a vulnerability factor for the development of psychopathology? Is personality changed by the experience of mental disorder? Does personality affect the way in which psychopathology is manifested? Widiger, Verhuel, and van den Brink (1999) ably explored many of these questions and noted, for example, that "personality and psychopathology at times fail to be distinct conditions" (p. 351; see also, Widiger & Smith, Chapter 30, this volume). One of us (Clark, 2005) reviewed the extensive literature relating personality and psychopathology and proposed an integrating hierarchical framework in which "adult personality traits emerge from three

biobehavioral dimensions ... and they share these genetic diatheses with later developing disorders" (p. 511), both those that currently are coded on Axis I (clinical syndromes, such as major depression or substance abuse) and Axis II (personality disorders; PDs).

In this model, for example, the well-established associations between (personality trait) N/NE and a wide range of psychopathology (Mineka, Watson, & Clark, 1998; Watson & Clark, 1994; Watson, Gamez, & Simms, 2005; Watson et al., 2006) result from a shared underlying temperament dimension of N/NE, certainly as a genetic diathesis, and perhaps also reflecting early environmental factors. Thus, N/NE is the primary component of a broad dimension of "internalizing" pathology—encompassing, at a minimum, the anxiety and depressive disorders—that has emerged repeatedly in large-scale studies of comorbidity (more precisely, co-occurrence, but the former term is used more typically) among common mental disorders (e.g., Kendler, Prescott, Myers, & Neale, 2003; see Clark, 2005). Similarly, the temperament dimension E/PE underlies both the corresponding personality trait and various types of psychopathology, particularly depression, anhedonia (e.g., in schizophrenia/schizotypy), and social phobia (for overviews, see Clark, 2005; Watson et al., 2005, 2006).

The personality dimension DvC has been linked with a second broad "externalizing" dimension of psychopathology, encompassing substance abuse/dependence and antisocial behavior/PD, that emerges in the aforementioned comorbidity studies (see Krueger & Markon, 2006; Krueger et al., 2002). Recent evidence also links this dimension (as well as N/NE) with attention-deficit/hyperactivity disorder (ADHD) and borderline personality disorder (e.g., Nigg et al., 2002; Nigg, Silk, Stavro, & Miller, 2005). In our model (Clark, 2005), a DvC temperament dimension again underlies both the personality trait and related mental disorders. Moreover, temperamental N/NE is posited to account for the moderate correlation between the internalizing and externalizing factors (e.g., Kendler et al., 2003). Finally, most recently, we (Watson, Clark, & Chmielewski, in press) and others (Tackett, Silberschmidt, Krueger, & Sponheim, in press) have proposed a sixth broad factor (i.e., beyond the FFM) of "oddity" or "peculiarity" that integrates schizotypal personality disorder and potentially other schizophrenia-spectrum disorders into an encompassing hierarchical model of personality and psychopathology. Thus, accumulating evidence increasingly appears to support the view that we proffered in the original edition of this chapter: It is more parsimonious to consider temperament dimensions as underlying both personality traits and various mental disorders than to view personality and psychopathology as separate domains that stand in some relation to each other.

Adopting this view of temperament in relation to psychopathology has far-ranging implications. First, it explains the extensive comorbidity among psychological disorders that has been a major challenge to the current categorical system of diagnosis (e.g., Clark, Watson, & Reynolds, 1995) as due to shared underlying temperaments (Clark, 2005, 2007). That is, persons with temperamentally high levels of N/NE are at increased risk for developing a broad range of internalizing, externalizing, and "odd" or "peculiar" disorders, so the likelihood that they will develop more than one disorder is increased as well. Similarly, individuals' temperamental level of DvC affects the probability of their developing one or more "externalizing" disorders, such as substance use disorders, psychopathy/antisocial PD, ADHD, or borderline PD. Furthermore, this view facilitates the generation of hypotheses regarding other Axis I and II disorder comorbidities. For example, if the comorbidity patterns of different types of eating disorders with other clinical syndromes and PD reflect common underlying temperament diatheses, the fact that patients with bulimia nervosa are higher in DvC than those with anorexia nervosa (Cassin & von Ranson, 2005) would lead to the prediction that bulimia patients have a higher rate of comorbid antisocial PD—which, in fact, is the case (Sansone, Levitt, & Sasone, 2005).

In turn, this approach raises the question of how best to conceptualize diagnoses. Clearly, it is untenable to argue that the DSM disorders represent distinct independent entities in the way that chicken pox is independent of measles. Given what appears to be a universal penchant for categorization, it is unlikely that the current diagnostic taxonomy will be replaced with a purely dimensional system in the immediate future. However, it is not improbable that temperament dimensions might provide the basis for a systematic reorganization of diagnoses, using the robust factors of internalizing, externalizing, and oddity as the foundation for a new taxonomy. In fact, such a proposal is being considered seriously by the DSM-V Task Force.

Diagnostic severity is the second major challenge to categorical systems of diagnosis that is addressed by adopting a temperament-based approach. Under the current system, a certain threshold of severity must be passed for an individual to receive any given diagnosis. However, in many domains of psychopathology, subclinical cases have been shown not only to exist with high prevalence but, more importantly, to represent a serious public health problem in terms of personal suffering, increased psychosocial dysfunction, and economic consequences such as unemployment, increased sick days, and lower productivity (e.g., Judd et al., 2000). Thus, the distinction between above-threshold and subclinical cases appears to be arbitrary and does not represent a true, natural boundary between disorder and nondisorder. This observed lack of a distinctive boundary is predicted, of course, from a temperament-based dimensional perspective.

In sum, the temperament-based model of personality that has emerged recently from the study of trait psychology is a powerful tool that has been fruitful in integrating diverse findings regarding personality structure and processes, the neurobiology of personality, child development, and psychopathology. No doubt the full specification of this model will be extraordinarily complex. Nonetheless, we are optimistic that the broad outlines of a temperament-based paradigm are clear, and that explicating the nature and scope of these temperamental systems will carry us well through the 21st century.

ACKNOWLEDGMENTS

We thank Richard Depue for his comments on a draft of an earlier version of this chapter and Leigh Wensman for her tireless efforts tracking down relevant new research to help us update it.

NOTES

1. It is important to acknowledge here that Block (e.g., Block & Block, 2006) earlier used the

terms "undercontrolled" and "overcontrolled" to characterize the contrasting poles of his construct *ego control*, which overlaps with both E and DvC.

REFERENCES

Ahadi, S. A., Rothbart, M. K., & Ye, R. (1993). Child temperament in the U.S. and China: Similarities and differences. *European Journal of Personality, 7,* 359–378.

Allport, G. W. (1937). *Personality: A psychological interpretation.* New York: Holt.

Balatsky, G., & Diener, E. (1993). Subjective well-being among Russian students. *Social Indicators Research, 28,* 21–39.

Barrick, M. R., & Mount, M. K. (1991). The Big Five personality dimensions and job performance: A meta-analysis. *Personnel Psychology, 44,* 1–26.

Beer, J. M., Arnold, R. D., & Loehlin, J. C. (1998). Genetic and environmental influences on MMPI factor scales: Joint model fitting to twin and adoption data. *Journal of Personality and Social Psychology, 74,* 818–827.

Block, J., & Block, J. H. (2006). Venturing a 30-year longitudinal study. *American Psychologist, 61,* 315–327.

Bouchard, T. J., Jr., & Loehlin, J. C. (2001). Genes, evolution, and personality. *Behavior Genetics, 31,* 243–273.

Buss, A., & Plomin, R. (1975). *A temperament theory of personality development.* New York: Wiley.

Carver, C. S., & White, T. L. (1994). Behavioral inhibition, behavioral activation, and affective responses to impending reward and punishment: The BIS/BAS scales. *Journal of Personality and Social Psychology, 67,* 319–333.

Caspi, A., Roberts, B. W., & Shiner, R. L. (2005). Personality development: Stability and change. *Annual Review of Psychology, 56,* 453–484.

Cassin, S. E., & von Ranson, K. M. (2005). Personality and eating disorders: A decade in review. *Clinical Psychology Review, 25,* 895–916.

Clark, L. A. (2005). Temperament as a unifying basis for personality and psychopathology. *Journal of Abnormal Psychology, 114,* 505–521.

Clark, L. A. (2007). Assessment and diagnosis of personality disorder: Perennial issues and emerging conceptualization. *Annual Review of Psychology, 58,* 227–258.

Clark, L. A., & Watson, D. (1988). Mood and the mundane: Relations between daily life events and self-reported mood. *Journal of Personality and Social Psychology, 54,* 296–308.

Clark, L. A., & Watson, D. (1990). *The General Temperament Survey.* Unpublished manuscript, University of Iowa, Iowa City.

Clark, L. A., & Watson, D. (1991). Affective dis-positions and their relation to psychological and physical health. In C. R. Snyder & D. R. Forsyth (Eds.), *Handbook of social and clinical psychology* (pp. 221–245). Elmsford, NY: Pergamon Press.

Clark, L. A., & Watson, D. (1999). Temperament: A new paradigm for trait psychology. In L. A. Pervin & O. P. John (Eds.), *Handbook of personality: Theory and research* (2nd ed., pp. 399–423). New York: Guilford Press.

Clark, L. A., Watson, D., & Leeka, J. (1989). Diurnal variation in the positive affects. *Motivation and Emotion, 13,* 205–234.

Clark, L. A., Watson, D., & Reynolds, S. (1995). Diagnosis and classification in psychopathology: Challenges to the current system and future directions. *Annual Review of Psychology, 46,* 121–153.

Cleckley, H. (1964). *The mask of sanity* (4th ed.). St. Louis, MO: Mosby.

Corr, P. J. (2004). Reinforcement sensitivity theory and personality. *Neuroscience and Biobehavioral Reviews, 28,* 317–332.

Costa, P. T., Jr., & McCrae, R. R. (1992). *Revised NEO Personality Inventory (NEO-PI-R) and NEO Five-Factor Inventory (NEO-FFI) professional manual.* Odessa, FL: Psychological Assessment Resources.

De Clercq, B., De Fruyt, F., Van Leeuwen, K., & Mervielde, I. (2006). The structure of maladaptive personality traits in childhood: A step toward an integrative developmental perspective for *DSM-V. Journal of Abnormal Psychology, 115,* 639–657.

Depue, R. A., & Collins, P. F. (1999). Neurobiology of the structure of personality: Dopamine, facilitation of incentive motivation, and extraversion. *Behavioral and Brain Sciences, 22,* 491–569.

Diener, E., Smith, H., & Fujita, F. (1995). The personality structure of affect. *Journal of Personality and Social Psychology, 69,* 130–141.

Digman, J. M. (1990). Personality structure: Emergence of the five-factor model. *Annual Review of Psychology, 41,* 417–440.

Digman, J. M. (1994). Child personality and temperament: Does the five-factor model embrace both domains? In C. F. Halverson, G. A. Kohnstamm, & R. P. Martin (Eds.), *The developing structure of temperament and personality from infancy to adulthood* (pp. 323–338). Hillsdale, NJ: Erlbaum.

Digman, J. M. (1997). Higher-order factors of the Big Five. *Journal of Personality and Social Psychology, 73,* 1246–1256.

Eid, M., Riemann, R., Angleitner, A., & Borkenau, P. (2003). Sociability and positive emotionality: Genetic and environmental contributions to the covariation between different facets of extraversion. *Journal of Personality, 71,* 319–346.

Epstein, S., & O'Brien, E. J. (1985). The person–situation debate in historical and current perspective. *Psychological Bulletin, 98,* 513–537.

Eysenck, H. J. (1967). *The biological bases of personality.* Baltimore: University Park Press.

Eysenck, H. J. (1990). Genetic and environmental contributions to individual differences: The three major dimensions of personality. *Journal of Personality, 58,* 245–261.

Eysenck, H. J. (1992). Four ways five factors are not basic. *Personality and Individual Differences, 13,* 667–673.

Eysenck, H. J. (1997). Personality and experimental psychology: The unification of psychology and the possibility of a paradigm. *Journal of Personality and Social Psychology, 73,* 1224–1237.

Eysenck, H. J., & Eysenck, S. B. G. (1975). *Manual of the Eysenck Personality Questionnaire.* San Diego, CA: Educational and Industrial Testing Service.

Finkel, D., & McGue, M. (1997). Sex differences and nonadditivity in heritability of the Multidimensional Personality Questionnaire scales. *Journal of Personality and Social Psychology, 72,* 929–938.

Fraley, R. C., & Roberts, B. W. (2004). Patterns of continuity: A dynamic model for conceptualizing the stability of individual differences in psychological constructs across the life course. *Psychological Review, 112,* 60–74.

Funder, D. C. (2006). Towards a resolution of the personality triad: Persons, situations, and behaviors. *Journal of Research in Personality, 40(1),* 21–34.

Goldsmith, H. H., Buss, K. A., & Lemery, K. S. (1997). Toddler and childhood temperament: Expanded content, stronger genetic evidence, new evidence for the importance of environment. *Developmental Psychology, 33,* 891–905.

Gough, H. G. (1987). *California Psychological Inventory* [Administrator's guide]. Palo Alto, CA: Consulting Psychologists Press.

Gray, E. K., & Watson, D. (2002). General and specific traits of personality and their relation to sleep and academic performance. *Journal of Personality, 70,* 177–206.

Gray, J. A. (1982). *The neuropsychology of anxiety: An enquiry into the functions of the septa-hippocampal system.* Oxford, UK: Clarendon Press.

Gray, J. A. (1987a). Perspectives on anxiety and impulsivity. *Journal of Research in Personality, 21,* 493–509.

Gray, J. A. (1987b). *The psychology of fear and stress* (2nd ed.). Cambridge, UK: Cambridge University Press.

Haig, J. (1997). *Sexual expectations and sexual behavior.* Unpublished manuscript, University of Iowa, Iowa City.

Hare, R. D. (1991). *The Hare Psychopathy Checklist—Revised Manual.* North Tonawanda, NY: Multi-Health Systems.

Horne, J. A., & Ostberg, O. (1977). A self-assessment questionnaire to determine morningness–eveningness in human circadian rhythms. *International Journal of Chronobiology, 4,* 97–110.

Jang, K. L., Livesley, W. J., Angleitner, A., Reimann, R., & Vernon, P. A. (2002). Genetic and environmental influences on the covariance of facets defining the five-factor model of personality. *Personality and Individual Differences, 33,* 83–101.

Jang, K. L., McCrae, R. R., Angleitner, A., Riemann, R., & Livesley, W. J. (1998). Heritability of facet-level traits in a cross-cultural twin sample: Support for a hierarchical model of personality. *Journal of Personality and Social Psychology, 74,* 1556–1565.

John, O. P., & Srivastava, S. (1999). The Big Five trait taxonomy: History, measurement, and theoretical perspectives. In L. A. Pervin & O. P. John (Eds.), *Handbook of personality: Theory and research* (2nd ed., pp. 102–138). New York: Guilford Press.

Jorm, A. F., Christensen, H., Henderson, A. S., Jacomb, P. A., Korten, A. E., & Rodgers, B. (1999). Using the BIS/BAS scales to measure behavioural inhibition and behavioural activation: Factor structure, validity and norms in a large community sample. *Personality and Individual Differences, 26,* 49–58.

Judd, L. L., Akiskal, H. S., Zeller, P. J., Paulus, M., Leon, A. C., Maser, J. D., et al. (2000). Psychosocial disability during the long-term course of unipolar major depressive disorder. *Archives of General Psychiatry, 57,* 375–380.

Keller, M. C., Coventry, W. L., Heath, A. C., & Martin, N. G. (2005). Widespread evidence for non-additive genetic variation in Cloninger's and Eysenck's personality dimensions using a twin plus sibling design. *Behavior Genetics, 35,* 707–721.

Kendler, K. S., Prescott, C. A., Myers, J., & Neale, M. C. (2003). The structure of genetic and environmental risk factors for common psychiatric and substance use disorders in men and women. *Archives of General Psychiatry, 60,* 929–937.

Kohnstamm, G. A., Halverson, C. F., Mervielde, I., & Avilla, V. (1998). *Parental descriptions of child personality: Developmental antecedents of the Big Five?* Mahwah, NJ: Erlbaum.

Krueger, R. F., Hicks, B. M., Patrick, C. J., Carlson, S. R., Iacono, W. G., & McGue, M. (2002). Etiologic connections among substance dependence, antisocial behavior, and personality: Modeling the externalizing spectrum. *Journal of Abnormal Psychology, 111,* 411–424.

Krueger, R. F., & Markon, K. E. (2006). Reinterpreting comorbidity: A model-based approach to understanding and classifying psychopathology. *Annual Review of Clinical Psychology, 2,* 111–133.

Lodi-Smith, J., & Roberts, B. W. (2007). Social investment and personality: A meta-analysis of the relationship of personality traits to investment in work, family, religion, and volunteerism. *Personality and Social Psychology Review, 11,* 1–19.

Loehlin, J. C., & Gough, H. G. (1990). Genetic and environmental variation on the California Psychological Inventory vector scales. *Journal of Personality Assessment, 54,* 463–468.

Loehlin, J. C., McCrae, R. R., Costa, P. T., Jr., & John, O. P. (1998). Heritabilities of common and measure-specific components of the Big Five personality factors. *Journal of Research in Personality, 32,* 431–453.

Loehlin, J. C., & Nichols, R. C. (1976). *Heredity, environment, and personality.* Austin: University of Texas Press.

Luciano, M., Wainwright, M. A., Wright, M. J., & Martin, N. G. (2006). The heritability of conscientiousness facets and their relationship to IQ and academic achievement. *Personality and Individual Differences, 40,* 1189–1199.

Mackinnon, A., Jorm, A. F., Christensen, H., Scott, L. R., Henderson, A. S., & Korten, A. E. (1995). A latent trait analysis of the Eysenck Personality Questionnaire in an elderly community sample. *Personality and Individual Differences, 18,* 739–747.

Markon, K. E., Krueger, R. F., & Watson, D. (2005). Delineating the structure of normal and abnormal personality: An integrative hierarchical approach. *Journal of Personality and Social Psychology, 88,* 139–157.

McCartney, K., Harris, M. J., & Bernieri, F. (1990). Growing up and growing apart: A developmental meta-analysis of twin studies. *Psychological Bulletin, 107,* 226–237.

McCrae, R. R., & Costa, P. T., Jr. (1987). Validation of a five-factor model of personality across instruments and observers. *Journal of Personality and Social Psychology, 52,* 81–90.

McCrae, R. R., & Costa, P. T., Jr. (1996). Toward a new generation of personality theories: Theoretical contexts for the five-factor model. In J. S. Wiggins (Ed.), *The five-factor model of personality* (pp. 51–87). New York: Guilford Press.

McCrae, R. R., & Costa, P. T., Jr. (1997). Personality trait structure as a human universal. *American Psychologist, 52,* 509–516.

McGue, M., Bacon, S., & Lykken, D. T. (1993). Personality stability and change in early adulthood: A behavioral genetic analysis. *Developmental Psychology, 29,* 96–109.

Measelle, J. R., John, O. P., Ablow, J. C., Cowan, P. A., & Cowan, C. P (2005). Can children provide coherent, stable, and valid self-reports on the Big Five dimensions? A longitudinal study from ages 5 to 7. *Journal of Personality and Social Psychology, 89,* 90–106.

Meyer, G. J., & Shack, J. R. (1989). Structural convergence of mood and personality: Evidence for old and new directions. *Journal of Personality and Social Psychology, 57,* 691–706.

Mineka, S., Watson, D. W., & Clark, L. A. (1998). Psychopathology: Comorbidity of anxiety and unipolar mood disorders. *Annual Review of Psychology, 49,* 377–412.

Mischel, W. (1968). *Personality and assessment.* New York: Wiley.

Mischel, W., & Peake, P. K. (1982). Beyond déjà vu in the search for cross-situational consistency. *Psychological Review, 89,* 730–755.

Nigg, J. T., John, O. P., Blaskey, L. G., Huang-Pollock, C. L., Willcutt, E. G., Hinshaw, S. P., et al. (2002). Big Five dimensions and ADHD symptoms: Link between personality traits and clinical syndromes. *Journal of Personality and Social Psychology, 83,* 451–469.

Nigg, J. T., Silk, K. R., Stavro, G., & Miller, T. (2005). Disinhibition and borderline personality disorder. *Development and Psychopathology, 17,* 1129–1149.

Oniszczenko, W., Zawadzki, B., Strelau, J., Riemann, R., Angleitner, A., & Spinath, F. M. (2003). Genetic and environmental determinants of temperament: A comparative study based on Polish and German samples. *European Journal of Personality, 17,* 207–220.

Pedersen, N. L. (1993). Genetic and environmental continuity and change in personality. In T. J. Bouchard & P. Propping (Eds.), *Twins as a tool of behavioral genetics* (pp. 147–162). New York: Wiley.

Plomin, R., Corley, R., Caspi, A., Fulker, D. W., & DeFries, J. (1998). Adoption results for self-reported personality: Evidence for nonadditive genetic effects? *Journal of Personality and Social Psychology, 75,* 211–218.

Plomin, R., & Daniels, D. (1987). Why are children in the same family so different from one another? *Behavioral and Brain Sciences, 10,* 1–16.

Revelle, W. (2008). The contribution of reinforcement sensitivity theory to personality theory. In P. J. Corr (Ed.), *The reinforcement sensitivity theory of personality* (pp. 508–527). Cambridge, UK: Cambridge University Press.

Riemann, R., Angleitner, A., & Strelau, J. (1997). Genetic and environmental influences on personality: A study of twins reared together using the self- and peer report NEO-FFI scales. *Journal of Personality, 65,* 449–475.

Roberts, B. W., & DelVecchio, W. F. (2000). The rank-order consistency of personality traits from childhood to old age: A quantitative review of longitudinal studies. *Psychological Bulletin, 126,* 3–25.

Roberts, B. W., Robins, R. W., Trzesniewski, K., & Caspi, A. (2003). Personality trait development in adulthood. In J. Mortimer & M. Shanahan (Eds.), *Handbook of the life course* (pp. 579–598). New York: Kluwer.

Roberts, B. W., Walton, K. E., & Viechtbauer, W. (2006). Patterns of mean-level change in personality traits across the life course: A meta-analysis of longitudinal studies. *Psychological Bulletin, 132,* 1–25.

Rothbart, M. K., & Ahadi, S. A. (1994). Temperament and the development of personality. *Journal of Abnormal Psychology, 103,* 55–66.

Rothbart, M. K., Ahadi, S. A., & Hershey, K. L. (1994). Temperament and social behavior in childhood. *Merrill–Palmer Quarterly, 40,* 21–39.

Sansone, R. A., Levitt, J. L., & Sansone, L. A. (2005). The prevalence of personality disorders among those with eating disorders. *Eating Disorders: The Journal of Treatment and Prevention, 13,* 7–21.

Shiner, R., & Caspi, A. (2003). Personality differences in childhood and adolescence: Measurement, development, and consequences. *Journal of Child Psychology and Psychiatry, 44,* 2–32.

Smith, C. S., Reily, C., & Midkiff, K. (1989). Evaluation of three circadian rhythm questionnaires with suggestions for an improved measure of morningness. *Journal of Applied Psychology, 74,* 728–738.

Strelau, J. (1983). *Temperament–personality–activity.* London: Academic Press.

Strelau, J., & Zawadzki, B. (1995). The Formal Characteristics of Behavior—Temperament Inventory (FCB-TI): Validity studies. *European Journal of Personality, 9,* 207–229.

Tackett, J., Silberschmidt, A., Krueger, R. F., & Sponheim, S. (in press). A dimensional model of personality disorder: Incorporating Cluster A characteristics. *Journal of Personality.*

Tellegen, A. (1985). Structures of mood and personality and their relevance to assessing anxiety, with an emphasis on self-report. In A. H. Tuma & J. D. Maser (Eds.), *Anxiety and the anxiety disorders* (pp. 681–706). Hillsdale, NJ: Erlbaum.

Tellegen, A., Lykken, D. T., Bouchard, T. J., Jr., Wilcox, K. J., Segal, N. L., & Rich, S. (1988). Personality similarity in twins reared apart and together. *Journal of Personality and Social Psychology, 54,* 1031–1039.

Thayer, R. E. (1989). *The biopsychology of mood and arousal.* New York: Oxford University Press.

Thomas, A., & Chess, S. (1977). *Temperament and development.* New York: Brunner/Mazel.

Thomas, A., Chess, S., & Birch, H. (1968). *Temperament and behavior: Disorders in children.* New York: New York University Press.

Vaidya, J. G., Gray, E. K., Haig, J., & Watson, D. (2002). On the temporal stability of personality: Evidence for differential stability and the role of life experiences. *Journal of Personality and Social Psychology, 83,* 1469–1484.

Viken, R. J., Rose, R. J., Kaprio, J., & Koskenvuo, M. (1994). A developmental genetic analysis of adult personality: Extraversion and neuroticism from 18 to 59 years of age. *Journal of Personality and Social Psychology, 66,* 722–730.

Watson, D. (1988). The vicissitudes of mood measurement: Effects of varying descriptors, time frames, and response formats on measures of positive and negative affect. *Journal of Personality and Social Psychology, 55,* 128–141.

Watson, D. (2000). *Mood and temperament.* New York: Guilford Press.

Watson, D. (2004). Stability versus change, dependability versus error: Issues in the assessment of personality over time. *Journal of Research in Personality, 38,* 319–350.

Watson, D. (2005). Rethinking the mood and anxiety disorders: A quantitative hierarchical model for *DSM-V. Journal of Abnormal Psychology, 114,* 522–536.

Watson, D., & Clark, L. A. (1984). Negative affectivity: The disposition to experience aversive emotional states. *Psychological Bulletin, 96,* 465–490.

Watson, D., & Clark, L. A. (1992a). Affects separable and inseparable: A hierarchical model of the negative affects. *Journal of Personality and Social Psychology, 62,* 489–505.

Watson, D., & Clark, L. A. (1992b). On traits and temperament: General and specific factors of emotional experience and their relation to the five-factor model. *Journal of Personality, 60,* 441–476.

Watson, D., & Clark, L. A. (1993). Behavioral disinhibition versus constraint: A dispositional perspective. In D. M. Wegner & J. W. Pennebaker (Eds.), *Handbook of mental control* (pp. 506–527). New York: Prentice Hall.

Watson, D., & Clark, L. A. (Eds.). (1994). Personality and psychopathology [Special issue]. *Journal of Abnormal Psychology, 103*(1).

Watson, D., & Clark, L. A. (1997). Extraversion and its positive emotional core. In R. Hogan, J. Johnson, & S. Briggs (Eds.), *Handbook of personality psychology* (pp. 767–793). San Diego, CA: Academic Press.

Watson, D., Clark, L. A., & Chmielewski, M. (in press). Structures of personality and their relevance to psychopathology: II. Further articulation of a comprehensive unified trait structure. *Journal of Personality.*

Watson, D., Clark, L. A., & Tellegen, A. (1984).

Cross-cultural convergence in the structure of mood: A Japanese replication and comparison with U.S. findings. *Journal of Personality and Social Psychology, 47,* 127–144.

Watson, D., Clark, L. A., & Tellegen, A. (1988). Development and validation of brief measures of positive and negative affect: The PANAS Scales. *Journal of Personality and Social Psychology, 54,* 1063–1070.

Watson, D., Gamez, W., & Simms, L. J. (2005). Basic dimensions of temperament and their relation to anxiety and depression: A symptom-based perspective. *Journal of Research in Personality, 39,* 46–66.

Watson, D., & Humrichouse, J. (2006). Personality development in emerging adulthood: Integrating evidence from self-ratings and spouse ratings. *Journal of Personality and Social Psychology, 91,* 959–974.

Watson, D., Klohnen, E. C., Casillas, A., Simms, E. N., Haig, J., & Berry, D. S. (2004). Match makers and deal breakers: Analyses of assortative mating in newlywed couples. *Journal of Personality, 72,* 1029–1068.

Watson, D., Kotov, R., & Gamez, W. (2006). Basic dimensions of temperament in relation to personality and psychopathology. In R. F. Krueger & J. L. Tackett (Eds.), *Personality and psychopathology* (pp. 7–38). New York: Guilford Press.

Watson, D., & Tellegen, A. (1985). Toward a consensual structure of mood. *Psychological Bulletin, 98,* 219–235.

Watson, D., Wiese, D., Vaidya, J., & Tellegen, A. (1999). The two general activation systems of affect: Structural findings, evolutionary considerations, and psychobiological evidence. *Journal of Personality and Social Psychology, 76,* 820–838.

Wechsler, J., Davenport, A., Dowdall, G., Moeykens, B., & Castillo, S. (1994). Health and behavioral consequences of binge drinking in college: A national survey of students in 140 campuses. *Journal of the American Medical Association, 272,* 1672–1677.

Widiger, T. A., Verhuel, R., & van den Brink, W. (1999). Personality and psychopathology. In L. Pervin & O. P. John (Eds.). *Handbook of personality* (2nd ed., pp. 347–366). New York: Guilford Press.

Wilson, G. D., Barrett, P. T., & Gray, J. A. (1989). Human reactions to reward and punishment: A questionnaire examination of Gray's personality theory. *British Journal of Psychology, 80,* 509–515.

Wilson, G. D., Gray, J. A., & Barrett, P. T. (1990). A factor analysis of the Gray–Wilson Personality Questionnaire. *Personality and Individual Differences, 11,* 1037–1045.

Zuckerman, M., Tushup, R., & Finner, S. (1976). Sexual attitudes and experience: Attitude and personality correlates and changes produced by a course in sexuality. *Journal of Consulting and Clinical Psychology, 44,* 7–19.

APPENDIX: A SELECTION OF RECENT REFERENCES ON THE BIOLOGICAL BASES OF TEMPERAMENT

Canli, T. (Ed.). (2006). *Biology of personality and individual differences.* New York: Guilford Press.

Corr, P. J. (Ed.). (2008). *Reinforcement sensitivity theory of personality.* New York: Cambridge University Press.

Davidson, R. J. (2003). Affective neuroscience and psychophysiology: Toward a synthesis. *Psychophysiology, 40,* 655–665.

Depue, R. A., & Lenzenweger, M. F. (2006). A multidimensional neurobehavioral model of personality disturbance. In R. F. Krueger & J. L. Tackett (Eds.), *Personality and psychopathology* (pp. 210–261). New York: Guilford Press.

Fox, N. A., Henderson, H. A., Marshall, P. J., Nichols, K. E., & Ghera, M. M. (2005). Behavioral inhibition: Linking biology and behavior within a developmental framework. *Annual Review of Psychology, 56,* 235–262.

McNaughton, H., & Corr, P. J. (2004). A two-dimensional neuropsychology of defense: Fear/anxiety and defensive distance. *Neuroscience and Biobehavioral Reviews, 28,* 285–305.

Plomin, R., DeFries, J. C., Craig, I. W., & McGuffin, P. (Eds.). (2003). *Behavioral genetics in the postgenomic era.* Washington, DC: American Psychological Association.

Smillie, L. D., Pickering, A. D., & Jackson, C. J. (2006). The new reinforcement sensitivity theory: Implications for personality measurement. *Personality and Social Psychology Review, 10,* 320–335.

Whittle, S., Allen, N. B., Lubman, D. I., & Yucel, M. (2006). The neurobiological basis of temperament: Towards a better understanding of psychopathology. *Neuroscience and Biobehavioral Reviews, 30,* 511–525.

Zuckerman, M. (2005). *Psychobiology of personality* (2nd ed.). New York: Cambridge University Press.

CHAPTER 10

Behavioral Genetics and Personality

A New Look at the Integration of Nature and Nurture

Robert F. Krueger
Wendy Johnson

If you enter the phrase "nature–nurture" into Google, the sorts of words that come up in the brief descriptions of the relevant webpages include "debates," "acrimonious," "versus," "controversy," and "dispute." This flavor of the Web presence of nature–nurture is not too surprising. Nature and nurture have been viewed as being at odds for as long as these words have been conjoined. The origin of the phrase "nature–nurture" can be traced to Shakespeare's *Tempest* (1611/1974), in which Prospero describes Caliban as "a born devil, on whose nature nurture can never stick" (IV.i.188–190), as well as to Francis Galton (1865), who is credited with coining the exact phrase "nature–nurture" in the context of studying hereditary contributions to human abilities. For Shakespeare and Galton, the idea was that nature and nurture were independent developmental forces, to be compared in their influence, with the aim of declaring one part of the equation more influential than the other.

Controversies and disputes can certainly be enormously helpful in advancing scientific inquiry. Consider how, in personality psychology, discussion surrounding the role of the person and the situation in producing behavior strengthened our understanding that persons bring underlying behavioral tendencies to situations, yet modify their behavior to conform to situational expectations (Kenrick & Funder, 1988). Nevertheless, controversy can also have unfortunate polarizing consequences, implying that scientists need to take sides or profess allegiance to one view versus another. A major goal of this chapter is to show that taking sides in the nature–nurture debate, as applied to personality research, is actually a scientific mistake. Both genetic and environmental factors are important to personality. The fundamental challenge we now face involves understanding how genetic and environmental factors work together in creating personality. Surmounting this challenge has proven difficult because doing so involves going beyond the traditional focus of behavioral genetic inquiry, which has been to document the magnitude of genetic and environmental influences on behavior. Hence, a related goal of this chapter is to convey the essence of recent methodological and conceptual advances that allow us to begin to understand how genetic and environmental influences actually come together to shape personality. Importantly, research incorporating these advances has just begun to appear in the literature. The "look" of behavioral genetics in psychological science has changed since the last edition of this handbook was published in 1999 (cf. Moffitt, 2005), and we hope to convey some of these important advances to a broad audience of personality researchers.

We have organized this chapter into three sections, starting with the most well-established aspects of the relevant literature, and moving toward the newest directions in personality research designed to understand the interplay of genetic and environmental influences. In the first of these sections, we describe some postulates based on well-established research findings. In the second section, we describe current directions in research as a set of propositions. We conclude by delineating questions for future research. The idea of specifying postulates and propositions is not to enshrine these as immutable laws, but rather to specify clearly what we see as the things we currently know, as backdrop for the final section, where we explain the things we would most like to understand better. In the process, we hope the reader will come to share our enthusiasm for genetically informed personality research, and will share our desire to relegate the controversy pitting nature against nurture to the historical backdrop for the development of a scientifically compelling account of how DNA and environmental inputs combine to create individual personalities.

POSTULATES BASED ON WELL-ESTABLISHED RESEARCH FINDINGS

Personality Results from Both Genetic and Environmental Influences

Evidence from Self-Reports of Twins

In one sense, Postulate I seems self-evident; how could personality come about, except through transactions between the blueprint for the construction of the organism (DNA) and the world outside the organism? In another sense, however, establishing this proposition was scientifically critical, especially in relation to the origins of individual differences in personality. Radical environmentalism was characteristic of psychology for much of its early history, as epitomized by J. B. Watson (1924). A direct quote from Watson's book *Behaviorism* (1924, p. 94) is worth providing because it conveys the extreme nature of this approach: "There is no such thing as an inheritance of capacity, talent, temperament, mental constitution, and characteristics. These things again depend on training that goes on mainly in the cradle."

J. B. Watson's (1924) view is incompatible with the results of behavioral genetic studies of self-reported personality variables, most of which were conducted in the decades since Watson was writing. Behavioral genetic studies parse individual differences in traits into at least three distinct sources: (1) genetic effects, (2) shared environmental effects, and (3) nonshared environmental effects. Genetic effects index the extent to which observed or "phenotypic" variation in a trait arises from genetic differences among people. The well-known heritability statistic is the ratio of variance from genetic sources to total variation in the trait, or the proportion of total trait variation linked to genetic variation. Importantly, it is a statistic indexing variance—the extent of differences among persons within a group. As a concept, it only applies at the level of a specific group of persons (a sample or population of persons, in statistical terms). When we speak of, for example, 50% of variance in extraversion being due to genetic effects, we are referring to differences *among individuals*. We do *not* mean that 50% of any individual's level of extraversion can be attributed to genetic effects.

Shared environmental effects index the extent to which people are similar, independent of genetic effects, because they grew up in the same household, thereby sharing factors such as parental socioeconomic status and religious traditions. Nonshared environmental effects index the extent to which family members are different, in spite of sharing genetic material and growing up together. Commonly used examples include having different teachers and friends, participating in different leisure activities such as sports, and receiving different parental treatment.

The distinction between shared and nonshared experiences is subtle. For example, people within a family may experience the same putatively objective event (e.g., a household move), but that event is only a shared environmental experience to the extent that it acts to make family members similar. If the event acts to make persons within the same family different, then it will

show up as nonshared environmental variation within the family. Measurement imprecision also gets categorized with nonshared
environmental effects, since such imprecision
acts to make every individual appear unique
(e.g., a specific person is sleepy when filling
out a questionnaire and does not pay close
attention). Like genetic effects, both kinds
of environmental effects are variance concepts, and they are commonly discussed as
proportions of total variance. For example,
akin to the heritability, the extent of shared
environmental contributions can be conceptualized as the ratio of shared environmental
variation to total variation in the trait, or the
proportion of total trait variation linked to
shared environmental variation.

The Big Five dimensions (John, Naumann, & Soto, Chapter 4, this volume) have
been major targets of research on the heritability of personality. After reviewing the
literature, Bouchard and Loehlin (2001)
concluded that, in adults on whom most of
the studies have been based, genetic effects
accounted for almost half of the variation in
each of the Big Five domains. Shared environmental effects accounted for essentially
no variation, so that the remaining variation was accounted for by nonshared environmental effects. This pattern of findings is
well-known and well-replicated at this point.
Indeed, Turkheimer (2000) went so far as
to describe this pattern as essentially applicable to all known human individual differences, and he enshrined it as a series of laws.
The pattern is also generally similar across
sexes, such that heritabilities are similar for
both men and women (Bouchard & Loehlin,
2001). Importantly, the pattern is also generally similar when models of personality structure other than the Big Five are considered.

Although the patterns of genetic and
environmental influence described above are
well known, there are still some things about
their law-like nature that seem remarkable.
First, it is striking that each of the Big Five
domains is similarly heritable. Consider the
breadth of human individual differences encompassed by the Big Five—from more temperamental features such as activity level and
emotional tone, encompassed by domains
such as extraversion and neuroticism, to
more attitudinal features such as interests in
art and literature, encompassed by the domain of openness. Across this breadth of hu-

man experience, genes play a major role in
explaining why people differ.

Second, genetic effects on personality
are not small, at least not in the aggregate;
accounting for 50% of the variance in any
psychological variable is unusual. Third,
the main effect of shared environment is remarkable for its absence. This finding has
been a source of much generative controversy (Rowe, 1994). Yet when one reflects
on what the shared environmental component of variance represents, its absence in
understanding adult personality may not be
too surprising. Recall that it reflects environmental effects that make people growing up
together the same, *independent* of genetic endowment. It reflects environments working
separately and independently from genetic
effects, in such a way as to make people the
same within families. If environments and
DNA work together to produce personality
in a more *transactional* (interactive and correlational) manner, their effects will tend to
appear in the genetic or nonshared environmental components of variation in personality (Purcell, 2002).

Finally, the effects of nonshared environment are as large as, if not larger than,
genetic effects. Although these nonshared environmental effects are not trivial, they have
been hard to link with specific psychological
constructs (Turkheimer & Waldron, 2000).
As with the absence of shared environmental
effects, the presence—but frustrating ano-
nymity—of nonshared environmental effects
may be profitably addressed by pursuing a
more transacting conception of genes and environments. We will return to and elaborate
the theme of articulating gene–environment
transactions throughout this chapter because
we consider this to be the forefront of research in personality genetics.

Evidence beyond Self-Reports in Twins

Self-reports are a mainstay of personality psychology, and deservedly so. Much of
what makes personality interesting is that it
reflects the uniqueness of the individual, and
individuals have the most direct experience
of their unique personalities. Nevertheless,
evidence for genetic influence on personality extends beyond self-report, into both the
reports of others and even into the realm of
direct observation.

Riemann, Angleitner, and Strelau (1997) studied self and peer ratings of the Big Five simultaneously, and found that self and peer ratings showed broadly similar levels of genetic influence. In addition, much of the variation was common to the self and peer ratings, which were highly correlated (.55 on average). This finding is important because it shows that the genetic signal picked up by specific reports of personality is not unique to the reporter. Rather, the self-report signal appears to be much the same signal picked up by peer reports. Personality traits are not simply in the minds of specific reporters, but rather, reflect heritable consistencies that can be detected from multiple vantage points.

These consistencies extend beyond reports of personality to direct behavioral observations. Behavioral observations are most commonly employed in research with children because very young children cannot report directly on their personality characteristics. Directly observed individual differences in children, such as behavioral inhibition (Matheny, 1989; Robinson, Kagan, Reznick, & Corley, 1992), shyness in the home and the laboratory (Cherny, Fuiles, Corley, Plomin, & DeFries, 1994), and activity level measured using actometers (Saudino & Eaton, 1991) have been shown to be heritable.

More recently, observational research has also been extended to the study of adults. This is a critical extension because the vast majority of our understanding of the genetics of personality is based solely on self-reports of personality traits (Brody, 1993). The work of Borkenau, Riemann, Angleitner, and Spinath (2001) in the German Observational Study of Adult Twins (GOSAT) fills this critical gap in the literature. Three hundred pairs of adult twins from throughout Germany were videotaped while engaging in 15 distinct tasks, and judges independently rated the twins' personalities from these videotapes, using bipolar rating scales corresponding with the Big Five. Assessed in this manner and modeled as latent phenotypes, the Big Five domains all showed notable heritability, with a median value of 41%. Interestingly, and in contrast to most self-report findings, the video-based observational assessments in GOSAT also showed nontrivial shared environmental effects, on average, with a median value across the Big Five of 26%.

Another recent report from the GOSAT group focused on genetic and environmental contributions to observers' personality ratings aggregated across the 15 tasks, as well as the extent to which there were residual genetic effects on task-specific ratings (Borkenau, Riemann, Spinath, & Angleitner, 2006). Task-specific genetic influences were found, independent of aggregate cross-task genetic influences. Put somewhat differently, genetic influences were documented not only on cross-situational consistency, but also on personality characteristics as manifested in specific tasks. Nevertheless, the cross-situational genetic effects were stronger.

Taken together, these recent reports from the GOSAT group are important because they extend the study of genetic and environmental influences on personality beyond its traditional focus on self-reports of traits. Evidence for genetic influences on personality in adults is not limited to self-reports but extends also to observations (Borkenau et al., 2001). Moreover, cross-situational consistency is not the only place where genetic influences are seen; such heritable influences are also seen on individual behavioral differences in specific tasks (Borkenau et al., 2006).

Evidence from Adoption Studies

Parsing personality variation into genetic and environmental components requires genetically informative sampling designs, that is, samples of people for which we understand the genetic relationships and thus can discern patterns of genetic and environmental transmission. In addition to twin samples, samples of adopted individuals can contribute to understanding genetic and environmental influences on personality. Adoption creates families in which the effects of genetics and environment can be distinguished. Consider, for example, families with both adoptive and biological children. All the children in those families, both biological and adopted, share a home environment, and the biological children share genetic effects both with each other and with their parents. However, the adoptive children do not share genetic effects with the biological children or with their common parents because they are genetically unrelated.

Adoption studies are rarer than twin studies, and they also come to somewhat different conclusions. Like twin studies, adoption studies show little influence of the shared environment, but they also yield smaller estimates for genetic influence on personality and temperament when compared with twin studies (Loehlin, Horn, & Willerman, 1981; Loehlin, Willerman, & Horn, 1982; Plomin, Coon, Carey, DeFries, & Fulker, 1991; Plomin, Corley, Caspi, Fulker, & DeFries, 1998; Scarr, Webber, Weinberg, & Wittig, 1981).

There are a number of possible reasons for disagreements between estimates of genetic influence on personality derived from twin and adoption studies. One possibility is that identical twins reared together assimilate or imitate each other. This possibility can be evaluated by comparing twin similarity in twins reared together with similarity in twins reared apart. Two major studies of twins reared apart reach somewhat different conclusions on this issue. A study from Sweden showed greater similarity among reared-together monozygotic (MZ) twins, when compared with reared-apart MZ twins (Pedersen, Plomin, McClearn, & Friberg, 1988)—a pattern of findings that suggests assimilation on the part of the twins reared together. However, another study showed the resemblance of MZ twins reared apart and together to be similar for personality traits (Tellegen et al., 1988).

Another possibility that receives more consistent support involves nonadditive genetic effects. Genetic effects can be additive, meaning that the multiple genes that contribute to observed variation in a characteristic are fungible, adding up their separate influences to create continuous variation in an observable characteristic, or phenotype. Genetic effects can also be nonadditive, meaning that the precise combination of relevant alleles (forms of genes) is important in understanding the resulting phenotype. The most common example of nonadditive genetic effects is simple Mendelian dominance, in which the heterozygous type resembles one but not the other of the homozygous types. MZ twins share both additive and nonadditive genetic effects completely because they share the same genotype. However, the resemblance between first-degree relatives, such as siblings, dizygotic (DZ) twins, and parents and their offspring, is greater for additive than nonadditive genetic effects. As a result, adoption studies that involve first-degree relatives, such as siblings or parents and their offspring, but not MZ twins will indicate less overall genetic influence on personality than

twin studies involving MZ twins if nonadditive genetic effects are important contributors to personality variation.

Loehlin, Neiderhiser, and Reiss (2003) recently provided a very informative analysis of the issue of nonadditive genetic effects on personality variation derived from data collected as part of the Nonshared Environment in Adolescent Development (NEAD) study (Reiss, Neiderhiser, Hetherington, & Plomin, 2000). The NEAD study was unique in including not just MZ and DZ twin pairs, but also full sibling pairs from intact families, full sibling pairs from remarried families, half-siblings in remarried families, and genetically unrelated siblings in remarried families. The existence of these other pairs, beyond just MZ and DZ twins, allowed Loehlin and colleagues to examine the impact of MZ pairs on heritability estimates for a series of dimensions of both adjustment and maladjustment, akin to personality constructs. In analyses excluding the MZ pairs, smaller estimates of genetic influence were obtained, suggesting the importance of nonadditive genetic effects in understanding personality (cf. Lykken, Bouchard, McGue, & Tellegen, 1992). This nonadditive complexity at the genomic level may well be part of the reason that linking specific alleles with behavior has proven very challenging, as we describe in greater detail below.

The Genetic Structure of Personality Closely Resembles the Phenotypic Structure of Personality

If we take the findings of numerous behavioral genetic studies of personality variation seriously, the nature–nurture debate is, to some extent, over, at least if the debate is framed in terms of radical positions about the dominance of either genetic or environmental influences. That is, every individual-differences characteristic that could be measured is probably at least somewhat heritable, but the influence of the environment is also typically as great as the influence of genes (Turkheimer, 2000). Does this mean that behavioral genetic studies of personality have outlived their usefulness?

The answer to this question is "no," because the study of *variation* is only one aspect of what can be learned by parsing the contributions of nature and nurture to personality. For example, much inquiry in personality psychology is focused not on variation but on covariation. An especially important topic has been the structure of personality, or the way in which individual differences in personality are organized. When this type of research is extended to the behavioral genetic context, investigators estimate not only genetic and environmental influences on personality variation, but also the extent to which covariation in pairs of traits reflects genetic and environmental sources. For example, the extent to which genetic effects are common to pairs of traits can be indexed by genetic correlations, which are interpreted in much the same way as phenotypic correlations (e.g., a genetic correlation of 1.0 means that the genetic effects on the two variables being correlated are entirely in common). A series of these correlations can be subjected to multivariate factor analyses of the same sort that are used to parse the observed, phenotypic structure of personality.

Although the Big Five have been influential constructs in behavioral genetic personality studies, recent work points to an even broader hierarchical structure that integrates various structural models involving two, three, four, and five "big traits" (Markon, Krueger, & Watson, 2005). At the two-trait level, Extraversion and Openness from the Big Five combine to form a broader factor of "Plasticity," and Agreeableness, Conscientiousness, and a lack of Neuroticism combine to form a broader factor of "Stability" (DeYoung, 2006; Digman, 1997). Behavioral genetic research supports the genetic basis of this organizational scheme, in the sense that genetic correlations among the Big Five reveal broadly similar Big Two genetic factors (Jang et al., 2006).

At the three-trait phenotypic level, Neuroticism breaks off from the broader stability factor, resulting in factors that reflect negative emotionality (neuroticism), positive emotionality (extraversion and openness), and disinhibition (disagreeableness and unconscientiousness). Primary personality traits that delineate the Big Three at the phenotypic level show this same Big Three structure at the genetic level (Krueger, 2000). The phenotypic four-trait level consists essentially of the Big Five without Openness, and this level has been influential in research linking personality and psychopathology (D. Watson, Clark, & Harkness, 1994), and related research on dimensional approaches to classifying

personality pathology (Widiger, Simonsen, Krueger, Livesley, & Verheul, 2005). Factor analyses of genetic correlations among scales delineating primary dimensions of personality pathology reveal essentially these same Big Four dimensions (Livesley, Jang, & Vernon, 1998). Finally, genetic correlations among scales designed to delineate the Big Five at the phenotypic level reveal the Big Five at the genetic level as well (McCrae, Jang, Livesley, Riemann, & Angleitner, 2001; Yamagata et al., 2006).

Taken together, these studies suggest that genetic influences on personality are not organized around one specific level of the personality hierarchy, such as the Big Five level. Rather, genetic influences are organized by the entire hierarchy and all of its multiple levels, in the same way that phenotypic individual differences are hierarchically organized. This hierarchical perspective on genetic–phenotypic correspondence in personality structure is also consistent with behavioral genetic research examining etiological influences on traits beneath the level of the Big Five. Jang, McCrae, Angleitner, Riemann, and Livesley (1998) examined the heritability of variance in facets of the Big Five that remained after the common Big Five variance was removed, and found nontrivial residual heritabilities. We (Johnson & Krueger, 2004) examined a related issue: the extent to which genetic influences on specific adjectives that delineate the Big Five are tightly clustered within each Big Five domain. We found evidence that genetic effects on Extraversion and Neuroticism were relatively more tightly clustered, whereas genetic effects on Conscientiousness, Agreeableness, and Openness were relatively more diffuse.

A potentially provocative implication of this body of work is that specific genetic effects may operate at different levels of the personality hierarchy. If true, thinking in terms of genes "for" broad phenotypic traits at specific levels may not map nature well in all cases. For example, genes involved in building brain systems that regulate emotion may map onto extraversion and neuroticism (cf. Canli, 2004, Chapter 11, this volume; Eid, Riemann, Angleitner, & Borkenau, 2003) in a manner consistent with our findings (Johnson & Krueger, 2004) regarding the relative genetic coherence of these domains at the Big Five level. Yet there may be other genetic effects that drive more specific, narrow individual differences at a level beneath the Big Five traits, such as characteristic responses to narrow classes of relevant stimuli (e.g., sociability vs. achievement striving within the domain of Positive Emotionality). Ultimately, a better understanding of the brain systems that underlie personality could help to constrain theories about how specific genetic effects translate into specific phenotypic personality structures at distinct hierarchical levels (Krueger & Markon, 2002). Even more direct would be finding functional genetic polymorphisms at any level in the trait hierarchy and evaluating empirically the extent to which these polymorphisms correlate with other levels, including their association with specific brain systems.

Personality Stability over Time Is Attributable More to Genetic Than to Environmental Influences

The multivariate approach to parsing genetic and environmental effects can also be extended to the study of personality over time in longitudinal studies. Perhaps not surprisingly, this literature tends to point to the role of genetic factors in maintaining stability, with environmental effects acting more to promote change (for a recent review, see Krueger, Johnson, & Kling, 2006). However, this general summary obscures the existence of periods of the life course during which genetic effects may contribute to change, and environmental effects may contribute to stability. For example, early in life, novel genetic effects may be important in understanding temperamental development. Plomin and colleagues (1993) examined change and continuity in temperament from 14 to 20 months of age and found evidence for novel genetic effects at 20 months. Later in life, the unique environmental niches people occupy may be important in understanding personality continuity. We (Johnson, McGue, & Krueger, 2005) studied twins who were 59 years old, on average, at a first assessment wave, and 64 years old, on average, at a second assessment wave. Consistent with other studies reviewed by Krueger and colleagues (2006), genetic effects on personality were essentially perfectly correlated across the two waves, emphasizing the role of genetic factors in explaining the stability of personality. However, nonshared environmental influences on person-

ality were also highly correlated across the two waves (.53 to .73). Importantly, because nonshared environmental influences on personality were somewhat greater than 50%, the relative contributions of environmental and genetic influences to personality stability were essentially equal, consistent with other longitudinal studies of personality (Krueger et al., 2006).

Measures of the Environment Are Partly Genetically Influenced and Much of the Genetic Effect on These Measures Is Shared with Personality

One important and provocative finding emerging from behavioral genetic research is that environmental influences are themselves shaped by genetics. For example, the seminal work of David Rowe (1981, 1983) showed that family experiences, such as adolescents' perceptions of their parents' acceptance and affection, are subject to genetic influence. People create much of their experience of the world partly through genetic mechanisms. This likely happens through perception of experience, but it also likely happens because genetically influenced patterns of behavior tend to elicit common patterns of responses from the environment, and because people gravitate toward environments that meet their psychological needs and avoid environments that do not. In combination, all of these processes act to make nurture partly attributable to nature (Plomin & Bergeman, 1991).

The evidence of genetic influence on environmental factors is now rather extensive, having been documented using a variety of assessment approaches and study designs (Kendler & Baker, 2007). Genetic effects extend beyond self-report and are seen, for example, in observational measures of the family environments of infants (Braungart, Fulker, & Plomin, 1992), children (Rende, Slomkowski, Stocker, Fulker, & Plomin, 1992), and adolescents (O'Connor, Hetherington, Reiss, & Plomin, 1995). Evidence for genetic effects also extends beyond twins reared together, to the environmental experiences of twins who were reared in different families, with identical twins generally reporting more similar family experiences than fraternal twins (Hur & Bouchard, 1995; Plomin, McClearn, Pedersen, Nesselrode,

& Bergeman, 1988). This research, taken together, provides relatively strong evidence for the impact of genetic endowment on the way people elicit, react to, and create their own family environments because the twins reared apart in these studies were rating their different rearing families. Moreover, as people grow up and have children of their own, they contribute to their family environments as parents, and parenting style also shows nontrivial genetic influence (Kendler, 1996; Losoya, Callor, Rowe, & Goldsmith, 1997; Perusse, Neale, Heath, & Eaves, 1994).

This work raises the question of why measures of environmental experiences show genetic influences. The answer seems to be at least partly that genetic effects on personality drive genetic effects on environmental experiences. One of us (R. F. K.; Krueger, Markon, & Bouchard, 2003) studied this question in twins reared apart who provided extensive data on both their personalities and their rearing family environments, from perceptions of the general family climate (characteristics such as warmth and discipline) to physical facilities available in the family home (e.g., books and tools). The twins' recollections of their rearing environments were partly heritable, and genetic effects on recalled environments were entirely accounted for by genetic effects on personality. These findings suggest that genes that affect personality also lead people to recall and/or interact with family members in specific ways, so that the way people are nurtured is fundamentally influenced by their nature (Plomin & Bergeman, 1991). Such common genetic effects on personality and environmental measures also extend beyond recalled family environments, to areas such as life events (Saudino, Pedersen, Lichtenstein, McClearn, & Plomin, 1997) and parenting styles (Chipuer, Plomin, Pedersen, McClearn, & Nesselroade, 1993; Losoya et al., 1997).

Most Environmental Influences on Personality Are Nonshared, But the Meaning of This Finding Remains Elusive

By definition, shared environmental influences act to make family members similar. We presented evidence from both twin and adoption studies that influences of this kind are of little importance in the development and manifestation of personality. Though

Plomin and Daniels's (1987) classic paper enumerating some of the likely mechanisms involved is now 20 years old, the absence of shared environmental influences continues to surprise and baffle theorists attempting to conceptualize the processes involved in personality development. This bafflement is partly due to the fact that the associations between offspring outcomes and environmental influences such as parental attitudes and rearing styles, religious involvement, and socioeconomic status continue to be robust. It is also because the search for the specific nonshared environmental influences that act to make siblings growing up in the same family so different that was spawned by Plomin and Daniels's paper has been rather disappointing.

Turkheimer and Waldron (2000) documented the results of this search in a well-known meta-analysis. They concluded that a broad range of specifically identified nonshared familial and peer environmental variables, considered theoretically important, accounted for little, if any, of the nonshared environmental variance in personality, at least as measured to date (cf. Plomin, Asbury, & Dunn, 2001). As they saw it, this was likely due to measurement difficulties and underlying stochastic processes that would elude our ability to detect and quantify the processes involved in personality development for some time to come.

Harris (1998, 2006) offered an alternative account for the absence of shared environmental influences. She argued that parents contribute little to the socialization of their offspring beyond the genes they pass along because (1) most socialization takes place in the context of peer, not family, interactions and (2) learning is context-dependent, so what is learned at home does not translate to those all-important situations outside the home.

Distinguishing between Objective and Effective Environments

To understand how specific environmental circumstances contribute to personality differences, it is important to distinguish between objective and effective measurement of environments (Goldsmith, 1993; Turkheimer & Waldron, 2000). "Objective measurement of environments" refers to the assessment of environmental circumstances as they appear to the researcher, regardless of the effects of these circumstances on the people who experience them. Thus, environmental circumstances are objectively shared within families when their measured values apply to more than one sibling in the family, regardless of whether the circumstances act to make the siblings similar or different. Many of the most commonly used variables that distinguish among families, such as parental socioeconomic status and relationship quality or residence neighborhood and school, are measured objectively. Environmental circumstances are objectively nonshared when each sibling within a family has a unique measured value for the circumstance, again regardless of whether the circumstance acts to make the siblings similar or different. Peer relationships and classroom assignments are common examples of nonshared environmental circumstances usually measured objectively. To emphasize, the shared and nonshared characterization of the objectively measured environment refers to the definition of measurement, not to the kinds of effects the environment may have.

"Effective measurement of environments" refers to the nature of the effects of those environments on the people who experience them, regardless of how they were measured. Environmental circumstances are effectively shared when they act to make family members more similar, and nonshared when they act to make family members different. The estimates of shared environmental variance resulting from behavioral genetic analyses refer, without actually specifying them, only to environmental circumstances that are effectively shared. This means that the objectively shared environmental circumstances that are so consistently associated with outcomes actually contribute to shared environmental variance only if they act to make family members more similar than they would be based on their shared genetic endowments.

Consider the example of parental education, often measured using the mid-parent average or the mother's education. Two siblings in an intact family will both grow up with, say, one parent who attended but did not graduate from college and another who did graduate from college. Measured objectively in this way, the siblings' parental educational environment is shared, and both will experience the effects of growing up with parents with these levels of education. To the extent that this matters for the outcomes in question, their parents' education is acting to make them more similar to each other than to siblings with other patterns of parental education. But one sibling may share more interests with the parent who graduated from college than the other sibling, and may therefore be more influenced by a higher level of parental education than the other sibling. If this is the case, then, measured effectively, at least some of the influence of parental education is nonshared. An estimate of variance due to shared environmental influence will pick up only the portion of influence of parental education acting to make the siblings more similar to each other than they are to siblings with other patterns of parental education.

In addition, whatever influence parental education has on offspring education is primarily indirect, which means that level of parental education is a very coarse measure of the forces of parental influence, such as exposure to knowledge, culture, and the intellectual activities and debate in which we are actually likely interested. Moreover, education levels tend to "bunch" around program graduation landmarks so that the distribution of education levels is not evenly continuous. Both of these factors, along with reporting and other inaccuracies, act to reduce the apparent influence of parental education, whether shared or nonshared, on offspring outcomes.

The point here is that the definition of shared environmental influences as those environmental circumstances that act to make family members more similar to each other than they are to members of other families is very narrow and potentially affected by restriction in sample range. To the extent that some environmental measure makes all sample members relatively similar to each other regardless of family membership, the ability to pick up greater similarities within families than between families will be reduced (Stoolmiller, 1999). For example, if socioeconomic status matters and its range is restricted in a sample, then all the families in that sample will be relatively similar, and within-family similarities can be observed only within the context of restricted between-family variation. In addition, subtle differences in the actual environment experienced by each sibling (due, e.g., to varying ages of siblings at the time of parental divorce) as well as in siblings' perspectives on that environment (e.g., one sibling blames herself for conflict between her parents and becomes depressed and isolated, whereas another throws himself into activities away from home in order to escape) will be picked up as nonshared environmental influences. Moreover, chance events and variations in the specific combinations of environmental circumstances that act in concert from individual to individual will all contribute to nonshared rather than shared environmental influences. This is one reason why perceptions of the environment may be more useful constructs for personality research, as opposed to putatively "objective" environmental circumstances.

Family Dynamics and the Meaning of Environmental Components of Variance

Family members may also act to establish their own individuality by differentiating from each other (Ansbacher & Ansbacher, 1956; Feinberg & Hetherington, 2000), creating correlations between genetic and nonshared environmental influences, to the extent that this differentiation process is at least initially driven by genetic factors. Schachter, Shore, Feldman-Rotman, Marquis, and Campbell (1976) suggested that this sibling de-identification process relieves competitive pressures between siblings and is most pronounced for siblings who are more similar in age or sex. The small volume of research in this area has tended to focus on systematic associations between family circumstances and the extent of differentiation between pairs of siblings. For example, Grotevant (1978) found that girls with sisters reported fewer feminine occupational interests than did girls with brothers. Feinberg and Hetherington (2000) examined relations between age differences between siblings and similarity of sibling outcomes, with the general observation that siblings who were closer in age tended to be less similar. Feinberg, Reiss, Neiderhiser, and Hetherington (2005) found that shared environmental influences, indicating greater sibling similarity, tended to be higher in families in which parents displayed greater negativity to their children.

In contrast, shared environmental influences tended to be lower, indicating greater sibling differentiation, in the presence of higher levels of conflict between parents.

Although these kinds of family dynamics may very well affect the degree of sibling similarity and thus estimates of shared environmental influences, motivation to differentiate from siblings may also be related to individual differences in personality. For example, the well-known twin researcher David Lykken once mentioned that his work with twins had led him to wish that he had had an MZ twin himself, so that he would have experienced the kind of psychological closeness he had observed in many pairs. In contrast, others might be glad to have been spared what feels like the psychological intrusion of growing up constantly presented with someone so similar. Individual differences of this kind should "wash out" from many univariate estimates of shared environmental influences in samples representative of the population. This will be the case, however, only when this response to the physical proximity of psychologically similar others is independent of the traits of interest. In addition, a sibling's particular characteristics may inspire admiration and emulation or scorn and the desire to differentiate. Some evidence, at least for the admiration and emulation process, has been provided by McGue and Iacono (2001), who found that older siblings' antisocial and substance use behavior contributed directly to similar behavior in younger siblings.

PROPOSITIONS BASED ON MAJOR DIRECTIONS IN CURRENT RESEARCH

Genetic and Environmental Influences on Personality Interact

The previous sections presented relatively well-established observations in personality genetics. The existence of substantial genetic effects on personality is robust to measurement approach and study design, and effectively shared environments seem to have little impact on personality. When environments are measured directly, they show genetic effects that are closely related to genetic effects on personality per se. Nonshared environments, emerging as anonymous components of variation from family research, are as important as genetic effects, but their psychological nature remains elusive.

As we noted above in discussing nonshared environmental effects, integrating these observations in a comprehensive theory of the origins of personality has proven challenging. Yet one often unrecognized assumption of the previously reviewed research may provide a key to advancing our understanding and thereby integrating nature and nurture. This often ignored assumption is that genes and environments are *additive*, as opposed to *interactive*. For example, research showing that personality is heritable has traditionally estimated heritability as a statistic that is applicable to an entire population, to which is added an analogous statistic representing environmental effects to account for the total variation in a personality characteristic—as if the two were completely independent. The roughly 50% heritability of the Big Five traits cited earlier is such a statistic, describing how much of the total variation in the Big Five can be traced to genetic variation at the level of the population. In theory, however, this 50% value could vary as a function of other variables. For example, in circumstances where people have the freedom to express their genetic proclivities, genetic influences might be enhanced, whereas circumstances that constrain individual freedoms might dampen genetic influences.

Recent developments in statistical modeling have rendered these conceptual possibilities empirically tractable. We can only provide a brief description of these developments here; one of us (R. F. K.; Krueger & Tackett, 2007) provides a more extensive primer on these developments aimed at personality researchers just getting into twin research, and the other (W. J.; Johnson, 2007) provides a detailed account of the ways in which these developments promise to provide a richer perspective on genetic and environmental influences on human individual differences.

Essentially, when genetic and environmental influences on personality are estimated using the traditional approach, the estimates are based on summary statistics that compare the overall similarity of pairs of people in specific groups, such as comparing the overall similarity of MZ twins to their twin siblings with the overall similarity of DZ twins to their twin siblings. This

approach results in an overall account of genetic and environmental influences on a personality construct. Recent developments go well beyond this approach because they do not model summary statistics; rather, they model the data obtained from specific individuals directly. As a result, genetic and environmental influences on personality can be quantified as moderated by, or contingent on, other individual characteristics.

These modeling developments have opened up major conceptual possibilities for personality genetics that are just beginning to be realized. A broad picture of how the genetic and environmental influences on personality are moderated by other characteristics of persons—and how personality can itself moderate the genetic and environmental influences on other characteristics—is difficult to generate because this research is in its infancy. Nevertheless, some examples from the recent literature serve to make the general point that genetic influences on personality seem to behave in a more nuanced manner than can be captured by classical approaches to the analysis of behavioral genetic data.

The major focus of this kind of work on personality to date has been on ways in which diverse aspects of family life, from relationships to family income, moderate genetic and environmental influences on personality. Characterizing genetic contributions to personality in terms of an overall heritability statistic entails summarizing across diverse family circumstances that may dampen or enhance genetic effects. This summarizing process may gloss over a range of scenarios, and understanding the limitations of the classical approach may be a key to reconciling the role of the family in shaping personality with evidence of substantial genetic effects on individual differences (W. A. Collins, Maccoby, Steinberg, Hetherington, & Bornstein, 2000). Rather than having direct and purely shared environmental effects that make people from the same families more similar than they would be based on genetic endowments, family variables may sometimes act indirectly, to moderate the impact of genes and environments on personality.

For example, Boomsma, de Geus, van Baal, and Koopmans (1999) presented evidence that a religious upbringing reduces the impact of genetic factors on disinhibitory personality characteristics. Jang and colleagues (2005) showed how a variety of factors, such as parental bonding, family functioning, and nonassaultive traumatic events, impacted genetic and environmental influences on emotional stability (the opposite of neuroticism), often by enhancing the impact of nonshared environmental factors. Similar to this research, we (Johnson & Krueger, 2006) showed that nonshared environmental factors had a greater impact on life satisfaction at lower levels of financial standing. Money appeared to buffer the impact of random environmental shocks on an individual's genetically influenced happiness setpoint (Lykken, 1999). We showed how adolescents' perceptions of their relationships with their parents impacted the relative importance of genetic and environmental effects on positive and negative emotionality (Krueger, South, Johnson, & Iacono, in press). For example, higher levels of perceived parental regard were associated with enhanced genetic effects on positive emotionality. Moderating effects on personality are not universal, however; Kendler, Aggen, Jacobson, and Neale (2003) found no evidence that family dysfunction moderated genetic and environmental effects on neuroticism.

These types of moderating effects might also work in the opposite direction, with personality constructs acting to moderate the etiology of various outcomes. It is tempting to characterize the phenomena described as "gene × environment interaction," or genetic control of sensitivity to different environments, but this rubric is conceptually problematic because, as described above, various aspects of "the environment" also show genetic influences; that is, the ways in which people perceive environments are also affected by the genetic endowments people bring to bear in interpreting the external world. "The environment" may sometimes be better conceived of as the person's psychological experience of the world, as opposed to some putatively objective aspect of the world entirely outside the person.

Along these lines, we (Johnson & Krueger, 2005) showed that a person's subjective sense of control moderates genetic and environmental effects on health in a manner similar to the more putatively objective environment provided by the person's income. A higher sense of control and a higher in-

come both acted to suppress genetic effects on physical health. We found that high levels of positive emotionality enhanced the genetic effects on parental regard (South, Krueger, Johnson, & Iacono, in press). The fact that high levels of parental regard also enhanced the genetic effects on positive emotionality (Krueger et al., in press) suggests a bidirectional feedback loop whereby adolescents with positive emotional dispositions elicit parental regard, a situation that allows for the enhanced expression of genetic effects on positive emotionality. Similar to Boomsma and colleagues' (1999) findings regarding the impact of a religious upbringing on disinhibition, Timberlake and colleagues (2006) showed that self-rated religiousness reduced the impact of genetic factors on initiating smoking.

In sum, there are now quite a few examples in the literature of how various circumstances, often related to some aspect of the individual's family situation, serve to change the relative influence of genetic and environmental influences on personality. It seems the family does indeed matter in understanding the origins of personality, but its effects involve enhancing or dampening genetic endowments. That is, rather than acting directly to make children in the same family more similar than they would be by virtue of the extent to which they share genes (i.e., through shared environmental main effects), families influence the magnitude of genetic effects.

Personality Is Linked to Outcomes through Correlational and Interactive Processes

As we have noted, the behavioral genetic methods generally used to estimate sources of genetic and environmental variance in personality and related variables are based on the assumption that genetic and environmental influences are independent. When we accept this assumption, we also assume that there are no gene–environment interactions or correlations that would act to create differing degrees of genetic and environmental influences within different subgroups of the population, of the kind that the new methods described above are starting to allow us to estimate. Gene–environment interactions (G × E) occur when genetic differences are moderated by environmental effects. For example, Caspi and colleagues (2002) observed that boys carrying the low-activity variant of the monoamine oxidase A (MAO-A) gene were more likely to display antisocial behavior in adolescence and young adulthood, but only if they had been exposed to severe parental maltreatment (see also Kim-Cohen et al., 2006). Gene–environment correlations (r_{GE}) occur when genetic differences are associated with differential exposure to environmental circumstances. For example, Jaffee and colleagues (2004) found that 25% of the variance in the corporal punishment children received at the hands of their parents could be attributed to genetic influences on the children's own misbehavior (see also Wade & Kendler, 2000).

Though the behavioral genetic models that assumed independence were a first step toward understanding genetic and environmental influences, it is becoming increasingly clear that G × E and r_{GE} are likely to be common and to be useful in understanding how nature and nurture transact. The efforts people undertake, to seek or create environments compatible with their genetic endowments, are fundamental to the process of evolution, and differences in response to the environment caused by genetic differences are the raw material for natural selection (Ridley, 2003). We may tend to think of evolution as a long-term process that took place in the long-distant past, but the day-to-day behavioral activities of response and adaptation to the environment—activities in which we all engage every day—are the stuff of which it is made. Behavior occurs through genetic expression, and genetic expression reflects the environment in which it takes place. There is a large body of evidence for genetic influences on all other areas of human biological, psychological, and behavioral functioning; it would be distinctly strange if there were no genetic influences on selection of, and responsiveness to, the environment.

Importantly, violations of the "independence assumption" do not invalidate traditional behavioral genetic methods. Rather, they render the estimates applicable only on an overall, average basis. In the presence of G × E or r_{GE}, the components of variance attributable to genetic and environmental influences are not static within the population: Genetic variance could be relatively large within one segment of the population

and relatively small in another, and the same is true for environmental variance (Johnson, 2007). The estimates are specific to the population in which they are developed for essentially the same reason: The differences in the components of variance may depend on other characteristics of the individuals in the population, characteristics that can vary from population to population, and within populations over time. These characteristics can be measured either categorically or continuously. For example, Rose, Dick, Viken, and Kaprio (2001) observed that genetic influences were more important in explaining alcohol-use patterns in adolescents residing in urban areas, whereas shared environmental influences were more important for adolescents residing in rural areas. We (Johnson & Krueger, 2005) found that genetic influences on physical health decreased continuously with increasing perceived control over life. Uncovering how these processes are involved in the development and manifestation of personality means identifying the relevant moderating variables and measuring them accurately (Rutter, Moffitt, & Caspi, 2006).

The presence of G × E or r_{GE} also introduces systematic distortions in the estimates of variance attributable to genetic and environmental influences from models that are based on the assumption that these influences are independent. These distortions have different effects, depending on the nature of the interaction or correlation that violates the independence assumption. Specifically, in twin studies, G × E between genetic and shared environmental influences acts to increase the estimate of genetic influence, whereas G × E between genetic and nonshared environmental influences acts to increase the estimate of nonshared environmental influence; r_{GE} between genetic and shared environmental influences acts to increase the estimate of shared environmental influence; and r_{GE} between genetic and nonshared environmental influences acts to increase the estimate of genetic influence (Purcell, 2002).

These principles can be used in combination with the typical results of behavioral genetic studies of personality to pinpoint likely mechanisms of G × E and r_{GE} involving personality. G × E between genetic and shared environmental influences may have exaggerated the apparent genetic influences on personality at the expense of the shared environmental influences typically absent in study results. In contrast, r_{GE} between genetic and shared environmental influences is unlikely, as it would increase apparent shared environmental influences on personality, and we typically observe none. This means, for example, that we might expect to find neighborhood effects on neuroticism that differ by genetic vulnerability to neuroticism, but we would not expect to find that family culture involving neuroticism influences how people make residential choices. G × E and r_{GE} involving genetic and nonshared environmental influences have offsetting effects and may be common. They both involve transactions between genetic influences and environmental circumstances unique to each individual. Thus, even r_{GE} between genetic and nonshared environmental influences, which acts to increase estimates of genetic influence, will tend to be idiosyncratic in form. Examples probably most commonly involve individual differences in taking advantage of opportunities or responses to trauma and individual differences in experience arising from individual differences in behavior.

Models that estimate genetic and environmental influences can contribute importantly to the amplification and illustration of theoretical principles of personality development. In particular, Caspi, Roberts, and Shiner (2005) have articulated the cumulative continuity and the co-responsive principles of personality development. The cumulative continuity principle states that personality stability increases with age. Stability peaks perhaps around age 60, though personality characteristics are never completely fixed. Genetic influences contribute to this stability in a straightforward way (Johnson et al., 2005; Pedersen & Reynolds, 1998; Viken, Rose, & Koskenvuo, 1994). We know this because the same genetic influences contribute to personality at earlier and later adult ages. However, as described earlier, straightforward nonshared environmental influences also contribute to stability in personality (Johnson et al., 2005). This finding likely reflects the fact that, for many people, many aspects of the environment, such as place of residence, spousal relationship, occupation, and leisure and social activities, remain relatively stable over long periods of time in adulthood (Johnson, 2007).

In addition to these contributions of straightforward genetic and nonshared envi-

ronmental influences to personality stability, transactions between genetic and environmental influences such as G × E and r_{GE} also make contributions. Caspi and colleagues (2005) have identified niche-building processes, in which individuals create, seek out, or end up in environments that are correlated with their personality traits, as fundamental to the stability of personality. Because of the genetic influences on personality traits, these niche-building processes are perfect examples of r_{GE} in action. In addition, as Caspi and colleagues noted, once people enter trait-correlated environments, those environments may have causal effects of their own, contributing to maintenance of the personality trait and preventing the development of opportunities for change. Such effects are often examples of G × E.

To date, few investigators have studied the emergence of niche-building processes, and none has done so in a behavioral genetic framework. The ideas are thus primarily theoretical at present. Two studies do touch on these issues, though in samples that were not informative about genetic and environmental influences (Roberts, Caspi, & Moffitt, 2003; Roberts & Robins, 2004). The first study was based on the Dunedin longitudinal study of an entire birth cohort in New Zealand, in which personality and work experiences were measured at ages 18 and 26. In general, lower levels of negative emotionality, reflecting lower Stress Reaction, Aggression, and Alienation, and higher levels of positive emotionality and constraint, reflecting especially greater Social Closeness, Social Potency, and Self-Control, were associated with greater occupational attainment, work satisfaction, work involvement, financial security, and work autonomy and stimulation (Roberts et al., 2003). In the second study, Roberts and Robins (2004) measured the fit between person and environment as the correlation between consensus ratings of qualities of a university environment and individual perceptions of the ideal university environment over a period of 4 years in 305 university students from the Berkeley Longitudinal Study; they found that greater academic aptitude and emotional stability, male gender, and lower agreeableness were associated with better fit. In combination with the knowledge that all of these traits show substantial genetic influence, these studies allow us to infer the transactions between genetic and environmental influences that allow stable personality traits to contribute to the emergence of individualized environmental niches.

But these transactions between genetic and environmental influences contribute to personality change as well as stability. Caspi and colleagues' (2005) co-responsive principle summarizes the process. According to this principle, life experiences tend to reinforce the personality characteristics that originally draw people to those experiences. The easygoing, cheerful child who expresses affection naturally is well received by others and quickly establishes friendships that build further social skills and a solid basis of positive emotional experience, developing and deepening the trait we think of as extraversion. In contrast, the stress-reactive, socially awkward child who is easily angered is frequently rebuffed by others and quickly becomes resentful and alienated, developing and deepening the trait we think of as aggression. In the language of life-course dynamics and the psychopathology literature, the co-responsive principle links the process of social selection, in which people seek experiences that are correlated with their personality traits, with the process of social causation, in which experiences affect personality traits. In the language of behavior genetics, the co-responsive principle links active r_{GE}, in which the correlation between environmental and genetic influences results from niche building, with passive and evocative r_{GE}, in which the correlation between environmental and genetic influences arises from growing up with family members similar to oneself and from the responses of others to genetically influenced behavioral displays.

The two studies described above addressed the co-responsive principle as well as niche building. In the Dunedin sample (Roberts et al., 2003), young adults at age 26 who attained higher-status jobs and jobs that involved acquisition of resource power became more socially dominant, harder working, happier, and more self-confident. Those who found more satisfying work tended to become less anxious and less prone to stress. Work involvement was associated with increases in willingness to work hard and support for conventional norms. Those who attained greater financial security tended to become less prone to stress and better adjusted socially. Confirmation of the co-responsive

principle was evidenced by the fact that these same personality characteristics at age 18 had predicted the age 26 occupational outcomes. In the Berkeley sample (Roberts & Robins, 2004), fit improved a little over the course of the study, primarily because students' views of the ideal university environment changed to more closely match the actual university environment. In addition, students who fit better with the university environment underwent less personality change, and fit between person and environment was associated with increases in emotional stability and decreases in agreeableness. In both of these studies, effects were not dramatic, but they were consistent, and the samples consisted of young adults. Most people are still just embarking on their occupational careers at age 26, so the actual career outcomes are far from clear, and college attendance is a period of transition for most people. Thus we could anticipate greater co-responsive effects and clearer indications of niche building over longer time frames.

The principles of niche building and co-responsiveness in personality development and the emerging evidence in support of them suggest the proposition that many life outcomes can be thought of as extensions of personality. Life experiences and the situations in which people find themselves do not descend randomly, bringing about transformations in personality over time and across situations. Rather, the traits that people already possess lead them to create situations and experiences that reinforce and elaborate on those same personality traits. Though the studies to date that have provided data supporting this proposition have not specifically addressed the roles of genetic and environmental influences in these processes, we can infer them from the general knowledge we have that both genetic and environmental influences on personality are pervasive, yet neither is deterministic. Future studies should be designed to address these roles directly, but we propose that, to paraphrase an old expression, genetic influences on personality affect the beds we make, and then we lie in them.

Finding Main Effects of Specific Genes on Personality Has Been Difficult

Ten years ago, personality researchers were dazzled by the prospect of the imminent discovery of the specific genes that contribute to population variation in personality. They anticipated that these discoveries would revolutionize personality research by making possible the use of individuals' specific genotypes to clarify causal relations from cells to social processes, thereby illuminating how genes influence personality development. These hopes have not materialized, despite many concerted gene searches, great improvements in the techniques used, the power to detect specific genetic effects, and great reductions in the costs of implementing these techniques. This is not because the studies, many of them published in prominent journals with high-impact factors, have not produced results. Rather, it is because the results that have been produced have not been convincingly and consistently replicated (Munafo et al., 2003). This situation is far from unique to personality research. It persists in many areas of psychological research as well as many areas of behavioral epidemiology and medical research.

There are many specific reasons for this lack of replication, but they can be summarized under one general heading: The traits involved are polygenic. This means that many genes, each with relatively small effect, are involved in the expression of each trait. We know this to be the case because, unlike the wrinkled and not wrinkled peas studied by Gregor Mendel, the offspring of, for example, a stress-reactive father and a calm and unflappable mother are not neatly described as either stress-reactive or calm and unflappable, as they would be if a single gene were involved in stress reactivity. Rather, the offsprings' relative stress reactivity can be ordered along a basically normally distributed continuum. Although most of the individual genes involved in personality may follow the basic Mendelian patterns of transmission and expression and their effects may even be neatly additive, no single gene is likely to be essential to trait expression, and possession of any one of them is unlikely to determine trait expression. This means that two family members who are relatively concordant for, say, level of aggression may share relatively few to none of the genes relevant to their level of aggression with two other family members who are similarly concordant and similarly aggressive but from another family. This is more likely to be true for more

complex and multifaceted traits; for example, conscientiousness compared with the tendency to pursue goal-directed behavior. To complicate the picture, most of the genes involved in commonly occurring personality traits are likely to be pleiotropic—which means that these genes have more than one function: They are likely involved in many different biochemical processes throughout the brain and thus may be associated with several different personality traits, no matter how independently those traits are construed.

The basic problem is that everyone has a unique personality, yet everyone also expresses all the basic personality traits to some degree in some situations. Moreover, there are likely many different pathways within the brain to actualize any behavior related to personality. This multiplicity may be the reason that personality structure is so richly hierarchical. In addition, regardless of the level of detail at which we measure personality, the traits we measure are amalgamations of different motivations and responses. For example, compliance, a facet of agreeableness in the five-factor model, may involve the perception that cooperation has some long-term reward, fear of punishment, actual enjoyment of the activities involved for their own sakes, lack of alternative activities and intolerance for boredom, and, in any case, the ability to comprehend requirements and activate appropriate behaviors. Activity, a facet of theoretically independent extraversion in the five-factor model, may involve many similar motivations and responses, to varying or even similar degrees. Obviously, experience will affect how one perceives one's situation with respect to these kinds of motivations and responses as well, but the point here is that it is very unlikely that certain genes will be involved in activity but not in compliance, or vice versa.

The universality of at least some level of expression of all basic personality traits suggests that variation in genetic expression may underlie much of the phenotypic variation in personality traits. Though genetic expression itself is at least partially under genetic control (York et al., 2005), work with experimental nonhuman animals makes clear that variation in genetic expression can also be triggered by environmental circumstances. For example, Weaver and colleagues (2004) described differential environmental effects on genetic expression in rats. Differences in maternal licking, grooming, and nursing practices were associated with long-term differences in offsprings' hypothalamic–pituitary–adrenal response to stress. These differences appeared to result from differences in DNA methylation of a glucocorticoid receptor gene promoter in the hippocampus. The differences in maternal treatment appeared to contribute to parental behavior by the offspring as well, leading to differences in stress response that were transmitted from generation to generation. Whether or not there are processes directly analogous to these in humans, it is highly likely that these kinds of general processes take place in humans, contributing to genetic variation that we can sometimes pick up through statistical decomposition of variance but not through examination of DNA samples.

In humans, MZ twins provide information about another mechanism that complicates the search for genes for multigenic traits such as personality. Though MZ twins share a common genetic background that tends to make them similar, significant variation in gene expression remains. The extent of this variation increases with age (Fraga et al., 2005), suggesting that it is subject to environmental influences. But postnatal environmental experiences are probably not the only sources of these epigenetic differences. MZ twins tend to be similar to the same degree regardless of whether they are reared together or apart (Wong, Gottesman, & Petronis, 2005). This "similarity of similarity" may be due to r_{GE}. It may also be the result of the tendency for additional resemblance due to shared rearing environments to be offset by differentiation, as described above.

Recently, several studies have identified specific genes involved in personality-related behavioral effects due to interdependence between specified DNA sequence variations and specific measured environments (Caspi et al., 2002, 2003; Caspi, Moffitt, et al., 2005). The phenomena characterized in these studies are examples of G × E. As noted above, Caspi and colleagues (2002) observed that a variant of the MAO-A gene was associated with antisocial behavior, but only in boys who had experienced maltreatment in childhood. Caspi and colleagues (2003) reported that a functional polymorphism in the sero-

tonin transporter gene was associated with greater depressive symptomatology, but only in people who had experienced stressful life events. Caspi, Moffitt, and colleagues (2005) found that adolescent cannabis use was a significant risk factor for psychotic symptoms and schizophreniform disorder in adulthood, but only for those carrying the valine allele of the COMT gene. These studies have replicated surprisingly well (Eley et al., 2004; Foley et al., 2004; Grabe et al., 2005; Haberstick et al., 2005; Kaufman et al., 2004; Kendler, Kuhn, Vittum, Prescott, & Riley, 2005; Wihelm et al., 2006; Zalsman et al., 2006), especially considering the longstanding tacit assumptions that main genetic effects would be the norm (e.g., Boomsma & Martin, 2002) and that G × E would be difficult to detect (e.g., Bergeman, Plomin, McClearn, Pedersen, & Friberg, 1988).

These studies are important because they provide specific examples of kinds of transactions between genes and environments that are likely common and have measurable effects on phenomena with large public health consequences (but see Eaves, 2006). They are also important specifically to personality researchers because the phenomena involved are among those that can be considered extensions of personality (Krueger, Caspi, & Moffitt, 2000). For example, antisocial behavior, problems with substances, and aggressive and impulsive personality traits form a genetically coherent spectrum of interrelated externalizing problems; genetic effects in this spectrum transcend a putative divide between "personality" and "outcomes" (Krueger et al., 2002).

In addition, unlike the main effects of specific genes on personality that have proved so inconsistent, replication of the specific G × E effects reported in these studies is less critical to their importance. This is because the early assumption that G × E and r_{GE} would be transitory and trivial in relation to main genetic effects (Bergeman et al., 1988) may have been at least partially correct. That is, G × E and r_{GE} involving any specific gene and environmental circumstance may be transitory, existing in some populations and circumstances and not others, even though the overall phenomena are common and far from trivial in the aggregate. On the other hand, there is another sense in which the original assumption about G × E and r_{GE}

may have been correct. That is, the effects involved in these reported G × E relations account for modest proportions of the total incidence of antisocial behavior, depressive symptomatology, and psychotic symptoms and schizophreniform disorder in adulthood. To understand the occurrence of these problems, we may need to look beyond these specific examples of G × E.

TWO BROAD QUESTIONS
TO FRAME FUTURE RESEARCH

This chapter began with well-established observations in personality genetics and moved to current trends in research. This closing section attempts to go one step further, to look just over the horizon and to be a bit provocative. We briefly outline two very challenging—but, in our view, important—questions that may be worth thinking about in pursuing personality genetics in the next few years.

Do We Need to Find Specific Genes and Specific Environmental Effects in Order to Understand Many Personality Processes?

For many, the purpose of demonstrating the presence of genetic influences on human personality and other behavioral traits has been primarily to provide evidence warranting a search for the specific genes involved. Though the fact that genes code for proteins rather than psychological characteristics, per se, is well established, the implications of this fact for understanding behaviors influenced by many genes have probably not been fully absorbed (Kendler, 2005). In particular, we cannot expect that any specific genes are necessary to manifest any specific level of any personality trait, and we cannot expect that the effects of any specific genes are necessarily limited to a specific personality trait. Moreover, we must expect that the effects of specific genes may be contingent on other factors such as environmental circumstances or the presence of other genes. Finally, we must expect that the proteins that are the direct products of gene expression are only initial steps in long series of transactions in the brain and metabolism that lead to manifested behavior. Interruptions and digressions that change the nature of the be-

havioral outcomes can occur at many stages in these transaction processes.

Everyone has a personality and manifests behaviors shared with all other humans across a broad range. Everyone becomes aggressive sometimes, just as everyone sometimes refrains from dangerous behavior. The idiosyncrasies that make each individual personality unique are in the details of the eliciting circumstances and particular constellations of behaviors. This general commonality of shared behavior underlying individual differences in personality makes possible some analogies to physical health. Everyone has cardiovascular, respiratory, and digestive systems that perform the same basic functions with varying degrees of efficiency. Health lies in the optimal functioning of these systems, and illness takes idiosyncratic forms depending on eliciting circumstances and particular constellations of genetic vulnerabilities.

For physical health as measured by numbers of chronic illnesses, we (Johnson & Krueger, 2005) demonstrated that genetic variance increased with decreasing monetary income and decreasing perceived control over life. In other words, under stressful environmental conditions that included psychological stress, genetic vulnerabilities to illness were more likely to be expressed—a form of G × E interaction. Importantly, these expressed genetic vulnerabilities took many different forms involving different physiological systems; without doubt they involved many different genes.

Also importantly, even in the most stressful environments, not everyone was ill, and some people were ill even in the most benign environments, indicating that expression of genetic vulnerabilities was not entirely due to level of income or perceived control over life. Though the results have some importance for medical practitioners interested in the development and treatment of particular diseases, their primary importance lies in the insight they provide into the more general process of health maintenance and disease manifestation, a process involving so many genes and physiological pathways that separate identification may not be very meaningful

We commonly measure and conceptualize broad personality trait domains (e.g., the Big Five) at levels of generality similar to that of physical health. Hence, we can expect to gain insight into the niche-building and co-responsive processes involved in personality development through quantitative approaches that examine the effects of genes and environments in an aggregate sense. In particular, research can illuminate patterns of expression and suppression of genetic and environmental effects both common and unique to personality traits and personal circumstances—without necessarily identifying the specific genes and environments involved. We can learn a lot about the origins and nature of personality without necessarily finding specific genes and specific environments by studying how genetic and environmental effects on personality are enhanced and suppressed by specific circumstances.

What Can We Learn from Pondering the Link between Quantitative and Molecular Genetic Research?

Having noted that finding specific genes and environments is not the only way to make behavioral genetic research interesting and relevant to understanding personality, we would still like to understand the biological mechanisms that lead from genes to behaviors. However, pretty much everything is heritable (Turkheimer, 2000), and with regard to personality, numerous traits are heritable to about the same extent (roughly 50%). These heritabilities are not trivial—50% is far from a "small effect size." Yet, as we have described, it has been frustratingly difficult to document reliable links between specific molecular genetic polymorphisms and specific personality traits (Ebstein, 2006). If everything is so heritable, why is it so hard to find the genes involved in personality?

The key to unraveling this riddle may lie in understanding just how much variation is glossed over by a general heritability statistic. As one example, we (Krueger et al., in press) examined how genetic and environmental contributions to personality traits might change as a function of the nature of adolescents' relationships with their parents. Across a range of parental regard (e.g., "I admire my parent and my parent admires me"), genetic contributions to positive emotionality (akin to extraversion) varied widely, from 34% at low levels of regard to 77% at high levels of regard. Fifty percent is a good "halfway point" (indeed, the heritability of positive emotionality was 52% when we estimated

it without modeling regard as a moderator). But this very general 52% value disguised a wide range of etiological scenarios, in which genetic effects on positive emotionality were markedly diminished and enhanced. In sum, we might ask not "how heritable is a trait" but rather "what are the circumstances in which genetic contributions to this trait are enhanced or suppressed?"—and look for specific polymorphism–personality associations in circumstances in which genetic contributions are enhanced.

Interestingly, this viewpoint is conceptually similar to the "genomic psychology" approach outlined by Canli (Chapter 11, this volume). At the core of Canli's approach is the idea that gene effects are usually contingent—that G × E interactions are the norm in relating specific polymorphisms to behavior. We suspect that this approach will prove more generative than the idea that genes have main effects on behavior, and it may also show us how to reconcile quantitative and molecular genetic research. In particular, we suspect that molecular genetic–behavior links will be stronger in circumstances where genetic variation is shown to be larger in quantitative genetic research. We look forward to the fourth edition of this chapter, in which we will see if this admittedly provocative prediction has borne empirical fruit.

ACKNOWLEDGMENTS

We wish to acknowledge helpful comments from Robert Plomin and Peter Borkenau on previous drafts, and we thank Megan Lucy for her assistance with preparing the chapter. We also acknowledge support for our collaborative work from National Institute on Aging Grant No. AG20166.

REFERENCES

Ansbacher, H. L., & Ansbacher, R. R. (1956). *The individual psychology of Alfred Adler*. New York: Basic Books.

Bergeman, C. S., Plomin, R., McClearn, G. E., Pedersen, N., & Friberg, L. T. (1988). Gene–environment interaction in personality development: Identical twins reared apart. *Personality and Aging*, 3, 399–406.

Boomsma, D. I., de Geus, E. J. C., van Baal, G. C. M., & Koopmans, J. R. (1999). A religious upbringing reduces the influence of genetic factors on disinhibition: Evidence for interaction between genotype and environment on personality. *Twin Research, 2,* 115–125.

Boomsma, D. I., & Martin, N. (2002). Gene–environment interactions. In H. D'haenen, J. A. den Boer, & P. Willner (Eds.), *Biological psychiatry* (pp. 181–187). New York: Wiley.

Borkenau, P., Riemann, R., Angleitner, A., & Spinath, F. M. (2001). Genetic and environmental influences on observed personality: Evidence from the German Observational Study of Adult Twins. *Journal of Personality and Social Psychology, 80,* 655–668.

Borkenau, P., Riemann, R., Spinath, F. M., & Angleitner, A. (2006). Genetic and environmental influences on person × situation profiles. *Journal of Personality, 74,* 1451–1479.

Bouchard, T. J., Jr., & Loehlin, J. C. (2001). Genes, evolution, and personality. *Behavior Genetics, 31,* 243–273.

Braungart, J. M., Fulker, D. W., & Plomin, R. (1992). Genetic mediation of the home environment during infancy: A sibling adoption study of the HOME. *Developmental Psychology, 28,* 1048–1055.

Brody, N. (1993). Intelligence and the behavior genetics of personality. In R. Plomin & G. E. McClearn (Eds.), *Nature, nurture, and psychology* (pp. 161–178). Washington, DC: American Psychological Association.

Canli, T. (2004). Functional brain mapping of extraversion and neuroticism: Learning from individual differences in emotion processing. *Journal of Personality, 72,* 1105–1132.

Caspi, A., McClay, J., Moffitt, T., Mill, J., Martin, J., Craig, I. W., et al. (2002). Role of genotype in the cycle of violence in maltreated children. *Science, 297,* 752–754.

Caspi, A., Moffitt, T., Cannon, M., McClay, J., Murray, R., Harrington, H., et al. (2005). Moderation of the effect of adolescent-onset cannabis use on adult psychosis by a functional polymorphism in the COMT gene: Longitudinal evidence of a gene × environment interaction. *Biological Psychiatry, 57,* 1117–1127.

Caspi, A., Roberts, B. W., & Shiner, R. L. (2005). Personality development: Stability and change. *Annual Review of Psychology, 56,* 453–484.

Caspi, A., Sugden, K., Moffitt, T., Taylor, A., Craig, I. W., Harrington, H., et al. (2003). Influence of life stress on depression: Moderation by a polymorphism in the 5-HTT gene. *Science, 301,* 386–389.

Cherny, S. S., Fuiles, D. W., Corley, R. P., Plomin, R., & DeFries, J. C. (1994). Continuity and change in infant shyness from 14 to 20 months. *Behavior Genetics, 24,* 365–379.

Chipuer, H. M., Plomin, R., Pedersen, N. L., McClearn, G. E., & Nesselroade, J. R. (1993). Genetic influence on family environment: The role

of personality. *Developmental Psychology, 29,* 110–118.

Collins, W. A., Maccoby, E. E., Steinberg, L., Hetherington, E. M., & Bornstein, M. H. (2000). Contemporary research on parenting: The case for nature and nurture. *American Psychologist, 55,* 218–232.

DeYoung, C. G. (2006). Higher-order factors of the Big Five in a multi-informant sample. *Journal of Personality and Social Psychology, 91,* 1138–1151.

Digman, J. M. (1997). Higher-order factors of the Big Five. *Journal of Personality and Social Psychology, 73,* 1246–1256.

Eaves, L. (2006). Genotype × environment interaction in psychopathology: Fact or artifact. *Twin Research and Human Genetics, 9,* 1–8.

Ebstein, R. P. (2006). The molecular genetic architecture of human personality: Beyond self-report questionnaires. *Molecular Psychiatry, 11,* 427–445.

Eid, M., Riemann, R., Angleitner, A., & Borkenau, P. (2003). Sociability and positive emotionality: Genetic and environmental contributions to the covariation between different facets of extraversion. *Journal of Personality, 71,* 319–346.

Eley, T. C., Sugden, K., Corsico, A., Gregory, A. M., Sham, P., McGuffin, P., et al. (2004). Gene–environment interaction analysis of serotonin system markers with adolescent depression. *Moelcular Psychiatry, 9,* 915–922.

Feinberg, M. E., & Hetherington, E. M. (2000). Sibling differentiation in adolescence: Implications for behavioral genetic theory. *Child Development, 71,* 1512–1524.

Feinberg, M. E., Reiss, D., Neiderhiser, J. M., & Hetherington, E. M. (2005). Differential association of family subsystem negativity on siblings' maladjustment: Using behavior genetic methods to test process theory. *Journal of Family Psychology, 19,* 601–610.

Foley, D. L., Wormley, B., Silberg, J., Maes, H. H., Hewitt, J. K., Eaves, L., et al. (2004). Childhood adversity, MAOA genotype, and risk for conduct disorder. *Archives of General Psychiatry, 61,* 738–744.

Fraga, M. F., Ballestar, E., Paz, M. F., Ropero, S., Setien, F., Ballestar, M. L., et al. (2005). Epigenetic differences arise during the lifetime of monozygotic twins. *Proceedings of the National Academy of Sciences, 102,* 10604–10609.

Galton, F. (1865). Heredity talent and character. *Macmillan's Magazine, 12,* 157–166, 318–327.

Goldsmith, H. H. (1993). Nature–nurture issues in the behavioral genetic context: Overcoming barriers to communication. In R. Plomin & G. E. McClearn (Eds.), *Nature, nurture, and psy-*

chology. Washington, DC: American Psychological Association.

Grabe, H. J., Lange, M., Volzke, H., Lucht, M., Freyberger, H. J., John, U., et al.. (2005). Mental and physical distress is modulated by a polymorphism in the 5-HT transporter gene interacting with social stressors and chronic disease burden. *Molecular Psychiatry, 10*, 220–224.

Grotevant, H. D. (1978). Sibling constellations and sex-typing of interests in adolescence. *Child Development, 49*, 540–542.

Haberstick, B. C., Lessem, M., Hopfer, C. J., Smolen, A., Ehringer, M. A., Timberlake, D., et al. (2005). Monoamine oxidase A (MAOA) and antisocial behaviors in the presence of childhood and adolescent maltreatment. *American Journal of Medical Genetics: Neuropsychiatric Genetics, 135B*, 996–998.

Harris, J. R. (1998). *The nurture assumption.* New York: The Free Press.

Harris, J. R. (2006). *No two alike: Human nature and human individuality.* New York: Norton.

Hur, Y., & Bouchard, T. J. (1995). Genetic influences on perceptions of childhood family environment: A reared apart twin study. *Child Development, 66*, 330–345.

Jaffee, S. R., Caspi, A., Moffitt, T., Polo-Thomas, M., Price, T. S., & Taylor, A. (2004). The limits of child effects: Evidence for genetically mediated child effects on corporal punishment but not on physical maltreatment. *Developmental Psychology, 40*, 1047–1058.

Jang, K. L., Dick, D. M., Wolf, H., Livesley, W. J., & Paris, J. (2005). Psychosocial adversity and emotional instability: An application of gene–environment interaction models. *European Journal of Personality, 19*, 359–372.

Jang, K. L., McCrae, R. R., Angleitner, A., Riemann, R., & Livesley, W. J. (1998). Heritability of facet-level traits in a cross-cultural twin sample: Support for a hierarchical model of personality. *Journal of Personality and Social Psychology, 74*, 1556–1565.

Johnson, W. (2007). Genetic and environmental influences on behavior: Capturing all the interplay. *Psychological Review, 114*, 423–440.

Johnson, W., & Krueger, R. F. (2004). Genetic and environmental structure of adjectives describing the domains of the Big Five model of personality: A nationwide U.S. twin study. *Journal of Research in Personality, 38*, 448–472.

Johnson, W., & Krueger, R. F. (2005). Higher perceived life control decreases genetic variance in physical health: Evidence from a national twin study. *Journal of Personality and Social Psychology, 88*, 165–173.

Johnson, W., & Krueger, R. F. (2006). How money buys happiness: Genetic and environmental processes linking finances and life satisfaction.

Journal of Personality and Social Psychology, 90, 680–691.

Johnson, W., McGue, M., & Krueger, R. F. (2005). Personality stability in late adulthood: A behavior genetic analysis. *Journal of Personality, 73*, 523–551.

Kaufman, J. C., Yang, B., Douglas-Palumberi, H., Houshyar, S., Lipschitz, D., Krystal, J. H., et al. (2004). Social supports and serontonin transporter gene moderate depression in maltreated children. *Proceedings of the National Academy of Sciences, USA, 101*, 17316–17321.

Kendler, K. S. (1996). Parenting: A genetic–epidemiologic perspective. *American Journal of Psychiatry, 153*, 11–20.

Kendler, K. S., Aggen, S. H., Jacobson, K. C., & Neale, M. C. (2003). Does the level of family dysfunction moderate the impact of genetic factors on the personality trait of neuroticism? *Psychological Medicine, 33*, 817–825.

Kendler, K. S., & Baker, J. H. (2007). Genetic influences on measures of the environment: A systematic review. *Psychological Medicine, 37*, 615–626.

Kendler, K. S., Kuhn, J. W., Vittum, J., Prescott, C. A., & Riley, B. (2005). Stressful life events, genetic liability and onset of an episode of major depression in women. *American Journal of Psychiatry, 159*, 1133–1145.

Kenrick, D. T., & Funder, D. C. (1988). Profiting from controversy: Lessons from the person–situation debate. *American Psychologist, 43*, 23–34.

Kim-Cohen, J., Caspi, A., Taylor, A., Williams, B., Newcombe, R., Craig, I. W., et al. (2006). MAOA, maltreatment, and gene–environment interaction predicting children's mental health: New evidence and a meta-analysis. *Molecular Psychiatry, 11*, 903–913.

Krueger, R. F. (2000). Phenotypic, genetic, and nonshared environmental parallels in the structure of personality: A view from the Multidimensional Personality Questionnaire. *Journal of Personality and Social Psychology, 79*, 1057–1067.

Krueger, R. F., Caspi, A., & Moffitt, T. (2000). Epidemiological personology: The unifying role of personality in population-based research on problem behaviors. *Journal of Personality, 68*(6), 967–997.

Krueger, R. F., Hicks, B. M., Patrick, C. J., Carlson, S. R., Iacono, W. G., & McGue, M. (2002). Etiologic connections among substance dependence, antisocial behavior, and personality: Modeling the externalizing spectrum. *Journal of Abnormal Psychology, 111*, 411–424.

Krueger, R. F., Johnson, W., & Kling, K. C. (2006). Behavior genetics and personality development. In D. K. Mroczek & T. D. Little (Eds.), *Hand-*

book of personality development (pp. 81–108). Mahwah, NJ: Erlbaum.

Krueger, R. F., & Markon, K. E. (2002). Behavior genetic perspectives on clinical personality assessment. In J. N. Butcher (Ed.), Clinical personality assessment: Practical approaches (2nd ed., pp. 40–55). New York: Oxford University Press.

Krueger, R. F., Markon, K. E., & Bouchard, T. J. (2003). The extended genotype: The heritability of personality accounts for the heritability of recalled family environments in twins reared apart. Journal of Personality, 71, 809–833.

Krueger, R. F., South, S., Johnson, W., & Iacono, W. (in press). Gene–environment interactions and correlations between personality and parenting: The heritability of personality is not always 50%. Journal of Personality.

Krueger, R. F., & Tackett, J. L. (2007). Behavior genetic designs. In R. W. Robins, R. C. Fraley, & R. F. Krueger (Eds.), Handbook of research methods in personality psychology (pp. 62–78). New York: Guilford Press.

Livesley, W. J., Jang, K. L., & Vernon, P. A. (1998). Phenotypic and genetic structure of traits delineating personality disorder. Archives of General Psychiatry, 55, 941–948.

Loehlin, J. C., Horn, J. M., & Willerman, L. (1981). Personality resemblance in adoptive families. Behavior Genetics, 11, 309–330.

Loehlin, J. C., Neiderhiser, J. M., & Reiss, D. (2003). The behavior genetics of personality and the NEAD study. Journal of Research in Personality, 37, 373–387.

Loehlin, J. C., Willerman, L., & Horn, J. M. (1982). Personality resemblances between unwed mothers and their adopted-away offspring. Journal of Personality and Social Psychology, 42, 1089–1099.

Losoya, S. H., Callor, S., Rowe, D. C., & Goldsmith, H. H. (1997). Origins of familial similarity in parenting: A study of twins and adoptive siblings. Developmental Psychology, 33, 1012–1023.

Lykken, D. T. (1999). Happiness. New York: Golden Books.

Lykken, D. T., Bouchard, T. J. Jr., McGue, M., & Tellegen, A. (1992). Emergenesis: Genetic traits that may not run in families. American Psychologist, 47, 1565–1577.

Markon, K. E., Krueger, R. F., & Watson, D. (2005). Delineating the structure of normal and abnormal personality: An integrative hierarchical approach. Journal of Personality and Social Psychology, 88, 139–157.

Matheny, A. P. (1989). Children's behavioral inhibition over age and across situations: Genetic similarity for a trait during change. Journal of Personality, 57, 215–235.

McCrae, R. R., Jang, K. L., Livesley, W. J., Riemann, R., & Angleitner, A. (2001). Sources of structure: Genetic, environmental, and artifactual influences on the covariation of personality traits. Journal of Personality, 69, 511–535.

McGue, M., & Iacono, W. G. (2001, July). Parent and sibling influences on adolescent alcohol use and misuse: Evidence from a U. S. adoption cohort. Paper presented at a meeting of the Behavior Genetics Association, Cambridge, UK.

Moffitt, T. E. (2005). The new look of behavioral genetics in developmental psychopathology: Gene–environment interplay in antisocial behaviors. Psychological Bulletin, 131, 533–554.

Munafo, M. R., Clark, T. G., Moore, L. R., Payne, E., Walton, R., & Flint, J. (2003). Genetic polymorphisms and personality in healthy adults: A systematic review and meta-analysis. Molecular Psychiatry, 8, 471–484.

O'Connor, T. G., Hetherington, E. M., Reiss, D., & Plomin, R. (1995). A twin-sibling study of observed parent–adolescent interactions. Child Development, 66, 812–829.

Pedersen, N. L., Plomin, R., McClearn, G. E., & Friberg, L. (1988). Neuroticism, extraversion, and related traits in adult twins reared apart and reared together. Journal of Personality and Social Psychology, 55, 950–957.

Pedersen, N. L., & Reynolds, C. A. (1998). Stability and change in adult personality: Genetic and environmental components. European Journal of Personality, 12, 365–386.

Perusse, D., Neale, M. C., Heath, A. C., & Eaves, L. J. (1994). Human parental behavior: Evidence for genetic influence and potential implication for gene–culture transmission. Behavior Genetics, 24, 327–335.

Plomin, R., Asbury, K., & Dunn, J. (2001). Why are children in the same family so different? Nonshared environment a decade later. Canadian Journal of Psychiatry, 46, 225–233.

Plomin, R., & Bergeman, C. S. (1991). The nature of nurture: Genetic influence on "environmental" measures. Behavioral and Brain Sciences, 14, 373–427.

Plomin, R., Coon, H., Carey, G., DeFries, J. C., & Fulker, D. W. (1991). Parent–offspring and sibling adoption analyses of parental ratings of temperament in infancy and childhood. Journal of Personality, 59, 705–732.

Plomin, R., Corley, R., Caspi, A., Fulker, D. W., & DeFries, J. (1998). Adoption results for self-reported personality: Evidence for nonadditive genetic effects? Journal of Personality and Social Psychology, 75, 211–218.

Plomin, R., & Daniels, D. (1987). Why are children in the same family so different from one another? Behavioral and Brain Sciences, 10, 1–60.

Plomin, R., Emde, R. N., Braungart, J. M., Campos, J., Corley, R., Fulker, D. W., et al. (1993). Genetic change and continuity from fourteen to twenty months: The MacArthur Longitudinal Twin Study. *Child Development, 64,* 1354–1376.

Plomin, R., McClearn, G. E., Pedersen, N. L., Nesselroade, J. R., & Bergeman, C. S. (1988). Genetic influence on childhood family environment perceived retrospectively from the last half of the life span. *Developmental Psychology, 24,* 738–745.

Purcell, S. (2002). Variance component models for gene–environment interaction in twin analysis. *Twin Research, 5*(6), 554–571.

Reiss, D., Neiderhiser, J. M., Hetherington, E. M., & Plomin, R. (2000). *The relationship code: Deciphering genetic and social influences on adolescent development.* Cambridge, MA: Harvard University Press.

Rende, R. D., Slomkowski, C. L., Stocker, C., Fulker, D. W., & Plomin, R. (1992). Genetic and environmental influences on maternal and sibling interaction in middle childhood: A sibling adoption study. *Developmental Psychology, 28,* 484–490.

Ridley, M. (2003). *Nature via nurture: Genes, experience, and what makes us human.* New York: HarperCollins.

Riemann, R., Angleitner, A., & Strelau, J. (1997). Genetic and environmental influences on personality: A study of twins reared together using the self- and peer-report NEO-FFI scales. *Journal of Personality, 65,* 449–475.

Roberts, B. W., Caspi, A., & Moffitt, T. (2003). Work experiences and personality development in young adulthood. *Journal of Personality and Social Psychology, 84,* 582–593.

Roberts, B. W., & Robins, R. W. (2004). Person–environment fit and its implications for personality development: A longitudinal study. *Journal of Personality, 72,* 89–110.

Robinson, J. L., Kagan, J., Reznick, J. S., & Corley, R. (1992). The heritability of inhibited and uninhibited behavior: A twin study. *Developmental Psychology, 28,* 1030–1037.

Rose, R. J., Dick, D. M., Viken, R. J., & Kaprio, J. (2001). Gene–interaction in patterns of adolescent drinking: Regional residency moderates longitudinal influences on alcohol use. *Alcoholism: Clinical and Experimental Research, 25,* 637–643.

Rowe, D. C. (1981). Environmental and genetic influences on dimensions of perceived parenting: A twin study. *Developmental Psychology, 17,* 203–208.

Rowe, D. C. (1983). A biometrical analysis of perceptions of family environment: A study of twin and singleton sibling kinships. *Child Development, 54,* 416–423.

Rowe, D. C. (1994). *The limits of family influ-*

ence: *Genes, experience, and behavior.* New York: Guilford Press.

Rutter, M., Moffitt, T., & Caspi, A. (2006). Gene–environment interplay and psychopathology: Multiple varieties but real effects. *Journal of Child Psychology and Psychiatry, 47,* 226–261.

Saudino, K. J., & Eaton, W. O. (1991). Infant temperament and genetics: An objective twin study of motor activity level. *Child Development, 62,* 1167–1174.

Saudino, K. J., Pedersen, N. L., Lichtenstein, P., McClearn, G. E., & Plomin, R. (1997). Can personality explain genetic influences on life events? *Journal of Personality and Social Psychology, 72,* 196–206.

Scarr, S., Webber, P. L., Weinberg, R. A., & Wittig, M. A. (1981). Personality resemblance among adolescents and their parents in biologically related and adoptive families. *Journal of Personality and Social Psychology, 40,* 885–898.

Schachter, F. F., Shore, E., Feldman-Rotman, S., Marquis, R. E., & Campbell, S. (1976). Sibling deidentification. *Developmental Psychology, 12,* 418–427.

Shakespeare, W. (1974). The Tempest. In G. B. Evans (Ed.), *The Riverside Shakespeare* (pp. 1606–1638). Boston: Houghton Mifflin. (Original work performed 1611)

South, S., Krueger, R. F., Johnson, W., & Iacono, W. G. (in press). Adolescent personality moderates the genetic and environmental influences on perceived relationships with parents. *Journal of Personality and Social Psychology.*

Stoolmiller, M. (1999). Implications of the restricted range of family environments for estimates of heritability and nonshared environment in behavior–genetic adoption studies. *Psychological Bulletin, 125,* 392–409.

Tellegen, A., Lykken, D. T., Bouchard, T. J., Wilcox, K., Segal, N., & Rich, A. (1988). Personality similarity in twins reared together and apart. *Journal of Personality and Social Psychology, 54,* 1031–1039.

Timberlake, D. S., Rhee, S. H., Haberstick, B. C., Hopfer, C., Ehringer, M., Lessem, J. M., et al. (2006). The moderating effects of religiosity on the genetic and environmental determinants of smoking initiation. *Nicotine and Tobacco Research, 8,* 123–133.

Turkheimer, E. (2000). Three laws of behavior genetics and what they mean. *Current Directions in Psychological Science, 9,* 160–164.

Turkheimer, E., & Waldron, M. (2000). Nonshared environment: A theoretical, methodological, and quantitative review. *Psychological Bulletin, 126*(1), 78–108.

Viken, R. J., Rose, R. J., & Koskenvuo, M. (1994). A developmental–genetic analysis of adult personality: Extraversion and neuroticism from 18 to 59. *Journal of Personality and Social Psychology, 67,* 722–730.

Wade, T. D., & Kendler, K. S. (2000). The genetic epidemiology of parental discipline. *Psychological Medicine, 30,* 1303–1313.

Watson, D., Clark, L. A., & Harkness, A. R. (1994). Structures of personality and their relevance to psychopathology. *Journal of Abnormal Psychology, 103,* 18–31.

Watson, J. B. (1924). *Behaviorism.* New York: Norton.

Weaver, I. C. G., Cervoni, N., Champagne, F. A., D'Alessio, A. C., Sharma, S., Seckl, J. R., et al. (2004). Epigenetic programming by maternal behavior. *Nature Neuroscience, 7,* 847–854.

Widiger, T. A., Simonsen, E., Krueger, R., Livesley, J. W., & Verheul, R. (2005). Personality disorder research agenda for the DSM-V. *Journal of Personality Disorders, 19,* 315–338.

Wihelm, K. A., Mitchell, P. B., Niven, H., Finch, A., Wedgewood, L., Scimone, A., et al. (2006). Life events, first depression onset, and the serotonin transporter gene. *British Journal of Psychiatry, 188,* 210–215.

Wong, A. H. C., Gottesman, I. I., & Petronis, A. (2005). Phenotypic differences in genetically identical organisms: The epigenetic perspective. *Human Molecular Genetics, 14,* R11–R18.

Yamagata, S., Suzuki, A., Ando, J., Ono, Y., Kijima, N., Yoshimura, K., et al. (2006). Is the genetic structure of human personality universal? A cross-cultural twin study from North America, Europe, and Asia. *Journal of Personality and Social Psychology, 90,* 987–998.

York, T. P., Miles, M. F., Kendler, K. S., Jackson-Cook, C., Bowman, M. L., & Eaves, L. (2005). Epistatic and environmental control of genomewide gene expression. *Twin Research, 8,* 5–15.

Zalsman, G., Huang, Y., Oquendo, M. A., Burke, A. K., Hu, X., Brent, D. A., et al. (2006). A triallelic serotonin transporter gene promoter polymorphism (5-HTTLPR), stressful life events, and severity of depression. *American Journal of Psychiatry, 163,* 1588–1593.

CHAPTER 11

Toward a "Molecular Psychology" of Personality

Turhan Canli

Biologically based theories of personality have always been shaped by the available technologies of neuroscience. In the modern history of the field, efforts to develop such theories began with the work of Eysenck, Gray, and their contemporaries (Eysenck, 1967; Fowles, 2006; Gray, 1970). Reflecting the cutting-edge tools of behavioral neuroscience available at the time, this work was largely based on animal studies and utilized electrical stimulation and lesion placements to identify neural circuits involved in individual differences in anxiety and arousal, and pharmacological manipulations to identify the neurochemistry underlying these circuits.

More recently, advances in noninvasive brain mapping have catalyzed new developments in the field, beginning with recordings of electroencephalograms (EEGs) from the scalp surface, and then advancing to brain imaging such as positron emission tomography (PET) and functional magnetic resonance imaging (fMRI). These methodologies have begun to be used to associate personality traits with individual differences in brain structure and function, conducted in healthy individuals (as opposed to brain-damaged patients).

Parallel to the developments in brain mapping, advances in molecular biology and genetics during the past decade have made it possible to identify common variations in genes that are related to personality traits. These genetic variations are now being mapped onto brain circuits by combining molecular genetics with noninvasive brain imaging in a field called "imaging genetics" (Hariri, Drabant, & Weinberger, 2006). The pace of discovery is breathtaking, and the most recent technological advances now make it possible to conduct whole-genome association studies that assess the potential functional contributions of many hundreds of thousands, and soon millions, of gene variations to behavior in a single experiment. For psychologists interested in the biological mechanisms of personality, this chapter serves as a snapshot of the field and its emerging molecular perspective, particularly with regard to the personality traits of extraversion and neuroticism.

THE EMERGENCE OF *MOLECULAR PSYCHOLOGY*

The field of quantitative behavioral genetics has provided a large body of evidence for the heritability of personality traits (Defries, McGuffin, McClearn, & Plomin, 2000; Dilalla & Gottesman, 2004; see also Krueger & Johnson, Chapter 10, this volume). Comparing mono- and dizygotic twins, adopted siblings, and other family members, investigators estimate that extraversion and neuroticism have a heritability of approximately 40–50%, leaving the remainder to environmental and unknown factors, of which the nonshared environment accounts for about 35% (Carey, 2003).

Molecular genetics has begun to identify common gene variations, called *polymorphisms* (found in more than 1% of the population). Some of these polymorphisms may be of interest to psychologists because they impart individual differences in the brain's structure or function and may thus contribute to individual differences in behavior. There are different kinds of polymorphisms. For example, SNPs (pronounced "snips") are single-nucleotide polymorphisms in which a single nucleotide base is substituted for another. (In DNA, there are four bases: adenine [A], cytosine [C], guanine [G], and thymine [T]; C and T, or A and G, may be substituted for one another.) VNTRs are "variable number of tandem repeats," in which certain sequences of nucleotides are repeated within a gene, but the number of repeats is variable across individuals. An insertion/deletion polymorphism is one in which a sequence of nucleotides is present in one variant, but absent in another.

Note that in the literature, the gene product is printed in regular font, whereas the gene that codes for it is printed in italic font. For example, the gene *5-HTT* contains the genetic code for creating the serotonin transporter 5-HTT. Another convention is that human genes are printed in capital letters, whereas nonhuman animal genes are printed using an initial capital followed by lowercase letters. Thus, *5-HTT* denotes the human serotonin transporter gene, whereas *5-Htt* denotes a nonhuman animal's serotonin transporter gene.

An alternative to studying individual candidate genes are genome-wide linkage and association studies. A linkage study is used to test the association (linkage) between genes. The underlying assumption is that genes (or other genetic markers, which can be any identifiable segment of the DNA) that are located close to one another are likely to be inherited together. By calculating the statistical odds of two genetic markers lying near each other, investigators can track the inheritance pattern of genes that have not

yet been identified but whose approximate location is known. In contrast, an association study seeks to relate genetic markers to phenotypes, including complex traits.

Genome-wide studies may be very well suited for complex traits, which are likely to be moderated by many genes of small effect size (known as quantitative trait loci, QTL), any single one of which may not be sufficient or necessary to reliably associate with the trait (Plomin, Owen, & McGuffin, 1994). Genome-wide scans have already been applied to complex traits such as intelligence (Craig & Plomin, 2006; Plomin et al., 2001), and several genome-wide linkage studies for neuroticism have been conducted (Fullerton et al., 2003; Kuo et al., 2007; Nash et al., 2004; Neale, Sullivan, & Kendler, 2005). These studies have identified QTLs on several chromosomes that await fine-mapping and further association study to identify specific genes that may be associated with neuroticism. Most recently, gene microarray technology has been developed that allows investigators to scan the entire genome for hundreds of thousands (soon a million) SNPs in a single experiment, to associate genetic variation with complex traits (Plomin & Schalkwyk, 2007). However, as of yet, this technology has not been applied to the study of traits such as extraversion or neuroticism.

Obviously, as is well known from quantitative behavioral genetics, complex traits are not all about genetics. The role of the environment, especially the nonshared unique environment and life experience of the individual, is almost equally important. Recent molecular studies of *epigenetic* processes have begun to shed light on the underlying mechanisms that may explain these gene-by-environment (G × E) interactions. Epigenetics is concerned with the regulation of genes (turning genes on or off, or altering the amount of protein they produce) and the transmission of genetic information that takes place without altering the nucleotide sequence of the genome itself. There are several mechanisms that accomplish this, one being DNA *methylation*. In DNA methylation, a methyl group is attached to the DNA without altering the nucleotide sequence. The effect of the presence of the methyl group is suppression (or silencing) of the gene's expression. The relevance of all this to psychologists is that *life experience can moderate DNA methylation* and therefore gene expression.

This effect was demonstrated in a study investigating epigenetic regulation of the stress response in rats (Weaver et al., 2004). Rat maternal behavior can moderate offsprings' later response to stress, with good rat maternal behavior (lots of licking and grooming of the pups) promoting greater stress resistance in the offspring. Weaver and colleagues asked whether the quality of maternal behavior would lead to differential methylation of the glucocorticoid receptor gene in the hippocampus of the offspring (both the glucocorticoid receptor and the hippocampus are involved in the stress response). Indeed, the pups that had experienced good maternal care showed less methylation than the pups that had experienced poor maternal care. Cross-fostering showed that the degree of methylation was determined by the foster mother's level of maternal care, not by the biological mother.

Taken together, there emerges a "molecular" perspective that looks at complex traits in terms of individual differences that represent the contributions, functions, and interactions between many genes of small effect across the entire genome. It is a perspective that looks at G × E interactions in terms of epigenetic mechanisms, by which environmental variables or an individual's life experience can moderate expression of these genes. The molecular perspective can be applied to any discipline within psychology. For example, studies of epigenetic programming of gene polymorphisms (discovered through whole-genome association scans) could be applied to questions that are of central interest to psychologists, such as the role of early childhood experiences, cognitive operations, emotional biases, social behavior, and vulnerability versus resilience for psychopathology.

For the remainder of this chapter, I limit the molecular perspective to complex personality traits, particularly extraversion and neuroticism. Given the infancy of this field, this review focuses on individual gene polymorphisms and studies of gene–environment interactions, as there is not (yet) data available that have identified other genes through whole-genome scanning.

The data reviewed below lead me to suggest this general framework: Extraversion and neuroticism are associated with individual differences in cognitive processes, particularly in the cognitive processing of valenced stimuli. These processes are mediated by a variety of brain circuits, including (but not limited to) limbic regions involved in emotion and prefrontal cortical regions involved in cognitive control and emotion regulation. Viewed from the bottom up, individual differences in extraversion and neuroticism can be regarded as arising from variation within an underlying neural circuitry, which itself reflects gene–environment interactions. Viewed from the top down, individuals exert control as active agents (Bandura, 1999) and thus contribute to the shaping of their own environment and experiences, which in turn can alter gene expression and modify neural circuitry. This molecular perspective can therefore accommodate a complex set of interactions between behavioral, neural, and genetic levels of analysis to attain a deeper understanding of the biological basis of personality.

TRAITS AND GENES

The field of molecular genetics of personality began in 1996 with the publication of three seminal papers reporting significant associations between specific gene polymorphisms and personality traits. Two of these publications focused on the association between the dopamine D4 receptor gene (*DRD4*) and extraversion (Benjamin et al., 1996) and the related trait of novelty seeking (Ebstein et al., 1996). The third publication focused on the association between the serotonin transporter gene (*5-HTT*) and neuroticism and harm avoidance (Lesch et al., 1996).

The *DRD4* is highly polymorphic, with variations located in regulatory, coding, and noncoding regions (Ebstein, 2006). One of these polymorphisms is a VNTR in exon III, which ranges from 2 to 10 repeats, with the 2-, 4-, and 7-repeat alleles being most common (Asghari et al., 1995). The 7-repeat allele of the dopamine D4 receptor gene is associated with less efficient function than the 2- or 4-repeat alleles, and the 10-repeat allele is more efficient than the 2-repeat allele (Asghari et al., 1995; Jovanovic, Guan, & Van Tol, 1999). The 7-repeat allele may result in a reduced, or suboptimal, response to dopamine (Swanson et al., 2000). The studies by Ebstein et al. and by Benjamin et al. found that presence of the 7-repeat allele is associated with higher extraversion and novelty seeking.

Another *DRD4* polymorphism is a SNP in the promoter region of the gene that features a C-to-T substitution (C-521T), resulting in a 40% reduction in the transcription of the gene's T allele compared to the C allele (Okuyama, Ishiguro, Toru, & Arinami, 1999; Ronai et al., 2001). The C allele of this SNP was reported to be associated with higher scores in novelty seeking (Okuyama et al., 2000) and extraversion (Bookman, Taylor, Adams-Campbell, & Kittles, 2002; Eichhammer et al., 2005).

Because both sets of findings inspired a number of replication studies, with inconsistent results, two meta-analyses assessed the publication record for these *DRD4* polymorphisms. One focused on associations with novelty seeking (Schinka, Letsch, & Crawford, 2002): It found no significant association with respect to presence of the 7-repeat allele of the VNTR exon III polymorphism (although a small positive effect was found when long repeats were contrasted against short repeats), but it did find a significant association with respect to the C-521T polymorphism. A second meta-analysis added publications that contained measures of extraversion as well as original data (Munafo, Yalcin, Willis-Owen, & Flint, 2008). These investigators found a significant association between approach-related traits (novelty seeking, impulsivity, and extraversion) and the C-521T polymorphism, but not the VNTR exon III polymorphism. Follow-up analysis showed that the association for the C-521T polymorphism was significant for novelty seeking and impulsivity, but not for extraversion. Furthermore, no association with extraversion was found when these investigators analyzed a new sample of 309 individuals who scored extremely high or low in extraversion (selected from a population-based sample of $N = 40,090$). Based on these analyses, Munafo and colleagues concluded that there was support for an association of the C-521T polymorphism and novelty seeking and impulsivity, which may account for about 3% of the observed variance, but no support for an association with extraversion.

Thus, despite being the first gene to be associated with extraversion, it now appears that there is no direct association between *DRD4* and this personality trait. A possible replacement candidate gene for extraversion could be the catechol-O-methyltransferase gene (*COMT*), which degrades dopamine (as well as epinephrine and norephinephrine). This gene contains a functional polymorphism (*COMT* Val[158]Met) that results in a G → A substitution, and a shift from production of the high-activity amino acid Valine (Val) to the low-activity amino acid Methionine (Met). Because the Met allele is associated with one-fourth the enzymatic activity of the Val allele in breaking down dopamine, this allele produces relatively higher levels of dopamine (Chen et al., 2004; Lotta et al., 1995; Mannisto & Kaakkola, 1999). It was recently reported that the *COMT* Val[158]Met polymorphism is associated with individual differences in extraversion in a healthy population sample of 363 individuals (Reuter & Hennig, 2005). Specifically, individuals homozygous for the Val allele had significantly higher extraversion scores than all other participants. No association with neuroticism was found in that study, although another study reported an association between harm avoidance and the Met allele (Enoch, Xu, Ferro, Harris, & Goldman, 2003). Still another study using extreme scorers, based on peer ratings, reported an overrepresentation of the Met allele in high-neuroticism females, but a complete absence of the Met allele in high-neuroticism males (Eley et al., 2003). Thus, whereas the Val allele is associated with extraversion, the Met allele may be associated with neuroticism or related traits, perhaps in interaction with an individual's sex.

The association with neuroticism is clearer for the serotonin transporter gene, which was first reported more than a decade ago by Lesch and colleagues (Lesch et al., 1996), and continues to be the most-studied gene associated with neuroticism (Reif & Lesch, 2003), although it may also play a larger role in social cognition (for detailed discussions, see Canli & Lesch, 2007). The serotonin transporter removes serotonin (also known as 5-hydroxytrypamine, or 5-HT) from the space between two nerve cells. A deletion/insertion polymorphism in the regulatory region of the serotonin transporter gene (*5-HTT*) produces a short and a long gene allele. The polymorphism is functional: The short allele produces about 65% less of the transporter than the long allele does. Of interest to personality psychologists, individuals who carry one or two copies of the *5-HTT* short allele (each individual carries two alleles, one from each parent) reported higher levels of neuroticism than individuals who carry only the long allele (Lesch et al., 1996). The polymorphism is quite common: For example, among European Americans, 32% only carry the long allele, 19% only carry the short allele, and 49% carry one of each allele type (Lesch et al., 1996). However, the observed association only accounted for 3–4% of the total observed variance, consistent with the view that complex traits such as neuroticism are likely regulated by many genes of small effect size.

Individual replication studies have produced mixed results and have been subjected to several meta-analyses. These meta-analyses have confirmed a small but significant role for *5-HTT* in neuroticism (Schinka, Busch, & Robichaux-Keene, 2004; Sen, Burmeister, & Ghosh, 2004), although the conclusions that can be drawn from these analyses are sensitive to methodological choices (Munafo, Clark, & Flint, 2005a, 2005b).

Although these association studies have identified some candidate gene polymorphisms associated with extraversion and neuroticism, it comes as somewhat of a surprise that after more than a decade of searching, so few candidates have been identified. This paucity suggests that the construct may be too broad to be useful, that the genetic effect sizes may be too small to replicate reliably, that the associations are more complex, perhaps involving additional moderating variables, or that these traits may be more strongly associated with variation within the epigenome than the genome itself.

ENDOPHENOTYPES OF EXTRAVERSION AND NEUROTICISM

The relatively subtle effects by which gene polymorphisms may moderate complex behaviors are, in part, due to the distance between the levels of analysis of the genotype, which operates at the molecular and cellular level, and the phenotype, which operates at the level of self-reported personality. A stronger association between genotype and phenotype should be expected if the level of analysis for the phenotype were moved closer to the level at which polymorphisms

regulate biological processes. Examples of such so-called *endo*-phenotypes are isolated cognitive processes or localized brain measures, and this approach is therefore known as the endophenotype approach (Congdon & Canli, 2005; de Geus, Wright, Martin, & Boomsma, 2001; Gottesman & Gould, 2003; Hasler, Drevets, Gould, Gottesman, & Manji, 2006).

Endophenotypes of complex traits such as extraversion and neuroticism can be conceptualized in terms of gene variations that are associated with individual differences in cognitive–affective processes and their associated neural substrates. Thus, extraversion and neuroticism can be deconstructed into constituent psychological processes, such as attention, perception, memory, or emotional arousal states (Canli, 2004). There are three advantages in using this approach when developing biological models of personality.

The first advantage is that cognitive psychology has already developed a number of task paradigms to quantify behavioral performance in cognitive–affective tasks. The second advantage is that cognitive neuroscience has made excellent progress mapping out the neural circuitry that mediates these processes, and a number of studies have begun to correlate patterns of brain activation with participants' extraversion and neuroticism scores. The third advantage is that measures of individual differences at the behavioral or neural level have already been shown to be more sensitive to genetic variation than measures based on self-reported traits (Hamer, 2002). Conceptualizing extraversion and neuroticism in terms of cognitive–affective processes makes it therefore possible to develop comprehensive theories of personality that integrate behavioral, neural, and genetic data. Next I illustrate this opportunity by focusing on one particular endophenotype: emotional attentional processing associated with extraversion and neuroticism.

ILLUSTRATIVE CASE: EMOTIONAL ATTENTION
Cognitive Endophenotype

Extraversion and neuroticism are associated with individual differences in attentional processing of emotional stimuli. For example, we conducted an attentional processing task, the dot-probe task, in which we related individual differences in extraversion to task performance (Amin, Constable, & Canli, 2004). In this reaction-time task, participants are instructed to respond to a dot-probe that is initially hidden behind one of two images but revealed when these images are simultaneously removed. If the participant's attention is drawn to the image that covers the probe, removal of that image should result in a faster identification of the probe stimulus than if the participant's attention is drawn to the other image. If the two images differ in emotional valence, this task can be used to reveal attentional biases toward, or away from, positive and negative stimuli. We presented image pairs, of which one was neutral and the other was emotionally positive or negative. We found that extraversion was correlated with significantly faster reaction times when the probe was placed behind the neutral than the negative image, suggesting that highly extraverted participants avoided attending to the negative item. In other studies, extraversion was associated with increased attention toward positive stimuli. For example, individuals who score high in extraversion show slower reaction times to shift attention away from locations associated with positive incentives (Derryberry & Reed, 1994).

Neuroticism is also associated with attentional bias, particularly in response to negative word and face stimuli, based on evidence from emotional Stroop and dot-probe tasks. In an emotional Stroop task, high-anxiety subjects showed an interference effect (as measured by slower reaction times) when processing anxiety-related words, compared to low-anxiety subjects (Richards, French, Johnson, Naparstek, & Williams, 1992). In another variant of the emotional Stroop task, called the word–face Stroop task (Haas, Omura, Constable, & Canli, 2006), we tested healthy normal volunteers and asked them to judge the valence of word stimuli (negative, positive, or neutral). Placed underneath these words were happy, sad, or neutral faces, generating word–face pairs that were either neutral (neutral word–neutral face), emotionally congruent (positive word–happy face or negative word–sad face), or emotionally incongruent (positive word–sad face or negative word–happy face). We found that neuroticism correlated with reaction time to incongruent but not

congruent pairs (Haas, Omura, Constable, & Canli, 2007). However, this behavioral outcome was limited to the anxious facet of neuroticism, suggesting attentional interference as a function of conflicting emotional signals that may be specific to some aspects of neuroticism, but not others.

Neural Endophenotype

Cognitive neuroscience has accomplished a fairly sophisticated understanding of the neural substrate mediating attentional processes. For example, Posner and colleagues conceptualize attentional processes in terms of alerting, orienting, and executive attention, each of which is associated with a distinct neural circuit (Fan, McCandliss, Fossella, Flombaum, & Posner, 2005; Posner & Rothbart, 2007). Of these three types of attentional processes and networks, executive attention is particularly relevant for the present discussion, because individual differences within its associated circuitry have been associated with extraversion and neuroticism, and with gene polymorphisms previously associated with these traits.

"Executive attention" refers to the ability to monitor and resolve conflicting information, instructions, emotions, or motor responses (Posner & Rothbart, 2007). Brain regions involved in executive attention involve the anterior cingulate cortex (ACC), lateral ventral and prefrontal cortex, and the basal ganglia. Of these, the ACC plays a significant role in a number of different cognitive processes, which can broadly be summarized as reflecting cognitive operations such as error detection, conflict monitoring, cognitive control, and decision making in the dorsal–caudal ACC (Botvinick, Braver, Barch, Carter, & Cohen, 2001; Botvinick, Cohen, & Carter, 2004; Rushworth, Behrens, Rudebeck, & Walton, 2007; Walton, Croxson, Behrens, Kennerley, & Rushworth, 2007) and emotional operations in the ventral and subgenual ACC (Drevets et al., 1997; Mayberg et al., 2005; Rauch et al., 1994). The lateral ventral and prefrontal cortical regions are actually activated across a diverse set of tasks involving perception, response selection, executive control, working memory, episodic memory, and problem solving (Duncan & Owen, 2000), and thus appear to play a broad role in so-called "executive function," with their specific roles still to be elucidated. The basal ganglia are primarily involved in motor control. In the context of probing this executive attentional network in the processing of *emotional* stimuli, one also needs to add the amygdala, an almond-shaped set of nuclei in the medial temporal cortex, to this circuit. The amygdala is a brain region that plays a central role in the processing of emotional stimuli (Aggleton, 2000).

As reviewed in the previous section, extraversion and neuroticism are associated with individual differences in attentional processes, including executive attention as measured with the emotional Stroop task. We have used two variants of the emotional Stroop to investigate the neural basis of executive attentional processes related to extraversion and neuroticism. One is the emotional word Stroop task. In our version of this task, the word stimuli were presented in green, blue, or yellow colors, and participants were asked to press a button corresponding to the color in which each word was printed. Prior work using the emotional Stroop task had identified the ACC as a region that is sensitive to the emotional meaning of the word (Whalen et al., 1998). There was also some evidence that the amygdala and the inferior parietal cortex were engaged during this task (Compton et al., 2003; Isenberg et al., 1999). Based on the first study to associate brain response to emotional stimuli with extraversion or neuroticism (Canli et al., 2001), we expected to find that ACC response to positive stimuli would vary as a function of extraversion. In that earlier study, there was no significant association between ACC activation to negative stimuli and neuroticism, but that null result may have reflected a ceiling effect, because all participants had experienced the emotional images as highly negative. Therefore, we remained open to the possibility that ACC activation to negative stimuli might vary as a function of neuroticism. Our prior work had also not accounted for the possibility that the activation differences ascribed to these personality traits might be moderated by mood state. We therefore sought to dissociate the contributions of extraversion and positive mood to ACC activation to positive stimuli, and dissociate the contributions of neuroticism and negative mood to ACC activation to negative stimuli.

Participants completed mood state and personality trait questionnaires and were scanned while they viewed negative, positive, and neutral words using the emotional Stroop task. Using a partial regression analysis approach, we found that ACC activation to positive, relative to neutral, words varied as a function of extraversion (controlling for positive mood), but not as a function of positive mood (controlling for extraversion). Thus, ACC activation to positive stimuli reflected stable interindividual differences. Surprisingly, the opposite pattern emerged for negative stimuli: ACC activation to negative, relative to neutral, words did *not* vary as a function of neuroticism (controlling for negative vote), but *did* vary as a function of negative mood (controlling for neuroticism). Thus, AC activation to negative stimuli may have reflected dynamic intraindividual differences that may vary, depending on the individual's mood state.

We also used the word–face Stroop task described in the previous section (Haas et al., 2006). As noted above, we found behavioral evidence for interference produced by incongruent emotional information, because participants had much slower reaction times in response to emotionally incongruent than emotionally congruent word–face pairs. This interference effect was associated with activation of the ACC. Specifically, we observed greater activation in the caudal region of the ACC during trials of high, relative to low, emotional conflict. This observation is consistent with a model that proposes that the caudal ACC plays a significant role in conflict monitoring (Botvinick et al., 2001, 2004).

In a subsequent set of analyses (Haas et al., 2007), we correlated ACC activation during the word–face Stroop task with participants' neuroticism scores. Neuroticism is a risk factor for mood and anxiety disorders (Bienvenu & Stein, 2003), which have been associated with dysfunction in the amygdala and the subgenual region of the ACC (Drevets, 2000; Drevets et al., 1997; Gotlib et al., 2005; Rauch et al., 1994; Rauch, Shin, & Wright, 2003). We found that neuroticism correlated with activation in both amygdala and subgenual ACC during trials of high, relative to low, emotional conflict (Figure 11.1). We verified the discriminant validity of this observation by confirming that this association was specific to self-reported neu-

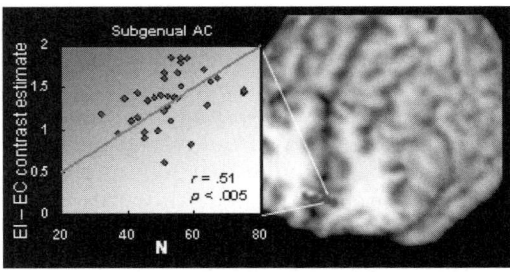

FIGURE 11.1. Changes in subgenual anterior cingulate (AC) activation associated with neuroticism in response to emotional conflict. The cluster of activation lies within the subgenual ACC. Data are plotted for this cluster of activation with the *x*-axis representing individuals' neuroticism scores and the *y*-axis representing the signal change difference between emotionally incongruent (EI) and emotionally congruent (EC) trials. From Haas, Omura, Constable, and Canli (2007). Copyright 2007 by the Psychonomic Society. Reprinted by permission.

roticism and not negative mood state, reaction time, or error rates. For the ACC, we confirmed that this association was specific to the subgenual region, because no other regions within the ACC showed a significant correlation with neuroticism.

Imaging Genetics

As reviewed above, cognitive and neuroimaging studies revealed that extraversion and neuroticism are associated with individual differences in attentional processes. Given prior reports of an association between polymorphisms of *COMT* with extraversion (as reviewed above, initial associations of *DRD4* and extraversion did not hold up to meta-analytic review), and of *5-HTT* with neuroticism, we may therefore hypothesize that individual differences associated with these personality traits in the neural circuitry of attention may reflect the moderating influence of *COMT* and *5-HTT*. Recent work in the emerging field of "imaging genetics" (Hariri et al., 2006) has begun to assess such hypotheses, and to identify other gene polymorphisms that may play a role in the neural circuitry of attentional processes.

There is considerable evidence that the *COMT* Val[158]Met polymorphism is associated with individual differences in a range of cognitive functions, including attentional processes (for reviews, see Goldberg & Weinberger, 2004; Heinz & Smolka, 2006; Weinberger et al., 2001; Winterer & Goldman, 2003). For example, participants in a fMRI study engaged in an attentional task involving perceptual conflict (Blasi et al., 2005). Task performance correlated with the number of low-activity Met alleles. There was also a significant correlation between the degree of ACC activation (as reviewed above, the ACC is a key region in attention and conflict monitoring) and *COMT* genotype: ACC activity was inversely correlated with the number of Met alleles. In light of better task performance associated with the Met allele, this reduction in ACC activation was interpreted to represent a more efficient neural system that can accomplish the same task with less oxygen consumption.

In addition to nonemotional cognitive processes, the *COMT* Val[158]Met polymorphism is also associated with individual differences in neural response to affective stimuli (Smolka et al., 2005). In an fMRI study in which participants viewed neutral and negatively and positively valenced images, it was reported that response to negative (but not positive) images, relative to neutral images, correlated positively with the number of Met[158] alleles in limbic brain regions (hippocampus, amygdala, and thalamus), as well as prefrontal regions (ventrolateral prefrontal cortex and dorsolateral prefrontal cortex), and regions associated with visuospatial attention (fusiform gyrus and inferior parietal lobule). In support of the endophenotype approach, it was reported that participants' genotype explained up to 38% of interindividual variance in brain activation to negative images, which is about an order of magnitude bigger than would be seen in studies using self-report measures.

Summarizing the data for the *COMT* Val[158]Met polymorphism, there is some evidence for an association with extraversion (associated with Val), and possibly neuroticism (associated with Met). Although extraversion is associated with attentional emotional processing of positive stimuli, which can be mapped onto ACC function, the imaging genetics evidence has not yet shown that this activation is associated with the Val[158] allele. Instead, it points to a role of the Met[158] allele in response to negative stimuli and a role in ACC activation in attention to conflict. Thus, although there may be some imaging genetics evidence for an attentional mechanism associated with neuroticism or related traits, a direct link between self-reported extraversion, biased attentional processing of positive stimuli, and ACC activation as a function of the *COMT* Val[158] allele has not yet been established. Given the small number of studies, it is clear that much more work is needed to determine whether the *COMT* genotype can account for cognitive processing biases of positive emotional stimuli associated with extraversion.

The previous discussion of *COMT*'s role in extraversion notwithstanding, the bulk of the imaging genetics literature has focused on the *5-HTT* genotype, neuroticism, and the brain's response to negative emotional stimuli. Hariri and colleagues (Hariri et al., 2002) were the first to use this endophenotype approach in a seminal study showing that presence of the *5-HTT* short allele was associated with increased activation in the amygdala in response to emotional faces, relative to a visuospatial control task. Highlighting the power of the endophenotype approach, the difference was statistically significant with a relatively small sample of 28 subjects, compared to the 500+ subjects included in the original study by Lesch and colleagues (Lesch et al., 1996). Indeed, the observed effect size in the study by Hariri et al. was six times greater, reflecting the power of the endophenotype approach to reveal genotype–phenotype associations.

We have used the emotional Stroop task to show an association between the *5-HTT* genotype and emotional attentional processes (Canli et al., 2005). We found a similar association between greater amygdalar activation to negative, relative to neutral, stimuli that was associated with presence of the *5-HTT* short allele. However, we provided additional evidence (Canli et al., 2005, 2006) to suggest that the mechanism by which the short allele operates on the amygdala may involve a steady-state level of high *tonic* activation, rather than a momentary increase in *phasic* activation. The difference between these two conceptualizations (illustrated in Figure 11.2) of *5-HTT* function is significant for two reasons. The first is that it would provide a genetic mechanism for a theory

about the so-called "default mode" of the brain (Raichle et al., 2001; Shulman et al., 1997), which may be elevated activation in the absence of cognitive constraints. The second is that there are significant long-term differences in the brain's response to tonic versus phasic stress (McEwen, 2007). Although our observations were replicated by two different groups (Heinz et al., 2007; Rao et al., 2007), the interpretation of these observations continues to be a matter of debate (Canli & Lesch, 2007).

Given the role of the ACC in attentional processes discussed above, it is interesting that the presence of the *5-HTT* short allele is associated with decreased connectivity between the amygdala and ACC (Pezawas et al., 2005). In light of evidence from animal work showing that the ACC can inhibit amygdalar function (Maren & Quirk, 2004; Rosenkranz, Moore, & Grace, 2003), Pezawas and colleagues proposed that vulnerability to mood disorders, which are associated with neuroticism and the *5-HTT* short allele, reflects an underlying dysfunctional emotion regulation circuit. To this, I would add that reduced connectivity between the ACC and amygdala during processing of negative emotional stimuli may be one underlying mechanism that may contribute to the behavioral phenotype of neuroticism.

Summarizing the data for the *5-HTT* genotype, there is evidence for an association with neuroticism, which is associated with attentional emotional processing (perhaps mediated by negative mood state in some brain regions) of negative stimuli, which can be mapped onto ACC and amygdalar function. Imaging genetics has shown that the presence of the *5-HTT* short allele is associated with greater activation in the amygdala in response to negative, relative to neutral, stimuli. However, the interpretation of this data is currently subject to debate. Analysis of the functional connectivity between the ACC and the amygdala suggests that the presence of the short allele may be associated with reduced connectivity within an emotion regulatory network that could reflect an underlying mechanism contributing to a neurotic phenotype.

In addition to *COMT* and *5-HTT*, a number of other gene polymorphisms have been identified that are associated with individual differences in cognitive or affective

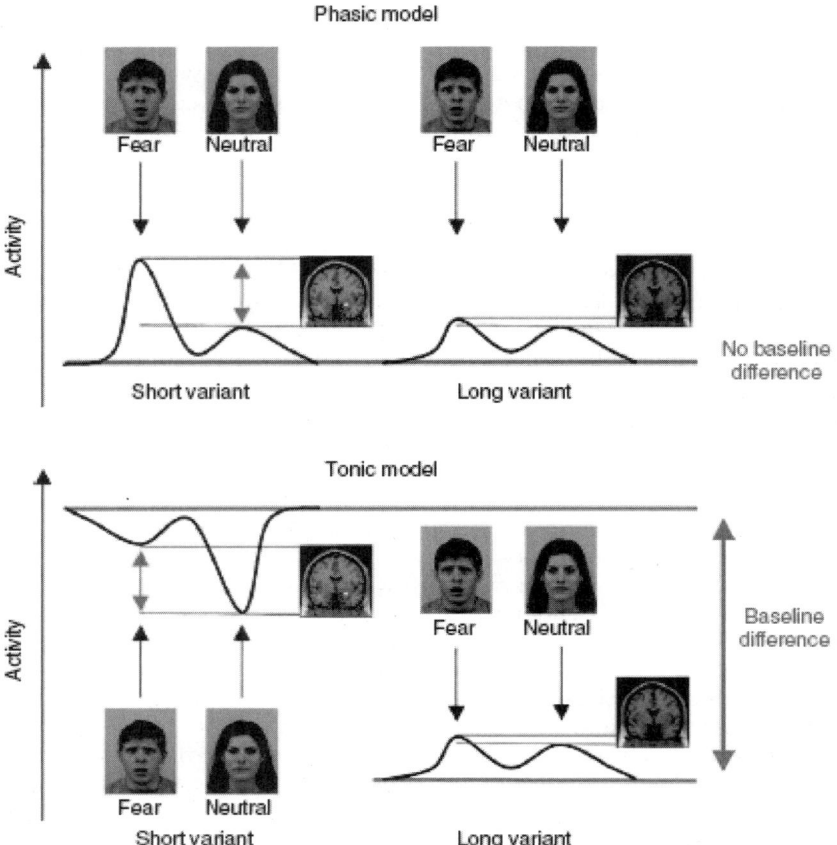

FIGURE 11.2. The standard "phasic" versus "tonic" model of *5-HTT*-dependent modulation of brain activity. The phasic model explains greater negative emotionality in carriers of the *5-HTT* short allele, compared with noncarriers, in terms of greater amygdala reactivity to negative stimuli. The tonic model explains greater negative emotionality in carriers of the *5-HTT* short allele, compared with noncarriers, in terms of greater baseline activation of the amygdala. From Canli and Lesch (2007). Copyright 2007 by Nature Publishing Group. Reprinted by permission.

processes (Ebstein, Zohar, Benjamin, & Belmaker, 2002; Goldberg & Weinberger, 2004; Hashimoto, 2007; Noblett & Coccaro, 2005; Reif & Lesch, 2003). For example, a polymorphism in the dopamine receptor 2 gene (*DRD2*) has been reported to interact with *COMT* in a Stroop task (Reuter et al., 2005). Variations within *DRD4* and the gene for monoamine oxidase A (*MAOA*, which breaks down monoaminergic neurotransmitters such as dopamine, serotonin, epinephrine, and norepinephrine), moderated executive attention in the attention network task (ANT) (Fan, McCandliss, Sommer, Raz, &

Posner, 2002). However, these studies used nonemotional stimuli, so it remains to be seen whether these polymorphisms are associated with differential attention to valenced stimuli in limbic and emotion regulatory regions. Many other studies implicating gene polymorphisms in affective processes have focused on patient populations and/or have not used cognitive–affective task paradigms optimized for studying emotional attentional processes. Thus, many of these candidate gene polymorphisms remain to be investigated as potential moderators of biased attentional processing of emotional stimuli.

INTERACTIONS WITH LIFE STRESS

Clinical Evidence

As stated earlier, the nonshared environment also plays a significant role in personality. One measure of such a nonshared environmental variable is an individual's unique life stress history. The interaction of genotype and life stress for genes relevant to extraversion or neuroticism is best illustrated by the *5-HTT* genotype, which was found to moderate the impact of life stress on depression. This effect was first demonstrated in a remarkable 23-year longitudinal study of over 1,000 participants, which documented individuals' stressful life experiences and the impact of these experiences on later depression as a function of the *5-HTT* genotype (Caspi et al., 2003). Caspi and colleagues (2003) reported that individuals who carried the *5-HTT* short allele showed twice as many instances of depressive symptoms, diagnosed depression, and suicidality as a function of stressful life events than did noncarriers.

Several replication studies have added further, albeit partial, support for the assertion that the *5-HTT* genotype moderates the impact of life stress on later depression or other mood disorders. Kendler and colleagues reported a significant difference between homozygous carriers of the *5-HTT* short allele and carriers of the long allele for the impact of life stress on later depression (Kendler, Kuhn, Vittum, Prescott, & Riley, 2005). However, two other studies reported significant interactions between the *5-HTT* genotype and life stress only in female participants (Eley et al., 2004; Grabe et al., 2005), and another two studies failed to replicate any G × E interaction for the *5-HTT* polymorphism (Gillespie, Whitfield, Williams, Heath, & Martin, 2005; Surtees et al., 2005). Because the nonreplication studies used an older sample than the other studies, some authors (Gillespie et al., 2005) suggested that age might be an important additional moderator of vulnerability to depression. Indeed, the impact of *5-HTT* genotype may be blunted by additional environmental factors. For example, depression scores of maltreated children who were homozygous carriers of the *5-HTT* short allele and who lacked social support had depression-related scores that were twice as high as those of other children

(Kaufman et al., 2004). On the other hand, depression scores were only minimally elevated for maltreated children who were homozygous carriers of the *5-HTT* short allele, but who did receive positive social support (Kaufman et al., 2004). Thus, several factors (*5-HTT* genotype, age, social support) may act in concert to moderate the effects of life stress on vulnerability toward later psychopathology.

Imaging Genetics

Following the endophenotype approach discussed above, we investigated neural correlates of these G × E interactions in a sample of healthy individuals (Canli et al., 2006). We were particularly interested in brain regions that responded to emotional stimuli as a function of the interaction between the *5-HTT* genotype and life stress. Two key regions of interest were the amygdala and hippocampus, which are moderated by the *5-HTT* genotype (see above) and by life stress (McEwen & Sapolsky, 1995), respectively.

Participants completed a self-report questionnaire, which we developed from items in the life-history calendar (Caspi, 1996). The questionnaire contained 28 items related to work, financial and legal problems, death and serious illness, family and relationships, and other stressful life events. We were interested in whether activation in the amygdala and hippocampus would correlate with life stress, and whether the correlation would be differentially expressed as a function of the *5-HTT* genotype (i.e., a G × E interaction). We demonstrated such an interaction both with fMRI, using a face-processing task in a sample of 48 participants, and with perfusion imaging in a sample of 21 participants. The perfusion data, in particular, showed that "resting" activation (i.e., activation when the participant is "at rest" and not engaged in any particular cognitive task—this does not mean that the participant's brain is not active) of the amygdala and hippocampus varied as a function of both the *5-HTT* genotype and life stress history. For carriers of the short allele, more life stress was associated with higher resting activation. For noncarriers of the short allele (i.e., those individuals who were homozygous for the long allele), more life stress was associated with *lower* resting activation. Given that amygdalar activation is associated with a state of vigilance (Davis & Whalen, 2001) and hippocampal activation with a stress response (McEwen, 2007), these findings suggest that the *5-HTT* genotype has a profound impact on how individuals respond to and process stressful life experiences.

To address this possibility more directly, we assessed the interaction between the *5-HTT* genotype and life stress on self-reported rumination, which is associated with neuroticism (Roberts, Gilboa, & Gotlib, 1998). Indeed, activation in the amygdala has been linked to rumination (Ray et al., 2005), although there are likely many brain regions that contribute to this behavior. As shown in Figure 11.3, there was a striking difference in the way that life stress affected self-reported rumination of carriers versus noncarriers of the *5-HTT* short allele. For homozygous long-allele carriers, more life stress is associated with *lower* levels of rumination, perhaps affirming the adage that "what doesn't kill you makes you stronger." For carriers of the *5-HTT* short allele, more life stress is associated with *higher* levels of rumination, perhaps because these individuals become sensitized to the effects of life stress.

The G × E data reviewed here suggest a neurogenetic mechanism by which neuroticism may be associated with increased rumination: Presence of the *5-HTT* short allele is associated with increased activation in

limbic brain regions and reduced connectivity to regulatory regions such as the ACC. Life stress further increases tonic limbic activation in the amygdala and hippocampus in carriers of the *5-HTT* short allele, which may contribute to increased rumination. The exact mechanisms by which this occurs are currently unknown. A top-down hypothesis is that the functional connectivity between cortical emotion regulatory regions and the amygdala is further reduced by accumulation of life stress experiences in *5-HTT* short-allele carriers, and that either emotion regulation itself or the relay of emotion regulatory signals to the limbic system becomes degraded. A bottom-up hypothesis is that molecular mechanisms affecting neural processing in the amygdala or hippocampus diminish local processing capacity, leading to a "burnt out" limbic system. These and other hypotheses remain to be evaluated in future work (Canli & Lesch, 2007).

CONCLUDING THOUGHTS ON INTEGRATING BIOLOGY AND PSYCHOLOGY

In this chapter, I presented a "molecular" perspective on personality traits that conceptualizes personality traits such as extraversion and neuroticism in terms of individual differences in cognitive processes of valenced stimuli. Viewed from the bottom up, these individual differences are believed to arise from G × E interactions between specific gene polymorphisms and unique life experiences (through epigenetic processes) that moderate neural circuits. Although the chapter focused on individual candidate genes, the technology exists, and work is underway, to conduct whole-genome association studies that can investigate many hundreds of thousands, and soon millions, of SNPs in a single experiment. These studies reflect the widely held belief that personality traits reflect the contributions of many genes of small effect size. In that sense, I refer to the *emergence* of molecular psychology, as opposed to its *arrival*. The biggest challenge in translating the molecular approach into real scientific progress will be the analysis of vast and complex datasets, the minimization of false-positive results, and the integration of convergent lines of evidence. A path-breaking study of this kind reported the discovery of a novel

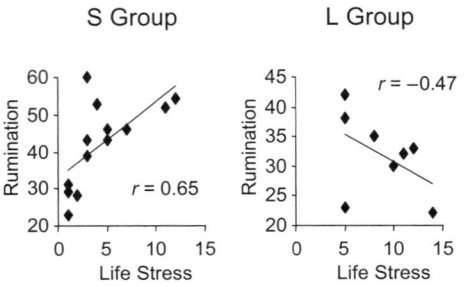

FIGURE 11.3. Self-reported rumination as a function of a G × E interaction of *5-HTT* genotype and life stress. S Group, carriers; L Group, noncarriers. From Canli et al. (2006). Copyright 2006 by the National Academy of Sciences. Reprinted by permission.

gene related to memory (Papassotiropoulos et al., 2006). It required multiple independent samples of several hundred subjects each, was conducted across multiple laboratories on two continents, contained two replication studies, and involved convergent evidence from whole-genome association studies, animal work, and fMRI. If this effort becomes the gold standard for biological studies of personality, then our field will enter the club of "Big Science" endeavors, changing the culture of personality psychology.

But in the excitement to use cutting-edge molecular biology and neuroimaging techniques to better understand the biological basis of personality, it is critical not to forget the top-down perspective of psychology. For example, none of what I described in this chapter explains why an individual may act aggressively in one domain of life but not another, although psychological theories of such situational contingencies have been developed (Mischel, 1999; Mischel & Shoda, 1998). Similarly, the work described in this chapter has treated the individual as a passive recipient of environmental and genetic input. Although one cannot change one's genetics (yet—it is possible that gene therapies will eventually allow individuals to do so), one can certainly change one's environment. This agentic view of personality (Bandura, 1999) has not yet been integrated into biological studies. There is a great need for psychologists, neuroscientists, and molecular biologists to collaborate. Without integrating the richness of psychological thought into these collaborations, they are doomed to fall short of their potential.

ACKNOWLEDGMENT

The work from our laboratory discussed in this review was supported by the National Science Foundation (Grant No. BCS-0224221).

REFERENCES

Aggleton, J. P. (Ed.). (2000). *The amygdala: A functional analysis* (2nd ed.). Oxford, UK: Oxford University Press.

Amin, Z., Constable, R. T., & Canli, T. (2004). Attentional bias for valenced stimuli as a function of personality in the dot-probe task. *Journal of Research in Personality, 38,* 15–23.

Asghari, V., Sanyal, S., Buchwaldt, S., Paterson, A., Jovanovic, V., & Van Tol, H. H. (1995). Modulation of intracellular cyclic AMP levels by different human dopamine D4 receptor variants. *Journal of Neurochemistry, 65*(3), 1157–1165.

Bandura, A. (1999). Social cognitive theory of personality. In L. A. Pervin & O. P. John (Eds.), *Handbook of personality: Theory and research* (2nd ed., pp. p. 154–196). New York: Guilford Press.

Benjamin, J., Li, L., Patterson, C., Greenberg, B. D., Murphy, D. L., & Hamer, D. H. (1996). Population and familial association between the D4 dopamine receptor gene and measures of novelty seeking. *Nature Genetics, 12,* 81–84.

Bienvenu, O. J., & Stein, M. B. (2003). Personality and anxiety disorders: A review. *Journal of Personality Disorders, 17*(2), 139–151.

Blasi, G., Mattay, V. S., Bertolino, A., Elvevag, B., Callicott, J. H., Das, S., et al. (2005). Effect of catechol-O-methyltransferase val158met genotype on attentional control. *Journal of Neuroscience, 25,* 5038–5045.

Bookman, E. B., Taylor, R. E., Adams-Campbell, L., & Kittles, R. A. (2002). DRD4 promoter SNPs and gender effects on extraversion in African Americans. *Molecular Psychiatry, 7*(7), 786–789.

Botvinick, M. M., Braver, T. S., Barch, D. M., Carter, C. S., & Cohen, J. D. (2001). Conflict monitoring and cognitive control. *Psychological Review, 108*(3), 624–652.

Botvinick, M. M., Cohen, J. D., & Carter, C. S. (2004). Conflict monitoring and anterior cingulate cortex: An update. *Trends in Cognitive Sciences, 8,* 539–546.

Canli, T. (2004). Functional brain mapping of extraversion and neuroticism: learning from individual differences in emotion processing. *Journal of Personality, 72*(6), 1105–1132.

Canli, T., & Lesch, K. P. (2007). Long story short: The serotonin transporter in emotion regulation and social cognition. *Nature Neuroscience, 10*(9), 1103–1109.

Canli, T., Omura, K., Haas, B. W., Fallgatter, A. J., Constable, R. T., & Lesch, K. P. (2005). Beyond affect: A role for genetic variation of the serotonin transporter in neural activation during a cognitive attention task. *Proceedings of the National Academy of Sciences, USA, 102*(34), 12224–12229.

Canli, T., Qiu, M., Omura, K., Congdon, E., Haas, B. W., Amin, Z., et al. (2006). Neural correlates of epigenesis. *Proceedings of the National Academy of Sciences, USA, 103,* 16033–16038.

Canli, T., Zhao, Z., Desmond, J. E., Kang, E., Gross, J., & Gabrieli, J. D. E. (2001). An fMRI study of personality influences on brain reactivity to emotional stimuli. *Behavioral Neuroscience, 115*(1), 33–42.

Carey, G. (2003). *Human genetics for the social sciences* (Vol. 4). Thousand Oaks, CA: Sage.

Caspi, A. (1996). A life-history calendar. *International Journal of Methods in Psychiatry Research, 6,* 101.

Caspi, A., Sugden, K., Moffitt, T. E., Taylor, A., Craig, I. W., Harrington, H., et al. (2003). Influence of life stress on Depression: Moderation by a polymorphism in the 5-HTT Gene. *Science, 301,* 386–389.

Chen, J., Lipska, B. K., Halim, N., Ma, Q. D., Matsumoto, M., Melhem, S., et al. (2004). Functional analysis of genetic variation in catechol-O-methyltransferase (COMT): Effects on mRNA, protein, and enzyme activity in postmortem human brain. *American Journal of Human Genetics, 75*(5), 807–821.

Compton, R. J., Banich, M. T., Mohanty, A., Milham, M. P., Herrington, J., Miller, G. A., et al. (2003). Paying attention to emotion: An fMRI investigation of cognitive and emotional stroop tasks. *Cognitive, Affective, and Behavioral Neuroscience, 3*(2), 81–96.

Congdon, E., & Canli, T. (2005). The endophenotype of impulsivity: Reaching consilience through behavioral, genetic, and neuroimaging approaches. *Behavioral and Cognitive Neuroscience Reviews, 4*(4), 262–281.

Craig, I., & Plomin, R. (2006). Quantitative trait loci for IQ and other complex traits: Single-nucleotide polymorphism genotyping using pooled DNA and microarrays. *Genes, Brain, and Behavior, 5*(Suppl. 1), 32–37.

Davis, M., & Whalen, P. J. (2001). The amygdala: Vigilance and emotion. *Molecular Psychiatry, 6*(1), 13–34.

de Geus, E. J., Wright, M. J., Martin, N. G., & Boomsma, D. I. (2001). Genetics of brain function and cognition. *Behavior Genetics, 31*(6), 489–495.

Defries, J. C., McGuffin, P., McClearn, G. E., & Plomin, R. (Eds.). (2000). *Behavioral genetics* (4th ed.). New York: Worth.

Derryberry, D., & Reed, M. A. (1994). Temperament and attention: Orienting towards and away from positive and negative signals. *Journal of Personality and Social Psychology, 66,* 1128–1139.

Dilalla, L. F., & Gottesman, I. I. (Eds.). (2004). *Behavior genetics principles: Perspectives in development, personality, and psychopathology.* Washington, DC: American Psychological Association.

Drevets, W. C. (2000). Neuroimaging studies of mood disorders. *Biological Psychiatry, 48*(8), 813–829.

Drevets, W. C., Price, J. L., Simpson, J. R., Jr., Todd, R. D., Reich, T., Vannier, M., et al. (1997). Subgenual prefrontal cortex abnormalities in mood disorders. *Nature, 386,* 824–827.

Duncan, J., & Owen, A. M. (2000). Common regions of the human frontal lobe recruited by diverse cognitive demands. *Trends in Neuroscience, 23,* 475–483.

Ebstein, R. P. (2006). The molecular genetic architecture of human personality: Beyond self-report questionnaires. *Molecular Psychiatry, 11*(5), 427–445.

Ebstein, R. P., Novick, O., Umansky, R., Priel, B., Osher, Y., Blaine, D., et al. (1996). Dopamine D4 receptor (D4DR) exon III polymorphism associated with the human personality trait of novelty seeking. *Nature Genetics, 12,* 78–80.

Ebstein, R. P., Zohar, A. H., Benjamin, J., & Belmaker, R. H. (2002). An update on molecular genetic studies of human personality traits. *Applied Bioinformatics, 1*(2), 57–68.

Eichhammer, P., Sand, P. G., Stoertebecker, P., Langguth, B., Zowe, M., & Hajak, G. (2005). Variation at the DRD4 promoter modulates extraversion in Caucasians. *Molecular Psychiatry, 10*(6), 520–522.

Eley, T. C., Sugden, K., Corsico, A., Gregory, A. M., Sham, P., McGuffin, P., et al. (2004). Gene–environment interaction analysis of serotonin system markers with adolescent depression. *Molecular Psychiatry, 9,* 908–915.

Eley, T. C., Tahir, E., Angleitner, A., Harriss, K., McClay, J., Plomin, R., et al. (2003). Association analysis of MAOA and COMT with neuroticism assessed by peers. *American Journal of Medical Genetics, 120B*(1), 90–96.

Enoch, M. A., Xu, K., Ferro, E., Harris, C. R., & Goldman, D. (2003). Genetic origins of anxiety in women: A role for a functional catechol-O-methyltransferase polymorphism. *Psychiatric Genetics, 13*(1), 33–41.

Eysenck, H. J. (1967). *The biological basis of personality.* Springfield, IL: Thomas.

Fan, J., McCandliss, B. D., Fossella, J., Flombaum, J. I., & Posner, M. I. (2005). The activation of attentional networks. *NeuroImage, 26,* 471.

Fan, J., McCandliss, B. D., Sommer, T., Raz, A., & Posner, M. I. (2002). Testing the efficiency and independence of attentional networks. *Journal of Cognitive Neuroscience, 14*(3), 340–347.

Fowles, D. C. (2006). Jeffrey Gray's contributions to theories of anxiety, personality, and psychopathology. In T. Canli (Ed.), *Biology of personality and individual differences* (pp. 7–36). New York: Guilford Press.

Fullerton, J., Cubin, M., Tiwari, H., Wang, C., Bomhra, A., Davidson, S., et al. (2003). Linkage analysis of extremely discordant and concordant sibling pairs identifies quantitative-trait loci that influence variation in the human personality trait neuroticism. *American Journal of Human Genetics, 72*(4), 879–890.

Gillespie, N. A., Whitfield, J. B., Williams, B., Heath, A. C., & Martin, N. G. (2005). The relationship between stressful life events, the serotonin transporter (5-HTTLPR) genotype and major depression. *Psychological Medicine*, *35*(1), 101–111.

Goldberg, T. E., & Weinberger, D. R. (2004). Genes and the parsing of cognitive processes. *Trends in Cognitive Science*, *8*(7), 325–335.

Gotlib, I. H., Sivers, H., Gabrieli, J. D. E., Whitfield-Gabrieli, S., Goldin, P., Minor, K. L., et al. (2005). Subgenual anterior cingulate activation to valenced emotional stimuli in major depression. *NeuroReport*, *16*(16), 1731–1734.

Gottesman, I. I., & Gould, T. D. (2003). The endophenotype concept in psychiatry: Etymology and strategic intentions. *American Journal of Psychiatry*, *160*(4), 636–645.

Grabe, H. J., Lange, M., Wolff, B., Volzke, H., Lucht, M., Freyberger, H. J., et al. (2005). Mental and physical distress is modulated by a polymorphism in the 5-HT transporter gene interacting with social stressors and chronic disease burden. *Molecular Psychiatry*, *10*(2), 220–224.

Gray, J. A. (1970). The psychophysiological basis of introversion–extraversion. *Behaviour Research and Therapy*, *8*, 249–266.

Haas, B. W., Omura, K., Constable, R. T., & Canli, T. (2006). Interference produced by emotional conflict associated with anterior cingulate activation. *Cognitive, Affective, and Behavioral Neuroscience*, *6*(2), 152–156.

Haas, B. W., Omura, K., Constable, R. T., & Canli, T. (2007). Emotional conflict and neuroticism: Personality-dependent activation in the amygdala and subgenual anterior cingulate. *Behavioral Neuroscience*, *121*(2), 249–256.

Hamer, D. (2002). Genetics: Rethinking behavior genetics. *Science*, *298*, 71–72.

Hariri, A. R., Drabant, E. M., & Weinberger, D. R. (2006). Imaging genetics: Perspectives from studies of genetically driven variation in serotonin function and corticolimbic affective processing. *Biological Psychiatry*, *59*(10), 888–897.

Hariri, A. R., Mattay, V. S., Tessitore, A., Kolachana, B., Fera, F., Goldman, D., et al. (2002). Serotonin transporter genetic variation and the response of the human amygdala. *Science*, *297*, 400–403.

Hashimoto, K. (2007). BDNF variant linked to anxiety-related behaviors. *Bioessays*, *29*(2), 116–119.

Hasler, G., Drevets, W. C., Gould, T. D., Gottesman, I. I., & Manji, H. K. (2006). Toward constructing an endophenotype strategy for bipolar disorders. *Biological Psychiatry*, *60*(2), 93–105.

Heinz, A., & Smolka, M. N. (2006). The effects of catechol O-methyltransferase genotype on brain activation elicited by affective stimuli and cognitive tasks. *Reviews in the Neurosciences*, *17*(3), 359–367.

Heinz, A., Smolka, M. N., Braus, D. F., Wrase, J., Beck, A., Flor, H., et al. (2007). Serotonin transporter genotype (5-HTTLPR): Effects of neutral and undefined conditions on amygdala activation. *Biological Psychiatry*, *61*(8), 1011–1014.

Isenberg, N., Silbersweig, D., Engelien, A., Emmerich, S., Malavade, K., Beattie, B., et al. (1999). Linguistic threat activates the human amygdala. *Proceedings of the National Academy of Sciences, USA*, *96*, 10456–10459.

Jovanovic, V., Guan, H. C., & Van Tol, H. H. (1999). Comparative pharmacological and functional analysis of the human dopamine D4.2 and D4.10 receptor variants. *Pharmacogenetics*, *9*(5), 561–568.

Kaufman, J., Yang, B. Z., Douglas-Palumberi, H., Houshyar, S., Lipschitz, D., Krystal, J. H., et al. (2004). Social supports and serotonin transporter gene moderate depression in maltreated children. *Proceedings of the National Academy of Sciences, USA*, *101*, 17316–17321.

Kendler, K. S., Kuhn, J. W., Vittum, J., Prescott, C. A., & Riley, B. (2005). The interaction of stressful life events and a serotonin transporter polymorphism in the prediction of episodes of major depression: A replication. *Archives of General Psychiatry*, *62*(5), 529–535.

Kuo, P. H., Neale, M. C., Riley, B. P., Patterson, D. G., Walsh, D., Prescott, C. A., et al. (2007). A genome-wide linkage analysis for the personality trait neuroticism in the Irish affected sibpair study of alcohol dependence. *American Journal of Medical Genetics B Neuropsychiatric Genetics*, *144*(4), 463–468.

Lesch, K. P., Bengel, D., Heils, A., Sabol, S. Z., Greenberg, B. D., Petri, S., et al. (1996). Association of anxiety-related traits with a polymorphism in the serotonin transporter gene regulatory region. *Science*, *274*, 1527–1531.

Lotta, T., Vidgren, J., Tilgmann, C., Ulmanen, I., Melen, K., Julkunen, I., et al. (1995). Kinetics of human soluble and membrane-bound catechol O-methyltransferase: A revised mechanism and description of the thermolabile variant of the enzyme. *Biochemistry*, *34*(13), 4202–4210.

Mannisto, P. T., & Kaakkola, S. (1999). Catechol-O-methyltransferase (COMT): Biochemistry, molecular biology, pharmacology, and clinical efficacy of the new selective COMT inhibitors. *Pharmacology Review*, *51*(4), 593–628.

Maren, S., & Quirk, G. J. (2004). Neuronal signalling of fear memory. *Nature Reviews Neuroscience*, *5*(11), 844–852.

Mayberg, H. S., Lozano, A. M., Voon, V., McNeely, H. E., Seminowicz, D., Hamani, C., et al.

(2005). Deep brain stimulation for treatment-resistant depression. *Neuron, 45*(5), 651–660.

McEwen, B. S. (2007). Physiology and neurobiology of stress and adaptation: Central role of the brain. *Physiology Review, 87*(3), 873–904.

McEwen, B. S., & Sapolsky, R. M. (1995). Stress and cognitive function. *Current Opinion in Neurobiology, 5*(2), 205–216.

Mischel, W. (1999). Personality coherence and dispositions in a Cognitive-Affective Personality System (CAPS) approach. In D. Cervone & Y. Shoda (Eds.), *The coherence of personality: Social-cognitive bases of consistency, variability, and organization* (pp. 37–60). New York: Guilford Press.

Mischel, W., & Shoda, Y. (1998). Reconciling processing dynamics and personality dispositions. *Annual Review of Psychology, 49,* 229–258.

Munafo, M. R., Clark, T. G., & Flint, J. (2005a). Does measurement instrument moderate the association between the serotonin transporter gene and anxiety-related personality traits? A meta-analysis. *Molecular Psychiatry, 10*(4), 415–419.

Munafo, M. R., Clark, T. G., & Flint, J. (2005b). Promise and pitfalls in the meta-analysis of genetic association studies: A response to Sen and Shinka. *Molecular Psychiatry, 10,* 895–897.

Munafo, M. R., Yalcin, B., Willis-Owen, S. A., & Flint, J. (2008). Association of the dopamine D4 receptor (DRD4) gene and approach-related personality traits: Meta-analysis and new data. *Biological Psychiatry, 63,* 197–206.

Nash, M. W., Huezo-Diaz, P., Williamson, R. J., Sterne, A., Purcell, S., Hoda, F., et al. (2004). Genome-wide linkage analysis of a composite index of neuroticism and mood-related scales in extreme selected sibships. *Human Molecular Genetics, 13*(19), 2173–2182.

Neale, B. M., Sullivan, P. F., & Kendler, K. S. (2005). A genome scan of neuroticism in nicotine dependent smokers. *American Journal of Medical Genetics B Neuropsychiatric Genetics, 132*(1), 65–69.

Noblett, K. L., & Coccaro, E. F. (2005). Molecular genetics of personality. *Current Psychiatry Report, 7*(1), 73–80.

Okuyama, Y., Ishiguro, H., Nankai, M., Shibuya, H., Watanabe, A., & Arinami, T. (2000). Identification of a polymorphism in the promoter region of DRD4 associated with the human novelty seeking personality trait. *Molecular Psychiatry, 5*(1), 64–69.

Okuyama, Y., Ishiguro, H., Toru, M., & Arinami, T. (1999). A genetic polymorphism in the promoter region of DRD4 associated with expression and schizophrenia. *Biochemical and Biophysical Research Communications, 258*(2), 292–295.

Papassotiropoulos, A., Stephan, D. A., Huentel-man, M. J., Hoerndli, F. J., Craig, D. W., Pearson, J. V., et al. (2006). Common kibra alleles are associated with human memory performance. *Science, 314,* 475–478.

Pezawas, L., Meyer-Lindenberg, A., Drabant, E. M., Verchinski, B. A., Munoz, K. E., Kolachana, B. S., et al. (2005). 5-HTTLPR polymorphism impacts human cingulate–amygdala interactions: A genetic susceptibility mechanism for depression. *Nature Neuroscience, 8*(6), 828–834.

Plomin, R., Hill, L., Craig, I. W., McGuffin, P., Purcell, S., Sham, P., et al. (2001). A genome-wide scan of 1842 DNA markers for allelic associations with general cognitive ability: A five-stage design using DNA pooling and extreme selected groups. *Behavior Genetics, 31*(6), 497–509.

Plomin, R., Owen, M. J., & McGuffin, P. (1994). The genetic basis of complex human behaviors. *Science, 264,* 1733–1739.

Plomin, R., & Schalkwyk, L. C. (2007). Microarrays. *Developmental Science, 10*(1), 19–23.

Posner, M. I., & Rothbart, M. K. (2007). Research on attention networks as a model for the integration of psychological science. *Annual Review of Psychology, 58*(1), 1–23.

Raichle, M. E., MacLeod, A. M., Snyder, A. Z., Powers, W. J., Gusnard, D. A., & Shulman, G. L. (2001). A default mode of brain function. *Proceedings of the National Academy of Sciences, USA, 98*(2), 676–682.

Rao, H., Gillihan, S. J., Wang, J., Korczykowski, M., Sankoorikal, G. M., Kaercher, K. A., et al. (2007). Genetic variation in serotonin transporter alters resting brain function in healthy individuals. *Biological Psychiatry, 62,* 600–606.

Rauch, S. L., Jenike, M. A., Alpert, N. M., Baer, L., Breiter, H. C., Savage, C. R., et al. (1994). Regional cerebral blood flow measured during symptom provocation in obsessive–compulsive disorder using oxygen 15-labeled carbon dioxide and positron emission tomography. *Archives of General Psychiatry, 51,* 62–70.

Rauch, S. L., Shin, L. M., & Wright, C. I. (2003). Neuroimaging studies of amygdala function in anxiety disorders. *Annals of the New York Academy of Sciences, 985,* 389–410.

Ray, R. D., Ochsner, K. N., Cooper, J. C., Robertson, E. R., Gabrieli, J. D., & Gross, J. J. (2005). Individual differences in trait rumination and the neural systems supporting cognitive reappraisal. *Cognitive, Affective, and Behavioral Neuroscience, 5*(2), 156–168.

Reif, A., & Lesch, K. P. (2003). Toward a molecular architecture of personality. *Behavioural Brain Research, 139*(1–2), 1–20.

Reuter, M., & Hennig, J. (2005). Association of the functional catechol-O-methyltransferase

VAL158MET polymorphism with the personality trait of extraversion. *NeuroReport*, *16*(10), 1135–1138.

Reuter, M., Peters, K., Schroeter, K., Koebke, W., Lenardon, D., Bloch, B., et al. (2005). The influence of the dopaminergic system on cognitive functioning: A molecular genetic approach. *Behavioural Brain Research*, *164*(1), 93–99.

Richards, A., French, C. C., Johnson, W., Naparstek, J., & Williams, J. (1992). Effects of mood manipulation and anxiety on performance of an emotional Stroop task. *British Journal of Psychology*, *83*, 479–491.

Roberts, J. E., Gilboa, E., & Gotlib, I. H. (1998). Ruminative response style and vulnerability to episodes of dysphoria: Gender, neuroticism, and episode duration. *Cognitive Therapy and Research*, *22*(4), 401–423.

Ronai, Z., Barta, C., Guttman, A., Lakatos, K., Gervai, J., Staub, M., et al. (2001). Genotyping the −521C/T functional polymorphism in the promoter region of dopamine D4 receptor (DRD4) gene. *Electrophoresis*, *22*(6), 1102–1105.

Rosenkranz, J. A., Moore, H., & Grace, A. A. (2003). The prefrontal cortex regulates lateral amygdala neuronal plasticity and responses to previously conditioned stimuli. *Journal of Neuroscience*, *23*(35), 11054–11064.

Rushworth, M. F. S., Behrens, T. E. J., Rudebeck, P. H., & Walton, M. E. (2007). Contrasting roles for cingulate and orbitofrontal cortex in decisions and social behaviour. *Trends in Cognitive Sciences*, *11*(4), 168–176.

Schinka, J. A., Busch, R. M., & Robichaux-Keene, N. (2004). A meta-analysis of the association between the serotonin transporter gene polymorphism (5-HTTLPR) and trait anxiety. *Molecular Psychiatry*, *9*(2), 197–202.

Schinka, J. A., Letsch, E. A., & Crawford, F. C. (2002). DRD4 and novelty seeking: Results of meta-analyses. *American Journal of Medical Genetics*, *114*(6), 643–648.

Sen, S., Burmeister, M., & Ghosh, D. (2004). Meta-analysis of the association between a serotonin transporter promoter polymorphism (5-HTTLPR) and anxiety-related personality traits. *American Journal of Medical Genetics*, *127B*(1), 85–89.

Shulman, G. L., Fiez, J. A., Corbetta, M., Buckner, R. L., Miezin, F. M., Raichle, M. E., et al. (1997). Common blood flow changes across visual tasks: II. Decreases in cerebral cortex. *Journal of Cognitive Neuroscience*, *9*, 648–663.

Smolka, M. N., Schumann, G., Wrase, J., Grusser, S. M., Flor, H., Mann, K., et al. (2005). Catechol-O-methyltransferase val158met genotype affects processing of emotional stimuli in the amygdala and prefrontal cortex. *Journal of Neuroscience*, *25*(4), 836–842.

Surtees, P. G., Wainwright, N. W., Willis-Owen, S. A., Luben, R., Day, N. E., & Flint, J. (2005). Social adversity, the serotonin transporter (5-HTTLPR) polymorphism and major depressive disorder. *Biological Psychiatry*, *59*, 224–229.

Swanson, J. M., Flodman, P., Kennedy, J., Spence, M. A., Moyzis, R., Schuck, S., et al. (2000). Dopamine genes and ADHD. *Neuroscience and Biobehavioral Reviews*, *24*(1), 21–25.

Walton, M. E., Croxson, P. L., Behrens, T. E., Kennerley, S. W., & Rushworth, M. F. (2007). Adaptive decision making and value in the anterior cingulate cortex. *NeuroImage*, *36*(Suppl. 2, T142–154.

Weaver, I. C., Cervoni, N., Champagne, F. A., D'Alessio, A. C., Sharma, S., Seckl, J. R., et al. (2004). Epigenetic programming by maternal behavior. *Nature Neuroscience*, *7*(8), 847–854.

Weinberger, D. R., Egan, M. F., Bertolino, A., Callicott, J. H., Mattay, V. S., Lipska, B. K., et al. (2001). Prefrontal neurons and the genetics of schizophrenia. *Biological Psychiatry*, *50*(11), 825–844.

Whalen, P. J., Bush, G., McNally, R. J., Wilhelm, S., McInerney, S. C., Jenike, M. A., et al. (1998). The emotional counting Stroop paradigm: A functional magnetic resonance imaging probe of the anterior cingulate affective division. *Biological Psychiatry*, *44*(12), 1219–1228.

Winterer, G., & Goldman, D. (2003). Genetics of human prefrontal function. *Brain Research and Brain Research Reviews*, *43*(1), 134–163.

CHAPTER 12

Personality in Animals

Tamara A. R. Weinstein
John P. Capitanio
Samuel D. Gosling

Consider the following hypothetical study of personality. A set of individuals, whose genetic lineage is known, is monitored from conception to birth and observed at regular intervals from birth to death. Because maternity and paternity are known for certain, a subset of the individuals can be cross-fostered at birth so that the effects of maternal postnatal social environment can be distinguished from the effects of biological inheritance and prenatal effects. The environments in which the individuals live can be carefully monitored and, if the researchers wish, manipulated. Numerous physiological measures can be taken, including regular blood samples, and samples of body and brain tissue can be collected at autopsy. On top of all this, several generations could be examined in the course of 10 years.

Although such a study could never be conducted on human participants, if it were done, it would permit investigators to address numerous foundational questions about the genetic, neurochemical, physiological, and environmental bases of personality. However, many of the features of this hypothetical study could be implemented in nonhuman animal research—indeed, many of them already are. There is now compelling evidence that personality traits can be assessed in nonhuman animals (Gosling & Vazire, 2002;

Vazire, Gosling, Dickey, & Schapiro, 2007), opening the way for animal studies to augment human personality research on such basic questions.

To illustrate the opportunities that animal research can bring to personality science, consider some features of one ongoing animal personality research program (the findings are presented in greater detail later in the chapter). One of us (J. P. C.) has collected personality data on over 175 rhesus monkeys since 1993. The animals' personalities were assessed at 5–10 years of age, and a four-factor structure was derived by factor analysis using one subsample and confirmed on a separate subsample using confirmatory factor analysis. Some of the animals were removed from the living situation in which personality was measured, and were tested in a variety of situations, both nonsocial and social (including with both familiar and unfamiliar companions). Behavioral and physiological measures were obtained in these situations for up to several years following the initial assessments. Persisting relationships were found between the personality factors and measures of social behavior and emotionality, plasma cortisol concentrations, tetanus- and herpes-virus-specific antibody responses, heart rate, and central nervous system functioning. One personality factor,

Sociability, reflecting a tendency to affiliate, was found to be related to variation in patterns of neural innervation of lymph nodes, to moderate the response to a social stressor and influence expression of genes associated with innate immune responses, and to relate to individual differences in progression of immunodeficiency virus disease (Capitanio, 1999, 2002, 2004; Capitanio, Mendoza, & Baroncelli, 1999; Capitanio, Mendoza, & Bentson, 2004; Capitanio & Widaman, 2005; Capitanio et al., in press; Maninger, Capitanio, Mendoza, & Mason, 2003; Ruys, Capitanio, & Mendoza, 2002; Sloan, Capitanio, Tarara, & Cole, in press).

As we shall see, providing animal models for human personality research is only one application of studies of animal personality. Animal research can also illuminate the evolutionary processes that shaped personality structure and promoted individual differences in personality. In addition, the assessment of personality in animals has numerous practical applications that can contribute to human and animal welfare. In this chapter, we provide an overview of the emerging field of animal personality, summarizing the major issues and findings, and pointing to the potential contributions to be made by this emerging cross-disciplinary field.

HISTORY

Over the past three decades, personality research in nonhuman animals has become increasingly common in the scientific literature, with particularly fast growth in the last 5 years. As a mark of the widespread interest in, and broad applicability of, animal personality research, studies have been conducted across a wide range of disciplines, including biological psychiatry, behavioral ecology, applied ethology (or animal welfare), animal behavior, primatology, behavioral genetics, and comparative psychology. Indeed, the strongest interest in individual differences in animal behavior has come from fields outside mainstream personality research. For example, the field of applied ethology has produced many studies examining personality in a broad range of domestic species, including cattle, pigs, sheep, dogs, and mink. In their attempts to solve practical issues (e.g., which individuals tend to become agitated when handled), applied ethologists have made great progress in developing methods for assessing individual differences in behavior.

Although many personality psychologists are just now becoming aware of the relevant nonhuman literature, historically there were closer ties between researchers studying individual differences in human and nonhuman species. In the formative days of social and personality psychology, investigators believed that studies of animals could inform research on the psychological processes underlying individual differences in social behavior in the same way animal research had informed most other areas of psychology (Domjan & Purdy, 1995). One early landmark in animal personality research was Nobel Laureate Ivan Pavlov's series of studies at the beginning of the 20th century (e.g., Pavlov, 1906); this research program identified four basic types of canine personality based on three properties of the nervous system: force, equilibrium, and mobility. Interest in animal personality continued with Yerkes's and Crawford's ape studies in the 1930s and with those of Hebb in the 1940s. At the time, such work was considered relevant to researchers in human social and personality psychology. Indeed, in the 1935 *Handbook of Social Psychology*, more than a third of the chapters were devoted to work on nonhuman subjects. But two decades later, in the 1954 handbook, the attention to nonhuman studies had faded significantly; already, Hebb and Thomson saw cause to draw attention to the importance of animal studies, warning in their chapter that social psychology will "be dangerously myopic if it restricts itself to the human literature" (p. 532). Fifteen years later Zajonc's text *Animal Social Psychology* (1969) again highlighted the value of research on nonhuman social behavior, revealing a large animal literature that was "entirely surprising in scope, quality, and significance" (p. v). Unfortunately, during the subsequent 30 years, with few notable exceptions (e.g., Buss, 1988), personality theory and research based on nonhuman animals largely disappeared from contemporary social and personality psychology—none of the chapters in the latest *The Handbook of Social Psychology* (Gilbert, Fiske, & Lindzey, 1998) or either *Handbooks of Personality* (Hogan, Johnson, & Briggs, 1997; Pervin & John, 1999) focused on nonhuman animals, and studies of nonhuman animals rarely appeared in mainstream personality journals. Yet there are myriad ways in which animal studies can inform human personality psychology research. This chapter reviews the basic issues in the recently reinvigorated field of animal personality and illustrates the varied and unique contributions that animal studies can make to our understanding of personality.

DEFINITIONS

What is meant by "personality"? There is no single definition of personality that would satisfy all personality psychologists, and most would be satisfied by only a very broad definition. For example, one way to define personality that captures most phenomena studied by personality psychologists is as those characteristics of individuals that describe and account for consistent patterns of feeling, cognition, and behaving. The phenomena studied by human personality psychologists include temperament and character traits, dispositions, goals, personal projects, abilities, attitudes, physical and bodily states, moods, and life stories. The vast majority of animal personality studies focus on just a subset of these constructs: behavioral traits. Although researchers do not rule out the possibility that behavioral traits are associated with characteristic patterns of cognition and affect, they tend to focus on cross-situational and cross-temporal patterns of behavior, which are easier to measure. Focusing on overt measures of consistency in behavioral patterns, rather than on underlying emotional processes, is often done to avoid inviting criticisms about anthropomorphism and lack of objectivity.

In animal personality research, terms such as "temperament" and "behavioral syndrome" or "style" are often used instead of "personality" for the very reason of avoiding the anthropomorphic connotations of the "*p*-word." In human research, temperament is considered a construct closely related to personality; it has often been defined as the inherited, early-appearing tendencies that continue throughout life and serve as the foundation for personality. This definition is not adopted uniformly by animal or even human researchers (McCrae et al., 2000), but

a similar definition of temperament that has gained acceptance among nonhuman primate researchers is that proposed by Clarke and Boinski (1995), who stated that temperament refers to behavioral styles or tendencies that show continuity over time and can be identified in early infancy, and which are reflected in the degree and nature of responsivity to novel or stressful stimuli. The term "behavioral syndrome" has gained recent popularity in the field of behavioral ecology (Sih, Bell, Johnson, & Ziemba, 2004). Behavioral syndromes are defined as suites of correlated behaviors expressed either within a given behavioral context or across different contexts. Clearly, this definition very closely matches the concept of personality in humans.

We prefer the term "personality" for three reasons. First, it is confusing to create new terms without a compelling conceptual reason to do so. Second, using the term "personality" facilitates connections with the enormous existing research on personality in humans. Third, we do not think it is useful, as some have suggested, to adopt the term "temperament" for nonhumans because to do so would entail a priori assumptions (e.g., about traits being inherited and appearing early) that may or may not be appropriate; for example, it is increasingly clear that individual differences in adult animal behavior are a function of both biological tendencies and experience, as is the case with humans.

METHODS

Methods for assessing personality in animals can be split into two broad categories: codings of overt behaviors and ratings of broader traits by knowledgeable observers. Behavior codings and trait ratings reflect different solutions to the apparent tradeoff between quantifying personality in terms of objective behaviors and using humans to record and interpret information more subjectively. Many animal behavior researchers regard behavior codings as intrinsically superior to global personality ratings. Historically, rating data obtained from observers have been derided as subjective and inappropriate for the objective requirements of scientific measurement. In contrast, many human researchers would argue that behavior codings actually deserve the closest scrutiny. They would point to research on human personality, where consensual observer ratings are often considered to be the sine qua non of personality traits (Gosling, Kwan, & John, 2003). Animal personality researchers who have chosen to sacrifice the objectivity supposedly gained from detailed behavior codings do so in favor of obtaining more comprehensive ratings on traits such as confidence, curiosity, and playfulness by people who are familiar with individual animals.

Behavior codings have been used widely in animal personality studies. In a comprehensive review, one of us (Gosling, 2001) found that 74% of the animal personality studies to that date had used behavior codings to assess personality. Behavior codings often require repeated observations of individuals, and thus can be performed only with animals whose behavior is easily visible or recorded. It is surprisingly difficult to summarize the specific methods and procedures used in the typical behavior coding study because the details are often not reported; for example, researchers seldom report how many observers coded each animal, who the observers were (e.g., experts vs. undergraduate research assistants), how the observers were trained, how many hours of observation were collected for each animal, or the interobserver reliabilities of the codings.

The choice of which behaviors to code is largely driven by the goals of the study, and much variation across studies exists with respect to the specific behaviors chosen to code. Once the behaviors have been chosen, the observers must be trained to recognize and record these behaviors. This can be done with basic paper-and-pencil techniques or by using more sophisticated computer-based data collection systems (e.g., Noldus, 1991). To facilitate the process of deciding which behaviors to code, researchers typically refer to published ethograms, which are lists of species-typical behaviors.

Trait ratings are used less commonly than behavior codings in animal personality studies. In Gosling's 2001 review, only 34% of the studies used trait ratings to measure animal personality; most of these examined dogs, cats, or primates. Typically, researchers have quantified impressions by asking observers who were familiar with the animals to rate each one on a number of personality traits. Usually these ratings were made

by more than one observer, and occasionally they were made at several points in time.

Both codings and ratings can be based on three possible sources of information: experimenter-defined behavioral tests, naturalistic behavior, and observers' knowledge of the animals. Behavioral tests involve exposing an individual to a specific situation or stimulus believed to elicit meaningful individual differences in behavior. For example, in study of social responsiveness in rhesus monkeys, one of us (Capitanio, 2002) exposed 12 adult males to videotapes of unfamiliar animals displaying aggressive, affiliative, or nonsocial behaviors. Wide variation in behavioral responses to the videotapes were seen, with individuals differing in the frequencies of behaviors such as yawning (which reflects tension), lipsmacking (which reflects appeasement), as well as durations of looking at the displayed images.

In typical studies of naturalistic behaviors, trained observers record the behavior of one animal at a time in "focal animal samples," in which frequencies and/or durations of virtually all (or, sometimes, a focused subset of) behaviors displayed are collected (Altmann, 1974). The number of observers for each animal varies across studies, but is usually as low as one or two. Focal samples can vary in duration from study to study (e.g., from 10 seconds to 30 minutes), as does the number of times each animal is sampled.

Personality assessments can also draw upon observers' familiarity with particular animals. For example, in the video playback study described above (Capitanio, 2002), personality assessments had been made on the animals using the rating methodology nearly 4 years prior to the playback experiment. Six of the twelve animals had been rated high in "Sociability," a dimension reflecting a tendency to affiliate, and the remaining six animals had been rated low on this dimension. The variation in responses that were found in this study was strongly related to the prior personality rating: Animals that were low in Sociability showed higher frequencies of yawning and lower frequencies of lipsmacking, and tended to have higher durations of looking at the videotapes. Importantly, when both high- and low-sociable animals saw a social signal (threat, lipsmack) displayed on the videotape, their most common response was to avert their gaze. High-sociable animals, however, gaze-averted in about half the time compared to low-sociable animals. Given the threatening nature of direct eye contact in this species, this suggested that high Sociability reflected greater social skill in managing potentially dangerous situations.

In theory, coding or rating methods could be applied to any of the three sources of information outlined above. In practice, however, the information available in behavioral tests and naturalistic observations is almost always gathered using coding methods, and the information accumulated by observers about individuals is almost always recorded using rating methods.

Vazire and colleagues (2007) compared codings and trait ratings in a study of chimpanzees that implemented both methods, evaluating each in terms of its reliability, subjectivity, and practicality. Their analyses showed that the widely supposed advantages of codings over trait ratings are often not borne out in practice. Specifically, trait-rating methods were more reliable and practical than behavior-coding methods and were not as subjective as many researchers believe. Trait ratings are reliable and hence well suited for detecting consistencies in animals' behavior, the very foundation of personality. Behavior codings, in contrast, can be difficult to measure reliably, particularly when observations are made across different times of day or under varying conditions. Even when behaviors are measured at the same time of day or under the same conditions, they may reflect other characteristics of the environment (e.g., situational influences), not just personality. Behavior can be used to infer personality, but personality and behavior are not the same thing (Capitanio, 2004): An individual's traits, dispositions, or proclivities combine with elements of the situation or environment to promote expression of particular behaviors. But those same behaviors can be expressed in very different situations and can be prompted by different proclivities. For example, in some contexts, a monkey's sexual presentation posture (rump elevated, legs braced, orientation toward another individual) can reflect friendliness, appeasement or subordination, or an invitation for sexual behavior. Behavior-coding methods may be better suited for experimental manipulations, where researchers are concerned with detecting the effects of situational variables on behavior.

Vazire and colleagues' (2007) findings indicate that researchers (1) cannot assume that behavior codings are reliable and (2) should compute and report reliabilities for behavior codings as they do with trait ratings. In addition, researchers using either method should take steps to improve the reliability of their measures. For example, behavior codings can be made more reliable by increasing the number and length of observation, providing specific definitions of the behaviors to be coded, and training observers extensively. Trait ratings can also be made more reliable by increasing the number of observers, ensuring that all observers are well-acquainted with the animals they are rating, and providing specific definitions of the traits being rated.

To estimate and reduce the effects of observer bias on both trait-rating and behavior-coding methods, researchers can perform variance-partitioning analyses such as intraclass correlations or the social relations model (Kenny, 1994). These analyses allow researchers to measure and statistically control for "perceiver effects," which are systematic idiosyncrasies in observers' ratings (Kwan, Gosling, & John, 2008).

An important additional advantage of trait ratings over behavioral codings is their relative practicality. In fact, the efficiency with which ratings can be applied suggests that studies of personality could be carried out in many contexts where researchers may be discouraged by the efforts associated with coding methods. These findings further suggest that rating studies of personality can piggyback on the many animal studies already underway.

Ultimately the choice of whether to use rating or coding methods should be driven by theoretical concerns because the two methods measure different things. Rating methods assess broader psychological traits, whereas behavioral-coding methods assess the observable results of these traits interacting with contextual factors.

SPECIES STUDIED

In the most comprehensive review to date, one of us (Gosling, 2001) identified 187 personality studies of one kind or another in 64 different species. It should be noted that these studies varied a great deal in quality, with some of them, especially the early studies, consisting of little more than a series of field observations. Furthermore, the species studied were far from representative of the species in existence. Eighty-four percent of the studies in Gosling's review focused on mammals (29% primates, 55% nonprimates), 8% focused on fish, 4% focused on birds, and the remaining 4% were divided among reptiles, amphibians, arthropods, and mollusks.

TRAITS STUDIED

This review (Gosling, 2001) also summarized the traits studied in past animal research. There are numerous conceptual challenges to defining traits and determining their equivalence across studies and across species. However, a number of dimensions have appeared consistently across multiple species. Many of the papers identified a dimension reflecting an individual's characteristic reaction to novel stimuli or situations. This dimension has been referred to with terms such as Reactivity, Emotionality, or Fearfulness, and has been measured by behavioral indicators such as defecation rate in open field tests and by ratings on traits such as "nervous." A second recurring dimension is the propensity to seek out novel stimuli or situations in the first place, and has been identified in several articles as Exploration. This dimension has been measured by behaviors such as approach to novel objects and by ratings on traits such as "curious." Several studies identified a dimension differentiating those individuals who sought out social interactions from those who preferred to remain solitary. This dimension, usually referred to as Sociability, has been measured by behaviors such as frequency of social encounters and by ratings on traits such as "affiliative." A number of studies identified an Aggression dimension derived from such behavioral measures as latency to attack another individual and by ratings of traits such as "aggressive." A fifth dimension to appear in several studies referred to an animal's general activity level and has been measured by behaviors such as the amount of enclosure covered by the animal's roaming and by ratings on traits such as "energetic." Several studies also identified a Dominance or Assertiveness dimension, which was usually related to the individual's

rank in the dominance hierarchy (e.g., Gosling, 1998; King & Figueredo, 1997; Sapolsky & Ray, 1989).

Most studies in the review (Gosling, 2001) had a narrow scope, focusing on only one or two dimensions. To get a better idea of the personality structures associated with different species, exploratory studies with a broader focus are needed. One of us (Gosling & John, 1999) reviewed 19 such studies, using the five-factor model (FFM; John, 1990; see also John, Naumann, & Soto, Chapter 4, this volume; McCrae & Costa, Chapter 5, this volume) as an organizing framework for the findings. The FFM dimensions of Extraversion, Neuroticism, and Agreeableness showed considerable generality across the 12 species included in their review. Of the 19 studies, 17 identified a factor closely related to Extraversion, capturing dimensions ranging from Surgency in chimpanzees; Sociability in pigs, dogs, and rhesus monkeys; Energy in cats and dogs; Vivacity in donkeys; to a dimension contrasting bold approach versus avoidance in octopuses. Of course, the way these personality dimensions are manifested depends on the species: Whereas the human scoring low on Extraversion stays at home on Saturday night or tries to blend into a corner at a large party, the octopus scoring low on Boldness stays in its protective den during feedings and attempts to hide itself by changing color or releasing ink into the water.

Factors related to Neuroticism appeared almost as frequently, capturing dimensions such as Fearfulness, Emotional Reactivity, Excitability, and low Nerve Stability. Factors related to Agreeableness appeared in 14 studies, with Affability, Affection, and Social Closeness representing the high pole, and Aggression, Hostility, and Fighting representing the low pole. Factors related to Openness were identified in all but 4 of the 12 species. The two major components defining this dimension were Curiosity–Exploration (interest in new situations and novel objects) and Playfulness (which is associated with Extraversion when social, rather than imaginative, aspects of play are assessed). Chimpanzees were the only species with a separate Conscientiousness factor, which was defined more narrowly than in humans but included the lack of attention and goal-directedness and erratic, unpredictable, and disorganized behavior typical of the low pole. Dominance emerged as a clear separate factor in 7 of the

19 studies reviewed (Gosling & John, 1999). A separate Activity dimension was identified in only two of the studies.

Overall, the past 10 years of research have shown that it is viable to assess at least some elements of personality in animals. This fact raises the question of whether animal research can be used to inform the field of personality psychology. In the following section we discuss examples of animal personality studies that, in our opinion, firmly establish the importance of animal research in the field of personality.

WHY STUDY ANIMAL PERSONALITY?

Animal personality research is useful in three broad domains, all of which are relevant to humans, although in very different ways. The first domain involves understanding a species for its own sake. All animals, including humans, must accomplish certain tasks in order to survive and reproduce, such as obtain food, protect themselves from predators, and secure a mate. At a fundamental level, understanding the personality structure within a species helps us understand the different strategies that animals employ in accomplishing these tasks. In this way, personality research in nonhuman animals parallels that in humans, by focusing on how individual-difference factors facilitate or constrain an animal's ability to solve the problems with which it is faced daily. Taking a comparative perspective on personality can, for example, highlight common solutions that different species have taken to solve common problems. Just as human personality research has enriched the field of animal personality research, this "behavioral ecology" approach to personality research may suggest novel ways of thinking about human personality. A second domain in which animal personality research is valuable concerns its utility in "animal model" research. The greater experimental control of both environmental and genetic factors in animal research, coupled with a greater ability to manipulate independent variables and assess dependent variables, provides a powerful way of exploring issues that are of fundamental importance to humans. Finally, there are practical applications of animal personality research relating to the interaction between humans and animals, including the welfare of animals used

in scientific experiments, animals as pets, and conservation of endangered species. Below, we describe examples in each of these three domains.

STUDYING ANIMALS TO ADDRESS SPECIES-SPECIFIC QUESTIONS OF BEHAVIOR

The primary goal of behavioral ecology studies of animal personality is to gain a better understanding of how individuals of a given species vary in their day-to-day behaviors, and to explore the adaptive function of such variation. Historically, behavioral ecologists, like many psychologists, have viewed individual differences in behavior as representing nonadaptive, random variation surrounding a presumably adaptive population mean. Recently, however, the notion that the differences themselves may represent nonrandom and possibly adaptive solutions to the challenges of survival and reproduction has become more widely accepted (Dall, Houston, & McNamara, 2004; Nettle, 2006). The existence of suites of correlated behaviors (i.e., behaviors that co-occur) could reflect variation in adaptive strategies among individuals within a population. Correlations among behaviors may be expressed either within a given context (e.g., correlations between activity and exploratory behaviors in a foraging context) or across different contexts (e.g., correlations among feeding, antipredator, and mating behaviors); as noted, in the field of behavioral ecology, these suites of behaviors are commonly referred to as behavioral syndromes (Sih et al., 2004). Such syndromes presumably reflect underlying genetic or physiological mechanisms and constrain the flexibility of individuals' behaviors. This constraint in behavioral flexibility can generate tradeoffs, in which a certain personality characteristic may prove advantageous for an animal in one situation but not another. For example, highly aggressive individuals of a given species may be successful in defending their territories and monopolizing valuable food sources against conspecifics, but these same individuals may act inappropriately aggressively toward predators, approaching them when fleeing might actually result in a greater probability of survival; the reverse would hold true for less aggressive individuals. The existence of variation in environments may thus have helped maintain individual differences in behavior during the course of evolution, because the fitness benefits associated with different personality characteristics change as environmental conditions fluctuate (Wilson, 1998). To continue the example, when predator densities were low, high aggressiveness may have been adaptive, and when predator densities were high, aggressiveness may have been less useful for individuals.

Compelling evidence supporting this idea is provided by a Netherlands research group that has been conducting long-term studies of personality in a natural population of a passerine bird species, the great tit, *Parus major*, over the last several years (see Groothuis & Carere, 2005, for a review). Birds have been found that differ consistently in exploratory behavior when placed in a novel environment, and these differences have been correlated with variation in a wide range of social and nonsocial behaviors (specific examples are discussed below). Notably, differences in exploratory tendency between individuals were related to variation in their annual survival as well as to survival of their offspring; the direction of the relationship, however, depended on the distribution and availability of food during the winter (Dingemanse, Both, Drent, & Tinbergen, 2004). Thus, fluctuations in environmental conditions may have led to fluctuations in competition for space and food, which in turn affected the survival and reproductive success of different personalities (reflecting alternative strategies); such variation in selection pressures is one mechanism that can maintain individual differences in personality in a population.

The understanding of how individuals differ in the behaviors they use to deal with the challenges of survival and reproduction, the constraints or tradeoffs that animals experience with respect to behavioral flexibility, and why evolution may have favored the maintenance of individual differences in personality in a given population or species are the key issues that behavioral ecologists seek to explore through the study of personality. Animals must accomplish many tasks in their daily lives. Although the specific challenges they encounter often depend on the species or population in question, common tasks include acquisition of food and territory, avoidance of predation, competition for mates, the rearing of offspring, and integration into a social group (which often includes establishing dominance rank among a hierarchy of individuals). Below we describe examples of studies that address how personality influences the way in which animals solve some of these challenges. As noted in our discussion above, animal studies primarily use the coding approach in order to assess individual variation in personality, and most behavioral ecology studies of personality have done so by measuring animals' responses to novel or threatening stimuli. As a result, much attention has been paid to the "shy–bold continuum," which comprises behaviors such as exploration, activity, and aggression (Wilson, Clark, Coleman, & Dearstyne, 1994).

Anti-Predator Behavior

Some studies of anti-predator behavior have demonstrated negative consequences associated with possessing certain personality traits. Quinn and Cresswell (2005) measured personality in wild chaffinches (*Fringilla coelebs*) by assessing activity level, and then related variation in activity level to anti-predator behavior when birds were presented with a model hawk. Anti-predator behavior was assessed in two situations: a low-risk or indirect threat situation, in which the model hawk flew 2 meters to the side of the chaffinch, and the presumed optimal response was to freeze to avoid detection; and a high-risk or direct threat situation, in which the model flew directly overhead, and the presumed optimal response was to escape. Activity level in the absence of a predator was negatively correlated with freezing behavior in both the low- and high-risk predator situations. Thus, individuals low in activity experienced a tradeoff in which they were more likely to perform the correct anti-predator response in the low-risk situation (i.e., to freeze), but were less likely to perform the correct response in the high-risk situation, where fleeing, rather than freezing, was presumed optimal. The opposite tradeoff occurred in highly active birds.

Competition for Mates

In many species of birds and fish, females prefer to mate with brightly colored males rather than males with duller coloration. One hypothesis that has been proposed to explain this phenomenon states that if the expression of preferred traits in males (such as conspicuous colors) is indicative of males' overall quality, females will choose to mate with males that express these traits in order to gain benefits such as access to a better territory or for transmission of better genes to their offspring. Godin and Dugatkin (1996) showed that in the Trinidadian guppy (*Poecilia reticulata*), the conspicuousness of males' coloration correlated positively with boldness toward a cichlid fish predator as well as their escape distance—that is, more colorful males approached a fish predator more often than did drab males, but when the predator began "stalking" them, the brightly colored males fled sooner, and from a greater distance, compared to the drab males. Godin and Dugatkin concluded from their experiments that bold males were more informed about nearby predators and more likely to survive encounters with them. In addition, they found that though females preferred more colorful males as mates, females actually preferred bolder males irrespective of coloration when given the opportunity to observe males' behavior toward a potential fish predator. By preferentially mating with colorful males, female guppies were thus choosing relatively bold, and perhaps more viable, individuals. If such viability is heritable, females may potentially gain fitness benefits from mating with these males by producing more viable offspring.

Parental Care/Reproductive Success

Some studies of personality and parental care have found behavioral inhibition, or shyness, to be associated with lower levels of parental behavior. One such example is demonstrated by Budaev, Zworykin, and Mochek's (1999) study of a captive group of convict cichlids, *Cichlasoma (Archocentrus) nigrofasciatum*. They assessed fish behavior in a novel area and in the presence of a novel fish. Individuals varied along an activity–inhibition dimension, such that active/uninhibited cichlids were quicker to enter the novel area and approach the novel fish, whereas inhibited individuals typically "froze" in the presence of the novel fish. Male cichlids that were more inhibited also engaged in less food provisioning of their brood. Females that were most inhibited spent the least amount of time near offspring when their broods were youngest,

and both males and females that were inhibited spent less time near their offspring during later brood stages.

Similarly, Reale, Gallant, Leblanc, and Festa-Bianchet (2000) found that in bighorn sheep, ewes that were bolder (i.e., those that were most likely to approach and remain for longer periods of time at a salt lick associated with the experimenters' trap) were most likely to start reproducing earlier and to have higher weaning success than shy ewes. Reale and colleagues' results suggest that ewes that were more willing to spend time feeding in a risky area may be obtaining important nutrients that enable them to reproduce earlier and have healthier offspring. In both of these examples, inhibition may be a safer, more effective strategy in novel, potentially dangerous situations, but in the context of parental care it is boldness that appears to be associated with behaviors that lead to increased offspring survival.

Behavioral inhibition (or shyness) is not always associated with poorer parental care, however. Both, Dingemanse, Drent, and Tinbergen (2005) measured exploratory behavior in a wild population of great tits during temporary capture and placement in a novel environment, which was a room consisting of five artificial trees. Exploration was measured using the number of movements between branches during the first 2 minutes after the individual entered the room; individuals were classified as either slow or fast explorers. Fledgling condition (as measured by mass) was affected by the interaction between both parents' exploratory behavior, with assortative pairs (i.e., slow–slow and fast–fast pairs) producing fledglings in the best condition. Offspring of both of these sets of parents may have been in similarly good condition because parents were able to specialize in one of two different behavioral strategies that each led to the same end result of heavier offspring: fast-exploring pairs may have been better able to obtain or defend a high-quality territory, whereas slow-exploring pairs may have been better parents (e.g., engaged in more food provisioning).

The three examples above demonstrate that any given trait, such as behavioral inhibition, is not uniformly "good" or "bad"— what is important is how that trait affects functioning in the environments that the individuals experience.

Dominance Rank/Integration into the Social Hierarchy

Becoming integrated into a social group, which usually involves establishing a place in the hierarchy, is a crucial task for socially living animals. Dominance rank has important consequences for fitness because it can affect territory acquisition, access to food, mating success, and survival of offspring. Data from the Netherlands great tit research program suggest that personality influences dominance interactions in complex ways. Verbeek, Boon, and Drent (1996) showed that in pairwise confrontations of juvenile male great tits, fast explorers started and won more fights than slow explorers. However, when tits were formed into aviary groups (which better modeled natural social dynamics than simple pairwise interactions), the relationship between personality and dominance rank varied according to the stability of the hierarchy (Verbeek, De Goede, Drent, & Wiepkema, 1999). That is, during the first day in the aviary, when dominance ranks had not yet stabilized, fast explorers averaged higher dominance ranks and initiated more fights than slow explorers. During this period of social instability, fast explorers took more risks in their fighting behavior (while slow explorers were more cautious), and also had more difficulty coping with defeat than slow explorers. Once the hierarchy stabilized, fast explorers either won or lost all fights with slow explorers—the end result being that slow explorers typically had intermediate dominance ranks, but on average were actually higher in dominance rank than fast explorers. These studies suggest that high levels of boldness or aggression, though often associated with success in agonistic encounters, may not always lead to high dominance rank if individuals are not able to cope with defeat or do not sufficiently temper risky behavior with caution.

Nonhuman primate researchers have found that the relationship between personality and dominance rank is similarly complex and dynamic. Fairbanks and colleagues (2004) administered an intruder challenge test to adolescent male vervet monkeys. In this test, a caged, unfamiliar adult male was placed at the periphery of the target individual's home enclosure. Individuals were found to differ in social impulsivity, reflecting variation in the tendency to approach rapidly, examine (by touching or sniffing), and challenge (through threats or displays) the intruder. Males with the highest impulsivity scores were most likely to become the alpha male upon introduction into a new group. However, impulsivity declined in all males from adolescence to adulthood. Interestingly, the decline in dominant males was most marked, such that their adult impulsivity scores equaled those of subordinate males 1 year following introduction into new groups. According to Fairbanks and colleagues, increased impulsivity during adolescence may motivate males to leave their natal groups and face the challenges of emigration and immigration. Upon entering a new group, however, the most successful males were the ones that responded with bold overconfidence during the intense initial competition, and then became more measured and conservative in their behavior as alpha males. This study provides additional support for the idea that high levels of aggression or boldness may initially benefit an individual in agonistic encounters, but in order for status to be maintained, caution must be exercised in the long term. The results of such studies of personality and dominance rank suggest new ways of examining normative patterns of personality development and change in many species, including humans.

Finally, an extensive research program conducted by Sapolsky and colleagues on wild olive baboons (*Papio anubis*) has shown that among males, reactivity to stressors (as measured by glucocorticoid function) does not relate to dominance rank in a straightforward manner (Ray & Sapolsky, 1992; Sapolsky & Ray, 1989; Virgin & Sapolsky, 1997). That is, the traditional notion that subordinate males are more stressed than dominant males does not necessarily hold true. Rather, it is styles of dominance (i.e., personality) that best predict glucocorticoid function. For example, high-ranking males that demonstrated behaviors suggesting high degrees of social skillfulness, control, and predictability over social contingencies appeared to be the least physiologically stressed in their daily lives (Sapolsky & Ray, 1989). Dominant males lacking these behavioral features, in contrast, had cortisol concentrations that were as high as those of subordinate males. Virgin and Sapolsky (1997) conducted a similar analysis of subordinate males and found that personality differences in these animals were also associated with variation in glucocorticoid function. One subset of subordinate males had significantly high rates of consortships (a behavior usually shown only by high-ranking males) and glucocorticoid responses to stress that were similar to those of dominant males. These animals turned out to be significantly more likely than other subordinates to move to the upper half of the hierarchy in subsequent years.

Population/Species Differences

A final important goal of behavioral ecology research on animal personality is to determine the taxonomic distribution of various personality traits, and to examine how personality differs between populations of a species according to variation in ecological factors (Fraley, Brumbaugh, & Marks, 2005). Employing such a comparative approach to personality research can help us (1) understand how certain traits may have evolved by looking at phylogenetic continuities, and (2) identify common traits across a variety of unrelated taxa that may have evolved independently in response to similar environmental conditions.

Interspecies differences in personality are thought to result from differences in population density, sex ratio, group composition, susceptibility to predation, and habitat and temporal differences in food distribution and availability during the course of evolution (Clarke & Boinski, 1995; Gosling & John, 1999). Mettke-Hofmann, Ebert, Schmidt, Steiger, and Stieb (2005) showed that the correlation between two behaviors typically indicative of boldness can differ between two closely related species of warbler. They compared neophobic and exploratory behaviors between the species at two different times of year: once at the end of the breeding season, and again 10 months later, at the beginning of the following breeding season. Nonmigratory Sardinian warblers showed consistency in personality over time, and neophobia and exploration were negatively related to one another. In contrast, the migratory garden warblers neither behaved consistently over time nor showed a correlation between neophobia and exploration. These results suggest that behavior is more flexible across

time and context in one species of warbler than in the other, and that such increased flexibility is likely necessitated by the variety of challenges presented by migration. In individuals of migratory species, the dimensions of personality so far studied may exert less of a constraining effect on behavior and therefore result in fewer tradeoffs. This lower constraint in turn may predispose individuals to be better able to survive the long migratory journey and subsequently make the rapid behavioral adjustments necessary to adapt to a new environment. In contrast, behavioral consistency or predictability may benefit individuals of nonmigratory species, for example, by facilitating the maintenance of long-term social relationships. If nonmigratory birds are more likely to encounter the same individuals regularly across their lifespan (whereas migratory birds may be more likely to experience frequent turnover in their associations), behavioral predictability will better allow individuals to remember and appropriately respond to one another, facilitating social stability.

Many studies of personality among nonhuman primates have compared different populations or species. Clarke and Boinski (1995) compared personality in three species of macaque—rhesus, bonnet, and longtailed—and found that long-tailed macaques were the most behaviorally responsive, but also rather fearful; bonnets were the most passive; and rhesus were the most active and hostile. de Waal and Luttrell (1989) compared the differing styles of social organization of rhesus and stump-tailed macaques (*Macaca arctoides*) and showed again that rhesus monkeys were more aggressive and less relaxed, tolerant, and socially cohesive than the stump-tails. One of us suggested that the marked behavioral and social organization differences between macaque species are not a result of differences in personality structure, per se, but of differences in where each species' modal "location" is along the dimensions that make up the structure (Capitanio, 2004). In the case of de Waal's data, for example, both stump-tailed and rhesus macaques may demonstrate the dimension Agreeableness, but stump-tails as a species may have a higher modal value for Agreeableness compared to rhesus. Within the genus *Macaca*, for example, evolution of the various species may have resulted from natural selection operating on a relatively fixed set of traits in the ancestral species. Complex species differences in personality and social organization may have resulted from straightforward differences in ecological pressures. If, for example, a group of animals occupied a habitat in which it was advantageous for individuals to exercise a high degree of vigilance and protectiveness in their daily actions (perhaps due to heavy predation pressure), the resulting social structure of the group may very likely exhibit stylistic differences compared to that of a group of individuals whose tendencies toward vigilance and protectiveness were less strong. With reproductive isolation, the different groups may eventually have evolved into different species.

Evidence for this phenomenon in nonhuman primates comes from intraspecific studies relating population differences in environment to those of personality. Johnson and Southwick (1984) found that maternal style of free-ranging rhesus macaques varied among three populations and was affected by the level of environmental risk for infant mortality, such that mothers in higher-risk environments were more protective of their infants than were mothers in lower-risk areas. Similarly, Hauser and Fairbanks (1988) found that in wild vervet monkeys, mothers that lived in groups with a higher-quality food supply were more rejecting toward, and had more conflict with, their infants than mothers in neighboring groups with poorer food quality. Given that nonhuman primate mothers exert a large degree of control over their infants' social interactions early in life, and variation in maternal style has been shown to have long-term consequences for a variety of behaviors exhibited by offspring (Fairbanks, 1996), it is not difficult to imagine how relatively simple differences in predation risk or food availability could lead to the differences in personality and social organization that distinguish different species.

The studies discussed above highlight the importance of considering ecological factors when attempting to relate personality to functionally important consequences. A particularly important consideration when interpreting individual differences in personality is that such differences are highly dependent on the ecological and social environment of the study population (Clarke & Boinski, 1995). In the following discussion of the use of animals in modeling personality traits of humans, we urge the reader to bear in mind the salient differences between humans and model species, as well as the importance of examining other (especially closely related) species in order to better understand the evolution of human personality.

ANIMAL MODEL RESEARCH

Since virtually the beginning of modern psychology, nonhuman animals have been used to model psychological and physiological processes, with a goal of elucidating analogous or homologous (Campbell & Hodos, 1970) processes in humans. Of course, in any area, a model is not exactly the same as the thing being modeled, so care must be taken to ensure the validity of the model (Crnic, Reite, & Shucard, 1982). While we recognize the value and importance of studying personality/temperament in a variety of species, in this section we review data from nonhuman primate studies that demonstrate some of the questions that have been asked in trying to understand psychological and physiological processes from an "animal model" perspective. Other chapters in this volume address many of these issues in human studies. We recognize that this review is not comprehensive, although it does summarize data from several laboratories that have long-standing research programs in primate personality. Other important research programs not covered in detail in this review include those by J. R. Kaplan, N. H. Kalin, and J. E. King and their colleagues (e.g., Kaplan, Manuck, Fontenot, & Mann, 2002; Nelson, Shelton, & Kalin, 2003; Pederson, King, & Landau, 2005).

Prenatal Contributions to Personality

The prenatal period is often overlooked when one considers the role of "experience" in shaping personality. In one sense this is odd, because inasmuch as personality is an emergent property of brain activity, the prenatal period is the principal time in an organism's life when brain development proceeds most rapidly, and developmental trajectories are most likely to be impacted by particular experiences. In another sense, however, the lack of attention paid to the prenatal period is not surprising, given the logistical difficulties in studying this developmental period in humans. Nonhuman primate studies have been important in understanding the role of prenatal experience in personality, owing not only to the ability to experimentally manipulate conditions and to obtain samples (both behavioral and physiological) more regularly, but also because of the ability to follow animals longitudinally in a time frame that is considerably accelerated compared to that for humans.

Schneider developed a paradigm for inducing prenatal stress in pregnant rhesus monkey females that was simple yet produced dramatic results. During mid- to late-gestation, pregnant females were relocated to a cage in an adjacent room for a 10-minute period, during which they experienced three randomly distributed noise bursts of 1-second duration each. This simple procedure was repeated 5 days per week for a few weeks. In comparison to control animals whose mothers were not exposed to this stressor during pregnancy, prenatally stressed (PNS) animals showed impaired neuromotor development and attentional deficits at birth (Schneider, 1992a); more disturbance and less exploratory behavior in a playroom setting at 6 months of age (Schneider, 1992b); continued deficits in exploration and increased disturbance behavior, as well as excessive clinging under stressful conditions assessed at 18 months of age (Clarke & Schneider, 1993); and impaired adaptability and sociability (as indexed by greater inactivity and less proximity) in a social setting at 4 years of age (Clarke, Soto, Bergholz, & Schneider, 1996). Behaviorally, these results suggested to the authors that prenatal stress appeared to result in an "inhibited" personality (Clarke & Schneider, 1997). Further results by this group suggested the neural substrates that might be involved. Specifically, this paradigm for inducing prenatal stress has been shown to result in persisting alterations in functioning of the hypothalamic–pituitary–adrenal axis (a major stress-response system; Clarke, Wittwer, Abbott, & Schneider, 1994), elevations in cerebrospinal fluid concentrations of dopamine and norepinephrine metabolites (Schneider et al., 1998), and reduced neurogenesis in the dentate gyrus (Coe et al., 2003). Finally, these prenatal stress-induced

biobehavioral changes have also been linked to impaired immune system function (Coe, Kramer, Kirschbaum, Netter, & Fuchs, 2002), suggesting possible health implications.

The Importance of Early Postnatal Social Experience

Many readers of this chapter are already aware of the contributions of nonhuman primate research to the study of personality: We refer to the studies of Harlow and Mason, dating from the 1950s, that examined the role of early social experience in the development of social and emotional competence. Although these studies were not framed as investigations into "personality," per se, the pervasive deficiencies in emotionality, social abilities, and overall responsiveness resulting from adverse early experience reflect psychological processes that are fundamental to personality (see Capitanio, 1986, for a comprehensive review of this literature). In the parlance of the FFM, adult rhesus monkeys that were reared with limited or no social opportunities (and in a restricted laboratory environment) for the first year of life could be described as showing little social interest and competence (very low Extraversion, Agreeableness, and Conscientiousness) as well as low adaptability and high volatility (high Neuroticism, low Openness).

Gene × Environment Interactions

While the above research suggests an important role for experience in the development of personality, even extreme reductions in socioemotional opportunities, exemplified by the studies of isolation rearing early in life, did not always produce uniform results. With recent advances in molecular genetic techniques, interest has grown in documenting how different patterns of responsiveness can result, even within the same environments, depending on the individual's genotype. The gene that has been studied most frequently is associated with the central nervous system monoamine neurotransmitter serotonin. Once released into the synaptic cleft, serotonin is drawn back inside the neuron in a process known as "reuptake." The gene that codes for the protein responsible for reuptake has a promoter region upstream of the gene itself that controls the transcription of the gene. The promoter has two forms (alleles) in both humans and rhesus monkeys. The short allele results in reduced efficiency in transcription of the reuptake protein, compared to the long form of the gene (Heils et al., 1996). Thus, three genotypes are possible: long–long, long–short, or short–short.

Research with humans has demonstrated personality correlates of variation in the serotonin transporter promoter polymorphism. For example, a meta-analysis revealed that possession of a short allele is associated with Neuroticism, as measured by the NEO Personality Inventory (Sen, Burmeister, & Ghosh, 2004). Moreover, interactions of genotype and life stress have been reported for depression and suicidality, such that individuals possessing a short allele who encounter life stress are at greater risk than those possessing two long alleles (Caspi et al., 2003). Experimental research with nonhuman primates has begun to explore such genotype-by-environment interactions, with much of the published data emerging from the National Institute of Health (NIH) laboratories of Suomi and Higley. The animal model permits exploration not only of the behavioral phenomena, but also the neural substrates of the behavior. In these studies, animals are typically reared either with their mothers (usually in a social group) or with peers in a nursery setting (Shannon, Champoux, & Suomi, 1998). On a neonatal assessment battery modeled after the Brazelton scale, nursery-reared (NR) infants showed higher scores on an Orientation cluster, reflecting better visual orientation and attention, than did mother-reared (MR) animals. Genotype interacted with rearing environment, however: A short allele was associated with lower Orientation scores, but only for NR animals, not for MR infants (Champoux et al., 2002). As juveniles, NR monkeys with a short allele also showed higher rates of aggressive behavior, compared to MR monkeys with a short allele (Barr et al., 2003). Impulsive aggressiveness has been associated with reduced concentrations in cerebrospinal fluid of the serotonin metabolite 5-HIAA in rhesus monkeys (Higley et al., 1992; similar results have been found for low serotonin function in humans: see Carver & Miller, 2006), and

in fact Bennett and colleagues (2002) reported that, although the serotonin genotype was not related to 5-HIAA concentrations in MR animals, there was an effect in NR animals: Possession of a short allele was associated with reduced 5-HIAA concentrations. Finally, in a study of alcohol consumption by adolescent female monkeys, genotype was again found to interact with early rearing experience, in that the greatest alcohol consumption was found for heterozygous animals that had been peer reared (Barr, Schwandt, Newman, & Higley, 2004). Together, these data demonstrate clearly the phenomenon of genotype-by-environment interactions, as well as the value of an experimental approach to studying the nature of such interactions on behavioral traits and later outcomes.

Health-Related Outcomes

The relationship between personality and health has been of interest for decades. Nonhuman primate personality research has explored both correlates of, and mechanisms associated with, health outcomes. Attention has focused on the trait Sociability. This is one of four personality dimensions identified in adult male rhesus monkeys (Capitanio, 1999; Capitanio & Widaman, 2005), using the rating methodology (see above). The emphasis in this research program has been on conducting the initial personality assessments in the familiar social groups into which the animals had been born, and then measuring behavioral and physiological outcomes in very different contexts and at time points that could be many years after the initial personality assessments. In these studies, Sociability has been found to reflect a tendency to affiliate, as indexed by greater frequencies of approaches, higher durations of social grooming, and lower durations of time spent alone (Capitanio, 1999). Centrally, Sociability is associated with greater sensitivity in dopaminergic function, a result reminiscent of data from humans for the trait Extraversion (e.g., Depue & Collins, 1999; Netter, 2006).

The first indication that Sociability might be associated with health-related outcomes was from a post hoc analysis of personality and immune measures taken from a study of simian immunodeficiency virus (SIV) disease progression (Capitanio et al., 1999). SIV infection in rhesus monkeys is widely considered the best animal model for AIDS, and results in a disease course that closely mimics the human disease, although at a more accelerated rate. In SIV-infected monkeys, animals higher in Sociability had a greater decline in SIV riboneucleic acid (RNA), which is a measure of viral load and is a strong predictor of survival in both humans and monkeys. Once humans or monkeys are infected with their respective immunodeficiency viruses, the ability of their immune systems to control already-present (i.e., latent) infections with herpesviruses can become impaired. We found that a decline in antibody to the latent herpesvirus cytomegalovirus (CMV) was associated with faster disease progression (Baroncelli et al., 1997), and it was animals that had been rated lower in Sociability years earlier that showed the greatest decline in the CMV antibody response (Capitanio et al., 1999).

The result that Sociabililty might be associated with disease-related outcomes prompted further prospective studies of animals selected as being high or low in Sociability. We assessed personality of adult male rhesus monkeys while they lived in their familiar outdoor social groups, and then relocated them to indoor housing. Our first hypothesis was that such a change in social environment might have a greater "meaning" to high- versus low-sociable animals, and result in different immune responses. Shortly after the move, we vaccinated the animals with tetanus toxoid, using a veterinary preparation of the same vaccine that humans receive about every 10 years. High-sociable animals had significantly higher tetanus-specific antibody responses to vaccination compared to low-sociable animals (Maninger et al., 2003), confirming our expectation. Later (Capitanio et al., in press), animals were inoculated with SIV to study disease progression; half of the animals experienced stable social conditions, and the other half unstable, stressful social conditions. Personality differences were again found. Within the first few weeks following infection, low-sociable monkeys showed indications of faster disease progression, but only if they were in the unstable social conditions—a personality-by-situation interaction. Specifically, low-sociable animals displayed a greater innate immune response compared to high-sociable monkeys. This immune response was an increase in the transcription of genes in immune system white blood cells that are associated with antiviral proteins called interferons. Normally, such an immune response would be beneficial, but in the context of SIV or HIV infection, it is not; this response reflects greater viral replication, and in fact is associated with higher viral load, itself a strong predictor of more rapid disease progression. Examination of the behavioral and hormonal responses of the animals again revealed personality-by-situation interactions. Low-sociable animals in unstable conditions coped by showing more sustained submissive behavior, and also displayed a plasma cortisol profile indicative of social stress, compared to high-sociable animals in unstable conditions. All of the relationships between Sociability and outcome measures (gene expression, submissive behavior, and cortisol) were statistically significant for animals in unstable social conditions; none of these relationships was significant for animals in stable conditions. Thus, these data demonstrate that early in immunodeficiency virus infection, personality factors can be influential in the body's ability to develop an immune response to the virus, and this action appears to be mediated by the effect of personality on coping processes, in particular (Capitanio et al., in press).

Personality was also found to be related to a potentially important mechanism that could mediate the effects on disease. Lymph nodes are structures dispersed throughout the body, and many of the body's immune responses take place there. Lymph nodes are innervated by fibers of the sympathetic nervous system, which secrete norepinephrine, and norepinephrine can have a significant adverse impact on immune function, especially in the context of HIV infection (e.g., Cole, Korin, Fahey, & Zack, 1998). This innervation provides one way in which the brain can communicate its state to the body's immune system. Working with lymph nodes from uninfected monkeys, Sloan and colleagues (in press) found that high- and low-sociable animals have lymph nodes that are "wired" differently. Specifically, low-sociable animals had a 2.8-fold greater density of catecholamine-secreting nerves compared to high-sociable monkeys. Because norepinephrine can accelerate HIV replication in vitro (Cole et al., 1998), these results provide a plausible mechanism for why SIV-infected animals that are low-sociable and that experience stressful circumstances should have evidence of accelerated disease progression (Capitanio et al., in press).

These studies demonstrate the range of questions that can be asked in an animal modeling context that would either be very difficult or impossible to perform with humans, yet, given the similarity in personality dimensions between monkeys and humans, also show direct relevance to human physical and mental health and suggest new avenues of research.

PRACTICAL APPLICATIONS OF ANIMAL PERSONALITY RESEARCH

There has been a growing interest in how an individual-differences approach can inform practical solutions to common challenges in working with animals. Here we briefly review some selected applications.

Training of Animals

In a nonhuman primate research laboratory, there are many situations in which training of animals is essential for their effective use in experimental research. For example, rhesus monkeys can be trained to extend their arms for phlebotomy, a practice that results in a substantial reduction in stress to the animal, compared to blood sampling that involves the more usual physical restraint or chemical immobilization. Coleman, Tully, and Mc-Millan (2005) used a simple assessment of temperament to identify animals that were more easily trained to perform a simple instrumental task. A human observer stood in front of the animal's cage and placed a novel food item within the animal's reach. Animals were classified as "exploratory" (inspected the novel food within 10 seconds), "moderate" (inspected the food within the 3-minute trial but not within the first 10 seconds), or "inhibited" (did not inspect the food within the 3-minute trial). Over 85% of the exploratory monkeys, and 75% of the moderate monkeys learned the instrumental task of touching a target. In contrast, only 22% of the inhibited monkeys performed the task consistently. While the authors readily acknowledged the caveat that excluding poten-

tial research subjects based on temperament can create problems for generalizability of results, the project does provide a quantitative approach to a phenomenon that everyone who has ever trained a rhesus monkey (or any animal) has experienced—namely, that some individuals learn tasks more readily than others.

Well-Being of Laboratory Animals

Just as there are individual differences in trainability that depend on personality processes, so too do such differences relate to other aspects of well-being in a laboratory environment. As described above, animals that display an inhibited temperamental style show deficiencies in social abilities and general adaptability. Boyce, O'Neill-Wagner, Price, Haines, and Suomi (1998) reported that such animals are also at greater risk for injuries. Owing to reconstruction of a rhesus monkey troop's outdoor 5-acre habitat, animals were confined for a 6-month period to a large (1,000 square feet) indoor enclosure. Veterinary records were examined and comparisons were made of preconfinement, confinement, and postconfinement periods. Approximately one-third of the animals were rated high on inhibition, and it was these animals that sustained the greatest increase in injuries during the confinement period.

An interesting approach to great ape personality has been taken by King and colleagues, who have developed an instrument based on the FFM. Recently, this approach was extended to the much understudied ape, the orangutan (Weiss, King, & Perkins, 2006). Five factors (Extraversion, Dominance, Neuroticism, Agreeableness, and Intellect) were found. In addition to conducting personality ratings, the zoo keepers also rated animals on a measure of "subjective well-being," which reflected items such as how pleasurable and satisfying the social interactions were for the target orangutan, and how happy the rater would be if he or she were the target orangutan for a week. The measure of well-being was positively correlated with Extraversion and Agreeableness and negatively correlated with Neuroticism.

Together, these data suggest that knowledge of an animal's personality characteristics could be valuable for management of an animal colony, a recognition that has prompted two laboratories to implement broad-based assessment programs aimed at quantifying personality for just this reason (Capitanio, Kyes, & Fairbanks, 2006; Fairbanks, 2001).

Personality-Based Selection for Working-Dog Occupations

It has been well documented in the field of personnel selection that some personalities are better suited than others to certain jobs (Hogan, Hogan, & Roberts, 1996). Selecting the right personality for the job improves the effectiveness with which the job is performed and the well-being and satisfaction of the individual in the job. The principles of personnel selection can also be applied to the animal domain. A dog that is fearful is not well suited to bomb detection, where it will be required to work in environments that are unusual, unpredictable, and noisy. Training a working dog requires a substantial investment of resources, so organizations that raise and place working dogs have a keen interest in directing those resources to the individuals best suited to the job. As a result, the vast majority of personality studies of dogs have been done by these organizations on the two most widely used breeds, Labrador retrievers and German shepherds (Jones & Gosling, 2005). One study of 2,655 German Shepherds and Belgian Tervurens showed that boldness assessed in a series of behavioral tests between 12 and 18 months of age predicted success in subsequent working-dog trials (Svartberg, 2002); although there were breed differences in boldness, these differences accounted for only part of the variance in performance. This study showed that some personalities are better suited than others to work-relevant tasks, and it demonstrated that these personalities can be identified through a reasonably straightforward battery of tests.

Personality assessments of domestic animals have also been developed to help potential owners identify a pet that matches their needs (Coren, 1998) and to assist with adoption decisions at animal shelters (Ledger & Baxter, 1996). In one study Ledger and Baxter (1996) showed that the behavioral responses of animal-shelter dogs to an unfamiliar person entering their kennel correlated 0.64 with ratings of excitability subsequently made by their new owners after adoption. Clearly, such information would be very useful in setting realistic owner expectations about their new dog and in matching dogs to suitable homes, both of which would reduce the rate of unsuccessful adoptions.

CONCLUSIONS

The review above has described three broad domains in which personality research in nonhumans is flourishing. Several points emerge from this review. First, there is now a reasonably broad base of personality research on animals, with much of it emanating from fields other than mainstream personality. This research base reflects a diversity of species and is notable in that many of the personality dimensions that have been studied are not only similar across species, but are remarkably similar to those found in our own species. Second, just as in other fields of psychology that have turned to animal models, animal personality researchers are studying animals because they make it possible to address questions that would not be possible to address in human studies. Advantages of studying nonhuman species include more rapid development, shorter generation time, greater experimental control, and greater access to tissue samples. Third, the studies conducted to date are just beginning to scratch the surface of the questions that can be addressed using animal subjects. There are many more questions pertaining to central nervous system function, health outcomes, the role of genetics, the importance of prenatal experience, and so on, that can be explored in nonhumans and that are relevant to similar questions that are being, or could be, asked about humans. Finally, animal personality research is providing links to fields hitherto unconnected to the field of human personality, such as behavioral ecology. Why is there something called "personality" in humans, and where did it come from? Certainly, it is more than just coincidental that human and nonhuman primates share many personality characteristics as well as underlying brain substrates. Does it make sense to think about human personality from the perspective of tradeoffs, as behavioral ecologists do? The study of nonhuman personality provides a rich context for understanding the natural world and humans' own place in it.

REFERENCES

Altmann, J. (1974). Observational study of behavior: Sampling methods. *Behaviour, 49,* 227–265.

Baroncelli, S., Barry, P. A., Capitanio, J. P., Lerche, N. W., Otsyula, M., & Mendoza, S. P. (1997). Cytomegalovirus and simian immunodeficiency virus coinfection: Longitudinal study of antibody responses and disease progression. *Journal of Acquired Immune Deficiency Syndromes and Human Retrovirology, 15,* 5–15.

Barr, C. S., Newman, T. K., Becker, M. L., Parker, C. C., Champoux, M., Lesch, K. P., et al. (2003). The utility of the non-human primate model for studying gene by environment interactions in behavioral research. *Genes, Brain, and Behavior, 2,* 336–340.

Barr, C. S., Schwandt, M. L., Newman, T. K., & Higley, J. D. (2004). The use of adolescent nonhuman primates to model human alcohol intake: Neurobiological, genetic, and psychological variables. *Annals of the New York Academy of Sciences, 1021,* 221–233.

Bennett, A. J., Lesch, K. P., Heils, A., Long, J. C., Lorenz, J. G., Shoaf, S. E., et al. (2002). Early experience and serotonin transporter gene variation interact to influence primate CNS function. *Molecular Psychiatry, 7,* 118–122.

Both, C., Dingemanse, N. J., Drent, P. J., & Tinbergen, J. M. (2005). Pairs of extreme avian personalities have highest reproductive success. *Journal of Animal Ecology, 74,* 667–674.

Boyce, W. T., O'Neill-Wagner, P., Price, C. S., Haines, M., & Suomi, S. J. (1998). Crowding stress and violent injuries among behaviorally inhibited rhesus macaques. *Health Psychology, 17,* 285–289.

Budaev, S. V., Zworykin, D. D., & Mochek, A. D. (1999). Individual differences in parental care and behaviour profile in the convict cichlid: A correlation study. *Animal Behaviour, 58,* 195–202.

Buss, A. H. (1988). *Personality: Evolutionary heritage and human distinctiveness.* Hillsdale, NJ: Erlbaum.

Campbell, C. B. G., & Hodos, W. (1970). The concept of homology and the evolution of the nervous system. *Behavior, Brain, and Evolution, 3,* 353–367.

Capitanio, J. P. (1986). Behavioral pathology. In G. Mitchell & J. Erwin (Eds.), *Comparative primate biology* (Vol. 2A, pp. 411–454). New York: Liss.

Capitanio, J. P. (1999). Personality dimensions in adult male rhesus macaques: Prediction of behaviors across time and situation. *American Journal of Primatology, 47,* 299–320.

Capitanio, J. P. (2002). Sociability and responses to video playbacks in adult male rhesus monkeys (*Macaca mulatta*). *Primates, 43,* 169–177.

Capitanio, J. P. (2004). Personality factors between and within species. In B. Thierry, M. Singh, & W. Kaumans (Eds.), *Macaque societies: A model for the study of social organization* (pp. 13–37). Cambridge, UK: Cambridge University Press.

Capitanio, J. P., Abel, K., Mendoza, S. P., Blozis, S. A., McChesney, M. B., Cole, S. W., et al. (in press). Personality and serotonin transporter genotype interact with social context to affect immunity and viral set-point in simian immunodeficiency virus disease. *Brain, Behavior, and Immunity.*

Capitanio, J. P., Kyes, R. C., & Fairbanks, L. A. (2006). Considerations in the selection and conditioning of Old World Monkeys for laboratory research: Animals from domestic sources. *ILAR Journal, 47,* 294–306.

Capitanio, J. P., Mendoza, S. P., & Baroncelli, S. (1999). The relationship of personality dimensions in adult male rhesus macaques to progression of simian immunodeficiency virus disease. *Brain, Behavior, and Immunity, 13,* 138–154.

Capitanio, J. P., Mendoza, S. P., & Bentson, K. L. (2004). Personality characteristics and basal cortisol concentrations in adult male rhesus macaques (*Macaca mulatta*). *Psychoneuroendocrinology, 29,* 1300–1308.

Capitanio, J. P., & Widaman, K. F. (2005). Confirmatory factor analysis of personality structure in adult male rhesus monkeys (*Macaca mulatta*). *American Journal of Primatology, 65,* 289–294.

Caspi, A., Sugden, K., Moffitt, T. E., Taylor, A., Craig, I. W., Harrington, H., et al. (2003). Influence of life stress on depression: Moderation by a polymorphism in the 5-HTT gene. *Science, 301,* 386–389.

Champoux, M., Bennett, A., Shannon, C., Higley, J. D., Lesch, K. P., & Suomi, S. J. (2002). Serotonin transporter gene polymorphism, differential early rearing, and behavior in rhesus monkey neonates. *Molecular Psychiatry, 7,* 1058–1063.

Clarke, A. S., & Boinski, S. (1995). Temperament in nonhuman primates. *American Journal of Primatology, 37,* 103–125.

Clarke, A. S., & Schneider, M. L. (1993). Prenatal stress has long-term effects on behavioral responses to stress in juvenile rhesus monkeys. *Developmental Psychobiology, 26,* 293–304.

Clarke, A. S., & Schneider, M. L. (1997). Effects of prenatal stress on behavior in adolescent rhesus monkeys. *Annals of the New York Academy of Sciences USA, 807,* 490–491.

Clarke, A. S., Soto, A., Bergholz, T., & Schneider, M. L. (1996). Maternal gestational stress alters adaptive and social behavior in adolescent rhesus monkey offspring. *Infant Behavior and Development, 19,* 451–461.

Clarke, A. S., Wittwer, D. J., Abbott, D. H., & Schneider, M. L. (1994). Long-term effects of prenatal stress on HPA axis activity in juvenile rhesus monkeys. *Developmental Psychobiology, 27,* 257–269.

Coe, C. L., Kramer, M., Czeh, B., Gould, E., Reeves, A. J., Kirschbaum, C., et al. (2003). Prenatal stress diminishes neurogenesis in the dentate gyrus of juvenile rhesus monkeys. *Biological Psychiatry, 54,* 1025–1034.

Coe, C. L., Kramer, M., Kirschbaum, C., Netter, P., & Fuchs, E. (2002). Prenatal stress diminishes the cytokines response of leukocytes to endotoxin stimulation in juvenile rhesus monkeys. *Journal of Clinical Endocrinology and Metabolism, 87,* 675–681.

Cole, S. W., Korin, Y. D., Fahey, J. L., & Zack, J. A. (1998). Norepinephrine accelerates HIV replication via protein kinase A-dependent effects on cytokine production. *Journal of Immunology, 161,* 610–616.

Coleman, K., Tully, L. A., & McMillan, J. L. (2005). Temperament correlates with training success in adult rhesus macaques. *American Journal of Primatology, 65,* 63–71.

Coren, S. (1998). *Why we love the dogs we do: How to find the dog that matches your personality.* New York: Free Press

Crnic, L. S. , Reite, M. L., & Shucard, D. W. (1982). Animal models of human behavior: Their application to the study of attachment. In R. N. Emde, & R. J. Harmon (Eds.), *Development of attachment and affiliative systems* (pp. 31–42). New York: Plenum Press.

Dall, S. R. X., Houston, A. I., & McNamara, J. M. (2004). The behavioural ecology of personality: Consistent individual differences from an adaptive perspective. *Ecology Letters, 7,* 734–739.

de Waal, F. B. M., & Luttrell, L. M. (1989). Toward a comparative socioecology of the genus *macaca:* Different Dominance styles in rhesus and stumptail monkeys. *American Journal of Primatology, 19,* 83–109.

Dingemanse, N. J., Both, C., Drent, P. J., & Tinbergen, J. M. (2004). Fitness consequences of avian personalities in a fluctuating environment. *Proceedings of the Royal Society of London Series B-Biological Sciences, 271,* 847–852.

Domjan, M., & Purdy, J. E. (1995). Animal research in psychology: More than meets the eye of the general psychology student. *American Psychologist, 50,* 496–503.

Fairbanks, L. A. (1996). Individual differences in maternal style: Causes and consequences for mothers and offspring. *Advances in the Study of Behavior, 25,* 589–611.

Fairbanks, L. A. (2001). Individual differences in response to a stranger: Social impulsivity as a dimension of temperament in vervet monkeys (*Cercopithecus aethiops sabaeus*). *Journal of Comparative Psychology, 115,* 22–28.

Fraley, R. C., Brumbaugh, C. C., & Marks, M. J. (2005). The evolution and function of adult attachment: A comparative and phylogenetic analysis. *Journal of Personality and Social Psychology, 89,* 731–746.

Gilbert, D. T., Fiske, S. T., & Lindzey, G. (1998). *The handbook of social psychology* (4th ed.). Oxford, UK: Oxford University Press.

Godin, J. G. J., & Dugatkin, L. A. (1996). Female mating preference for bold males in the guppy, *Poecilia reticulata. Proceedings of the National Academy of Sciences USA, 93,* 10262–10267.

Gosling, S., Kwan, V. S. Y, & John, O. P. (2003). A dog's got personality: A cross-species comparative approach to personality judgments in dogs and humans. *Journal of Personality and Social Psychology, 85,* 1161–1169.

Gosling, S. D. (1998). Personality dimensions in spotted hyenas (*Crocuta crocuta*). *Journal of Comparative Psychology, 112,* 107–118.

Gosling, S. D. (2001). From mice to men: What can we learn about personality from animal research? *Psychological Bulletin, 127,* 45–86.

Gosling, S. D., & John, O. P. (1999). Personality dimensions in nonhuman animals: A cross-species review. *Current Directions in Psychological Science, 8,* 69–75.

Gosling, S. D., & Vazire, S. (2002). Are we barking up the right tree? Evaluating a comparative approach to personality. *Journal of Research in Personality, 36,* 607–614.

Groothuis, T. G. G., & Carere, C. (2005). Avian personalities: Characterization and epigenesis. *Neuroscience and Biobehavioral Reviews, 29,* 137–150.

Hauser, M. D., & Fairbanks, L. A. (1988). Mother offspring conflict in vervet monkeys: Variation in response to ecological conditions. *Animal Behaviour, 36,* 802–813.

Heils, A., Teufel, A., Petri, S., Stober, G., Riederer, P., Bengel, D., et al. (1996). Allelic variation of human serotonin transporter gene expression. *Journal of Neurochemistry, 66,* 2621–2624.

Higley, J., Mehlman, P., Taub, D., Higley, S., Suomi, S., Vickers, J., et al. (1992). Cerebrospinal fluid monoamine and adrenal correlates of aggression in free-ranging rhesus monkeys. *Archives of General Psychiatry, 49,* 436–441.

Hogan, R., Hogan, J., & Roberts, B. W. (1996). Personality measurement and employment decisions: Questions and answers. *American Psychologist, 51,* 469–477.

Hogan, R., Johnson, J. A., & Briggs, S. R. (1997). *Handbook of personality psychology.* New York: Academic Press.

John, O. P. (1990). The "Big Five" factor taxonomy: Dimensions of personality in the natural language and in questionnaires. In L. A. Pervin (Ed.), *Handbook of personality: Theory and research* (pp. 66–100). New York: Guilford Press.

Johnson, R. L., & Southwick, C. H. (1984). Structural diversity and mother–infant relations among rhesus-monkeys in India and Nepal. *Folia Primatologica*, *43*, 198–215.

Jones, A. C., & Gosling, S. D. (2005). Temperament and personality in dogs (*Canis familiaris*): A review and evaluation of past research. *Applied Animal Behaviour Science*, *95*, 1–53.

Kaplan, J. R., Manuck, S. B., Fontenot, M. B., & Mann, J. J. (2002). Central nervous system monoamine correlates of social dominance in cynomolgus monkeys (*Macaca fascicularis*). *Neuropsychopharmacology*, *26*, 431–443.

Kenny, D. A. (1994). *Interpersonal perception: A social relations analysis*. New York: Guilford Press.

King, J., & Figueredo, A. (1997). The five-factor model plus dominance in chimpanzee personality. *Journal of Research in Personality*, *31*, 257–271.

Kwan, V. S. Y., Gosling, S. D., & John, O. P. (2008). Anthropomorphism as a special case of social perception: A cross-species comparative approach and a new empirical paradigm. *Social Cognition*, *26*, 129–142.

Ledger, R. A., & Baxter, M. (1996). A validated test to assess the temperament of dogs. In I. J. H. Duncan, T. M. Widowski, & D. B. Haley (Eds.), *Proceedings of the 30th International Congress of the ISAE* (p. 111). Guelph, ON, Canada: Colonel K. L. Campbell Centre for the Study of Animal Welfare.

Maninger, N., Capitanio, J. P., Mendoza, S. P., & Mason, W. A. (2003). Personality influences tetanus-specific antibody response in adult male rhesus macaques after removal from natal group and housing relocation. *American Journal of Primatology*, *61*, 73–83.

McCrae, R. R., Costa, P. T., Jr., Ostendorf, F., Angleitner, A., Hrebickova, M., Avia, M. D., et al. (2000). Nature over nurture: Temperament, personality, and life span development. *Journal of Personality and Social Psychology*, *78*, 173–186.

Mettke-Hofmann, C., Ebert, C., Schmidt, T., Steiger, S., & Stieb, S. (2005). Personality traits in resident and migratory warbler species. *Behaviour*, *142*, 1357–1375.

Nelson, E. E., Shelton, S. E., & Kalin, N. H. (2003). Individual differences in the responses of naive rhesus monkeys to snakes. *Emotion*, *3*, 3–11.

Netter, P. (2006) Dopamine challenge tests as an indicator of psychological traits. *Human Psychopharmacology: Clinical and Experimental*, *21*, 91–99.

Nettle, D. (2006). The evolution of personality variation in humans and other animals. *American Psychologist*, *61*, 622–631.

Noldus, L. P. J. J. (1991). The observer: A software system for collection and analysis of observational data. *Behavior Research Methods, Instruments and Computers*, *23*, 415–429.

Pavlov, I. P. (1906). The scientific investigation of the psychical faculties or processes in the higher animals. *Science*, *24*, 613–619.

Pederson, A. K., King, J. E., & Landau, V. I. (2005). Chimpanzee (*Pan troglodytes*) personality predicts behavior. *Journal of Research in Personality*, *39*, 534–549.

Pervin, L. A., & John, O. P. (1999) *Handbook of personality: Theory and research*. New York: Guilford Press.

Ray, J. C., & Sapolsky, R. M. (1992). Styles of male social behavior and their endocrine correlates among high-ranking wild baboons. *American Journal of Primatology*, *28*, 231–250.

Reale, D., Gallant, B. Y., Leblanc, M., & Festa-Bianchet, M. (2000). Consistency of temperament in bighorn ewes and correlates with behaviour and life history. *Animal Behaviour*, *60*, 589–597.

Ruys, J. D., Capitanio, J. P., & Mendoza, S. P. (2002). Individual differences in personality and neuroendocrine responses to pharmacological treatment in adult male rhesus macaques (*Macaca mulatta*). *American Journal of Primatology*, *57*(S1), 78.

Sapolsky, R. M., & Ray, J. C. (1989). Styles of dominance and their endocrine correlates among wild olive baboons (*Papio anubis*). *American Journal of Primatology*, *18*, 1–13.

Schneider, M. L. (1992a). The effect of mild stress during pregnancy on birthweight and neuromotor maturation in rhesus monkey infants (*Macaca mulatta*). *Infant Behavior and Development*, *15*, 389–403.

Schneider, M. L. (1992b). Prenatal stress exposure alters postnatal behavioral expression under conditions. *Developmental Psychobiology*, *25*, 529–540.

Schneider, M. L., Clarke, A. S., Kraemer, G. W., Roughton, E. C., Lubach, G. R., Rimm-Kaufman, S., et al. (1998). Prenatal stress alters brain biogenic amine levels in primates. *Development and Psychopathology*, *10*, 427–440.

Sen, S., Burmeister, M., & Ghosh, D. (2004). Meta-analysis of the association between a serotonin transporter promoter polymorphism (5-HTTLPR) and anxiety-related personality traits. *American Journal of Medical Genetics: Part B, Neuropsychiatric Genetics*, *127B*, 85–89.

Sih, A., Bell, A. M., Johnson, J. C., & Ziemba,

R. E. (2004). Behavioral syndromes: An integrative overview. *Quarterly Review of Biology, 79*(3), 241–277.

Sloan, E. K., Capitanio, J. P., Tarara, R. P., & Cole, S. W. (in press). Social temperament and lymph node innervation. *Brain, Behavior, and Immunity.*

Svartberg, K. (2002). Shyness–boldness predicts performance in working dogs. *Applied Animal Behaviour Science, 79*, 157–174.

Vazire, S., Gosling, S. D., Dickey, A. S., & Schapiro, S. J. (in press). Measuring personality in nonhuman animals. In R. W. Robins, R. C. Fraley, & R. F. Krueger (Eds.), *Handbook of research methods in personality psychology* (pp. 190–206). New York: Guilford Press.

Verbeek, M. E. M., Boon, A., & Drent, P. J. (1996). Exploration, aggressive behavior and dominance in pair-wise confrontations of juvenile male great tits. *Behaviour, 133*, 945–963.

Verbeek, M. E. M., De Goede, P., Drent, P. J., &

Wiepkema, P. R. (1999). Individual behavioural characteristics and dominance in aviary groups of great tits. *Behaviour, 136*, 23–48.

Virgin, C. E., & Sapolsky, R. M. (1997). Styles of male social behavior and their endocrine correlates among low-ranking baboons. *American Journal of Primatology, 42*, 25–39.

Weiss, A., King, J. E., & Perkins, L. (2006). Personality and subjective well-being in orangutans (*Pongo pygmaeus* and *Pongo abelii*). *Journal of Personality and Social Psychology, 90*, 501–11.

Wilson, D. S. (1998). Adaptive individual differences within single populations. *Philosophical Transactions of the Royal Society of London, Series B, 353*, 199–205.

Wilson, D. S., Clark, A. B., Coleman, K., & Dearstyne, T. (1994). Shyness and boldness in humans and other animals. *Trends in Ecology and Evolution, 9*, 442–446.

Zajonc, R. B. (1969). *Animal social psychology.* New York: Wiley.

PART IV

Developmental Approaches

CHAPTER 13

Parents' Role in Children's Personality Development

The Psychological Resource Principle

Eva M. Pomerantz
Ross A. Thompson

As has been noted by numerous scholars of personality, there are remarkable differences among individuals on a host of psychological dimensions. Elucidating the key differences (e.g., John, Chapter 4, this volume; Robins, Chapter 16, this volume), the nature of these differences (e.g., McCrae & Costa, Chapter 5, this volume; Schultheiss, Chapter 24, this volume), and their consequences (e.g., Fraley & Shaver, Chapter 20, this volume; Lucas & Diener, Chapter 32, this volume) are fundamental endeavors to understanding personality. However, insight into personality cannot be fully achieved without also elucidating its development—that is, how differences among individuals evolve (see Pomerantz & Newman, 2000). There is now much evidence that the development of psychological functioning is shaped by multiple forces ranging from the biological to the familial to the cultural (for a review, see Bugental & Grusec, 2006). Despite some arguments to the contrary (e.g., Harris, 1995; Scarr & McCartney, 1983), socialization by parents is key (see Baumrind, 1993; Collins, Maccoby, Steinberg, Hetherington, & Bornstein, 2000). A number of diverse strands of theo-

ry and research indicate that from the very first days of children's lives onward, parents' socialization practices play a central role in shaping children's psychological trajectories (for reviews, see Bornstein, 2006; Parke & Buriel, 2006).

Throughout our species' evolution, children have depended on the resources parents provide, making parents unique influences on virtually all aspects of development (Clutton-Brock, 1991; Thompson et al., 2005). The most fundamental relationships in children's lives are often those they have with their parents. Even as peers become increasingly prominent in children's lives, parents continue to be central (e.g., Offer & Offer, 1975). Thus from infancy through adolescence, and perhaps beyond, children look to parents to provide important psychological resources. We take the perspective that parents' provision of such resources shapes children's personality development (see also Eccles, Early, Frasier, Belansky, & McCarthy, 1997; Grolnick, Deci, & Ryan, 1997). When parents create a psychologically positive environment, children flourish; when parents fail to do so, children suffer.

As a consequence of their genetic heritage, as well as their experiences outside the home, children come to their interactions with parents varying in their psychological resources. Because such resources influence parents' practices, as well as children's responses to those practices, the role of parents in children's personality development is shaped, in part, by children themselves (see Pomerantz, Wang, & Ng, 2005b). Hence, as a number of scholars have argued, although parents are a central influence in the socialization process, children are active agents in the process as well (e.g., Belsky, 1984; Collins et al., 2000; Grusec & Goodnow, 1994).

The goal of this chapter is to explicate the role of parents in shaping children's personality development. To this end, we focus on a central principle of parents' socialization of their children: Parents shape children's personality development through their provision of psychological resources. Because of controversy over whether parents actually contribute to children's development beyond their genetic legacy, we begin by making the case that despite the support for the role of genetics, there is also support for the role of socialization by parents. We then discuss the major models and methods guiding research on parental influence. In the subsequent section, we explicate the psychological resource principle. In this context, we discuss the psychological resources important to children's personality development and how parents facilitate the growth of such resources. We then turn to the implications of the psychological resource principle for understanding how parents and children jointly contribute to the socialization process as well as contextual variations in this process.

DO PARENTS REALLY MATTER?

Asking whether socialization by parents really makes a difference in children's personality development would have struck previous generations of investigators as odd or even as naive, but current developmental scientists are asking this question with considerable seriousness. The reason for their concern is research in developmental behavioral genetics that uses twin and adoption studies to estimate the genetic contribution to human characteristics, including personality attributes in children (for reviews, see Plomin, DeFries, McClearn, & Rutter, 1997; Rutter, 2006; Rutter, Silberg, O'Connor, & Simonoff, 1999). Based on such research, some investigators argue that traditional conclusions about the profound influence of parents' behavior (e.g., nurturance, sensitivity, and punitiveness) on children's personality must be reconsidered to reflect the more profound influence of shared genes as the basis for both parental and child personality and the characteristics they share.

Because identical twins are genetically identical and fraternal twins share only about half their genes, developmental behavioral genetics research can estimate genetic and environmental contributions to a wide range of human characteristics. Similar estimates can also be derived from studies of adopted children. Several conclusions have emerged from a large body of twin and adoption studies. First, the proportion of variability owing to genetic differences among individuals on many dimensions of psychological functioning—expressed as a "heritability" estimate—can be high. Heritability estimates for many personality attributes range from .20 to .80, often at, or above, .50, indicating that from 20 to 80% of the variance in these attributes is due to genetic influences. Second, research also shows that parents respond differentially to children's hereditary characteristics, treating temperamentally easy offspring much differently, for example, than temperamentally difficult children. Thus parenting practices are adapted in response to, and sometimes evoked by, hereditary characteristics of children. This influence is called the "gene–environment correlation," and it reflects one way in which genetic processes alter the environmental influences that children experience (Scarr & McCartney, 1983; see also Roberts, Wood, & Caspi, Chapter 14, this volume).

Third, in studies of the association between parenting and children's personality, most traditional socialization research confounds the influence of parents' socialization practices with the contributions of their genes to children's personality development. Children may become prone to aggressive behavior, for example, not only because of a home environment in which parents are punitive and are thus models of aggressive conduct, but also because of shared genes that contribute to aggression in both parents and children. Indeed, parents' practices may arise in response to the attributes of children that have a hereditary basis. When traditional research measures only the association between parents' practices and children's subsequent personality, the assumption is often that earlier parenting *caused* children's personality without consideration that shared genes may be underlying the association.

Based on the conclusions from the developmental behavioral genetics research, several scholars have argued that parents have much less—and very different—influence on the development of personality in children than traditional socialization theories portray (e.g., Harris, 1995; Rowe, 1994; Scarr, 1992). They argue that parents are important for providing an adequately supportive environment in which children's genetically based individual attributes can develop. Differences in parents' practices within the normal range do not influence children's attributes to a great extent, they conclude, because of the preeminence of heredity. Indeed, research in developmental behavioral genetics indicates that the most important kind of environmental influence on children is "nonshared" rather than "shared." Shared environmental influences are those that individuals, such as siblings, have in common and that contribute to their similarities—for example, the influence of parents' childrearing styles, the availability of books in the home, or familial economic resources—consistent with traditional socialization views. By contrast, nonshared environmental influences are those that contribute to differences among individuals in the same environment. To some developmental scholars, the preeminence of the non-shared environment points to influences outside the home—specifically, the peer environment—as the source of the nonshared influences that contribute to the distinctive personality attributes of children within a family (Harris, 1995).

Taken together, the critique of traditional parent–child socialization research from developmental behavioral genetics has provoked a reconsideration of the relative importance of genes and parenting practices in children's personality development. It has caused greater numbers of developmental scientists to enlist genetically sensitive research designs in their work. As a consequence, an expanding body of research can now begin to address the relative influence of genes and the environment, as well as their interaction, on children's development (see Collins et al., 2000). But there are several reasons why the conclusion that genes, rather than parenting practices, are determinative is premature and somewhat misleading. Indeed, for these reasons, we believe the conclusion that traditional socialization research findings are uninterpretable is also incorrect.

First, heritability estimates are not stable, generalizable human attributes but, rather, are relative to the populations and contexts studied (Plomin et al., 1997). As a population statistic expressed as a proportion of explained variance, in other words, heritability depends on the genetic and environmental characteristics of the particular population studied. Heritability estimates tend to be lower in populations characterized by considerable environmental diversity and higher in genetically more heterogeneous populations. To illustrate, Turkheimer and colleagues (Turkheimer, Haley, Waldron, D'Onofrio, & Gottesman, 2003) found that whereas genetic differences explained more than 80% of the variance in IQ for 7-year-old twins growing up in affluent families, environmental (shared and nonshared) influences explained the same proportion of variance in IQ for twins growing up in impoverished families. *Environment was a greater influence on IQ in homes characterized by greater variability in resources.*

Partly for this reason, heritability estimates are not indications of the malleability of human characteristics (Maccoby, 2000; Plomin et al., 1997). First, interventions that alter relevant aspects of the environment, such as changes in parents' practices (but also educational opportunities, therapeutic support, and improved nutrition) can significantly change attributes that have a strong genetic basis. Although individual differences in height are highly heritable, for example, there have been considerable increases in average height in many populations during the past century owing to improved nutrition, medical care, and other environmental influences; children rescued from impoverished environments likewise exhibit impressive gains in height (and weight) with therapeutic assistance. For these and other reasons, many developmental scholars have abandoned reliance on heritability estimates because they provide a misleadingly precise quantitative index of genetic influence that is ambiguous when interpreted (see Rutter, 2006).

Second, research studies show that efforts to modify parenting practices can change the behavior of parents, which, in turn, influences children in ways that cannot be explained by the hereditary characteristics they share (for reviews, see Baumrind, 1993; Shonkoff & Phillips, 2000). As one example, van den Boom (e.g., 1994) enlisted mothers of irritable infants into an intervention study designed to improve mothers' sensitivity through individualized training sessions. At the end of the training, mothers in the intervention group were more responsive to their children than control group mothers, and their infants were also more sociable, exploratory, and securely attached. Findings such as these are the foundation for an extensive range of intervention efforts to improve parenting; the findings document that changes in parenting can create predictable changes in the functioning of children (Shonkoff & Phillips, 2000). Taken together, such findings offer strong evidence that parenting substantially influences children's personality development in ways predicted by traditional socialization theory.

Third, although the distinction between shared and nonshared environment is conceptually important, its relevance to a critique of traditional socialization research is misunderstood. Indeed, we would argue that most parenting practices should be conceptualized as contributing to *nonshared* environmental influences because parents develop unique relationships with each of their offspring, treat siblings distinctively because of their individual attributes (e.g., age, sex, and temperament), and change their parenting practices with time and experience (Grusec & Goodnow, 1994; Holden & Miller, 1999). This perspective is consistent with traditional socialization theory: Although some of these adaptations result from the gene–environment correlations discussed above, research shows that gene–environment correlations typically account for only a small part of the variability in children's attributes, with parents' behavior remaining a large, independent influence (Rutter et al., 1999).

Finally, research in developmental behavior and molecular genetics shows that the most important influences on children likely derive from an *interaction* of genes with environment (Plomin & Rutter, 1998; Rutter et al., 1997; Rutter, Moffitt, & Caspi, 2006; Rutter & Silberg, 2002). In particular, as molecular genetics enables investigators to identify markers for specific genes and their associations with behavior, they are discovering that hereditary influences are polygenic and multifactorial, involving the impact of multiple genes co-acting with environmental influences to increase the probability of certain behavioral attributes (Plomin & Rutter, 1998). Contrary to traditional views of genetic influence, in other words, gene action has probabilistic (not static) effects on behavior, based on the action of other genes and the environmental conditions in which genes function. As one simple illustration of gene–environment interaction, Caspi and colleagues (2002) found that in a large sample of men followed longitudinally, a childhood history of maltreatment predicted adult antisocial behavior, but these effects were moderated by activity of a gene encoding the monoamine oxidase A (MAO-A) enzyme, which had been previously linked to aggressive behavior. Although the main effect of MAO-A activity on antisocial behavior was not evident, men with a history of maltreatment and low MAO-A activity exhibited heightened risk for antisocial conduct, whereas those with a maltreatment history and high MAO-A activity did not. For men growing up in well-functioning homes, there were no differences according to MAO-A activity.

Indeed, the interaction between genes and environment has been traced to the level of environmental influences on biochemical factors that alter gene expression, showing that variations in the maternal care of rat pups, for example, alters gene expression in brain regions governing endocrine and autonomic reactivity to stress, causing offspring to respond with fearful, anxious reactions to environmental events—but that postnatal experience can reverse these effects (Kaffman & Meaney, 2007; Meaney & Szyf, 2005; Parent et al., 2005). Such an interactive process at multiple levels of analysis underscores the conclusion of a National Academy of Sciences report that "the long-standing debate about the importance of nature *versus* nurture … is overly simplistic and scientifically obsolete" (Shonkoff & Phillips, 2000, p. 6).

What does the findings from the work on genetics mean for the study of parental influences on children's personality development? First, genetically informed research designs should be enlisted whenever possible to better understand genetic and environmental influences, as well as their interaction, on personality growth. Second, the interpretation of research findings not so designed can be aided by an expanding body of research on genetic and environmental sources of variability underlying central dimensions of parent and child functioning. For example, recent studies indicate that heritability is low and shared and nonshared environmental influences high for parental sensitivity, parent–child relationship quality, and the security of attachment in the early years (see Bokhorst et al., 2003; O'Connor & Croft, 2001; Roisman & Fraley, 2006). Awaiting further studies of this kind, and acknowledging the reciprocal influences that occur in parent–child interaction, we can proceed with the assumption that children's personality development is affected by *both* parental genes and behavior—and indeed, that the influence of one does not undermine the importance of the other. We now turn to a discussion of the major theoretical models and empirical methods guiding the bulk of research on socialization by parents.

MODELS AND METHODS

Models

Theory and research on the role of parents in children's personality development has been guided by three general models of the socialization process: unidirectional, interactive, and transactional models (see Sameroff, 1975). In the early years of concern with understanding parents' role, parents were considered to have a unidirectional influence on children (e.g., Baldwin, 1955; Sears, Maccoby, & Levin, 1957). Although originally emerging out of the Freudian perspective, such *unidirectional models* are consistent with the social learning perspective in which children's psychological development is viewed as shaped almost exclusively by children's environment through parents' modeling and reinforcement (e.g., Bandura, 1986;

Mischel, 1966). For example, when parents use harsh disciplinary practices with their children, they model aggressive behavior, which children in turn adopt in interacting with others (see McCord, 1988; Patterson & Capaldi, 1991). Most contemporary theories, however, are guided by unidirectional models positing that parents influence children through a host of more complex psychological mechanisms (e.g., Glasgow, Dornbusch, Troyer, Steinberg, & Ritter, 1997; Kochanska, 2002; Laible & Thompson, 2002; Pomerantz et al., 2005b). For example, parents' conversations with children about everyday experiences provide children with insight into others' emotions and expectations, as well as into the self; such insight may shape children's subsequent behavior (Thompson, Laible, & Ontai, 2003).

Although models depicting the socialization process as a unidirectional transmission from parents to children guide much contemporary theory and research, there is general consensus that children also play a role in the socialization process. Indeed, owing, in part, to developmentalists' awareness of the importance of children's genotypic individuality, children are thought to play a role in shaping how parents influence them (e.g., Bugental & Grusec, 2006; Collins et al., 2000; Parke & Buriel, 2006). *Interactive models* of socialization describe the effects of parenting as contingent on what children bring to their interactions with parents. The earliest version of such a model is Thomas and Chess's (1977) idea of "goodness of fit." Thomas and Chess suggested that the fit between parenting practices and children's temperament is critical to children's subsequent development. This idea that parenting does not have a uniform impact on children, but instead depends on what children bring to their interactions with parents, is consistent with the concept of gene–environment interaction discussed above, but also drives a number of contemporary theories of parental socialization (e.g., Bugental, 2004; Pomerantz et al., 2005b; Schwartz, Dodge, Pettit, Bates, & Conduct Problems Prevention Research Group, 2000). For example, Kochanska (e.g., 1993) argues that gentle discipline is most effective in promoting internalization of parents' rules among temperamentally fearful children because it fosters optimal anxious arousal among such children, thereby sensitizing them to their parents' messages; gentle discipline is much less effective with temperamentally fearless children, as it fosters little anxious arousal in such children. Although what children bring to their interactions with parents may be biologically based, it may also depend on prior socialization experiences (e.g., Grusec & Goodnow, 1994; Pomerantz et al., 2005b).

In *transactional models* of socialization, children are viewed as active agents who shape the parenting they receive, which in turn shapes them (see Sameroff, 1975; Scarr & McCartney, 1983; Thomas, Chess, & Birch, 1970). Some versions of the transactional model of socialization have implicated children's genetically based attributes as central in evoking responses from parents that in turn maintain such attributes, so that there is continuity within children over time (see Lytton, 2000; Scarr & McCartney, 1983). In this vein, several scholars have made the case that the problems for children who have aggression issues may spiral out of control over the course of development, because such children elicit negative responses from parents that further contribute to children's aggression (e.g., Lytton, 2000; Patterson, Bank, & Stolmiller, 1990). However, parents' responses to children's attributes may also change children (see Bell & Chapman, 1986). In this vein, Pomerantz and Eaton (2001) provide evidence consistent with the idea that parents respond to children's poor performance in school through heightened assistance with homework, which in turn facilitates, rather than undermines, children's subsequent performance. Other transactional models incorporate the mutual influences of parents and children into relationship-oriented formulations by characterizing parent–child dyads as mutually responsive or securely attached (e.g., Bowlby, 1969; Thompson et al., 2005). Such characterizations recognize that although each partner makes important contributions to the quality of the relationship (e.g., through parental sensitivity and child temperament), the interaction of these characteristics over time results in a dyadic quality that is "more than the sum of the parts" (Laible & Thompson, 2007). The value of this approach is reflected in a large body of research documenting how attachment security predicts personality development (for a review, see Thompson, 2006).

Methods

Parenting Assessment

A key challenge in assessing parenting is that investigators cannot unobtrusively monitor the daily interactions between parents and children in the home around the clock. Hence, investigators have had to satisfy themselves with the use of multiple assessments that, taken together, provide a holistic appraisal of parenting. Three forms of assessment are common: Observations, parent reports, and child reports. Observational methods are often used in the laboratory and, less frequently, in the home. Such methods generally involve the observation of parents and children interacting in the context of a setting constructed to reflect real-life activities. For example, in her research with mothers and toddlers, Kochanska (e.g., Kochanska, Aksan, Penney, & Boldt, 2007) observed parents cleaning up as well as making cupcakes in both the home and laboratory. In an effort to create tasks mirroring academic activities, Grolnick and colleagues (Grolnick, Gurland, DeCourcey, & Jacob, 2002), for example, had parents and children create a map or write a poem. Observational techniques are also used in unstructured settings, most commonly in the form of free play tasks in which parents and children play with a set of toys (e.g., Askan, Kochanska, & Ortmann, 2006; Deci, Driver, Hotchkiss, Robbins, & Wilson, 1993).

Observational methods have a number of strengths. First, they allow for an objective assessment of parents' actual behavior because individuals who code parents' behavior do not harbor social desirability concerns. Second, structured settings allow for control over the activities in which parents and children engage, thereby ensuring that differences in parenting do not reflect differences in activities. Even in unstructured settings, there is some control over the activities, given that the same stimuli are available to all parents and children. Third, observational methods are ideal for assessing the minute-by-minute interactions between parents and children. On the negative side, observational techniques do not necessarily capture parenting during the ins and outs of daily life (see Pomerantz & Ruble, 1998b). Parents may attend more to children during observational tasks than they do on a day-today basis. In addition, some of the activities used for observations are ones that may not reflect parents' and children's daily activities. Parents' social desirability concerns may also influence parents' and children's behavior, as they often know they are being videotaped.

Parents frequently serve as reporters of their own parenting. Indeed, there are a number of measures designed to assess parents' beliefs about parenting as well as their actual parenting (for a review, see Holden & Edwards, 1989). These measures often ask parents to rate their agreement with multiple statements about parenting. For example, the Parenting Stress Index developed by Abidin (1995) asks parents to directly report the demands and problems they experience in the parental role. Another popular approach is to present parents with a series of scenarios and ask them to rate how likely they would be to respond in a variety of ways. The Coping with Children's Negative Emotions Scale (Fabes, Poulin, Eisenberg, & Madden-Derdich, 2002) asks parents to identify how they would respond to children's negative emotions as described in 12 commonly occurring, hypothetical scenarios. Such questionnaires are useful in that they can assess parenting across a wide range of situations that may not be captured in observational settings.

However, parents' reports may be problematic in that they reflect parents' beliefs about what they should do rather than what they actually do (see Holden & Edwards, 1989; Pomerantz & Ruble, 1998b). To address this issue, some investigators rely on reports from parents in which they report on their interactions with children each day (e.g., Crouter, Helms-Erikson, Updegraff, & McHale, 1999; Patterson & Stouthamer-Loeber, 1984). For example, to examine how parents respond to their children's small failures in daily life, Ng, Kenney-Benson, and Pomerantz (2004) had mothers report every day for 10 days on whether their children had a failure and how they responded to it. These reports may be less prone to bias by parents' beliefs because parents must think specifically about what happened that particular day. However, there may still be some social desirability issues as parents are reporting on their own behavior (for the strengths and weaknesses of daily reports, see Bolger, Davis, & Rafaelli, 2003).

Many investigators working with children old enough to report on the parenting they receive use children's reports. Most commonly, children rate their agreement with statements about how their parents treat them. For example, in Schaefer's (1965) Child Report of Parental Behavior Inventory, which is frequently used in contemporary research (e.g., Barber, Stolz, & Olsen, 2006), children indicate their agreement with statements such as "My mom lets me do anything I would like" and "My mother lets me go any place I please without asking." Such reports can be valuable because they index children's *interpretations* of parents' practices, which may be more important in understanding the influence of parenting than direct observations of parents alone. Children's reports are not only associated with parents' reports (e.g., Pomerantz, 2001; Smetana, 1995), but actually appear to be more accurate than are parents' reports in that they are more strongly associated with observers' ratings of parenting (Sessa, Avenevoli, Steinberg, & Morris, 2001). Children's reports also allow for a broader sample of participants because it is often easier to recruit children on their own to participate during school hours than to meet with parents and children together outside of school hours.

Unfortunately, children's reports are problematic in that they may be confounded with their functioning; for example, depressed children may be particularly likely to view their parenting experiences in a negative light. Many investigators have addressed this issue by using longitudinal designs that partial out children's functioning at the point at which parenting was assessed, then predicting children's functioning at a later time point (e.g., Barber et al., 2006; Steinberg, Lamborn, Darling, Mounts, & Dornbusch, 1994; Wang, Pomerantz, & Chen, 2007).

Research Designs

The early research aimed at understanding the role of parents in children's personality development used concurrent, correlational designs in which parenting was assessed at one time point and linked to children's functioning at that same time point (e.g., Baumrind, 1971; Sears et al., 1957). Although such a design is still used (e.g., Davidov & Grusec, 2006; Nelson, Hart, Chongming, Olsen, &

Shenghua, 2006), acknowledgment of children's influence on parents (and the critique of genetically informed scientists) has led to greater reliance on longitudinal designs, in which parenting is assessed at one time point and used to predict, sometimes in interaction with children's attributes, children's functioning at a later time point (e.g., Kochanska, 1997; Pettit, Bates, & Dodge, 1997; Pomerantz, Wang, & Ng, 2005a). Such a design provides insight into whether parenting actually foreshadows children's personality. As noted, longitudinal designs commonly adjust for children's functioning at the initial time point, which takes investigators one step closer to ruling out the possibility that children's functioning is the driving effect of parenting. However, such adjustments are not always recommended because they may overcontrol for antecedent influences (children's prior functioning is affected by parenting as well as heredity) and may not be possible if aspects of children's functioning are not present early in development or cannot be measured comparably. Even more sophisticated designs allow for the simultaneous examination of parent and child effects (e.g., Eisenberg et al., 2003; Stice & Barrera, 1995; Wang et al., 2007), thereby identifying transactional processes (for additional methods of examining transactional processes, see Sameroff & Macenzie, 2003).

Although longitudinal, correlational designs provide windows into the direction of effects, they are still characterized by third-variable problems. That is, other (often unmeasured) variables may be influencing both parents' and children's behavior and their association over time. Investigators have addressed this possibility to some extent by adjusting for a variety of potential third variables, such as parents' socioeconomic status, educational attainment, and psychopathology, and using genetically informed research designs (e.g., Caspi et al., 2002; Dodge, Pettit, Bates, & Valente, 1995; Madon, Guyll, Spoth, Cross, & Hilbert, 2003). However, because it is impossible to take into account all potential third variables, it is important to complement correlational designs with experimental ones. Unfortunately, this approach is all too infrequent in work on parenting. However, when such an approach has been used, it has proved quite fruitful.

Three major strategies can be employed experimentally. First, investigators can cre-ate interventions to change parenting practices; they may then examine whether these changes influence children's functioning. As noted earlier, van den Boom (e.g., 1994) taught mothers of irritable infants sensitive parenting skills, which not only enhanced their parenting compared to mothers of irritable infants who were not taught such skills, but also enhanced children's functioning. Second, investigators can examine whether the practices used by parents actually exert a causal effect by manipulating them in the laboratory. For example, the wide body of research demonstrating that parental control foreshadows negative functioning in children (e.g., Barber, 1996; Frodi, Bridges, & Grolnick, 1985; Pettit et al., 1997) is supported by experimental studies manipulating the exertion of control by an experimenter in the laboratory (e.g., Lepper & Greene, 1975; Ryan, Mims, & Koestner, 1983; Vansteenkiste, Simons, Lens, Soenens, & Matos, 2005). A third strategy, guided by transactional models of socialization, manipulates the behavior of children and examines how adults respond to such behavior (e.g., Bugental, Lyon, Krantz, & Cortez, 1997; Keller & Bell, 1979). Bugental, Caporael, and Shennum (1980), for example, assessed women's physiological arousal while interacting with computer-simulated children who behaved either responsively or unresponsively. Women's arousal was different in each condition, underscoring the important influences that children's responsiveness can have on adult practices.

Summary

In sum, theory and research concerned with parents' role in children's personality development is guided by a set of models that vary in the extent to, and manner in which, parents and children contribute to such development. Taken together, these models suggest that although parents shape children's functioning, children are also active agents in the process. Methodological strategies guided by these models have relied mainly on correlational designs, with the most sophisticated research using longitudinal methods to determine not only the role of parenting in the socialization process, but also the role of children. We now turn to an explication of the mechanisms by which parents contribute to children's functioning.

THE PSYCHOLOGICAL RESOURCE PRINCIPLE

Children's biological predispositions, often in the form of temperament, lay the foundation for their subsequent personality development. However, through their provision of psychological resources, parents can also shape the course of such development. In doing so, parents can strengthen children's initial predispositions and the developmental trajectories that ensue, or they can weaken such predispositions, redirecting children onto a new trajectory. The psychological resource principle embodies the idea that parents facilitate the growth of psychological resources that serve as building blocks for children's competent functioning. In this section, we first discuss three key psychological resources—affective, behavioral, and cognitive—and their role in children's competence. We then turn to how parents can encourage the development of such resources, focusing on the affective, behavioral, and cognitive dimensions of parenting.

The ABCs of Psychological Resources: Affect, Behavior, and Cognition

What are the hallmarks of competent functioning in children? We draw from Masten and Coatsworth (1998) in defining competence as success at major developmental tasks. Although there are many such tasks that children encounter throughout their lives, we focus here on three critical ones that emerge early in life (see Roisman, Masten, Coatsworth, & Tellegen, 2004; Shiner, Masten, & Tellegen, 2002). First, competence is evident in children's ability to control their behavior in response to societal rules. This includes complying with the requests of adults, such as parents and teachers, and involves refraining from antisocial behavior as reflected in aggression, delinquency, and other externalizing problems. Second, competent functioning is reflected in children's ability to create positive social relations with adults and peers. In the context of this developmental task, competence involves maintaining relationships of mutual cooperation with adults and acceptance by peers, including the development of friendships. Third, a key developmental task for children (especially once they reach school) is academic achievement, with competent functioning reflected in academic performance. Developmental foundations

for academic achievement emerge in the growth of cognitive skills in early childhood. We now turn to a description of the salient affective, cognitive, and behavioral resources required for children to achieve competence at these tasks. Although children's competent functioning involves an interaction of these resources, this threefold delineation helps to highlight features of parents' contributions to the resources that children require.

Affective Resources

Affective resources include the heightened experience of positive emotions, such as happiness, love, and pride, and the dampened experience of negative emotions, such as sadness, anger, and shame; such resources also involve the capacity for emotion regulation. Although children's emotional experiences are often considered important in and of themselves (for reviews, see Hammen & Rudolph, 2003; Rudolph, Hammen, & Daley, 2006), they also play a role in the development of children's competent functioning. Children's experience of positive emotions signals to them that there is little immediate danger in their environment (for this point in regard to adults, see Lyubomirsky, King, & Diener, 2005). As a consequence, children feel safe to pursue new goals, thereby developing new psychological capabilities that ultimately lead to competent functioning (see Lyubomirsky et al., 2005). In pursuing a new goal, for example, children may cultivate new behavioral repertoires (e.g., strategies for controlling their impulses, harmoniously interacting with peers, and constructively studying) that promote competence at the important developmental tasks with which they are faced.

As is evident from Lyubomirsky and colleagues' (2005) comprehensive review, there is much research linking positive emotions to competent functioning in the social and academic arenas, albeit mainly among adults. Notably, positive emotions foreshadow competence, with experimental studies demonstrating their causal role (for a review, see Lyubomirsky et al., 2005). For example, using experimental methods to induce positive affect in adults, Isen and others (e.g., Hirt, Melton, McDonald, & Harackiewicz, 1996; Isen & Geva, 1987) demonstrated that such affect heightens creativity. Conversely, there is a wealth of evidence linking negative emotions, as well as limited emotion regulation, to a lack of competent functioning in multiple arenas (for reviews, see Rudolph, 2005; Rudolph, Flynn, & Abaied, 2008). Such emotions have been identified as a precursor to dampened competence. For example, in the social arena, depressed children generate heightened interpersonal stress (e.g., Rudolph et al., 2000). In the academic arena, children's depression predicts dampened performance in school over time (e.g., Roeser, Eccles, & Sameroff, 1998).

Behavioral Resources

Although affective resources are important, children also need a behavioral repertoire on which to draw. We use the term "behavioral resources" to refer to the variety of functional strategies that children use in their day-to-day lives to accomplish the goals they are pursuing. These involve constructive tactics for, among other things, delaying gratification, dealing with challenge, and interacting with peers. Behavioral resources such as these are critical to successful goal attainment; without the appropriate actions, even the best of intentions go awry. Moreover, children's behavioral resources are observable. As such, they shape how others respond to them. Influencing others' responses to them may often be the goal of children's behaviors—for example, when children share with their peers so that their peers will like them. Such positive responses may also be a byproduct of children's behavior—for example, when children adopt a mastery orientation in dealing with challenging academic work, teachers respond positively.

In line with the idea that behavioral resources play a key role in children's competent functioning, a wealth of research from different areas indicates that the strategies children adopt play an influential role in such functioning. For example, self-control from an early age has been linked to competent functioning, as manifested in heightened internalization of mothers' rules and decreased externalizing problems (e.g., Eisenberg et al., 2005; Kochanska, Murray, & Coy, 1997). Children's heightened control also appears to enhance performance in school (e.g., Duckworth & Seligman, 2006; Mischel, Shoda, & Rodriguez, 1989). Other behavioral resources are important as well. For example, chil-

dren whose behavioral repertoire includes cooperation, helpfulness, and the initiation of social interactions are well accepted by their peers, often establishing positive friendships beginning in early childhood (e.g., Coie, Dodge, & Kupersmidt, 1990; Parke et al., 1997). In the academic arena, children who focus on mastering their schoolwork rather than becoming helpless in the face of challenge subsequently are protected from affective problems (e.g., Nolen-Hoeksema, Girgus, & Seligman, 1992) and do quite well in school (e.g., Fincham, Hokoda, & Sanders, 1989).

Cognitive Resources

The cognitive resources children possess are also influential in the development of their competent functioning. Children's cognitive resources are manifest in their mental representations of themselves, others, and the world in which they reside. Such representations include, but are not limited to, their perceptions of themselves and others, the attributions they make for their own and others' behavior, the reasons they have for goal pursuit, and the value they place on different goals. Children's mental representations guide their interpretation of their world, which in turn influences their affect and behavior (e.g., Bretherton & Munholland, 1999; Dweck & London, 2004; Eccles, 1983), ultimately shaping how important others respond to them (e.g., Crick & Dodge, 1994; Thompson, 2000).

The empirical evidence for the power of children's cognitive resources in the development of competent functioning is impressive. Mental representations deriving from secure or insecure parent–child attachments (i.e., "internal working models"; Bowlby, 1973) predict young children's social and behavioral competence (for a review, see Thompson, 2000). Children who believe that their peers harbor hostile intentions toward them engage in heightened aggressive behavior that is likely to lead their peers to reject them (for a review, see Crick & Dodge, 1994). Children's perceptions of themselves also foreshadow their competent functioning in the academic arena (for a review, see Guay, Marsh, & Boivin, 2003). The reasons children have for pursuing their goals in the academic arena appear to be of import as well:

When faced with challenge, children who are engaged in academic work to learn rather than to demonstrate that they are smart improve their strategies, refrain from making negative statements about themselves, and ultimately perform better (e.g., Elliott & Dweck, 1988; Kenney-Benson, Pomerantz, Ryan, & Patrick, 2006).

The ABCs of Parents' Provision of Psychological Resources: Affective, Behavioral, and Cognitive Dimensions of Parenting

Given the centrality of parents in children's lives, parents can facilitate or inhibit the growth of the affective, behavioral, and cognitive resources children need for competent functioning. When parents create environments rich in such resources, children may flourish and become competent, constructive members of society; when parents fail to create such environments, children may flounder in developing competence. In this section, drawing from Pomerantz, Grolnick, and Price (2005), we focus on how parents support the growth of children's psychological resources through affective, behavioral, and cognitive avenues of parenting (for more comprehensive reviews of parental socialization, see Bornstein, 2006; Parke & Buriel, 2006). Although each of these avenues of parenting is likely to exert its major influence on children's competence through the corresponding psychological resource in children (e.g., parents' affect contributes to children's affective resources and parents' behavior contributes to children's behavioral resources), each is also likely to influence the other psychological resources.

The Affective Dimension of Parenting

Since the inception of the formal study of parenting, parents' affect toward children has been identified as a central dimension of parenting (e.g., Baldwin, 1955; Sears et al., 1957). Indeed, as Dix (1991) emphasized, parenting is an inherently affective endeavor. As such, it may be characterized by positive affect manifested in parents' enjoyment, warmth, and praise while interacting with their children (e.g., Denham et al., 2000; Nolen-Hoeksema, Wolfson, Mumme, & Guskin, 1995). Although this positive affect may often emanate from parents, it may

also be part of what Maccoby (1992) labels "mutual responsivity" in which parents and children reciprocate shared positive affect (see also Kochanska, 1997). Parents' involvement in children's lives, whereby parents provide support to children and their endeavors, has been included as a dimension of parental warmth as well (e.g., Grolnick, Kurowski, & Gurland, 1999; Steinberg et al., 1994). Parents' interactions with children can also be characterized by negative affect, as manifested in their annoyance, hostility, and criticism while interacting with children (e.g., Denham et al., 2000; Nolen-Hoeksema et al., 1995). Such negative affect may sometimes emerge in response to children's negative affect—a pattern that can lead to escalating spirals of negative affect (e.g., P. M. Cole, Teti, & Zahn-Waxler, 2003; Patterson, 1982).

From infancy, parents directly transmit their affect to their children, thereby contributing to children's affective resources. When parents are affectively positive (vs. negative) in their interactions with infants and children, they sustain and even foster positive emotions in them. In contrast, when parents express negative affect, they transmit negative emotions. In line with this idea, using experience-sampling methods, Larson and Gillman (1999) showed that in single-parent households, mothers' expression of negative emotions, such as anxiety, foreshadowed their adolescents' experience of such emotions 2 hours later. Mothers' emotional expressions toward children have also been linked to ongoing emotional distress in children (e.g., Denham et al., 2000). For example, mothers' high positive and low negative affect while assisting their elementary school children with homework, as assessed in daily interviews, predicts increased positive and decreased negative emotional functioning in children 6 months later (Pomerantz et al., 2005a). Importantly, parents' negative affect—especially when it is directed at children—appears to affect not only children's immediate emotions, but also their capacity for emotion regulation; thus parents' affect influences children's affective resources in multiple ways (Thompson & Meyer, 2007).

Although the major role of parents' affect in the socialization process may be to shape children's affective resources, parents' affect may also shape children's behavioral resources. Parents' negative (vs. positive) affectivity may overarouse children, and this overarousal may interfere with their attentional and processing abilities, thereby inhibiting the development of such behavioral resources as effortful control (see Hoffman, 2000). Moreover, several investigators have made the case that parents' positive (vs. negative) affect predisposes children to internalize parents' requests, instructions, and values (see Dix, 1991; Grusec & Goodnow, 1994), so that children are motivated and able to learn from their parents' scaffolding (see Eisenberg et al., 2005). Through their positive affect, parents also model constructive responses to challenge, conveying to children that although the situation with which they are confronted (e.g., awaiting their turn, a disagreement with a peer, or a difficult homework assignment) may be frustrating, it can be overcome (Eisenberg et al., 2005; Pomerantz et al., 2005a). In contrast, when parents become irritated and frustrated in the face of challenge, they may convey to children that giving up or venting bad feelings is the best strategy (Thompson & Meyer, 2007).

Consistent with the idea that parents' affect contributes to children's behavioral resources, Eisenberg and colleagues (e.g., Eisenberg et al., 2003) found that parents' expression of positive affect during interactions with children at early adolescence foreshadows children's heightened self-control. In addition, parents' high positive and low negative affect while working with children on challenging tasks, such as homework, has been linked to reduced helplessness in children (e.g., Nolen-Hoeksema et al., 1995; Pomerantz et al., 2005a). It is possible, indeed likely, that the link documented between parents' affect and children's behavioral resources is not a direct one, but rather mediated by the affective resources fostered by parents' affect (see Eisenberg et al., 2005; Pomerantz et al., 2005a).

Parents' affect may shape children's cognitive resources in several ways. When they demonstrate positive (vs. negative) affect toward their children, parents convey that their children are worthy. Such an affective parental style also conveys to children that they live in a world in which others are well intentioned. As a consequence, children may develop positive perceptions of themselves and others. This is the view underlying attachment theorists' belief that from secure early attachments, young children create mental working models of relationships that cause them to approach others in a more trusting manner—a view that is supported by research findings that securely attached children function more positively in other close relationships, such as with peers and teachers (for a review, see Thompson, 2006). Third, by demonstrating heightened positive affect, even when they might be frustrated, parents convey to children that challenges are not necessarily threatening and can even create opportunities for enjoyable learning experiences—an attitude that may influence, in turn, children's goal orientation. Consistent with this idea, mothers' heightened positive and reduced negative affect in the context of assisting their elementary schoolchildren with their homework predicts increased mastery orientation toward schoolwork and intrinsic reasons for doing schoolwork in children 6 months later (Pomerantz et al., 2005a).

The Behavioral Dimension of Parenting

Parents' behavior during their interactions with children plays an important role in the development of children's psychological resources. Although a number of practices (e.g., conversational style, mastery focus, sensitivity, and responsivity) have been deemed significant in parents' socialization of their children (e.g., Gottfried, Fleming, & Gottfried, 1994; Kochanska & Coy, 2002; Laible & Thompson, 2002), we focus on two that have been identified as central: parents' autonomy support versus control and their provision of structure versus chaos (see Baumrind, 1971; Grolnick et al., 1997).

In conjunction with their affect, parents' autonomy support versus control was identified as a key dimension in early work on parenting (e.g., Baldwin, 1955; Schaefer, 1959). Hence, an extensive body of theory and research has focused on multiple forms of parental autonomy support and control (for reviews, see Barber, 2002; Pomerantz & Ruble 1998a; Rollins & Thomas, 1979). Here, we draw on Deci and Ryan's (1987) self-determination theory, in which autonomy support is defined as allowing children to explore their environment, initiate their own behavior, take an active role in solving their own problems, and independently express themselves. Controlling behavior, in contrast, involves the exertion of pressure by parents to channel children toward particular outcomes (e.g., doing well in school). Such pressure often takes the form of directives, commands, and love withdrawal.

When parents are autonomy supportive rather than controlling, they provide children with the experience of solving problems and challenges on their own, which may facilitate children's development of behavioral resources. In the context of solving problems on their own, children may develop strategies to deal with the difficulties with which they are confronted (e.g., Ng et al., 2004; Nolen-Hoeksema et al., 1995). In contrast, when parents are controlling, children have fewer opportunities to develop such strategies. In line with this analysis, parents' autonomy support (vs. control), assessed using a variety of methods, predicts enhanced self-control, mastery behavior, and constructive learning strategies during the toddler through adolescent years (e.g., Frodi et al., 1985; Kochanska & Knaack, 2003; Nolen-Hoeksema et al., 1995; Steinberg, Elmen, & Mounts, 1989; Wang et al., 2007). Moreover, maternal sensitivity—which can be viewed as an age-appropriate manifestation of autonomy support for infants and toddlers—is associated with enhanced cognitive and language development and more advanced play in very young children (e.g., Bornstein & Tamis-LeMonda, 1997; Damast, Tamis-LeMonda, & Bornstein, 1996). Investigators concerned with the role of parents in children's peer relations have documented that parents' heightened control, often in the form of harsh discipline, predicts dampened social skills and heightened aggressive behavior in children (e.g., Dodge, Pettit, & Bates, 1994; Pettit et al., 1997), which may be due not only to the lack of opportunity to solve problems on their own, but also to messages that exerting control (often in the form of aggression) is acceptable (McCord, 1988) and that others have hostile, rather than supportive, intentions (Weiss, Dodge, Bates, & Pettit, 1992).

When parents support children's autonomy, they allow children to take initiative and express their opinions, thereby cultivating cognitive resources in them. Parents' support for autonomy communicates to children that they are competent and au-

tonomous individuals. As a consequence, children may develop positive mental representations of themselves and others, as well as intrinsic reasons for pursuing their goals (see Grolnick et al., 1999; Pomerantz et al., 2005b). In contrast, when parents are controlling, they communicate to children that they lack the competence and autonomy to do things on their own, thereby undermining children's perceptions of themselves and reinforcing extrinsic reasons for pursing goals. Consistent with this idea, much research links parents' heightened autonomy support to positive perceptions of competence and intrinsic motivation in children throughout the school years (e.g., Ginsburg & Bronstein, 1993; Grolnick, Ryan, & Deci, 1991). In addition, children may develop positive representations of others when parents are autonomy supportive, because such an orientation is responsive to children's needs and desires, whereas controlling parents privilege their own needs and desires over their children's. Indeed, when parents refrain from using harsh discipline, children are less likely to see their peers as harboring hostile intent toward them (e.g., Weiss et al., 1992).

Although parents' autonomy support (vs. control) has been linked to enhanced affective resources in children (for a review, see Gerlsma, Emmelkamp, & Arrindell, 1990), often foreshadowing such resources (e.g., Barber et al., 2006; Wang et al., 2007), this link is likely to be indirect, mediated by the effects of such parenting on children's behavioral and cognitive resources. For example, parents' autonomy support (vs. control) is associated with diminished depressive symptoms in children, but this link is accounted for by the tendency of children with autonomy supportive parents to hold few extrinsic reasons for pursuing perfectionistic standards (Kenney-Benson & Pomerantz, 2005).

Another important parenting behavior, albeit one that has received less attention than parents' support for autonomy, is the extent to which parents create a structured versus chaotic environment for children. Structure entails the provision of a systematic framework oriented toward the development of children's competence through the use of clear and consistent guidelines, expectations, and rules (Grolnick & Ryan, 1989; Skinner, Johnson, & Snyder, 2005). Structure also involves predictable consequences for children's actions and clear feedback, thereby making the relations between children's actions and outcomes apparent to them. Such an environment allows children to anticipate consequences and plan behavior accordingly (Grolnick & Ryan, 1989; Skinner et al., 2005). In contrast, some parents provide a chaotic environment in which guidelines, expectations, and rules are unclear and inconsistent as well as arbitrary—a situation that may obscure children's recognition of the consequences of their behavior (Skinner et al., 2005).

The structure (vs. chaos) that parents provide is likely to contribute to the development of children's behavioral and cognitive resources. On the behavioral front, a structured environment helps children learn what the standards are and how to fulfill them, which may assist them in developing useful strategies. In contrast, a chaotic environment may give children little information that is relevant to developing such strategies. Research focusing on the quality of parental assistance and instruction to children suggests that it has benefits for children's behavioral resources (e.g., Pianta, Smith, & Reeve, 1991). For example, using observations of mothers with their preschool children, Pianta, Nimetz, and Bennett (1997) showed that the more that mothers' instruction involved teaching, including an initial orienting instruction and well-timed hints, the better were children's work habits in school during kindergarten. Mothers' structured instruction with children when they were in preschool also predicted enhanced frustration management and social skills during kindergarten. In addition, when parents monitor children's behavior, by checking on their whereabouts and making rules for their safety, children are less likely to develop externalizing symptoms (for a review, see Weisz, Sweeney, Proffitt, & Carr, 1993).

Parental structure may also promote cognitive resources (Grolnick & Ryan, 1989; Skinner et al., 2005). When expectations and guidelines are clear and consistent, children can foresee the effects of their actions, which allows them to develop a sense of control. In contrast, when parents create an environment that is haphazard, unpredictable, or chaotic, children do not have a basis from which to be or feel effective. In general, when parents create structured, rather than chaot-

ic, environments, children display enhanced cognitive resources (for a review, see Pomerantz et al., 2005). For example, Grolnick and Ryan (1989) found that the more structure (e.g., clear and consistent provision of rules, expectations, and guidelines for children) parents provided their middle school children, the more children felt in control of their performance in school (see also Skinner et al., 2005).

The Cognitive Dimension of Parenting

The influence of parents' affect and behavior on children is accompanied by that of parents' cognition. Several aspects of parents' beliefs about themselves and their children have received attention over the last three decades, including parents' perceptions of control over children, self-efficacy in regards to parenting, and attributions of the intentions of others (for a review, see Bornstein, 2006). One of the most studied dimensions of parents' cognitions, which we focus on in this section, has been parents' perceptions of children's competence, particularly in the academic arena.

Such cognitions shape children's cognitive resources. There is a rich body of research indicating that through their perceptions of children's competence, parents act as interpreters of reality for children, thereby guiding them toward the niches for which they are suited and ultimately shaping their self-perceptions (see Eccles, 1983). In essence, parents' perceptions of children's competence may act as self-fulfilling prophecies because parents communicate such perceptions to children, which in turn influence children's self-perceptions. Much research shows that parents' perceptions of children's competence, which are often based in reality, foreshadow children's perceptions of their competence (for a review, see Wigfield, Eccles, Schiefele, Roeser, & Davis-Kean, 2006). For example, Frome and Eccles (1998) demonstrated that children's grades in math and English predicted, over time, parents' perceptions of children's competence in these school subjects, such that the higher children's achievement, the more positive parents' perceptions. These investigators also found that above and beyond children's actual achievement, parents' perceptions of children's competence in math and English predicted children's subsequent perceptions of their own competence. Parents' perceptions also appear to contribute to children's reasons for pursuing their schoolwork, with more positive parental perceptions foreshadowing children holding intrinsic rather than extrinsic reasons (Pomerantz & Dong, 2006).

Above and beyond their influence on children's perceptions of competence, parents' perceptions of children's competence may play a part in children's behavioral and affective resources as well, although little attention has been directed to this issue. In terms of behavioral resources, when children feel that parents believe in them, they may be more likely to engage in active goal pursuit, developing important strategies for goal attainment. Research by Madon and colleagues (2003) is consistent with this notion: Above and beyond children's own expectations for their drinking behavior, when parents expected adolescents to refrain from such behavior, adolescents were more likely to do so.

In terms of affective resources, even if children themselves do not believe in their own competence, it can be valuable to know that parents believe in them, potentially buffering children against emotional distress. Parents' positive perceptions of children's competence in multiple arenas are associated with better emotional functioning in children (e.g., D. A. Cole, Martin, & Powers, 1997). Mothers' positive perceptions are particularly likely to foreshadow better emotional functioning in children when mothers also believe that children's competence is stable (Pomerantz & Dong, 2006). However, the extent to which such effects are independent of children's perceptions of their own competence has not received attention.

Summary

The psychological resource principle involves two key notions. First, affective, behavioral, and cognitive resources are essential to the development of competent functioning in children. Much research links these psychological resources to children's competent functioning, with a sizeable portion showing that they actually foreshadow it. Second, although there are other sources of psychological resources, parents are a major source. Parents can facilitate or inhibit the growth of children's psychological resources through their affect, behavior, and cognition in the socialization process. Indeed, there is much evidence consistent with the notion that these dimensions of parenting are influential. The research we have reviewed has identified the dimensions of parenting that are important for the psychological resources that contribute to children's personality development. However, this research is only a first step. We now turn our attention to consider how the effects of parents may be shaped by children's need for psychological resources.

IMPLICATIONS OF THE PSYCHOLOGICAL RESOURCE PRINCIPLE

A key feature of the psychological resource principle is that it depicts parents as facilitating the growth of psychological resources in children, thereby shaping children's subsequent competent functioning. This formulation suggests that the role of parents is dependent on children's need for such resources. Children may vary in their need because of variation in the extent to which their biological and social histories have facilitated or inhibited the growth of their psychological resources. Children may also vary in their need for psychological resources because their environments vary in the extent to which they challenge such resources. Hence, as we elaborate below, the effects of parental provision of psychological resources on children may depend partly on (1) the extent to which children already possess psychological resources, and (2) the extent to which their environment is challenging, and thus demanding, of psychological resources (for a review of additional child–parent interactions, see Rothbart & Bates, 2006).

The Joint Role of Parents and Children in the Socialization Process

As a consequence of their hereditary characteristics as well as socialization experiences with adults and peers, some children lack important psychological resources, whereas others already possess them. Those who are lacking depend on parents to provide the resources they need. When parents fail to do so, instead creating environments that undermine the growth of their children's psychological resources, these children are particularly likely to suffer. By contrast, children who are well endowed may not look to parents to the same extent to provide them with such resources, and parents may thus not have as large an influence on them.

Several studies are in line with the idea that children's affective resources moderate the role that parents play in their subsequent development. In general, this research suggests that children, particularly boys, who have problems regulating their negative emotions are more sensitive to parents' practices than are their counterparts who do not have such problems. In longitudinal research on boys during the toddler years, Belsky and colleagues (Belsky, Hsieh, & Crnic, 1998; Park, Belsky, Putnam, & Crnic, 1997) found that negative, intrusive parenting was more predictive of subsequent externalizing and inhibition problems in boys high in negative emotionality than in boys low in negative emotionality. Moreover, the more children in the early elementary school years view their parents as controlling, the more likely they are to have internalizing symptoms (Morris et al., 2002).

In a similar manner, children who lack behavioral resources are particularly sensitive to variations in parental support. In the social arena, Schwartz and colleagues (2000) proposed that children's positive interactions with friends might buffer the effects of negative parenting on subsequent victimization by peers, by enhancing children's self-regulation skills and facilitating the development of other core social skills. In two longitudinal studies beginning in the preschool and kindergarten years and following children into the middle elementary school years, these investigators tested their hypothesis that children's friendships moderate the influence of parents' negative affect and control. Across the two studies, the negative effects of these aspects of parenting on children's subsequent victimization were stronger in children with few reciprocated friendships than in children with many such friendships (see also Criss, Pettit, Bates, Dodge, & Lapp, 2002; Lansford, Criss, Pettit, Dodge, & Bates, 2003). In the academic arena, Pomerantz and colleagues (2005a) used a daily interview method to examine mothers' affect on the days their elementary and middle school children had homework. When mothers' affect was positive on days children had homework, children demonstrating heightened helplessness (as reported by teachers, mothers, and children) experienced enhanced motivational and emotional functioning 6 months later to a greater extent than did children demonstrating less helplessness (see also Ng et al., 2004).

There is also evidence consistent with the notion that children's cognitive resources influence how parenting shapes children. Using a longitudinal design, Pomerantz (2001) had children report on their mental representations of their competence, as reflected in their estimates of competence and their attributional style in the academic and social arenas. Children with negative mental representations of themselves were particularly vulnerable to parents' control efforts. Parents' control foreshadowed heightened depressive symptoms in children with negative mental representations, but not in children with positive mental representations (see also Pomerantz, Ng, & Wang, 2006).

Contextual Variations in the Socialization Process

Children's need for psychological resources may fluctuate as a function of contextual influences. Contexts that are challenging demand additional affective, behavioral, and cognitive resources from children. As a consequence, when operating in such contexts, children may be in particular need of parents' support. Even children who are already rich in psychological resources may rely on their parents' provisioning as challenging contexts tax their resources. In contexts that are not characterized by challenge, in contrast, children may rely less on their parents to provide such resources. As a consequence, although the quality of parents' affect, behavior, and cognition when interacting with children may always be important, it may be particularly so when children are operating in a challenging context—whether it be an ongoing or temporary one.

Children may be exposed to chronic challenge because they reside in a stressful environment. Such environments may include homes characterized by family conflict or a lack of economic resources, poor neighborhoods with residential instability, and classrooms with a harsh teacher in a school unable to supply children with basic learning materials. Such environments are likely to demand heightened psychological resources from children, and may even deplete such resources over time. Parents may be able to counteract these effects. Several studies are consistent with this analysis. Indeed, as earlier noted, Turkheimer and colleagues (2003) found that environmental rather than genetic sources of variability were paramount in IQ for children growing up in socioeconomically stressed families compared to affluent families. In addition, longitudinal research conducted by Pettit and colleagues (1997) indicates that supportive affective and behavioral parenting, assessed when children were just entering kindergarten, foreshadowed diminished externalizing problems 7 years later in children from poor and divorced families, but not necessarily for their counterparts with financially stable, married parents (see also Beyers, Bates, Pettit, & Dodge, 2003; Brody, Dorsey, Forehand, & Armistead, 2002; Pettit et al., 1999).

Although how parents provide care in the context of chronic challenge is of much import, parenting in the context of temporary challenge is also significant. Temporary challenge manifests itself in the myriad of difficult situations in which children find themselves on a daily basis (e.g., the completion of homework and resolving a dispute with a peer). Given that homework is often a challenging context in which children experience negative affect (e.g., Fuligni, Yip, & Tseng, 2002), Pomerantz and colleagues (2005) examined mothers' affect in such a context in a study of elementary and middle school children and their mothers. In this study, mothers' affect was assessed every day in the context of a daily interview. Mothers' affect on the days children had homework and the days children did not have homework was compared; mothers had higher negative affect on the days children had homework, but not necessarily lower positive affect. Of major interest for current purposes, however, is that mothers' affect on the days children had homework was predictive of children's academic and emotional functioning 6 months later, but this was not the case for mothers' affect on the days children did not have homework.

Summary

Consistent with the psychological resource principle, the quality of parenting matters most when children are most in need of psychological resources. Evidence suggests that this is the case especially when children lack affective, behavioral, or cognitive resources, perhaps because of their prior socialization or biological history. Because children who lack such resources often elicit negative parenting (e.g., Thomas & Chess, 1977), parents who are able to provide psychological resources may be particularly sensitive parents who can adjust their parenting to create a "good fit" with their children's needs. The psychological resource principle also suggests that when children are in challenging situations that deplete their psychological resources, they are in greater need of parents' support. In line with this notion, a number of studies suggest that parenting matters most when it takes place in challenging situations.

CONCLUSION

There is clear evidence that parents shape children's personality. In line with the psychological resource principle, a sizeable body of research supports the notion that parents' provision of psychological resources contributes to children's competent functioning. Parents have the potential to provide affective, behavioral, and cognitive resources that serve as the foundation for the development of competence in children. There is growing evidence that the greater children's need for such resources, the more parents matter. Thus, parents' influence on children's personality is determined partly by the psychological resources that children possess; although such resources may be based in children's biology, they may also be based in children's prior experiences, which may be shaped, to some extent, by the environment in which they reside. Key for future theory and research is to elucidate the extent to which personality during adulthood has been shaped by the contributions of parents to personality during childhood.

ACKNOWLEDGMENT

Work on this chapter was partially supported by Grant No. R01 MH57505 from the National Institute of Mental Health.

REFERENCES

Abidin, R. R. (1995). *Parenting Stress Index* (3rd ed.). Odessa, FL: Psychological Assessment Resources.

Askan, N., Kochanska, G., & Ortmann, M. R. (2006). Mutually responsive orientation between parents and their young children: Toward methodological advances in the science of relationships. *Developmental Psychology, 42,* 833–848.

Baldwin, A. L. (1955). *Behavior and development in childhood.* New York: Dryden.

Bandura, A. (1986). *Social foundations of thought and action: A social-cognitive theory.* Englewood Cliffs, NJ: Prentice Hall.

Barber, B. K. (Ed.). (2002). *Intrusive parenting.* Washington, DC: American Psychological Association.

Barber, B. K., Stolz, H. E., & Olsen, J. A. (2006). Parental support, psychological control, and behavioral control: Assessing relevance across time, culture, and method. *Monographs of the Society for Research in Child Development, 70*(Serial No. 282).

Baumrind, D. (1971). Current patterns of parental authority. *Developmental Psychology Monograph, 1*(4, Pt. 2).

Baumrind, D. (1993). The average expectable environment is not good enough: A response to Scarr. *Child Development, 64,* 1299–1317.

Bell, R. Q., & Chapman, M. (1986). Child effects in studies using experimental or brief longitudinal approaches to socialization. *Developmental Psychology, 22,* 595–603.

Belsky, J. (1984). The determinants of parenting: A process model. *Child Development, 55,* 83–96.

Belsky, J., Hsieh, K., & Crnic, K. (1998). Mothering, fathering, and infant negativity as antecedents of boys' externalizing problems and inhibition at age 3 years: Differential susceptibility to rearing experience? *Development and Psychopathology, 10,* 301–319.

Beyers, J. M., Bates, J. E., Pettit, G. S., & Dodge, K. A. (2003). Neighborhood structure, parenting processes, and the development of youths' externalizing behaviors: A multilevel analysis. *American Journal of Community Psychology, 31,* 35–53.

Bokhorst, C., Bakermans-Kranenburg, M., Pasco Fearon, R., van IJzendoorn, M., Fonagy, P., & Schuengel, C. (2003). The importance of shared environment in mother–infant attachment security: A behavioral genetic study. *Child Development, 74,* 1769–1782.

Bolger, N., Davis, A., & Rafaelli, E. (2003). Diary methods. *Annual Review of Psychology, 54,* 579–616.

Bornstein, M. H. (2006). Parenting science and practice. In K. A. Renninger & I. E. Sigel (Eds.), *Handbook of child psychology: Vol. 4. Child psychology in practice* (6th ed., pp. 893–949). Hoboken, NJ: Wiley.

Bornstein, M. H., & Tamis-LeMonda, C. S. (1997). Maternal responsiveness and infant mental abilities: Specific predictive relations. *Infant Behavior and Development, 20,* 283–296.

Bowlby, J. (1969). *Attachment and loss: Vol. 1. Attachment.* New York: Basic Books.

Bowlby, J. (1973). *Attachment and loss: Vol. 2. Separation, anxiety, and anger.* New York: Basic Books.

Bretherton, I., & Munholland, K. A. (1999). Internal working models in attachment relationships: A construct revisited. In J. Cassidy & P. R. Shaver (Eds.), *Handbook of attachment: Theory, research, and clinical applications* (pp. 89–111). New York: Guilford Press.

Brody, G. H., Dorsey, S., Forehand, R., & Armistead, L. (2002). Unique and protective contributions of parenting and classroom processes to the adjustment of African American children living in single-parent families. *Child Development, 73,* 274–286.

Bugental, D. B. (2004). Thriving in the face of early adversity. *Journal of Social Issues, 60,* 219–235.

Bugental, D. B., Caporael, L., & Shennum, W. A. (1980). Experimentally produced child uncontrollability: Effects on the potency of adult communication patterns. *Child Development, 51,* 520–528.

Bugental, D. B., & Grusec, J. E. (2006). Socialization processes. In N. Eisenberg (Ed.), *Handbook of child psychology: Vol. 3. Social, emotional, and personality development* (6th ed., pp. 366–428). Hoboken, NJ: Wiley.

Bugental, D. B., Lyon, J. E., Krantz, J., & Cortez, V. (1997). Who's the boss? Differential accessibility of dominance ideation in parent–child relationships. *Journal of Personality and Social Psychology, 72,* 1297–1309.

Carver, C., & Miller, C. (2006). Relations of serotonin function to personality: Current views and a key methodological issue. *Psychiatry Research, 144*(1), 1–15.

Caspi, A., McClay, J., Moffitt, T. E., Mill, J., Martin, J., Craig, I. W., et al. (2002). Role of genotype in the cycle of violence in maltreated children. *Science Education, 297,* 851–854.

Clutton-Brock, T. H. (1991). *The evolution of pa-

rental care. Princeton, NJ: Princeton University Press.

Coie, J. D., Dodge, K. A., & Kupersmidt, J. B. (1990). Peer group behavior and social status. In S. R. Asher & J. D. Coie (Eds.), *Peer rejection in childhood* (pp. 17–59). New York: Cambridge University Press.

Cole, D. A., Martin, J. M., & Powers, B. (1997). A competency-based model of child depression: A longitudinal study of peer, parent, teacher, and self-evaluations. *Journal of Psychology and Psychiatry*, *38*, 505–514.

Cole, P. M., Teti, L. O., & Zahn-Waxler, C. (2003). Mutual emotion regulation and the stability of conduct problems between preschool and early school age. *Development and Psychopathology*, *15*, 1–18.

Collins, W. A., Maccoby, E. E., Steinberg, L., Hetherington, E. M., & Bornstein, M. (2000). Contemporary research on parenting: The case for nature and nurture. *American Psychologist*, *55*, 218–232.

Crick, N. R., & Dodge, K. A. (1994). A review and reformulation of social information-processing mechanisms in children's social adjustment. *Psychological Bulletin*, *115*, 74–101.

Criss, M. M., Pettit, G. S., Bates, J. E., Dodge, K. A., & Lapp, A. L. (2002). Family adversity, positive peer relationships, and children's externalizing behavior: A longitudinal perspective on risk and resilience. *Child Development*, *73*, 1220–1237.

Crouter, A. C., Helms-Erikson, H., Updegraff, K., & McHale, S. M. (1999). Conditions underlying parents' knowledge about children's daily lives in middle childhood: Between- and within-family comparisons. *Child Development*, *70*, 246–259.

Damast, A. M., Tamis-LeMonda, C. S., & Bornstein, M. H. (1996). Mother–child play: Sequential interactions and the relation between maternal beliefs and behaviors. *Child Development*, *67*, 1752–1766.

Davidov, M., & Grusec, J. (2006). Untangling the links of parental responsiveness to distress and warmth to child outcomes. *Child Development*, *77*, 44–58.

Deci, E. L., Driver, R. E., Hotchkiss, L., Robbins, R. J., & Wilson, I. M. (1993). The relation of mothers' controlling vocalizations to children's intrinsic motivation. *Journal of Experimental Child Psychology*, *55*, 151–162.

Deci, E. L., & Ryan, R. M. (1987). The support of autonomy and the control of behavior. *Journal of Personality and Social Psychology*, *53*, 1024–1037.

Denham, S. A., Workman, E., Cole, P. M., Weissbrod, C., Kendziora, K. T., & Zahn-Waxler, C. (2000). Prediction of externalizing behavior problems from early to middle childhood: The role of parental socialization and emotion expression. *Development and Psychopathology*, *12*, 23–45.

Depue, R. A., & Collins, P. F. (1999). Neurobiology of the structure of personality: Dopamine, facilitation of incentive motivation, and extraversion. *Behavioral and Brain Sciences*, *22*, 491–517.

Dix, T. (1991). The affective organization of parenting: Adaptive and maladaptive processes. *Psychological Bulletin*, *110*, 3–25.

Dodge, K. A., Pettit, G. S., & Bates, J. E. (1994). Socialization mediators of the relation between socioeconomic status and child conduct problems. *Child Development*, *65*, 649–665.

Dodge, K. A., Pettit, G. S., Bates, J. E., & Valente, E. (1995). Social information-processing patterns partially mediate the effect of early physical abuse on later conduct problems. *Journal of Abnormal Psychology*, *104*, 632–643.

Duckworth, A. L., & Seligman, M. E. (2006). Self-discipline gives girls the edge: Gender in self-discipline, grades, and achievement test scores. *Journal of Educational Psychology*, *98*, 198–208.

Dweck, C. S., & London, B. (2004). The role of mental representation in social development. *Merrill–Palmer Quarterly*, *50*, 428–444.

Eccles, J. S. (1983). Expectancies, values and academic behaviors. In J. T. Spence (Ed.), *Achievement and achievement motives* (pp. 75–146). San Francisco: Freeman.

Eccles, J. S., Early, D., Frasier, K., Belansky, E., & McCarthy, K. (1997). The relation of connection, regulation, and support for autonomy to adolescents' functioning. *Journal of Adolescent Research*, *12*, 263–289.

Eisenberg, N., Zhou, Q., Losoya, S. H., Fabes, R. A., Shepard, S. A., Murphy, B. C., et al. (2003). The relations of parenting, effortful control, and ego control to children's emotional expressivity. *Child Development*, *74*, 875–895.

Eisenberg, N., Zhou, Q., Spinrad, T. L., Valiente, C., Fabes, R. A., & Liew, J. (2005). Relations among positive parenting, children's effortful control, and externalizing problems: A three-wave longitudinal study. *Child Development*, *76*, 1055–1071.

Elliott, E. S., & Dweck, C. S. (1988). Goals: An approach to motivation and achievement. *Journal of Personality and Social Psychology*, *54*, 5–12.

Fabes, R. A., Poulin, R. E., Eisenberg, N., & Madden-Derdich, D. A. (2002). The Coping with Children's Negative Emotions Scale (CCNES): Psychometric properties and relations with children's emotional competence. *Marriage and Family Review*, *34*, 285–310.

Fairbanks, L. A., Jorgensen, M. J., Huff, A., Blau, K., Hung, Y. Y., & Mann, J. J. (2004). Adolescent impulsivity predicts adult dominance attainment in male vervet monkeys. *American Journal of Primatology, 64*(1), 1–17.

Fincham, F. D., Hokoda, A., & Sanders, R. (1989). Learned helplessness, test anxiety, and academic achievement: A longitudinal analysis. *Child Development, 60,* 138–145.

Frodi, A., Bridges, L., & Grolnick, W. S. (1985). Correlates of mastery-related behavior: A short-term longitudinal study of infants in their second year. *Child Development, 56,* 1291–1298.

Frome, P. M., & Eccles, J. S. (1998). Parents' influence on children's achievement-related perceptions. *Journal of Personality and Social Psychology, 74,* 435–452.

Fuligni, A. J., Yip, T., & Tseng, V. (2002). The impact of family obligation on the daily activities and psychological well-being of Chinese American adolescents. *Child Development, 73,* 302–314.

Gerlsma, C., Emmelkamp, P. M., & Arrindell, W. A. (1990). Anxiety, depression, and perception of early parenting: A meta-analysis. *Clinical Psychology Review, 10,* 251–277.

Ginsburg, G. S., & Bronstein, P. (1993). Family factors related to children's intrinsic/extrinsic motivational orientation and academic performance. *Child Development, 64,* 1461–1474.

Glasgow, K. L., Dornbusch, S. M., Troyer, L., Steinberg, L., & Ritter, P. L. (1997). Parenting styles, adolescents' attributions, and educational outcomes in nine heterogeneous high schools. *Child Development, 68,* 507–529.

Gottfried, A. E., Fleming, J. S., & Gottfried, A. W. (1994). Role of parental motivational practices in children's academic intrinsic motivation and achievement. *Journal of Educational Psychology, 86,* 104–113.

Grolnick, W. S., Deci, E. L., & Ryan, R. M. (1997). Internalization within the family: The self-determination theory perspective. In J. Grusec & L. Kuczynski (Eds.), *Parenting and children's internalization of values: A handbook of contemporary theory* (pp. 135–161). New York: Wiley.

Grolnick, W. S., Gurland, S. T., DeCourcey, W., & Jacob, K. (2002). Antecedents and consequences of mothers' autonomy support: An experimental investigation. *Developmental Psychology, 38,* 143–154.

Grolnick, W. S., Kurowski, C. O., & Gurland, S. T. (1999). Family processes and the development of children's self-regulation. *Educational Psychologist, 34,* 3–14.

Grolnick, W. S., & Ryan, R. M. (1989). Parent styles associated with children's self-regulation and competence in school. *Journal of Educational Psychology, 81,* 143–154.

Grolnick, W. S., Ryan, R. M., & Deci, E. L. (1991).

Inner resources for school achievement: Motivational mediators of children's perceptions of their parents. *Journal of Educational Psychology, 83,* 508–517.

Grusec, J. E., & Goodnow, J. J. (1994). Impact of parental discipline methods on the child's internalization of values: A reconceptualization of current points of view. *Developmental Psychology, 30,* 4–19.

Guay, F., Marsh, H. W., & Boivin, M. (2003). Academic self-concept and academic achievement: Developmental perspectives on their causal ordering. *Journal of Educational Psychology, 95,* 124–136.

Hammen, C., & Rudolph, K. D. (2003). Childhood mood disorders. In E. J. Mash & R. A. Barkley (Eds.), *Child psychopathology* (2nd ed., pp. 233–278). New York: Guilford Press.

Harris, J. R. (1995). Where is the child's environment?: A group socialization theory of development. *Psychological Review, 102,* 458–489.

Hirt, E. R., Melton, R. J., McDonald, H. E., & Harackiewicz, J. M. (1996). Processing goals, task interest, and the mood–performance relationship: A mediational analysis. *Journal of Personality and Social Psychology, 71,* 245–261.

Hoffman, M. L. (2000). *Empathy and moral development: Implications for caring and justice.* Cambridge, UK: Cambridge University Press.

Holden, G. W., & Edwards, L. A. (1989). Parental attitudes toward child rearing: Instruments, issues, and implications. *Psychological Bulletin, 106,* 29–58.

Holden, G. W., & Miller, P. C. (1999). Enduring and different: A meta-analysis of the similarity in parents' child rearing. *Psychological Bulletin, 125,* 223–254.

Isen, A. M., & Geva, N. (1987). The influence of positive affect on acceptable level of risk: The person with a large canoe has a large worry. *Organizational Behavior and Human Decision Processes, 39,* 145–154.

Kaffman, A., & Meaney, M. J. (2007). Neurodevelopmental sequelae of postnatal maternal care in rodents: Clinical and research implications of molecular insights. *Journal of Child Psychology and Psychiatry, 48,* 224–244.

Keller, B. B., & Bell, R. Q. (1979). Child effects on adult's method of eliciting altruistic behavior. *Child Development, 50,* 1004–1009.

Kenney-Benson, G. A., & Pomerantz, E. M. (2005). The role of mothers' use of control in children's perfectionism: Implications for the development of children's depressive symptoms. *Journal of Personality, 73,* 23–46.

Kenney-Benson, G. A., Pomerantz, E. M., Ryan, A., & Patrick, H. (2006). Sex differences in math performance: The role of children's approach to school work. *Developmental Psychology, 42,* 11–26.

Kochanska, G. (1993). Toward a synthesis of parental socialization and child temperament in early development of conscience. *Child Development, 64*, 325–347.

Kochanska, G. (1997). Mutually responsive orientation between mothers and their young children: Implications for early socialization. *Child Development, 68*, 94–112.

Kochanska, G. (2002). Committed compliance, moral self, and internalization: A mediational model. *Developmental Psychology, 38*, 339–351.

Kochanska, G., Aksan, N., Penney, S. J., & Boldt, L. J. (2007). Parental personality as an inner resource that moderates the impact of ecological adversity on parenting. *Journal of Personality and Social Psychology, 92*, 136–150.

Kochanska, G., & Coy, K. C. (2002). Child emotionality and maternal responsiveness as predictors of reunion behaviors in the Strange Situation: Links mediated and unmediated by separation distress. *Child Development, 73*, 228–240.

Kochanska, G., & Knaack, A. (2003). Effortful control as a personality characteristic of young children: Antecedents, correlates, and consequences. *Journal of Personality, 71*, 1087–1112.

Laible, D. J., & Thompson, R. A. (2002). Mother–child conflict in the toddler years: Lessons in emotion, morality, and relationships. *Child Development, 73*, 1187–1203.

Laible, D. J., & Thompson, R. A. (2007). Early socialization: A relational perspective. In J. E. Grusec & P. D. Hastings (Eds.), *Handbook of socialization: Theory and research* (pp. 181–207). New York: Guilford Press.

Lansford, J. E., Criss, M. M., Pettit, G. S., Dodge, K. A., & Bates, J. E. (2003). Friendship quality, peer group affiliation, and peer antisocial behavior as moderators of the link between negative parenting and adolescent externalizing behavior. *Journal of Research on Adolescence, 13*, 161–184.

Larson, R. W., & Gillman, S. (1999). Transmission of emotions in the daily interactions of single-mother families. *Journal of Marriage and the Family, 61*, 21–37.

Lepper, M. R., & Greene, D. (1975). Turning play into work: Effects of adult surveillance and extrinsic rewards on children's intrinsic motivation. *Journal of Personality and Social Psychology, 31*, 579–486.

Lytton, H. (2000). Toward a model of family-environmental and child-biological influences on development. *Developmental Review, 20*, 150–179.

Lyubomirsky, S., King, L., & Diener, E. (2005). The benefits of frequent positive affect: Does happiness lead to success? *Psychological Bulletin, 131*, 803–855.

Maccoby, E. E. (1992). The role of parents in the socialization of children: An historical overview. *Developmental Psychology, 28*, 1006–1017.

Maccoby, E. E. (2000). Parenting and its effects on children: On reading and misreading behavior genetics. *Annual Review of Psychology, 51*, 1–27.

Madon, S., Guyll, M., Spoth, R. L., Cross, S. E., & Hilbert, S. (2003). The self-fulfilling influence of mothers' expectations on children's underage drinking. *Journal of Personality and Social Psychology, 84*(6), 1188–1205.

Masten, A. S., & Coatsworth, J. D. (1998). The development of competence in favorable and unfavorable environments: Lessons from research on successful children. *American Psychologist, 53*, 205–220.

McCord, J. (1988). Parental behavior in the cycle of aggression. *Psychiatry, 51*, 14–23.

Meaney, M. J., & Szyf, M. (2005). Maternal care as a model for experience-dependent chromatin plasticity? *Trends in Neuroscience, 28*, 456–463.

Mischel, W. (1966). A social-learning view of sex differences in behavior. In E. E. Maccoby (Ed.), *The development of sex differences* (pp. 57–81). Stanford, CA: Stanford University Press.

Mischel, W., Shoda, Y., & Rodriguez, M. L. (1989). Delay of gratification in children. *Science, 244*, 933–938.

Morris, A. S., Silk, J. S., Steinberg, L., Sessa, F. M., Avenevoli, S., & Essex, M. J. (2002). Temperamental vulnerability and negative parenting as interacting predictors of child adjustment. *Journal of Marriage and the Family, 64*, 461–471.

Nelson, D. A., Hart, C. H., Chongming, Y., Olsen, J. A., & Shenghua, J. (2006). Aversive parenting in China: Associations with child physical and relational aggression. *Child Development, 77*, 554–572.

Ng, F. F., Kenney-Benson, G. A., & Pomerantz, E. M. (2004). Children's achievement moderates the effects of mothers' use of control and autonomy support. *Child Development, 75*, 764–780.

Nolen-Hoeksema, S., Girgus, J. S., & Seligman, M. E. (1992). Predictors and consequences of childhood depressive symptoms: A 5-year longitudinal study. *Journal of Abnormal Psychology, 101*, 405–422.

Nolen-Hoeksema, S., Wolfson, A., Mumme, D., & Guskin, K. (1995). Helplessness in children of depressed and nondepressed mothers. *Developmental Psychology, 31*, 377–387.

O'Connor, T., & Croft, C. (2001). A twin study of attachment in preschool children. *Child Development, 72*, 1501–1511.

Offer, D., & Offer, J. B. (1975). *Teenage to young*

manhood: A psychological study. New York: Basic Books.

Parent, C., Zhang, T.-Y., Caldji, C., Bagot, R., Champagne, F. A., Pruessner, J., et al. (2005). Maternal care and individual differences in defensive responses. *Current Directions in Psychological Science, 14*, 229–233.

Park, S.-Y., Belsky, J., Putnam, S., & Crnic, K. (1997). Infant emotionality, parenting, and 3-year inhibition: Exploring stability and lawful discontinuity in a male sample. *Developmental Psychology, 33*, 218–227.

Parke, R. D., & Buriel, R. (2006). Socialization in the family: Ethnic and ecological perspectives. In N. Eisenberg (Ed.), *Handbook of child psychology: Vol. 3. Social, emotional, and personality development* (6th ed., pp. 429–504). Hoboken, NJ: Wiley.

Parke, R. D., O'Neil, R., Spitzer, S., Isley, S., Welsh, M., Wang, S., et al. (1997). A longitudinal assessment of sociometric stability and the behavioral correlates of children's social acceptance. *Merrill–Palmer Quarterly, 43*, 635–662.

Patterson, G. R. (1982). *Coercive family process*. Eugene, OR: Castalia.

Patterson, G. R., Bank, L., & Stolmiller, M. (1990). The preadolescent's contributions to disrupted family process. In R. Montemayor, G. R. Adams, & T. P. Gullotta (Eds.), *From childhood to adolescence: A transitional period* (pp. 107–133). Newbury Park, CA: Sage.

Patterson, G. R., & Capaldi, D. M. (1991). Antisocial parents: Unskilled and vulnerable. In P. A. Cowan & E. M. Hetherington (Eds.), *Family transitions* (pp. 195–218). Hillsdale, NJ: Erlbaum.

Patterson, G. R., & Stouthamer-Loeber, M. (1984). The correlation of family management practices and delinquency. *Child Development, 55*, 1299–1307.

Pettit, G. S., Bates, J. E., & Dodge, K. A. (1997). Supportive parenting, ecological context, and children's adjustment: A seven-year longitudinal study. *Child Development, 68*, 908–923.

Pettit, G. S., Bates, J. E., Dodge, K. A., & Meece, D. W. (1999). The impact of after-school peer contact on early adolescent externalizing symptoms as moderated by parental monitoring, perceived neighborhood safety, and prior adjustment. *Child Development, 70*, 768–778.

Pianta, R. C., Nimetz, S. L., & Bennett, E. (1997). Mother–child relationships, teacher–child relationships, and school outcomes in preschool and kindergarten. *Early Childhood Research Quarterly, 12*, 263–280.

Pianta, R. C., Smith, N., & Reeve, R. (1991). Observing mother and child behavior in a problem solving situation at school entry: Relations with classroom adjustment. *School Psychology Quarterly, 56*, 1–16.

Plomin, R., DeFries, J. C., McClearn, G. E., & Rutter, M. (1997). *Behavioral genetics* (3rd ed.). New York: Freeman.

Plomin, R., & Rutter, M. (1998). Child development, molecular genetics, and what to do with genes once they are found. *Child Development, 69*, 1223–1242.

Pomerantz, E. M. (2001). Parent × child socialization: Implications for the development of depressive symptoms. *Journal of Family Psychology, 15*, 510–525.

Pomerantz, E. M., & Dong, W. (2006). The effects of mothers' perceptions of children's competence: The moderating role of mothers' theories of competence. *Developmental Psychology, 42*, 950–961.

Pomerantz, E. M., & Eaton, M. M. (2001). Maternal intrusive support in the academic context: Transactional socialization processes. *Developmental Psychology, 37*, 174–186.

Pomerantz, E. M., Grolnick, W. S., & Price, C. E. (2005). The role of parents in how children approach achievement: A dynamic process perspective. In A. J. Elliot & C. S. Dweck (Eds.), *The handbook of competence and motivation* (pp. 259–278). New York: Guilford Press.

Pomerantz, E. M., & Newman, L. S. (2000). Looking in on the children: Using developmental psychology as a tool for hypothesis testing and model building in social psychology. *Personality and Social Psychology Review, 4*, 300–316.

Pomerantz, E. M., Ng, F., & Wang, Q. (2006). Mothers' mastery-oriented involvement in children's homework: Implications for the well-being of children with negative perceptions of competence. *Journal of Educational Psychology, 98*, 99–111.

Pomerantz, E. M., & Ruble, D. N. (1998a). The multidimensional nature of control: Implications for the development of sex differences in self-evaluation. In J. Heckhausen & C. S. Dweck (Eds.), *Motivation and self-regulation across the life-span* (pp. 159–184). New York: Cambridge University Press.

Pomerantz, E. M., & Ruble, D. N. (1998b). The role of maternal control in the development of sex differences in child self-evaluative factors. *Child Development, 69*, 458–478.

Pomerantz, E. M., Wang, Q., & Ng, F. F. (2005a). Mothers' affect in the homework context: The importance of staying positive. *Developmental Psychology, 42*, 414–427.

Pomerantz, E. M., Wang, Q., & Ng, F. F. (2005b). The role of children's competence experiences in the socialization process: A dynamic process framework for the academic arena. In R. Kail (Ed.), *Advances in child development and behavior* (Vol. 33, pp. 193–227). San Diego, CA: Academic Press.

Quinn, J. L., & Cresswell, W. (2005). Personality, anti-predation behaviour and behavioural plasticity in the chaffinch *Fringilla coelebs*. *Behaviour, 142*, 1377–1402.

Roeser, R. W., Eccles, J. S., & Sameroff, A. (1998). Academic and emotional functioning in early adolescence: Longitudinal relations, patterns, and prediction by experience in middle school. *Development and Psychopathology, 10*, 321–352.

Roisman, G. I., & Fraley, R. C. (2006). The limits of genetic influence: A behavior–genetic analysis of infant–caregiver relationship quality and temperament. *Child Development, 77*, 1656–1667.

Roisman, G. I., Masten, A. S., Coatsworth, D., & Tellegen, A. (2004). Salient and emerging developmental tasks in the transition to adulthood. *Child Development, 75*, 123–133.

Rollins, B. C., & Thomas, D. L. (1979). Parental support, power, and control techniques in the socialization of children. In W. R. Burr, R. Hill, F. I. Nye, & I. L. Reiss (Eds.), *Contemporary theories about the family* (pp. 317–364). New York: Free Press.

Rothbart, M. K., & Bates, J. E. (2006). Temperament. In N. Eisenberg (Ed.), *Handbook of child psychology: Vol. 3. Social, emotional, and personality development* (6th ed., pp. 99–166). Hoboken, NJ: Wiley.

Rowe, D. C. (1994). *The limits of family influence: Genes, experience, and behavior*. New York: Guilford Press.

Rudolph, K. D. (2005). A self-regulation approach to understanding adolescent depression in the school context. In T. Urdan & F. Pajares (Eds.), *Educating adolescents: Challenges and strategies* (Vol. 4, pp. 33–64). Greenwich, CT: Information Age.

Rudolph, K. D., Flynn, M., & Abaied, J. L. (2008). A developmental perspective on interpersonal theories of youth depression. In J. R. Z. Abela & B. L. Hankin (Eds.), *Handbook of depression in children and adolescents* (pp. 79–102). New York: Guilford Press.

Rudolph, K. D., Hammen, C., Burge, D., Lindberg, N., Herzberg, D., & Daley, S. E. (2000). Toward an interpersonal life-stress model of depression: The developmental context of stress generation. *Development and Psychopathology, 12*, 215–234.

Rudolph, K. D., Hammen, C., & Daley, S. E. (2006). Mood disorders. In D. A. Wolfe & E. J. Mash (Eds.), *Behavioral and emotional disorders in adolescents: Nature, assessment, and treatment* (pp. 300–342). New York: Guilford Press.

Rutter, M. (2006). *Genes and behavior: Nature–nurture interplay explained*. Oxford, UK: Blackwell.

Rutter, M., Dunn, J., Plomin, R., Simonoff, E., Pickles, A., Maughan, B., et al. (1997). Integrating nature and nurture: Implications of person–environment correlations and interactions for developmental psychology. *Development and Psychopathology, 9*, 335–364.

Rutter, M., Moffitt, T. E., & Caspi, A. (2006). Gene–environment interplay and psychopathology: Multiple varieties but real effects. *Journal of Child Psychology and Psychiatry, 47*, 226–261.

Rutter, M., & Silberg, J. (2002). Gene–environment interplay in relation to emotional and behavioral disturbance. *Annual Review of Psychology, 53*, 463–490.

Rutter, M., Silberg, J. L., O'Connor, T. G., & Simonoff, E. (1999). Genetics and child psychiatry: I. Advances in quantitative and molecular genetics. *Journal of Child Psychology and Psychiatry, 40*, 3–18.

Ryan, R. M., Mims, V., & Koestner, R. (1983). Relation of reward contingency and interpersonal context to intrinsic motivation: A review and test using cognitive evaluation theory. *Journal of Personality and Social Psychology, 45*, 736–750.

Sameroff, A. (1975). Transactional models in early social relations. *Human Development, 18*, 65–79.

Sameroff, A., & Macenzie, M. J. (2003). Research strategies for capturing transactional models of development: The limits of the possible. *Development and Psychopathology, 15*, 613–640.

Scarr, S. (1992). Developmental theories for the 1990s: Development and individual differences. *Child Development, 63*, 1–19.

Scarr, S., & McCartney, K. (1983). How people make their own environments: A theory of genotype environment effects. *Child Development, 54*, 424–435.

Schaefer, E. S. (1959). A circumplex model for maternal behavior. *Journal of Abnormal and Social Psychology, 59*, 226–235.

Schaefer, E. S. (1965). Children's reports of parental behavior: An inventory. *Child Development, 36*, 413–424.

Schwartz, D., Dodge, K. A., Pettit, G. S., Bates, J. E., & the Conduct Problems Prevention Research Group. (2000). Friendship as a moderating factor in the pathway between early harsh home environment and later victimization in the peer group. *Developmental Psychology, 36*, 646–662.

Sears, R. R., Maccoby, E. E., & Levin, H. (1957). *Patterns of child rearing*. Evanston, IL: Row, Peterson.

Sessa, F. M., Avenevoli, S., Steinberg, L., & Morris, A. S. (2001). Correspondence among informants on parenting: Preschool children, mothers, and observers. *Journal of Family Psychology, 15*, 53–68.

Shannon, C., Champoux, M., & Suomi, S. J. (1998). Rearing condition and plasma cortisol in rhesus monkey infants. *American Journal of Primatology, 46*(4), 311–321.

Shiner, R. L., Masten, A. S., & Tellegen, A. (2002). A developmental perspective on personality in emerging adulthood: Childhood antecedents and concurrent adaptation. *Journal of Personality and Social Psychology, 83,* 1165–1177.

Shonkoff, J., & Phillips, D. (Eds.). (2000). *From neurons to neighborhoods: The science of early childhood development.* Washington, DC: National Academy Press.

Skinner, E., Johnson, S., & Snyder, T. (2005). Six dimensions of parenting: A motivational model. *Parenting: Science and Practice, 5,* 175–235.

Smetana, J. G. (1995). Parenting styles and conceptions of parental authority during adolescence. *Child Development, 66,* 299–316.

Steinberg, L., Elmen, J. D., & Mounts, N. S. (1989). Authoritative parenting, psychosocial maturity, and academic success among adolescents. *Child Development, 60,* 1424–1436.

Steinberg, L., Lamborn, S. D., Darling, N., Mounts, N. S., & Dornbusch, S. (1994). Over-time changes in adjustment and competence among adolescents from authoritative, authoritarian, indulgent, and neglectful homes. *Child Development, 65,* 754–770.

Stice, E., & Barrera, M. (1995). A longitudinal examination of the reciprocal relations between perceived parenting and adolescents' substance use and externalizing behaviors. *Developmental Psychology, 31,* 322–334.

Thomas, A., & Chess, S. (1977). *Temperament and development.* New York: Brunner/Mazel.

Thomas, A., Chess, S., & Birch, H. G. (1970). The origin of personality. *Scientific American, 223,* 102–109.

Thompson, R. A. (2000). The legacy of early attachments. *Child Development, 71,* 145–152.

Thompson, R. A. (2006). Conversation and developing understanding: Introduction to the special issue. *Merrill–Palmer Quarterly, 52,* 1–16.

Thompson, R. A., Braun, K., Grossmann, K. E., Gunnar, M. R., Heinrichs, M., Keller, H., et al. (2005). Early social attachment and its consequences: The dynamics of a developing relationship. In C. S. Carter, L. Ahnert, K. E. Grossmann, M. Lamb, S. Porges, & N.

Sachser (Eds.), *Attachment and bonding: A new synthesis (Dahlem Workshop Report 92)* (pp. 349–383). Cambridge, MA: MIT Press.

Thompson, R. A., Laible, D. J., & Ontai, L. L. (2003). Early understandings of emotion, morality, and self: Developing a working model. In R. V. Kail (Ed.), *Advances in child development and behavior* (Vol. 31, pp. 137–171). San Diego, CA: Academic Press.

Thompson, R. A., & Meyer, S. (2007). Socialization of emotion regulation in the family. In J. J. Gross (Ed.), *Handbook of emotion regulation* (pp. 249–268). New York: Guilford Press.

Turkheimer, E., Haley, A., Waldron, M., D'Onofrio, B., & Gottesman, I. I. (2003). Socioeconomic status modifies heritability of IQ in young children. *Psychological Science, 14,* 623–628.

van den Boom, D. C. (1994). The influence of temperament and mothering on attachment and exploration: An experimental manipulation of sensitive responsiveness among lower-class mothers with irritable infants. *Child Development, 65,* 1457–1477.

Vansteenkiste, M., Simons, J., Lens, W., Soenens, B., & Matos, L. (2005). Examining the motivational impact of intrinsic versus extrinsic goal framing and autonomy-supportive versus internally controlling communication style on early adolescents' academic achievement. *Child Development, 76,* 483–501.

Wang, Q., Pomerantz, E. M., & Chen, H. (2007). The role of parents' control in early adolescents' psychological functioning: A longitudinal investigation in the United States and China. *Child Development, 78,* 1592–1610.

Weiss, B., Dodge, K. A., Bates, J. E., & Pettit, G. S. (1992). Some consequences of early harsh discipline: Child aggression and a maladaptive social information processing style. *Child Development, 63,* 1321–1335.

Weisz, J. R., Sweeney, L., Proffitt, V., & Carr, T. (1993). Control-related beliefs and self-reported depressive symptoms in late childhood. *Journal of Abnormal Psychology, 102,* 411–418.

Wigfield, A., Eccles, J. S., Schiefele, U., Roeser, R. W., & Davis-Kean, P. (2006). Development of achievement motivation. In N. Eisenberg (Ed.), *Handbook of child psychology: Vol. 3. Social, emotional, and personality development* (6th ed., pp. 933–1002). Hoboken, NJ: Wiley.

The Development of Personality Traits in Adulthood

Brent W. Roberts
Dustin Wood
Avshalom Caspi

Personality traits are defined as the relatively enduring patterns of thoughts, feelings, and behaviors that distinguish individuals from one another. The crux of personality trait development lies in one's interpretation of the two words "relatively enduring." For many years, the implicit assumption was that traits were "enduring enough" to ignore the issue of development. Recently, more nuanced developmental questions about traits have arisen because a critical mass of longitudinal studies showed that personality traits do change. These more nuanced questions center on both continuity and change and are the focus of this chapter.

Our first section addresses the basic question, what do we mean by *continuity* and *change*? In the context of defining what is meant by continuity and change, we also review the findings related to each type of continuity and/or change. Then we attempt to answer three related questions. First, why are personality traits consistent? Second, why do personality traits change, especially in adulthood? And, third, why don't personality traits change more than they do? Along the way, we point out major principles that we have derived from the body of empirical and theoretical work on personality development (Table 14.1) and mechanisms that we believe to be responsible for both continuity and change in personality (Tables 14.2 and 14.3).

TYPES OF CONTINUITY AND CHANGE OBSERVED IN LONGITUDINAL RESEARCH

The assertion that an individual's personality has changed or remained the same over time is ambiguous. Likewise the claim that personality traits are both consistent and changeable is seemingly contradictory. A further ambiguity arises when a claim of continuity or change rests on observations not of an individual but of a sample of individuals. The continuity or change of an attribute at the group level may be partially independent of changes at the individual level. Moreover, different forms of continuity and change, either at the sample or individual level, may be entirely independent of one another, making it not only possible but inevitable that there is both continuity and change in personality traits. There are, in short, a number of meanings denoted by the terms "continuity" and "change." The purpose of this section is to disentangle some of those meanings.

First we discuss the main statistical approaches to studying continuity and change in longitudinal research and then touch on one conceptual definition of change that does

TABLE 14.1. Principles of Personality Development

Cumulative continuity principle:	Personality traits increase in rank-order consistency throughout the lifespan.
Maturity principle:	People become more socially dominant, agreeable, conscientious, and emotionally stable with age.
Plasticity principle:	Personality traits are open systems that can be influenced by the environment at any age.
Role continuity principle:	Consistent roles rather than consistent environments are the cause of continuity in personality over time.
Identity development principle:	With age, the process of developing, committing to, and maintaining an identity leads to greater personality consistency.
Social investment principle:	Investing in social institutions, such as age-graded social roles, outside of the self is one of the driving mechanisms of personality development, in general, and greater maturity, in particular.
Correspondsive principle:	The effect of life experience on personality development is to deepen the characteristics that lead people to those experiences in the first place.

not correspond strongly with any particular statistic. Figure 14.1 provides a schematic of the different types of statistical change. At the foundation is structural continuity, which refers to the persistence of correlational patterns among a set of variables over time or across age groups. Typically, structural continuity is evaluated using either exploratory or confirmatory factor analysis. It is the foundation of any research on continuity and change because establishing structural continuity is the first step that should be taken in all such investigations, regardless of whether the focus is the development of personality traits or other constructs (Baltes, Reese, & Nesselroade, 1977). Structural continuity is important because it establishes whether the same construct is being measured at different time points or ages (Little, 1997). Tracking the remaining types of continuity and change in a construct without first establishing structural continuity is, by definition, a pointless endeavor.

The remaining types of development can be organized nicely in a two-by-two table, with the organizing dimensions being whether the development of a characteristic is examined at the individual or population level, and whether the focus is on absolute or relative standing on the dimension. The population-level examination of relative ranking of individuals is often referred to as "rank-order stability." We prefer "rank-order consistency," largely because the term "stability" denotes an absence of change, which may be

misleading. The population-level examination of absolute change is described as mean-level change, which tracks whether samples or populations as a whole increase, decrease, or remain the same on their average score over time and age. At the individual level, the analogue to rank-order consistency is ipsative consistency. The latter tracks the relative ordering of constructs within an individual over time and age. Finally, change examined at the level of the individual in absolute terms is often referred to as "intra-individual differences in individual change" (Nesselroade, 1991), which we typically shorten to "individual differences in change." Individual differences in change capture each person's unique pattern of increasing, decreasing, or not changing at all on any given dimension.

In the following sections we go into more detail about each type of continuity/

	Relative	Absolute
Population	Rank-order consistency	Mean-level change
Individual	Ipsative consistency	Individual differences in change

Structural Consistency

FIGURE 14.1. Organizationl scheme for the basic indices of continuity and change.

change, the evidence for each, and some of the ancillary questions related to each concept. We close this section with a discussion of one type of conceptual change that is not strongly associated with a specific statistic: heterotypic continuity.

Structural Continuity/Change

At the time of our last review (Caspi & Roberts, 1999), there was a surprising lack of evidence either *for* or *against* the structural continuity of personality across time and age. Since 1999, examining the structural continuity of personality has become much more common. First, the Big Five structure tends to emerge in late childhood and become clarified in adolescence (Allik, Laidra, Realo, & Pullman, 2004; Lamb, Chuang, Wessels, Broberg, & Hwang, 2002). For example, the Big Five appear to emerge out of early childhood temperament dimensions, such as inhibition (Deal, Halverson, Havill, & Martin, 2005). Presumably, then, if a child was rated on a Big Five measure in childhood, the scores among the five would correlate more highly, because these dimensions have yet to fully differentiate from one another. It is possible that with age, the personality of young children, which is relatively undifferentiated, may become more complex both because of cognitive changes and because children acquire a larger set of roles and identities as they age (Block, 1982).

From late adolescence through late middle age, the evidence for the structural continuity of personality traits appears to be strong, with most studies showing little if any serious changes in the factor structure of the Big Five across time or age groups (e.g., Allemand, Zimprich, & Hertzog, 2007; Costa & McCrae, 1992; Robins, Fraley, Roberts, & Trzesniewski, 2001). The same appears to be true of personality structure in old age, though there are some studies that raise questions concerning the comparability of personality structure in old age to young adulthood (Mroczek, Ozer, Spiro, & Kaiser, 1998). Therefore it remains unclear whether the structure of personality traits remains consistent in old age and old-old age (e.g., over 80).

One interesting question that remains to be investigated is whether personality traits become less differentiated, like cognitive abilities, in old age (Baltes, Lindenberger, & Staudinger, 2006). Facets of cognitive ability show signs of becoming more highly correlated in old age (e.g., Deary, Whiteman, Star, Whalley, & Fox, 2004). This de-differentiation is thought to result from a decrease in the integrity of the physiological systems related to cognitive ability, which reduces the specificity of particular skills. A similar idea could be tested with personality traits, for example, by examining whether the higher-order structure of the Big Five, in which the five traits are captured by two dimensions of alpha and beta (Digman, 1997), becomes clearer with age.

The second way in which differentiation may occur is not captured by existing statistical methods. This form of differentiation entails adding new behaviors into one's repertoire for a trait, or more knowledge about existing behaviors. For example, representations of the self become more complex with age (Labouvie-Vief, Chiodo, Goguen, & Diehl, 1995). This added complexity means that more underlying nodes and facets of personality traits develop with time. That is, people may become more sophisticated consumers of their own personality, knowing when and with whom they are outgoing or shy, and in what situations they feel comfortable or anxious. This elaboration of personality may serve as a buffer to global change, as people become more attuned to specific aspects of their personality and determine that change in one relationship or context will not affect the larger network of thoughts, feelings, and behaviors tied to a personality trait. Unfortunately, this type of change has been ignored by most researchers because typical approaches to personality assessment use measures that do not change in content over time.

Rank-Order Consistency/Change

Since the earliest reviews of rank-order consistency, researchers have reported the same two findings: Personality traits demonstrate moderate to high rank-order consistency (e.g., correlations between .4 and .6) over reasonably long periods of time (e.g., 4–10 years), and the longer one tracks rank-order consistency, the lower it gets (e.g., Fraley & Roberts, 2005). Four reviews/meta-analyses on the topic (Ardelt, 2000; Bazana & Stelmack, 2004; Roberts & DelVecchio, 2000; Schuerger, Zarrella, & Hotz, 1989) have come to similar conclusions, with some elaborations and caveats. Specifically, rank-order consistency increases with age and does not appear to plateau until after age 50. Moreover, rank-order consistency does not vary markedly across the Big Five traits, assessment method (i.e., self-reports, observer ratings, and projective tests), or gender.

Several conclusions can be drawn from these reviews and meta-analyses. First, the magnitude of rank-order consistency, although not perfectly "stable," is still remarkably high, especially within windows of 3–10 years. Second, the level of rank-order consistency in childhood and adolescence is much higher than originally expected, especially after age 3. Even more impressive is the fact that the level of rank-order consistency increases in a relatively linear fashion through adolescence and young adulthood. Adolescence is stereotypically considered a time of storm and stress. In turn, young adulthood is the most demographically dense period of the life course, because it involves more life-changing roles and identity decisions than any other period (Arnett, 2000). Yet, despite these dramatic contextual changes, personality traits show no marked decline in rank-order consistency during this time period. Third, rank-order consistency peaks later in adulthood than expected. According to one prominent perspective, personality traits are essentially fixed and unchanging after age 30 (McCrae & Costa, 1994). However, the meta-analytic findings show that rank-order consistency peaks some time after age 50, and at a level well below unity. Finally, the levels of consistency found in recent meta-analyses replicated smaller studies dating back over a half century (e.g., Crook, 1941). Apparently, there have been few, if any, cohort shifts in the level of rank-order stability in personality traits over the past 60 years.

Although personality traits show some degree of change at all ages, they also demonstrate a clear pattern of increasing continuity across the life course. We describe this as the *cumulative continuity principle* (see Table 14.1). People demonstrate higher levels of rank-order consistency with age across all personality traits (Roberts & DelVecchio, 2000). We believe that people exhibit this pattern of increasing continuity throughout

the life course for several reasons, including gene–environment correlations and the processes surrounding identity development (see section below on why personality is consistent).

One of the most interesting secondary questions about differential continuity is whether it exists across long periods of time. This question can be further refined into two critical questions for personality psychology: (1) Does childhood personality predict adult personality, reflecting the twin maxims of the "child is the father to the man" and "give me a child at 7 and I will show you the adult"?; and (2) Is there truly long-term continuity in personality across the vast expanse of adulthood—that is, is the 20-year-old recognizable in the 70-year old?

There is increasing evidence that child temperament can predict a broad range of outcomes much later in the individual's life, but at relatively modest levels of predictive validity. In one of the first studies to examine the continuity of child personality into adulthood (Caspi & Silva, 1995), temperament measured at age 3 predicted personality trait measures collected at age 18. Relative to children categorized as "well-adjusted," children who were categorized as "undercontrolled" at age 3 were found, at age 18, to score higher on aggression, alienation, and stress reaction (similar to neuroticism) and lower on self-control and harm avoidance. Children who were categorized as "inhibited" typically scored higher on harm avoidance and lower on aggression and social potency. All of these effects were approximately in the range of .2–.4 standard deviations—thus small, but not negligible, effects. These differences were largely replicated without any noticeable decrease in magnitude when the same participants were resurveyed at age 26 (Caspi et al., 2003). Similar relationships have been found between infant and adult attachment styles, with classifications of attachment made in the first year of life showing a meta-analytic estimate of $r = .27$ in their ability to predict adult attachment styles (Fraley, 2002).

Personality assessed in later childhood (around the period of 6–12 years) also shows moderate relations with adult personality and life outcomes. In one study, childhood activity and inhibition level, as rated by teachers, showed moderate associations ($rs > .30$) with self-reported or parent-reported

Big Five dimensions assessed at about age 18 (Deal et al., 2005). Personality traits assessed in children at ages 8–10 (by self-report, or teacher or parent reports) have also been found to correlate moderately (rs ≈ .20) with comparable personality dimensions assessed in middle age (Hampson & Goldberg, 2006; Laursen, Pulkkinen, & Adams, 2002; Shiner, Masten, & Roberts, 2003).

The important message here is that the behavioral patterns observed in early childhood are linked to personality traits in adulthood. The significance of this link lies in how much importance one places on small or modest effect sizes (e.g., correlations between .1 and .3). It should be remembered that the typical assessment of childhood temperament is made by parents or teachers, and the typical adult assessment is a self-report. This methodological heterogeneity results in more inherent sources of unreliability than those generally used to assess personality in adulthood (wherein the same person generally completes the same questionnaire on two occasions) and consequently should make the finding of *any* longitudinal relationship all the more impressive. On the other hand, long-term rank-order consistency of analogous constructs, such as intelligence, is much higher from childhood to old age (Deary et al., 2004). The question of whether childhood behavioral tendencies have anything to say about adult personality should be considered solved: They do. The question becomes not so much *whether* we are able to forecast adult behavior from childhood, but what the modest effect sizes mean in terms of practical and theoretical significance (Fraley & Roberts, 2005).

The findings on the long-term rank-order consistency of personality traits in adulthood parallel the findings from childhood to adulthood: The continuity over decades, rather than years, is quite modest. For example, the test–retest correlation in a 50-year longitudinal study of architects ranged from 0 to above .5, with the modal correlation hovering around .2–.4 (Feist & Barron, 2003). The average long-term consistency (e.g., 40 years) of neuroticism averages about .2 (Fraley & Roberts, 2005). The fact that consistency is not zero is conceptually interesting, but such a weak correlation means that we might not recognize the 70-year-old from what we knew when he or she was 20. There has been

little or no discussion of why personality trait consistency diminishes to this level or what types of changes occur over that long of a period. We should assume that there are substantive personality changes occurring across a lifetime, and some effort should be made to investigate what these changes are and why they come about.

Mean-Level Change

"Mean-level change" refers to changes in the quantity or amount of an attribute over time in a sample or population of individuals. Changes in mean levels of personality traits were recently examined in a meta-analysis of 92 different longitudinal studies (Roberts, Walton, & Viechtbauer, 2006). Across these studies, it was found that people became more socially dominant (a facet of extraversion), especially in young adulthood, and they became more conscientious and emotionally stable through midlife. Although much of the change on agreeableness was positive, the increase was only statistically significant in old age. Finally, individuals demonstrated gains in social vitality (a second facet of extraversion) and openness to experience in adolescence and then equivalent declines in old age for both of these trait domains. Many of these patterns are also discernible in cross-sectional studies (Labouvie-Vief, Diehl, Tarnowski, & Shen, 2000; Srivastava, John, Gosling, & Potter, 2003).

Much like the meta-analyses of longitudinal consistency (e.g., Roberts & DelVecchio, 2000), several conspicuous factors did not affect patterns of mean-level change across the life course. First, men and women did not differ in their patterns of mean-level change in personality traits. Although reliable sex differences exist on several personality trait dimensions (Feingold, 1994), it appears that there are few reliable sex differences in the way these traits develop over time.

Interestingly, like rank-order consistency, time was related to change in mean levels. Longitudinal studies that followed participants for a longer period of time reported larger mean-level change estimates. The positive association between time and mean-level change is important for theoretical models of human nature. A common assumption is that personality traits act like metabolic set-points. People may stray briefly from their biological propensity, but they will then drift back to their genetically driven setpoint. Under these types of models, one would expect to find a negative or null association between time and mean-level change because any change would represent short-term fluctuations that disappear as people return to their biologically driven setpoint. However, time is positively associated with personality trait change, which indicates that a strong setpoint model does not apply to personality trait development. That is, when people change, then tend to retain the changes in personality traits for long periods of time.

We also found that cohort standing was related to differential patterns of mean-level change. Younger cohorts had larger standardized mean-level changes in terms of social dominance. The changes in social dominance were consistent with the cross-sectional patterns that indicate that younger cohorts are more assertive (e.g., Twenge, 2001). In addition, a curvilinear relationship was found between cohort standing and both agreeableness and conscientiousness. This pattern indicated that studies focusing on samples from the 1950s and 1960s tended not to increase as much as samples from before and after this period of the 20th century, a pattern first identified by Helson, Jones, and Kwan (2002). These cohort findings point to the importance both of social context and the more inclusive social climate or culture of the people living in a particular period of history. Presumably, social climate affects the way roles are enacted and the behaviors rewarded in those roles, which then affect personality trait development.

We describe the general pattern of personality trait change as the *maturity principle* (Table 14.1) because it corresponds quite closely to definitions of maturity that are functional in nature (Roberts & Wood, 2006). Functional or social maturity is characterized by those qualities that serve to facilitate functioning in society—mature people are more liked, respected, and admired in their communities, social groups, and interpersonal relationships (Hogan & Roberts, 2004). This definition is quite similar to Allport's (1961) characterization of the mature person as happy, showing fewer traces of neurotic and abnormal tendencies, and having the capacity for warm and com-

passionate relationships. From this perspective, maturity is marked by higher levels of emotional stability, conscientiousness, and agreeableness. Research suggests that people do become more mature with age, increasing in assertiveness, self-control, responsibility, and emotional stability, especially between the ages of 20 and 40.

Several other features of the Roberts and colleagues (2006) meta-analysis are important to point out. Most of the patterns of change were heterogeneous and the effect sizes were small for studies tracking development for periods of less than 6 years. Heterogeneity in effect sizes indicates that there is significant variability in the effects across studies. Pragmatically speaking, this means that in some situations, longitudinal studies would find patterns that largely replicate the meta-analysis (e.g., Blonigen, Hicks, Krueger, Patrick, & Iacono, 2006; Donnellan, Conger, & Burzette, 2007), whereas in other situations apparently contradictory findings will emerge (e.g., Watson & Humrichouse, 2006). This is to be expected when heterogeneity combines with small effect sizes, especially in short-term studies. On the other hand, the potential long-term patterns of personality trait change were larger, indicating that studies that follow or track individuals for longer periods of time will reap more compelling evidence for or against the average patterns discovered through meta-analytic aggregation.

Another glaring omission identified in the meta-analytic review is a distinct lack of multimethod research on mean-level change in personality over time. Unlike the evidence for rank-order consistency, we cannot say with confidence that the patterns of mean-level change will replicate across method. This omission was highlighted in a recent longitudinal study of newlywed couples (Watson & Humrichouse, 2006), which found that many personality traits thought to increase in young adulthood, such as agreeableness and conscientiousness, actually decreased over time when assessed by observers. Of course, in this case the observer was a spouse and the sample was drawn from newlyweds, which leads to the inevitable conclusion that the decreases were the result of the honeymoon effect, in which spouses viewed each other through "rose-colored glasses" when they were first married and only came to realize that their spouse was less than perfect after spending a few years with them. None-theless, this study highlights the interesting findings that may emerge when researchers move beyond mono-method studies of per-sonality trait development.

Ipsative Continuity

Structural, differential, and mean-level con-tinuities are indexed by statistics that char-acterize a sample of individuals. However, continuity at the group level may not mir-ror continuity at the individual level. For this reason, some researchers examine "ipsative continuity," which refers to continuity in the configuration of variables within an individ-ual across time.

In Block's seminal work, described in *Lives through Time* (1971), he analyzed ipsative continuity using the California Q-sort. Block's analysis showed that aggregate indices of continuity mask large individual differences in personality continuity. For ex-ample, the average-ipsative correlation be-tween early and late adolescence exceeded .70, but the intraindividual Q-correlations ranged from moderately negative to the maximum imposed by measurement error. Other studies of personality continuity and change between childhood and adolescence report average ipsative correlations ranging from .43 to .71, with considerable variabil-ity in the distribution of these scores (from –.44 to .92), indicating that from childhood to adolescence people vary widely in how much ipsative continuity or change they ex-hibit (Asendorpf & van Aken, 1991; Ozer & Gjerde, 1989). Recent studies have reported similar levels of average ipsative consistency. In a 3-year longitudinal study of children and adolescence, the average profile corre-lation within individuals across a Big Five measure was above .8 (De Fruyt, Bartels, et al., 2006). Slightly lower levels of ipsative consistency across Big Five measures and the (MPQ) have been found in college stu-dents (Robins et al., 2001) and young adults (Donnellan et al., 2007; Roberts, Caspi, & Moffitt, 2001).

Of course, ipsative analyses can be used to study change also. Block (1971) focused on ipsative change in personality by identify-ing groups of men and women marked by specific patterns of change. More recently,

Morizot and Le Blanc (2003, 2005) replicat-ed and extended these findings in a 36-year longitudinal study of men. In a subsample of men who were not jailed as adolescents, they found four developmental groups: com-munals (became less neurotic and impulsive with age), agentics (increased on extraver-sion; decreased on neuroticism and impulsiv-ity), undercontrolled (higher on impulsivity and neuroticism to start), and overcontrolled (no personality change with age; Morizot & Le Blanc, 2005). These four groups par-tially replicate the developmental groups first identified by Block and show the potential of tracking a full profile of personality traits over time. The broader message of these ip-sative studies is that traits can interact with one another to direct the expected pattern of development over time.

Possibly the most interesting work to come out of the ipsative approach is the re-search showing that higher profile stability is associated with mean levels of personal-ity traits themselves. In an 8-year longitudi-nal study, men and women who were more controlled, less neurotic, and more proso-cially oriented demonstrated less change in personality traits and greater profile consis-tency across personality traits (Roberts et al., 2001). These findings were largely replicat-ed, using parent ratings of personality in a 10-year longitudinal study of Iowans (Don-nellan et al., 2007). Therefore, it appears that once people attain high levels of traits associated with maturity—e.g., emotional stability, agreeableness, and conscientious-ness—they keep these qualities in place more readily than people who score lower on these indices. This enhanced stability may be a re-sult of many factors, but most likely these personality traits are reinforced by society in person–environment transactions because they are so often seen as desirable or reward-ing by others.

The advantage of these ipsative indices of continuity is that they reflect the continu-ity of each individual within the sample. This is the type of consistency that most individu-als think about when confronted with the question of whether their "personality" has changed. If the overall organization of one's character remains essentially intact, then changes on individual dimensions may not impact a person's opinion or perspective on whether his or her personality has changed.

Individual Differences in Change

The phrase "individual differences in change" refers to the gains or losses in absolute levels of a personality trait that each individual experiences over time (Nesselroade, 1991). These are changes that deviate from the population mean-level pattern of change. Historically, personality psychologists have not concerned themselves with individual differences in change and have focused disproportionately on population indices of development (Mroczek & Spiro, 2003). This oversight is puzzling, given the fact that personality psychology as a field prides itself on understanding the individual. What could be more intrinsic to understanding personality development than the ability to account for and understand each individual's unique pattern of development?

Of course, one important empirical hurdle needs to be surmounted to imbue the study of individual differences in change with any significance. One must overcome the inference that any deviation around the general pattern of change is simply error (Watson, 2004). The most direct way to confront this inference is to test whether there are people who change more than would be expected, given the level of reliability of any given measure. Individual-level change has been the focus of psychotherapy outcome research for years, and so has the issue of whether changes that occur in therapy are real or simply meaningless fluctuations of an unreliable measure (Jacobson & Truax, 1991). In order to bolster the argument that therapy works at the individual level, psychotherapy outcome researchers developed the Reliable Change Index (RCI) to gauge changes in dimensions related to therapeutic intervention. The RCI gauges the amount of change that occurs against the amount of change that could be expected, given the unreliability of the measure. We introduced this index to personality development researchers in two longitudinal studies (Roberts et al., 2001; Robins et al., 2001) that tracked personality development in young adulthood. In both studies, we found that a greater-than-chance proportion of individuals in our samples showed reliable change, suggesting that reliable individual differences in change existed.

The RCI index has now been used widely in longitudinal studies of personality trait development. Using this index, researchers have replicated the existence of reliable individual differences in change during childhood and adolescence (De Fruyt, Bartels, et al., 2006; Pullman, Raudsepp, & Allik, 2006), young adulthood (Donnellan et al., 2007; Vaidya, Gray, Haig, & Watson, 2002; Watson & Humrichouse, 2006), middle age (Branje, van Lieshout, & van Aken, 2004; van Aken, Denissen, Branje, Dubas, & Goossens, 2006), and old age (Steunenberg, Twisk, Beekman, Deeg, & Kerkhof, 2005).

The use of the RCI has provided unambiguous evidence that individual differences in personality trait change exist and are not attributable to measurement error. On the other hand, the RCI is fundamentally flawed. First, it is grossly conservative. It requires that people move more than two standard errors on a trait in order to categorize them as changing reliably. It is quite possible that smaller changes are important and reliable. Second, it is applicable to studies that track change over two waves of assessment. It is now clear that two-wave longitudinal studies provide unreliable and imprecise assessments of change (Singer & Willett, 2003). The optimal way to track personality change is to gather multiple assessments over time and apply growth-modeling techniques to estimate individual differences in change over time. Using these techniques, researchers have shown that reliable individual differences in personality trait change occur across young adulthood, middle age, and old age (Jones, Livson, & Peskin, 2003; Mroczek & Spiro, 2003; Roberts & Chapman, 2000; Scollon & Diener, 2006; Small, Hertzog, Hultsch, & Dixon, 2003).

The second way of establishing both the existence and the importance of individual differences in personality trait change is to test whether life experiences are associated with changes in personality traits. For example, if people who experience more satisfying work grow happier and more emotionally stable with time, this indicates that not everyone changes in this way and that work experiences may be a causal force for personality trait change. It also provides a potential explanation for why most people might change in a normative fashion, as we discuss below in the section on social investment. We review this material in more detail below in the section on why personality traits change. Suffice it to say that certain life experiences are associated with distinctive patterns of trait development (Roberts & Mroczek, 2008).

Finally, it should be noted that individual differences in change may be important from a practical standpoint. Studies have shown that modest changes in personality traits can result in profound consequences for health. Specifically, men and women who showed increased levels of hostility experienced increased obesity, inactivity, social isolation, and worse physical health compared to those who did not show increased levels of hostility (Siegler et al., 2003). In the case of neuroticism, men who increased one half of a standard deviation in neuroticism in old age suffered a 32% increase in mortality compared to men who did not change in neuroticism (Mroczek & Spiro, 2007). These studies point to the fact that relatively modest changes in personality traits may have significant consequences for individuals.

Personality Coherence

The kinds of continuity and change discussed so far refer to statistical indices of continuity and change in identical constructs over time. The concept of coherence enlarges the definition of continuity and change to include "heterotypic continuity," which entails identifying relations between different sets of behavior across different ages. For instance, individuals who hurt animals as children might engage in more criminal behavior in adulthood. It is important to emphasize that coherence and heterotypic continuity refer to conceptual rather than statistical continuity among behaviors. When relationships are found between different behaviors over time, these heterotypic connections need to be explained by an underlying dispositional attribute that (1) is related to both behaviors at different time points, and (2) shows a sizable degree of rank-order consistency. For instance, hurting animals as children and adult criminal activity might be indicators of underlying, consistent antisocial tendencies. Accordingly, the investigator who claims to have discovered coherence must have a theory—no matter how rudimentary or implicit—that specifies the latent construct or provides the basis on which the diverse behaviors and attributes can be said to belong to the same equivalence class.

The argument that coherence requires a theoretical framework and not just a statistic means that heterotypic continuity remains an alluring, if difficult, concept to prove. Research has shown that childhood personality is linked to adult outcomes, which, at first blush, look like heterotypic continuity. Shy children leave their parental home at an older age and delay their assumption of adult social roles, such as marriage and work (Caspi, Elder, & Bem, 1988). Anxious, stress-prone children grow up to become conventional, moralistic conservatives (Block & Block, 2006). Children who are more agreeable grow up to smoke fewer cigarettes in adulthood (Hampson, Goldberg, Vogt, & Dubanoski, 2007). Inhibited children become adults who are seen as more neurotic and less extraverted, agreeable, conscientious, and open to experience (Deal et al., 2005).

Although these examples provide unequivocal evidence linking childhood personality to later adult phenomena, it is unclear whether they are examples of heterotypic continuity. The implicit theory behind these results would be best approximated by trait theory or five-factor theory, which posits that traits are latent temperaments that are unaffected by experience (e.g., McCrae et al., 2000). Invoking this theoretical framework invites skepticism, however. Is conservatism simply a manifestation of neuroticism? The findings connecting childhood inhibition to all of the Big Five pose even more difficulties for a trait model. Clearly, inhibition is linked to all of the Big Five in adulthood. Yet, in adulthood, the Big Five are only modestly correlated, indicating that inhibition must be differentiated into multiple domains that result in the Big Five. Therefore, it would be difficult to conclude that the Big Five exist in temperamental form early in life and progress in an undifferentiated form into adult versions of traits.

As these examples illustrate, the theories behind claims of coherence often amount to appeals to the reader's intuition. Often they are post hoc interpretations of empirical relations discovered in large correlation matrices (Moss & Susman, 1980). With the notable exception of the psychoanalytic theory of psychosexual stages and their adult sequelae, few personality theories specify links between personality variables at different developmental periods. That is to say, the field of personality development remains without a coherent theory of development (Roberts, 2005).

WHY ARE PERSONALITY TRAITS BOTH CONSISTENT AND CHANGEABLE?

Given the evidence that has emerged in the last decade, it is now an unavoidable conclusion that personality traits show both continuity and change. Adding the small phrase "and change" to the term continuity may seem subtle, but it dramatically shifts the theoretical sands on which personality psychology rests. First, it leads us to another basic principle of personality development, the *plasticity principle* (Table 14.1 on page 376). This principle states that personality traits are open systems that can be influenced by the environment at any age. This principle undermines the assumption that personality traits do not change—an assumption that many continue to hold. By assuming that personality traits do not change, researchers can simplify their view of human nature: One component, personality traits, is stable and unchanging. Making this assumption allows researchers to use personality traits in a straightforward, if limited, manner as predictors of outcomes, not as outcomes themselves. Expanding the conceptualization of

personality traits to one that subsumes both continuity and change makes the world a much more interesting place—it necessitates that we explain why personality is consistent, for example. For the remainder of this chapter we address the questions of why personality is consistent, why it changes, and why it does not change more than it does.

Why Are Personality Traits Consistent?

The mechanisms responsible for personality trait continuity can be organized into several categories, including genetic, environmental, person–environment transactions, and identity structure (see Table 14.2). In the following section, we outline the primary mechanisms we believe facilitate increasing consistency in personality traits across the life course.

Genetic and Environmental Mechanisms

Genetic factors could be contributors to continuity over time because the genome itself is relatively unchanging.[1] The best evidence for the role of genes in maintaining consistency has been provided by longitudinal studies that track identical and fraternal twins over time. For example, McGue, Bacon, and Lykken (1993) administered personality tests to monozygotic and dyzygotic twins over a 10-year period. Their estimates of overall consistency were similar to other studies (ranging from .4 to .7), showing that there was a balance

TABLE 14.2. Why Are Personality Traits Consistent?

Genetic effects:	Genes provide a continuous physiological substrate.
Role continuity/ environment:	Consistent perceptions of environment maintain continuity.
Person × environment transactions:	
Attraction:	People are attracted to environments that are consistent with their personality.
Selection:	People are selected into roles that are consistent with their personality.
Reactance:	People selectively attend to information relevant to preexisting dispositions.
Evocation:	People evoke reactions from others that reinforce existing dispositions.
Manipulation:	People change their environment to better fit their personality.
Attrition:	People leave environments that call for too much change.
Identity clarity:	A clearer sense of identity facilitates selection, evocation, and reaction.

of consistency and change. Most interestingly, the authors estimated that 80% of the personality consistency demonstrated by their sample of twins was attributable to genetic influences (see also, Lykken & Tellegen, 1996). Since this research, several other longitudinal twin studies have produced more moderate findings. In a 3-year longitudinal study of child and adolescent twins, personality continuity was associated with genetic effects as well as shared and nonshared environmental factors (De Fruyt, Bartels, et al., 2006). Similarly, in midlife, personality consistency results from both genetic and environmental factors (Johnson, McGue, & Krueger, 2005). Clearly, one of the reasons for consistency in personality has to be the genetic foundation of human behavior.

Ironically, the best evidence for the fact that the "environment" contributes to personality continuity over time comes from these very same behavioral genetics studies. The evidence that both shared and nonshared environmental factors contribute to personality continuity over time provides support for the effect of environments as analogous to the effect of genetics. That is, just as behavioral genetics studies do not measure actual genes yet infer genetic effects, they also do not measure actual environments, and yet they infer environmental effects. As behavioral genetic studies indicate the existence of nongenetic effects on stability in this way, the next order of business is to identify what these effects are.

We believe that the ideal environment to consider when investigating the association of environmental experiences and personality development is the social role (Roberts, 2007). Social roles capture the component of the environment that is most likely related to continuity: a consistent subjective environment in the form of roles that people enact across time and place. We describe this as the *role continuity principle* (see Table 14.1 on page 376). For example, adolescents who play specific roles in high school, such as being a "jock" or a "brain," tend to adopt similar roles in later life stages, such as in college or in their chosen occupation or leisure interests (Barber, Eccles, & Stone, 2001). We believe that it is this coherence of social roles that transcends the physical environment and facilitates personality consistency over time.

Person–Environment Transactions

Person–environment transactions capture a third set of mechanisms that promote consistency (Caspi & Roberts, 1999; Roberts, 2006). These mechanisms reflect the environmental and individual difference factors that combine to promote continuity. There are at least six types of person–environment transactions that should contribute to continuity: attraction, selection, reactance, evocation, manipulation, and attrition (see Table 14.2). Attraction transactions, or "active niche picking," reflect the processes by which people are drawn to and choose experiences whose qualities are consistent with their own personalities. For example, people who are more extraverted prefer jobs that are described as social or enterprising, such as teaching or business management (Ackerman & Heggestad, 1997). In terms of dating and marital partners, individuals tend to enter relationships with mates who prefer their personality traits (Botwin, Buss, & Schackelford, 1997). Thus, continuity may be enhanced to the extent that individuals can select personality-reinforcing situations.

Second, continuity may be enhanced through selection effects, whereby people are selected into situations and given preferential treatment on the basis of their personality characteristics. These recruitment effects begin to appear early in development. For example, children's personality traits influence their emerging relationships with teachers at a young age (Birch & Ladd, 1998). In adulthood, job applicants who are more extraverted, conscientious, and less neurotic are liked better by interviewers and are more often recommended for the job (Cook, Vance, & Spector, 2000). In terms of relationship partners, there is strong evidence that people who are more agreeable, less neurotic, and more open to experience are preferred by most people (Watson et al., 2004).

Third, reactive transactions may contribute to consistency because these transactions lead individuals to extract a subjective psychological environment from the objective surroundings based on their personality. Peoples' conscious and unconscious schemas, based in part on their personality traits, act as filters for social information. These personality-based cognitive filters help to create an idiosyncratic, personal reality for each individual that is unique to his or her own personality. Typically, these cognitive schemas help individuals selectively respond to information that is congruent with their expectations and self-views (Fiske & Taylor, 1991). Persistent ways of perceiving, thinking, and behaving are preserved, in part, by features of the cognitive system, and because of these features the course of personality is likely to be quite conservative and resistant to change (Westen, 1991).

Fourth, evocative processes may also engender greater personality consistency over time (Caspi & Roberts, 1999). That is, people tend to evoke personality-consistent responses from others, and this process can occur outside of conscious awareness. For example, aggression typically evokes hostility from others (Dodge & Tomlin, 1987). Likewise, dominant behavior is typically met with submissive responses (Thorne, 1987). Thus, dominant people, by evoking more submissive responses from others, find the world full of people willing to follow their lead. Given that people make up the primary "environment," evocative transactions would be one of the strongest contributors to personality trait continuity.

Fifth, people can manipulate their environment. If they do not like their work or their relationship partner, people can change (manipulate) either for the better. In work settings, success and power bring with it the opportunity to shape the nature of the organization by hiring, firing, and promoting workers. Individuals also may shape their work to better fit themselves through job crafting (Wrzesniewski & Dutton, 2001) or job sculpting (Bell & Staw, 1989). They can change their day-to-day work environments through changing the tasks they do, organizing their work differently, or changing the nature of the relationships they maintain with others (Wrzesniewski & Dutton, 2001). Presumably these changes in work environments lead to an increase in the fit between personality and work. In turn, increased fit with one's environment is associated with elevated consistency (Roberts & Robins, 2004).

Sixth, continuity can be maintained as consequences of "attrition" or "de-selection pressures," whereby people leave settings (e.g., jobs, marriages) that do not fit with their personality, or they are released from

these settings because of their trait-correlated behaviors (Cairns & Cairns, 1994). For example, longitudinal evidence from different countries shows that children who exhibit a combination of high irritability/antagonism and poor self-control are at heightened risk of unemployment as young adults (Caspi, Wright, Moffitt, & Silva, 1998; Kokko & Pulkkinen, 2000). Moreover, people who are disagreeable, neurotic, and low in conscientiousness experience elevated levels of divorce (Roberts, Kuncel, Shiner, Caspi, & Goldberg, 2007), presumably because these individuals often create hostile, dissatisfying relationships (Watson et al., 2004). Being forced out of situations that might bring pressure to change allows people to maintain a consistent personality, even if it is a maladaptive one.

Identity Mechanisms

A final set of factors that facilitates increasing personality consistency has to do with a person's meta-perceptions of his or her own personality, which have been nominally described as identity structures (Roberts & Wood, 2006). Specifically, with age, the process of developing, committing to, and maintaining an identity leads to greater personality consistency (Roberts & Caspi, 2003). We describe this as the *identity development principle* (see Table 14.1 on page 376). Embedded in this principle is the process of finding one's niche. People select roles that appear to fit with their dispositions, values, and abilities, and this selection process should facilitate continuity over time (Roberts & DelVecchio, 2000). Assuming that most roles do not fit perfectly, people are likely motivated to shape the features of their roles so that they do fit better than before. Thus, through building an optimal or satisfying niche, people inevitably create an environment that supports continuity over time.

Although identity is made up of constituent elements, such as traits and goals, it also consists of meta-cognitive factors that reflect people's perceptions of their own attributes (Roberts & Wood, 2006). For example, with age people become clearer about their personality attributes, interests, abilities, and life story (Helson, Stewart, & Ostrove, 1995). This increase in identity clarity may also contribute to increasing consistency with age. For example, having an achieved identity was found to be related to higher levels of psychological well-being (Helson et al., 1995). Similarly, self-concept clarity is associated with higher levels of self-esteem (Campbell, 1990). Therefore, identity, and aspects of identity such as achievement, certainty, and clarity are linked to higher levels of psychological well-being and adjustment, which in turn are related to higher levels of personality trait consistency (Donnellan et al., 2007; Roberts et al., 2001).

In sum, it is clear that numerous factors contribute to the increase in personality continuity observed over the life course. Genetic factors, the environment, person–environment transactions, and identity development are all implicated in the inevitable stabilization of personality traits that comes with age.

Why Do Personality Traits Change with Age?

As we have seen, personality trait change is systematic and real, not simply random. How does personality change come about? First, people might change in response to contingencies in the environments found in social roles (see Table 14.3). For example, parents reward and punish their children in an effort to shape their behavior. Presumably, long-term exposure to specific reward and punishment schedules should result in personality differences among people. The second and third change mechanisms are watching ourselves and watching others, especially in new contexts. Personality change may come about by adopting new behaviors through watching others (e.g., modeling), or by watching ourselves do things differently, often in the context of a new role or in response to new role demands (Caspi & Roberts, 1999). Another change mechanism reflects listening to others. Thus, spouses may inevitably point out to their partners the existence of some characterological flaws that were previously unrecognized. This feedback, if willingly acknowledged, may facilitate change in personality.

Several longitudinal studies have demonstrated that experiences in work and marriage are associated with changes in personality traits. Work-related experiences, such as working more than others or attaining higher status, are associated with increases in the social dominance facet of extraversion and traits from the domain of conscientiousness (Clausen & Gilens, 1990; Elder, 1969; Roberts, 1997; Roberts, Caspi, & Moffitt, 2003). Achieving higher status at work is also associated with increases in masculinity and decreases in femininity (Kasen, Chen, Sneed, Crawford, & Cohen, 2006). In addition, positive experiences in work are associated with increases in traits tied to the domain of emotional stability (Roberts & Chapman, 2000; Scollon & Diener, 2006; van Aken et al., 2006).

Marital and family experiences also are associated with changes in personality traits.

TABLE 14.3. Why Do Personality Traits Change with Age and Why Don't They Change More?

Why do personality traits change with age?	
Role contingencies:	Roles provide reinforcements and punishments for specific behaviors.
Watching ourselves:	Seeing changes in our own behaviors leads to changes in perceptions of ourselves or changes in reputation.
Watching others:	Change comes about through modeling others' behavior.
Listening to others:	People provide feedback on how we should change.
Role expectations and demands:	Roles communicate behaviors that will be reinforced and punished.

Why don't personality traits change more?	
Filibustering:	Waiting out the press to change in the hope that the catalyst will lose steam.
Identity structure:	Complexity of identity buffers dispositions from environmental turbulence.
Dispositions:	Certain traits may predispose people to be less receptive to demands to change.
Social-cognitive mechanisms:	Accommodation, optimization, selection, immunization, and defense mechanisms shape information in order to deflect the press to change.

For example, women experiencing stable, satisfying, and fulfilling relationships become more emotionally stable and conscientious (Lehnart & Neyer, 2006; Roberts & Bogg, 2004; Roberts & Chapman, 2000; Robins, Caspi, & Moffitt, 2002; Scollon & Diener, 2006). Similarly, engaging in a serious partnership for the first time in young adulthood is associated with decreases in neuroticism and increases in conscientiousness (Neyer & Asendorpf, 2001; Neyer & Lehnart, 2007), and receiving more support from family members during adolescence is associated with increases in agreeableness (Asendorpf & van Aken, 2003; Branje, van Lieshout, van Aken, & Haselager, 2004). Finally, getting married or remarried in late middle age and old age is associated with decreases in neuroticism over time in men (Mroczek & Spiro, 2003). These longitudinal studies demonstrate that experiences in the conventional roles of work and relationships can explain, in part, the increases in agreeableness, conscientiousness, and emotional stability found in young and middle adulthood.

It is most common to assume that environments cause changes in psychological functioning. Nonetheless, to infer that environments are causal forces requires either (1) evidence for the prospective effects of social context on personality trait change, or (2) evidence for personality trait change that arises from interventions. In terms of the prospective effects of social context on personality trait change, there are now a handful of studies demonstrating this type of pattern. For example, remaining in an intact marriage and not smoking marijuana were both prospectively related to changes in responsibility (Roberts & Bogg, 2004). Specifically, experiences of an intact marriage and low marijuana use in young adulthood predicted increases in social responsibility in midlife. Analogously, Lehnart and Neyer (2006) found that higher levels of relationship security predicted increases in conscientiousness, and higher levels of relationship dependency predicted decreases in neuroticism. Interestingly, these effects held only for people who did not change relationships, highlighting the fact that for contexts to have an effect on personality trait development, it may be critical that the context does not change over time (Roberts, 2006). Of course, prospective effects are rare, and a number of studies have

failed to detect such effects (e.g., Scollon & Diener, 2006; Watson & Humrichouse, 2006). Nonetheless, the fact that some prospective effects do exist bolsters the inference that social contexts can and do affect personality trait change.

The best evidence for the effect of environmental experiences on personality trait development comes from intervention studies that actively attempt to change personality. There have been several recent attempts to track personality trait changes in individuals receiving some form of active intervention, such as psychotherapy or drug therapy. The few studies that do exist are quite provocative. In the first study, a sample of chronic substance users was tracked for over a year while receiving wide-ranging treatments to improve vocational skills, coping abilities, and spiritual development (Piedmont, 2001) and change in personality traits above and beyond changes in symptomology was tested in these individuals. Positive changes in all of the Big Five personality traits were found on the order of one-quarter to one-half of a standard deviation from pretreatment to posttreatment. In the second study a large sample of patients with depression received a wide variety of treatments. It was found that neuroticism scores decreased one-half of a standard deviation over a 6-month period (De Fruyt, Van Leeuwen, Bagby, Rolland, & Rouillon, 2006).

These two studies dovetail with earlier research showing similar levels of personality trait change that resulted from therapeutic interventions (Bagby, Joffe, Parker, Kalemba, & Harkness, 1995; Trull, Useda, Costa, & McCrae, 1995). These studies are notable for the fact that they show quite clearly that personality traits *can be changed*. Moreover, when compared to the magnitude of personality trait change that occurs across the life course, which appears to be around one full standard deviation (Roberts et al., 2006), the magnitude of the change is quite dramatic. Through 6 months of therapy, people can achieve change equal to 20 years of natural progression in personality development. One caveat should be mentioned. Both of these studies relied on self-report personality assessments, which beg the question of whether patients were responding to demand characteristics of the intervention. Future research should track change in more objective measures of personality traits, such as observer ratings or behavioral observations.

One of the most salient features of the longitudinal studies examining mean-level change in personality is the fact that young adulthood—the years from ages 20 to 40—are the critical years for personality trait development. Presumably, people are confronted with more role contingencies and more opportunities to watch others, themselves, and receive feedback during this period of the life course. We have attempted to explain the fact that this age period is the fulcrum for personality trait development with the *social investment principle* (see Table 14.1 on page 376), which states that investing in social institutions, such as age-graded social roles, is one of the primary reasons for personality trait development in young adulthood (Lodi-Smith & Roberts, 2007; Roberts, Wood, & Smith, 2005). Three assumptions underlie this principle. First, people build identities by making psychological commitments to social institutions in the form of social roles, such as work, marriage, family, and community. Second, social roles come with their own set of expectations and contingencies that promote a reward structure that calls for becoming more socially dominant, agreeable, conscientious, and less neurotic. Third, the dominant pattern of role investments seen in quasi-universal tasks of social living, such as developing a family and career (Helson et al., 2002), occurs in young adulthood. In turn these quasi-universal transitions in young adulthood help to explain the normative patterns of personality change that result from role investments during this time of the life course.

The key personality changing element within the social investment experience lies in committing oneself to social institutions outside of one's existing identity structure. This act exposes a person to the contingencies contained in the new social role, expressed in the form of role expectations for appropriate behavior (Sarbin, 1964). For example, people come to their first job with a set of expectations about how they should act that are derived from their experiences watching significant others, such as parents, mentors, friends, and other influential people, in the same types of roles (Caspi & Roberts, 1999). Such role expectations can affect change either through punishing inappropriate behav-

ior or rewarding appropriate behavior. Role expectations exert social control over behavior, such that people who violate the expectations are punished and those who conform to the expectations are rewarded with social regard.

Another key ingredient of social investment that should help to facilitate change is the commitment to the organization, institution, or relationship (Lodi-Smith & Roberts, 2007). This is better explained in the converse situation, in which people are not invested. These individuals do not respond to role expectations and socialization forces within the social roles and relationships to which they are exposed because they do not care about, or see rewards in responding to, the demands of the situation. By committing to social roles and relationships, people make investments that they believe will suit their life and possibly reflect their preferred niche. If a niche subsequently calls for change, a person will be more likely to respond if he or she has an emotional and long-term perspective on that investment. In contrast, lack of commitment should lead to indifference or skepticism in the face of demands for change.

The social investment principle captures the key transition in the age-graded nature of roles in young adulthood. Specifically, people move from dependency on others in adolescence to simultaneous autonomy and increasing accountability to others as young adults (e.g., to their company and their family). The dual demands of increasing self-sufficiency and increasing responsibility to others naturally press people to behave in a more communal manner and become more self-controlled with age (Wood & Roberts, 2006a). Thus, investments in conventional social institutions should be related to increasing scores on measures of agreeableness, conscientiousness, and emotional stability.

In sum, we propose that people change by responding to contingencies, modeling others, and receiving persistent feedback that contradicts closely held views of the self (Table 14.3). Moreover, the most likely source of these forces of change arises via investment in social institutions such as marriage, work, and community. These institutions, embodied in social roles, bring with them expectations and demands for confidence, prosocial behaviors, responsibility, and emotional stability. Of course, sometimes people select new identities in order to change (Snyder & Ickes, 1985). But we believe that this is the least likely pathway through which personality traits change. Rather, change is most likely the result of the long-term press of social environments that are chosen for reasons other than personality trait development (e.g., interests, abilities, or goals).

Why Don't Personality Traits Change More?

One of the most striking features of the longitudinal studies that track the relationship between life experiences and personality change is the relatively small effect that environmental contingencies have on personality trait change. Despite robust shifts in environments, people do not demonstrate dramatic shifts in terms of personality traits. Rather, individuals demonstrate significant shifts on a minority of traits and small-to-moderate shifts on the remaining traits (e.g., Roberts et al., 2001). This invites our last question of personality development, why don't we find more evidence of personality trait change?

The first reason for the modest changes that occur in personality traits may be that the influence of continuity mechanisms outweighs the impact of change mechanisms. That is, if people are successful in selecting, evoking, and shaping environments, then the environments themselves will not bring with them pressures to reconstruct personality. People may also be motivated to remain consistent. As Block (1982) wrote: "Through the course of evolution, individuals have been programmed to follow the adaptive imperative: Assimilate if you can; accommodate if you must. Assimilatory efforts are the first line of adaptation" (p. 286).

Moreover, if there is a press to change, the press will be in the direction of the personality qualities that drew the person to that environment in the first place. Thus, the most common effect of life experiences on personality development is to deepen the characteristics that lead people to specific environments (Roberts & Caspi, 2003; Roberts et al., 2003; Roberts, O'Donnell, & Robins, 2004; Roberts & Robins, 2004). We describe this as the *correspensive principle* (Table 14.1 on page 376). Specifically, life experiences that are correspensive (i.e., that elicit behaviors that are consistent with their dispositions) will be viewed as validating and

thus rewarding to a person, resulting in an elaboration of the dispositions being rewarded by experience. Correspensiveness helps to explain one of the key features of personality trait development in adulthood: its modest nature. Typically, individuals do not go through dramatic transformation in terms of personality traits. Change seems to occur at a modest rate over long periods of time in a minority of traits within each person's profile of dispositions and often in the direction of the traits that led that individual to a particular social context in the first place.

The question of why we do not see as much change as we might expect, given the shifts in environments, points to mechanisms that intervene between changes in environments and changes in personality. We see four sets of mechanisms that people use mostly in response to environmental contingencies that demand change. These mechanisms tend to preclude change because of how they affect the information gleaned from the experience in the environment (see Table 14.3 on page 387). The first set concerns actively avoiding new environments or avoiding making the social and emotional investment that would result in change. The second set is the effect of identity structures and negotiations on experience. The third set involves individual-difference characteristics that seem to buffer or enhance susceptibility to environmental contingencies. The fourth set encompasses social-cognitive factors that inoculate or diminish the significance, relevance, or meaningfulness of the environmental press to change.

In most socialization theories, the assumption is that the path from the environment to the person is direct. Clearly, the path is not direct. First, situations affect behavior directly and broad-level phenomena indirectly (Roberts, 2005). Second, experiences that occur early in the process of acquiring the role may not be internalized because of the identity negotiations that take place. People do not simply respond to the press to change. They may try to shape the role to fit themselves better, and it may take time before these strategies are exhausted and they to come to terms with a set of expectations that contradicts their strongly held self-perceptions. Third, people may simply try to wait out a press to change. We describe this strategy as "filibustering," in which people attempt to delay what might seem to be the inevitable by ignoring it and hoping it will go away. For example, a new administrator may come to a job and demand that employees become more service oriented (e.g., accommodating, friendly, polite). An employee could simply wait out the new supervisor in hope that either the system will crush the supervisor's desire for climate change or that the supervisor will be replaced.

Another reason why personality traits may not change dramatically is that the effects of molecular changes in environments are filtered through multiple levels of the trait hierarchy (Roberts, 2006; Wood & Roberts, 2006b). Specifically, role identities and other mid-level psychological structures may play a particularly important mediating role between life experiences and personality trait change. Due to their closer proximity to role experiences, role identities may change substantially because of role-relevant experiences, even while these experiences only lightly affect a person's general identity (Wood, 2007; Wood & Roberts, 2006b). For example, after becoming a parent, it might be presumed that a man would see himself as a more conscientious person. However, he may report that he has not changed in terms of conscientiousness because the change is only localized to a specific role identity—the parent role—and not his entire personality. In essence, the effect of the experience in one role is muted at the general personality level, which considers not just the identity one has as a parent, but also self-views about oneself as a friend, child, worker, and so on.

An additional set of factors that mollify the press to change are dispositions themselves. Certain people are less inclined than others to respond to environmental contingencies. For example, in work settings, people who were uncooperative were less likely to adopt a competitive stance when the organizational culture demanded it (Chatman & Barsade, 1995). Similarly, unconventional, less adjusted women were less likely to change in ways consistent with the changing cultural climate of the 1960s, 70s, and 80s (Roberts & Helson, 1997). Accordingly, one would assume that people suffering from certain personality disorders, such as narcissistic personality disorder, would not have the necessary psychological skills to respond to role contingencies and would thus change

less in response to role expectations or feedback than others—unless, of course, the role expectations call for the person to become more narcissistic (Robins & Paulhus, 2001).

An additional set of identity-related factors that would moderate the effect of environmental demands for change are a person's existing cognitive and emotional schemas that are designed to protect identity when it is threatened. These social-cognitive factors subsume a wide range of conscious and unconscious information-processing factors while sharing one thing in common: They all act to reconfigure the meaning of experience, not experience itself (Cramer, 1998).

The first set of social-cognitive mechanisms, drawn from lifespan developmental theory, are termed "accommodative" strategies (Brandtstadter & Greve, 1994) and refer to the adjustments one makes in goals or self-evaluative standards in order to maintain consistent self-views. Brandtstadter (1992) showed that people increase the use of flexible goal adjustment with age and simultaneously diminish their tenacious goal pursuit. Thus, with age, people recalibrate their goals rather than persist in attempting to achieve specific outcomes (e.g., earning enough for retirement rather than earning enough to become rich). By recalibrating goals, people can maintain consistent self-views (e.g., "I am successful").

Similarly, the optimization and compensation strategies from the selection, optimization, and compensation model (SOC; Baltes & Baltes, 1990) can be seen as continuity-promoting mechanisms. "Optimization" refers to emphasizing goals and activities that reflect a person's strengths rather than emphasizing something new or untested (e.g., selection). Compensation reflects the inevitable tailoring of goals and activities to make up for the natural degradation of abilities in old age. Both of these mechanisms entail emphasizing, if not fostering, existing characteristics or skills. Applied to the sphere of personality traits, one can easily see that the successful utilization of optimization and compensation strategies would facilitate the maintenance of personality traits. For example, a person with a propensity to work hard, despite decreasing his or her expenditure of energy at work, can maintain a self-impression that he or she is conscientious by emphasizing other facets of conscientiousness, such as his or her organization skills or ability to be efficient.

Brandtstadter and Greve (1994) described a fourth information-processing factor, immunization, which is defined as processes that protect the self from self-discrepant evidence. These mechanisms include de-emphasizing the personal relevance of an experience, searching for and finding an alternative interpretation, and questioning the credibility of the source of information. In relation to personality consistency, one may imagine a person receiving feedback from a friend that he or she is hostile and mean. If this person feels that he or she is not hostile, then immunizing mechanisms may be employed to discount the friend's opinion. In order to maintain a consistent self-perception, this person may attempt to trivialize the importance of the relationship, attribute the feedback to the friend's own issues (alternative interpretation), or question the friend's ability to make such interpretations (question credibility). All of these strategies would serve to maintain the person's self-perception that he or she is not hostile or at least not as hostile as the friend claims.

Accommodation, optimization, and immunization mechanisms are assumed to be available to conscious awareness. Defense mechanisms are assumed to perform similar functions to the conscious information-processing mechanisms identified above, but do so outside of conscious awareness. Contemporary perspectives define defense mechanisms as unconscious mental operations that function to protect the individual from experiencing excessive anxiety (Cramer, 1998). Defense mechanisms are seen not only in the classical psychoanalytic sense as acting to filter unacceptable internal thoughts, impulses, or wishes, but also in the contemporary sense as filtering out experiences and information that threaten one's self-esteem or self-integration (Cramer, 1998). The filtering of undesirable experiences/information is seen as leading to more adaptive behavior (Davidson, MacGregor, Johnson, Woody, & Chaplin, 2004).

If we assume that, in part, personality change results from experiencing events that contradict closely held views of the self, or from receiving feedback from others that we are different from our self-perceptions, then defense mechanisms should buffer the effect of these episodes. Being told that one's personality must change would be quite stressful (Block, 1982). In fact, research shows that people become anxious when presented with information that contradicts their self-perceptions, even if that new information is more positive than their closely held self-concept (Swann, Pelham, & Krull, 1989).

Accommodation, optimization, compensation, immunization, and defense mechanisms serve the agenda of maintaining continuity in personality in response to environmental contingencies that normally would result in change. Combined with identity negotiations and individual differences in personality traits themselves, people are potentially well defended against environmental presses to change their personality. This is even truer when we see that changes in behaviors, thoughts, and feelings at the lower level of abstraction must negotiate the path upward to broader attributions about the self. Thus, we also see why change is typically modest in relation to putatively dramatic environmental contingencies. Unfortunately, to our knowledge, the buffering of these mechanisms has not been tested in longitudinal studies of personality trait development.

CONCLUSIONS

In this chapter we have attempted to address four fundamental questions about personality trait development: How do personality traits develop in adulthood? Why do personality traits become more consistent with age? Why do personality traits change with age? Why don't personality traits change more than they do? Looking back since the last installment of this chapter, it is most gratifying to see the research on personality trait development come of age. It is no longer an anomaly to report longitudinal data, and the shear number and quality of studies emerging in the last decade bodes well for the continued development of the field.

With these recent accomplishments in mind, we would like to make several recommendations about where we would like to see the field of personality development move in the coming decade and what questions need answering. The first handbook chapter on personality development (Caspi & Bem, 1990) ended with a *mea culpa* that the chapter had not addressed the issue of personality change. The subsequent installments have rectified this oversight, but similarly have left a number of issues untouched themselves.

First, this chapter has focused exclusively on personality traits. Personality psychology encompasses more concepts than personality traits. The development of other, clearly important domains and constructs are in dire need of attention. How do goals and motives develop with age? Are narrative structures as consistent as personality traits? Do the same mechanisms and processes derived from the study of personality traits apply to other types of constructs? Some initial research has shown that goal ratings are more consistent over time than previously suspected (Roberts et al., 2004). Moreover, interests are more consistent than personality traits at a younger age (Low, Yoon, Roberts, & Rounds, 2005), and narrative structures, though consistent, are less so than personality traits (McAdams et al., 2006). These and other related issues, such as the interplay between different domains (e.g., goals and traits over time), deserve greater attention.

Second, we need a better understanding of the process-oriented mechanisms that explain continuity and change. These mechanisms are absent in most trait theories but are key components of social-cognitive approaches to personality. For example, many of the reasons why personality traits remain consistent over time rest on social-cognitive processes, such as the filtering effect of schemas or the evocative effects of behaviors. Understanding personality change entails understanding the growth of self-knowledge and the opportunities to recognize change in one's own behavior. Future research should integrate trait and social-cognitive models of personality development and test them in well-run longitudinal studies in order to better understand the processes of personality development.

Third, the most glaring omission in this review is a complete lack of understanding of how people come to have personality traits in the first place. How does a trait such as conscientiousness emerge from the stew of temperament and early childhood experience to become a full-fledged disposition in adulthood? What are the key developmental experiences that shape conscientiousness

and other traits? The typical answer to these questions alludes to genetics, temperament, and a little hand waving. Simply assuming that the Big Five emerge like some premature adult doppelganger in children is an insufficient and unsatisfying portrait of what has to be a much more dynamic story. Future research needs to develop a coherent theoretical framework and accounting for the development of personality traits from childhood, to adulthood, and into old age.

In conclusion, the field of personality trait development has surged forward in the last decade to a state of maturity unlike any point in the past. It is now time to move past simple questions of whether personality is stable or changeable to the harder questions of why and how personality traits, and other personality constructs, develop.

NOTE

1. Although genes may be unchanging, their effects may change over the life course because of epigenetic effects, such as methylation, which change the expression of genes (Roberts & Jackson, in press).

REFERENCES

Ackerman, P. L., & Heggestad, E. D. (1997). Intelligence, personality, and interests: Evidence for overlapping traits. *Psychological Bulletin, 121*, 219–245.

Allemand, M., Zimprich, D., & Hertzog, C. (2007). Cross-sectional age differences and longitudinal age changes of personality in middle adulthood and old age. *Journal of Personality, 75*, 1–36.

Allik, J., Laidra, K., Realo, A., & Pullman, H. (2004). Personality development from 12 to 18 years of age: Changes in mean levels and structure of traits. *European Journal of Personality, 18*, 445–462.

Allport, G. W. (1961). *Pattern and growth in personality*. New York: Holt, Rinehart & Winston.

Ardelt, M. (2000). Still stable after all these years? Personality stability theory revisited. *Social Psychology Quarterly, 63*, 392–405.

Arnett, J. J. (2000). Emerging adulthood: A theory of development from the late teens through the twenties. *American Psychologist, 55*, 469–480.

Asendorpf, J. B., & van Aken, M. A. G. (1991). Correlates of the temporal consistency of personality patterns in childhood. *Journal of Personality*, 59, 689–703.

Asendorpf, J. B., & van Aken, M. A. G. (2003). Validity of Big Five personality judgements in childhood: A 9 year longitudinal study. *European Journal of Personality*, 17, 1–17.

Bagby, R. M., Joffe, R. T., Parker, J. D. A., Kalemba, B., & Harkness, K. L. (1995). Major depression and the five-factor model of personality. *Journal of Personality Disorders*, 9, 224–234.

Baltes, P. B., & Baltes, M. M. (1990). Psychological perspectives on successful aging: The model of selective optimisation with compensation. In P. B. Baltes & M. M. Baltes (Eds.), *Successful aging: Perspectives from the behavioural sciences* (pp. 1–34). New York: Cambridge University Press.

Baltes, P. B., Lindenberger, U., & Staudinger, U. M. (2006). Life span theory in developmental psychology. In W. Damon & R. M. Lerner (Eds.), *Handbook of child psychology: Vol. 1. Theoretical models of human development* (6th ed., pp. 569–664). New York: Wiley.

Baltes, P. B., Reese, H. W., & Nesselroade, J. R. (1977). *Life-span developmental psychology: Introduction to research methods.* Oxford, UK: Brooks/Cole.

Barber, B. L., Eccles, J. S., & Stone, M. R. (2001). Whatever happened to the jock, the brain, and the princess? Young adult pathways linked to adolescent activity involvement and social identity. *Journal of Adolescent Research*, 16, 429–455.

Bazana, P. G., & Stelmack, R. M. (2004). Stability of personality across the life span: A meta-analysis. In R. M. Stelmack (Ed.), *On the psychobiology of personality* (pp. 113–144). New York: Elsevier.

Bell, N. E., & Staw, B. M. (1989). People as sculptors versus sculpture: The roles of personality and personal control in organizations. In M. B. Arthur, D. T. Hall, & B. S. Lawrence (Eds.), *Handbook of career theory* (pp. 232–251). New York: Cambridge University Press.

Birch, S. H., & Ladd, G. W. (1998). Children's interpersonal behaviors and the teacher–child relationship. *Developmental Psychology*, 34, 934–946.

Block, J. (1971). *Lives through time.* Berkeley, CA: Bancroft.

Block, J. (1982). Assimilation, accommodation, and the dynamics of personality development. *Child Development*, 53, 281–295.

Block, J., & Block, J. H. (2006). Nursery school personality and political orientation two decades later. *Journal of Research in Personality*, 40, 734–749.

Blonigen, D. M., Hicks, B. M., Krueger, R. F., Patrick, C. J., & Iacono, W. G. (2006). Continuity and change in psychopathic traits as measured via normal-range personality: A longitudinal-biometric study. *Journal of Abnormal Psychology*, 115, 85–95.

Bollen, K. A. (1989). *Structural equations with latent variables.* New York: Wiley.

Botwin, M., Buss, D. M., & Shackelford, T. (1997). Personality and mate preferences: Five factors in mate selection and marital satisfaction. *Journal of Personality*, 65, 107–136.

Brandtstadter, J. (1992). Person control over development: Some developmental implications of self-efficacy. In R. Schwarzer (Ed.), *Self-efficacy: Thought control of action* (pp. 127–145). Washington, DC: Hemisphere.

Brandtstadter, J., & Greve, W. (1994). The aging self: Stabilizing and protective processes. *Developmental Review*, 14, 52–80.

Branje, S. J., van Lieshout, C. F., & van Aken, M. A. (2004). Relations between Big Five personality characteristics and perceived support in adolescents' families. *Journal of Personality and Social Psychology*, 86, 615–628.

Branje, S. J., van Lieshout, C. F., van Aken, M. A., & Haselager, G. J. (2004). Perceived support in sibling relationships and adolescent adjustment. *Journal of Child Psychology and Psychiatry*, 45, 1385–1396.

Cairns, R. B., & Cairns, B. D. (1994). *Lifelines and risks: Pathways of youth in our time.* New York: Cambridge University Press.

Campbell, J. D. (1990). Self-esteem and clarity of the self-concept. *Journal of Personality and Social Psychology*, 59, 538–549.

Caspi, A. (2000). The child is father of the man: Personality continuities from childhood to adulthood. *Journal of Personality and Social Psychology*, 78, 158–172.

Caspi, A., & Bem, D. J. (1990). Personality continuity and change across the life course. In L. A. Pervin (Ed.), *Handbook of personality: Theory and research* (pp. 549–575). New York: Guilford Press.

Caspi, A., Elder, G. H., & Bem, D. J. (1988). Moving away from the world: Life-course patterns of shy children. *Developmental Psychology*, 24, 824–831.

Caspi, A., Harrington, H., Milne, B., Amell, J. W., Theodore, R. F., & Moffitt, T. E. (2003). Children's behavioral styles at age 3 are linked to their adult personality traits at age 26. *Journal of Personality*, 71, 495–513.

Caspi, A., & Roberts, B. W. (1999). Personality continuity and change across the life course. In L. A. Pervin & O. P. John (Eds.), *Handbook of personality: Theory and research* (2nd ed., pp. 300–326). New York: Guilford Press.

Caspi, A., & Silva, P. A. (1995). Temperamental qualities at age three predict personality traits in young adulthood: Longitudinal evidence from a birth cohort. *Child Development, 66*, 486–498.

Caspi, A., Wright, B. R. E., Moffitt, T. E., & Silva, P. A. (1998). Early failure in the labor market: Childhood and adolescent predictors of unemployment in the transition to adulthood. *American Sociological Review, 63*, 424–451.

Chatman, J. A., & Barsade, S. G. (1995). Personality, organizational culture, and cooperation: Evidence from a business simulation. *Administrative Science Quarterly, 40*, 423–443.

Clausen, J. A., & Gilens, M. (1990). Personality and labor force participation across the life course: A longitudinal study of women's careers. *Sociological Forum, 5*, 595–618.

Cook, K. W., Vance, C. A., & Spector, P. E. (2000). The relation of candidate personality with selection interview outcomes. *Journal of Applied Social Psychology, 30*, 867–885.

Costa, P. T., Jr., & McCrae, R. R. (1992). Four ways five factors are basic. *Personality and Individual Differences, 13*, 653–665.

Cramer, P. (1998). Defensiveness and defense mechanisms. *Journal of Personality, 66*, 879–894.

Cramer, P., & Tracy, A. (2005). The pathway from child personality to adult adjustment: The road is not straight. *Journal of Research in Personality, 39*, 369–394.

Crook, M. N. (1941). Retest correlations in neuroticism. *Journal of General Psychology, 24*, 173–182.

Davidson, K. W., MacGregor, M. W., Johnson, E. A., Woody, E. Z., & Chaplin, W. F. (2004). The relation between defense use and adaptive behavior. *Journal of Research in Personality, 38*, 105–129.

Deary, I. J., Whiteman, M. C., Starr, J. M., Whalley, L. J., & Fox, H. C. (2004). The impact of childhood intelligence on later life: Following up the Scottish mental surveys of 1932 and 1947. *Journal of Personality and Social Psychology, 86*, 130–147.

De Fruyt, F., Bartels, M., Van Leeuwen, K. G., De Clercq, B., Decuyper, M., & Mervielde, I. (2006). Five types of personality continuity in childhood and adolescence. *Journal of Personality and Social Psychology, 91*, 538–552.

De Fruyt, F., Van Leeuwen, K., Bagby, R. M., Rolland, J., & Rouillon, F. (2006). Assessing and interpreting personality change and continuity in patients treated for major depression. *Psychological Assessment, 18*, 71–80.

Deal, J. E., Halverson, C. F., Havill, V., & Martin, R. P. (2005). Temperament factors as longitudinal predictors of young adult personality. *Merrrill–Palmer Quarterly, 51*, 315–334.

Digman, J. M. (1997). Higher-order factors of the Big Five. *Journal of Personality and Social Psychology, 73*, 1246–1256.

Dodge, K. A., & Tomlin, A. M. (1987). Utilization of self-schemas as a mechanism of interpretational bias in aggressive children. *Social Cognition, 5*, 280–300.

Donnellan, M. B., Conger, R. D., & Burzette, R. G. (2007). Personality development from late adolescence to young adulthood: Differential stability, normative maturity, and evidence for the maturity–stability hypothesis. *Journal of Personality, 75*, 237–263.

Elder, G. H. (1969). Occupational mobility, life patterns, and personality. *Journal of Health and Social Behavior, 10*, 308–323.

Feingold, A. (1994). Gender differences in personality: A meta-analysis. *Psychological Bulletin, 116*, 429–456.

Feist, G. J., & Barron, F. X. (2003). Predicting creativity from early to late adulthood: Intellectual, potential, and personality. *Journal of Research in Personality, 37*, 62–88.

Fiske, S. T., & Taylor, S. E. (1991). *Social cognition* (2nd ed.). New York: McGraw-Hill.

Fraley, R. C. (2002). Attachment stability from infancy to adulthood: Meta-analysis and dynamic modelling of developmental mechanisms. *Personality and Social Psychology Review, 6*, 123–151.

Fraley, R. C., & Roberts, B. W. (2005). Patterns of continuity: A dynamic model for conceptualizing the stability of individual differences in psychological constructs across the life course. *Psychological Review, 112*, 60–74.

Hampson, S. E., & Goldberg, L. R. (2006). A first large cohort study of personality trait stability over the 40 years between elementary school and midlife. *Journal of Personality and Social Psychology, 91*, 763–779.

Hampson, S. E., Goldberg, L. R., Vogt, T. M., & Dubanoski, J. P. (2007). Mechanisms by which childhood personality traits influence adult health status: Educational attainment and healthy behaviors. *Health Psychology, 26*, 121–125.

Helson, R., Jones, C., & Kwan, V. S. Y. (2002). Personality change over 40 years of adulthood: Hierarchical linear modeling analyses of two longitudinal samples. *Journal of Personality and Social Psychology, 83*, 752–766.

Helson, R., Stewart, A. J., & Ostrove, J. (1995). Identity in three cohorts of midlife women. *Journal of Personality and Social Psychology, 69*, 544–557.

Hogan, R., & Roberts, B. W. (2004). A socioanalytic model of maturity. *Journal of Career Assessment, 12*, 207–217.

Jacobson, N. S., & Truax, P. (1991). Clinical significance: A statistical approach to defining meaningful change in psychotherapy research. *Journal of Consulting and Clinical Psychology, 59*, 12–19.

Johnson, W., McGue, M., & Krueger, R. F. (2005). Personality stability in late adulthood: A behavioral genetic analysis. *Journal of Personality, 73*, 523–551.

Jones, C. J., Livson, N., & Peskin, H. (2003). Longitudinal hierarchical linear modeling analyses of California Psychological Inventory data from age 33 to 75: An examination of stability and change in adult personality. *Journal of Personality Assessment, 80*, 294–308.

Kasen, S., Chen, H., Sneed, J., Crawford, T., & Cohen, P. (2006). Social role and birth cohort influences on gender-linked personality traits in women: A 20-year longitudinal analysis. *Journal of Personality and Social Psychology, 91*, 944–958.

Kokko, K., & Pulkkinen, L. (2000). Aggression in childhood and long-term unemployment in adulthood: A cycle of maladaptation and some protective factors. *Developmental Psychology, 36*, 463–472.

Labouvie-Vief, G., Chiodo, L. M., Goguen, L. A., & Diehl, M. (1995). Representations of self across the life span. *Psychology and Aging, 10*, 404–415.

Labouvie-Vief, G., Diehl, M., Tarnowski, A., & Shen, J. (2000). Age differences in adult personality: Findings from the United States and China. *Journal of Gerontology: Psychological Sciences, 55B*, 4–17.

Lamb, M. E., Chuang, S. S., Wessels, H., Broberg, A. G., & Hwang, C. P. (2002). Emergence and construct validation of the Big Five factors in early childhood: A longitudinal analysis of their ontogeny in Sweden. *Child Development, 73*, 1517–1524.

Laursen, B., Pulkkinen, L., & Adams, R. (2002). The antecedents and correlates of agreeableness in adulthood. *Developmental Psychology, 38*, 591–603.

Lehnart, J., & Neyer, F. J. (2006). Should I stay or should I go? Attachment and personality in stable and instable romantic relationships. *European Journal of Personality, 20*, 475–495.

Little, T. D. (1997). Mean and covariance structures (MACS) analyses of cross-cultural data: Practical and theoretical issues. *Multivariate Behavioral Research, 32*, 53–76.

Lodi-Smith, J. L., & Roberts, B. W. (2007). Social investment and personality: A meta-analytic analysis of the relationship of personality traits to investment in work, family, religion, and volunteerism. *Personality and Social Psychology Review, 11*, 68–86.

Low, D. K. S., Yoon, M., Roberts, B. W., & Rounds, J. (2005). The stability of interests from early adolescence to middle adulthood: A quantitative review of longitudinal studies. *Psychological Bulletin, 131*, 713–737.

Lykken, D., & Tellegen, A. (1996). Happiness is a stochastic phenomenon. *Psychological Science, 7*, 186–189.

McAdams, D. P., Bauer, J. J., Sakaeda, A. R., Anyidoho, N. A., Machado, M. A., Magrino-Failla, K., et al. (2006). Continuity and change in the life story: A longitudinal study of autobiographical memories in emerging adulthood. *Journal of Personality, 74*, 1372–1400.

McCrae, R. R., & Costa, P. T., Jr. (1994). The stability of personality: Observation and evaluations. *Current Directions in Psychological Science, 3*, 173–175.

McCrae, R. R., Costa, P. T., Jr., Ostendorf, F., Angleitner, A., Hrebickova, M., Avia, M. D., et al. (2000). Nature over nurture: Temperament, personality, and life span development. *Journal of Personality and Social Psychology, 78*, 173–186.

McGue, M., Bacon, S., & Lykken, D. T. (1993). Personality stability and change in early adulthood: A behavioral genetic analysis. *Developmental Psychology, 29*, 96–109.

Morizot, J., & Le Blanc, M. (2003). Searching for a developmental typology of personality and its relations to antisocial behavior: A longitudinal study of adjudicated men sample. *Criminal Behavior and Mental Health, 13*, 241–277.

Moss, H. A., & Susman, E. J. (1980). Longitudinal study of personality development. In O. G. Brim & J. Kagan (Eds.), *Constancy and change in human development* (pp. 530–595). Cambridge, MA: Harvard University Press.

Mroczek, D. K., Ozer, D. J., Spiro, A., III, & Kaiser, R. T. (1998). Evaluating a measure of the five-factor model of personality. *Assessment, 5*, 287–301.

Mroczek, D. K., & Spiro, A. (2003). Modeling intraindividual change in personality traits: Findings from the Normative Aging Study. *Journals of Gerontology: Series B: Psychological Sciences and Social Sciences, 58B*, 305–306.

Mroczek, D. K., & Spiro, A. (2007). Personality change influences mortality in older men. *Psychological Science, 18*, 371–376.

Nesselroade, J. R. (1991). Interindividual differences in intraindividual change. In L. M. Collins & J. L. Horn (Eds.), *Best methods for the analysis of change* (pp. 92–105). Washington, DC: American Psychological Association.

Neyer, F. J., & Asendorpf, J. B. (2001). Personality-relationship transaction in young adulthood. *Journal of Personality and Social Psychology, 81*, 1190–1204.

Neyer, F. J., & Lehnart, J. (2007). Relationships matter in personality development: Evidence from an 8-year longitudinal study across young adulthood. *Journal of Personality, 75*, 535–568.

Ozer, D. J., & Gjerde, P. F. (1989). Patterns of

personality consistency and change from childhood through adolescence. *Journal of Personality, 57,* 483–507.

Piedmont, R. L. (2001). Cracking the plaster cast: Big Five personality change during intensive outpatient counseling. *Journal of Research in Personality, 35,* 500–520.

Pullman, H., Raudsepp, L., & Allik, J. (2006). Stability and change in adolescents' personality: A longitudinal study. *European Journal of Personality, 20,* 447–459.

Roberts, B. W. (1997). Plaster or plasticity: Are adult work experiences associated with personality change in women? *Journal of Personality, 65,* 205–231.

Roberts, B. W. (2005). Blessings, banes, and possibilities in the study of childhood personality. *Merrill–Palmer Quarterly, 51,* 367–378.

Roberts, B. W. (2006). Personality development and organizational behavior. In B. M. Staw (Ed.), *Research in organizational behavior* (Vol. 27, pp. 1–40). New York: Elsevier Science/JAI Press.

Roberts, B. W. (2007). Contextualizing personality psychology. *Journal of Personality, 75,* 1071–1081.

Roberts, B. W., & Bogg, T. (2004). A 30-year longitudinal study of the relationships between conscientiousness-related traits and the family structure and health–behavior factors that affect health. *Journal of Personality, 72,* 325–354.

Roberts, B. W., & Caspi, A. (2003). The cumulative continuity model of personality development: Striking a balance between continuity and change in personality traits across the life course. In R. M. Staudinger & U. Lindenberger (Eds.), *Understanding human development: Lifespan psychology in exchange with other disciplines* (pp. 183–214). Dordrecht, Netherlands: Kluwer.

Roberts, B. W., Caspi, A., & Moffitt, T. (2001). The kids are alright: Growth and stability in personality development from adolescence to adulthood. *Journal of Personality and Social Psychology, 81,* 670–683.

Roberts, B. W., Caspi, A., & Moffitt, T. E. (2003). Work experiences and personality development in young adulthood. *Journal of Personality and Social Psychology, 84,* 582–593.

Roberts, B. W., & Chapman, C. N. (2000). Change in dispositional well-being and its relation to role quality: A 30-year longitudinal study. *Journal of Research in Personality, 34,* 26–41.

Roberts, B. W., & DelVecchio, W. F. (2000). The rank-order consistency of personality traits from childhood to old age: A quantitative review of longitudinal studies. *Psychological Bulletin, 126,* 3–25.

Roberts, B. W., & Helson, R. (1997). Changes in culture, changes in personality: The influence of individualism in a longitudinal study of women. *Journal of Personality and Social Psychology, 72,* 641–651.

Roberts, B. W., & Jackson, J. J. (in press). The power of personality: Biological models, personality traits, and human nature. *Journal of Personality.*

Roberts, B. W., Kuncel, N., Shiner, R. N., Caspi, A., & Goldberg, L. (2007). The power of personality: A comparative analysis of the predictive validity of personality traits, SES, and IQ. *Perspectives in Psychological Science, 2,* 313–345.

Roberts, B. W., & Mroczek, D. (2008). Personality trait change in adulthood. *Current Directions in Psychological Science, 17,* 31–35.

Roberts, B. W., O'Donnell, M., & Robins, R. W. (2004). Goal and personality trait development in emerging adulthood. *Journal of Personality and Social Psychology, 87,* 541–550.

Roberts, B. W., & Robins, R. W. (2004). A longitudinal study of person–environment fit and personality development. *Journal of Personality, 72,* 89–110.

Roberts, B. W., Walton, K., & Viechtbauer, W. (2006). Patterns of mean-level change in personality traits across the life course: A meta-analysis of longitudinal studies. *Psychological Bulletin, 132,* 1–25.

Roberts, B. W., & Wood, D. (2006). Personality development in the context of the neo-socioanalytic model of personality (pp. 11–39). In D. Mroczek & T. Little (Eds.), *Handbook of personality development* (pp. 11–40). Mahwah, NJ: Erlbaum.

Roberts, B. W., Wood, D., & Smith, J. L. (2005). Evaluating five factor theory and social investment perspectives on personality trait development. *Journal of Research in Personality, 39,* 166–184.

Robins, R. W., Caspi, A., & Moffitt, T. E. (2002). It's not just who you're with, it's who you are: Personality and relationship experiences across multiple relationships. *Journal of Personality, 70,* 925–964.

Robins, R. W., Fraley, R. C., Roberts, B. W., & Trzesniewski, K. (2001). A longitudinal study of personality change in young adulthood. *Journal of Personality, 69,* 617–640.

Robins, R. W., & Paulhus, D. L. (2001). The character of self-enhancers: Implications for organizations. In B. W. Roberts & R. T. Hogan (Eds.), *Personality psychology in the workplace: Decade of behavior* (pp. 193–219). Washington, DC: American Psychological Association.

Sarbin, T. R. (1964). Role theoretical interpretation of psychological change. In P. Worchel

& D. Byrne (Eds.), *Personality change* (pp. 176–219). New York: Wiley.

Schuerger, J. M., Zarrella, K. L., & Hotz, A. S. (1989). Factors that influence the temporal stability of personality by questionnaire. *Journal of Personality and Social Psychology, 56,* 777–783.

Scollon, C. N., & Diener, E. (2006). Love, work, and changes in extraversion and neuroticism over time. *Journal of Personality and Social Psychology, 91,* 1152–1165.

Shiner, R. L., Masten, A. S., & Roberts, J. M. (2003). Childhood personality foreshadows adult personality and life outcomes two decades later. *Journal of Personality, 71,* 1145–1170.

Siegler, I. C., Costa, P. T., Brummett, B. H., Helms, M. J., Barefoot, J. C., Williams, R. B., et al. (2003). Patterns of change in hostility from college to midlife in the UNC Alumni Heart Study predict high-risk status. *Psychosomatic Medicine, 65,* 738–745.

Singer, J. D., & Willett, J. B. (2003). *Applied longitudinal analysis: Modeling change and event occurrence.* New York: Oxford University Press.

Small, B. J., Hertzog, C., Hultsch, D. F., & Dixon, R. A. (2003). Stability and change in adult personality over 6 years: Findings from the Victoria Longitudinal Study. *Journal of Gerontology: Psychological Sciences, 58,* 166–176.

Snyder, M., & Ickes, W. (1985). Personality and social behavior. In E. Aronson & G. Lindzey (Eds.), *Handbook of social psychology* (pp. 248–305). New York: Random House.

Srivastava, S., John, O. P., Gosling, S. D., & Potter, J. (2003). Development of personality in early and middle adulthood: Set like plaster or persistent change? *Journal of Personality and Social Psychology, 84,* 1041–1053.

Steunenberg, B., Twisk, J. W., Beekman, A. T., Deeg, D. J., & Kerkhof, A. J. (2005). Stability and change in neuroticism in aging. *Journal of Gerontology: Psychological Sciences, 60,* 27–33.

Swann, W. B., Pelham, B. W., & Krull, D. S. (1989). Agreeable fancy or disagreeable truth? Reconciling self-enhancement and self-verification. *Journal of Personality and Social Psychology, 57,* 782–791.

Thorne, A. (1987). The press of personality: A study of conversations between introverts and extraverts. *Journal of Personality and Social Psychology, 53,* 718–726.

Trull, T. J., Useda, D., Costa, P. T., Jr., & McCrae, R. R. (1995). Comparison of the MMPI-2 personality psychopathy five (PSY-5), the NEO PI, and the NEO PI-R. *Psychological Assessment, 7,* 508–516.

Twenge, J. M. (2001). Changes in women's assertiveness in response to status and roles: A cross-temporal meta-analysis, 1931–1993. *Journal of Personality and Social Psychology, 81,* 133–145.

Vaidya, J. G., Gray, E. K., Haig, J., & Watson, D. (2002). On the temporal stability of personality: Evidence for differential stability and the role of life experiences. *Journal of Personality and Social Psychology, 83,* 1469–1484.

Van Aken, M. A., Denissen, J. J., Branje, S. J., Dubas, J. S., & Goossens, L. (2006). Midlife concerns and short-term personality change in middle adulthood. *European Journal of Personality, 20,* 497–513.

Watson, D. (2004). Stability versus change, dependability versus error: Issues in the assessment of personality over time. *Journal of Research in Personality, 38,* 319–350.

Watson, D., & Humrichouse, J. (2006). Personality development in emerging adulthood: Integrating evidence from self-ratings and spouse ratings. *Journal of Personality and Social Psychology, 91,* 959–974.

Watson, D., Klohnen, E. C., Casillas, A., Nus Simms, E., Haig, J., & Berry, D. S. (2004). Match makers and deal breakers: Analyses of assortative mating in newlywed couples. *Journal of Personality, 72,* 1029–1068.

Westen, D. (1991). Social cognition and object relations. *Psychological Bulletin, 109,* 429–455.

Wood, D. (2007). Using the PRISM to compare the explanatory value of general and role-contextualized trait ratings. *Journal of Personality, 75,* 1103–1126.

Wood, D., & Roberts, B. W. (2006a). Cross-sectional and longitudinal tests of the personality and role identity structural model (PRISM). *Journal of Personality, 74,* 779–809.

Wood, D., & Roberts, B. W. (2006b). The effect of age and role information on expectations for Big Five personality traits. *Personality and Social Psychology Bulletin, 32,* 1482–1496.

Wrzesniewski, A., & Dutton, J. E. (2001). Crafting a job: Revisioning employees as active crafters of their work. *Academy of Management Review, 26,* 179–201.

CHAPTER 15

Challenges and Opportunities at the Interface of Aging, Personality, and Well-Being

Carol D. Ryff

This chapter brings together three literatures that have typically been examined as independent twosomes. First are studies of personality and aging, which are concerned with questions of stability and change in individual-difference characteristics as individuals move across the adult life course. Second are studies of well-being and aging, which also focus on stability and change in reported levels of happiness, satisfaction, and life engagement from early adulthood through midlife and old age. Third, is research on personality and well-being, which addresses the comparative influence of personal characteristics (e.g., basic traits) versus life circumstances in predicting reported levels of well-being. The latter inquiries have been largely unconcerned with life-course dynamics.

The objective herein is to summarize and evaluate prior research from each of the above twosomes as well as to call for simultaneous consideration of all three topics. Scientific advances in integrating these areas require, however, that certain thorny issues be addressed, such as the problem of construct redundancy and measurement overlap in assessment of personality and well-being. Other challenges pertain to limitations in the kinds of questions that guide these inquiries as well as the methodologies used to answer them. Thus, a further objective of the chapter is to delineate possible future inquiries that are less bound by entrenched dichotomies (e.g., change vs. stability, top-down vs. bottom-up approaches) as well as less constrained by single summary indices (e.g., means, correlation coefficients) that impede delineation of diverse trajectories of personality change and continuity. Similarly, longstanding practices of investigating longitudinal dynamics one variable at a time have undermined knowledge of whole persons as they age. Alternative approaches emphasizing the integration of personality, well-being, and aging via "multiple pathways" are advanced.

The chapter is divided into two primary sections. The first provides overviews of studies and findings exemplifying each of the above three twosomes. The limited numbers of investigations that have worked simultaneously on all three levels are also described. The second section addresses challenges in putting these realms together, most of which are foreshadowed in the literature described in the first section. Building on these, opportunities for future research are outlined, including new scientific agendas that transcend pervasive dichotomies and novel methodologies that facilitate integrative understanding of how and why people age as they do.

PROMINENT TWOSOMES AND AN OCCASIONAL THREESOME

Personality and Aging

Considerable research has been amassed on the question of whether personality is stable or changing as people age, as summarized in numerous reviews (e.g., Caspi, Roberts, Shiner, 2005; Helson, Soto, & Cate, 2006; Roberts & DelVecchio, 2000; Roberts, Walton, & Viechtbauer, 2006; Ryff, Kwan, & Singer, 2001). As it has unfolded in time, this work reveals diverse "storylines" that are described below. It should be noted that another chapter in this volume (see Roberts, Wood, & Caspi, Chapter 14) addresses some of the same literature, albeit with less of a focus on aging.

Bernice Neugarten, a premier leader in the nascent field of personality and aging, was explicitly concerned with whether personality *develops* in the second half of life. Proposing that it does, she put forth novel suggestions about the "executive processes" of personality in the middle years, which involve managing complexity, exercising leadership, and being engaged in decision-making roles (Neugarten, 1973). Her classic text, *Middle Age and Aging* (1968), also gave shape to an emergent field of inquiry explicitly concerned with differences in various psychological processes between midlife and older-age adults, many assessed with projective techniques. Other early formulations of mid- and later-life development included Erikson's (1959) psychosocial stages, Bühler and Massarik's (1968) description of basic life tendencies that work toward the fulfillment of life, and Jung's (1933) characterization of turning inward in later life as well as gender differences in psychological changes with aging. Viewed collectively, the storyline of this initial body of work was largely one of generating conceptual ideas about how personality develops in the second half of life.

The next most notable storyline, exemplified by the work of Costa and McCrae (1980, 1988), offered a sharp critique of the above literature, construing it as little more than personal impressions in need of a cor-

rective "look at the facts" (McCrae & Costa, 1990, p. 17). Hence, a rich era of empirical productivity ensued, built around the factor-analytically derived trait model of personality. Using multiple designs (cross-sectional, longitudinal, sequential) and primarily data from the Baltimore Longitudinal Study of Aging, their comprehensive findings, summarized in McCrae and Costa (2003), emphasized the stability of personality, measured in terms of mean-level changes and cross-time time correlations. Such stability was evident across the traits that comprised the five-factor model: neuroticism, extraversion, agreeableness, conscientiousness, and openness to experience.

Nonetheless, while trait psychology was being revitalized with its resounding message of stability, others were reporting evidence of personality change. For example, Whitbourne and colleagues used both longitudinal and sequential designs to document psychological changes consistent with Erikson's stage model, specifically the young-adult transition from identity to intimacy (Whitbourne & Waterman, 1979; Whitbourne, Zuschlag, Elliot, & Waterman, 1992). Others, using primarily cross-sectional designs, examined Erikson's midlife challenge of generativity (Keyes & Ryff, 1998; McAdams & de St. Aubin, 1998; Peterson & Klohnen, 1995). By far, however, it was the longitudinal research of Helson and colleagues that most sharply challenged the stability perspective by documenting extensive personality change from early adulthood into midlife (Helson & Moane, 1987; Helson & Roberts, 1994; Helson & Soto, 2005; Helson & Wink, 1992). This work drew guidance from the early formulations of adult development, described above, as well as showed abiding interest in the life contexts (e.g., the roles and statuses, life transitions) surrounding those under study.

For example, using 30 years of data from the Mills Longitudinal Study of women, Roberts, Helson, and Klohnen (2002) showed mean increases in norm orientation (e.g., being considerate of others and less impulsive) and complexity (e.g., having tolerance for human diversity and fallibility) from ages 21 to 52. Increases in dominance (consistent with changing sex roles) as well as changes in femininity and masculinity (linked with life circumstances such as marital tension, divorce, and participation in the paid labor force) were also reported, despite relatively high rank-order consistency in many of these areas. Helson and Soto (2005) added other evidence of change in positive and negative emotionality, defenses, and affect complexity, drawing theoretical guidance from the Labouvie-Vief and González (2004) formulation of emotion regulation. Taken together, these studies depicted multiple forms of change (in traits, emotionality, coping, goals, motivation) that comprised evidence for personality development from young adulthood through middle age (Helson et al., 2006).

Drawing on analytic advances (hierarchical linear modeling), Helson, Jones, and Kwan (2002) combined California Personality Inventory (CPI) data from the Mills sample with two other longitudinal studies (Oakland Growth Study, Berkeley Guidance Study) to further document increases with age in norm adherence, decreases with age in social vitality, and midlife peaks on dominance and independence—all over a 40-year period. Their findings also underscored the importance of period effects, as illustrated by low scores on responsibility linked to the culture of individualism that was prominent from the late 1950s to the late 1970s. An important prior study, also using latent curve analyses with the Oakland and Berkeley samples (Jones & Meredith, 1996), had further underscored individual differences in the direction and degree to which individuals changed with age (e.g., in self-confidence, cognitive commitment, outgoingness, and dependability).

Growth-curve modeling techniques were also employed in the Normative Aging Study, which followed midlife and older-age men over a 12-year period (Mroczek & Spiro, 2003). This investigation brought the competing stability-versus-change narratives into high relief because of its focus on two of the big five traits: neuroticism and extraversion. Although little change was evident *on average* for extraversion, individual differences in rate of change were nonetheless prominent, showing that older men became slightly less extraverted over time, whereas younger men became slightly more extraverted. Neuroticism, in turn, showed both decline on average with age as well as individual differences, wherein younger men showed more marked decline than older men. Importantly, life

events, such as marriage or remarriage and death of spouse, were found to account for such differences in rates of decline in neuroticism with age.

Another methodological variant, latent-change analysis, was employed by Small, Hertzog, Hultsch, and Dixon (2003) with Victoria Longitudinal Study, which followed midlife and older adults over a six-year period. Using the five-factor model (Costa & McCrae, 1985), they documented an invariant factor structure over time and high-stability coefficients for all five factors. Nonetheless, they also showed that all five dimensions indicated significant individual differences in personality change. Some of these changes were related to age and gender (e.g., women were more likely to show decreases in neuroticism and increases in agreeableness than men, whereas older persons were more likely to show increases in neuroticism compared to younger adults).

Finally, meta-analyses of longitudinal studies have been increasingly adopted in an effort to distill primary empirical storylines across multiple studies. Roberts and colleagues (Fraley & Roberts, 2005; Roberts & DelVecchio, 2000) used such methods to show considerable evidence for rank-order stability of the Big Five traits (measured both by self-report and observer ratings). However, it was further emphasized that these correlations increased with age, for example, from .41 in childhood to .55 at age 30 and then reaching a plateau around .70 between ages 50 and 70. They also noted that rank-order stability decreases as time interval between observations increases. Overall, this work indicated that personality stabilizes at a later period in the life course than had been claimed by McCrae and Costa (1994). Using longitudinal twin data from ages 59–64, Johnson, McGue, and Krueger (2005) further clarified that such stability had a strong genetic foundation, supplemented by the stability of environmental effects.

Meta-analyses of mean-level change in personality traits (Roberts et al., 2006) tell a somewhat different story. Evidence from 92 longitudinal samples indicated that four of six traits demonstrated significant change in middle and old age. For example, increases in social dominance (a facet of extraversion), conscientiousness, and emotional stability were observed, especially in young adulthood (ages 20–40). In contrast, on measures of social vitality (another facet of extraversion) and openness, the data showed increases in adolescence followed by decreases in both of these domains in old age. Agreeableness showed change only in old age. These patterns were depicted as showing "normative change" in personality—that is, when most people change in the same way during a specific period within the life course. Costa and McCrae (1997) had argued that personality traits do not demonstrate mean-level change after around age 30 but noted that if such change occurs, it is likely attributable to genetic factors (McCrae et al., 2000).

Efforts to formulate a theory of "personality trait development" have built on the above meta-analyses (Roberts & Caspi, 2003; Roberts & Wood, 2006). The central idea in this conceptualization is that making normative commitments to conventional social institutions creates identities needed in adult work, family, and community contexts. Thus, it is investment in conventional social institutions that gives rise to increases in traits such as agreeableness, conscientiousness, and emotional stability. Caspi and colleagues (2005), in fact, equate maturity with the above trait changes thought to accompany the capacity to become productive and involved contributor to society. Curiously, this formulation signals a return to the distant past—namely, Havighurst's (1948) formulation of "developmental tasks," which were described over a half century ago as the routes through which individuals become worthy, responsible members of society. A colleague of Neugarten's at the University of Chicago, Havighurst delineated the key tasks of adulthood to be those of selecting a mate, starting a family, committing to an occupation, and taking on civic responsibility. Research on adult personality development has, it seems, come full circle.

Summary

To recap, the above literature reveals a changing cross-time narrative, beginning with early perspectives that were conceptually rich but empirically lacking in their proposed progressions of adult development well into later life. These were followed by empirically rigorous but theoretically lacking trait perspectives, which depicted personality as stable after early adulthood and offered genetics as the putative explanation for such effects. Along the way, others used longitudinal designs and psychometrically sound assessments of diverse characteristics to assemble mean-level evidence of personality change. These outcomes were frequently in substantive areas that bore some connection to early conceptual formulations of adult development.

Methodological advances related to modeling intraindividual change have contributed a prominent new narrative, which speaks strongly to individual differences in profiles of personality change and continuity. This literature has also begun to identify factors that predict such variants in rate and direction of change, such as age, birth cohort, and life events. Paralleling these findings have been meta-analyses of longitudinal studies using traits and facets of the Big Five dimensions of personality. These analyses document increasing rank-order stability with age, while simultaneously showing evidence of mean-level changes in some areas thought to be linked to normative role commitments.

Well-Being and Aging

There are also multiple storylines accompanying research on well-being and aging, beginning with early national survey data that showed that fewer older persons reported themselves to be very happy compared to younger adults (Gurin, Veroff, & Feld, 1960). Neugarten, however, again featured prominently in this realm with her classic study of life satisfaction among the elderly (Neugarten, Havighurst, & Tobin, 1961). Lawton (1975), another notable early leader in the psychology of aging, studied a similar construct, namely, later-life morale. To the surprise of many, these investigations, and others built on them (Cameron, 1975; Larson, 1978), generated evidence that old age was not inevitably characterized by declining well-being. Apparently, social scientists brought more negative expectations to the study of aging than was reported by those living through the experience of growing old.

Subsequent studies continued to evaluate later-life well-being using measures of life satisfaction and happiness, along with ratings of positive and negative affect (e.g., Diener, Sandvik, & Larsen, 1985; Diener & Suh, 1997; Herzog & Rogers, 1981; Liang, 1984; Malatesta & Kalnok, 1984; Shmotkin, 1990). In the main, these investigations, most of which were cross-sectional in nature, showed either negligible age differences in well-being or age increments in life satisfaction and positive affect, concomitant with age decrements in negative affect. In effect, the storyline continued that later-life well-being was, on average, quite positive. For example, using data from a national study of Americans known as MIDUS (Midlife in the U.S.), Mroczek and Kolarz (1998) showed cross-sectional increments (curvilinear) in positive affect from ages 25–74 and concomitant decrements (linear) in negative affect across these same decades of adult life. The patterns were somewhat qualified by gender, marital status, and personality characteristics (a point revisited later). Using the same study, Prenda and Lachman (2001) also documented a positive linear relationship between age and life satisfaction. Because cohort differences rather than aging (maturational) processes constitute a rival interpretation of these apparent gains in later-life well-being, the 23-year study of Charles, Reynolds, and Gatz (2001) offered important longitudinal evidence of stability in positive affect with aging, along with longitudinal decreases in negative affect.

Given the recurrent evidence that life satisfaction, happiness, and contentment do not show downward trajectories with aging, many became interested in what factors might account for this generally upbeat story. Some have considered the intentional actions older persons may take, such as flexibly adjusting their goal pursuits, to maintain high levels of well-being (Brandtstädter, Wentura, & Rothermund, 1999). Others have examined "selectivity" processes; that is, older persons become more selective in their social interaction partners so as to optimize their emotional experience in the final years of life (Carstensen, 1995), or they selectively focus resources in certain domains so as to optimize functioning and compensate for loss (Freund & Baltes, 2002). Efforts to understand affect regulation in later life have emphasized two independent principles, each of which shows a different relation with age (Labouvie-Vief & Gonzalez,

2004; Labouvie-Vief & Medler, 2002). Affect optimization—the tendency to constrain affect to positive values—shows increments until old age, whereas affect complexity—the amplification of affect in search of differentiation and objectivity—seems to peak in middle age. Juxtaposed to the above psychological accounts are more biologically based explanations, such as that aging itself is linked with reduced physiological arousal to negative events (Panksepp & Miller, 1996), thereby creating a different neurobiological stance for responding to stress or adversity.

The above storylines pertain in large part to "hedonic" aspects of well-being, such as enjoyment, contentment, and happiness (Kahneman, Diener, & Schwarz, 1999). However, the study of well-being has increasingly emphasized "eudaimonic" aspects of positive functioning as well (Ryan & Deci, 2001). These involve engagement with existential challenges, such as finding purpose and meaning in one's life as well as experiencing self-realization and growth over time (Ryff, 1985, 1989). These ideas originate with Aristotle, who considered eudaimonia to be the highest of all human goods and defined it as striving to realize the best that is within us (see Ryff & Singer, 2008). To articulate the substantive specifics of self-realization, numerous accounts of human growth and development (Bühler, 1935; Bühler & Massarik, 1968; Erikson, 1959; Neugarten, 1968, 1973), as well as ideas from existential and humanistic psychology (Allport, 1961; Frankl, 1959/1992; Maslow, 1968; Rogers, 1962) and clinical psychology (Jahoda, 1958; Jung, 1933) were distilled into a multidimensional formulation of well-being (Ryff, 1985, 1989). Included in it are six distinct aspects of well-being: autonomy, environmental mastery, personal growth, positive relations with others, purpose in life, and self-acceptance (Ryff & Keyes, 1995).

The empirical storyline linked to eudaimonic aspects of well-being diverges notably from the positive portrayal of hedonic well-being described above. Multiple studies, including those based on community samples as well as nationally representative samples, have shown sharply downward profiles from young adulthood to old age for self-rated purpose in life and personal growth (Clarke, Marshall, Ryff, & Rosenthal, 2000; Ryff, 1989, 1991; Ryff & Keyes, 1995).

Other aspects of well-being in this formulation, such as autonomy and environmental mastery, have shown incremental age profiles, whereas others, such as positive relations with others and self-acceptance, have shown little age variation. The latter finding is, however, at odds with lifespan studies of self-esteem (Robins & Trzesniewski, 2005; Robins, Trzesniewski, Tracy, Gosling, & Potter, 2002), which, across multiple cross-sectional studies, have shown relatively high levels in childhood, followed by drops in adolescence, then increments in adulthood, but sharp declines in old age. Curiously, eudaimonic self-acceptance probes more critical self-awareness, drawn theoretically from Jungian notions of the shadow (see Ryff, 1985; Ryff & Singer, 2008), but nonetheless shows less cross-sectional decline in later life than traditional measures of self-esteem.

In one of the few investigations to examine psychological (eudaimonic) and subjective (hedonic + life satisfaction) well-being in the same study, Keyes, Shmotkin, and Ryff (2002) used data from MIDUS to document that the two are related but distinct constructs, and further that they are differentially related to other factors. For example, older adults with lower levels of education showed higher levels of subjective but lower levels of psychological well-being, whereas younger adults with more education and higher levels of openness to experience showed higher levels of psychological and lower levels of subjective well-being. Their focus on sociodemographic correlates illustrates an alternative approach to accounting for variation in reported well-being.

That is, rather than look to other psychological variables, such as goal pursuits, selectivity, or compensation processes, to account for declining life engagement among older adults, social structural influences have been invoked. Sharply downward age trajectories for purpose in life and personal growth have been linked to contemporary societal challenges in providing older persons with meaningful roles and opportunities for continued growth. Sociologists have termed this phenomenon the "structural lag" problem, which suggests that social institutions lag behind the added years of life many now experience (Riley, Kahn, & Foner, 1994). Illustrating such ideas, Greenfield and Marks (2004) used MIDUS data and focused on older persons who occupied few major roles. They found that those who engaged in formal volunteering, an aspect of active life engagement, had higher levels of purpose in life than those lacking both major roles and volunteer experiences.

How eudaimonic well-being is influenced by one's standing in the socioeconomic (SES) hierarchy has also been of interest. When self-rated well-being is arrayed according to educational attainment among men and women in MIDUS, the story is clear: All aspects of psychological well-being and educational standing are strongly positively correlated, with the associations being especially pronounced for personal growth and purpose in life, the two pillars of eudaimonia (Ryff & Singer, 2008). These findings bring into high relief further sociological observations: namely, that the opportunities for self-realization are not equally distributed across the social order but occur via the allocation of resources, which enables some to make the most of their talents and capacities (Dowd, 1990). Other analyses on educational disparities in psychological well-being (Marmot, Ryff, Bumpass, Shipley, & Marks, 1997; Marmot et al., 1998) add to this story by showing that those at the low end of the SES hierarchy are not only more likely to succumb to disease and disability, they are also more likely to suffer from diminished opportunities to make the most of their lives.

In addition to social structural influences on eudaimonic well-being, others have examined proximal life experiences, such as early parental loss or parental divorce (Maier & Lachman, 2000), growing up with an alcoholic parent (Tweed & Ryff, 1991), trauma disclosure (Hemenover, 2003), community relocation (Smider, Essex, & Ryff, 1996), caregiving (Marks, 1998), and change in marital status (Marks & Lambert, 1998). Among other things, these investigations have demonstrated that psychological well-being does, indeed, change with aging, particularly as individuals negotiate life challenges and life transitions. Longitudinal studies have documented dynamic shifts in eudaimonic well-being as individuals go through discrete life transitions, such as community relocation (e.g., Kling, Ryff, & Essex, 1997; Kwan, Love, Ryff, & Essex, 2003), or deal with chronic life challenges, such as caregiving (Kling, Seltzer, & Ryff, 1997).

Summary

Aging and well-being involve diverse storylines. Studies of life satisfaction and hedonic well-being reveal a largely positive portrayal of aging, using both cross-sectional and longitudinal designs. Efforts to account for such profiles have cited psychosocial processes such as goal orientations, selectivity processes, or consciously oriented affect regulation. Eudaimonic well-being, in contrast, has shown older adults to be vulnerable to diminished levels of life purpose and growth, perhaps linked to the societal insufficiency in roles and opportunities for meaningful engagement. Educational standing has also been shown to be a strong correlate of eudaimonic well-being. Variation in existential life engagement, furthermore, has been linked with life experiences and life transitions, some normative and others non-normative. Like much of the previously reviewed personality research, the preceding work has revolved largely around studies of mean-level differences and correlational stability. As such, what is known pertains essentially to the average story on aging and well-being rather than the variants around it.

Personality and Well-Being

The storylines linking personality to well-being (see also Lucas & Diener, Chapter 32, this volume) involves subsets of the above variables. In the main, this work has shown little emphasis on life-course dynamics, such that reported links between particular traits and various aspects of well-being are not studied as possibly differing as people age. Neuroticism is, by far, the trait most strongly associated with poor well-being, typically assessed in terms of negative affect (e.g., DeNeve & Cooper, 1998; Diener & Lucas, 1999; McCrae & Costa, 1991; Schmutte & Ryff, 1997). Neuroticism also predicts increased distress in response to daily stressors (Bolger & Schilling, 1991; Mroczek & Almeida, 2004). Using a longitudinal sample, Kling, Ryff, Love, and Essex (2003) found that neuroticism predicted increased depression 8 months after community relocation. On the positive side, extraversion has consistently been found to predict higher well-being, defined primarily in terms of positive affect (e.g., DeNeve & Cooper, 1998; Diener & Lucas, 1999; Fleeson, Malanos, & Archille,

2002; McCrae & Costa, 1991; Schmutte & Ryff, 1997. Extraversion also predicted increased self-esteem 8 months after relocation (Kling et al., 2003).

DeNeve and Cooper (1998) conducted a large meta-analysis to test the scope of support for the top-down perspective on personality and well-being (reflected in the above work), which asserts that people have a global tendency, derived from stable personality traits thought to be rooted in psychobiology (Gray, 1991), to experience life in a positive or negative manner (Diener, 1984). Neuroticism was found to be the strongest predictor of life satisfaction, happiness, and negative affect, whereas positive affect was predicted equally well by extraversion and agreeableness. (There was wide age variation in the studies assembled for this meta-analysis, although it was not considered in the overall summary of findings.) In addition, the findings were contrasted with bottom-up formulations of personality and well-being, which focus on contextual influences (e.g., sociodemographic standing, work and family life, health). Such indices have been of limited value in predicting well-being, as revealed by national survey studies (Andrews & Withey, 1976; Campbell, Converse, & Rodgers, 1976).

A notable problem with the top-down approach, particularly as it pertains to neuroticism and extraversion, is construct redundancy. Schmutte and Ryff (1997) detailed the duplication that exists between facets of neuroticism (e.g., depression, anxiety, vulnerability to distress) (Costa & McCrae, 1985) and items used to measure negative affect (Bradburn, 1969; Watson, Clark, & Tellegen, 1988). Similarly, facets of extraversion include positive emotion and activity and thus are blurred with the assessment of positive affect (Bradburn, 1969; Watson et al., 1988). This overlap obscures the meaning of significant correlations between the above two traits and affect, suggesting artifactual results due to overlapping item content. Source overlap (i.e., the same respondent is rating his or her traits and well-being) is a further problem, which can be obviated, to some extent, by use of spousal ratings (see Schmutte & Ryff, 1997).

Moving to other traits, a small number of studies have shown that agreeableness and conscientiousness, although less strongly linked to well-being compared with neuroticism and extraversion, nonetheless show positive links to well-being (DeNeve & Cooper, 1998; Diener & Lucas, 1999; McCrae & Costa, 1991; Schmutte & Ryff, 1997). Openness, in contrast, has been found to have different links to various aspects of well-being (e.g., Diener & Lucas, 1999; McCrae & Costa, 1991; Schmutte & Ryff, 1997), showing positive associations with both positive and negative affect. McCrae and Costa (1991) suggested that openness may amplify the experience of both kinds of affect. Longitudinal support for this idea was evident in our study (Kling et al., 2003), which found that openness predicted longitudinal increases in both self-esteem and depression 8 months after relocation.

Despite the limited variance in subjective well-being explained by sociodemographic variables (e.g., age, gender, race, martial status, education, income) (Andrews & Withey, 1976; Campbell et al., 1976; DeNeve & Cooper, 1998; Diener, 1984; Diener & Biswas-Diener, 2002), some have nonetheless attempted to integrate top-down and bottom-up perspectives. Feist, Bodner, Jacobs, Miles, and Tan (1995) frame the bottom-up approach as a kind of tabula rasa model molded by experience and link it to the summing of well-being across particular life domains (marriage, work, family), augmented by objective life circumstances, such as health. Their top-down formulation is Kantian, in the sense of the mind being an active interpreter of experience. Using a four-wave study of young adults and measures of health, daily hassles, world assumptions, and constructive thinking, they found that both bottom-up and top-down models provided a good fit for the data, with neither being better than the other. The findings were interpreted with an emphasis on bidirectional links between personality and situational influences.

Summary

Efforts to link personality and well-being have centered primarily on links between neuroticism with negative affect or depressive symptoms and extraversion with positive affect. Top-down formulations are said to reflect biologically based temperament models, but these claims are rarely accompanied by supportive genetic evidence. Top-down models have also been portrayed as

being more consequential for well-being than bottom-up contextual formulations, although evidence supporting the former is likely inflated by problems of construct redundancy (e.g., using facets of neuroticism, such as depression, anxiety, and distress, to predict negative affect; using facets of extraversion, such as positive emotion and activity, to predict positive affect). Increasingly, other mediating influences between personality traits and well-being (e.g., goals, cognitive processes, emotion socialization) are being considered (Diener & Lucas, 1999; Lucas & Diener, Chapter 32, this volume). Contextual influences, in turn, have been shown to have little influence in accounting for variation in well-being, but these levels of influences have typically been poorly conceptualized as well as thinly assessed. How standing in the socioeconomic hierarchy makes its way to well-being undoubtedly involves intervening mechanisms, such as social comparison processes or perceptions of inequality (Ryff, Magee, Kling, & Wing, 1999), but these have rarely been considered in the above literature.

Personality, Well-Being, and Aging

A limited number of investigations have simultaneously considered personality traits, well-being, and aging. At the conceptual level, Staudinger and Kunzman (2005) distinguished between age changes in personality adjustment versus personality growth, defining the former in terms of select traits and select aspects of eudaimonic well-being, and deeming the latter a mix of select aspects of eudaimonic well-being, emotion regulation, and wisdom. Others have attempted empirical integration by employing personality traits as *control variables* to assess whether the links between aging and well-being hold after individual differences in traits have been adjusted for, or as *interaction terms* to assess whether links between aging and well-being are evident only among those with particular personality traits. For example, Mroczek and Kolarz (1998) considered traits and contextual influences as "controls" in their multivariate models linking age to positive and negative affect. However, they also examined possible interactions and found that age interacted with extraversion in predicting positive affect in men—older introverted men showing higher levels of positive affect than younger introverted men, whereas the relationship was not as strong among extra-verted men.

The previously described longitudinal investigation of aging and affect (Charles et al., 2001) used latent-curve analyses to document high variability around the pattern of decline in negative affect over time. That is, those scoring high on neuroticism were less likely to exhibit these cross-time decreases. Positive affect, in turn, showed cross-time stability, but this pattern also varied by traits: Those scoring high on neuroticism were more likely to show decline in positive affect over time, whereas those scoring high on extraversion were more likely to have higher levels of stable positive affect. Both investigations thus emphasized how individual-difference variables modified patterns of aging and affect.

The previously noted study (Keyes et al., 2002) considered the role of personality traits, along with age and education, in predicting different combinations of psychological (eudaimonic) and subjective (hedonic plus life satisfaction) well-being. Using a typological approach, they found that the on-diagonal types (i.e., those with high or low levels of both types of well-being) were strongly differentiated by their levels of neuroticism, extraversion, and conscientiousness, whereas the off-diagonal types (e.g., high psychological well-being, low subjective well-being) were most strongly differentiated by their levels of openness to experience, and less so by neuroticism and conscientiousness.

Each of the preceding investigations examined the influence of traits on well-being one at a time, but of course, all individuals are combinations of traits. To consider how traits work together in predicting longitudinal change in well-being and distress, Bardi and Ryff (2007) examined two-way interactions among select Big Five traits. As hypothesized, they found that openness to experience amplified the negative versus positive emotional tendencies of neuroticism and extraversion, respectively, to predict gains or losses in eudaimonic well-being and distress following community relocation. In addition, extraversion also interacted with conscientiousness and agreeableness to predict changes in psychological distress. The time course of these effects also varied, with some occurring shortly after the relocation transition and others appearing many months later.

Finally, in a notably innovative analysis (both for its longitudinal sweep as well as its use of techniques for modeling intraindividual change), Mroczek and Spiro (2005) examined change in life satisfaction over a 22-year period in a large sample of men (Normative Aging Study). Life satisfaction was found to peak at age 65 and then decline, but there were individual differences in such patterns. Extraversion, in turn, predicted the variability in such change, with higher levels of extraversion associated with a flat but high life satisfaction trajectory, compared to a more curved trajectory (high in midlife but lower at younger and older ages) for those with lower levels of extraversion. In addition to this dispositional (top-down) prediction of life satisfaction, their analyses also incorporated contextual influences (bottom-up) and found that both marital status and health were linked with time-varying life satisfaction. Being married and having better health, both assessed statically and dynamically, were linked with high levels of life satisfaction (but not the shape of the change trajectories). Such findings challenged previous claims that subjective well-being improves with age, while also creatively integrating both ipsative and normative perspectives on personality change.

Beyond the scientific findings described above, the integration of aging, personality, and well-being also has significant clinical implications. Years ago, Costa and McCrae (1986) offered grim observations on this issue, suggesting that if happiness reflects personality, to a large extent, and if personality is stable in adulthood, then one's good or bad fate is largely sealed in the early years of adulthood. For those who are emotionally unstable, withdrawn, antagonistic, and disorganized, the "news is not so good" (Costa, Metter, & McCrae, 1994, p. 55). They noted that the philosopher Schopenhauer also recognized the sad fact that "we cannot all be happy" (p. 56).

Fortunately, some in the treatment realm disagree. Fava and colleagues have focused on those who would seem to personify the above sad news above—that is, individuals who suffer from recurrent major depression. Relevant to the present chapter, the therapeutic intervention provided to such individuals involved the promotion of well-being (Fava, 1999; Fava et al., 2004). Clients are required to keep daily diaries in which they are instructed to record *only* the positive experiences of the day. Treatment sessions then focus on elaboration of these experiences, along with clarification of maladaptive thought patterns that prematurely curtail experiences of the positive. Those receiving "well-being therapy" have shown dramatically improved remission profiles compared to clients receiving standard clinical management (Fava, Rafanelli, Grandi, Conti, & Belluardo, 1998), and more importantly, such effects have been shown to endure over a 6-year period (Fava et al., 2004). Thus, there appears to be some element of hope for those suffering from entrenched forms of emotional distress, and interestingly enough, it hinges on the promotion of experiences of well-being.

Summary

The above studies have shown how aging and well-being are linked after adjusting for traits or by invoking them as moderators or predictors. Extraversion is clearly a plus factor for the likelihood of experiencing positive affect and life satisfaction as people age. In addition, those who have both high eudaimonic and hedonic well-being tend to be people who are low on neuroticism and high on extraversion and conscientiousness. Alternatively, those who are high on openness to experience tend to have greater eudaimonic than hedonic well-being. Recent inquiries have also clarified how traits interact to predict longitudinal change in well-being and distress, with openness serving to amplify the positive or negative effects of extraversion and neuroticism, respectively. Methodological innovations, using growth-curve modeling, have facilitated the simultaneous assessment of individual differences in how traits and well-being come together as well as delineated different intraindividual trajectories through time. Clinical applications suggest that the long-term fate of highly neurotic individuals may not be so inevitably sealed as was once assumed.

CHALLENGES AND FUTURE OPPORTUNITIES

Building on observations from the preceding review, this section distills key challenges involved in linking personality and well-being as people age from early adulthood to later life. These, in turn, point to future opportunities, both conceptually and methodologically, for advancing the integration of the multiple domains described above.

The Outlived Usefulness of Pervasive Dichotomies

Three prominent dichotomies are evident in the preceding review. The first pertains to whether personality, broadly defined, is characterized by *change* versus *stability* as individuals grow older. Initial theories and organizing ideas pointed to change—indeed, psychological development, in the second half of life—but these were sharply disputed by the renaissance in trait research launched by Costa and McCrae, whose overwhelming message was one of stability. Others nonetheless found evidence of longitudinal change in areas informed by early developmental arenas (e.g., norm orientation, complexity, emotion regulation). Most recently, meta-analyses of traits add further support to the narrative of longitudinal change, as observed in facets of particular traits, with such patterns depicted as reflecting maturity processes, presumably tied to the assumption of adult roles. Evidence of mean-level change in trait facets is all the more remarkable, given the factor-analytic origins of traits (i.e., they have no conceptual grounding in ideas of development, or any other theory) as well as scale-construction processes surrounding them, which purged as unreliable items showing sensitivity to cross-time change (Costa & McCrae, 1985, 1989).

Evidence of mean-level change in personality with aging is importantly augmented with findings from multilevel modeling techniques, which emphasize wide *individual differences* in patterns of change or stability for both traits and well-being. Thus, the wisdom issued decades ago by Block (1971)—namely, that some people change with time, and others do not—seems all the more compelling as it has played out across many studies of adulthood and later life. Also encouraging is the growing number of studies focused on identification of factors that predict such differential trajectories. The field will be notably advanced by maintaining this emphasis on who changes, who does not, and why, than by engaging in fruitless debate about whether personality change or stability is the more dominant narrative.

A second pervasive dichotomy is the distinction between *top-down* versus *bottom-up* approaches to personality and well-being. The putative explanation for top-down formulations (i.e., traits predict well-being) is genetics, whereas bottom-up models emphasize environmental influences (i.e., contextual factors predict well-being), thus invoking another time-worn either–or choice. Based on the literature assembled above, there is good reason to view both top-down and bottom-up approaches as operative in understanding life-course variation in well-being. That is, both traits and sociodemographic status variables (e.g., age, gender, marital status, SES, race/ethnicity) account for variance in well-being outcomes (Andrews & Withey, 1976; Campbell et al., 1976; DeNeve & Cooper, 1998; Diener, 1984; Diener & Lucas, 1999; Keyes et al., 2002; Mroczek & Kolarz, 1998; Mroczek & Spiro, 2005; Ryff & Singer, 2008), albeit to differing degrees. The comparative advantage ascribed to traits appears premature, given duplication in what is being assessed under the heading of traits and well-being, along with problems of source overlap.

Beyond these measurement issues, it is perhaps even more imperative to recognize that contextual/environmental influences are fundamentally implicated in defining the conditions under which genetic predispositions are, or are not, to be expressed (Caspi et al., 2002, 2003). That is, contextual variables are essential for making sense of how particular genotypes (e.g., variants in serotonin transporter genes) progress to behavioral phenotypes (e.g., depression). Many, it should be noted, have both genetic and environmental risk but do *not* progress to disease symptomatology (see Ryff & Singer, 2005). This observation only further underscores the importance of integrating complex risk and protective factors, reflecting both genetic (top-down) and environmental (bottom-up) influences.

In calling for joint emphasis on personality and contextual factors, it should be acknowledged that some who have studied adult development and aging, most notably Helson and colleagues (e.g., Helson, Soto, & Cate, 2006), have incorporated such combinations of variables into their predictions of psychological change for many years. As described above, proximal life challenges, such as caregiving, or standing in the socioeconomic hierarchy have also been examined as environmental inputs that shape reported levels of well-being. Thus, the message to combine top-down and bottom-up perspectives offers nothing novel; rather the observation is about a needed shift of emphasis toward more integrative work of this variety.

A third less explicit, but nonetheless relevant, dichotomy pertains to *normative* versus *non-normative* influences on personality and well-being. Roberts and colleagues suggest that assuming adult roles and responsibilities shapes "normative personality change," thus, paralleling ideas put forth by a life-course researcher (i.e., Havighurst) over 50 years ago. However, even then, there was little appreciation of counterpoint experiences—namely, non-normative phenomena that represent atypical happenings, and sometimes even the "non-happenings," of adult life. To illustrate, some adults do not marry or have children, or if they do, the experience is not what they expected it would be. For example, Ryff and Seltzer (1996) illustrated many variants in the parental experience, including having a child with mental retardation or mental illness, and examined subsequent links to parents' well-being. Many such parents also have nondisabled children as well, and thus are engaged in both normative and non-normative parenting simultaneously. Being single in a society where most adults marry represents yet another non-normative status that social scientists have linked with prejudice, discrimination, and stigma (e.g., Byrne & Carr, 2005; DePaulo & Morris, 2005)—all relevant influences on well-being.

Beyond these example are numerous others obvious in the contemporary world around us—young adults go off to fight in dangerous wars, middle-age adults lose their jobs during economic downturns, spouses leave or become ill and require caregiving, and so on. Thus, many individuals pursue well-being in the face of an adverse, if not hostile, world (Shmotkin, 2005). For those who study how personality and well-being are entwined in time, there is a need to incorporate the full scope of what is occurring— both the expected, typical, and planned events of adult life, along with experiences that are unexpected, atypical, and unplanned.

Viewed collectively, these observations call for research on aging, personality, and well-being that puts multiple realities together, rather than forces either–or choices. Varieties of psychological change *and* stability (in both personality and well-being) must be considered, with diverse mixes among them likely to be explained by combinations of biological *and* environmental influences, the latter including both normative *and* non-normative life experiences. Put another way, the science we pursue needs to come closer to the novels we read in capturing the variety and complexity of adult life. This admonition calls for extension of, and refinement in, methods used to carry out these inquiries, as discussed below.

Beyond Single-Summary Indices, Studied One Variable at a Time

The injunction to embrace complexity in studying how people age, via the integration of multiple levels of analysis (e.g., traits, life experiences, sociodemographic characteristics, well-being) is impeded by the use of single-summary indices (typically means and correlation coefficients), studied one variable at a time. Multilevel modeling techniques are greatly advancing our understanding of individual differences in rate and direction of change in traits and well-being, although these approaches also tend to focus averages in change trajectories for limited subgroups. Efforts to assess antecedents to life-course changes in well-being have similarly adopted single antecedents (e.g., neuroticism *or* extraversion *or* income *or* marital status), again typically examining one at a time. The net effect is a body of research that dissembles people into component parts, and then not surprisingly, ends up accounting for limited variance in whatever outcomes are under investigation. These method-driven limitations need to be augmented by innovations that allow for (1) more variants in the data than can be discerned from single- or limited-summary indices, and that can address (2) multiway interactions—that is, *combinations of factors*—to account for variation in particular outcomes (e.g., well-being). This is a call for integrative, person-centered methods.

Typologies constitute an obvious direction for pursuing these objectives, examples of which readily come to mind, such as Block's (1971) pioneering work on types of personality development from adolescence

to early adulthood. Robins, John, and Caspi (1998) provided a useful historical summary of personality typologies and then delineated how to generate them through univariate, bivariate, or multivariate procedures (e.g., using factor or cluster analyses). They also discuss numerous empirical examples, including their own research (Robins, John, Caspi, Moffitt, & Stouthamer-Loeber, 1996), which differentiated adolescents into three types (resilients, overcontrollers, undercontrollers) and further distinguished among them by examining their profiles on personality traits as well as other variables (e.g., IQ, school performance and conduct, internal and externalizing behaviors).

In adulthood and aging research, typologies of well-being have received considerable attention, such as how differing combinations of psychological (eudaimonic) and subjective (hedonic + life satisfaction) well-being (Keyes et al., 2002), or affective, cognitive, and temporal aspects of well-being (Shmotkin, 1998), come together. The latter comprise various "adaptational options," wherein some are happy or unhappy in multiple ways (congruous types), whereas others reveal mixes of well-being (incongruous types), possibly reflective of compensation processes (Shmotkin, 2005). How well-being varies over time has also been differentiated according to various types (e.g., ascending, descending, stable, curvilinear, fluctuating, divergent). Another typology pertains to retrospective ratings of happiness and suffering among older Israelis (Shmotkin, Berkovich, & Cohen, 2006). Respondents reported on "anchor periods" (e.g., the happiest period, the most difficult period) in their lives. Findings showed that women tended to report both high happiness and high suffering, whereas men tended to report low happiness and low suffering. Other variables were found to discriminate among the well-being types in various anchor periods, such as educational status and whether or not respondents were Holocaust survivors.

Focused on person-centered longitudinal trajectories, Ryff, Singer, and Radler (2007) used two waves of data from the MIDUS national survey to differentiate among those who were stable, at high or low levels, as well as those who improved or declined (a little or a lot) over a 9- to 10-year period. This was done by cross-classifying individuals based on their standing in the distribution of psychological well-being (divided into quintiles) at baseline and a decade later. The analysis thus augmented conventional cross-time indices (change in mean level, stability coefficients) with diverse person-centered trajectories of change, which were found to vary considerably by age (e.g., young adults and the elderly were more likely to show decline than middle-age adults).

Types of personalities and/or types of well-being also need to be integrated with sociodemographic and experiential variables. The art of such integration is to find the right balance that allows for multiple variants, but does not descend into case study analyses. An example pertains to the use of sociodemographic background variables, along with personal characteristics and diverse life experiences, to delineate life-history pathways to midlife resilience, defined as having high psychological well-being at age 52–53, despite having previously experienced major depression (Singer, Ryff, Carr, & Magee, 1998). Boolean algebra was employed to extract multiple co-occurring conditions within particular subgroups that corresponded to differing combinations of adversity factors (e.g., growing up poor, having an alcoholic parent) and advantage factors (e.g., having high intelligence, a good job, a supportive spouse). These constituted differing life-history pathways to both depression and recovery from it. Examples of other complex typologies and the methods used to generate them, such as grade of membership analysis, were subsequently elaborated by Singer and Ryff (2001).

A final example pertains to the use of recursive partitioning, which is a tree-structured type of regression that is useful for identifying combinations of variables implicated in particular outcomes. How differing combinations of biomarkers predict later-life mortality among distinct subgroups provides one illustration of the methodology (Gruenewald, Seeman, Ryff, Karlamangia, & Singer, 2006). A more recent application (Gruenewald, Mroczek, Ryff, & Singer, 2008) is more relevant to the present chapter. In this investigation, the objective was to combine different personality traits, demographic status variables, and work and family contextual influences to account for differing levels of positive and negative affect among young,

middle, and old-age adults. To demonstrate the gains in integrative understanding that are afforded by recursive partitioning, the method was applied to the study of Mroczek and Kolarz (1998), described above. That study had used data from MIDUS to show differing age profiles for positive and negative affect and for how they interacted with other variables in the analysis (considering only two-way interactions). Recursive partitioning, in contrast, allows for multiway, nonlinear interactions, the combinations of which may further vary by particular subgroups, for example, defined by age or gender. Although neuroticism was a strong predictor of negative affect (as prior analyses had shown), the recursive partitioning approach showed how it combined with other factors, depending on the age of respondents. For example, among young adults, it was neuroticism combined with work stress and financial control that accounted for different levels of negative affect, whereas for middle-age adults, it was neuroticism combined with extraversion and financial control that mattered; meanwhile, for older adults, neuroticism interacted with health status, gender, and financial control. The most novel finding for positive affect was that it was predicted by both extraversion *and* neuroticism, in combination with other factors that again varied by age (i.e., financial control for young adults; relationship quality and financial control for midlife adults; marital status and financial control for older adults). The robustness of these patterns was documented via parallel findings using split-sample analyses. Taken together, the findings provided strong support for both top-down and bottom-up approaches to affective well-being. Essential to generating them, however, was the use of analytic methods that are well suited to identifying integrative pathways.

In addition to alternative methods, it is also essential to build theories and conceptual frameworks that put multiple levels of analysis together. Ideas of resilience and vulnerability may prove useful in this regard, as they allow for delineation of differing combinations of risk and protective factors that culminate in various well- or ill-being outcomes. For example, although low SES is frequently linked with *average* profiles of health and well-being that are below those with higher levels of education, income, and occupational status (Adler, Marmot, McEwen,

& Stewart, 1999), there is considerable variability around such means, and in fact, the variability is greater at the low end of the SES hierarchy (Ryff & Singer, 2002). This observation paves the way for probing high well-being among those who lack socioeconomic advantage (Markus, Ryff, Curhan, & Palmersheim, 2004; Ryff, Singer, & Palmersheim, 2004; Singer & Ryff, 1997, 1999). Such psychological resilience (defined as the capacity to maintain or regain high well-being in the face of adversity) has also been observed among racial/ethnic minorities (Ryff, Keyes, & Hughes, 2003). These studies are useful for explicating the meaning-making and possibly growth-producing effects of adversity, as poignantly portrayed years ago by Frankl (1959/1992).

In addition, Shmotkin's (2005) work on "happiness in the face of adversity" offers a comprehensive and conceptually rich formulation on how well-being is regulated so as to maintain a favorable psychological environment in the face of a hostile world. Subjective well-being is thus seen as a dynamic system involving multiple modules, including how well-being is introspectively experienced (experiential function), how it is communicated to others (declarative function), how it is organized (differential function), and how it is temporally patterned (narrative function). Collectively, these functions comprise the adaptational processes that make it possible to achieve high well-being, despite the various challenges and adversity that life entails.

To reiterate the key point of this section, research at the interface of aging, personality, and well-being needs to go beyond analytic methods that involve single-summary indices of variables, studied one at a time. Person-centered typologies offer a useful route to exploiting the middle territory between strongly nomothetic and idiographic approaches—what others have referred to as *idiothetic* research (Jones & Meredith, 1996; Lamiell, 1981)—and thus, serve to enrich our understanding of varieties of personality and well-being. In addition, alternative forms of data analysis, based on such techniques as recursive partitioning, offer new directions for integrating the complex array of factors (personality traits, sociodemographic status variables, contextual influences) that contribute to, and perhaps also follow from, differing profiles of well-being in the journey from early adulthood to old age.

Context Is Imperative, but What Is It?

Throughout this chapter emphasis has been given to the importance of incorporating contextual factors into the study of life-course changes in well-being. Personality psychologists, of course, have abiding interests in situational influences on people's attitudes and behavior, but the meaning of situations varies considerably depending on one's disciplinary orientation, or subspeciality, within psychology. Experimentalists, for example, study laboratory situations that are amenable to manipulation, whereas life-course researchers examine proximal situations related to work and family life, examples of which are evident in some of the above investigations. Longitudinal personality researchers have also focused on social–relational aspects of context, tracking how quality of social relationships predicts personality change over time, and vice versa (Neyer & Asendorpf, 2001; Robins, Caspi, & Moffitt, 2002).

However, it is important to note that lifespan developmental perspectives have also drawn extensively on sociology in formulating the meaning of context (see Baltes, 1987; Caspi, 1987; Ryff, 1987). This, in turn, calls for consideration of yet more influences, such as social roles, norms, socialization processes, and macro-level influences (e.g., economic disparities). The latter meanings of context have, in general, been given less attention in the literature reviewed above, although interest in them (e.g., roles, educational standing, well-being) is growing (Ahrens & Ryff, 2006), along with greater attention to the task of integrating macro- and micro-level influences on well-being (Ryff et al., 1999).

CONCLUSION: GOING FOR THE WHOLE GEMISH

A perhaps uncharitable characterization of research on personality and well-being in adulthood and later life is that it is an arcane literature in which people cannot recognize themselves or make sense of others in the world around them. That is, the focus on single variables and average stories within them may have culminated in a body of knowledge that many find uninformative, if not uninteresting. One alternative is to pursue a new era of science that puts the separate pieces of personality, well-being, and context together in order to describe whole people and the multiple forces, internal and external, impinging on them. Going for the whole story, despite the inevitable complexities involved, will help generate findings that are responsive to the variability in the world around us—including the reality, for example, of those who succumb to greed and corruption in midlife (e.g., corporate tycoons, lobbyists, and members of Congress who increasingly appear in the media) rather than ascend to adults roles of maturity, responsibility, and enriched well-being.

The above admonition parallels the message of McAdams and Pals (2006), who also advocate an integrative framework. Drawing on the vision of early leaders in the field, such as Allport (1937) and Murray (1938), they emphasize that personality psychology is the arena that should facilitate understanding of the whole person. Their proposed integration, among other things, calls for putting dispositional traits together with characteristic adaptations that include "motives, goals, plans, strivings, strategies, values, virtues, schemas, self-images, mental representations of significant others, development tasks, and many other aspects of human individuality that speak to motivational, social-cognitive and developmental concerns" (p. 208). So doing most assuredly constitutes a much needed and valuable stride forward, although it will require careful attention to the problem of construct redundancy, described above. Despite their distinctive labels, many individual-difference variables exist within a hair's distance from each other. Meaningful integration will thus require working out where constructs and measures address distinctive versus overlapping phenomena.

Beyond combining variables about the person, the integration advocated herein also emphasizes the importance of including contextual variables, including proximal situations related to work, family life, and other social ties, as well as broader social-structural influences, such as economic and political forces and standing in the socioeconomic hierarchy. The central message in embracing this wide territory is that aging, personality, and well-being come together in different ways for different people, depending on many other factors. The knowledge we generate needs to capture this complexity, and thereafter, assess its functional significance, for example, with regard to health

(Ryff, Singer, & Love, 2004), another topic for another time.

ACKNOWLEDGMENTS

The writing of this chapter and the research reported herein was supported by the National Institute on Aging (Grant No. P01-AG020166) as well as by earlier support from the National Institute of Mental Health (Grant No. P50-MH61083) and the National Institute on Aging (Grant No. R01-AG08979). I would like to thank Dan Mroczek, Rick Robins, Dov Shmotkin, and an anonymous reviewer for very helpful suggestions on an earlier version of the chapter.

REFERENCES

Adler, N. E., Marmot, M., McEwen, B. S., & Steward, J. (Eds.). (1999). Socioeconomic status and health in industrialized nations: Social, psychological, and biological pathways [Special issue]. *Annals of the New York Academy of Sciences, 896.*

Allport, G. W. (1937). *Personality: A psychological interpretation.* New York: Holt, Rinehart & Winston.

Allport, G. W. (1961). *Pattern and growth in personality*. New York: Holt, Rinehart & Winston.

Ahrens, C. C., & Ryff, C. D. (2006). Multiple roles and well-being: Sociodemographic and psychological moderators. *Sex Roles, 55,* 801–815.

Andrews, F. M., & Withey, S. B. (1976). *Social indicators of well-being: America's perception of life quality*. New York: Plenum Press.

Baltes, P. B. (1987). Theoretical propositions of life-span developmental psychology: On the dynamics between growth and decline. *Developmental Psychology, 23,* 611–626.

Bardi, A., & Ryff, C. D. (2007). Interactive effects of traits on adjustment to a life transition. *Journal of Personality, 75,* 1–29.

Block, J. H. (1971). *Lives through time.* Berkeley, CA: Bancroft Books.

Bolger, N., & Schilling, E. A. (1991). Personality and the problems of everyday life: The role of neuroticism in exposure and reactivity to daily stressors. *Journal of Personality, 59,* 355–386.

Bradburn, N. M. (1969). *The structure of psychological well-being.* Chicago: Aldine.

Brandtstädter, J., Wentura, D., & Rothermund, K. (1999). Intentional self-development through adulthood and later life: Tenacious pursuit and flexible adjustment of goals. In J. Brandtstädter & R. M. Lerner (Eds.), *Action and self-development: Theory and research through the life span* (pp. 373–400). Thousand Oaks, CA: Sage.

Bühler, C. (1935). The curve of life as studied in biographies. *Journal of Applied Psychology, 43,* 653–673.

Bühler, C., & Massarik, F. (Eds.). (1968). *The course of human life.* New York: Springer.

Byrne, A., & Carr, D. S. (2005). Caught in the cultural lag: The stigma of singlehood. *Psychological Inquiry, 16,* 84–91.

Cameron, P. (1975). Mood as indicant of happiness: Age, sex, social class, and situational differences. *Journal of Gerontology, 30,* 216–224.

Campbell, A., Converse, P. E., & Rodgers, W. L. (1976). *The quality of American life: Perceptions, evaluations, and satisfactions.* New York: Sage Foundation.

Carstensen, L. L. (1995). Evidence for a life-span theory of socioemotional selectivity. *Current Directions in Psychological Science, 4*(5), 151–156.

Caspi, A. (1987). Personality in the life course. *Journal of Personality and Social Psychology, 53,* 1203–1213.

Caspi, A., McClay, J., Moffitt, T. E., Mill, J., Martin, J., Craig, I. W., et al. (2002). Role of genotype in the cycle of violence in maltreated children. *Science, 297,* 851–854.

Caspi, A., Roberts, B. W., & Shiner, R. L. (2005). Personality development: Stability and change. *Annual Review of Psychology, 56,* 453–484.

Caspi, A., Sugden, K., Moffitt, T. E., Taylor, A., Craig, I. W., Harrington, H., et al. (2003). Influence of life stress on depression: Moderation by polymorphism in the 5-HTT gene. *Science, 301,* 386–389.

Charles, S. T., Reynolds, C. A., & Gatz, M. (2001). Age-related differences and change in positive and negative affect over 23 years. *Journal of Personality and Social Psychology, 80*(1), 136–151.

Clarke, P. J., Marshall, V. W., Ryff, C. D., & Rosenthal, C. J. (2000). Well being in Canadian seniors: Findings from the Canadian study of health and aging. *Canadian Journal on Aging, 19*(2), 139–159.

Costa, P. T., Jr., & McCrae, R. R. (1980). Influence of extraversion and neuroticism on subjective well-being: Happy and unhappy people. *Journal of Personality and Social Psychology, 38,* 668–678.

Costa, P. T., Jr., & McCrae, R. R. (1985). *The NEO Personality Inventory manual.* Odessa, FL: Psychological Assessment Resources.

Costa, P. T., Jr., & McCrae, R. R. (1986). Personality stability and its implications for clinical psychology. *Clinical Psychology Review, 6,* 407–423.

Costa, P. T., Jr., & McCrae, R. R. (1988). Per-

sonality in adulthood: A six-year longitudinal study of self-reports and spouse ratings on the NEO personality inventory. *Journal of Personality and Social Psychology, 54*(5), 853–863.

Costa, P. T., Jr., & McCrae, R. R. (1989). *The NEO-PI/NEO-FFI manual supplement.* Odessa, FL: Psychological Assessment Resources.

Costa, P. T., Jr., & McCrae, R. R. (1997). Longitudinal stability of adult personality. In R. Hogan, J. A. Johnson, & S. R. Briggs (Eds.), *Handbook of personality psychology* (pp. 269–290). San Diego, CA: Academic Press.

Costa, P. T., Jr., Metter, E. J., & McCrae, R. R. (1994). Personality stability and its contribution to successful aging. *Journal of Geriatric Psychiatry, 27,* 41–59.

DeNeve, K. M., & Cooper, H. (1998). The happy personality: A meta-analysis of 137 personality traits and subjective well-being. *Psychological Bulletin, 124*(2), 197–229.

DePaulo, B. M., & Morris, W. L. (2005). Singles in society and in science. *Psychological Inquiry, 16*(2–3), 57–83.

Diener, E. (1984). Subjective well-being. *Psychological Bulletin, 95,* 542–575.

Diener, E., & Biswas-Diener, R. (2002). Will money increase subjective well-being? *Social Indicators Research, 57*(2), 119–169.

Diener, E., & Lucas, R. E. (1999). Personality and subjective well-being. In D. Kahneman, E. Diener, & N. Schwarz (Eds.), *Well-being: The foundations of hedonic psychology* (pp. 213–229). New York: Sage Foundation.

Diener, E., Sandvik, E., & Larsen, R. J. (1985). Age and sex differences for emotional intensity. *Developmental Psychology, 21,* 542–546.

Diener, E., & Suh, E. M. (1997). Measuring quality of life: Economic, social, and subjective indicators. *Social Indicators Research, 40,* 189–216.

Dowd, J. J. (1990). Ever since Durkheim: The socialization of human development. *Human Development, 33,* 138–159.

Erikson, E. H. (1959). Identity and the life cycle: Selected papers [Special issue]. *Psychological Issues, 1,* 1–171.

Fava, G. A. (1999). Well-being therapy: Conceptual and technical issues. *Psychotherapy and Psychosomatics, 68,* 171–179.

Fava, G. A., Rafanelli, C., Grandi, S., Conti, S., & Belluardo, P. (1998). Prevention of recurrent depression with cognitive behavioral therapy. *Archives of General Psychiatry, 55,* 816–821.

Fava, G. A., Ruini, C., Rafanelli, C., Finos, L., Conti, S., & Grandi, S. (2004). Six-year outcome of cognitive behavior therapy for prevention of recurrent depression. *American Journal of Psychiatry, 161*(10), 1872–1876.

Feist, G. J., Bodner, T. E., Jacobs, J. F., Miles, M., & Tan, V. (1995). Integrating top-down and bottom-up structural models of subjective well-being: A longitudinal investigation. *Journal of Personality and Social Psychology, 68,* 138–150.

Fleeson, W., Malanos, A. B., & Archille, N. M. (2002). An intraindividual process approach to the relationship between extraversion and positive affect: Is acting extraverted as "good" as being extraverted? *Journal of Personality and Social Psychology, 83*(6), 1409–1422.

Fraley, R. C., & Roberts, B. W. (2005). Patterns of continuity: A dynamic model for conceptualizing the stability of individual differences in psychological constructs across the life course. *Psychological Review, 112*(1), 60–74.

Frankl, V. E., & Lasch, I. (1992). *Man's search for meaning: An introduction to logotherapy.* Boston: Beacon Press. (Original work published 1959)

Freund, A. M., & Baltes, P. B. (2002). Life-management strategies of selection, optimization, and compensation: Measurement by self-report and construct validity. *Journal of Personality and Social Psychology, 82*(4), 642–662.

Gray, J. A. (1991). Neural systems, emotion, and personality. In J. Madden, IV (Ed.), *Neurobiology of learning, emotion, and affect* (pp. 273–306). New York: Raven Press.

Greenfield, E. A., & Marks, N. (2004). Formal volunteering as a protective factor for older adults' psychological well-being. *Journals of Gerontology: Series B: Psychological Sciences and Social Sciences, 59B*(5), S258–S264.

Gruenewald, T. L., Mroczek, D. K., Ryff, C. D., & Singer, B. H. (2008). Pathways to negative and positive affect: An integrative approach using recursive partitioning. *Developmental Psychology, 44,* 330–343.

Gruenewald, T. L., Seeman, T. E., Ryff, C. D., Karlamangia, A. S., & Singer, B. H. (2006). Combinations of biomarkers predictive of later life mortality. *Proceedings of the National Academy of Sciences, 103,* 14158–14163.

Gurin, G., Veroff, J., & Feld, S. (1960). *Americans view their mental health.* New York: Basic Books.

Havighurst, R. J. (1948). *Developmental tasks and education.* Chicago: University of Chicago.

Helson, R., Jones, C., & Kwan, V. S. Y. (2002). Personality change over 40 years of adulthood: Hierarchical linear modeling analyses of two longitudinal samples. *Journal of Personality and Social Psychology, 83,* 752–766.

Helson, R., & Moane, G. (1987). Personality change in women from college to midlife. *Journal of Personality and Social Psychology, 53,* 176–186.

Helson, R., & Roberts, B. W. (1994). Ego development and personality change in adulthood.

Journal of Personality and Social Psychology, 66(5), 911–920.

Helson, R., & Soto, C. J. (2005). Up and down in middle age: Monotonic and nonmonotonic changes in roles, status, and personality. *Journal of Personality and Social Psychology, 89*(2), 194–204.

Helson, R., Soto, C. J., & Cate, R. A. (2006). From young adulthood through the middle ages. In D. K. Mroczek & T. D. Little (Eds.), *Handbook of personality development* (pp. 337–352). Mahwah, NJ: Erlbaum.

Helson, R., & Wink, P. (1992). Personality change in women from the early 40s to the early 50s. *Psychology and Aging, 71*(1), 46–55.

Hemenover, S. H. (2003). The good, the bad, and the healthy: Impacts of emotional disclosure of trauma on resilient self-concept and psychological distress. *Personality and Social Psychology Bulletin, 29,* 1236–1244.

Herzog, A. R., & Rodgers, W. L. (1981). Age and satisfaction: Data from several large surveys. *Research on Aging, 3*(2), 142–165.

Jahoda, M. (1958). *Current concepts of positive mental health.* New York: Basic Books.

Johnson, W., McGue, M., & Krueger, R. F. (2005). Personality stability in late adulthood: A behavioral genetic analysis. *Journal of Personality, 73*(2), 523–551.

Jones, C. J., & Meredith, W. (1996). Patterns of personality change across the life span. *Psychology and Aging, 11,* 57–65.

Jung, C. G. (1933). *Modern man in search of a soul* (W. S. Dell & C. F. Baynes, Trans.). New York: Harcourt, Brace & World.

Kahneman, D., Diener, E., & Schwarz, N. (Eds.). (1999). *Well-being: The foundations of hedonic psychology.* New York: Sage Foundation.

Keyes, C. L. M., & Ryff, C. D. (1998). Generativity in adult lives: Social structural contours and quality of life consequences. In D. P. McAdams & E. de St. Aubin (Eds.), *Generativity and adult development: Psychosocial perspectives on caring for and contributing to the next generation.* Washington, DC: American Psychological Association.

Keyes, C. L. M., Shmotkin, D., & Ryff, C. D. (2002). Optimizing well-being: The empirical encounter of two traditions. *Journal of Personality and Social Psychology, 82*(6), 1007–1022.

Kling, K. C., Ryff, C. D., & Essex, M. J. (1997). Adaptive changes in the self-concept during a life transition. *Personality and Social Psychology Bulletin, 23*(9), 981–990.

Kling, K. C., Ryff, C. D., Love, G., & Essex, M. (2003). Exploring the influence of personality on depressive symptoms and self-esteem across a significant life transition. *Journal of Personality and Social Psychology, 85*(5), 922–932.

Kling, K. C., Seltzer, M. M., & Ryff, C. D. (1997). Distinctive late-life challenges: Implications for coping and well-being. *Psychology and Aging*, *12*(2), 288–295.

Kwan, C. M. L., Love, G. D., Ryff, C. D., & Essex, M. J. (2003). The role of self-enhancing evaluations in a successful life transition. *Psychology and Aging*, *18*(1), 3–12.

Labouvie-Vief, G., & Gonzallez, M. M. (2004). Dynamic integration: Affect optimization and differentiation in development. In D. Y. Dai & R. J. Sternberg (Eds.), *Motivation, emotion, and cognition: Integrative perspectives on intellectual functioning and development* (pp. 237–272). Mahwah, NJ: Erlbaum.

Labouvie-Vief, G., & Medler, M. (2002). Affect optimization and affect complexity: Modes and styles of regulation in adulthood. *Psychology and Aging*, *17*(4), 571–587.

Lamiell, J. T. (1981). Toward an idiothetic psychology of personality. *American Psychologist*, *36*, 276–289.

Larson, R. (1978). Thirty years of research on the subjective well-being of older Americans. *Journals of Gerontology: Medical Sciences*, *33*, 109–125.

Lawton, M. P. (1975). The Philadelphia Geriatric Center Morale Scale: A revision. *Journal of Gerontology*, *30*, 85–89.

Liang, J. (1984). Dimensions of the Life Satisfaction Index A: A structural formulation. *Journal of Gerontology*, *39*, 613–622.

Maier, E. H., & Lachman, M. E. (2000). Consequences of early parental loss and separation for health and well-being in midlife. *International Journal of Behavioral Development*, *24*(2), 183–189.

Malatesta, C. Z., & Kalnok, M. (1984). Emotional experience in younger and older adults. *Journal of Gerontology*, *39*, 301–308.

Marks, N. F. (1998). Does it hurt to care?: Caregiving, work–family conflict, and midlife well-being. *Journal of Marriage and the Family*, *60*(4), 951–966.

Marks, N. F., & Lambert, J. D. (1998). Marital status continuity and change among young and midlife adults: Longitudinal effects on psychological well-being. *Journal of Family Issues*, *19*, 652–686.

Markus, H. R., Ryff, C. D., Curhan, K. B., & Palmersheim, K. A. (2004). In their own words: Well-being at midlife among high school-educated and college-educated adults. In O. G. Brim, C. D. Ryff, & R. C. Kessler (Eds.), *How healthy are we?: A national study of well-being at midlife* (pp. 273–319). Chicago: University of Chicago Press.

Marmot, M. G., Fuhrer, R., Ettner, S. L., Marks, N. F., Bumpass, L. L., & Ryff, C. D. (1998). Contribution of psychosocial factors to socioeconomic differences in health. *Milbank Quarterly*, *76*(3), 403–448.

Marmot, M. G., Ryff, C. D., Bumpass, L. L., Shipley, M., & Marks, N. F. (1997). Social inequalities in health: Next questions and converging evidence. *Social Science and Medicine*, *44*(6), 901–910.

Maslow, A. H. (1968). *Toward a psychology of being* (2nd ed.). New York: Van Nostrand.

McAdams, D. P., & Pals, J.L. (2006). The new Big Five: Fundamental principles for an integrative science of personality. *American Psychologist*, *61*, 204–217.

McAdams, D. P., & St. de Aubin, E. (Eds.). (1998). *Generativity and adult development: How and why we care for the next generation*. Washington, DC: American Psychological Association.

McCrae, R. R., & Costa, P. T., Jr. (1990). *Personality in adulthood*. New York: Guilford Press.

McCrae, R. R., & Costa, P. T., Jr. (1991). Adding *liebe und arbeit*: The full five-factor model and well-being. *Personality and Social Psychology Bulletin*, *17*, 227–232.

McCrae, R. R., & Costa, P. T., Jr. (1994). The stability of personality: Observation and evaluations. *Current Directions in Psychological Science*, *3*(6), 173–175.

McCrae, R. R., & Costa, P. T., Jr. (Eds.). (2003). *Personality in adulthood: A five-factor theory perspective* (2nd ed.). New York: Guilford Press.

McCrae, R. R., Costa, P. T., Jr., Ostendorf, F., Angleitner, A., Hrebickova, M., Avia, M. D., et al. (2000). Nature over nurture: Temperament, personality, and life span development. *Journal of Personality and Social Psychology*, *78*(1), 173–186.

Mroczek, D. K., & Almeida, D. M. (2004). The effect of daily stress, personality, and age on daily negative affect. *Journal of Personality and Social Psychology*, *72*(2), 355–378.

Mroczek, D. K., & Kolarz, C. M. (1998). The effect of age on positive and negative affect: A developmental perspective on happiness. *Journal of Personality and Social Psychology*, *75*(5), 1333–1349.

Mroczek, D. K., & Spiro, A., III. (2003). Modeling intraindividual change in personality traits: Findings from the Normative Aging Study. *Journals of Gerontology: Psychological Sciences*, *58B*, P153–P165.

Mroczek, D. K., & Spiro, A., III. (2005). Change in life satisfaction during adulthood: Findings from the veterans affairs normative aging study. *Journal of Personality and Social Psychology*, *88*(1), 189–202.

Murray, H.A. (1938). *Explorations in personality*. New York: Oxford University Press.

Neugarten, B. L. (1968). *Middle age and aging*. Chicago: University of Chicago Press.

Neugarten, B. L. (1973). Personality change in late life: A developmental perspective. In C. Eisodorfer & M. P. Lawton (Eds.), *The psychology of adult development and aging* (pp. 311–335). Washington, DC: American Psychological Association.

Neugarten, B. L., Havighurst, R. J., & Tobin, S. S. (1961). The measurement of life satisfaction. *Journal of Gerontology, 16,* 134–143.

Neyer, F. J., & Asendorpf, J. B. (2001). Personality-relationship transactions in young adulthood. *Journal of Personality and Social Psychology, 81,* 1190–1204.

Panksepp, J., & Miller, A. (1996). Emotions and the aging brain: Regrets and remedies. In C. Magai & S. H. McFadden (Eds.), *Handbook of emotion, adult development, and aging* (pp. 3–26). San Diego, CA: Academic Press.

Peterson, B. E., & Klohnen, E. C. (1995). Realization of generativity in two samples of women in midlife. *Psychology and Aging, 10,* 20–29.

Prenda, K. M., & Lachman, M. E. (2001). Planning for the future: A life management strategy for increasing control and life satisfaction in adulthood. *Psychology and Aging, 16*(2), 206–216.

Riley, M. W., Kahn, R. L., & Foner, A. (1994). *Age and structural lag .* New York: Wiley.

Roberts, B. W., & Caspi, A. (2003). The cumulative continuity model of personality development: Striking a balance between continuity and change in personality traits across the life course. In U. M. Staudinger & U. Lindenberger (Eds.), *Understanding human development: Dialogues with lifespan psychology* (pp. 183–214). Dordrecht, Netherlands: Kluwer.

Roberts, B. W., & DelVecchio, W. F. (2000). The rank-order consistency of personality traits from childhood to old age: A quantitative review of longitudinal studies. *Psychological Bulletin, 126*(1), 3–25.

Roberts, B. W., Helson, R., & Klohnen, E. C. (2002). Personality development and growth in women across 30 years: Three perspectives. *Journal of Personality, 70*(1), 79–102.

Roberts, B. W., Walton, K. E., & Viechtbauer, W. (2006). Patterns of mean-level change in personality traits across the life course: A meta-analysis of longitudinal studies. *Psychological Bulletin, 132*(1), 1–25.

Roberts, B. W., & Wood, D. (2006). Personality development in the context of the neosocioanalytic model of personality. In D. K. Mroczek & T. D. Little (Eds.), *Handbook of personality development* (pp. 11–39). Mahwah, NJ: Erlbaum.

Robins, R. W., Caspi, A., & Moffitt, T. E. (2002). It's not just who you're with, it's who you are: Personality and relationship experiences across multiple relationships. *Journal of Personality, 70,* 925–964.

Robins, R. W., John, O. P., & Caspi, A. (1998). The typological approach to studying personality. In R. B. Cairns, L. R. Bergman, & J. Kagan (Eds.), *Methods and models for studying the individual* (pp. 135–160). Thousand Oaks, CA: Sage.

Robins, R. W., John, O. P., Caspi, A., Moffitt, T. E., & Stouthamer-Loeber, M. (1996). Resilient, overcontrolled, and undercontrolled boys: Three replicable personality types. *Journal of Personality and Social Psychology, 70,* 157–171.

Robins, R. W., & Trzesniewski, K. H. (2005). Self-esteem development across the lifespan. *Current Directions in Psychological Science, 14,* 158–162.

Robins, R. W., Trzesniewski, K. H., Tracy, J. L., Gosling, S. D., & Potter, J. (2002). Global self-esteem across the life-span. *Psychology and Aging, 17,* 423–434.

Rogers, C. R. (1962). The interpersonal relationship: The core of guidance. *Harvard Educational Review, 32*(4), 416–429.

Russell, B. (1958). *The conquest of happiness.* New York: Liveright. (Original work published 1930)

Ryan, R. M., & Deci, E. L. (2001). On happiness and human potentials: A review of research on hedonic and eudaimonic well-being. *Annual Review of Psychology, 52,* 141–166.

Ryff, C. D. (1985). Adult personality development and the motivation for personal growth. In D. Kleiber & M. Maehr (Eds.), *Advances in motivation and achievement: Vol. 4. Motivation and adulthood* (pp. 55–92). Greenwich, CT: JAI Press.

Ryff, C. D. (1987). The place of personality and social structure research in social psychology. *Journal of Personality and Social Psychology, 53*(6), 1192–1202.

Ryff, C. D. (1989). Happiness is everything, or is it?: Explorations on the meaning of psychological well-being. *Journal of Personality and Social Psychology, 57*(6), 1069–1081.

Ryff, C. D. (1991). Possible selves in adulthood and old age: A tale of shifting horizons. *Psychology and Aging, 6*(2), 286–295.

Ryff, C. D., & Keyes, C. L. M. (1995). The structure of psychological well-being revisited. *Journal of Personality and Social Psychology, 69*(4), 719–727.

Ryff, C. D., Keyes, C. L. M., & Hughes, D. L. (2003). Status inequalities, perceived discrimination, and eudaimonic well-being: Do the challenges of minority life hone purpose and growth? *Journal of Health and Social Behavior, 44*(3), 275–291.

Ryff, C. D., Kwan, C. M. L., & Singer, B. H. (2001). Personality and aging: Flourishing agendas and future challenges. In J. E. Birren

& K. W. Schale (Eds.), *Handbook of the psychology of aging* (5th ed., pp. 477–499). San Diego, CA: Academic Press.

Ryff, C. D., Magee, W. J., Kling, K. C., & Wing, E. H. (1999). Forging macro-micro linkages in the study of psychological well-being. In C. D. Ryff & V. W. Marshall (Eds.), *The self and society in aging processes* (pp.247–278). New York: Springer.

Ryff, C. D., & Seltzer, M. M. (Eds.). (1996). *The parental experience in midlife*. Chicago: University of Chicago Press.

Ryff, C. D., & Singer, B. H. (2005). Social environments and the genetics of aging: Advancing knowledge of protective health mechanisms. *Journals of Gerontology: Series B, 60B*(Special Issue I), 12–23.

Ryff, C. D., & Singer, B. H. (2008). Know thyself and become what you are: A eudaimonic approach to psychological well-being. *Journal of Happiness Studies, 9,* 13–39.

Ryff, C. D., Singer, B., & Love, G. D. (2004). Positive health: Connecting well-being with biology. *Philosophical Transactions of the Royal Society of London B, 359,* 1383–1394.

Ryff, C. D., Singer, B. H., & Palmersheim, K. A. (2004). Social inequalities in health and well-being: The role of relational and religious protective factors. In O. G. Brim, C. D. Ryff, & R. C. Kessler (Eds.), *How healthy are we?: A national study of well-being at midlife* (pp. 90–123). Chicago: University of Chicago Press.

Ryff, C. D., Singer, B. H., & Radler, B. (2007). *Longitudinal trajectories of well-being: Findings from the MIDUS national study*. Unpublished manuscript.

Schmutte, P. S., & Ryff, C. D. (1997). Personality and well-being: Reexamining methods and meanings. *Journal of Personality and Social Psychology, 73*(3), 549–559.

Shmotkin, D. (1990). Subjective well-being as a function of age and gender: A multivariate look for differentiated trends. *Social Indicators Research, 23,* 201–230.

Shmotkin, D. (1998). Declarative and differential aspects of subjective well-being and implications for mental health in later life. In J. Lomranz (Ed.), *Handbook of aging and mental health: An integrative approach* (pp. 15–43). New York: Plenum Press.

Shmotkin, D. (2005). Happiness in the face of adversity: Reformulating the dynamic and modular bases of subjective well-being. *Review of General Psychology, 9*(4), 291–325.

Shmotkin, D., Berkovich, M., & Cohen, K. (2006). Combining happiness and suffering in a retrospective view of anchor periods in life: A differential approach to subjective well-being. *Social Indicators Research, 77,* 139–169.

Singer, B. H., & Ryff, C. D. (1997). Racial and ethnic equalities in health: Environmental, psychosocial, and physiological pathways. In B. Devlin, S. E. Feinberg, D. Resnick, & K. Roeder (Eds.), *Intelligence, genes, and success: Scientists respond to the bell curve* (pp. 89–122). New York: Springer-Verlag.

Singer, B. H., & Ryff, C. D. (1999). Hierarchies of life histories and associated health risks. In N. E. Adler & M. Marmot (Eds.), *Socioeconomic status and health in industrial nations: Social, psychological, and biological pathways* (Vol. 896, pp. 96–115). New York: New York Academy of Sciences.

Singer, B. H., & Ryff, C. D. (2001). Understanding aging via person-centered methods and the integration of narratives and numbers. In R. H. Binstock & L. K. George (Eds.), *Handbook of aging and the social sciences* (5th ed., pp. 44–65). San Diego, CA: Academic Press.

Singer, B. H., Ryff, C. D., Carr, D., & Magee, W. J. (1998). Life histories and mental health: A person-centered strategy. In A. Raftery (Ed.), *Sociological methodology* (pp. 1–51). Washington, DC: American Sociological Association.

Small, B. J., Hertzog, C., Hultsch, D. F., & Dixon, R. A. (2003). Stability and change in adult personality over 6 years: Findings from the Victoria Longitudinal Study. *Journal of Gerontology: Psychological Sciences, 58B,* P166–P176.

Smider, N. A., Essex, M. J., & Ryff, C. D. (1996). Adaptation to community relocation: The interactive influence of psychological resources and contextual factors. *Psychology and Aging, 11*(2), 362–372.

Staudinger, U. M., & Kunzmann, U. (2005). Positive adult personality development: Adjustment and/or growth? *European Psychologist, 10,* 320–329.

Tweed, S., & Ryff, C. D. (1991). Adult children of alcoholics: Profiles of wellness and distress. *Journal of Studies on Alcohol, 52,* 133–141.

Watson, D., Clark, L. A., & Tellegen, A. (1988). Development and validation of brief measures of positive and negative affect: The PANAS scales. *Journal of Personality and Social Psychology, 54,* 1063–1070.

Whitbourne, S. K., & Waterman, A. S. (1979). Psychosocial development during the adult years: Age and cohort comparisons. *Developmental Psychology, 15,* 373–378.

Whitbourne, S. K., Zuschlag, M. K., Elliot, L. B., & Waterman, A. S. (1992). Psychosocial development in adulthood: A 22-year sequential study. *Journal of Personality and Social Psychology, 63*(2), 260–271.

PART V

Self and Social Processes

CHAPTER 16

Naturalizing the Self

Richard W. Robins
Jessica L. Tracy
Kali H. Trzesniewski

Late in his life, Michelangelo began carving what many art historians consider his most mature and provocative sculpture, the *Florentine Pieta*, an enormous 8-foot statue he intended to place at the top of his own tomb. After working intensely for a decade on this monumental project, the artist entered his studio one day and, in a fit of rage, assaulted the sculpture with a sledgehammer. He broke off the hands and legs and nearly shattered the work before his assistants dragged him away. Why would Michelangelo attempt to destroy one of his greatest creations, a sculpture that has been described as among the finest works of the Renaissance?

How would a personality psychologist answer this question? A trait researcher might say that Michelangelo was highly impulsive and dispositionally prone to negative emotionality. A biologically oriented researcher might speculate that he had a deficiency in the monoamine oxidase A gene, low levels of serotonin, and an atypical pattern of activation in the frontal and temporal lobes. A motivational researcher might assume that Michelangelo's personal projects shifted and the *Florentine Pieta* came into conflict with other important goals. Yet none of these

explanations provides a completely satisfactory account of Michelangelo's seemingly irrational act. In our view, it is only through a consideration of self-processes—identity, self-esteem, and self-regulation—that one can begin to understand Michelangelo's behavior. An analysis of Michelangelo's "self" allows us to formulate hypotheses concerning a heightened sense of perfectionism and shame that likely accompanied his reputed narcissistic tendencies, a failure to live up to his own expectations and those of his father (who equated sculpting with manual labor), a breakdown in self-regulation, and an identity crisis due to his impending death.

Many aspects of human behavior are inexplicable without the notion that people have a self. In fact, an understanding of the self is necessary for a complete understanding of personality processes—the processes that generate and regulate thoughts, feelings, and behaviors. An understanding of the self helps explain not only such exceptional behaviors as Michelangelo's destructive act, but also many aspects of everyday social life: Why do some individuals feel shy in social contexts whereas others do not? Why are some individuals boastful in some situations but insecure in others? Why are some individuals preoccupied by achievement concerns whereas others crave intimacy?

PSYCHOLOGY'S MOST PUZZLING PUZZLE

In *Principles of Psychology*, William James (1890) referred to the self as psychology's "most puzzling puzzle" (p. 330). For the past century, psychologists have debated whether it is a puzzle worth puzzling about. In an article titled "Is the concept of self necessary?", Allport raised the possibility that the self is "an impediment in the path of psychological progress" (1955, p. 25). Skinner (1990, p. 1209) argued that "there is no place in a scientific analysis of behavior for a mind or self." Pinker (1997) described self-awareness as an intractable problem that we as a species are not sufficiently evolved to grasp. And, Ramachandran (2007) characterized the "problem of self" as "science's greatest riddle."

Faced with this daunting level of pessimism, we propose the perhaps overly optimistic thesis that a scientific understanding of the self is not only possible but is, in fact, fundamental to a science of personality. Research over the past few decades has documented many ways in which the self influences how people act, think, and feel in particular situations, the goals they pursue in life, and the ways they cope with and adapt to new environments. Many currently prominent areas of personality research assume a central role for the self, including the study of self-conscious emotions such as pride and shame (e.g., Tracy, Robins, & Tangney, 2007), traits such as narcissism (e.g., Morf & Rhodewalt, 2001), internal working models of attachment (e.g., Collins & Allard, 2004), autobiographical memories (e.g., Mclean, Pasupathi, & Pals, 2007; Sutin & Robins, 2005), self-regulation (Gailliot, Mead, & Baumeister, Chapter 18, this volume), and goals and motivation (e.g., Carver, Scheier, & Fulford, Chapter 29, this volume).

A NATURALIST VIEW OF THE SELF

In the early days of scientific psychology, the self was an integral part of many general theories of the person. Indeed, many "classic" readings on the self come from the writings of the most influential theorists of the first half of the 20th century: James (1890), Baldwin (1897), Cooley (1902), Mead (1934), McDougall (1908/1963), Murphy (1947), Hilgard (1949), and Allport (1955). Three basic themes recur in these broad conceptions of the person. First, the self was seen as fundamental to understanding social behavior and personality processes, and many early theorists attempted to link self-processes to other basic psychological processes. Specifically, the self was seen as an executive body coordinating the thoughts, feelings, and behavior of a highly complex, dynamic organism. Second, many of these perspectives emphasized the interplay between biological and social forces: The self is constructed out of the raw materials endowed by nature and shaped by nurture. Third, the self was conceptualized from an evolutionary and functionalist perspective. The early theorists were working in the immediate aftermath of Darwin, and many drew heavily on evolutionary thinking. In particular, James (1890) was committed to a *naturalistic* explanation of the origin and function of self-awareness, assuming that conscious mental life "emerged by way of natural selection because it gave our species certain survival, and therefore reproductive, advantages" (p. 52).

For most of the latter half of the 20th century, research on the self moved away from these three themes, as researchers came to conceptualize the self as a social and cultural construction. In the past decade, however, there has been renewed interest in a naturalist view of the self, spearheaded by neuroscientists such as Crick (1994), Gazzaniga (1998), Ramachandran (2004), Koch (2004), Edelman (2005), and others, who study the neural mechanisms underlying consciousness in an attempt to understand how a sense of self emerges from the activity of the brain. Similarly, in their search for the neural bases of affective experience, emotion researchers such as Damasio (2003) and LeDoux (2003) have discovered basic facts about how the brain is wired, which have profound implications for self researchers. Memory researchers have linked various forms of memory to the conscious experience of self (e.g., Tulving, 2005), and this work has been used to examine neural activation during processing of self-relevant information in normal populations (Kelley et al., 2002; Magno & Allan, 2007) and in people with amnesia (Klein, Loftus, & Kihlstrom, 1996). Baron-Cohen (2008) and other neurologists (e.g., Feinberg & Paul, 2005) provide vivid illustrations of how neurological disorders such as autism can produce profound deficits in self and identity.

Thus, researchers from a wide range of perspectives outside of the traditional boundaries of personality and social psychology are grappling with basic issues about the self. Moreover, within personality and social psychology, an explosion of recent research has linked brain mechanisms to self-related processes. Indeed, many of the topics mentioned above as integrating the study of self and personality have now been studied from a neuroscience perspective, including the neural bases of pride (Takahashi et al., 2008), attachment (Gillath, Bunge, Shaver, Wendelken, & Mikulincer, 2005), autobiographical memory (Levine, 2004), and self-regulation (Inzlicht & Gutsell, 2007). Building on this emerging biological account, researchers have also discussed the evolutionary origins of the self (Sedikides & Skowronski, 2003) and explored the genetics of self-esteem and

other self processes (e.g., Neiss et al., 2005; Neiss, Sedikides, & Stevenson, 2006).

What unites many of these perspectives is a naturalist view of the self—a belief that the self can be studied like any other natural phenomenon. One goal of this chapter is to help self research recover its roots by reconnecting it with broader scientific concerns. We return to a set of foundational issues that preoccupied William James when he formulated his naturalist perspective of the mind.

OVERVIEW OF THE CHAPTER

The literature on the self is enormous. In a recent survey of personality psychologists (Robins, Tracy, & Sherman, 2007), 43% of respondents indicated that they study the self-concept and 35% study self-esteem. A PsycINFO search for the keyword "self" identified 265,161 articles.[1] Even restricting the search to the past 30 years and to a single journal—the *Journal of Personality and Social Psychology*—yielded 2,411 articles with the keyword "self" (33% of all articles published in the journal from 1970 to 2007). As Figure 16.1 shows, research on the self

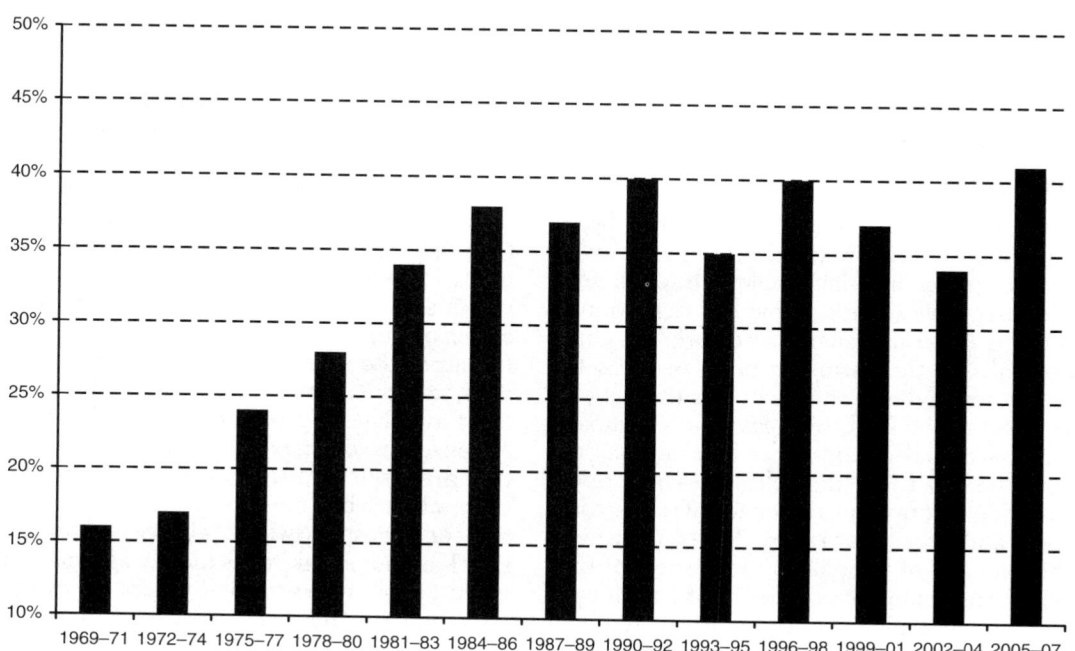

FIGURE 16.1. Percentage of articles in *JPSP* with "self" as a keyword.

surged in the 1970s—probably reflecting the rise of cognitive psychology and its emphasis on mental events—and then maintained a high level up to the present.

In this chapter, we do *not* attempt to provide a comprehensive review of the voluminous literature on the self. Several recent books and chapters provide such reviews: see Pickett, Chen, and Gardner (in press), Leary (2004), and Sedikides and Spence (2007) for general overviews of the self literature; Harter (2006) and Robins and Trzesniewski (2005) for research on the development of the self; Tracy and colleagues (2007) for research on self and emotions; Gailliot and colleagues (Chapter 18, this volume) for research on self-regulation; Swann and Bosson (Chapter 17, this volume) for research on the role of the self in social interaction; and Byrne (1996) for an overview of self-concept measures. Instead, our goal is to step back and reflect on some broader questions about the self: What is the self? When does the self first emerge and how does it change over time? Is the self distinctive to humans? How does the brain build a sense of self? Is the self a product of evolution? What are the adaptive functions of the self? These questions return us to James's initial set of concerns when he formulated his naturalist perspective on self and consciousness.

BASIC QUESTIONS ABOUT THE SELF

What Is the Self?: Definitional and Conceptual Issues

The question—what is the self?—has been an abiding concern of philosophers, writers, scientists, and laypeople. Although self theorists have offered numerous definitions, there is no consensual framework for conceptualizing the various aspects of the self. Some researchers embrace the theoretical richness of the field, whereas others bemoan its conceptual muddiness. One source of confusion is that "the self" does not refer to a single entity but rather to myriad structures and processes (Leary, 2004). Consider the example of happiness. One aspect of the self is the feeling or experience of happiness. This is what philosophers refer to as qualia or sentience. A second aspect is the conscious recognition that my feeling of happiness belongs to me—it is I who feels happy.

As Flanagan (1991) observed, "thoughts, feelings, and the like do not sit around disembodied. All thoughts and feelings are 'owned,' that is, all thoughts and feelings occur to someone" (p. 31). A third aspect refers to attentional focus—I can be aware (i.e., conscious) or not aware of my current state of happiness. For example, I could be feeling happy but not pay attention to this because I am focused on skiing down the mountain. Finally, I can have a stable representation of myself as happy—that is, I can think of myself as a generally happy person or have the belief that "I always feel happy when I am skiing." These four examples are only a sampling of the many ways the self has been defined in the literature.

Self-Awareness and Self-Representations

In our view, however, all of the definitions boil down to two basic classes of phenomena: (1) an ongoing sense of self-awareness and (2) stable mental representations. These two aspects of the self correspond to James's (1890) classic distinction between the self-as-perceiver (the "I") and the self-as-object of perception (the "Me").

Figure 16.2 shows some of the phenomena that relate to these two aspects of the self. What unites the different conceptions listed under *ongoing sense of self-awareness* is a view of the self as an active agent that processes information and regulates behavior. Our ongoing sense of awareness is the one psychological phenomenon for which we seem to have direct and irrefutable evidence—we all know what consciousness feels like from the inside. As Farthing (1993) notes, "Casual introspection seems to reveal a self: the unique entity that is the perceiver of our perceptions, the thinker of our thoughts, the feeler of our emotions and desires, and the agent of our actions" (p. 139). "Self-awareness" refers to a particular form of consciousness in which the object of attention is the self. Thus, I can be conscious that I am talking, but my consciousness becomes self-consciousness when I reflect on the fact that I am not speaking as lucidly as usual, or when I begin to worry that others are evaluating how intelligent I sound.

A second class of self-phenomena involve *stable mental representations* (see Figure 16.2). The self as mental representation is a product of reflexive activity ("Me") rather than the reflexive activity itself ("I"). These mental representations can be of the person as a physical, social, psychological, or moral being in the past, present, or future. This is what contemporary researchers mean by a self-concept, and what Sedikides and Skowronski (2003) refer to as the symbolic self, and Leary (2007) as the conceptual self.

Self-representations can vary in their degree of abstractness. At the most specific level are personal or autobiographical memories, such as "I remember feeling shy when I was with this person," which are related to episodic memory. At the next level are semantic representations or generalized knowledge about the self, such as "I am a shy person." Finally, at the most abstract or conceptual level are theories about the self, including personal narratives (Mclean et al., 2007) and more specific self-theories such as the *entity theorist* belief that "My shyness is fixed and I will always be shy" and the *incremental theorist* belief that "I can overcome my shyness if I really try" (Dweck, 1999).

Both self-awareness ("I") and self-representations ("Me") have been conceptualized as personality variables. That is, people vary in the degree to which they are chronically self-aware, and their self-representations vary in content, structure, stability, clarity, and complexity. Thus, there are meaningful individual differences in both aspects of the self, although, as we argue, the basic capacity for self-awareness and self-representation is common to all humans.

Another important definitional issue concerns self-esteem. In our ongoing sense of self-awareness we are continually evaluating ourselves (the "I" evaluates the "Me"). At the same time, we also form stable mental representations that have an evaluative component. The former can be thought of as the self-evaluation process (e.g., feeling competent while working on a task) whereas the latter can be thought of as self-esteem (e.g., stable representation of the self as competent or likable). This distinction raises the question of what is the "Me" that is being evaluated. From our perspective it is largely (but not exclusively) one's personality, that is, one's tendency to think, feel, and act in certain ways. However, our self-representations may or may not accurately reflect our personality characteristics (Robins & John, 1997).

Structure of the Self

Some theorists question the assumption that each person has a unique stable self that represents his or her distinctive personal experiences and traits (Brewer & Chen, 2007; Turner & Onorato, 1999; Tyler, Kramer, & John, 1999). Instead, these theorists see the self as a socially constructed entity, arguing that society enmeshes the individual in multiple specific social contexts, each imposing a role that confers a distinctive sense of self. From this "social self" perspective, people have multiple selves reflecting their various group memberships and associated identities. Consistent with this view, when answering the question "Who am I?," people come up with a vast array of responses that encompass everything from beliefs about private thoughts and feelings, to their place in the larger nexus of relationships, social roles, and cultural institutions (Gordon, 1968).

Within psychology, the idea that we have multiple selves dates back to James's

Ongoing Sense of Self-Awareness	**Stable Self-Representations**
• "I"	• "Me"
• Self as subject	• Self as object
• Self as perceiver	• Self as perceived
• Sentience	• Personal (episodic) memories
• Qualia	• Self-knowledge (semantic memory)
• Phenomenology	• Linguistic/symbolic self
• Subjective experience	• Self-concept
• Agent/homunculus	• Self-representation
• Self-awareness	• Self-theories
• Self-consciousness	• Ideal/ought/possible selves

FIGURE 16.2. Two classes of self phenomena.

The Principles of Psychology (1890), which included a summary table classifying the levels and structures of the self (p. 329). Table 16.1 shows our revised and expanded version of this table (see also Brewer & Gardner, 1996; Brown, 1998; Greenwald & Breckler, 1985). The first row shows the *personal* or individual self, which reflects people's beliefs about their private self, including their traits, values, and abilities. The second row shows the *relational* self, which reflects how people see themselves in intimate relationships. The third row shows the *social* self, which reflects how people see themselves in more general interpersonal contexts, including their social roles and reputation. The fourth row shows the *collective* self, which reflects people's identities concerning their various reference groups, such as their religion, ethnicity, and nationality. Some aspects of identity, such as gender, permeate all levels of the self from the personal (e.g., perceptions of feminine characteristics) to the collective (e.g., one's identity as a "feminist").

Interestingly, research suggests that information about the personal self (e.g., "altruistic") may be represented in memory separately (and thus encoded and retrieved separately) from information about the social and collective self (e.g., "peace activist"; Trafimow, Triandis, & Goto, 1991). People derive self-regard differently depending on which level of the self they are representing. For example, when an individual is focused on the personal self, self-esteem is rooted in meeting personal aspiration. However, when an individual is focused on the collective self, self-esteem is rooted in the accomplishments and prestige of the social groups to which the person belongs (Rubin & Hewstone, 1998).

A great deal of recent research has demonstrated cross-cultural differences in the de-

TABLE 16.1. Layers and Structures of the Self

Levels/ locus of audience	Orientation	Description	Example	Basis of self-regard	Cultural differences	Individual differences
Personal	Private	Traits, values, and abilities	"I am a sensitive person."	Personal aspirations and standards	Independent/ individualistic	• Personal Identity Orientation • Rosenberg Self-Esteem Scale • Authentic and Hubristic Pride Scales • Private Self-Consciousness • Individualism Scale
Relational	Intimate	Other people with whom we have direct personal contact	"I am Amy's close friend."	Mutual regard; pride in oneself as a relationship partner; validation from intimate others		• Inclusion of Other in Self Scale • Mutuality Scale • Interdependent Self-Construal Scale • Internal Working Models
Social	Inter-personal	Social roles and reputation	"I am a popular professor."	Public recognition; praise from others; pride in role		• Social Identity Orientation • Public Self-Consciousness Scale • Social Self-Confidence (vs. Shyness)
Collective	Communal	Social categories to which we belong	"I am Irish."	Ethnic pride; pride in one's social groups	Interdependent/ collectivistic	• Collective Identity Orientation • Collective Self-Esteem Scale • Inclusion of Other in Group Scale • Collectivism Scale

gree of emphasis on these various levels of the self. Specifically, Western cultures (e.g., United States) tend to be more focused on the personal self, whereas Eastern cultures (e.g., China, Japan) tend to be more focused on the collective self (e.g., Triandis, 1997). These differences appear to be socialized early in life and persist throughout the lifespan (e.g., Wang, 2006). However, it is important not to overemphasize these cultural differences, given the substantial individual differences that exist within groups. For example, even within Western cultures, women have more collectivistic, interdependent selves, whereas men tend to have more personal, independent selves (Josephs, Markus, & Tafarodi, 1992). Moreover, reviews of the literature on individualism–collectivism have failed to show consistent cultural differences, and, in some contexts, individuals from Western cultures do not appear to be any more individualistic or less collectivistic than individuals from Asian cultures (del Prado et al., 2007; Oyserman, Coon, & Kemmelmeier, 2002, but see Schimmack, Oishi, & Diener, 2005). For example, Japanese tend to focus on the personal self (e.g., their personality traits) to the same extent as Americans when they are asked to provide self-descriptions in specific contexts such as at home (Kanagawa, Cross, & Markus, 2001). Findings such as these have led to calls for refining the collectivism construct, including the need to distinguish between relational and group aspects of the collective self (Brewer & Chen, 2007).

Nonetheless, the individualism–collectivism distinction does predict differences in self-views. Individuals from East Asian cultures tend to accept and value negative information about the self more than individuals from Western cultures (Oyserman et al., 2002; Spencer-Rodgers, Peng, Wang, & Hou, 2004). Similarly, individuals from East Asian cultures tend to have lower self-esteem than those from most other cultures (Schmitt & Allik, 2005). Interestingly, this difference is only observed for explicit (i.e., self-report) measures of self-esteem, not implicit measures such as the implicit association test or preferences for the initials in one's own name (Heine & Hamamura, 2007; Yamaguchi et al., 2007). Thus, it is possible that East Asians report lower levels of explicit self-esteem because they are less prone to self-enhancement and instead adopt a more

modest self-presentation strategy. A related possibility is that individuals from both cultures engage in self-enhancement biases, but Easterners tend to self-enhance on collectivistic attributes and Westerners tend to self-enhance on individualistic attributes, which are more common on explicit self-esteem scales (Sedikides, Gaertner, & Vevea, 2005).

It appears that the structure of the self is not the same as the structure of personality, as embodied in models such as the five-factor model (FFM; John, Naumann, & Soto, Chapter 4, this volume; McCrae & Costa, Chapter 5, this volume). Clearly our self-representations include far more than just beliefs about personality traits, as research using the "Who am I?" test has revealed. The FFM was not intended as a complete model of personality, but rather as a model of individual personality traits. Thus, relational, social, and collective aspects of the self were not included in the research that led to the discovery of the FFM, and most lexical studies of personality structure have explicitly excluded social roles and relationships. Moreover, many aspects of the self do not reflect content domains such as the Big Five but rather how the content of the self is organized, including the degree of differentiation, complexity, and compartmentalization (Donahue, Robins, Roberts, & John, 1993; Rafaeli-Mor & Steinberg, 2002; Showers & Kling, 1996; Suh, 2002). Consequently, although the FFM effectively captures the trait-relevant aspects of the personal self, it fails to capture many other important aspects of the self, including its organizational structure and features of the relational, social, and collective self.

When Does the Self Emerge and How Does It Change across the Lifespan?

Our beliefs about ourselves seem to be relatively enduring. When we wake up in the morning we have the sense that we are the same person we were the previous day. It is unlikely that a person will think he or she is shy and introverted one day and socially bold and extraverted the next. Where does this enduring sense of self come from? At what age does it develop?

Infants, and virtually all animals, have at least one basic aspect of self-awareness: They can distinguish self from non-self and consequently do not eat themselves when they are hungry. However, it is difficult to determine whether infants and young children have more complex forms of self-awareness and self-representations because they cannot clearly communicate what they are thinking and feeling. Instead, researchers must infer the presence of a self from overt behavioral markers. Hart and Karmel (1996) described three classes of evidence for the existence of a sense of self: linguistic markers, cognitive-behavioral markers, and emotional markers.

Linguistic markers include self-referencing (e.g., use of personal pronouns), narrative language use (e.g., reference to events of personal significance that happened in the past), and declarative labeling speech. These behaviors begin to emerge around the second birthday (e.g., Kagan, 1998). For example, starting around age 2, children will label the self as "me" and identify objects as "mine."

Cognitive-behavioral markers include mirror self-recognition, imitation, and role taking. Mirror self-recognition (assessed in young children with the "rouge test") has been interpreted as evidence for objective self-awareness, subjective self-awareness, and self-representation. When a child sees its image with an unexpected mark on it, the child needs to focus attention on and identify itself in the mirror and become aware that the current image differs from some stable representation of its typical appearance. Children generally pass the rouge test by 18 months. Importantly, self-recognition seems to be rooted in the capacity to construct a psychological, not a physical, representation of the self; Priel and de Schonen (1986) found that Bedouin children without previous exposure to mirrors showed mirror self-recognition at the same age as children habitually exposed to mirrors. However, the stability of the self-representation in young children is limited. Using a version of the rouge test in which stickers were covertly placed on a child, researchers have found that children younger than 4 can find and remove the sticker from their body when presented with a live video of themselves, but not when the video is delayed as little as 2 seconds, suggesting that they do not have a representation of the self as continuous over time (Myazaki & Hiraki, 2006; Povinelli, & Simon, 1998). This research suggests that children younger than 5 are unable to hold a dual representation

of the self in mind—that is, a representation of the present and future or past self—suggesting that young children do not gain a sense of personal continuity until around age 5.

Emotional markers include self-conscious emotions and empathy. Self-conscious emotions such as shame, pride, guilt, and embarrassment require a sense of self. Pride, for example, occurs when individuals construe a positive outcome as relevant to their personal goals and aspirations (i.e., relevant to their identity) and as caused by their own actions or attributes (Tracy & Robins, 2004a). Thus, to feel a sense of pride (or, conversely, shame), a child must have stable self-representations that include knowledge of his or her goals and identity concerns, and the capacity to make internal attributions (e.g., to understand that "something about me or my actions caused that to happen"). These capacities seem to emerge around the age of 2½–3 years (Lagattuta & Thompson, 2007). Three-year-olds show signs of pride after success on a difficult, but not easy, task, and signs of shame after failing to complete an easy, but not a difficult, task (Lewis, Alessandri, & Sullivan, 1992). Similarly, after failing a task, children as young as 4 show a lack of persistence, view their failure as indicating that they lack the ability to complete the task, and report low expectations for their future performance (Dweck, 1999). These findings suggest that children as young as 3 or 4 can make internal attributions about their failures, and such attributions require the presence of a stable self-representational system.

Thus, children appear to have the cognitive skills needed to form specific and stable self-representations around age 4. Does this mean that young children also have a stable *evaluation* of their overall worth as a person (i.e., global self-esteem)? It is difficult to address this question because young children have obvious verbal limitations and there is no nonverbal test such as the mirror self-recognition task. Instead, the typical approach is to use self-report measures, sometimes aided by pictures or puppets, in which children are asked to report on their beliefs about their general competence and likableness. This research suggests that children as young as 4 can provide reliable evaluations of themselves, but only when they evaluate themselves in specific domains (e.g., Marsh, Ellis, & Craven, 2002; Measelle, John, Ablow, Cowan, & Cowan, 2005). It is not until later in childhood, sometime between ages 6 and 9, that children can reliably report on their *global* self-esteem, using standard self-report measures. These findings suggest that younger children lack the cognitive capacity to integrate their domain-specific evaluations into a generalized, global concept of the self (Harter, 2006). We believe this is the case because global self-esteem requires a representation of the self as a coherent, integrated entity—a representation that may take longer to develop than individual self-representations. However, it is possible that young children have a rudimentary evaluation of the self as generally good or bad. One study found that 5-year-old children who talked positively about themselves in a puppet interview had significantly higher scores at age 8 on a traditional self-report measure of self-esteem (Verschueren, Buyck, & Marcoen, 2001).

Although a coherent sense of self-worth emerges in childhood, it continues to evolve throughout the lifespan. Individuals who have relatively high (or low) self-esteem at one point in time tend to have high (or low) self-esteem years later, but the stability of self-esteem is relatively low in childhood and far from perfect across the entire lifespan (Trzesniewski, Donnellan, & Robins, 2003). Interestingly, self-esteem and personality show similar levels of stability and follow the same developmental trajectory through much of life: lower stability during childhood and increasingly high stability across adulthood. However, in contrast to personality traits, self-esteem becomes less stable in old age; this developmental shift may be due to greater self-reflection, resulting in questioning and reformulation of longstanding self-views, as one approaches the end of life.

In addition to examining the stability of individual differences, researchers have also examined whether self-esteem shows aggregate (or mean-level) increases or decreases over time. As we go through life, our self-esteem inevitably waxes and wanes over time, as part of the process of development. These fluctuations in self-esteem reflect changes in our social environment and maturational changes such as puberty and cognitive declines in old age. When these changes are normative, age-dependent, and influence individuals in a similar manner, they will produce aggregate (i.e., population-level) shifts in self-esteem across developmental periods.

A number of aggregate changes in self-esteem occur from childhood to old age (see Robins & Trzesniewski, 2005, for a review). On average, young children have relatively high self-esteem, which gradually declines over the course of childhood. Researchers have speculated that children have high self-esteem because it is artificially inflated, and that the subsequent decline reflects an increasing reliance on more realistic information about the self. Self-esteem continues to decline in adolescence, producing a substantial cumulative drop from childhood to adolescence. The adolescent decline has been attributed to physical and neurological changes associated with puberty, cognitive changes associated with the emergence of formal operational thinking, and social–contextual changes associated with the transition from grade school to junior high school (Harter, 2006).

Self-esteem increases gradually throughout adulthood, peaking sometime around the late 60s. Over the course of adulthood, individuals increasingly occupy positions of power and status, which might promote feelings of self-worth. However, self-esteem declines again in old age, beginning around age 70. This decline may be due to the dramatic confluence of changes that occur in old age, including changes in roles (empty nest, retirement), relationships (spousal loss, decreased social support), and physical functioning (declining health, memory loss, reduced mobility). The old age decline may also reflect a shift toward a more modest, humble, and balanced view of the self (Erikson, 1985). That is, as individuals grow old, they may increasingly accept their faults and limitations and become less concerned about inflating their self-worth, which artificially boosts reports of self-esteem earlier in life. Consistent with this interpretation, narcissism also tends to decline with age (Foster, Campbell, & Twenge, 2003).

Overall, men and women follow essentially the same developmental trajectory: Both genders tend to have high self-esteem in childhood, decline during adolescence, rise gradually throughout adulthood, and then decline in old age. Despite these similarities,

larities, there are three important differ-ences. First, men report slightly higher levels of self-esteem at almost every stage of life. Second, girls show a much steeper decline in self-esteem during adolescence. The ado-lescent gender gap has been attributed to maturational changes associated with pu-berty (e.g., changes in body shape and im-age) and social–contextual changes associ-ated with the differential treatment of boys and girls in the classroom and in society at large. Third, men show a sharper decline in old age, perhaps because they are more likely to experience, or are more adversely affected by, health problems, retirement, and diminished social support.

The absence of perfect stability of indi-vidual differences in self-esteem, combined with normative shifts in average self-esteem levels from childhood to old age, compels researchers to search for factors—both psy-chological and social–contextual—that pro-mote change in the self across the lifespan. In our view, the best way to understand self-esteem change is to understand the self-evaluative mechanisms that drive the self system; that is, the processes that underlie the way self-evaluations are formed, main-tained, and changed. Although experimen-tal research has linked a number of self-evaluative processes to short-term changes in self-evaluation, little is known about the influence of such processes on self-esteem change over longer periods of time and in real-world contexts.

We have explored how two self-evaluative factors impact self-esteem change: (1) implicit self theories and (2) positive illu-sions. In one study, we found that individuals who believe that their intelligence is a fixed quantity (i.e., entity theorists) tend to de-cline in self-esteem over the course of college relative to those who believe that their intel-ligence can improve (i.e., incremental theo-rists; Robins & Pals, 2002); thus, the college experience had an adverse impact on the self-esteem of entity theorists but bolstered the self-esteem of incremental theorists. This divergence was mediated by differences in helpless versus mastery-oriented responses, with entity theorists declining in self-esteem because they tend to become helpless in chal-lenging achievement contexts, whereas in-cremental theorists become mastery oriented in the same contexts. In a second study, we found that students who entered college with

unrealistically positive beliefs about their academic ability had higher self-esteem at first but then decreased in self-esteem over the course of college, compared to those with more accurate self-views (Robins & Beer, 2001). Thus, individuals with more objective beliefs about their ability were better able to maintain their self-esteem during college. These two examples illustrate the need to understand the motives and beliefs that regu-late self-evaluative processes and ultimately contribute to developmental changes in self-esteem. Conversely, as Roberts, Wood, and Caspi (Chapter 14, this volume) have argued, changes in self and identity constitute one critical mechanism through which changes occur in more basic aspects of personality, such as traits.

The previous sections have shown that the self emerges fairly early in life, is relative-ly stable, and has universal aspects. These conclusions suggest that self-esteem and oth-er aspects of the self may be a product of our evolutionary history. If so, we might expect to see early forms of self in nonhuman ani-mals with a shared phylogenetic history.

Is the Self Distinctive to Humans?

If omniscient beings from another planet were to study the inhabitants of the earth, what would stand out about the human spe-cies? Our use of tools? Our leisure time and range of creative endeavors? Our complex social organization and interactions? Cer-tainly all of these. But what would be per-haps most salient about the human species would be our inner world—the richness of our mental life. Tapping into the inner life of other species is unlikely to reveal the same rich stream of thoughts, feelings, intentions, and so on.

The capacity for self-awareness and self-representations seems to be a universal characteristic of humans. In all human cul-tures, people have an awareness of their own thoughts and feelings and have relatively sta-ble mental representations of themselves. The universality of these basic aspects of the self is a striking and highly significant fact that is often overlooked in light of the substantial individual and cross-cultural variability that exists in the way the self is manifested.

Whenever universal (i.e., species-typical) characteristics are found, scientists generally proceed to comparative, cross-species studies. The self may be part of human nature, but is it unique to humans? Comparative psychologists have discovered that a number of other species show advanced forms of self-awareness, including the same three indicators of a sense of self seen in young children: linguistic, cognitive-behavioral, and emotional markers.

Linguistic Markers

Language-trained great apes (chimps, gorillas, orangutans) show all three linguistic markers (self-referencing, narrative language use, and declarative labeling speech). Koko the gorilla, for example, displayed the capacity for reflexive self-referencing and narrative language use when she signed "me love happy Koko there" after being shown a picture of herself at a birthday party (Patterson & Linden, 1981, p. 86). As Koko's statement suggests, gorillas might also have personal memories that serve as the basis for some forms of linguistic self-referencing. Monkeys and nonprimates do not show any of these linguistic markers.

Cognitive-Behavioral Markers

In a series of seminal studies, Gallup (1970) showed that chimpanzees have the capacity to recognize themselves in a mirror. Gallup allowed chimps to view themselves in a mirror for a few days and then marked their faces with dye while they were anesthetized. Upon subsequently seeing their image in the mirror, the chimps often touched the marks on their face rather than touching the mirror itself. Based on these findings, Gallup (1977) concluded that "man may not be evolution's only experiment in self-awareness" (p. 14).

In subsequent research, dozens of animal species have been subjected to the mark test, but only chimpanzees (Gallup, 1970), orangutans (Suarez & Gallup, 1981), gorillas (Parker, 1994; Patterson & Cohn, 1994), dolphins (Reiss & Marino, 2001), and Asian elephants (Plotnik, de Waal, Reiss, 2006) have demonstrated the capacity for self-recognition. Interestingly, the first reactions to mirrors by all of these animals are social in nature—smiling, kissing, and vocalizing to their mirror image (Plotnik et al., 2006). Gallup (1977) found that chimpanzees reared in complete isolation from other chimps do not show mirror self-recognition, consistent with

Cooley's (1902) and Mead's (1934) theories that the self develops through social interaction and the experience of seeing oneself from the perspective of others.

The other two cognitive-behavioral markers—imitation and role taking—are present in humans by 2 years of age but extremely rare in other primates. Nonetheless they have been observed in a few cases, suggesting that chimps, orangutans, gorillas, and possibly monkeys have at least some capacity for imitation and role taking.

Emotional Markers

Like human children, nonhuman primates exhibit behaviors that suggest the capacity to experience self-conscious emotions and related social emotions such as compassion and empathy. Much of this evidence, however, is anecdotal. In one incident, Supinah, an orangutan, was observed attempting the difficult task of hanging a hammock from two trees. After successfully hanging the hammock, Supinah "threw herself back in the hammock" and "hugged herself with both arms" in apparent pride (Hayes, 1951, p. 188). In the primate literature, researchers have described dominant, or alpha male, chimpanzees walking with a "cocky" gait, upright posture, and piloerected fur, suggesting the possibility of a precursor to the pride display among these animals (de Waal, 1989). However, more controlled studies are needed.

The evidence for empathy in primates is also mostly anecdotal. Nonhuman primates clearly show helping behaviors. For example, it is not uncommon for a wounded chimp to be attended to—fed, groomed, and protected—by other members of the social group. Dominant adult males even chase away playing infants or noisy group members to keep them from disturbing the injured chimp (Boesch, 1992). A recent series of experiments provides more direct support for empathy and altruism in chimps (Warneken & Tomasello, 2006). After observing an experimenter "drop" an object and act as if she could not reach it, chimps were found to help out by retrieving the object and giving it to the experimenter, suggesting that they understood the experimenter's dilemma and empathized. However, in tasks where the experimenter's goal was more difficult to understand (e.g., trying to get around physical obstacles), chimps failed to provide help, whereas children as young as 18 months did. Thus, like other aspects of human psychology—personality, memory, attachment—we share many capacities with our phylogenetic cousins, but we differ in the complexity and frequency with which we display these capacities.

The findings of cross-species research on the self have several implications. First, they illustrate the value of a comparative perspective in personality psychology (Weinstein, Capitanio, & Gosling, Chapter 12, this volume). Comparative research helps identify which aspects of the self are uniquely human and which are common across species. Second, the finding that other species share certain aspects of the human self implies that self-awareness and self-recognition may be evolved capacities. Any capacity that is common to several species of primates is probably not crucially dependent on any species-specific factors, such as culture or language. Correspondingly, the fact that certain aspects of the self, such as the experience of guilt, seem to be unique to humans raises the question of whether these aspects are newly evolved differences, or the products of human culture. Third, comparisons with other species reveal what our conscious mental life might have been like at an early period in our evolutionary history; that is, our evolutionary ancestors may have had the same level of self-awareness as chimps. A phylogenetic perspective suggests that the self may have evolved from the most basic form of self-awareness (distinguishing self and non-self) to more complex forms of self-awareness seen in nonhuman primates (e.g., self-recognition) to the most complex forms of human self-representations (e.g., identity).

Finally, the existence of cross-species similarities and differences suggests one route to understanding the neural bases of the self. Can we identify brain regions or neural activation patterns that humans share with other animals who also show evidence of having a self?

How Does the Brain Build a Sense of Self?

The self is clearly dependent, in some manner, on the brain. If we did not have a brain, we would not have a self. But, as Hofstadter and Dennett (1981) pondered, "Who, or what, is the you that has the brain?" (p. 5).

At the heart of the mind–body debate is the puzzle of how a mass of tissue and the firing of brain cells can possibly produce a mind that is aware of itself and that can experience the color orange, the feeling of pride, and a sense of agency. Historically, the primary philosophical stance was to accept the mind–body distinction and assume that the self is not a physical entity but rather arises from a soul or spirit. For example, van Leeuwenhoek (1632–1723) believed that the brain contains a special vital animal spirit that embodies consciousness.

Most scientists, however, have rejected dualism and generally champion some form of materialism. Francis Crick (1994) illustrates this position: "You, your joys and your sorrows, your memories and your ambitions, your sense of personal identity and free will, are in fact no more than the behavior of a vast assembly of nerve cells and their associated molecules" (p. 3). Similarly, LeDoux (2003) states that "your 'self,' the essence of who you are, reflects patterns of interconnectivity between neurons in your brain" (p. 2), and Ramachandran (2007) asserts that "the self is not a holistic property of the entire brain; it arises from the activity of specific sets of interlinked brain circuits" (p. 1). Reflecting the central message of these quotes, Dennett (2005) asserts that, ultimately, a mechanistic approach to consciousness will explain it just as deeply and completely as other seemingly more concrete natural phenomena, such as metabolism and reproduction.

Unfortunately, attempts to understand exactly how the brain builds a sense of self have not been particularly successful, and speculative accounts abound. For example, two Nobel laureates—Crick (1994) and Edelman (1989, 2005)—have each provided accounts of the neural substrates of consciousness, but these accounts have little in common. This problem persists in more recent accounts of the neural bases of the self (e.g., Koch, 2004).

Those adopting a computational view of the mind believe that at least some aspects of the self can be explained by neural information processing (Sejnowski, 2003): "Computation has finally demystified mentalist terms. Beliefs are inscriptions in memory, desires are goal inscriptions, thinking is computation, perceptions are inscriptions triggered by sensors, trying is executing operations triggered by a goal" (Pinker, 1997, p. 78).

From this perspective, self-representations, self-awareness, self-regulation, and other self processes can be explained through the same neural mechanisms that account for the way the mind encodes, stores, retrieves, and manipulates information about the world. The computational view of the mind has also spawned the provocative thesis that the self is an illusion—there is no central executive coordinating our thoughts and feelings (Dennett, 2005). Artificial intelligence pioneer Marvin Minsky (1985) describes the mind as a "society of agents"—the agents of the brain are organized hierarchically into nested subroutines with a set of master decision rules. Although it may seem like there is an agent running the "society," in fact it is just the collective action of neural information processing in multiple parts of the brain. Similarly, some researchers believe that consciousness emerges as different groups of neurons—dealing with vision, memory, or touch—are activated. From this perspective, "There is no seat of consciousness, no internal theater where consciousness is a permanent spectator. Instead, what we experience as consciousness is this constant procession of waxing and waning of neuronal groupings" (Greenfield, 1996, p. 159).

Clearly, our current understanding of the neural mechanisms underlying the self is woefully inadequate. If we accept the materialist position and search for the proximate neural mechanisms involved in self processes, we need to go further than grand speculation about a "society of agents" or the "waxing and waning of neuronal groups." We need to approach the problem of how the brain produces a sense of self using the full array of methods used by cognitive neuroscientists. Below we discuss several neuroscientific methods that have been used to study the self and self-related phenomena.

Neuroanatomical Studies

An understanding of the gross anatomy of the brain can help us to better understand cross-species comparisons in self processes. For example, what distinguishes the brains of chimps (who show evidence of mirror self-recognition) from the brains of monkeys (who do not)? Which neuroanatomical areas are common to animals that show the capacity for self-recognition, or linguistic self-referencing, or self-conscious emotions? One

clue is that humans begin to show evidence of mirror self-recognition around 18–24 months of age, which is when the prefrontal cortex begins to mature in structure and function. Although there are likely many reasons why the neuroanatomy of two species might be similar or different, cross-species comparisons can at least identify possible anatomical regions that merit further exploration.

Functional Neurosurgery and Brain Lesioning

As with other intrusive techniques, the intentional lesioning of a particular brain region cannot be performed on humans. However, researchers could lesion nonhuman primates to determine whether damage to a particular area eliminates the capacity for mirror self-recognition and other markers of a sense of self. One kind of brain lesioning that traditionally has been performed on humans is functional neurosurgery. The dramatically altered behavior of lobotomized individuals demonstrates how removing brain tissue can destroy what we normally think of as a person's self. Another example is split-brain (commisurotomized) patients, whose corpus collosum has been severed, and who consequently suffer a host of deficits related to self processes (Gazzaniga, 1970).

Although intentional lesioning of humans is unethical, researchers can now create temporary "lesions" using transcranial magnetic stimulation (TMS), which uses a powerful yet noninvasive magnet to alter or suppress activity in specific brain regions. One important advantage of TMS is that it provides a stronger basis for making causal inferences than brain imaging techniques, which can only demonstrate correlations with neural activation. To date, we know of only one study that has used this promising method to study self processes; Kwan and colleagues (2007) showed that TMS (which serves to suppress activity) of the medial prefrontal cortex reduces the degree to which participants engaged in self-enhancement, defined as perceiving themselves more positively than they perceive others.

Neurological Disorders and Brain Damage

Some of the most fascinating avenues for understanding the self have come from the study of neurological patients in whom brain damage has produced cognitive, affective, and behavioral deficits. The complete loss of a sense of self is extremely rare, but many neurological disorders, including autism, Alzheimer's, Parkinson's, and epilepsy, produce profound changes in the self (Feinberg & Paul, 2005). There are also a host of neurological disorders characterized by bizarre distortions in body image, including macropsia and micropsia (an Alice-in-Wonderland-like feeling of having either grown incredibly large or incredibly small in size), asomatognosia (e.g., denial that the left side of one's body is part of oneself and assertions that any actions by one's left side were caused by someone else), and exosomesthesia (a pathological extension of the body image in which touches to the body are experienced as touches to nearby physical objects, and vice versa). Sufferers of Lesch–Nyhan syndrome have a pathological tendency toward self-harm, engaging in dramatic self-injurious behaviors such as biting off their fingers and poking out their eyes; they often feel as if their hands and mouth do not belong to them and are under the control of someone or something else, suggesting that their sense of agency—the feeling that "I" am the one controlling my body—is severely distorted.

Studies of patients with brain damage due to strokes or accidents suggest that the frontal lobes are involved in self-regulation. Phineas Gage is perhaps the most well-known example. He had frontal lobe damage after an iron rod penetrated his skull, and showed a diminished capacity to self-regulate as well as dramatic personality changes, including becoming more irreverent, obstinate, and impatient. In general, patients suffering from frontal lobe damage show deficits in the capacity to monitor and reflect on their own mental states (Beer, Shimamura, & Knight, 2004), suggesting that aspects of the self related to self-awareness (the "I") may be associated with activity in the frontal lobes. For example, Pinker (1997) describes the case of a 15-year-old boy with frontal lobe damage who would stay in the shower for hours at a time, unable to decide whether to get out. Patients with damage to a specific region of the frontal lobes, known as the orbitofrontal cortex, often show highly inappropriate social behaviors that are believed to be caused by impairments in self-insight, in the capacity to experience self-conscious emotions such

as embarrassment, and in the ability to use emotional information in the service of self-regulation (Beer, 2007; Beer, John, Scabini, & Knight, 2006). Patients with damage to the right parietal or prefrontal cortex are unable to recognize themselves in the mirror even after coaching, suggesting that they have lost the capacity for self-recognition (Keenan, Wheeler, Gallup, & Pascual-Leone, 2000).

Another provocative set of studies has examined self-awareness and self-representations in patients with amnesia. Tulving (1993) relates the story of K.C., an amnesic patient who lost the capacity to form new episodic memories. K.C. has a sense of self-awareness but not autonoetic awareness (autobiographical remembering, or the feeling that one "owns" one's memories). K.C. may be conscious in a similar way that a dog is conscious, but not in the same way as individuals without neurological damage. Interestingly, K.C. seems to have the capacity to revise his self-representations even without episodic memories of his specific behaviors and experiences: K.C.'s self-descriptions converge with his mother's descriptions of his current personality more closely than with her descriptions of his preamnesic personality (Tulving, 1993). Similarly, Klein, Loftus, and Kihlstrom (1996) found evidence that another amnesic patient, W.J., showed stable and seemingly accurate self-ratings of personality over a period of time during which she lacked the capacity to remember any personally experienced events. These findings suggest that one's current self-representations are not dependent on memories about personal experiences and thus have important implications for research on the personality judgment process. In particular, they suggest that trait self-ratings reflect different cognitive and neural mechanisms than self-ratings of specific past behaviors.

Despite the promise of patient studies to elucidate self processes, there are several caveats to generalizing from such studies, including (1) nonrandom assignment (e.g., patients with brain damage may differ on certain personality dimensions such as risk taking); (2) the brain damage associated with neurological disorders or lesions is often highly diffuse, making it difficult to pinpoint the specific brain region involved in any observed deficits; and (3) it is impossible to determine whether the damaged region is responsible for receiving or sending the necessary neural signals, or whether the damaged area simply blocks messages from being relayed between two adjacent brain areas that actually regulate the aspect of self-functioning that is showing a deficit (Beer & Lombardo, 2007).

Studies of Neural Functioning in Healthy Individuals

Recent advances in neuroimaging techniques, including methods based on electrical signals (EEG, ERP, MEG) and those based on functional imaging (PET, fMRI), permit more precise measurement of the structure and function of the brain. Although these methods are essentially correlational and thus unable to elucidate causal relations, they allow researchers to see which part of the brain becomes particularly active when someone performs a cognitive, affective, or behavioral task. Recently, personality and social psychologists have begun to adopt neuroimaging methods to study self-related processes, including self-recognition, self-referential encoding, self-reflection, self-regulation, and self-conscious emotions. Together with patient studies, new studies on the brain correlates of the self provide converging evidence that several regions within the frontal and temporal lobes, including the medial prefrontal cortex (MPFC), dorsolateral prefrontal cortex, orbitofrontal cortex, and anterior cingulate, are more heavily recruited when individuals engage in self-related processes (Beer, 2007). For example, there is now considerable evidence that the MPFC plays a critical role in self-referential processing (Kelley et al., 2002); specifically, activity in this region is associated with encoding information in reference to the self (e.g., "Does conscientious describe you?") but not encoding information in reference to others (e.g., "Does conscientious describe George Bush?") or encoding of general meaning (e.g., "Does *conscientious* have the same meaning as *responsible*?").

In another study on the neural bases of the self, Inzlicht and Gutsell (2007) used EEG to identify the neural correlates of subjects' capacity to control and restrain impulses. Their findings show that after engaging in one act of self-control (trying to control their emotions), participants performed worse at a subsequent task requiring self-control and showed decreased activity in a region

of the frontal lobes called the anterior cingulate cortex, suggesting that self-regulation depletes rather than strengthens the brain mechanisms that regulate this important aspect of personality. Sharot, Riccardi, Raio, and Phelps (2007) used fMRI to show that enhanced activity in the anterior cingulate cortex and amygdala are associated with optimistic beliefs about the self. Another provocative study showed that activity in the right middle frontal cortex was greater when participants viewed their own rather than familiar faces, and this difference became larger after their "independent selves" were primed by having them read essays containing first-person singular pronouns (e.g., *I*, *mine*), compared to when their "interdependent selves" were primed by essays containing second-person pronouns (e.g., *we*, *ours*) (Sui & Han, 2007).

One interesting question emerging from this research is what happens in the brain when participants are not performing any mental tasks, but are simply engaging in self-reflection. It turns out that a set of brain regions in the frontal, parietal, and medial temporal lobes consistently become active when people let their minds wander and engage in self-reflection, mentally traveling back and forth through time to learn from the past and plan for the future (Mason et al., 2007). Neuroscientists refer to this activity as the brain's "default mode," suggesting that we spend much of our time exploring past and future selves.

Together, these examples illustrate various ways in which the brain can affect self processes as well as other aspects of personality functioning. The ultimate goal of neuroscience research on the self is to understand how the brain generates self-awareness and self-representations. This goal is complicated because, like other higher-order mental functions, self processes probably emerge out of a complex interplay among multiple brain regions. Moreover, there is a crucial issue of determining the direction of causal relations; for example, does conscious self-reflection cause behavior, or is behavior initiated through unconscious brain processes that the conscious mind then watches and reflects? Finally, the research to date does not conclusively demonstrate that there are any brain states or structures that are *distinctively* linked to self processes; after reviewing the relevant literature, Gillihan and Farah (2005) concluded that there is little compelling evidence for brain networks devoted to the self that are physically and functionally distinct from those used for more general-purpose cognitive processing.

At least in principle, new knowledge about the brain can help us refine our theoretical conception of the self and self-related processes. Specifically, the way we conceptualize the self should be consistent with, and constrained by, what we know about how the brain works (e.g., memory researchers used to think that a sense of familiarity was simply a weaker form of recollection memory, but research suggests that familiarity and recollection involve distinct brain regions). For example, if one function of the self is to coordinate and tregulate internal body signals and behavioral responses (i.e., self-regulation), then the brain should be doing something different when the self is "in control" than when it is "out of control." If one motive governing the self system is self-enhancement, then there must be some neural mechanism that "tags" the valence of a self-relevant event and causes positive events to be encoded more deeply than negative ones; similarly, if there is selective retrieval of positive autobiographical memories, then there should be identifiable neural process that enables this to occur (e.g., preferential pathways to representations tagged as positively valenced).

Clearly, we have a long way to go before we truly understand the neural mechanisms underlying these and other aspects of the self. However, we believe that the new methods of brain science hold a great deal of promise and could ultimately lead to discoveries that provide a foundation for a naturalist view of the self.

Is the Self a Product of Evolution?

The eminent geneticist Theodosius Dobzhansky (1964) remarked that the self is the chief evolutionary novelty possessed by humans. Consistent with this view, behavioral genetic studies have documented the heritability of self-esteem and other self processes (e.g., Neiss et al., 2005, 2006). Evidence of heritability supports an evolutionary account of the self, but there are four possible interpretations. First, the self may be "genetic junk"; a characteristic that neither contributes to nor detracts from the organism's fitness but is nonetheless passed on to succeeding generations. A second possibility is that the self is a functionless byproduct of another adaptation that does not solve any adaptive problems on its own but is carried along with the more functional characteristic. For example, the self has been described as an incidental by-product of high-level intelligence and complex sensory processing associated with large brains.

However, it is difficult to write off the self as an evolutionary accident or a functionless by-product. As much as any other component of the mind, the self fulfills the criteria of an adaptive design as outlined by Williams (1966): It is universal, complex, reliably developing, well-engineered, and reproduction promoting. Aspects of the self are clearly universal (i.e., species-typical); although there is individual variability in self-awareness and self-representations, all humans have both capacities. The self is also clearly complex, reliably developing, and, as we argue subsequently, promotes survival and reproduction.

Yet, even if we accept that the self meets the criteria of adaptive design, it may not be an adaptation in the technical sense of the word. Instead, the self may be an "exaptation"—a feature that did not arise as an adaptation for its present use, but was subsequently co-opted for its current function (Gould, 1991); for example, a fly's wings were originally selected for thermoregulation but were later used for flying. However, it seems unlikely that the self is an exaptation because the environmental features (e.g., complex social interaction) that likely created selection pressures for a self existed in our ancestral, as well as our current, environment.

Finally, the self may be a full-fledged adaptation that is part of our genetic programming. If self-related processes serve an adaptive function, then the mechanisms that underlie these processes should be hardwired into the brain. Thus, to the extent that researchers can identify neural mechanisms that seem to support highly specialized self-processes, this work provides further support for an evolutionary account. The strongest version of this account is that just as the brain has an evolved module governing language acquisition, it may also have a module governing aspects of the self such as self-awareness and self-deception (Pinker, 1997). A more moderate position is that people have a genetic blueprint for the basic parts of the self, but the self is assembled through interaction with the current environment. It is possible that we share with other great apes the same neurologically rudimentary self, but through language development and complex social interaction we simply do more with the raw materials. This position nicely integrates universalist and cultural relativist positions on the self.

The assumption that the self is an adaptation leads to the question: What function does it serve? What reproductive or survival advantage is conferred by the capacity to reflect on one's internal states and form stable self-representations?

Why Do We Have a Self? What Are Its Adaptive Functions?

How did the self facilitate survival and reproduction during our evolutionary history? The two fundamental aspects of the self, self-awareness and self-representations, are believed to be adaptive solutions to the complex social problems that emerged when our ancestors began living in large, flexibly structured social groups (Sedikides & Skowronski, 2003). Individuals who survived and reproduced in our ancestral environment were able to navigate an intricate social structure in which they had to participate in negotiating dyadic and group-level coalition; address cheating and detection of cheaters; and deal with intergroup and intragroup (particularly intrasexual) competition.

How does the self help an individual solve these adaptive problems? In our view, the various functions of the self can be subsumed within four broad categories: self-regulation, information-processing filter, understanding others, and identity processes. Below we describe each category and discuss how it might be linked to adaptive outcomes.

Self-Regulation

One of the unique aspects of human nature is that we are goal directed, and not just toward proximal goals such as grabbing the food in front of us, but toward long-term

goals such as succeeding at work, finding a romantic partner, and being a good, moral person. These long-term goals are represented in the self system as various forms of self-representations—ideal selves (e.g., "to be a good father"), possible selves (e.g., "to be an artist"), dreaded selves (e.g., "to become like my mother"), and so on. These goal representations serve as reference points for self-regulation, motivating us to engage in behaviors that move us toward the attainment of desired identities and away from undesired or feared identities; they function as both goals to be pursued and standards against which outcomes are measured.

Self-awareness also plays a role in self-regulation, providing a sense of volition that facilitates goal-directed behavior and a means to evaluate goal-relevant outcomes (e.g., awareness of discrepancies between actual and ideal selves). Self-awareness provides a mechanism for greater flexibility of response in a social environment filled with competing and often conflicting goals; it allows us to monitor and regulate not only our overt behavioral responses but also our internal responses (e.g., fear, shame, optimism) to external stimuli and circumstances. Together, the two aspects of the self enable us to prioritize and organize goal-directed behavior amidst a complex and multiply-nested structure of goals and subgoals. Interestingly, recent research suggests that chimpanzees, our close evolutionary cousins, are also able to engage in fairly complex forms of self-regulation: For example, they use various strategies such as distraction to resist the temptation to eat right away when they know they will get more food later on (Evans & Beran, 2007).

Clearly the capacity for self-regulation does not guarantee problem-free and effective pursuit of goals. Humans often engage in self-defeating and maladaptive behaviors. Apparent failures of self-regulation may tell us a great deal about how the self system functions, as in the case of self-handicapping, in which individuals set themselves up for failure in a way that, somewhat paradoxically, protects self-esteem.

Information-Processing Filter

In a complex social environment it is inefficient for individuals to attend to and encode all of the information that is constantly bombarding them. The self addresses this dilemma by serving as a filter, or lens, through which the world is experienced. Our self-representations consist of cognitive structures, or schemas, that organize and direct processing of information about the self. Thus, the self serves as a top-down information filter that is guided by four basic motives: accuracy, consistency, popularity (i.e., social status and acceptance), and enhancement. These motives influence which information the self attends to, encodes, retrieves, and acts upon. We have described these motivational orientations in terms of four basic metaphors (Robins & John, 1997).

According to the *scientist* metaphor, individuals are driven to acquire *accurate* information about themselves and the world (Bem, 1972; Kelly, 1955; Trope, 1986). Just as the scientist develops empirically based theories, people use facts and observations to develop theories about themselves, engaging in a dispassionate search for accurate self-knowledge. Clearly accurate self-representations can serve an adaptive function, helping us to formulate realistic goals and act in accordance with our actual social status, mate value, and other objectively based self-representations. However, as Pinker (1997) notes, "our brains were shaped for fitness, not for truth" (p. 305); consequently, we sometimes adopt somewhat biased information processing strategies.

According to the *consistency seeker* metaphor, individuals strive to see themselves in a *consistent* manner, confirming their preexisting self-views regardless of reality (Swann, 1997; Swann & Bosson, Chapter 17, this volume). In fact, there is considerable evidence that people actively seek out and create contexts in which their self-views will be confirmed, even when these views are inaccurate and/or negative. Similarly, people selectively remember life events that are consistent with current self-representations, reconstructing their past to fit the present (Ross, 1989). Although consistency seeking may lead to information-processing errors, it can be a useful and efficient heuristic in a highly chaotic social environment. Consistency also serves an interpersonal function, ensuring that people will honor the identities they negotiated in previous social interactions and act similarly over time.

According to the *politician* metaphor, people strive to present themselves in ways that create the most favorable impressions on others, thereby enhancing their *social status* and *acceptance*. This perspective highlights the reciprocal nature of social interaction: Social reality is constructed and negotiated through interactions with others, in which behaviors represent public performances that "present images of the self for the social world to see and evaluate" (Schlenker, 1985, p. 21). Like politicians, people target their public performances to different audiences (or constituencies), which place multiple and often conflicting demands and expectations on them. The person-as-politician seeks to "maintain the positive regard of important constituencies to whom he or she feels accountable" (Tetlock, 1992, p. 332), which should increase status, reduce conflict, and facilitate coalition building.

Finally, according to the *egotist* metaphor, people narcissistically distort information to *enhance* their self-worth. Virtually every self theory posits some variant of the motive to protect and enhance self-worth, and a large body of research has documented numerous positivity biases in self-perception, including unrealistically positive self-conceptions, self-serving attributions for success and failure, and excessive optimism about the future (Dunning, 2005; Taylor & Brown, 1988). These self-enhancement biases may facilitate goal striving, emotional well-being, mate attraction, and other adaptive behaviors, at least in the short term (e.g., Lockard & Paulhus, 1988; Robins & Beer, 2001; Taylor & Brown, 1988). For example, in terms of mate selection, evolutionary psychologists view self-esteem as a way of gauging our value to prospective partners (e.g., our mate value). Individuals with higher self-perceived mate value may demand more in a partner and consequently pair up with partners who have higher mate value.

Together the four motives that drive processing of self-relevant information—accuracy, consistency, social status/acceptance, and enhancement—provide a flexible arsenal of tools that help us (and presumably our evolutionary ancestors) adapt to a complex, multistructured social environment. From an evolutionary perspective, the ideal mind would be able to convince itself that it is better, smarter, and faster than it really is when this view facilitates survival and reproduction, but switch to a reality mode when needed for increased fitness. Consistent with this perspective, Swann and Schroeder (1995) proposed that the various self-evaluative motives can be organized into a hierarchical system in which different motives are prioritized at different stages in the processing of self-relevant information. Specifically, enhancement may drive the first stage ("Does it make me feel good?"), consistency the second stage ("Is it consistent with how I see myself?"), and more deliberate and effortful cost–benefit analyses the third stage ("Is it accurate? Does it facilitate my social goals?"). This possibility makes sense from an evolutionary perspective and shows how processing of information about the self may indeed reflect the workings of a specialized adaptive design.

Understanding Others' Minds

In a complex social environment, survival and reproduction depend partly on the ability to explain, predict, and manipulate others. Children with autism show deficits in the ability to understand what other people know, want, or feel, and correspondingly they have dramatically diminished social interaction skills (Baron-Cohen, 2008). The capacity for self-awareness facilitates introspectively based social strategies such as empathy, sympathy, gratitude, deception, and pretense. Some theorists have even argued that subjective awareness evolved for the specific purpose of helping us to understand others (e.g., Leary, 2007). For example, children may learn to understand others by reflecting on their own internal states, feelings, and intentions, and simulating what might be happening in the mind of others (e.g., Harris, 1992). Consistent with these views, recent research suggests that people use the same neural circuits to understand themselves as they use to understand others (Decety & Jackson, 2006).[2]

The capacity to reflect on our internal states and feelings and project them onto others contributes to another capacity: the experience of self-conscious emotions, which requires the ability to evaluate oneself from the perspective of actual or imagined others. Self-conscious emotions are assumed to have evolved because they motivate indi-

viduals to protect, defend, and enhance their social reputation and self-image by engaging in behaviors that facilitate social status and acceptance and avoid social rejection (Keltner & Buswell, 1997; Tracy & Robins, 2007b). For example, researchers have argued that embarrassment and shame evolved for purposes of appeasement and avoidance of social approbation, guilt for encouraging communal relationships, and pride for attaining social dominance (Gilbert, 2007; Keltner & Buswell, 1997; Miller, 2007; Tangney & Dearing, 2002; Tracy & Robins, 2004c).

Self-conscious emotions guide individual behavior by compelling us to do things that are socially valued and to avoid doing things that lead to social approbation. We strive to achieve, to be a "good person," or to treat others well because doing so makes us feel proud of *ourselves*, and failing to do so makes us feel guilty or ashamed of *ourselves*. Society tells us what kind of person we should be; we internalize these beliefs in the form of actual and ideal self-representations; and self-conscious emotions motivate behavioral action toward the goals embodied in these self-representations. Thus, although we might understand cognitively that working hard is a good thing to do, it sometimes takes the psychological force of emotions such as guilt and pride to make us do so. By reinforcing adaptive social behaviors—encouraging us to act in ways that promote social status (getting ahead) and acceptance (getting along)—self-conscious emotions facilitate interpersonal reciprocity, a social arrangement that is highly beneficial in the long term (Trivers, 1971). In summary, self-conscious emotions help us thrive in a social world where attaining status and acceptance is essential to our ability to survive and reproduce. As Kemeny, Gruenwald, and Dickerson (2004) stated, emotions such as shame and pride "may be one way that individuals feel their place in the social hierarchy" (p. 154).[3]

Although self-conscious emotions can be linked to adaptive social behaviors, they can also be maladaptive. For example, the tendency to become anxiously preoccupied in social situations and excessively worried about being negatively evaluated can contribute to decreased social competence in the form of shyness. Yet shyness can also be functional when it motivates preparation and rehearsal for important interpersonal events, such as planning ahead for the first day of teaching a new class. Moreover, a moderate amount of wariness regarding strangers and unfamiliar or unpredictable situations undoubtedly had adaptive value in our evolutionary history; Wilson, Coleman, Clark, and Biederman (1993) have argued, based on their studies of the pumpkin sunfish, that it is adaptive for all species to have a mix of shyness and boldness.

The self-conscious emotion of pride also seems to be adaptive in some contexts and maladaptive in others. In the Greek myth, Narcissus ultimately dies from his excessive pride. From an evolutionary perspective, he acted in a particularly maladaptive manner because he spent all of his time gazing at his own reflection and ignored the love of a beautiful nymph with whom he could have produced offspring. Research suggests that narcissistic pride, in the form of inflated beliefs about the self, can have short-term adaptive benefits but long-term negative consequences (Robins & Beer, 2001). Moreover, narcissistic individuals are more inclined to cheat on their partners (Hunyady, Josephs, & Jost, in press), which could lead to lower relationship stability but also to higher numbers of offspring.[4]

One way to resolve the seeming paradox of pride's combination of beneficial and detrimental effects is to distinguish between two facets of pride. Several lines of research provide converging support for conceptualizing pride in terms of a "hubristic" or narcissistic facet (defined by terms such as "arrogant" and "conceited") and an authentic or achievement-based facet (defined by terms such as "confident" and "accomplished"; Tracy & Robins, 2007b). These two facets do not simply reflect good versus bad, high versus low arousal, or trait versus state aspects of pride. Moreover, they are not distinguished by the *kinds* of events that elicit the pride experience; both occur after success in a range of domains (e.g., academic, romantic relationships). Rather, it is the way in which success is appraised that determines which facet of pride occurs: Successes attributed to effort and hard work tend to promote authentic pride, whereas successes attributed to more stable (and less controllable) abilities tend to promote hubristic pride.

Authentic and hubristic pride have highly divergent personality correlates. Authentic pride is positively associated with adaptive traits such as Extraversion, Agreeableness, Conscientiousness, and genuine self-esteem, whereas hubristic pride is negatively related to these traits but positively associated with self-aggrandizing narcissism, shame proneness, and aggression. This pattern suggests that authentic pride is the more pro-social, adaptive facet of the emotion (Tracy, Chang, Robins, & Trzesniewski, in press).

The examples of shyness and narcissistic pride illustrate the complexities of the evolutionary perspective—certain aspects of the self may be adaptive in some ways but maladaptive in others. These opposing selection pressures lead to individual differences. Shyness and narcissism may be two ways of approaching the conflict between the dominant social goals of getting along and getting ahead: Shy individuals choose to focus on getting along and seeking approval, whereas narcissistic individuals focus on getting ahead (Roberts & Robins, 2000). Each may be a viable strategy from an evolutionary perspective. In fact, the two facets of pride may solve unique adaptive problems regarding the acquisition of status. Authentic pride might motivate behaviors geared toward long-term status attainment, whereas hubristic pride may provide a "short-cut" solution, granting status that is more immediate but fleeting—and, in some cases, unwarranted. A related possibility is that the second facet (hubristic pride) evolved as a "cheater" attempt to convince others of one's success in the absence of real accomplishments (Tracy & Robins, 2007a).

Identity Processes

Human social life may be viewed as a series of games; the rules are reflected in cultural norms and the parts that individuals play are defined by their social roles. Winning this game requires that humans form dyadic and group coalitions and generally navigate within a social structure that, more so than any other species, has complex layers of multiple, overlapping, and sometimes nontransitive social hierarchies (e.g., the highest-status hunters were not always the highest-status warriors). Imagine living in such a complex social environment without a self—that is, without any stable awareness of your position in the social structure and the roles you play in different contexts and with different interaction partners.

As discussed earlier, people's self-representations are comprised of multiple identities—personal, relational, social, and collective. All forms of identity allow us to differentiate ourselves from others, provide a sense of continuity and unity over time, and help us adapt to and navigate complex social structures and hierarchies by prescribing specific values and role-appropriate behaviors. Social identities also facilitate identification with the social group to which a person belongs. In any social group, the young, low-status members are tempted to defect to other groups. A sense of identity—and associated ingroup biases and outgroup derogation—may help prevent individuals from leaving their social group and disrupting their kinship network. Finally, stable identities are also efficient. It is more adaptive to have social interactions that are predictable, structured, and even ritualized, and to have identities that internalize the rules of each social context so that individuals do not have to relearn their social roles each day. In some ways, the self provides a bridge between the individual (and his or her personality characteristics) and the collective (and its associated social roles). For example, by eliciting collective feelings of pride when the group with which one identifies has an achievement (e.g., in the Olympic Games, or a high school football team), the self promotes solidarity among group members and helps reinforce the social inclusion of each proud group member.

In summary, we are proposing that the two aspects of the self—self-awareness and self-representations—are evolved mechanisms that serve four adaptive functions: self-regulation, information-processing filter, understanding others, and identity formation. It seems plausible that these four functions helped our evolutionary ancestors survive, reproduce, and attain social status and acceptance in a complex social environment characterized by long-term kinship relationships. Yet one may question what an evolutionary perspective, with its emphasis on ultimate function, can contribute beyond more proximate functional accounts. Thus, one challenge facing researchers working toward a naturalist account of the self is to provide more precise empirical demonstrations of how the specific functions of the self enhance aspects of fitness such as reproductive success.

TOWARD A NATURALIST APPROACH TO UNDERSTANDING THE SELF

We hope that this review of theory and research on the self has demonstrated that our understanding of many personality processes would be impoverished without the concept of self. Personality psychology is an unusually broad field because it covers a wide spectrum of phenomena and levels of analysis, from genetic markers of behavioral traits to neural mechanisms underlying emotions, to lexical studies of trait adjectives, to motives in personal life stories, to sociocultural perspectives on the formation of values. What provides coherence to these diverse themes is an emphasis on understanding consistencies in people's thoughts, feelings, and behaviors, and the mechanisms that underlie these consistencies. From our perspective, it is the self that ties together these various personality processes and, as Allport (1960) aptly put it, "makes the system cohere in any one person" (p. 308).

In this chapter we have attempted to outline a naturalist approach to the self. We have reviewed the current state of the field with regard to several fundamental questions concerning the structure, development, and function of the self. Our review of the literature was guided by a particular stance toward the self. In particular, we believe that research on the self should be (1) central to any theory of personality; (2) informed by an evolutionary perspective and organized around functionalist explanations; (3) informed by comparative, cross-species research; and (4) linked to basic psychological processes such as attention, memory, and emotion, and their associated neural mechanisms. Although the self continues to be a "puzzling puzzle," we believe that much progress is being made in the field and that a scientific understanding of the self is fundamental to a science of personality.

The psychology of the self has an important role to play in the integration of evolutionary biology and neuroscience into personality psychology. The self sits in a privileged position, encompassing and integrating all levels of the person from the biological to the social. This privileged position is fundamentally inclusionary: There is ample room, and indeed serious need, for a variety of approaches to understanding the structure and function of the self and its relation to other psychological processes.

An evolutionary perspective on the self was central to many early theories of personality and social behavior, and it must be considered a central issue for contemporary personality theories. The naturalist agenda outlined by James (1890) remains a worthwhile path for the next century of research on the science of the self. By naturalizing the self, we move the field of personality toward a truly biosocial perspective.

NOTES

1. The keyword "self" is clearly overinclusive and will detect articles examining psychological phenomena beyond the scope of research on the self. However, any other keyword (e.g., self-esteem, self-concept, self-awareness) is necessarily underinclusive and would fail to detect important aspects of the self literature.
2. In contrast to the idea that self-understanding is linked to an understanding of others, Klein, Cosmides, Murray, and Tooby (2004) described the case of an individual with autism who has developed normal, consensually accurate knowledge of his own traits but is unable to differentiate accurately between the personalities of his various family members.
3. The communication of self-conscious emotions to others may also serve an adaptive function. The nonverbal expression of embarrassment draws forgiveness and increases sympathy and liking from onlookers after a social transgression (Keltner & Buswell, 1997; Miller, 2007), and the pride expression may promote social status by increasing an individual's visibility to others following a socially valued achievement (Tracy & Robins, 2004b).
4. Narcissistic behavior also seems to be present and in some cases adaptive in nonhuman animals. Sapolsky (1997) describes an orangutan named Hobbes—the "cocky son of a high-ranking female" (p. 83)—who immediately began acting like the alpha male after migrating to a new troop. To Sapolsky's surprise, Hobbes was quickly treated by others as a high-status animal, despite his initial low status in the group. Although we clearly do not know whether Hobbes had an overly positive self-representation, his narcissistic behavior does seem to have served the adaptive function of helping him attain social status and consequently mates. Similar benefits may accrue to humans who believe they are more brilliant and powerful than they really are. An interesting point relevant to the positive illusions debate is that Hobbes had unusually high cortisol levels; as Sapolsky pointed out, "it doesn't come cheap to be a bastard twelve hours a day—a couple of months of this sort of thing is likely to exert a physiological toll" (p. 86).

REFERENCES

Allport, G. W. (1955). Is the concept of self necessary? In *Becoming: Basic considerations for a psychology of personality* (Chapter 10). New Haven, CT: Yale University Press.

Allport, G. W. (1960). The open system in personality theory. *Journal of Abnormal and Social Psychology, 61,* 301–310.

Baldwin, J. M. (1897). *Social and ethical interpretations in mental development.* New York: Macmillan.

Baron-Cohen, S. (2008). *Autism and Asperger's syndrome (the facts).* Oxford, UK: Oxford University Press.

Beer, J. S. (2007). Neural systems for self-conscious emotions and their underlying appraisals. In J. L. Tracy, R. W. Robins, & J. P. Tangney (Eds.), *The self-conscious emotions: Theory and research* (pp. 53–67). New York: Guilford Press.

Beer, J. S., John, O. P., Scabini, D., & Knight, R. T. (2006). Orbitofrontal cortex and social behavior: Integrating self-monitoring and emotion–cognition interactions. *Journal of Cognitive Neuroscience, 18,* 871–879.

Beer, J. S., & Lombardo, M. V. (2007). Patient and neuroimaging methodologies. In R. W. Robins, R. C. Fraley, & R. F. Krueger (Eds.), *Handbook of research methods in personality psychology* (pp. 360–369). New York: Guilford Press.

Beer, J. S., Shimamura, A. P., & Knight, R. T. (2004). Frontal lobe contributions to executive control of cognitive and social behavior. In M. S. Gazzaniga (Ed.), *The newest cognitive neurosciences* (3rd ed., pp. 1091–1104). Cambridge, MA: MIT Press.

Bem, D. J. (1972). Self-perception theory. In L. Berkowitz (Ed.), *Advances in experimental social psychology* (Vol. 6, pp. 1–62). New York: Academic Press.

Boesch, C. (1992). New elements of a theory of mind in wild chimpanzees. *Behavioral and Brain Sciences, 15,* 149–150.

Brewer, M. B., & Chen, Y. (2007). Where (Who)

are collectives in collectivism? Toward conceptual clarification of individualism and collectivism. *Psychological Review, 114,* 133–151.

Brewer, M. B., & Gardner, W. (1996). Who is this "we"? Levels of collective identity and self representations. *Journal of Personality and Social Psychology, 71,* 83–93.

Brown, J. D. (1998). *The self.* New York: McGraw-Hill.

Byrne, B. M. (1996). *Measuring self-concept across the life span: Issues and instrumentation.* Washington, DC: American Psychological Association.

Collins, N. L., & Allard, L. M. (2004). Cognitive representations of attachment: The content and function of working models. In M. B. Brewer & M. Hewstone (Eds.), *Social cognition: Perspectives on social psychology* (pp. 60–85). Malden, MA: Blackwell.

Cooley, C. H. (1902). *Human nature and the social order.* New York: Scribner.

Crick, F. H. C. (1994). *The astonishing hypothesis: The scientific search for the soul.* New York: Scribner.

Damasio, A. R. (2003). Feelings of emotion and the self. In J. Ledoux, J. Debiec, & H. Moss (Eds.), The self: From soul to brain. *Annals of the New York Academy of Sciences, 1001,* 253–261.

de Waal, F. B. M. (1989). *Chimpanzee politics: Power and sex among apes.* Baltimore: Johns Hopkins University Press.

Decety, J., & Jackson, P. L. (2006). A social–neuroscience perspective on empathy. *Psychological Science, 15,* 54–58.

del Prado, A. M., Church, A. T., Katigbak, M. S., Miramontes, L. G., Whitty, M. T., Curtis, G. J., et al. (2007). Culture, method, and the content of self-concepts: Testing trait, individual–self-primacy, and cultural psychology perspectives. *Journal of Research in Personality, 41,* 1119–1160.

Dennett, D. C. (2005). *Sweet dreams: Philosophical obstacles to a science of consciousness.* Cambridge, MA: MIT Press.

Dobzhansky, T. (1964). *Heredity and the nature of man.* New York: New American Library.

Donahue, E. M., Robins, R. W., Roberts, B. W., & John, O. P. (1993). The divided self: Concurrent and longitudinal effects of psychological adjustment and social roles on self-concept differentiation. *Journal of Personality and Social Psychology, 64,* 834–846.

Dunning, D. (2005). *Self-insight: Roadblocks and detours on the path to knowing thyself.* New York: Psychology Press.

Dweck, C. S. (1999). *Self-theories: Their role in motivation, personality, and development.* Philadelphia: Psychology Press.

Edelman, G. M. (1989). *The remembered present: A biological theory of consciousness.* New York: Basic Books.

Edelman, G. M. (2005). *Wider than the sky: The phenomenal gift of consciousness.* New Haven, CT: Yale University Press.

Erikson, E. H. (1985). *The life cycle completed: A review.* New York: Norton.

Evans, T. A., & Beran, M. J. (2007). Chimpanzees use self-distraction to cope with impulsivity. *Biology Letters, 3,* 599–602.

Farthing, G. W. (1993). The self paradox in cognitive psychology and Buddhism: Review of "The embodied mind: Cognitive science and human experience." *Contemporary Psychology, 38,* 139–140.

Feinberg, T. E., & Paul, J. (Eds.). (2005). *The lost self: Pathologies of the brain and identity.* Oxford, UK: Oxford University Press.

Flanagan, O. J. (1991). *The science of the mind.* Cambridge, MA: MIT Press.

Foster, J. D., Campbell, W. K., & Twenge, J. M. (2003). Individual differences in narcissism: Inflated self-views across the lifespan and around the world. *Journal of Research in Personality, 37,* 469–486.

Gallup, G. G. (1970). Chimpanzees: Self-recognition. *Science, 167,* 86–87.

Gallup, G. G. (1977). Self-recognition in primates: A comparative approach to the bidirectional properties of consciousness. *American Psychologist, 32,* 329–338.

Gazzaniga, M. S. (1970). *The bisected brain.* New York: Appleton-Century-Crofts.

Gazzaniga, M. S. (1998). *The mind's past.* Berkeley: University of California Press.

Gilbert, P. (2007). The evolution of shame as a marker for relationship security: A biopsychosocial approach. In J. L. Tracy, R. W. Robins, & J. P. Tangney (Eds.), *The self-conscious emotions: Theory and research* (pp. 283–309). New York: Guilford Press.

Gillath, O., Bunge, S. A., Shaver P. R., Wendelken, C., & Mikulincer, M. (2005). Attachment-style differences in the ability to suppress negative thoughts: Exploring the neural correlates. *Neuroimage, 28,* 835–847.

Gillihan, S. J., & Farah, M. J. (2005). Is self special? A critical review of evidence from experimental psychology and cognitive neuroscience. *Psychological Bulletin, 131,* 76–97.

Gordon, C. (1968). Self-conceptions: Configurations of content. In C. Gordon & K. J. Gergen (Eds.), *The self in social interaction* (pp. 115–136). New York: Wiley.

Gould, S. J. (1991). Exaptation: A crucial tool for evolutionary psychology. *Journal of Social Issues, 47,* 43–65.

Greenfield, S. A. (Ed.). (1996). *The human mind explained.* New York: Holt.

Greenwald, A. G., & Breckler, S. J. (1985). To

whom is the self presented? In B. R. Schlenker (Ed.), *The self and social life* (pp. 126–145). New York: McGraw-Hill.

Harris, P. L. (1992). From simulation to folk psychology: The case for development. *Mind and Language, 7*, 120–144.

Hart, D., & Karmel, M. P. (1996). Self-awareness and self-knowledge in humans, apes, and monkeys. In A. E. Russon, K. A. Bard, & S. T. Parker (Eds.), *Reaching into thought: The minds of the great apes* (p. 325–347). Cambridge, UK: Cambridge University Press.

Harter, S. (2006). The self. In W. Damon & R. M. Lerner (Series Eds.) & N. Eisenberg (Vol. Ed.), *Handbook of child psychology: Vol. 3. Social, emotional, and personality development* (6th ed., pp. 646–718). New York: Wiley.

Hayes, C. (1951). *The ape in our house.* New York: Harper.

Heine, S. J., & Hamamura, T. (2007). In search of East Asian self-enhancement. *Personality and Social Psychology Review, 11*, 4–27.

Hilgard, E. R. (1949). Human motives and the concept of the self. *American Psychologist, 4*, 374–382.

Hofstadter, D. R., & Dennett, D. C. (1981). *The Mind's I: Fantasies and reflections on self and soul.* New York: Bantam.

Hunyady, O., Josephs, L., & Jost, J. T. (in press). Priming the primal scene: Betrayal trauma, narcissism, and attitudes toward sexual infidelity. *Self and Identity.*

Inzlicht, M., & Gutsell, J. N. (2007). Running on empty: Neural signals for self-control failure. *Psychological Science, 18*, 933–937.

James, W. (1890). *The principles of psychology.* Cambridge, MA: Harvard University.

Josephs, R. A., Markus, H. R., & Tafarodi, R. W. (1992). Gender and self-esteem. *Journal of Personality and Social Psychology, 63*, 391–402.

Kagan, J. (1998). Is there a self in infancy? In M. Ferrari & R. J. Sternberg (Eds.), *Self-awareness: Its nature and development* (pp. 137–147). New York: Guilford Press.

Kanagawa, C., Cross, S. E., & Markus, H. R. (2001). "Who am I?" The cultural psychology of the conceptual self. *Personality and Social Psychology Bulletin, 27*, 90–103.

Keenan, J. P., Wheeler, M. A., Gallup, G. G., & Pascual-Leone, A. (2000). Self-recognition and the right prefrontal cortex. *Trends in Cognitive Sciences, 4*, 338–344.

Kelley, W. M., Macrae, C. N., Wyland, C. L., Caglar, S., Inati, S., & Heatherton, T. F. (2002). Finding the self?: An event-related fMRI study. *Journal of Cognitive Neuroscience, 14*, 785–794.

Kelly, G. A. (1955). *The psychology of personal constructs.* New York: Norton.

Keltner, D., & Buswell, B. N. (1997). Embarrass-

ment: Its distinct form and appeasement functions. *Psychological Bulletin, 122*, 250–270.

Kemeny, M. E., Gruenewald, T. L., & Dickerson, S. (2004). Shame as the emotional response to threat to the social self: Implications for behavior, physiology, and health. *Psychological Inquiry, 15*, 153–160.

Klein, S. B., Cosmides, L., Murray, E. R., & Tooby, J. (2004). On the acquisition of knowledge about personality traits: Does learning about the self engage different mechanisms than learning about others? *Social Cognition, 22*, 367–390.

Klein, S. B., Loftus, J., & Kihlstrom, J. F. (1996). Self-knowledge of an amnesic patient: Toward a neuropsychology of personality and social psychology. *Journal of Experimental Psychology: General, 125*, 250–260.

Koch, C. (2004). *The quest for consciousness: A neurobiological approach.* Woodbury, NY: Roberts.

Kwan, V. S. Y., Barrios, V., Ganis, G., Gorman, J. Lange, C., Kumar, M., et al. (2007). Assessing the neural correlates of self-enhancement bias: A transcranial magnetic stimulation study. *Experimental Brain Research, 182*, 379–385.

Lagattuta, K. H., & Thompson, R. A. (2007). The development of self-conscious emotions: Cognitive processes and social influences. In J. L. Tracy, R. W. Robins, & J. P. Tangney (Eds.), *The self-conscious emotions: Theory and research* (pp. 91–113). New York: Guilford Press.

Leary, M. R. (2004). What is the self?: A plea for clarity. *Self and Identity, 3*, 1–3.

Leary, M. R. (2007). How the self became involved in affective experience: Three sources of self-reflective emotions. In J. L. Tracy, R. W. Robins, & J. P. Tangney (Eds.), *The self-conscious emotions: Theory and research* (pp. 38–52). New York: Guilford Press.

LeDoux, J. (2003). *Synaptic self: How our brains become who we are.* New York: Penguin.

Levine, B. (2004). Autobiographical memory and the self in time: Brain lesion effects, functional neuroanatomy, and lifespan development. *Brain and Cognition, 55*, 54–68.

Lewis, M., Alessandri, S. M., & Sullivan, M. W. (1992). Differences in shame and pride as a function of children's gender and task difficulty. *Child Development, 63*, 630–638.

Lockard, J. S., & Paulhus, D. L. (1988). *Self-deception: An adaptive mechanism?* Englewood Cliffs, NJ: Prentice-Hall.

Magno, E., & Allan, K. (2007). Self-reference during explicit memory retrieval: An event-related potential analysis. *Psychological Science, 18*, 272–277.

Marsh, H. W., Ellis, L. A., & Craven, R. G. (2002). How do preschool children feel about themselves? Unraveling measurement and multidimensional self-concept structure. *Developmental Psychology, 38*, 376–393.

Mason, M. F., Norton, M. I., Van Horn, J. D., Wegner, D. M., Grafton, S. T., & Macrae, C. N. (2007). Wandering minds: The default network and stimulus-independent thought. *Science, 315*, 393–395.

Mclean, K. C., Pasupathi, M., & Pals, J. L. (2007). Selves creating stories creating selves: A process model of self development. *Personality and Social Psychology Review, 11*, 262–278.

McDougall, W. (1963). *An introduction to social psychology* (31st ed.). London: Methuen. (Original work published 1908)

Mead, G. H. (1934). *Mind, self, and society from the standpoint of a social behaviorist.* Chicago: University of Chicago Press.

Measelle, J. R., John, O. P., Ablow, J. C., Cowan, P. A., & Cowan, C. P. (2005). Can children provide coherent, stable, and valid self-reports on the Big Five dimensions? A longitudinal study from ages 5 to 7. *Journal of Personality and Social Psychology, 89*, 90–106.

Miller, R. S. (2007). Is embarrassment a blessing or a curse? In J. L. Tracy, R. W. Robins, & J. P. Tangney (Eds.), *The self-conscious emotions: Theory and research* (pp. 245–262). New York: Guilford Press.

Minsky, M. (1985). *The society of mind.* New York: Simon & Schuster.

Morf, C. C., & Rhodewalt, F. (2001). Unraveling the paradoxes of narcissism: A dynamic self-regulatory processing model. *Psychological Inquiry, 12*, 177–196.

Murphy, G. (1947). *Personality: A biosocial approach to origins and structure.* New York: Harper.

Myazaki, M., & Hiraki, K. (2006). Delayed intermodal contingency affects young children's recognition of their current self. *Child Development, 77*, 736–750.

Neiss, M. B., Sedikides, C., & Stevenson, J. (2006). Genetic influences on level and stability of self-esteem. *Self and Identity, 5*, 247–266.

Neiss, M. B., Stevenson, J., Sedikides, C., Kumashiro, M., Finkel, E. J., & Rusbult, C. E. (2005). Executive self, self-esteem, and negative affectivity: Relations at the phenotypic and genotypic level. *Journal of Personality and Social Psychology, 89*, 593–606.

Oyserman, D., Coon, H. M., & Kemmelmeier, M. (2002). Rethinking individualism and collectivism: Evaluation of theoretical assumptions and meta-analyses. *Psychological Bulletin, 128*, 3–72.

Parker, S. T. (1994). Incipient mirror self-recognition in zoo gorillas and chimpanzees. In S. T. Parker, R. W. Mitchell, & M. L. Boccia (Eds.), *Self-awareness in animals and humans:*

Developmental perspectives (pp. 301–307). New York: Cambridge University Press.

Patterson, F. G. P., & Cohn, R. H. (1994). Self-recognition and self-awareness in lowland gorillas. In S. T. Parker, R. W. Mitchell, & M. L. Boccia (Eds.), *Self-awareness in animals and humans: Developmental perspectives* (pp. 273–290). New York: Cambridge University Press.

Patterson, F. G. P., & Linden, E. (1981). *The education of Koko.* New York: Holt, Rinehart & Winston.

Pickett, C. L., Chen, S., & Gardner, W. L. (in press). *The self.* New York: Guilford Press.

Pinker, S. (1997). *How the mind works.* New York: Norton.

Plotnik, J. M., de Waal, F. B. M., & Reiss, D. (2006). Self-recognition in an Asian elephant. *Proceedings of the National Academy of Sciences, 103*, 17053–17057.

Povinelli, D. J., & Simon, B. B. (1998). Young children's understanding of briefly versus extremely delayed images of self: Emergence of an autobiographical stance. *Developmental Psychology, 34*, 188–194.

Priel, B., & de Schonen, S. (1986). Self-recognition: A study of a population without mirrors. *Journal of Experimental Child Psychology, 41*(2), 237–250.

Rafaeli-Mor, E., & Steinberg, J. (2002). Self-complexity and well-being: A research synthesis. *Personality and Social Psychology Review, 6*, 31–58.

Ramachandran, V. S. (2004). *A brief tour of human consciousness.* New York: Pi Press.

Ramachandran, V. S. (2007). *The neurology of self-awareness.* Retrieved January 8, 2007, from *www.edge.org.*

Reiss, D., & Marino, L. (2001). Mirror self-recognition in the bottlenose dolphin: A case of cognitive convergence. *Proceedings of the National Academy of Sciences, 98*, 5937–5942.

Roberts, B. W., & Robins, R. W. (2000). Broad dispositions, broad aspirations: The intersection of personality and major life goals. *Personality and Social Psychology Bulletin, 26*, 1284–1296.

Robins, R. W., & Beer, J. S. (2001). Positive illusions about the self: Short-term benefits and long-term costs. *Journal of Personality and Social Psychology, 80*, 340–352.

Robins, R. W., & John, O. P. (1997). The quest for self-insight: Theory and research on accuracy and bias in self-perception. In R. Hogan, J. Johnson, & S. Briggs (Eds.), *Handbook of personality psychology* (pp. 649–679). New York: Academic Press.

Robins, R. W., & Pals, J. L. (2002). Implicit self-theories in the academic domain: Implications for goal orientation, attributions, affect, and self-esteem change. *Self and Identity, 1,* 313–336.

Robins, R. W., Tracy, J. L., & Sherman, J. W. (2007). What kinds of methods do personality psychologists use?: A survey of journal editors and editorial board members. In R. W. Robins, R. C. Fraley, & R. F. Krueger (Eds.), *Handbook of research methods in personality psychology* (pp. 673–678) New York: Guilford Press.

Robins, R. W., & Trzesniewski, K. H. (2005). Self-esteem development across the lifespan. *Current Directions in Psychological Science, 14,* 158–162.

Ross, M. (1989). Relation of implicit theories to the construction of personal histories. *Psychological Review, 96,* 341–357.

Rubin, M., & Hewstone, M. (1998). Social identity theory's self-esteem hypothesis: A review and some suggestions for clarification. *Personality and Social Psychology Review, 2,* 40–62.

Sapolsky, R. M. (1997). *The trouble with testosterone: And other essays on the biology of the human predicament.* New York: Scribner.

Schimmack, U., Oishi, S., & Diener, E. (2005). Individualism: A valid and important dimension of cultural differences between nations. *Personality and Social Psychology Review, 9,* 17–31.

Schlenker, B. R. (1985). Introduction: Foundations of the self in social life. In B. R. Schlenker (Ed.), *The self and social life* (pp. 1–28). New York: McGraw-Hill.

Schmitt, D. P., & Allik, J. (2005). Simultaneous administration of the Rosenberg Self-Esteem Scale in 53 nations: Exploring the universal and culture-specific features of global self-esteem. *Journal of Personality and Social Psychology, 89,* 623–642.

Sedikides, C., Gaertner, L., & Vevea, J. L. (2005). Pancultural self-enhancement reloaded. *Journal of Personality and Social Psychology, 89,* 539–551.

Sedikides, C., & Skowronski, J. J. (2003). Evolution of the symbolic self: Issues and prospects. In M. R. Leary & J. P. Tangney (Eds.), *Handbook of self and identity* (pp. 594–609). New York: Guilford Press.

Sedikides, C., & Spence, C. (Eds.). (2007). *The self in social psychology: Frontiers of social psychology.* New York: Psychology Press.

Sejnowski, T. (2003). The computational self. In J. LeDoux, J. Debiec, & H. Moss (Eds.), The self: From soul to brain. *Annals of the New York Academy of Sciences, 1001,* 262–271.

Sharot, T., Riccardi, A. M., Raio, C. M., & Phelps, E. A. (2007). Neural mechanisms mediating optimism bias. *Nature, 450,* 102–105.

Showers, C. J., & Kling, K. C. (1996). The organization of self-knowledge: Implications for mood regulation. In L. L. Martin & A. Tesser (Eds.), *Striving and feeling: Interactions among goals, affect, and self-regulation* (pp. 151–173). Mahwah, NJ: Erlbaum.

Skinner, B. F. (1990). Can psychology be a science of the mind? *American Psychologist, 45,* 1206–1210.

Spencer-Rodgers, J., Peng, K., Wang, L., & Hou, Y. (2004). Dialectical self-esteem and East–West differences in psychological well-being. *Personality and Social Psychology Bulletin, 30,* 1416–1432.

Suarez, S. D., & Gallup, G. G. (1981). Self-recognition in chimpanzees and orangutans, but not gorillas. *Journal of Human Evolution, 10,* 175–188.

Suh, E. M. (2002). Culture, identity consistency, and subjective well-being. *Journal of Personality and Social Psychology, 83,* 1378–1391.

Sui, J., & Han, S. (2007). Self-construal priming modulates neural substrates of self-awareness. *Psychological Science, 18,* 861–866.

Sutin, A. R., & Robins, R. W. (2005). Continuity and correlates of emotions and motives in self-defining memories. *Journal of Personality, 73,* 793–824.

Swann, W. B., Jr. (1997). The trouble with change: Self-verification and allegiance to the self. *Psychological Science, 8,* 177–180.

Swann, W. B., & Schroeder, D. G. (1995). The search for beauty and truth: A framework for understanding reactions to evaluations. *Personality and Social Psychology Bulletin, 21,* 1307–1318.

Takahashi, H., Matsuura, M., Koeda, M., Yahata, N., Suhara, T., Kato, M., et al. (2008). Brain activations during judgments of positive self-conscious emotion: Pride and joy. *Cerebral Cortex, 18,* 898–903.

Tangney, J. P., & Dearing, R. L. (2002). *Shame and guilt.* New York: Guilford Press.

Taylor, S. E., & Brown, J. (1988). Illusion and well-being: A social psychological perspective on mental health. *Psychological Bulletin, 103,* 193–210.

Tetlock, P. E. (1992). The impact of accountability on judgment and choice: Toward a social contingency model. In M. P. Zanna (Ed.), *Advances in experimental social psychology* (Vol. 25, pp. 331–376). New York: Academic Press.

Tracy, J. L., Chang, J. T., Robins, R. W., & Trzesniewski, K. H. (in press). Authentic and hubristic pride: The affective core of self-esteem and narcissism. *Self and Identity.*

Tracy, J. L., & Robins, R. W. (2004a). Putting the self into self-conscious emotions: A theoretical model. *Psychological Inquiry, 15,* 103–125.

Tracy, J. L., & Robins, R. W. (2004b). Show your pride: Evidence for a discrete emotion expression. *Psychological Science, 15,* 194–197.

Tracy, J. L., & Robins, R. W. (2007a). The nature

of pride. In J. L. Tracy, R. W. Robins, & J. P. Tangney (Eds.), *The self-conscious emotions: Theory and research* (pp. 263–282). New York: Guilford Press.

Tracy, J. L., & Robins, R. W. (2007b). The psychological structure of pride: A tale of two facets. *Journal of Personality and Social Psychology, 92,* 506–525.

Tracy, J. L., & Robins, R. W. (2007c). Self-conscious emotions: Where self and emotion meet. In C. Sedikides & S. Spence (Eds.), *The self in social psychology: Frontiers of social psychology series* (pp. 187–209). New York: Psychology Press.

Tracy, J. L., Robins, R. W., & Tangney, J. P. (Eds.). (2007). *The self-conscious emotions: Theory and research.* New York: Guilford Press.

Trafimow, D., Triandis, H. C., & Goto, S. G. (1991). Some tests of the distinction between the private self and collective self. *Journal of Personality and Social Psychology, 60,* 649–655.

Triandis, H. C. (1997). Cross-cultural perspectives on personality. In R. Hogan, J. Johnson, & S. Briggs (Eds.), *Handbook of personality psychology* (pp. 439–464). New York: Academic Press.

Trivers, R. L. (1971). The evolution of reciprocal altruism. *Quarterly Review of Biology, 46,* 35–57.

Trope, Y. (1986). Self-enhancement and self-assessment in achievement behavior. In R. M. Sorrentino & E. T. Higgins (Eds.), *Handbook of motivation and cognition: Foundations of social behavior* (pp. 350–378). New York: Guilford Press.

Trzesniewski, K. H., Donnellan, M. B., & Robins, R. W. (2003). Stability of self-esteem across the lifespan. *Journal of Personality and Social Psychology, 84,* 205–220.

Tulving, E. (1993). Self-knowledge of an amnesic patient is represented abstractly. In T. K. Srull & R. S. Wyer (Eds.), *The mental representation of trait and autobiographical knowledge about the self: Advances in social cognition* (Vol. 5, pp. 147–156). Hillsdale, NJ: Erlbaum.

Tulving, E. (2005). Episodic memory and autonoesis: Uniquely human? In H. S. Terrace & J. Metcalfe (Eds.), *The missing link in cognition: Origins of self-reflective consciousness* (pp. 3–56). New York: Oxford University Press.

Turner, J. C., & Onorato, R. S. (1999). Social identity, personality, and the self-concept: A self-categorization perspective. In T. R. Tyler, R. M. Kramer, & O. P. John (Eds.), *The psychology of the social self* (pp. 11–46). Mahwah, NJ: Erlbaum.

Tyler, T. R., Kramer, R. M., & John, O. P. (Eds.). (1999). *The psychology of the social self.* Mahwah, NJ: Erlbaum.

Verschueren, K., Buyck, P., & Marcoen, A. (2001). Self-representations and socioemotional competence in young children: A 3-year longitudinal study. *Developmental Psychology, 37,* 126–134.

Wang, Q. (2006). Culture and the development of self-knowledge. *Current Directions in Psychological Science, 15,* 182–187.

Warneken, F., & Tomasello, M. (2006). Altruistic helping in human infants and young chimpanzees. *Science, 311,* 1301–1303.

Williams, G. C. (1966). *Adaptation and natural selection: A critique of some current evolutionary thought.* Princeton, NJ: Princeton University Press.

Wilson, D. S., Coleman, K., Clark, A. B., & Biederman, L. (1993). Shy–bold continuum in pumpkinseed sunfish (*Lepomis gibbosus*): An ecological study of a psychological trait. *Journal of Comparative Psychology, 107,* 250–260.

Yamaguchi, S., Greenwald, A. G., Banaji, M. R., Murakami, F., Chen, D., Shiomura, K., et al. (2007). Apparent universality of positive implicit self-esteem. *Psychological Science, 18,* 498–500.

CHAPTER 17

Identity Negotiation
A Theory of Self and Social Interaction

William B. Swann, Jr.
Jennifer K. Bosson

Only in man does man know himself.
—Goethe, *Torquato Tasso*, Act 2, Scene 3

The survival of people's identities rests not only in their own hands but in the hands of others. Whereas people who enjoy a steady supply of nourishment for their identities will retain those identities, those who repeatedly fail to receive such nourishment will ultimately relinquish their identities. The term "identity negotiation" refers to the processes through which people work to obtain such nourishment. This chapter offers a rudimentary theory of identity negotiation.

By "identity" we mean thoughts and feelings about the self, or self-views. Two broad classes of identities or self-views exist. "Personal self-views" refer to qualities that make people unique and distinct from others (e.g., intelligence, dominance). "Social self-views" refer to roles, group memberships, and other qualities that people share with others (e.g., American, Democrat).[1] These dual components of identity are integrated by personal narratives that organize and contextualize people's self-knowledge into a dynamic, coherent, and internally consistent whole (McAdams, 1999; see also Chapter 8, this volume). Thus, identity can be concep-

tualized at varying levels of specificity, ranging from relatively specific self-views to the larger self-narrative that is "more than the sum of its parts" (cf. Bosson & Swann, in press).

But identities are not merely historical repositories of past actions, accomplishments, and liaisons; they also regulate action. In particular, identities systematically influence the personas people assume in specific contexts, as well as the conditions under which they assume them. Generally speaking, people avoid personas that are disjunctive with important identities, preferring instead personas that exemplify their enduring conceptions of who they are.

The process of identity negotiation has several components, one of which includes those self-presentation processes people perform in the service of establishing who they are. Identity negotiation cannot be equated with self-presentation, however. Self-presentational activity represents a collection of behavioral tactics designed to achieve various interaction goals (e.g., Jones & Pittman, 1982). In contrast, the process of identity negotiation refers to a much broader set of processes through which people strike a balance between achieving their interaction goals and satisfying their identity-related goals, such as the needs for agency, communion, and psychological coherence. To this end, people generally conform to various principles of identity negotiation (discussed later in this chapter) that not only facilitate smooth interpersonal interactions but also promote intrapersonal harmony. Furthermore, the motivational forces that regulate identity negotiation processes remain operative well beyond the cessation of self-presentational activity. When, for example, people encounter identity-discrepant evaluations or are compelled to behave in identity-discrepant ways, they may "see" the experience as offering more support for their identity than it actually does. In this way, biases in people's modes of thinking can ensure the survival of identities that have been challenged. As a result, these identities may guide behavior once again.

IDENTITY NEGOTIATION IN HISTORICAL PERSPECTIVE

The intellectual seeds of the identity negotiation formulation were sown by several influential sociologists during the middle of the last century. Goffman (1959, 1961), for example, asserted that the first order of business in social interaction is establishing a "working consensus" or agreement regarding the roles each person will assume. Weinstein and Deutschberger (1964) and later McCall and Simmons (1966) elaborated these early themes. Within psychology, ideas related to identity negotiation were introduced by Secord and Backman (1965) and expanded upon by Swann (1983) and Schlenker (1985). I (W. B. S.) used the phrase "identity negotiation" to refer to the process of reconciling two competing forces in social interaction (Swann, 1987). One influence originates with "perceivers," who use their expectancies to guide their behavior toward "targets," thereby encouraging targets to provide behavioral confirmation for their expectancies (e.g., D. T. Miller & Turnbull 1986; Rosenthal & Jacobson, 1968; Snyder & Swann, 1978; Snyder, Tanke, & Berscheid, 1977). A counter-influence originates

with targets, who strive to bring perceivers to treat them in a manner that provides verification for their identities (Secord & Backman, 1965; Swann, 1983, 1999).

The mutual give and take that occurs between perceivers and targets means that the process of identity negotiation is a fundamentally interactionist phenomenon. As do other interactionist approaches, the process of identity negotiation merges two competing themes that dominated psychology during the last century: behaviorism and personality theory.

Behaviorist Approaches

Behaviorist approaches emphasize the roles of environmental and situational factors in shaping behavioral tendencies. In psychology, this emphasis is exemplified by Pavlov's and Watson's work on classical conditioning, as well as Skinner's (1974) work on operant conditioning, and, within personality, the work of Hull (1943) and N. E. Miller and Dollard (1941). Although the various behaviorist approaches differ in the attention they devote to internal processes such as genetic endowment, basic drives, and cognitions, they share an assumption that most (if not all) behavior is under the control of the external environment. Thus, to understand stable behavior, these perspectives suggest that one must look to the individual's particular history of conditioned, reinforced, and punished reactions.

In sociology, the behaviorist perspective appears in Cooley's (1902) and Mead's (1934) symbolic interactionist approaches, as well as Goffman's (1955) dramaturgical approach and the behavioral sociology approach to interaction (Burgess & Bushell, 1969; Homans, 1974). According to symbolic interactionism, personality is constructed through social interactions in which people internalize feedback from significant relationship partners. As such, personality is shaped largely by external forces, especially the reactions of others to the self. Similarly, according to the dramaturgical approach, people are performers who play out various social roles as if on stage. Rather than reflecting inherent dispositional qualities, personality reflects the roles that people enact within specific contexts, as well as the techniques that they use to manage the impression they make on observers. Related ideas can be found in the writings of sociological role theorists (Stryker & Statham, 1985), as well as behavioral sociologists who apply Skinnerian principles of reinforcement and exchange principles of asset negotiation to the study of human social interaction.

Behaviorist themes emerged with renewed vigor in the late 1960s. Within social psychology, Bem (1967) critiqued dissonance theory; within personality psychology, Mischel (1968) criticized trait approaches. Mischel's critique was especially influential, triggering the decades-long "person–situation" debate (see Kenrick & Funder, 1988).

Personality Approaches

In contrast to behaviorism, personality approaches emphasize the role of dispositions in shaping people's behaviors. Aristotle presaged modern personality approaches by proposing that all objects possessed a natural "essence," or fundamental set of properties that guided their activity (Lewin, 1931/1999). According to Aristotle, an object's behavior was driven entirely by its essence. From this perspective, although changing situations might "disturb and obscure the essential nature" of the object (Lewin, p. 57), they do not explain its behavior.

Contemporary theorists are unlikely to invoke Aristotle, but echoes of essentialism can be found in some modern trait theories (for a discussion, see Haslam, Bastian, & Bissett, 2004). Proponents of the Big Five model, for example, suggest that, to a degree, extraversion, neuroticism, openness to experience, agreeableness, and conscientiousness reflect genetically heritable tendencies that are expressed in predictable emotional and behavioral patterns (Costa & McCrae, 1994; Goldberg, 1981; John, 1990). By focusing on inborn (genetic) qualities that shape personality patterns across the lifespan, contemporary trait approaches reveal essentialist assumptions that are generally absent from behaviorist and situationist approaches.

As do personality theorists, self theorists generally emphasize the role of stable psychological structures in shaping individuals' behaviors and outcomes. Indeed, people's self-views constitute an important component of personality. As examples, self-verification theory (Swann, 1983, 1990,

1999) and its predecessors (Lecky, 1945; Secord & Backman, 1965) hold that people are strongly motivated to preserve their chronic self-views. To this end, people prefer and seek evaluations and relationship partners that confirm their beliefs about the self, and perceive the world in a manner that maintains a stable sense of self. As a result, once people's self-views are formed, these self-views may continue to guide and shape behavior.

Interactionist Approaches

Interactionist approaches view behavior as arising from an interaction of persons and situations. As noted by Jones (1998), some threads of interactionist thinking have been evident in most psychological theorizing since the inception of the field. Still, some theorists have clearly been more influential than others in promoting and popularizing the idea of the person–situation interaction.

Lewin's (1951) field theory proposed the interactionist assumption that behavior is a function of the "life space," or the interdependent relationship between the person and his or her environment. Lewin's thinking was influenced by a Galilean approach to science, in which both an object and its surroundings are considered equally important determinants of the object's behavior (see Lewin, 1931/1999). In Lewin's conceptualization, behavior is "always derived from the relation of the concrete individual to the concrete situation" (p. 65). Such interactionist assumptions can be found in the work of personality and social psychologists alike, including Erikson (1959), Sullivan (1953), Endler and Magnusson (1976), Swann (1983), Snyder and Ickes (1985), John and colleagues (John, Hampson, & Goldberg, 1991), Michel and Shoda (1999), and McAdams (1999). Within sociology, interactionism is evident in the work of Thomas, who argued that people both shape and are shaped by their experiences (Thomas & Thomas, 1928), and McCall and Simmons (1966), who emphasized the tendency for people to maximize interpersonal harmony by gravitating toward social settings that are likely to offer support for their identities. Although these theorists differ in the extent to which they explicitly invoke the language of interactionism, all emphasize the interplay of stable features of persons and the immediate pressures of situations in shaping identity and behavior (see Swann & Seyle, 2005).

The identity negotiation formulation follows in the interactionist tradition in that it assumes that behavior grows out of the interplay between self, situation, and other. This approach is exemplified in the merger of (1) self-verification theory with (2) the symbolic interactionist and expectancy theory approaches. In the tradition of self-verification theory, we assume that people's identities (especially their stable self-views) guide their choices of social partners and situations, the relationship goals they pursue in their social interactions, and their interpretations of, and reactions to, the feedback they receive. In the tradition of the symbolic interactionist and expectancy theory approaches, we assume that the reactions of others to the self exert a powerful influence on people's identities, both in the short term and more permanently.

THE NATURE OF IDENTITY NEGOTIATION

For most people, the word "negotiation" calls to mind those processes that occur when people strive to reach agreements regarding the exchange of materials, expertise, or services. Such "asset negotiations" have been the subject of several decades of careful analysis by researchers within both social psychology (e.g., Rubin & Brown, 1975) and organizational behavior and decision making (Lempert, 1972–1973; Thompson, 2005). Here we detail some of the primary similarities and differences between asset and identity negotiations.

Function and Ubiquity

The most striking difference between asset and identity negotiation is in the function that the two sets of processes serve. Whereas asset negotiations regulate the exchange of commodities, identity negotiation establishes the personas that each person will assume in a relationship. Usually, asset negotiations require that identity negotiation has already occurred. That is, before assets can be negotiated, negotiators must first initiate a process of identity negotiation. Once established, the mutual identities of the negotiators channel and constrain their subsequent response op-

tions. From this vantage point, identity negotiation is a critically important prelude to asset negotiations. In fact, identity negotiation processes are typically the first step in the formation of *all* relationships, including those that involve no asset negotiation whatsoever. For this reason, identity negotiation processes are far more common than asset negotiations.

In addition to these differences in functional properties and relative ubiquity, asset and identity negotiation also have different structural properties. Differences in underlying motivation, communication channel, and longevity are especially important.

Motivation

Because asset negotiations are designed to accomplish a specific material goal (e.g., establishing the price that a buyer will pay a seller for a product), the motives that fuel such negotiations are typically explicit and easy to recognize. In highly competitive contexts, asset negotiations may involve a zero-sum dynamic, in which one party maximizes his or her own personal outcomes at the expense of the other. In these cases, both parties may be preoccupied with "looking out for #1." More often, however, at least some modicum of cooperation benefits both parties. Even in business contexts, which are often stereotyped as "ruthless," negotiators are typically motivated to cooperate (Thompson, 2005; Walton & McKersie, 1965).

The motivations that fuel identity negotiations as compared to asset negotiations are generally far less explicit. In part, this lack of explicitness may reflect the fact that the "resources" being exchanged during identity negotiations are abstract psychological qualities that cannot be quantified or readily compared. That is, whereas asset negotiators are tasked with reaching agreements on tangibles such as the market value of merchandise, identity negotiators must agree on the personas that each person will assume in the interaction. Furthermore, the motivations that drive asset versus identity negotiations also differ in how distant they are from the resources being negotiated. Whereas agreeing on the resources that each party will receive is the ultimate goal of asset negotiations, agreeing on the personas that each party will assume is *not* the ultimate goal of the identity negotiation process. Instead, negotiating a public persona is merely a means to the larger ends of maintaining and nourishing one's self-views as well as meeting other important identity-related needs.

Although identity negotiations are potentially influenced by a wide range of motives, three identity-related needs may play especially important roles in the identity negotiation process: *agency* (which encompasses feelings of autonomy and competence), *communion* (which encompasses feelings of belonging and interpersonal connectedness), and *psychological coherence* (which encompasses feelings of regularity, predictability, and control). The basic human needs for agency and communion are assumed to underlie many aspects of personality and social behavior (Baumeister & Leary, 1995; Wiggins & Broughton, 1985), and theories of optimal functioning emphasize the importance of meeting both needs (e.g., Ryff, 1989). Similarly, humans have a need for psychological coherence (Guidano & Liotti, 1983; Popper, 1963); indeed, the mental and physical health of those who lack coherence tends to suffer (e.g., Swann, Chang-Schneider, & Angulo, 2007).

It is easy to see how people might gratify each of these motives through the process of identity negotiation. For example, to gratify their desire for agency, people will negotiate identities that reflect the self-views that make them unique from others (i.e., their personal self-views). To satisfy their desire for communion, people will negotiate identities that reflect the self-views that link them to other people (i.e., their social self-views). Finally, to gratify their desire for coherence, people will seek identity-consistent feedback and experiences (i.e., information that fits with their stable self-views).

Of course, people cannot always meet all of these needs simultaneously, nor is it always essential that they do so. For example, people who recognize their powerlessness in a given situation may (wisely) refrain from pursuing their agency needs, whereas those who are suspicious of their partner's motives may refrain from pursuing their desire for communion. Furthermore, conflicts may sometimes emerge between various motives, as when an identity linked to a personal self-view (e.g., "independent") clashes with

an identity linked to a social self-view (e.g., "family man"). The identity negotiation formulation suggests that most people learn to negotiate identities in ways that minimize tensions between their needs for agency, communion, and coherence. For example, the family man may meet his need for agency by negotiating a self-reliant identity in the context of his business, and at the same time meet his need for communion by negotiating a warm and involved identity in his relationships with his family. In each context, he may also meet his need for coherence by seeking verification of the (independent or warm) identity that he negotiates.

Communication Channel

The channels of communication through which asset versus identity negotiations flow will often vary in explicitness. Generally speaking, asset negotiations are quite explicit and purposeful, often occurring during interactions that have clearly demarcated beginnings, end points, and agendas. In contrast, the process of identity negation is often implicit, informal, and open-ended. Moreover, whereas asset negotiators emphasize verbal over nonverbal communications and commitments, identity negotiators are likely to use both communication channels (Swann, Stein-Seroussi, & McNulty, 1992).

Related to this point, because identity negotiations take place during everyday social interactions wherein many behaviors are overlearned and automatic (Bargh & Williams, 2006), people may engage in identity negotiations without consciously realizing that they are doing so. Thus, whereas asset negotiators are most likely consciously aware of the negotiation process from start to finish, identity negotiators may instead shift into and out of awareness of their ongoing negotiations. This point is reflected in Swann's (1987) notion of routine versus crisis self-verification, as well as McAdams's (1999) ideas regarding the waxing and waning of the self-narrative process. Both authors note that the process of establishing identities tends to become routine and recedes from consciousness once identities have been successfully negotiated, only to return to consciousness during times of change, disruption, and/or challenge.

Thus, people may only become aware that they want others to recognize and validate a given identity when they receive information that suggests that others see them in an identity-discrepant manner. From this vantage point, feedback that causes an individual to question his or her identity, rapid and unpredicted life changes, and novel environments or negotiation partners may all bring identity negotiations to the fore of an individual's consciousness. In this sense, the motives that drive identity negotiations may resemble those psychological and physical need states (e.g., hunger, thirst, loneliness) that enter awareness only when the relevant need is not being met.

Longevity

On balance, asset negotiations will persist only as long as the agreements and exchanges that they are designed to support. Sometimes these negotiations may remain in effect for very short periods; sometimes they may last for years or even decades. In contrast, identity negotiations should persist as long as the relationships between the relevant parties persist. As noted above, however, ongoing identity negotiations may be imperceptible to outsiders if the identity-relevant behaviors of the interaction partners are routinized. Even the interaction partners themselves may not realize that an identity negotiation is underway, given the tendency for such negotiations to become automatic and to fade from consciousness.

PRINCIPLES OF IDENTITY NEGOTIATION PROCESSES

The foregoing discussion suggests that identity negotiation is a special case of negotiation processes that is unique in its function, ubiquity, and structural properties. Given these distinctive qualities, it is not surprising that a unique set of principles governs the identity negotiation process. People presumably learn these principles in the same way that they learn all rules of social interaction: through a process of trial and error (Athay & Darley, 1980; Goffman, 1959). As noted above, people routinely conform to these principles even though they are seldom aware of them.

Rather, their adherence to these principles typically occurs automatically and implicitly (Jones & Pittman, 1982). Although there could be many such principles, we focus here on four of the most fundamental.

Clarity

Ambiguity regarding matters of identity and relationship goals can be misleading, put partners off balance, undermine trust, and produce disappointing outcomes. Hence, the first principle of interpersonal identity negotiation: One should clearly communicate one's desired identity and relationship goals to one's partner. To ensure clarity, identity negotiators should know the content and importance of their desired identity and interaction goal(s), and communicate these to their partner as early in the interaction as possible. Moreover, identity negotiators should communicate their desired identity and relationship goals via as many channels of communication as possible, because redundancy provides partners with corroborating information and thereby diminishes the probability of misunderstanding and conflict. Thus, for example, people may simultaneously communicate their identities through verbalizations and through the display of *identity cues*: overt signs and symbols of who they are (Goffman, 1959; Schlenker, 1980; Swann, 1983). Such cues may range from T-shirts to titles and honorifics (e.g., "Dr."), to bedroom and office décor (Gosling, Ko, Mannarelli, & Morris, 2002). The use of such redundant cues can facilitate the clarity with which identities are communicated.

Of course, maximal clarity is only possible or desirable insofar as people are certain about the identity that they want to negotiate. If someone is uncertain of a given identity, either for situational reasons (e.g., the situation is a novel one) or dispositional reasons (e.g., the individual is low in self-concept certainty) (Pelham, 1991), then clarity may suffer. In such circumstances, people can often achieve clarity by looking to their interaction partner for cues regarding the identity that he or she expects them to assume. When this occurs, people are particularly likely to adopt identities that provide behavioral confirmation of their partners' expectations (e.g., Snyder & Klein, 2005; Snyder & Swann, 1978).

Cooperation

Identity negotiators should cooperate with their partners by honoring the identities that they negotiate, as well as the identities that their partners proffer. One obvious way to uphold the cooperation principle is to behave in an identity-consistent manner throughout a given interaction. In this way, negotiators can avoid identity renegotiation, which can be highly disruptive and may undermine the interaction goals of one or both partners.

For identity negotiators to convey the impression that they are following the cooperation principle, the timing of their behaviors can be critical. Often, identity negotiations resemble asset negotiations in that people may bargain back and forth in an offer–counteroffer fashion (e.g., Athay & Darley, 1980; Goffman, 1959; Homans, 1974). In such scenarios, people may uphold the cooperation principle by following each concession on their partner's part with a concession of their own (Axelrod & Hamilton, 1981). For example, after receiving feedback indicating that one's partner accepts one's desired identity, one should reciprocate by accepting the identity that one's partner offers. Such reciprocal concessions should reinforce the mutual confirmation of identities that provides the basis for successful identity negotiation.

Although the foregoing discussion may imply that identity negotiations typically consist of equally weighted contributions on the part of each negotiator, this is often not the case. At times, negotiators are strongly invested in identities that their partners are reluctant to honor. At other times, negotiators may enter interactions with strongly held expectations about a partner's identity, only to discover that their partner has different ideas about who he or she is. In such cases, cooperation is still possible, provided that both parties are able and willing to be flexible. In general, to the extent that a negotiator's investment in a given identity is high, cooperation is facilitated by the partner's willingness to acquiesce and offer identity-consistent appraisals. Conversely, to the extent that the partner is strongly invested in his or her expectations, cooperation is facilitated by the negotiator's willingness to conform to those expectations. When both the negotiator and his or her partner are strongly invested in conflicting perceptions of one another's identities, cooperation may not be possible, and both parties are likely to be dissatisfied with the outcome of the negotiation.

Continuity

People expect their relationship partners to be fairly predictable and consistent across time (Athay & Darley, 1981; Rempel, Holmes, & Zanna, 1985). Thus, in addition to honoring the identity that one negotiates within the context of a given interaction (the cooperation principle), people will maximize interpersonal harmony if they also negotiate a consistent identity, within a given relationship, across time. That is, people should remain faithful to the identities that they negotiate in the context of ongoing relationships with specific others.

A challenge to the continuity principle may occur when people mature, shift status, or change in some way. Such changes can pose problems for relationship partners, because they will be forced to choose between assimilating the new identity to an existing one, renegotiating a new identity, or leaving the relationship. Often, such transitions are finessed through cognitive gymnastics that are designed to maximize the apparent overlap between the old and new identities (at least from the perspective of the one undergoing the change). One such strategy is discussed by McAdams (1996, 1999), who suggests that people may organize multiple identities around overarching cognitive or affective themes. For example, themes of cooperation may characterize many of the identities people strive to negotiate with close relationship partners, providing cognitive unity to the multiple roles that they enact. Similarly, people may imbue their various identities with a common affective tone, such as optimism, humor, pessimism, or passive acceptance. Using such higher-level cognitive and affective schemas, people may perceive continuity between two or more identities that outside observers might construe as conflicting. We elaborate upon this idea in the next section.

Cognitive gymnastics notwithstanding, problems may emerge when sudden identity changes occur that cannot be finessed, or when interaction partners do not perceive the continuity that individuals are able to impose on their own identities. For example, when one partner suddenly loses an interpersonal asset such as a job or status, that partner may become financially dependent on the other partner. Such reversals may turn the power dynamic in the relationship on its head, and this shift may have important reverberations for the respective identities of each partner. If such identity discontinuity cannot be repaired fairly quickly, partners will be forced to renegotiate the relevant identities.

Compatibility

Often, people know one another in two or more contexts that call for distinct identities. For example, married people may know one another not only as spouses but also as parents, colleagues, and tennis partners. When negotiating distinct identities with a given partner, negotiators should ensure that these identities are compatible with one another and with previously negotiated identities. Given the premium that people place on predictability and consistency in their relationship partners, someone who elicits appraisals of "bookworm" in one context and "college girl gone wild" in another context may be perceived as unreliable and therefore undesirable as a partner. If people want to negotiate different identities with the same partners, they can do so successfully only insofar as the appraisals associated with the different identities are not inconsistent either logically (e.g., Democrat vs. Republican) or emotionally (e.g., friend vs. adversary).

INTRAPSYCHIC MECHANISMS THAT HELP SUSTAIN IDENTITIES

Accompanying identity negotiation processes are a host of intrapsychic processes that shape how individuals interpret and react to the outputs of their identity negotiations. For the most part, these intrapsychic mechanisms enable people to maintain a sense of personal continuity even in the face of identity-discrepant feedback from others. Thus, both within a given negotiation and across different negotiations, people tend to perceive stability and regularity in their own identities and those of others. For example, as noted above, people who undergo identity change may perceive continuity between the old and new identities by organizing both identities

according to certain cognitive or affective themes. In this section of the chapter, we identify seven intrapsychic mechanisms that foster identity continuity and regularity by shaping how identity negotiation processes unfold.

Selective Attention

In general, people pay more attention to interpersonal feedback when they expect it to confirm their identity than they do when they expect it to disconfirm their identity (Swann & Read, 1981). As such, people may fail to notice feedback that is inconsistent with their identity and relationship goals. Moreover, when people are confronted with identity-threatening feedback that cannot be ignored, they respond by focusing more attention on their firmly held self-views (e.g., Dodgson & Wood, 1998). This tendency may serve to reinforce identities that have been challenged during identity negotiations, thus reducing the likelihood of identity change.

Discounting

When confronted with feedback that is inconsistent with their self-views, people tend to discount both the validity of the feedback (Korman, 1968; Markus, 1977) and the credibility of the evaluators who offer it to them (Shrauger & Lund, 1975; Swann, Griffin, Predmore, & Gaines, 1987). In some cases, such discounting might allow identity negotiators to remain untroubled by inconsistent feedback. In other cases, discounting may motivate identity negotiators to break off relations with the source of the identity-discrepant feedback, as when an interaction partner repeatedly displays such poor judgment.

Biased Interpretation

People's need for coherence and regularity may compel them to "see" more identity-consistent feedback than they actually receive during identity negotiations. Indeed, humans possess a powerful ability to interpret incoming information in a manner that is consistent with their prior knowledge. Interestingly, some propose that a particular region of the brain is responsible for such activity. Gazzaniga (1998), for example, suggests that a "left-hemisphere interpreter" drives humans' tendency to impose coherence and continuity on their conscious experiences (see also McAdams, 1997).

Anxiety as Information

Of course, if interpersonal evaluations are to be internalized, they must fall within the individual's latitude of acceptance (Jones, Rhodewalt, Berglas, & Skelton, 1981). Information that falls within the latitude of rejection will garner extra scrutiny. If the discrepant information pertains to a highly certain and central self-view or comes from a highly credible source, it may produce anxious arousal (Lundgren, & Schwab, 1977; Mendes & Akinola, 2006; Wood, Heimpel, Newby-Clark, & Ross, 2005), which will motivate behaviors designed to neutralize the threat posed to the identity in question (Burke, 1991; Swann, Chang-Schneider, & Angulo, 2007). Anxiety can thus signal to individuals that a given interaction partner poses a threat to their enduring beliefs about themselves.

Biased Recall

In general, people show better recall for identity-consistent feedback than they do for inconsistent feedback (Crary, 1966; Greenwald, 1980; Swann & Read, 1981), and they tend to recall past feedback as being more consistent with their self-views than it really was (Story, 1998). Thus, even if people receive identity-inconsistent feedback that they cannot ignore, discount, or reinterpret, they may still sustain their self-views—and thus meet their need for coherence—by forgetting the threatening feedback or misremembering its content.

Thematic Coherence

When individuals negotiate multiple identities in the context of a single relationship or across multiple different relationships, they may increase the underlying coherence and logic of the various identities through a process that McAdams (1996, 1999) refers to as "selfing." As noted earlier, people may increase compatibility by structuring their multiple identities around underlying themes

and narrative tones. For example, themes of agency and communion are prevalent in many people's identities, providing cognitive unity to the multiple roles that they enact. In a similar manner, distinct identities often share a common affective tone, such as optimism, humor, pessimism, or sorrow. Thus, the person who behaves somewhat differently and pursues different relationship goals across his or her various identity negotiations with a given partner may still maintain intrapsychic coherence by linking all of his or her identities to underlying concerns about competence and connectedness, or by imbuing the different identities with a similar affective tone.

Compartmentalization

Cognitive compartmentalization may be another mechanism through which some people achieve continuity among the different identities that they negotiate. People differ in the extent to which they organize their self-views into different cognitive compartments or *self-aspects* (Linville, 1985; Showers, 1992). Whereas some people's self-concepts contain a few broad self-aspects that encompass most of their specific self-views, other people organize the contents of their self-concept into numerous, nonredundant self-aspects (e.g., "student self," "religious self," "self at home"). Importantly, experiences that activate a given self-aspect should prime associated self-views. Therefore, people higher in self-complexity—those who organize their self-views into numerous nonredundant self-aspects—may find it easier to negotiate multiple distinct identities without experiencing threats to their sense of continuity.

For instance, if a professor's "self at work" self-aspect contains the qualities "introverted" and "submissive," whereas her "self at home" contains the qualities "outgoing" and "exuberant," she may find it relatively easy to negotiate each of these disparate identities in its own context. For this woman, even though her work and home identities differ, interactions in each separate context will activate primarily those self-views that are relevant to the current negotiation. Thus, when people negotiate very different identities with their different relationship partners, those with more complex self-structures should be less troubled by feelings of incompatibility. At present, however, this idea remains speculative.

A PROCESS MODEL OF IDENTITY NEGOTIATION

In this section we highlight some of the key links in the chain of events that make up the identity negotiation process. The process model of identity negotiation depicted in Figure 17.1 will guide our excursion. This model explicates the dynamically interrelated roles of self-views, relationship goals, situations, and others' appraisals in guiding identity negotiations and their outcomes. Along the way, we also illustrate how identity negotiators apply the interpersonal principles and intrapsychic mechanisms described above. Note that the processes described here presumably operate both in new relationships and in long-term, enduring relationships.

The Person's Initial Identity and Relationship Goals

The model begins with the initial identity and relationship goals. As noted earlier, "identity" refers to personal and social self-views, along with the narratives that people superimpose on their self-knowledge to foster a more consistent and coherent sense of self. "Relationship goals" are the desired end states for which people strive when they enter social interactions. These goals can be defined at various levels of specificity. At the broadest level, people strive to meet their needs for agency, communion, and psychological coherence. Depending on the nature of the relationship (e.g., Kelley & Thibaut, 1978), these broadly defined goals may also give rise to various midlevel goals such as self-verification, ingratiation, and self-promotion (Jones & Pittman, 1982), as well as specific goals such as garnering the affections of a particular person.

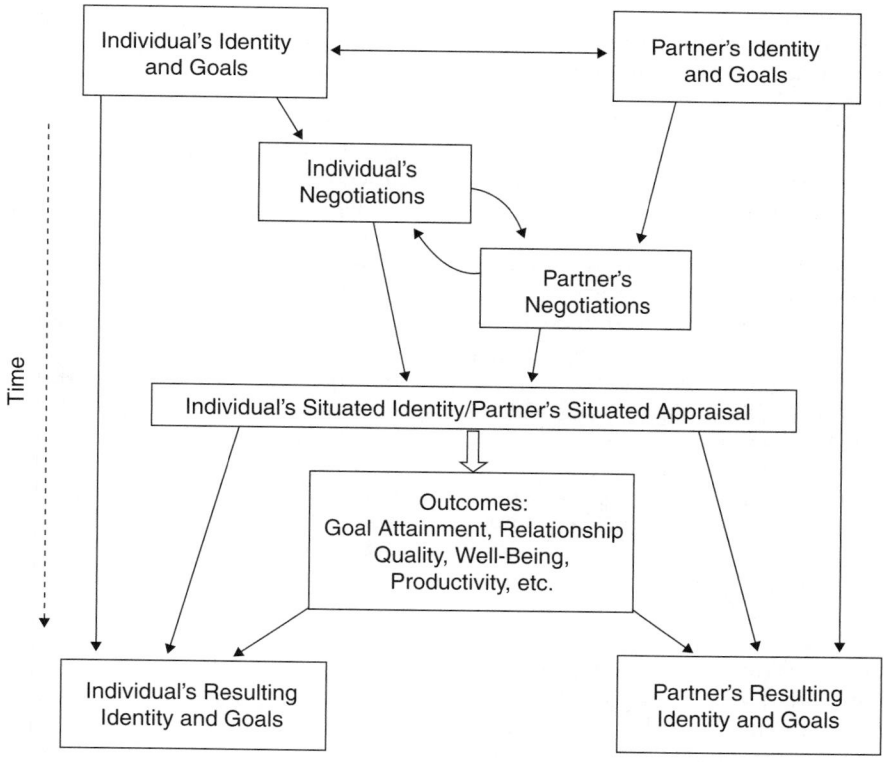

FIGURE 17.1. A process model of identity negotiation across time.

Peoples' initial identities and relationship goals should guide them toward certain environments and situations. Indeed, all organisms gravitate toward environments—or "opportunity structures" (e.g., Hawley, 1950; McCall & Simmons, 1966)—that routinely satisfy their needs (e.g., Clarke, 1954; Odum, 1963). For example, people's identities may guide them toward certain vocations, living environments, hobbies, and leisure activities, thereby ensuring that the experiences they routinely encounter are ones that support and buttress their chronic identities (cf. Caspi & Roberts, 1999). Moreover, people may choose interaction partners who seem similar to them (Byrne, 1971; Pinel, Long, Landau, Alexander, & Pyszczynski, 2006) or who seem to like them (Lowe & Goldstein, 1970; Sprecher, 1998).

Interestingly, the evidence that people prefer partners who like them may reflect a desire for appraisals that verify people's identities. Because the majority of people in unselected samples have positive self-views, for most people positive evaluations (e.g., appraisals that indicate that one is liked) will be more self-verifying than will negative evaluations. When researchers *do* measure participants' self-views, evidence of self-verification strivings emerges even among people with negative self-views. For example, a recent meta-analysis of self-verification in marriage relationships revealed that people enjoyed superior relationship quality if their spouses perceived them in a self-verifying manner (Chang-Schneider & Swann, 2007), and this was true whether people's self-views were positive or negative. Furthermore, people display such strivings at the level of personal self-views (Swann, Pelham, & Krull, 1989), collective self-views (Chen, Chen, & Shaw, 2004; Chen, Shaw, & Jeung, 2006), and group identities (e.g., Gómez, Seyle, Huici, & Swann, 2007; Lemay & Ashmore, 2004).

The Partner's Initial Identity and Relationship Goals

Because negotiations involve (at least) two individuals, all identity negotiations are shaped by the joint contributions of both parties. Thus, the partner's initial identity and relationship goals play integral roles in determining the outcomes of identity nego-

tiations. For instance, as noted above, partners' identities and goals will compel them to enter certain environments and opportunity structures, and to avoid others. Once both parties have entered the relationship, the identity negotiation process can begin in earnest. To this end, people will systematically deploy a host of interpersonal identity negotiation strategies.

Negotiations between the Person and the Partner

People may communicate their identities before they even open their mouths by displaying identity cues. For example, flashy sports cars that communicate wealth and confidence or ripped jeans that convey a laid-back and nonmaterialistic approach to life will project a particular identity to one's partner. Moreover, consciously or not, people tend to arrange and design their dorm rooms, offices (Gosling et al., 2002), homes (Sadalla, Vershure, & Burroughs, 1987), and personal websites (Vazire & Gosling, 2004) in ways that elicit identity-consistent evaluations from others. Of course, people also convey their identities to others through direct verbal communications. For example, the shy, unadventurous bookworm who wants her new college roommate to see her as such may note that "I'm not much of a partygoer. I'll probably spend most nights studying in the library."

Upon communicating their identities, negotiators must wait for their partner's counteroffer and then respond accordingly. If a negotiator's roommate responds to her displays of her introverted identity with "Don't be shy! Come to the party with me and I'll introduce you to people," the negotiator must then decide whether to utilize a more forceful behavioral strategy or acquiesce to the partner's counteroffer. One possibility is to reassert her introversion by behaving in an even more introverted fashion (Stets & Burke, 2003). For example, it was found that self-proclaimed submissives exaggerated their submissiveness when interacting with a confederate who ostensibly perceived them as dominant (Swann & Hill, 1982). Specifically, self-proclaimed submissives who thought they were perceived as dominant behaved in a substantially more submissive manner than did submissives who thought they were perceived as submissive.

According to the clarity principle discussed earlier, identity negotiators should use as many channels of communication as possible to convey their desired identities to interaction partners. The use of multiple channels may be especially helpful when people encounter resistance in bringing others to see them congruently. Returning to the example above, the introverted negotiator may increase the likelihood that her roommate will come to see her as shy if she supplements her verbalizations with nonverbal cues such as speaking in hushed tones, allowing her hair to fall into her face, and adopting an anxious expression each time her roommate invites her to a party. Moreover, the shy negotiator may communicate her intention to "power study" by stacking piles of books on her desk, sprinkling study guides and daily organizers throughout the apartment, and highlighting exam dates and paper deadlines on her calendar.

In response to the negotiator's amplified efforts to elicit an identity-consistent appraisal, her roommate must now make another counteroffer. In keeping with the cooperation principle, the roommate should acquiesce to the negotiator's wishes and offer behaviors that validate her preferred (i.e., introverted) identity. For example, the roommate may back down and stop insisting that they attend social events together. Furthermore, both parties may cooperate by following each concession on the other's part with a concession of her own. For example, if her roommate agrees to view her as an introvert, the negotiator may reciprocate by redoubling her efforts to honor the roommate's extraverted identity.

As their relationship unfolds across time, both parties should uphold the continuity principle by remaining faithful to their negotiated identities. Thus, the negotiator should continue to play the role of the introvert in her dealings with her roommate. Were she to host a wild, drunken party one night, this behavior could justifiably be viewed by the roommate as a breach of their interpersonal contract, and the roommate might "retaliate" by refusing to accept the negotiator's claim to an introvert identity.

The fourth principle of identity negotiation states that people should strive to maintain compatibility among the various identi-

ties that they negotiate with a given partner. In our ongoing example, this means that the identity the shy individual negotiates with her roommate in their apartment should be compatible with the identities that she negotiates with her roommate elsewhere. Insofar as the negotiator wishes to negotiate a more outgoing identity with her roommate in other contexts, she may maintain compatibility by seeking appraisals of herself that are only slightly more outgoing than the appraisals she seeks from her roommate when they are at home.

Intrapsychic Mechanisms

As noted earlier, the identity negotiation processes described above work hand-in-hand with a parallel set of intrapsychic mechanisms. These cognitive (e.g., attention, interpretation, and recall) and affective (e.g., anxiety in response to challenges to an important identity) mechanisms both accompany and sustain people's identity negotiations.

Consider the scenario in which a shy woman tells her roommate that she dislikes parties, and her roommate nonetheless encourages her to attend the evening's soiree ("Don't be shy! Come to the party with me and I'll introduce you to people"). In this case, the negotiator may interpret her roommate's offer to introduce her to people at the party as an acknowledgment of her social awkwardness rather than as a refusal to view her as introverted. Because interpersonal feedback is often ambiguous and open to interpretation, most people have little difficulty maintaining coherent and stable identities even when faced with interaction partners who view them in identity-inconsistent ways. If the inconsistency is too great to ignore, however, it will threaten the negotiator's need for coherence, which will produce unsettling feelings of anxiety. Such feelings should prompt identity negotiation strategies that are designed to correct the partner's inaccurate appraisals.

Intrapsychic processes facilitate continuity not only between a negotiator's self-views and the appraisals he or she receives from others, but also between the different identities that a person negotiates with the same partner. Consider a person who negotiates a highly introverted identity with her roommate in their home environment, and a mildly introverted identity with her roommate in the context of their larger social group. Despite this discrepancy, she may nonetheless maintain intrapsychic coherence by linking both of these identities to her underlying concerns about connectedness and intimacy or personal competence and academic achievement. Such cognitive gymnastics can even harmonize strikingly distinct identities. If a negotiator is outgoing and exuberant around her mother but shy and retiring around her roommate, she may increase the compatibility of these divergent identities by imbuing both of them with a tone of ironic humor. Furthermore, the negotiator may cognitively compartmentalize her different identities such that the specific self-views associated with each identity become salient primarily during interactions with the relevant partner.

The Person's Situated Identity

As shown in Figure 17.1, the identity negotiation processes and intrapsychic mechanisms described above jointly produce people's situated identities. A "situated identity" is a person's identity within a specific, circumscribed situation (Alexander & Knight, 1971). This idea is related to the notion of the working self-concept (Markus & Kunda, 1986), in that it is the currently active portion of a person's identity.

Note that people's situated identities reflect not only their own behavioral, cognitive, and affective contributions to the identity negotiation process, but also the contributions (e.g., feedback, verbal and nonverbal reactions) made by their partner, as well as the constraints imposed by the situation. Therefore, a negotiator's situated identity will sometimes overlap minimally with his or her initial identity. The discrepancy between a negotiator's initial and situated identities may be greater to the extent that the negotiator (1) is uncertain or unclear about the identity being negotiated (Campbell et al., 1996; Maracek & Mettee, 1972; Pelham & Swann, 1994; Swann & Ely, 1984; Swann, Pelham, & Chidester, 1988); (2) places relatively little importance on the negotiated identity (Markus, 1977; Pelham, 1991; Swann & Pelham, 2002); or (3) is low in self-awareness or self-consciousness (Ma-

jor, Cozzarelli, Testa, & McFarlin, 1988). Similarly, identity-discrepant feedback from a partner who is high in certainty or credibility should be particularly powerful in shaping a negotiator's situated identity (e.g., Josephs, Bosson, & Jacobs, 2003; Swann & Ely, 1984). Finally, situational influences that are exceptionally strong (e.g., emergencies, powerful authority figures or interaction goals, novel environments) or that provide unambiguous self-relevant information (e.g., obvious failure at a task, repeated doses of credible feedback) can also foster significant discrepancies between a negotiator's initial and situated identities. In part, situations can influence the overlap between initial and situated identities by activating people's communion needs. Those whose situation elicits a powerful need to belong may be willing to negotiate situated identities that differ substantially from their initial identities. We return to this idea shortly.

The Partner's Situated Appraisal

"Situated appraisals" are the impressions of negotiators that their partners develop as a result of identity negotiation processes. In general, identity negotiation processes will unfold more smoothly to the extent that partners' situated appraisals match negotiators' situated identities, because partners who achieve such matches will be better able to predict negotiators' reactions and behaviors within the circumscribed context of their relationship (Swann, 1984). Nevertheless, at times partners' situated appraisals will clash with negotiators' situated identities. In such instances, the identity negotiation process may end in a stalemate, with neither party willing (or able) to broker an agreement regarding the identity that the negotiator is to assume (Major et al., 1988). When this occurs, both parties are likely to feel dissatisfied with the outcome of the interaction.

In cases in which the criterion for the success of the identity negotiation process is the quality of the relationship between the negotiator and his or her partner, the match between the negotiator's situated identity and the partner's situated appraisal may be more important than the match between the negotiator's situated and initial identities. If, for example, the well-being of a relationship depends on one partner eliciting from the other uncharacteristically positive evaluations on a given dimension, negotiators may temporarily seek such evaluations and forgo their need for verification of their chronic self-views. In such cases, people may prioritize feedback that matches their "better than normal" situated identity over feedback that matches the identity they assume in most of their relationships.

A case in point is represented by people involved in short-term, relatively tenuous dating relationships. The very survival of such provisional relationships hinges on maintaining the interest of the partner. For this reason, people in dating relationships may negotiate whatever identity they feel is necessary to keep the relationship alive, even if it requires seeking feedback that is more favorable than the feedback they typically seek. That is, identity negotiations in dating relationships may be driven powerfully by people's communal needs, even at the expense of other important motives.

Consistent with this reasoning, Swann, Bosson, and Pelham (2002) found that when people held the goal of winning the love of a romantic partner, they sought appraisals of their physical attractiveness that were more positive than their chronic self-perceived attractiveness would warrant. More interestingly, people who negotiated highly attractive situated identities tended to elicit matching (i.e., highly attractive) situated appraisals from their partners. They did so, in part, by presenting themselves to their partners in a physically attractive manner. Thus, when people's relationship goals demand that they prioritize the fit between their situated identity and situated appraisal by seeking highly favorable feedback, they accordingly arrange it so that their partners develop—and they thus deserve—such positive evaluations.

In the short run, such harmony between the negotiator's situated identity and the partner's situated appraisal ensures that the identity negotiation process unfolds smoothly. In the long run—for example, in marriage relationships—a situated identity that receives reinforcement may become part of the negotiator's permanent identity. Alternatively, negotiators in long-term relationships may renegotiate identities that better reflect their stable self-views (e.g., Swann, De La Ronde, & Hixon, 1994).

Negotiation Outcomes

Once negotiators and their partners have established situated identities and appraisals, they will have achieved a "working consensus" (Goffman, 1959). At this point, the stage is set for people to work toward the goals that initially brought them into the interaction, such as collaborating on a work project, forging a romantic relationship, cohabitating peacefully, or negotiating assets. To the extent that negotiators' situated identities are consistent with their initial relationship goals and their partner's situated appraisal of them, they should be well positioned to achieve the outcomes they desire. Several such outcomes are relationship quality, psychological well-being, and work productivity.

Relationship Quality

With regard to relationship quality, the self-verification literature shows that people's satisfaction with their long-term relationships increases to the extent that their partners view them in an identity-confirming manner (i.e., their situated identity corresponds closely to both their initial identity and their partner's situated appraisal of them). For example, when married people's spouses see them as they see themselves, they are more intimate and satisfied with their spouses and are less likely to get divorced (for a review, see Swann, Chang-Schneider, & Angulo, 2007). Presumably, congruent appraisals foster predictability and manageability in the relationship, which may not only improve the likelihood that people can achieve their relationship goals (e.g., raising children), it may also be psychologically comforting. Such psychological comfort may, in turn, reap physiological dividends in the form of reduced anxiety. From this vantage point, self-verification has an affective regulatory function that may be well served by the identity negotiation process.

Well-Being

There is some indication that a lack of correspondence between people's situated identities and their partners' situated appraisals increases negative emotions and promotes maladaptive psychological and physiological outcomes. For example, Burke (2004) reported that identity-disconfirming events in the context of marital relationships increased people's distress for up to 2 days following the events. Similarly, Wood and colleagues (2005) found that low self-esteem participants felt anxious and concerned when confronted with success, apparently because success feedback was inconsistent with their identity (cf. Lundgren, & Schwab, 1977). Finally, Mendes and Akinola (2006) observed participants' cardiovascular responses to positive and negative evaluations that either confirmed or disconfirmed their self-views. When people received positive feedback, those with negative self-views became physiologically "threatened" (distressed and avoidant). In contrast, when they received negative feedback, people with negative self-views became physiologically "challenged" or galvanized (i.e., aroused, but in a manner associated with approach motivation). People with positive self-views displayed the opposite pattern.

If positive but nonverifying experiences are stressful for people with negative self-views, then over an extended period such experiences might prove to be physically debilitating. Sure enough, several independent investigations support this proposition. An initial pair of prospective studies (Brown & McGill, 1989) examined the impact of positive life events on the health outcomes of people with low and high self-esteem. For high-self-esteem participants, positive life events (e.g., improvement in living conditions, getting very good grades) predicted increases in health; among people low in self-esteem, positive life events predicted *decreases* in health. This finding was recently replicated and extended by Shimizu and Pelham (2004). These researchers discovered that positive life events predicted increased illness among people low in self-esteem, even when controlling for negative affectivity, thereby undercutting the rival hypothesis that negative affect influenced both self-reported self-esteem and reports of symptoms. Apparently, for people with negative self-views, the disjunction between positive life events and their chronically negative identity may be so psychologically threatening that it undermines physical health (cf. Iyer, Jetten, & Tsivrikos, in press).

Work Productivity, Job Retention, and Absenteeism

Recent research suggests that identity negotiation processes can influence outcomes in the workplace. For example, studies of small work groups suggest that, to the extent that individual group members bring their compatriots' appraisals of them in line with their identities, both individuals and groups benefit. Specifically, individuals who elicited identity-congruent appraisals were more committed to the group and performed better than those who did not (Swann, Kwan, Polzer, & Milton, 2003; Swann, Milton, & Polzer, 2000; see also London, 2003). Furthermore, when workers' identities are disconfirmed by the appraisals that their superiors offer them, they may actually leave their jobs. In a large-scale field study of workers in Texas, the investigators found that among employees with high self-esteem, those who received no pay raises were most apt to quit their jobs. In contrast, among employees with low self-esteem, attrition was highest among those who received raises (Schroeder, Josephs, & Swann, 2006). Apparently, employees become dissatisfied and leave their jobs when they receive professional feedback—in the form of financial compensation—that is inconsistent with their long-standing identities. People's identities may even influence their reactions to justice in the workplace. Whereas people with high self-esteem responded to high levels of procedural justice with high commitment and low rates of absenteeism, people with low self-esteem showed no such preferences (Wiesenfeld, Swann, Brockner, & Bartel, 2007).

In short, the outcome of the identity negotiation process, in general, and the fit between a person's situated identity and his or her partner's situated appraisal, in particular, have important implications. When people are seen as they see themselves, they enjoy superior relationship quality and duration, exhibit heightened psychological and physical well-being, and are even more productive and satisfied in the workplace.

Resulting Identity and Relationship Goals

The final step in the model depicted in Figure 17.1 consists of both parties' identities and relationship goals at the conclusion of a given iteration of the identity negotiation process. Although both the negotiator's and partner's resulting identities will usually resemble their initial identities, to a large degree, it is also possible for an identity to shift during the identity negotiation process. In this sense, the identity negotiation model allows for and explains both identity stability and identity change.

The foregoing discussion points to at least five conditions that will increase the probability of permanent (or at least long-term) identity change: (1) the aspect of identity being negotiated is relatively unimportant or uncertain to the person; (2) interpersonal feedback or experiences fall outside the negotiator's or partner's latitude of acceptance (and thus cannot easily be assimilated into preexisting identity); (3) feedback or experiences are difficult or impossible to dismiss (e.g., feedback comes from a highly credible source or is patently obvious); (4) feedback or experiences that are inconsistent with the person's initial identity nonetheless produce outcomes that are perceived as highly desirable; and (5) the social environment lacks opportunity structures (e.g., social networks, physical and psychological resources) that are necessary to sustain a given identity. In the next section, we discuss several factors that precipitate these conditions.

IDENTITY NEGOTIATION AND IDENTITY CHANGE

Up to this point in the chapter we have emphasized the importance of congruence in the perceptions of identity negotiators and their partners, especially when these perceptions match the negotiator's chronic (initial) identity. By implication, changes in identity appear to be unwelcome phenomena that can confuse or even derail the process of identity negotiation. Yet as disruptive and painful as identity changes may sometimes be, they are a natural, unavoidable, and critically important part of life (Marcia, 1980; Robins, Noftle, Trzesniewski, & Roberts, 2005; Whitbourne, 1986). In fact, although some changes in identity are triggered by events over which the negotiator has no control, other changes are triggered by changes in the negotiator him- or herself, some of which are intentional. Here, we consider several different cases of volitional and nonvoli-

tional identity change that reflect, to varying degrees, the five conditions of change listed above.

Sociocultural and Idiosyncratic Contextual Changes

Changes in widespread normative expectations may have a profound impact on how people construe their identity. For example, the civil rights and women's liberation movements in the United States altered cultural expectations and behavioral norms for blacks and women, respectively. Such changed expectations and norms subsequently impacted the identities of members of these groups, as happened when the women's liberation movement led men and women alike to relinquish stereotyped conceptions of women as weak and dependent (e.g., Spence, Deaux, & Helmreich, 1985). These widespread changes in gender stereotypes produced corresponding changes in girls' and women's identity-relevant feedback, experiences, opportunity structures, and outcomes.

People may also encounter changed expectations and behavioral norms when their immediate culture changes rapidly. A particularly dramatic example of such idiosyncratic culture change occurs when people enter "total institutions" (Goffman, 1961), or institutions such as prisons, mental hospitals, and military bases in which all aspects of personal life are controlled and regulated by authorities. In total institutions, those in power theoretically isolate people from their families and friends and systematically program their environments so as to encourage adoption of a new identity (Berger & Luckman, 1966). In general, such institutions are rarely successful in transforming the core identities of those who are disinclined to change (Schein, 1961). Rather, the success of this approach is limited to relatively modest, short-term alterations of behaviors and identities that are of a more peripheral nature.

Environmental Changes

Dramatic identity changes can occur when people shift their social networks by, for example, entering college or moving to a new town or country (e.g., Iyer et al., in press). Such shifts produce identity change for a variety of reasons (see Hormuth, 1990). First, as with the contextual changes described above, new environments inevitably provide people with new expectations and behavioral norms that can produce corresponding changes in identity. Furthermore, novel environments tend to increase people's self-focused attention, which over time can bring about identity change as new self-knowledge is acquired and new self-standards are applied.

Finally, new environments may not afford the opportunity structures that once nurtured and sustained an identity. In such cases, people who (for whatever reasons) fail to *remoor* their identity to a new social structure that resembles the old one will most likely experience identity change (Ethier & Deaux, 1994). For example, some (Sageman, 2004) have speculated that the initial link in the chain of events that led to the terrorist attacks on the World Trade Center in 2001 was set in place when a group of foreign students visited Europe and failed to receive the warm reception that their past successes had led them to expect. So rebuffed, they sought refuge by affiliating with a group of fellow visitors who happened to embrace political views that were far more radical than their own moderate views. Over time, they gradually became more and more aligned with a jihadist group, culminating in the fusion of their personal identities with the social identities associated with this new group (e.g., Swann et al., 2008). The consequences of this identity fusion process were catastrophic.

Developmental Growth and Role Changes

One common source of identity change is set in motion when the larger community recognizes a significant change in the individual. Such changes, for example, may entail the person's age (e.g., when adolescents become adults), status (e.g., when graduate students become professors), or social role (e.g., when singles get married). When such transformations occur, the community may abruptly alter the way that it treats the person. Usually, targets of such differential treatment will eventually become less invested in maintaining their initial identities and become willing to bring their identities into harmony with the treatment they currently receive. Support for such scenarios comes from theories

and research suggesting that late adolescence marks a developmental period during which changing treatment and expectations often prompt significant identity change (Arnett, 2000; Erikson, 1959; Pals, 1999).

Acquisition/Loss of Abilities

At various times in life people acquire new competencies or lose established ones. Although both gains and losses can occur at any point, gains tend to be concentrated during the early years (e.g., acquiring the ability to play sports, drive a car) and losses tend to be concentrated during the later years (e.g., *losing* the ability to play sports, drive a car). Whether people gain or lose an ability, the experience can have important implications for their identity. One especially powerful influence on people's abilities and related capacities is their physical health. Indeed, because serious illnesses have ramifications for so many aspects of people's lives, the shift from "healthy person" to "patient" may be one of the most psychologically wrenching identity transformations that people undergo. In a related vein, the physical changes that inevitably accompany aging can produce profound identity change even in healthy persons (Whitbourne, 1996).

Strategic Self-Verification

When people realize, either explicitly or implicitly, that their chronic identity could prevent them from achieving a valued goal, they may negotiate a situated identity that promotes the attainment of that goal. Over an extended period of time, such negotiations may produce permanent identity change. Consider, for example, a woman who decides that her negative conception of her attractiveness will prevent her from retaining the affections of her lover. Recognizing the problem, she may strive to be more attractive than usual in the context of her relationship with her lover. If her lover recognizes her heightened attractiveness, she may internalize his positive reactions and come to see herself as more attractive than she did originally (Swann et al., 2002). Notably, research shows that positive feedback from an interaction partner can encourage a person to internalize a new self-view (Jones, Gergen, &

Davis, 1962), thus increasing the likelihood that the negotiator's situated identity will become relatively permanent.

Self-Initiated Changes

On a related note, people may initiate an identity change either to address or repair an unsatisfying life situation or because they aspire to self-improvement. People may, for example, decide that they are dissatisfied with their standard of living and take systematic steps to adopt an identity that will accommodate a more lucrative profession. Some research suggests that such intentional identity change requires a self-focused state of mental preparedness or *subjective readiness to change* (Anthis & LaVoie, 2006). Even those who feel prepared for change, however, will likely find it difficult to alter deeply entrenched aspects of their identity simply because they want to (e.g., Swann, 1999). Indeed, for self-initiated identity change to take root successfully, people should change not only their own self-views and/or narratives, but also other aspects of the identity negotiation process that sustained their former identity, such as specific relationship partners and social contexts.

Gateway Identities

At times, people may engage in behavior but resist internalizing an identity that befits the behavior. For example, in recent years smoking rates stabilized at around 21% of U.S. adults (Centers for Disease Control and Prevention, 2005) but the stigma associated with smoking has increased steadily (Kim & Shanahan, 2003). An outgrowth of these trends is that many people take their smoking behavior underground or identify merely as "social smokers," even though they may smoke as energetically and frequently as self-acknowledged smokers. This "pseudo-nonsmoker" identity may be a *gateway identity*, a transitional identity that is relatively safe and nonthreatening but that can lull people into behaviors that eventually precipitate full-blown addiction. Once addiction takes hold, it will promote behaviors that produce lasting identity change.

Gateway identities may help people rationalize a wide range of socially questionable behaviors as well. For example, behaviors that range from mistreating a spouse to accepting a bribe and even murder may all be justified by individuals who acknowledge the behavior yet refuse to accept its identity implications. Although the behaviors justified by the gateway identity might be quite different, they all share the common effect of allowing people to cling to their established identities while engaging in behaviors that conflict with that identity. If the behaviors persist, it will become increasingly likely that the individual will be forced to recognize the behavior for what it is and update the identity in question.

In short, although we believe that identities tend to remain fairly stable, there are several mechanisms that can contribute to identity change. If there is a single quality that all of these mechanisms share, it is that they are either triggered by or lead to changes in the social environment. In this respect, identity negotiation theory shares the assumption of both self-categorization theory (e.g., Turner, Oakes, Haslam, & McGarty, 1994) and self-perception theory (Bem, 1972) that stability in people's interpersonal relations fosters stability in identity. Despite this similarity, however, identity negotiation theory does not assume that people's sense of identity is computed on an ad hoc basis from current inputs from the social environment. Identity negotiation theory rejects this "empty self" assumption, arguing instead that people derive a sense of self not only from currently available social inputs but also from chronically activated beliefs about the self that influence, as well as reflect, social inputs. This feature of identity negotiation theory bolsters its ability to explain the stability as well as changeability of self-knowledge.

SUMMARY AND CONCLUSIONS

"Identity negotiation processes" refer to those activities through which people establish, maintain, and change their identities. This chapter offers a rudimentary theory of identity negotiation. We assume that the identity negotiation process begins when people enter social interactions and strive to establish "who is who." To this end, people follow (largely without awareness or intention) a host of behavioral principles. Generally, these principles encourage people to negotiate identities that are compatible with their chronic self-views. Under some conditions, however, people may reorganize or transform their identity to accommodate new social realities. As a result, although identity negotiation processes and their accompanying intrapsychic mechanisms usually stabilize identities, they can lead to identity change under specifiable conditions.

To help define identity negotiation, we began by noting the ways in which it is related to, but distinct from, other negotiation processes such as asset negotiations. We then elaborated the interpersonal principles and intrapsychic mechanisms that guide identity negotiation processes, and we explained how these processes unfold during each of several successive stages of social interaction. Although our emphasis was on the ways in which the identity negotiation process can foster stable identities, we pointed to some specific conditions under which identity negotiation processes can lead to identity change.

Identity negotiation processes play a critically important role in peoples' relationships by making them predictable and manageable, which in turn allows people to meet their needs and accomplish their goals. Simply put, just as identities define people and make them viable as human beings, the identity negotiation process defines relationships and makes them viable as a foundation for organized social activity.

As a model that emphasizes the interactive influence of personal and social situational antecedents of behavior, identity negotiation theory joins the relatively recent spate of interactionist theories of personality (e.g., Carver & Scheier, 2003; Cervone, 2004; Dweck & Leggett, 1988; Higgins, 1990; Mischel & Shoda, 1999; see Swann & Seyle, 2005, for a discussion). Nevertheless, the theory is unique in its focus on the role of the self, which represents a key component of personality. In addition, by merging two approaches (self-verification theory and symbolic interactionism) that have heretofore received little attention from personality theorists, identity negotiation theory may open up new domains of inquiry regarding the social nature of personality.

ACKNOWLEDGMENTS

We are grateful to Tammy English and Jen Pals for their comments on an earlier version of this chapter.

NOTE

1. Further distinctions can be made between various subtypes of social self-views. Brewer and Gardner (1996), for example, distinguish relational self-views (e.g., personal qualities associated with role relationships) from collective self-views (e.g., personal qualities associated with group memberships, as "sensitive" is for women). Similarly, Gómez et al. (2007) have documented the impact of group identities (e.g., convictions about the groups with which people are aligned, such as "Spaniards are feisty").

REFERENCES

Alexander, C. N., & Knight, G. W. (1971). Situated identities and social psychological experimentation. *Sociometry, 34*, 65–82.

Anthis, K., & LaVoie, J. C. (2006). Readiness to change: A longitudinal study of changes in adult identity. *Journal of Research in Personality, 40*, 209–219.

Arnett, J. J. (2000). Emerging adulthood: A theory of development from the late teens through the twenties. *American Psychologist, 55*, 469–480.

Athay, M., & Darley, J. M. (1981). Towards an interpersonal action-centered theory of personality. In N. Cantor & J. Kihlstrom (Eds.), *Personality, cognition and social interactions* (pp. 281–307). Hillsdale, NJ: Erlbaum.

Axelrod, R., & Hamilton, W. D. (1981). The evolution of cooperation. *Science, 211*, 1390–1396.

Bargh, J. A., & Williams, E. L. (2006). The automaticity of social life. *Current Directions in Psychological Science, 15*, 1–4.

Baumeister, R., & Leary, M. (1995). The need to belong: Desire for interpersonal attachments as a fundamental human motivation. *Psychological Bulletin, 117*, 497–529.

Bem, D. J. (1967). Self-perception: An alternative interpretation of cognitive dissonance phenomena. *Psychological Review, 74*, 183–200.

Bem, D. J. (1972). Self-perception theory. In L. Berkowitz (Ed.), *Advances in experimental social psychology* (Vol. 6, pp. 1–62). New York: Academic Press.

Berger, P. L., & Luckman, T. (1966). *The social construction of reality*. Garden City, NY: Doubleday-Anchor.

Bosson, J. K., & Swann, W. B., Jr. (in press). Self-esteem: Nature, origins, and consequences. In R. Hoyle & M. Leary (Eds.), *Handbook of individual differences in social behavior.* New York: Guilford Press.

Brewer, M. B., & Gardner, W. (1996). Who is this "we"?: Levels of collective identity and self representations. *Journal of Personality and Social Psychology, 71,* 83–93.

Brown, J. D., & McGill, K. J. (1989). The cost of good fortune: When positive life events produce negative health consequences. *Journal of Personality and Social Psychology, 55,* 1103–1110.

Burgess, R. L., & Bushell, D. (1969). *Behavioral sociology: The experimental analysis of social process.* New York: Columbia University Press.

Burke, P. J. (1991). Identity processes and social stress. *American Sociological Review, 56,* 836–849.

Burke, P. J. (2004). Identities, events, and moods. In J. H. Turner (Ed.), *Advances in group processes: Vol. 21. Theory and research on human emotions* (pp. 25–49). New York: Elsevier.

Byrne, D. (1971). *The attraction paradigm.* New York: Academic Press.

Campbell, J. D., Trapnell, P. D., Heine, S. J., Katz, I. M., Lavallee, L. F., & Lehman, D. R. (1996). Self-concept clarity: Measurement, personality correlates, and cultural boundaries. *Journal of Personality and Social Psychology, 70,* 141–156.

Carver, C. S., & Scheier, M. A. (2003). Self-regulatory perspectives on personality. In T. Millon & M. J. Lerner (Eds.), *Handbook of psychology: Personality and social psychology* (Vol. 5, pp. 185–208). New York: Wiley.

Caspi, A., & Roberts, B. W. (1999). Personality continuity and change across the life course. In L. A. Pervin & O. P. John (Eds.), *Handbook of personality: Theory and research* (2nd ed., pp. 300–326). New York: Guilford Press.

Centers for Disease Control and Prevention. (2005). Cigarette smoking among adults: United States, 2004. *Morbidity and Mortality Weekly Report, 54,* 1121–1124.

Cervone, D. (2004). The architecture of personality. *Psychological Review, 111,* 183–204.

Chang-Schneider, C., & Swann, W. B., Jr. (2007). [Self-verification in marital relationships]. Unpublished raw data.

Chen, S., Chen, K. Y., & Shaw, L. (2004). Self-verification motives at the collective level of self-definition. *Journal of Personality and Social Psychology, 86,* 77–94.

Chen, S., Shaw, L., & Jeung, K. Y. (2006). Collective self-verification among members of a naturally-occurring group: Possible antecedents and long-term consequences. *Basic and Applied Social Psychology, 28,* 101–115.

Clarke, G. I. (1954). *Elements of ecology.* New York: Wiley.

Cooley, C. S. (1902). *Human nature and the social order.* New York: Scribner.

Costa, P. T., Jr., & McCrae, R. R. (1994). "Set like plaster"?: Evidence for the stability of adult personality. In T. Heatherton & J. Weinberger (Eds.), *Can personality change?* (pp. 21–40). Washington, DC: American Psychological Association.

Crary, W. G. (1966). Reactions to incongruent self-experiences. *Journal of Consulting Psychology, 30,* 246–252.

Dodgson, P. G., & Wood, J. V. (1998). Self-esteem and the cognitive accessibility of strengths and weaknesses after failure. *Journal of Personality and Social Psychology, 75,* 178–197.

Dweck, C. S., & Leggett, E. L. (1988). A social × cognitive approach to motivation and personality. *Psychological Review, 95,* 256–273.

Endler, N., & Magnusson, D. (1976). Toward an interactional psychology of personality. *Psychological Bulletin, 83,* 956–974.

Erikson, E. H. (1959). *Identity and the life cycle.* New York: International University Press.

Ethier, K. A., & Deaux, K. (1994). Negotiating social identity when contexts change: Maintaining identification and responding to threat. *Journal of Personality and Social Psychology, 67,* 243–251.

Gazzaniga, M. S. (1998). *The mind's past.* Berkeley: University of California Press.

Goffman, E. (1955). On face-work: An analysis of ritual elements in social interaction. *Psychiatry, 18,* 213–231.

Goffman, E. (1959). *The presentation of self in everyday life.* Garden City, NY: Doubleday-Anchor.

Goffman, E. (1961). *Asylums: Essays on the social situation of mental patients and other inmates.* Garden City, NY: Doubleday-Anchor.

Goldberg, L. R. (1981). Language and individual differences: The search for universals in personality lexicons. In L. Wheeler (Ed.), *Review of personality and social psychology* (pp. 141–165). Beverly Hills: Sage.

Gómez, Á., Seyle, C. D., Huici, C., & Swann, W. B., Jr. (2007). *Seeking verification of one's group identity.* Unpublished manuscript, University of Texas at Austin.

Gosling, S. D., Ko, S. J., Mannarelli, T., & Morris, M. E. (2002). A room with a cue: Personality judgments based on offices and bedrooms. *Journal of Personality and Social Psychology, 82,* 379–398.

Greenwald, A. G. (1980). The totalitarian ego: Fabrication and revision of personal history. *American Psychologist, 35,* 603–618.

Guidano, V. F., & Liotti, G. (1983). *Cognitive processes and emotional disorders: A structural approach to psychotherapy.* New York: Guilford Press.

Haslam, N., Bastian, B., & Bissett, M. (2004). Essentialist beliefs about personality and their implications. *Personality and Social Psychology Bulletin, 30,* 1661–1673.

Hawley, A. H. (1950). *Human ecology.* Oxford, UK: Ronald Press.

Higgins, E. T. (1990). Personality, social psychology, and cross-situation relations: Standards and knowledge activation as a common language. In L. A. Pervin (Ed.), *Handbook of personality: Theory and research* (pp. 301–338). New York: Guilford Press.

Homans, G. C. (1974). *Social behavior: Its elementary forms* (rev. ed.). New York: Harcourt Brace Jovanovich.

Hormuth, S. E. (1990). *The ecology of the self: Relocation and self-concept change.* Cambridge, UK: Cambridge University Press.

Hull, C. L. (1943). *Principles of behavior.* New York: Appleton.

Iyer, A., Jetten, J., & Tsivrikos, D. (in press). Torn between identities: Predictors of adjustment to identity change. In F. Sani (Ed.), *Individual and collective self-continuity.* Mahwah, NJ: Erlbaum.

John, O. P. (1990). The "Big Five" factor taxonomy: Dimensions of personality in the natural language and in questionnaires. In L. A. Pervin (Ed.), *Handbook of personality: Theory and research* (pp. 66–100). New York: Guilford Press.

John, O. P., Hampson, S. E., & Goldberg, L. R. (1991). The basic level in personality-trait hierarchies: Studies of trait use and accessibility in different contexts. *Journal of Personality and Social Psychology, 60,* 348–361.

Jones, E. E. (1998). Major developments in five decades of social psychology. In D. T. Gilbert, S. T. Fiske, & G. Lindzey (Eds.), *The handbook of social psychology* (4th ed., Vol. 1, pp. 3–57). Boston: McGraw-Hill.

Jones, E. E., Gergen, K. J., & Davis, K. E. (1962). Some determinants of reactions to being approved or disapproved as a person. *Psychological Monographs, 76,* 17.

Jones, E. E., & Pittman, T. (1982). Toward a general theory of strategic self-presentation. In J. Suls (Ed.), *Psychological perspectives on the self* (Vol. I, pp. 231–262). Hillsdale, NJ: Erlbaum.

Jones, E. E., Rhodewalt, F., Berglas, S., & Skelton, J. A. (1981). Effects of strategic self-presentation on subsequent self-esteem. *Journal of Personality and Social Psychology, 41,* 407–421.

Josephs, R. A., Bosson, J. K., & Jacobs, C. G. (2003). Self-esteem maintenance processes: Why low self-esteem may be resistant to change. *Personality and Social Psychology Bulletin, 29,* 920–933.

Kelley, H. H., & Thibaut, J. W. (1978). *Interpersonal relations: A theory of interdependence.* New York: Wiley.

Kenrick, D. T., & Funder, D. C. (1988). Profiting from controversy: Lessons from the person × situation debate. *American Psychologist, 43,* 23–34.

Kim, S., & Shanahan, J. (2003). Stigmatizing smokers: Public sentiment toward cigarette smoking and its relationship to smoking behaviors. *Journal of Health Communication, 8,* 343–367.

Korman, A. K. (1968). Task success, task popularity, and self-esteem as influences on task liking. *Journal of Applied Psychology, 52,* 484–490.

Lecky, P. (1945). *Self-consistency: A theory of personality.* New York: Island Press.

Lemay, E. P., Jr., & Ashmore, R. D. (2004). Reactions to perceived categorization by others during the transition to college: Internalization and self-verification processes. *Group Processes and Intergroup Relations, 7,* 173–187.

Lempert, R. (1972–1973). Norm-making in social exchange: A contract law model. *Law and Society Review, 7,* 1–32.

Lewin, K. (1999). The conflict between Aristotelian and Galileian modes of thought in contemporary psychology (D. K. Adams, Trans.). In M. Gold (Ed.), *The complete social scientist: A Kurt Lewin reader* (pp. 37–66). Washington, DC: APA.

Lewin, K. (1951). *Field theory in social science.* (D. Cartwright, Ed.). New York: Harper.

Linville, P. W. (1985). Self-complexity and affective extremity: Don't put all of your eggs in one cognitive basket. *Social Cognition, 3,* 94–120.

London, M. (2003). Antecedents and consequences of self-verification: Implications for individual and group development. *Human Resource Development Review, 2,* 273–293.

Lowe, C. A., & Goldstein, J. W. (1970). Reciprocal liking and attributions of ability: Mediating effects of perceived intent and personal involvement. *Journal of Personality and Social Psychology, 16,* 291–297.

Lundgren, D. C., & Schwab, M. R. (1977). Perceived appraisals by others, self-esteem, and anxiety. *Journal of Psychology, 97,* 205–213.

Major, B., Cozzarelli, C., Testa, M., & McFarlin, D. B. (1988). Self-verification versus expectancy confirmation in social interaction: The impact of self-focus. *Personality and Social Psychology Bulletin, 14,* 346–359.

Maracek, J., & Mettee, D. R. (1972). Avoidance of continued success as a function of self-esteem, level of esteem certainty, and responsibility for success. *Journal of Personality and Social Psychology, 22,* 90–107.

Marcia, J. E. (1980). Identity in adolescence. In J. Abelson (Ed.), *Handbook of adolescent psychology* (pp. 159–187). New York: Wiley.

Markus, H. (1977). Self-schemas and processing information about the self. *Journal of Personality and Social Psychology, 35,* 63–78.

Markus, H., & Kunda, Z. (1986). Stability and malleability of the self-concept. *Journal of Personality and Social Psychology, 51,* 858–866.

McAdams, D. P. (1996). Personality, modernity, and the storied self: A contemporary framework for studying persons. *Psychological Inquiry, 7,* 295–321.

McAdams, D. P. (1997). The case for unity in the (post)modern self: A modest proposal. In R. Ashmore & L. Jussim (Eds.), *Self and identity: Fundamental issues* (pp. 46–78). New York: Oxford University Press.

McAdams, D. P. (1999). Personal narratives and the life story. In L. A. Pervin & O. P. John (Eds.), *Handbook of personality: Theory and research* (2nd ed., pp. 478–500). New York: Guilford Press.

McCall, G. J., & Simmons, J. L. (1966). *Identities and interactions.* New York: Free Press.

Mead, G. H. (1934). *Mind, self, and society.* Chicago: University of Chicago Press.

Mendes, W. B., & Akinola, M. (2006). *Getting what you expected: How self-verifying information reduces autonomic and hormonal responses related to threat.* Manuscript in preparation, Harvard University.

Miller, D. T., & Turnbull, W. (1986). Expectancies and interpersonal processes. *Annual Review of Psychology, 37,* 233–256.

Miller, N. E., & Dollard, J. (1941). *Social learning and imitation.* New Haven, CT: Yale University Press.

Mischel, W. (1968). *Personality and assessment.* New York: Wiley.

Mischel, W., & Shoda, Y. (1999). Integrating dispositions and processing dynamics within a unified theory of personality: The Cognitive–Affective Personality System. In L. A. Pervin & O. John (Eds.), *Handbook of personality: Theory and research* (2nd ed., pp. 197–218). New York: Guilford Press.

Odum, E. P. (1963). *Ecology.* New York: Holt, Rinehart & Winston.

Pals, J. L. (1999). Identity consolidation in early adulthood: Relations with ego-resiliency, the context of marriage, and personality change. *Journal of Personality, 67,* 295–329.

Pelham, B. W. (1991). On confidence and consequence: The certainty and importance of self-knowledge. *Journal of Personality and Social Psychology, 60,* 518–530.

Pelham, B. W., & Swann, W. B., Jr. (1994). The juncture of intrapersonal and interpersonal knowledge: Self-certainty and interpersonal congruence. *Personality and Social Psychology Bulletin, 20,* 349–357.

Pinel, E. C., Long, A. E., Landau, M. J., Alexander, K., & Pyszczynski, T. (2006). Seeing I to I: A pathway to interpersonal connectedness. *Journal of Personality and Social Psychology, 90,* 243–257.

Popper, K. R. (1963). *Conjectures and refutations.* London: Routledge.

Rempel, J. K., Holmes, J. G., & Zanna, M. P. (1985). Trust in close relationships. *Journal of Personality and Social Psychology, 49,* 95–112.

Robins, R. W., Noftle, E. E., Trzesniewski, K. H., & Roberts, B. W. (2005). Do people know how their personality has changed?: Correlates of perceived and actual personality change in young adulthood. *Journal of Personality, 73,* 489–521.

Rosenthal, R., & Jacobson, L. (1968). *Pygmalion in the classroom: Teacher expectations and pupils' intellectual development.* New York: Holt, Rinehart & Winston.

Rubin, J. Z., & Brown, B. R. (1975). *The social psychology of bargaining and negotiation.* New York: Academic Press.

Ryff, C. D. (1989). Happiness is everything, or is it?: Explorations on the meaning of psychological well-being. *Journal of Personality and Social Psychology, 57,* 1069–1081.

Sadalla, E. K., Vershure, B., & Burroughs, J. (1987). *Environment and Behavior, 19,* 569–587.

Sageman, M. (2004). *Understanding terror networks.* Philadelphia: University of Pennsylvania Press.

Schein, E. (1961). *Coercive persuasion: A sociopsychological analysis of the "brainwashing" of American civilian prisoners by the Chinese Communists.* New York: Norton.

Schlenker, B. R. (1980). *Impression management.* Monterey, CA: Brooks/Cole.

Schlenker, B. R. (1985). *Identity and self-identification.* In B. R. Schlenker (Ed.), *The self and social life* (pp. 65–99). New York: McGraw-Hill.

Schroeder, D. G., Josephs, R. A., & Swann, W. B., Jr. (2006). *Foregoing lucrative employment to preserve low self-esteem.* Unpublished manuscript.

Secord, P. E., & Backman, C. W. (1965). An interpersonal approach to personality. In B. Maher (Ed.), *Progress in experimental personality research* (Vol. 2, pp. 91–125). New York: Academic Press.

Shimizu, M., & Pelham, B. W. (2004). The unconscious cost of good fortune: Implicit and explicit self-esteem, positive life events, and health. *Health Psychology, 23,* 101–105.

Showers, C. J. (1992). Compartmentalization of positive and negative self-knowledge: Keeping bad apples out of the bunch. *Journal of Personality and Social Psychology, 62,* 1036–1049.

Shrauger, J. S., & Lund, A. (1975). Self-evaluation and reactions to evaluations from others. *Journal of Personality, 43,* 94–108.

Skinner, B. F. (1974). *About behaviorism.* New York: Knopf.

Snyder, M., & Ickes, W. (1985). Personality and social behavior. In G. Lindzey & E. Aronson (Eds.), *Handbook of social psychology* (3rd ed., Vol. 2, pp. 833–947). Reading, MA: Addison-Wesley.

Snyder, M., & Klein, O. (2005). Construing and constructing others: On the reality and the generality of the behavioral confirmation scenario. *Interaction Studies, 6,* 53–67.

Snyder, M., & Swann, W. B., Jr. (1978). Behavioral confirmation in social interaction. *Journal of Experimental Social Psychology, 14,* 148–162.

Snyder, M., Tanke, E. D., & Berscheid, E. (1977). Social perception and interpersonal behavior: On the self-fulfilling nature of social stereotypes. *Journal of Personality and Social Psychology, 35,* 656–666.

Spence, J. T., Deaux, K., & Helmreich, R. L. (1985). Sex roles in contemporary American society. In G. Lindzey & E. Aronson (Eds.), *Handbook of social psychology* (3rd ed., pp. 149–178). New York: Random House.

Sprecher, S. (1998). Insiders' perspectives on reasons for attraction to a close other. *Social Psychology Quarterly, 61,* 287–300.

Stets, J. E., & Burke, P. J. (2003). A sociological approach to self and identity. In M. R. Leary & J. P. Tangney (Eds.), *Handbook of self and identity* (pp. 128–152). New York: Guilford Press.

Story, A. L. (1998). Self-esteem and memory for favorable and unfavorable personality feedback. *Personality and Social Psychology Bulletin, 24,* 51–64.

Stryker, S., & Statham, A. (1985). Symbolic interaction and role theory. In G. Lindzey & E. Aronson (Eds.), *Handbook of social psychology* (3rd ed., pp. 311–378). New York: Random House.

Sullivan, H. S. (1953). *The interpersonal theory of psychiatry.* New York: Norton.

Swann, W. B., Jr. (1983). Self-verification: Bringing social reality into harmony with the self. In J. Suls & A. G. Greenwald (Eds.), *Psychological perspectives on the self* (Vol. 2, pp. 33–66). Hillsdale, NJ: Erlbaum.

Swann, W. B., Jr. (1984). The quest for accuracy in person perception: A matter of pragmatics. *Psychological Review, 91,* 457–477.

Swann, W. B., Jr. (1987). Identity negotiation: Where two roads meet. *Journal of Personality and Social Psychology, 53,* 1038–1051.

Swann, W. B., Jr. (1990). To be adored or to be known: The interplay of self-enhancement and self-verification. In R. M. Sorrentino & E. T. Higgins (Eds.), *Handbook of motivation and cognition: Foundations of social behavior* (Vol. 2, pp. 408–448). New York: Guilford Press.

Swann, W. B., Jr. (1999). *Resilient identities: Self, relationships, and the construction of social reality.* New York: Basic Books.

Swann, W. B., Jr., Bosson, J. K., & Pelham, B. W. (2002). Different partners, different selves: The verification of circumscribed identities. *Personality and Social Psychology Bulletin, 28,* 1215–1228.

Swann, W. B., Jr., Chang-Schneider, C., & Angulo, S. (2007). Self-verification in relationships as an adaptive process. In J. Wood, A. Tesser, & J. Holmes (Eds.), *Self and relationships* (pp. 49–72). New York: Psychology Press.

Swann, W. B., Jr., Chang-Schneider, C., & McClarty, K. L. (2007). Do our self-views matter?: Self-concept and self-esteem in everyday life. *American Psychologist, 62,* 84–94.

Swann, W. B., Jr., De La Ronde, C., & Hixon, J. G. (1994). Authenticity and positivity strivings in marriage and courtship. *Journal of Personality and Social Psychology, 66,* 857–869.

Swann, W. B., Jr., & Ely, R. J. (1984). A battle of wills: Self-verification versus behavioral confirmation. *Journal of Personality and Social Psychology, 46,* 1287–1302.

Swann, W. B., Jr., Griffin, J. J., Predmore, S., & Gaines, B. (1987). The cognitive–affective crossfire: When self-consistency confronts self-enhancement. *Journal of Personality and Social Psychology, 52,* 881–889.

Swann, W. B., Jr., & Hill, C. A. (1982). When our identities are mistaken: Reaffirming self-conceptions through social interaction. *Journal of Personality and Social Psychology, 43,* 59–66.

Swann, W. B., Jr., Kwan, V. S. Y., Polzer, J. T., & Milton, L. P. (2003). Fostering group identification and creativity in diverse groups: The role of individuation and self-verification. *Personality and Social Psychology Bulletin, 29,* 1396–1406.

Swann, W. B., Jr., Milton, L. P., & Polzer, J. T. (2000). Should we create a niche or fall in line?: Identity negotiation and small group effectiveness. *Journal of Personality and Social Psychology, 79,* 238–250.

Swann, W. B., Jr., & Pelham, B. W. (2002). Who wants out when the going gets good?: Psychological investment and preference for self-verifying college roommates. *Self and Identity, 1,* 219–233.

Swann, W. B., Jr., Pelham, B. W., & Chidester, T. (1988). Change through paradox: Using self-verification to alter beliefs. *Journal of Personality and Social Psychology, 54,* 268–273.

Swann, W. B., Jr., Pelham, B. W., & Krull, D. S. (1989). Agreeable fancy or disagreeable truth?: Reconciling self-enhancement and self-verification. *Journal of Personality and Social Psychology, 57,* 782–791.

Swann, W. B., Jr., & Read, S. J. (1981). Self-verification processes: How we sustain our self-conceptions. *Journal of Experimental Social Psychology, 17,* 351–372.

Swann, W. B., Jr., & Seyle, C. D. (2005). Personality psychology's comeback and its emerging symbiosis with social psychology. *Personality and Social Psychology Bulletin, 31,* 155–165.

Swann, W. B., Jr., Seyle, C. D., Gómez, Á., Gaviria, E., Morales, A., & Huici, C. (2008). *Fighting and dying for one's group: The interplay of personal and social selves in extreme group behavior.* Unpublished manuscript, University of Texas at Austin.

Swann, W. B., Jr., Stein-Seroussi, A., & McNulty, S. (1992). Outcasts in a white lie society: The enigmatic worlds of people with negative self-conceptions. *Journal of Personality and Social Psychology, 62,* 618–624.

Thomas, W. I., & Thomas, D. S. (1928). *The child in America: Behavior problems and programs.* New York: Knopf.

Thompson, L. L. (2005). *The mind and heart of the negotiator* (3rd ed.). Upper Saddle River, NJ: Pearson Prentice Hall.

Turner, J. C., Oakes, P., Haslam, S. A., & McGarty, C. (1994). Self and collective: Cognition and social context. *Personality and Social Psychology Bulletin, 20,* 454–463.

Vazire, S., & Gosling, S. D. (2004). e-Perceptions: Personality impressions based on personal websites. *Journal of Personality and Social Psychology, 87,* 123–132.

Walton, R. E., & McKersie, R. B. (1965). *A behavioral theory of labor negotiation.* New York: McGraw-Hill.

Weinstein, E. A., & Deutschberger, P. (1964). Tasks, bargains, and identities in social interaction. *Social Forces, 42,* 451–455.

Whitbourne, S. K. (1986). *The me I know: A study of adult identity.* New York: Springer-Verlag.

Whitbourne, S. K. (1996). Psychosocial perspectives on emotions: The role of identity in the aging process. In C. Magai & S. H. McFadden (Eds.), *Handbook of emotion, adult development, and aging* (pp. 83–98). San Diego, CA: Academic Press.

Wiesenfeld, B. M., Swann, W. B., Jr., Brockner, J., & Bartel, C. (2007). Is more fairness always preferred?: Self-esteem moderates reactions to procedural justice. *Academy of Management Journal, 50,* 1235–1253.

Wiggins, J. S., & Broughton, R. (1985). The interpersonal circle: A structural model for the integration of personality research. In R. Hogan & W. H. Jones (Eds.), *Perspectives in personality* (Vol. 1, pp. 1–47). Greenwich, CT: JAI Press.

Wood, J. V., Heimpel, S. A., Newby-Clark, I., & Ross, M. (2005). Snatching defeat from the jaws of victory: Self-esteem differences in the experience and anticipation of success. *Journal of Personality and Social Psychology, 89,* 764–780.

CHAPTER 18

Self-Regulation

Matthew T. Gailliot
Nicole L. Mead
Roy F. Baumeister

Imagine two individuals who aim to study hard while attending college, save money regularly, and eventually land a good job. One individual successfully meets these goals. When friends invite her to a cookout the day before a big exam, she declines to stay home and study instead. At the grocery store, she resists purchasing the more expensive and tastier name-brand foods and instead buys generic foods. The other individual, however, is not so successful at meeting her goals. Although she plans to study before the big exam, she instead gives into the temptation of partying with friends, succumbs to peer pressure to drink, and then fails to stop drinking and ends up thoroughly intoxicated. Shopping at the mall, she spots several gifts for her friends that are too expensive for her budget, yet she cannot resist purchasing them.

What is the difference between these two individuals? The difference between them is that they vary in their ability to self-regulate. Self-regulation (also commonly referred to as self-control) is the capacity to override one's thoughts, emotions, impulses, and automatic or habitual behaviors. Self-regulation is a vital capacity throughout the entire lifespan. People must constantly adapt and adjust their behavior to new environments and demands by self-regulating. From the student who

must resist partying with friends to study, to the spouse feigning enjoyment at the conversation with the in-laws, life requires frequent self-regulation.

Self-regulation is a prominent component of personality. Early on, Freud (1923/1961) theorized that personality consisted of three components: the id, ego, and superego. The id gave rise to many impulsive and often inappropriate desires, whereas the superego dictated the morally or socially appropriate course of action. It was the role of the ego, however, to ultimately appease both the motives of the id and superego, and thus self-regulate by overriding the hedonistic urges of the id in favor of appeasing the superego. More recent theorizing portrays self-regulation in a similar light, though researchers rarely speak in Freudian terms. Self-regulation allows the individual to resist behaviors such as engaging in unsafe or promiscuous sex, abusing drugs and alcohol, overeating, overspending, fighting or acting violently, procrastinating, and making lewd or negative remarks toward others. In one sense, self-regulation can be seen as a process that allows the influence of personality to outshine the influence of the situation and other factors. A dieter with good self-regulation, for instance, should be able to refrain from eating dessert, even though the server might place a tray of delicious cakes, puddings, and other sweets directly in front of his or her table.

In this chapter we first describe the importance of self-regulation and how good self-regulation often benefits others, perhaps as much as it benefits the individual. We then cover both trait and state self-regulation. That is, self-regulation varies from person to person, as well as from situation to situation. Next, we describe how self-regulation operates, the factors that influence it, its nonconscious aspects, and the biology of it. Last, we present evidence demonstrating the benefits of good self-regulation across a variety of domains, including executive functioning and intellectual performance, interpersonal relationships, prejudice and stereotypes, social rejection, controlling emotions, dieting, drinking alcohol, and consumer behavior.

THE IMPORTANCE OF SELF-REGULATION

There are several reasons to regard self-regulation as highly important. In terms of practical applications, self-regulation is an important contributor to success in life. People with good self-regulation do better in work and in social life, and they have less psychopathology and other problems (Duckworth & Seligman, 2005; Mischel, Shoda, & Peake, 1988; Shoda, Mischel, & Peake, 1990; Tangney, Baumeister, & Boone, 2004).

Self-regulation influences many of the major problems faced by people individually and by society collectively. For instance, poor self-regulation can undermine drinking restraint, thereby possibly contributing to alcoholism and other harmful effects, such as drunk driving, impaired social relationships, and poor work performance. As another example, poor self-regulation can increase the spread of sexually transmitted diseases. All those diseases are, after all, known to be avoidable, provided one either abstains from sex or takes appropriate precautions against infection.

Poor self-regulation also contributes to crime and indeed is regarded as one of its most important causes (Gottfredson & Hirschi, 1990; Pratt & Cullen, 2000). In the movies, criminals often are portrayed as being highly intelligent and skilled at a particular task (e.g., breaking into intricate safes),

yet research depicts a very different picture. Criminals tend to lack self-discipline and to be highly impulsive. Rather than work long hours and save money, for instance, a criminal might lounge around at home and drink beer. Without money when the rent is due, the criminal then might decide impulsively to rob a convenience store. The trait aspect of low self-regulation is apparent in the fact that criminals tend to behave impulsively and erratically even with legal matters, such as having poor driving records, smoking cigarettes, and being involved in unplanned pregnancies (Gottfredson & Hirschi, 1990).

Drug and alcohol abuse is another area in which self-regulation is important. It can be very difficult to abstain from drug and alcohol use after one has established a routine of regular use. Many societal ills abound from such abuse, such as parental neglect, martial conflict, poverty, and crime. Self-regulation can, in theory, allow individuals to resist drug and alcohol abuse, thereby reducing the various problems associated with such abuse.

Self-regulation can also help prevent unhealthy or disordered eating. Bulimia and binge eating, for instance, can be viewed as failures of self-regulation insofar as the individual is overcome by the impulse to binge and fails to refrain from doing so. Self-regulation can also allow people to adhere to their dietary goals and maintain a healthy weight.

Other benefits of self-regulation include controlling monetary spending, performing well in school, and refraining from aggressive or violent behavior. Each of these benefits is important to society. Overspending, for example, is a major problem in modern society, causing individuals to accumulate relatively large debts that can interfere with their ability to pay for necessities, such as food or shelter. The U.S. government spends billions of dollars each year in hopes of improving academic performance—which can be thwarted by poor self-regulation in the form of procrastination, reduced persistence, and an inability to set and reach goals. Likewise, aggression and violence are major obstacles toward an efficient and harmonious social climate, resulting in harmful behaviors such as child, elderly, or spousal abuse. In sum, the costs of poor self-regulation are high, and improved self-regulation likely would reduce or eliminate numerous social ills. A more detailed description of these benefits is included toward the end of the chapter.

A different reason to be interested in self-regulation is its central importance to the psychology of self. Whereas self researchers had long focused on self-concept and self-esteem issues, during the 1980s they came to appreciate self-regulation as one of the most important functions of the self that contains an important key to understanding how the self operates (Baumeister, 1998; Higgins, 1996).

THE SOCIAL NATURE OF SELF-REGULATION

When many people think about self-regulation, they might focus on how good self-regulation benefits the individual. A person with good self-regulation, for instance, can maintain an attractive physique, succeed at school and work, and avoid self-destructive behaviors (e.g., drug addiction). Still other benefits of self-regulation are experienced at the interpersonal level. When the individual successfully self-regulates, it is often others who benefit. For example, good self-regulation should (1) help angry married spouses refrain from yelling at one another (Finkel & Campbell, 2001), (2) reduce the chances of a prejudice boss discriminating against employees of a different race (see Gordijn, Hindriks, Koomen, Dijksterhuis, & Van Knippenberg, 2004; Richeson & Shelton, 2003), and (3) increase monetary donations to charity (Gailliot, Baumeister, Maner, & de Waal, 2006).

That self-regulation benefits everyone is consistent with the idea that humans have evolved to be not only social but also cultural animals (Baumeister, 2005). Prehuman hominids that were able to cooperate with one another and participate in culture probably were far more likely to survive and pass along their genes than their counterparts who were unable to take part in culture. For instance, a "cultural animal" would reap the benefits of sharing food, tools, and knowledge in the group. Culture requires that people override (self-regulate) their own selfish impulses to cooperate with others and adhere to morals, laws, social norms, and other rules. Hence, the capacity for self-regulation probably evolved by facilitating participation

in culture. In this sense, human personality evolved to become less reactive and impulsive and more regulated or controlled.

DISPOSITIONAL ABILITIES IN SELF-REGULATION

Trait Self-Regulation

Personality represents stable, internal dispositions to think and behave in certain ways. In this sense, the ability to self-regulate can be considered a personality trait, insofar as individual differences in self-regulatory ability appear to be at least somewhat stable across the lifespan. Some people tend to be very effective self-regulators throughout the years, whereas other people are not. For instance, Mischel and colleagues (e.g., Mischel, Ebbesen, & Zeiss, 1972; Mischel et al., 1988; Shoda et al., 1990) have conducted studies on the ability to delay gratification. In these studies, children are presented with a marshmallow or other tempting treat and told that they can have the treat immediately or wait until later to receive an additional marshmallow or treat. Some children experience great difficulty resisting the treat and eat it right away, whereas other children are able to wait the full amount of time (e.g., 20 minutes) required to receive the additional treat. Follow-up studies on these same children have shown that those more capable of delaying gratification experience numerous benefits years later, even during adulthood. They perform better on the Scholastic Aptitude Test (SAT), cope better with stress, exhibit better mental health, and are more popular and socially competent. These findings are remarkable in view of the difficulty of predicting any sort of adult behavior based on measurements or observations taken at age 4, and they suggest that there is important continuity in personality from childhood into adulthood on this crucial dimension.

Other evidence on dispositional abilities in self-regulation paints a similar picture. Compared to college students with low-trait self-regulation, those with high-trait self-regulation earn better grades, maintain healthier relationships with others and experience less conflict in those relationships, engage in fewer unlawful acts, and experience better mental health, such as higher self-esteem, better emotion regulation abilities, and fewer impulse control problems, eating disorders, and drug and alcohol disorders. People with high-trait self-regulation also make better relationship partners, in the sense that they are less likely to yell and respond negatively to their partners, threaten to leave the relationship, or avoid discussing important relationship issues. In sum, self-regulation constitutes a stable and enduring personality trait that appears to be highly valuable to both the individual and society.

Conscientiousness

Almost all personality traits are related to one of the five major dimensions of individual differences in personality (the Big Five or five-factor model). Self-regulation is most closely related to the trait of conscientiousness. Like self-regulation, conscientiousness has been conceptualized as comprised of both proactive and inhibitive aspects (e.g., Costa, McCrae, & Dye, 1991). Many different factors are encapsulated by the dimension of conscientiousness, including self-regulation (Conn & Rieke, 1994), constraint, and will to achieve (Digman & Takemoto-Chock, 1981). Unlike trait self-regulation, which emerges and remains predictive of future behavior early in childhood, conscientiousness is fairly low during adolescence, but then it increases and remains stable in later adulthood.

Like self-regulation, conscientiousness has been shown to predict life outcomes, such as high academic achievement and good job performance (e.g., Luciano, Wainwright, Wright, & Martin, 2006). Personality psychologists have devoted attention to examining both conscientiousness and self-regulation, but mainly in terms of the facets underlying the trait of conscientiousness (e.g., Conn & Rieke, 1994). Otherwise, little attention has been paid to understanding the specific link between the two. It could be possible, however, that self-regulation is the acting force ensuring that one's behavior is in accordance with one's values and standards (which are determined partly by conscientiousness). Thus, one moderating variable of outcomes based on self-regulation could be the extent to which one is conscientious. In short, self-regulation and consciousness are clearly related, and both seem to be highly beneficial. Future research would benefit by examining the link between the two more thoroughly.

HOW SELF-REGULATION OPERATES

The TOTE Model

How exactly do people go about self-regulating? Researchers have developed what is known as the *test–operate–test–exit* (TOTE) model (Carver & Scheier, 1981; see Powers, 1973). As an example of the TOTE model, a person might step onto a scale and decide to lose some weight. Then he would perhaps start exercising and eating healthily. After a few weeks, he might step onto the scale again to see if he's made any progress toward his weight loss goals. If he has lost a satisfactory amount of weight, then he might stop dieting and exercising. In this case, weighing himself constitutes the *test* phase because he is testing how close he is to his self-regulatory goals. Exercising and eating healthily constitute the *operate* phase because he is taking action toward pursuing his goals. Finally, deciding to stop dieting and exercise constitute the *exit* phase because he stops paying attention to his weight and trying to lose weight.

Standards

In the previous example, the man had a desired weight in mind. The target weight or goal is referred to as his *standard*. Other examples of standards include the number of hours one hopes to work or study each week or the maximum amount of alcohol it would be socially appropriate to consume in a night. Standards are concepts of possible and usually desirable states, including ideals, expectations, values, and goals. Problems with setting standards, such as when people form vague, ambiguous, or conflicting standards, can undermine self-regulation, (Baumeister, Heatherton, & Tice, 1994). For example, a person might desire both to exercise regularly and to work long hours each week; given the limited amount of time available each day, these two goals could become incompatible insofar as satisfying one prevents him or her from reaching the other.

There are different types of standards. *Ideal* standards reflect hopes and aspirations, whereas *ought* standards reflect duties and obligations (Higgins, 1987; Higgins, Roney, Crowe, & Hymes, 1994; Shah, Higgins, & Friedman, 1998). Chronic orientations toward ideal or ought standards constitute a personality trait, with some people being chronically focused on ideal standards and others chronically focused on ought standards. People are more likely to meet their goals when their chronic focus matches the focus of the situation than when they mismatch (e.g., Freitas, Liberman, & Higgins, 2002). For example, people who are chronically focused on ideal standards would perform better on an exam that stressed the importance of solving as many questions correctly as possible (e.g., an exam for extra credit), that is, the ideal performance, whereas people chronically focused on ought standards would perform better on an exam that stressed the importance of avoiding mistakes.

Monitoring

In the dieting example used above, the man had to pay attention to the extent to which he followed his dietary goals. This focus of attention is referred to as *monitoring*. It's not enough to simply form goals, of course; one must also monitor the extent to which steps are being taken to achieve those goals and the extent to which they bring success or at least progress toward it.

Some researchers have argued that the primary purpose of self-awareness might be to benefit self-regulation via improved monitoring (Carver & Scheier, 1981). People pay attention to the self so as to achieve their goals. Good monitoring generally improves self-regulation, so factors that make monitoring difficult or impair it will generally harm self-regulation. For example, alcohol is associated with a host of self-regulatory failures, and it also reduces self-awareness and hence monitoring (Hull, 1981). With respect to personality, some people may be better monitors than others, and their self-regulatory abilities probably benefit from this monitoring facility.

Self-Regulatory Strength

For successful self-regulation, it is not enough for one simply to form standards and monitor progress toward them. Instead, one must actively exert effort toward achieving those goals. In other words, the *operate* phase of the TOTE model requires effort. Evidence indicates that the ability to self-regulate is limited, such that it seems to rely on a finite energy source or operate like a muscle. More specifically, self-regulation uses up this energy or fatigues the muscle, so that afterward people are less able to self-regulate. In one illustrative study, hungry participants first were presented with a bowl of radishes and some chocolate sweets (Baumeister, Bratslavsky, Muraven, & Tice, 1998). Some participants were asked to eat only the radishes and avoid eating the sweets. Hence, these participants had to self-regulate. Other participants were allowed to eat freely; they did not have to self-regulate. Afterward, the researchers measured how long participants persisted on an impossible figure tracing task. (Persistence requires self-regulation insofar as one must override the urge to quit and instead keep working on the task, even when repeated failures are discouraging and frustrating.) Consistent with the idea that their self-regulatory energy had been used up, participants who had initially avoided the sweets quit much sooner on the figure tracing task than did participants who ate freely. In another study, completing a thought suppression exercise, compared to completing math problems, undermined participants' ability to refrain from drinking free beer later on (Muraven, Collins, & Nienhaus, 2002)—even when they were expecting a driving test. Again, the initial act of self-regulation (suppressing thoughts) presumably depleted the self-regulatory energy needed for the subsequent task. Several other studies have produced similar results. For instance, after coping with a stressful workday, people are less likely to exercise and more likely to choose low-effort activities (e.g., watching television; Sonnentag & Jelden, 2005).

Moreover, the depletion of self-regulation seems to influence personality, such that the influence of some personality traits on behavior increases. For example, people with low self-esteem tend to underestimate and people with high self-esteem tend to overestimate the extent to which other people like them. One study found that completing an initial act of self-regulation amplified these tendencies (Geyer, Gailliot, & Baumeister, 2006). Apparently, self-regulation allows people with high self-esteem to keep their egotism in check, whereas it allows people with low self-esteem to maintain a positive self-image. When their self-regulatory energy has been depleted, however, they appear less able to do so.

Other studies have found that self-regulatory depletion increased (1) the willingness to engage in sexual infidelity among men and sexually promiscuous women (Gailliot & Baumeister, 2007); (2) the amount of food consumed by individuals who regularly try to limit what they eat (Kahan, Polivy, & Herman, 2003; Vohs & Heatherton, 2000); (3) the use of stereotypes among individuals low in motivation to avoid using stereotypes (Gordijn et al., 2004); (4) the amount of alcohol consumed by people scoring high in the temptation to drink (Muraven et al., 2002); and (5) the tendency of individuals with an anxious–ambivalent attachment style (see Hazan & Shaver, 1987) to divulge too much and individuals with an avoidant attachment style to divulge too little personal information when meeting someone new (Vohs, Baumeister, & Ciarocco, 2005). The idea is that people with certain personality types are prone to engage in certain behaviors (e.g., using stereotypes), but are less likely to do so when their self-regulatory resources have been depleted. As a result, their personality shines through, overpowering situational and other demands. In other cases, however, self-regulation facilitates the expression of personality. Hence, in these cases, the influence of personality on behavior is reduced. In one study, for instance, self-regulatory depletion caused participants scoring low in social anxiety to become more passive during a social interaction (Vohs, Gailliot, & Baumeister, 2006). Social interactions often require self-regulatory effort (see the section below), so presumably these participants no longer had the resources required to exert such effort.

Increasing Self-Regulatory Strength

Given that self-regulation is an important ability, it is unfortunate that the capacity for it is limited. Fortunately, however, it might be possible to increase one's self-regulatory stamina, that is, to avoid having one's self-regulatory resources being used up while self-regulating. Specifically, some evidence suggests that regularly self-regulating reduces or prevents self-regulatory depletion (though other studies have failed to replicate these effects). In one study, for instance, some participants self-regulated for 2 weeks (e.g., by continuously maintaining good posture), whereas other participants were not asked to self-regulate over the 2 weeks (Muraven, Baumeister, & Tice, 1999). Participants then completed two self-regulation tasks consecutively in the laboratory: namely, a thought suppression task followed by a persistence task. Participants who had completed the regular exercises participated longer on the persistence task than those who had not exercised (when also taking into account baseline performance at an earlier experimental session). The 2 weeks of self-regulatory exercise presumably improved participants' self-regulatory stamina, such that their self-regulatory "muscle" did not tire as easily.

Other studies have provided converging evidence (for review, see Baumeister, Gailliot, DeWall, & Oaten, in press). In one, a 2-month-long physical exercise program reduced impairments on a visual tracking task after a thought suppression task (Oaten & Cheng, 2006b). Completing the program also caused a decrease in smoking cigarettes, drinking alcohol, eating junk food, consuming caffeine, spending impulsively, watching television, and leaving dirty dishes in the sink, as well as an increase in eating healthily, studying, and controlling emotions. Participants in other studies have exhibited similar improvements after completing a 4-month program aimed at improving spending behaviors (Oaten & Cheng, 2004) and a program on study habits (Oaten & Cheng, 2006a). Furthermore, in a series of studies by Gailliot, Plant, Butz, and Baumeister (2007), some participants who completed 2 weeks of self-regulatory exercises (e.g., altering their habitual speaking patterns, using their nondominant hand for various tasks) performed better on self-regulatory tasks after having suppressed stereotypes or racial remarks (e.g., while interacting with a gay man), compared to participants who did not complete the exercises. Hence, there is a growing body of evidence suggesting that the capacity for self-regulation can be increased with regular exercise.

Counteracting Depletion

Though the ability to self-regulate is limited, self-regulatory resources are, of course, eventually replenished. Otherwise, everyone would run out of self-regulation forever and turn into undisciplined heathens. There appear to be a couple routes to replenishment (also, see below on biology).

One route is via sleep and rest, which seem to restore the ability to self-regulate. Self-regulatory failure is much more frequent during times when people are likely to be tired or fatigued. For instance, people are more likely to break their diets, go on drug or alcohol binges, or commit crimes as the day progresses into the evening (Baumeister et al., 1994). When people rest and recover after work (e.g., during the weekend), they seem to be more effective at self-regulation during the next workday, such as by performing better and taking more initiative (Sonnentag, 2003). Children who lack adequate sleep (due to sleeping disorders) display several signs of poor self-regulation, including externalizing problems, hyperactivity, emotional liability, aggressive behavior, and social difficulties (Rosen et al., 2004). Likewise, there is some evidence that certain forms of rest (i.e., meditation) can replenish self-regulatory strength after it has been depleted (Smith, 2002).

Another means of counteracting ego depletion seems to be experiencing a positive event or emotion. For instance, a series of studies by Tice, Baumeister, Shmueli, and Muraven (2007) found that an initial act of self-regulation impaired performance on later acts of self-regulation, consistent with the idea that self-regulation operates akin to a muscle. A boost of positive emotion, however, eliminated the self-regulatory impairments. For example, after the initial self-regulation task, participants in one study who watched a funny film performed relatively well on the final self-regulation task. Other work by Schmeichel, Vohs, and Baumeister (2005) has found that self-affirmation (see Steele, 1988) produced similar effects. An initial self-regulation task impaired performance on a second task, but not if participants had self-affirmed by thinking and writing about what was important to them.

To be sure, it is far from clear whether these manipulations actually replenish the depleted resource or merely motivate the person to make the exertion despite being depleted. We do think sleep manages to restore the resource in some way. But whether positive affect and self-affirmation actually replenish the depleted resource is hard to say. The comparison to a muscle is instructive. Tired muscles can be restored to their full powers via rest, but short-term incentives can also cause a person to exert strength even with a tired muscle.

Conservation, Motivation, and Acquiescence

Though self-regulation is limited and can be replenished, people do not appear to exhaust their self-regulatory resources. Rather, they appear to conserve their energy, especially when some of it has already been used up. For instance, performance on self-regulation tasks tends to be impaired when participants anticipate having to self-regulate later, compared to when they do not anticipate having to self-regulate, especially when they have already depleted some of their self-regulatory energy (Muraven, Shmueli, & Burkley, 2006). Presumably, individuals conserve their resources as needed.

Motivation, however, also influences one's ability to muster up self-regulatory energy (and indeed the effects of positive affect and self-affirmation, described in the preceding section, may well operate by increasing motivation rather than by replenishing the depleted resource). Muraven and Slessareva (2003) found that an initial self-regulation task (e.g., suppressing thoughts) impaired performance on a second task (e.g., forcing oneself to drink an unpleasant tasting but healthy beverage), consistent with previous findings. The self-regulatory impairments were, however, eliminated when participants were highly motivated to self-regulate on the second task, such as when they were paid for performing well or when they believed that their performance would benefit society (i.e., by helping cure Alzheimer's disease). Hence, it appears that individuals possess limited self-regulatory resources that are generally conserved, but the tendency to conserve can be overridden by motivation. As another simile, self-regulating is like spending money. The amount of money in any given bank account is reduced every time the person makes a purchase, so most people generally try to avoid buying everything they would like, especially when they have little money in their account (or so one would hope!). Given a good reason (motivation) to part from his or her limited cash, however, a person will dip into savings and spend.

The relationship between self-regulation and motivation suggests that self-regulatory depletion might reduce motivation. Specifically, motivation rises and falls in response to situational factors, such as the likelihood that a person believes he or she will successfully meet a goal (Brehm & Self, 1989). Depleted self-regulatory strength makes it less likely that a person will meet his or her goals, so it is plausible that depletion might reduce motivation, thereby impairing self-regulation.

That motivation can make up for the temporary lack of self-regulatory resources suggests that individuals fail to self-regulate because they acquiesce. Indeed, a review of the literature on self-regulation suggested a link between self-regulatory failures and insufficient motivation (Baumeister et al., 1994). A dieter ends up devouring a pack of pop tarts not necessarily because the frosted treats were impossible to resist but rather because resisting seemed too difficult—so the dieter gave up and gave in. During a self-regulatory struggle, the individual experiences an impulse to engage in some undesirable behavior and must restrain this impulse. Hence, the strength of the restraint has to overpower that of the impulse, or else the impulse wins out. For example, someone suffering from nymphomania might have a strong desire to have sex with a particular individual; his inner restraints must override this desire if he is to avoid the sexual liaison. Eventually, people abandon their restraints and acquiesce. Some urges (e.g., the desire to sleep, sit down, or urinate) are probably irresistible, but most others do not seem to be.

In support of the idea that people acquiesce, Hursh and Winger (1995) found that people addicted to drugs used more drugs when prices decreased and fewer drugs when prices increased. The drug users probably had some control over their addiction if they were able to use fewer drugs when prices were too high (though it is plausible that these results are attributable to their spending all of their money on drugs). Thus, drug users might acquiesce when drug prices are too low to resist. Other examples of acquiescence include American soldiers who were addicted to

heroin in Vietnam, yet gave up heroine with apparent ease upon returning to the United States; serial killers never killing others in front of police officers (Douglas, 1996), suggesting that they are capable of restraining themselves when sufficiently motivated; and the Malay of the Indian Archipelago no longer "running amok" (i.e., going on a violent rampage after being treated unfairly) after strict rules were imposed against such behavior. Though people commonly say that they were unable to resist certain behaviors, such as a shopper contending the he or she was unable to resist the purchase of a new outfit, this likely is not the case.

The evidence regarding acquiescence is not definitive, however, and it is somewhat plausible (in theory, at least) that an urge could be irresistible. For example, an urge could be powerful enough that it could not be overridden by weakened restraints. An individual with dispositionally poor self-regulation might be unable to resist his or her impulses in a state of extreme depletion, and perhaps while also being sleep deprived or malnourished (see below). Self-regulation requires higher-order thought and high-level symbolic representations (e.g., imagining the consequences of committing a crime). In the absence of cues signaling the need for self-regulation (e.g., the police), reasons underlying the need for self-regulation might not come to mind in an extremely depleted mental state. In other words, the will of the individual might be dictated entirely by the power of the immediate situation.

NONCONSCIOUS SELF-REGULATION

Being overcome by the power of the situation raises the possibility (albeit slight) that the automatic or nonconscious system (i.e., processes occurring outside of conscious awareness) might take over in a state of extreme depletion, and so the individual is unable to exert self-regulation. From this perspective, the nonconscious system can be a hindrance to successful self-regulation by activating harmful urges. In contrast to this view, a fair amount of evidence suggests that nonconscious processes might often benefit self-regulation. Though self-regulation has been portrayed thus far as relying extensively on controlled or conscious operations, successful self-regulation does not necessarily have to involve the active self.

More specifically, some have argued that goal attainment, from setting goals to completing them, can occur entirely outside of conscious awareness (Bargh, 1990; Bargh, Gollwitzer, Lee-Chai, Barndollar, & Trotschel, 2001). People might achieve their goals without even realizing that they set them! For example, participants in one study who had been unconsciously primed with the concepts of *achievement* or *cooperation* performed better on a subsequent task and were more likely to cooperate with another person, compared to participants who had not been primed (Bargh et al., 2001). This suggests that self-regulatory goals to do well or to get along with others can be activated and satisfied without the conscious mind.

Nonconscious self-regulation can also occur through the goals other people have for a person. Fitzsimons and Bargh (2003) found that priming the concept of *mother* caused participants to perform better on a verbal achievement task, but only among participants whose mothers placed high importance on their children's academic success. Apparently, the nonconscious system helps people to self-regulate for others, and people do not even realize that this occurs. Other research has shown that unpleasant emotions (e.g., sadness) increase activation of thoughts inconsistent with the unpleasant emotion (e.g., happy thoughts; Forgas & Ciarrocchi, 2002). These findings have been interpreted as evidence for nonconscious mood regulation (Gilbert, Pinel, Wilson, Blumberg, & Wheatley, 1998). When harmful thoughts and feelings arise, the nonconscious system can take charge and dispel them, thereby allowing the conscious system to pursue other endeavors.

Though both the conscious and non-conscious systems allow for successful self-regulation, the two likely work together most of the time. Indeed, sometimes the conscious system can transfer its self-regulatory demands to the nonconscious system, such as when forming an implementation intention. An implementation intention is an if–then statement (e.g., "If I think a stereotypical thought, then I will think of something else instead") that tends to improve self-regulation, such as reducing the use of stereotypes (Gollwitzer, 1999; Gollwitzer,

Achtziger, Schaal, & Hammelbeck, 2002; Gollwitzer & Brandstätter, 1997). Implementation intentions might even prevent the depletion of self-regulatory resources (Webb & Sheeran, 2002). Specifically, participants in one study completed the Stroop task, a task that requires an inhibition of the tendency to read words by stating aloud the ink color of color words (e.g., the word *red* printed in blue ink). Prior to completing the task, some participants formed the implementation intention of ignoring the meaning of the words, whereas other participants did not. On a later self-regulatory task, participants who had formed the implementation intentions performed well, whereas those without the implementation intentions did poorly (thus demonstrating the typical effect of self-regulatory depletion). Presumably, the implementation intention allowed the non-conscious system to carry out the effortful aspects of the Stroop task, thereby conserving self-regulatory resources.

Other evidence converges on the idea that the nonconscious system can reduce the effects of self-regulatory depletion. Specifically, participants in one study first were nonconsciously primed with either achievement-related words or neutral words (Weiland, Lassiter, Daniels, & Fisher, 2004). They then completed a task that either did or did not require self-regulation, and finally completed a task requiring persistence toward solving (unsolvable) puzzles. Participants whose self-regulatory resources had been depleted by the initial task quit sooner on the puzzles task—but only when they had been primed with neutral words. The nonconscious activation of *achievement* apparently reduced the workload of the conscious system.

In sum, self-regulation does not necessarily require conscious operations and can occur nonconciously. With respect to personality, some people might have better non-conscious self-regulatory abilities than other people, or their nonconscious system might be more easily influenced or activated to self-regulate. These possibilities await further exploration.

The Biology of Self-Regulation

In line with the emerging importance of biological research in psychological theory, researchers have made several advances in studying the physiological underpinnings of self-regulation. In the brain, the primary region responsible for self-regulation is the prefrontal cortex or frontal lobes. Individuals with damage to this brain region exhibit various self-regulatory deficits, such as being highly impulsive and showing poor and erratic judgment (Damasio, 1994). A classic example dates back to 1847, when an explosion at a railroad construction site shot a metal rod into the frontal lobes of a worker named Phineas Gage. Before the accident, Phineas was a calm, rationale, and decisive person. After the accident, however, he became highly impulsive, indecisive, and temperamental, and he ended up as a homeless drifter.

One brain region important for self-regulation within the prefrontal cortex is the dorsolateral prefrontal cortex (DLPFC), which helps modulate attention. Two studies by Richeson and colleagues (2003) found that the DLPFC might play an important role in the self-regulation of racial prejudice. Specifically, after interacting with a black person, white participants completed the Stroop task as a measure of self-regulation. Participants who held more negative nonconscious attitudes toward blacks performed worse on the Stroop than participants who held more positive attitudes. This effect, however, was mediated by the extent to which the DLPFC was activated (in a separate experimental session) while viewing black faces. In other words, participants whose DLPFC was highly active performed worse on the Stroop task after interacting with someone of a different race. A second study showed that DLPFC activation did not predict Stroop performance after a same-race interaction. It appears that the effects of self-regulatory depletion might be at least partly attributable to the DLPFC's involvement in attentional processes.

This neurobiological evidence shows more specifically how personality can be shaped by biology. Factors that interfere with the neurobiological underpinnings of self-regulation impair behavioral self-regulation. Hence, an individual's personality might be marked by poor self-regulation because certain brain regions are relatively ineffective.

Though pinpointing specific brain regions involved in self-regulation is most certainly an important scientific advancement, the broad generalization that the brain is involved in self-regulation is, of course, not surprising. Perhaps more surprising is research suggesting that body tissue outside of the brain also influences self-regulation. Specifically, it appears that self-regulation relies extensively on glucose available in the bloodstream (Gailliot et al., 2006). A single act of self-regulation reduces the amount of available glucose, thereby impairing later attempts at self-regulation. Moreover, restoring glucose to optimal levels restores self-regulation. For instance, Gailliot and colleagues (2006) found that glucose dropped in participants who controlled their attention while watching a video or interacted with someone of a different race, whereas glucose levels did not change in participants who watched the video as they would normally or interacted with someone of the same race. Low glucose after an initial self-regulation task (i.e., the Stroop, emotion regulation, attention control) predicted poorer performance on a subsequent self-regulation task (i.e., an effortful persistence task, the Stroop task). Furthermore, the effects of self-regulatory depletion were eliminated by a drink that contained glucose. In one illustrative study, an initial self-regulation task caused participants to volunteer for fewer hours to help a woman who had ostensibly been through a recent tragedy. Presumably, helping requires self-regulation (perhaps to override any selfish urges), and so depletion reduced helping. This effect was eliminated, however, when participants drank lemonade sweetened with sugar (glucose) rather than artificial sugar (no glucose). In other words, the glucose drink restored the capacity for self-regulation.

Other evidence converges on the notion that self-regulation relies heavily on glucose, much more so than most other mental process unrelated to self-regulation. For instance, several studies have linked criminal behavior to problems with the use of glucose (Bolton, 1979; Virkkunen & Huttunen, 1982), and poor self-regulation is one of the most prominent causes of criminal behavior. Problems with glucose or low glucose have been linked with several other signs of poor self-regulation, including aggression, impulsivity, deficits in attention control and emotion regulation, troubles coping with stress, and difficulties quitting smoking (Benton & Owens, 1993; Benton, Owens, & Parker, 1994; Donohoe & Benton, 1999; Lustman,

Frank, & McGill, 1991; Simpson, Cox, & Rothschild, 1974; West, 2001). Alcohol consumption impairs self-regulation (Baumeister et al., 1994), and it also reduces glucose in both the body and brain (Altura, Altura, Zhang, & Zakhari, 1996).

Moreover, as already noted, people are more likely to fail at self-regulation as the day progresses into the evening (Baumeister et al., 1994), which parallels declines in the efficiency with which people use glucose (Van Cauter, Polonsky, & Scheen, 1997), as well as the general pattern of metabolic rates, which are higher during the day than at night (Campbell, 1996). Even research on aromatherapy suggests a tie between self-regulation and glucose (Howard, 2006). Aromatherapy has been found to increase metabolism and likewise, to improve self-regulation in several ways, such as by improving vigilance and task performance, as well as increasing agreeableness, cooperation, and helping behavior (though some studies have produced null or conflicting results). Other factors related to glucose and its transportation to the brain (e.g., heart or blood circulatory problems) could very well influence self-regulation.

Nutrition might also influence self-regulation. Both subjectively and in metabolic terms, self-regulation is a demanding process, and it is plausible that effective self-regulation requires healthy nutrition for optimal brain functioning. In support of this view are studies show that giving prisoners and juvenile delinquents vitamin supplements improves their self-regulation by making them better behaved and less violent, whereas placebos do not (Gesch, Hammon, Hampson, Eves, & Crowder, 2002; Schoenthaler et al., 1997). In addition, malnourishment in children has been linked to a host of self-regulatory difficulties, including behavioral, emotional, and academic problems, and especially increased aggression and anxiety (Kleinman et al., 1998).

In short, biology and diet could potentially have a profound impact on self-regulation and hence personality. A stable and consistent diet of healthy foods should lead to consistently good self-regulation, whereas erratic eating and poor nutritional intake should cause fluctuations in self-regulatory abilities. The undisciplined coworker might be verbally aggressive and impulsive not necessarily because he or she is dispositionally unpleasant, but rather because he or she eats Ding-Dongs for breakfast and candy bars for lunch (without being motivated to eat more healthily).

SELF AND EXECUTIVE FUNCTIONING

The part of the self that is responsible for individuals' actions is referred to as the executive function of the self. Put another way, the phrase "executive function of the self" refers to the active, intentional aspects of the personality (see Baumeister, 1998; Gazzaniga, Ivry, & Mangun, 1998). One major executive function is that of self-regulation.

Self-regulation is consistent with the dual-process view of control (see Rothbaum, Weisz, & Snyder, 1982), in which it is posited that people seek harmony between themselves and the environment by trying either to change the world to accommodate the self (primary control) or by trying to change the self to fit with the world (secondary control). We believe that regulation of the self to fit with the environment is probably the most successful strategy for achieving and maintaining harmony between the self and the world. In other words, despite any pejorative connotations of the term "secondary control," it is often of primary importance. As we elaborate in forthcoming sections, when self-regulatory resources are temporarily depleted, people have a difficult time keeping their behavior in check, and vital decision making and thought processes are hindered.

Cognitive Processing

Guidance by the self is often needed to perform complex cognitive functions. These effortful thought processes may consume the same resources as self-regulation. In line with this idea, Schmeichel, Vohs, and Baumeister (2003) found that participants who had previously self-regulated (either by controlling their emotions or attention) subsequently performed worse on tasks requiring complex reasoning compared to participants who had not engaged in a self-regulatory task. For instance, they performed more poorly on logic and reasoning tasks, showed poorer reading comprehension, and had more difficulty when required to complete tasks that required extrapolation of information. Notably, decrements in performance observed when participants are depleted are specific to complex thinking that requires active attention and guidance by the self. Simpler mental activities, such as tests of general knowledge or recall of nonsense syllables, do not seem to be impaired by prior acts of self-regulation (see also Schmeichel, Demaree, Robinson, & Pu, 2006).

Memory

Recent research has begun focusing on the impact of self-regulation on memory. One line of research has specifically examined how self-regulation may impact memory processes that are influenced by involvement of the self. For example, previous work on the *self-choice effect* has shown that when people are able to choose the stimuli they are asked to remember, they are better able to recall that information than participants who are not able to choose the stimuli themselves (Kuhl & Kazén, 1994). If the self has the ability to influence memory, then self-regulation should theoretically have an influence on memory processes. It was found that when people's self-regulatory resources have been depleted, the self-choice effect is eliminated (Schmeichel, Gailliot, & Baumeister, 2005). That is, people whose resources are depleted do not show superior recall of stimuli when they are allowed to choose. Rather, they seem to choose in a more superficial manner, which interrupts the encoding of information and hence, memory. Depleted participants perform just as well as nondepleted participants when self-choice is not involved, such as when the experimenter tells them to remember some items and forget others. Thus, because effortful self-regulation can rob the self of precious resources needed to guide intentional behavior that involves the self, processes influenced by the self (e.g., memory) can become impaired.

Persuasion

If self-regulatory resources are needed to perform complex processes successfully, such as reading comprehension and extrapolation, they may also be required to evaluate, or resist, arguments presented to the self. Research conducted by Knowles, Brennan, and Linn

(2004), in which participants were presented with political advertisements, found that participants' level of skepticism diminished over time. Participants were most skeptical of the first political advertisement with which they were presented and were the least skeptical of the last advertisement with which they were presented. That participants' skepticism diminishes over time suggests that skepticism, and by extension resistance to persuasive attempts, depends on a limited resource that gets used up over time. When self-regulatory resources are used up, people are less able to resist persuasion.

In sum, self-regulation has important implications for cognitive processing, including memory, complex thought, and resisting persuasion. Presumably, self-regulation and the amount of resources available to engage in self-regulation influence these processes because self-regulation is one of the main components of executive functioning—that is, controlling intentional, action oriented behaviors performed by the self.

APPLICATIONS

In this next section we examine several main applications of self-regulation and attempt to clarify how research based primarily on the self-regulatory strength model demonstrates the influence of self-regulation on thought and behavior.

Interpersonal Processes

Picture the last time you met with a boss. Chances are that you automatically acted in a professional and socially appropriate way. Now imagine acting with your boss the same way you act with your friends. Most likely, you would have to make an intentional effort to override the normal, professional way you act with your boss (sometimes this happens at parties, which is probably why alcohol consumption can help!). Hence, self-regulatory resources allow people to monitor the situation and override their natural inclinations in the service of behaving most appropriately. In fact, research has found that participants who are instructed to act in ways that run contrary to their appropriate self-presentational patterns (e.g., presenting oneself very positively to a friend, rather than the more typical behavior of presenting oneself modestly), in comparison to ways that are in accordance with appropriate self-presentational patterns, perform more poorly on subsequent tasks that require self-regulation (Tice, Butler, Muraven, & Stillwell, 1995).

Other research has found that successful self-presentation requires self-regulatory resources. To elaborate, it has been suggested that people have a natural inclination to self-enhance, referred to as "automatic egotism" (Paulhus & Levitt, 1987). Yet, typically, people do not like to interact with others who self-enhance too much. Thus, automatic egotism must be kept in check in order to make a good impression and be liked by others. Egotistical ways of behaving involve an effortful process and should therefore take self-regulatory resources to override. In a series of studies, Vohs and colleagues (2005) found that participants who had engaged in previous acts of effortful self-regulation later become more egotistical, which was indicated by scoring higher on a narcissism scale, relative to participants who had not engaged in effortful self-regulation. Essentially, self-regulatory resources are needed to keep one's automatic egotism in check. When resources are low, people become more narcissistic and less likeable.

With respect to personality, it is likely that the day-to-day self-regulatory demands an individual faces can have an important influence on the impression the individual will make on others. While frequently experiencing stress or other demands, for instance, people might routinely behave in narcissistic ways. It is even probable that poor self-presentational abilities caused by temporary self-regulatory demands (e.g., quitting smoking over 1 month) can turn into enduring, dispositional patterns if they become automatized or engrained into one's personality.

Relationships

Self-regulation is beneficial to social interactions. As we have tried to emphasize, contextually appropriate self-regulation promotes harmonious interactions with others. It is unlikely, however, that all interactions require the same amount of self-regulation. Some interpersonal interactions likely require effortful and consuming self-regulation. In a series of studies, Finkel and colleagues (2006) confirmed the hypothesis that different interactions require differing amounts of self-regulation. More specifically, the researchers found that effortful, high-maintenance interactions with a confederate required more self-regulation than less effortful, low maintenance interactions. Participants who engaged in high-maintenance interactions with a confederate showed decrements in self-regulation on a subsequent task, relative to participants who engaged in effortless, low-maintenance interpersonal interactions.

As we indicated previously, self-regulation is conceptualized as a secondary control process, such that people change the self to be more harmonious with their surroundings. One realm where this can be important is in the maintenance of close romantic relationships. Particularly when faced with a partner who is acting in a negative or destructive manner, it is essential to not respond in kind. Finkel and Campbell (2001) investigated how self-regulation influences individuals' responses to partners who had engaged in potentially destructive behaviors. People can either inhibit the tendency to engage in similar destructive behavior in response to a partner's destructive behavior, or override this response and implement a more constructive response. Thus, self-regulation is needed to override a tendency to reciprocate the destructive behavior and implement a more desirable, harmonious response. In general, self-regulation is positively associated with the tendency to respond in an accommodating manner.

In another study, participants were asked to write about times when they were accommodating and times when they were not accommodating. Behaviors that were indicative of depletion, such as dieting, were more common prior to instances in which participants did not act in an accommodating way to their partner. Presumably, participants were less likely to act in an accommodating manner because they were depleted of the resources needed to implement a more desirable response (Finkel & Campbell, 2001). To follow up these general results, the researchers conducted a laboratory study. They found that participants who were temporarily depleted of self-regulatory resources after an emotion suppression task were more likely to indicate that they would engage in behaviors harmful to a relationship, such as picking a fit or distrusting the partner, and less likely to engage in behaviors helpful to the relationship, such as talking about problems or "letting go" of problems.

Not looking at potentially more attractive partners also could influence one's satisfaction with, and therefore maintenance of, one's romantic relationship. Vohs and Baumeister (2006) found that self-regulation plays an important role in whether one chooses to look at attractive others. They found that, among participants in a committed relationship, self-regulatory depletion increased the amount of time spent looking at magazines featuring scantily clad individuals. Moreover, these results were not simply due to passivity because the increase in time spent looking at magazines was specific to magazines containing pictures of opposite-sex individuals.

In sum, getting along with others requires self-regulation. If people encounter relatively high self-regulatory demands in their lives, then they are more likely to experience interpersonal problems. These problems might create the illusion that the individual's underlying disposition is inherently socially uncooperative. Conversely, people who experience few self-regulatory demands should get along well with others. In this sense, regular self-regulatory demands might shape internal dispositions toward interacting with others.

Prejudice and Stereotypes

When interacting with someone of a different race, stereotypes and expectations about outgroup members come to mind automatically or unintentionally (e.g., Devine, 1989). Trying to keep these thoughts out of mind may require self-regulatory resources, especially if one hopes to have a pleasant interaction. Research conducted on interracial interactions and self-regulation by Richeson and Shelton (2003) found that after highly prejudiced white participants interacted with a black participant, they performed more poorly on a cognitive control task (the Stroop task), compared to participants who interacted with a white participant or participants scoring low in prejudice.

Other contexts, aside from interracial interactions, also seem to require self-regulation. Gordjin and colleagues (Gordijn et al., 2004) found that suppressing stereotypes while writing a narrative about an outgroup member led to self-regulatory depletion. They also found that people who were low in internal motivation to suppress stereotypes (see Plant & Devine, 1998) showed the most pronounced depletion effects when suppressing stereotypes and subsequently showed an increased reliance on stereotypes while writing about the elderly. Apparently, stereotypic thoughts increased after writing the narrative because the resources needed to suppress stereotypical thoughts had been depleted, leading to a general rebound of stereotypic thoughts.

Having a stigmatized identity and then having the identity threatened also influences self-regulation. For example, Inzlicht, McKay, and Aronson (2003) found that black participants who were told that the Stroop task was indicative of intellectual ability performed more poorly on the task than black participants who were not told that the Stroop task was diagnostic of intellectual ability.

Rejection and Ostracism

Self-regulation keeps one's behavior in check with social standards. Humans have a fundamental need to belong. Self-regulation may have evolved with humans and culture because it enabled humans to live harmoniously with one another and reap the benefits of culture. One monitors one's own behavior, and compares it to inner standards as well as to social standards. As mentioned previously, behavior that is rewarded in society often requires successful self-regulation. If there is a break in one's implicit contract with society, one should show decrements in self-regulation. An example of this concerns interpersonal rejection. Baumeister, DeWall, Ciarocco, and Twenge (2005) demonstrated that when people believed they would be alone later in life, or when they had been rejected by peers, they performed worse on tasks that required self-regulation. Additional studies indicated that, after social rejection, individuals are able to self-regulate effectively if given a self-interested reason or incentive to do so. Thus, it is plausible that rejection might undermine the willingness rather than the ability to self-regulate (though it is also plausible that the increased willingness could have made up for a lack of self-regulatory resources). After all, why should people put forth the effort and suffer consequences for the self (e.g., depletion of resources), when doing so will not profit them socially (DeWall, Baumeister, & Vohs, 2007)?

Conversely, it appears that self-regulation may also be needed to reject other people. After all, since humans have a need for attachments, it should be difficult to sever the attachments. Indeed, Ciarocco, Sommer, and Baumeister (2001) found that participants who actively ignored another person showed decrements in self-regulatory performance on a subsequent physical stamina task and a persistence task, compared to those who had not actively ignored another person.

In short, both being rejected and rejecting others impairs self-regulation. Hence, individuals who are chronically rejected or who chronically ostracize others might display dispositionally poor self-regulation. Conversely, popular, well-liked individuals might have fewer factors draining their self-regulatory energy, thus allowing them to maintain positive relationships.

OTHER APPLICATIONS

Emotion Regulation

Self-regulatory resources likely are needed to help control emotions. Research has found that controlling emotions is impaired when one is depleted of self-regulatory resources. For example, Muraven and colleagues (1999) had one group of participants suppress a forbidden thought, whereas another group of participants were able to think whatever they liked. Participants were then shown a funny film clip and were instructed to stifle their emotional response (i.e., avoid laughing or smiling) while watching. Participants who had previously engaged in a thought suppression task were less able to prevent themselves from laughing while watching the film clip, compared to participants who were allowed to think freely. Hence, individuals who experience frequent self-regulatory demands should exhibit personalities marked by negative emotions (e.g., anger, sadness) more so than individuals who experience fewer self-regulatory demands.

Conversely, controlling one's emotions can deplete self-regulatory resources. For instance, after having controlled their emotions, participants have been shown to give up sooner on difficult or impossible tasks (Baumeister et al., 1998; Muraven et al., 1999), be less likely to accommodate to romantic partners' negative behavior (Finkel & Campbell, 2001), drink less of a healthy but bad tasting beverage (Muraven & Slessareva, 2003), and perform more poorly on analytical tasks (Schmeichel et al., 2003).

Dieting

Dieters impose external limits on, and regulations for, food intake. From a resource depletion model perspective, during a tempting situation, ensuring that one's behavior is in accordance with the standards set should consume resources, because one is actively trying to inhibit intake. Hence, there is evidence that people have a stronger desire to consume tasty but unhealthy products after they have engaged in an act of self-regulation (Vohs & Mead, 2006).

Research conducted by Vohs and Heatherton (2000) investigated chronic dieting within the self-regulatory strength model. One study exposed chronic dieters and nondieters to tempting foods. One group was told that the foods were not to be touched because they were for a future experiment, whereas another group was told that the foods were available for eating. Dieters, who are presumably regulating their intake, should have to actively self-regulate more to overcome the desire to eat the available tempting food than would nondieters. Indeed, when subsequently given the opportunity to sample ice cream, dieters in the available food condition ate significantly more ice cream than dieters in the "don't touch" condition. Nondieters were unaffected by these manipulations. A further study found that tempting dieters with food led them to give up sooner than nondieters on a persistence task. Dieters who engaged in an emotion regulation task also subsequently ate more ice cream.

Alcohol

When people have a high temptation to drink, and they are depleted, they drink more (Muraven et al., 2002). For example, participants who had engaged in a thought suppression activity and were subsequently given the opportunity to imbibe, drank more than those who had not self-regulated prior to the task. Notably, participants were told that they would be given a driving test after the task so as to ensure that they were actively trying to limit their alcohol intake. Using ecological momentary sampling methods, Muraven, Collins, Shiffman, and Paty (2005) found that underage participants were more likely to violate their alcohol intake limit on days that were more demanding in terms of self-regulation. Moreover, this was especially true for people with low-trait self-regulation. Thus, alcohol intake may be, in part, a function of self-regulatory strength.

Consumer Behavior

Hoch and Loewenstein (1991) posited that two factors determine whether a person makes a purchase at any given time: One is the strength of the desire to make the purchase, and the other is the amount of self-regulation one has to overcome that desire. A series of laboratory studies conducted by Vohs and Faber (in press) found that participants who had previously exerted self-regulation spent more in an impulsive buying scenario (e.g., at the bookstore) than participants who had not previously engaged in self-regulation. Thus, self-regulation can influence peoples' situational ability to spend or save money.

Passivity

Another study examined whether self-regulatory depletion would cause participants to become more passive during social interactions (Gailliot, Vohs, & Baumeister, 2006). Depleted participants were perceived by others as being more passive (e.g., less active, friendly, talkative, hostile) than were nondepleted participants while instructing others how to perform a task (i.e., how to putt in golf). Depletion increased social passivity only among participants low in social anxiety, however. Among nondepleted participants, low social anxiety was associated with high levels of social activity. Among depleted participants, low social anxiety was associated with low levels of social activity. Presumably, interacting in social situations

requires self-regulatory effort (e.g., impression management; Vohs et al., 2005). When depleted, people are less able or willing to exert such effort and consequently become more passive. People low in social anxiety are typically able to expend such effort, but when depleted, they appear to withdraw from social interactions, as do people high in social anxiety.

CLOSING REMARKS

A growing body of evidence suggests that self-regulation is beneficial for both the individual and society. Some individuals are dispositionally better at self-regulating than others. Moreover, it is plausible that good self-regulation allows the influence of personality to override that of the situation. When self-regulatory abilities are poor, situational factors might mask people's underlying dispositions. We also raise the possibility that temporary self-regulatory demands might have an enduring impact on personality. Self-regulation can be temporarily depleted and hence alter the individual's behavior. The unregulated behaviors might become engrained into personality, thereby shaping personality even in the absence of the self-regulatory depletion. In this sense, the relationship between self-regulation and personality might be cyclical. Impaired self-regulation can influence personality (e.g., social rejection makes people less willing to self-regulate for others and perhaps more dispositionally selfish), which ends up influencing self-regulation (e.g., a selfish individual is probably more likely to be rejected by others, thereby impairing self-regulation). It seems likely that personality and self-regulatory abilities operate in tandem.

REFERENCES

Altura, B. M., Altura, B. T., Zhang, A., & Zakhari, S. (1996). Effects of alcohol on overall brain metabolism. In H. Begleiter & B. Kissin (Eds.), *The pharmacology of alcohol and alcohol dependence: Alcohol and alcoholism* (Vol. 2, pp. 145–180). New York: Oxford University Press.

Bargh, J. A., Gollwitzer, P. M., Lee-Chai, A., Barndollar, K., & Trotschel, R. (2001). The automated will: Nonconscious activation and pursuit of behavioral goals. *Journal of Personality and Social Psychology, 81,* 1014–1027.

Baumeister, R. F. (1998). The self. In D. T. Gilbert, S. T. Fiske, & G. Lindzey (Eds.), *Handbook of social psychology* (4th ed., pp. 680–740). New York: McGraw-Hill.

Baumeister, R. F. (2005). *The cultural animal: Human nature, meaning, and social life.* New York: Oxford University Press.

Baumeister, R. F., Bratslavsky, E., Muraven, M., & Tice, D. M. (1998). Self-control depletion: Is the active self a limited resource? *Journal of Personality and Social Psychology, 74,* 1252–1265.

Baumeister, R. F., DeWall, C. N., Ciarocco, N. J., & Twenge, J. M. (2005). Social exclusion impairs self-regulation. *Journal of Personality and Social Psychology, 88,* 589–604.

Baumeister, R. F., Gailliot, M., DeWall, C. N., & Oaten, M. (in press). Self-regulation and personality: How interventions increase regulatory success, and how depletion moderates the effects of traits on behavior. *Journal of Personality.*

Baumeister, R. F., Heatherton, T. F., & Tice, D. M. (1994). *Losing control: How and why people fail at self-regulation.* San Diego, CA: Academic Press.

Benton, D., & Owens, D. S. (1993). Blood glucose and human memory. *Psychopharmacology, 113,* 83–88.

Benton, D., Owens, D. S., & Parker, P. Y. (1994). Blood glucose influences memory and attention in young adults. *Neuropsychologia, 32,* 595–607.

Bolton, R. (1979). Hostility in fantasy: A further test of the hypoglycemia–aggression hypothesis. *Aggressive Behavior, 2,* 257–274.

Brehm, J., & Self, E. A. (1989). The intensity of motivation. *Annual Review of Psychology, 40,* 109–131.

Campbell, N. A. (1996). *Biology.* Menlo Park, CA: Benjamin/Cummings.

Carver, C. S., & Scheier, M. F. (1981). *Attention and self-regulation: A control theory approach to human behavior.* New York: Springer-Verlag.

Ciarocco, N. J., Sommer, K. L., & Baumeister, R. F. (2001). Ostracism and ego depletion: The strains of silence. *Personality and Social Psychology Bulletin, 27,* 1156–1163.

Conn, S. R., & Rieke, M. L. (1994). *The 16PF fifth edition technical manual.* Champaign, IL: Institute for Personality and Ability Testing.

Costa, P. T., McCrae, R. R., & Dye, D. A. (1991). Facet scales for agreeableness and conscientiousness: A revision of the NEO Personality Inventory. *Personality and Individual Differences, 12,* 887–898.

Damasio, A. R. (1994). The brain binds entities and events by multiregional activation from convergence zones. In H. Gutfreund & G. Toulouse (Eds.), *Biology and computation: A physicist's choice* (pp. 749–758). River Edge, NJ: World Scientific.

Devine, P. G. (1989). Stereotypes and prejudice: Their automatic and controlled components. *Journal of Personality and Social Psychology, 56,* 5–18.

DeWall, C. N., Baumeister, R. F., & Vohs, K. D. (2007). *Recovering from rejection: Undoing the self-regulation deficits stemming from social exclusion.* Manuscript submitted for publication.

Digman, J. M., & Takemoto-Chock, N. K. (1981). Factors in the natural language of personality: Re-analysis, comparison, and interpretation of six major studies. *Multivariate Behavioral Research, 16,* 149–170.

Donohoe, R. T., & Benton, D. (1999). Blood glucose control and aggressiveness in females. *Personality and Individual Differences, 26,* 905–911.

Douglas, J. E. (1996). *Mindhunter: Inside the FBI's elite serial crime unit.* New York: Pocket Books.

Duckworth, A. L., & Seligman, M. E. P. (2005). Self-discipline outdoes IQ in predicting academic performance of adolescents. *Psychological Science, 16,* 939–944.

Finkel, E. J., & Campbell, W. K. (2001). Self-control and accommodation in close relationships: An interdependence analysis. *Journal of Personality and Social Psychology, 81,* 263–277.

Finkel, E. J., Campbell, W. K., Brunell, A. B., Dalton, A. N., Scarbeck, S. J., & Chartrand, T. L. (2006). High-maintenance interaction: Inefficient social coordination impairs self-regulation. *Journal of Personality and Social Psychology, 91*(3), 456–475.

Fitzsimons, G. M., & Bargh, J. A. (2003). Thinking of you: Nonconscious pursuit of interpersonal goals associated with relationship partners. *Journal of Personality and Social Psychology, 84,* 148–164.

Forgas, J. P., & Ciarrocchi, J. W. (2002). On managing moods: Evidence for the role of homeostatic cognitive strategies in affect regulation. *Personality and Social Psychology Bulletin, 28,* 336–345.

Freitas, A. L., Liberman, N., & Higgins, T. E. (2002). Regulatory fit and resisting temptation during goal pursuit. *Journal of Experimental Social Psychology, 38,* 291–298.

Freud, S. (1961). The ego and the id. In J. Strachey (Ed. & Trans.), *The standard edition of the complete psychological works of Sigmund Freud* (Vol. 19, pp. 12–66). London: Hogarth Press. (Original work published 1923)

Gailliot, M. T., & Baumeister, R. F. (2007). Self-regulation and sexual restraint: Dispositionally and temporarily poor self-regulatory abilities contribute to failures at restraining sexual behavior. *Personality and Social Psychology Bulletin, 33,* 173–186.

Gailliot, M. T., Baumeister, R. F., Maner, J. K., DeWall, C. N., Plant, E. A., Tice, D. M., et al. (2006). *Helping behavior is reduced by prior self-regulation and increased by glucose-containing drinks.* Unpublished manuscript.

Gailliot, M. T., Plant, E. A., Butz, D. A., & Baumeister, R. F. (2007). Increasing self-regulatory strength can reduce the depleting effect of suppressing stereotypes. *Personality and Social Psychology Bulletin, 33,* 281–294.

Gailliot, M. T., Vohs, K., & Baumeister, R. F. (2006). [Ego depletion increases passivity.] Unpublished data, Florida State University.

Gazzaniga, M. S., Ivry, R. B., & Mangun, G. R. (1998). *Cognitive neuroscience: The biology of the mind.* New York: Norton.

Gesch, C. B., Hammond, S. M., Hampson, S. E., Eves, A., & Crowder, M. J. (2002). Influence of supplementary vitamins, minerals and essential fatty acids on the antisocial behaviour of young adult prisoners: Randomised, placebo-controlled trial. *British Journal of Psychiatry, 181,* 22–28.

Geyer, A. L., Gailliot, M. T., & Baumeister, R. F. (2006). *Self-control depletion influences perceived self-liability as a function of self-esteem.* Manuscript in preparation.

Gilbert, D. T., Pinel, E. C., Wilson, T. D., Blumberg, S. J., & Wheatley, T. (1998). Immune neglect: A source of durability bias in affective forecasting. *Journal of Personality and Social Psychology, 75,* 617–638.

Gollwitzer, P. M. (1999). Implementation intentions: Strong effects of simple plans. *American Psychologist, 54,* 493–503.

Gollwitzer, P. M., Achtziger, A., Schaal, B., & Hammelbeck, J. P. (2002). *Intentional control of stereotypical beliefs and prejudicial feelings.* Unpublished manuscript, University of Konstanz, Germany.

Gollwitzer, P. M., & Brandstätter, V. (1997). Implementation intentions and effective goal pursuit. *Journal of Personality and Social Psychology, 73,* 186–199.

Gordijn, E. H., Hindriks, I., Koomen, W., Dijksterhuis, A., & Van Knippenberg, A. (2004). Consequences of stereotype suppression and internal suppression motivation: A self-regulation approach. *Personality and Social Psychology Bulletin, 30,* 212–224.

Gottfredson, M. R., & Hirschi, T. (1990). *A general theory of crime.* Stanford, CA: Stanford University Press.

Hazan, C., & Shaver, P. (1987). Romantic love conceptualized as an attachment process. *Journal of Personality and Social Psychology, 52,* 511–524.

Higgins, E. T. (1987). Self-discrepancies: A theory relating self and affect. *Psychological Review, 94,* 319–340.

Higgins, E. T. (1996). The "self digest": Self-knowledge serving self-regulatory functions. *Journal of Personality and Social Psychology, 71,* 1062–1083.

Higgins, E. T., Roney, C. J., Crowe, E., & Hymes, C. (1994). Ideal versus ought predilections for approach and avoidance distinct self-regulatory systems. *Journal of Personality and Social Psychology, 66,* 276–286.

Hoch, S. J., & Loewenstein, G. F. Time-inconsistent preferences and consumer self-control. *Journal of Consumer Research, 17,* 492–507.

Howard, P. J. (2006). *The owner's manual for the brain.* Austin, TX: Bard.

Hull, J. G. (1981). A self-awareness model of the causes and effects of alcohol consumption. *Journal of Abnormal Psychology, 90,* 586–600.

Hursh, S. R., & Winger, G. (1995). Normalized demand for drugs and other reinforcers. *Journal of the Experimental Analysis of Behavior* [Special issue: Behavioral economics], *64,* 373–384.

Inzlicht, M., McKay, L., & Aronson, J. (2006). Stigma as ego depletion: How being the target of prejudice affects self-control. *Psychological Science, 17,* 262–269.

Kahan, D., Polivy, J., & Herman, C. P. (2003). Conformity and dietary disinhibition: A test of the ego-strength model of self-regulation. *International Journal of Eating Disorders, 32,* 165–171.

Kleinman, R. E., Murphy, J. M., Little, M., Pagano, M., Wehler, C. A., Regal, K., et al. (1998). Hunger in children in the United States: Potential behavioral and emotional correlates. *Pediatrics, 101,* 3.

Knowles, E. S., Brennan, M., & Linn, J. A. (2004). *Consuming resistance to political ads.* Manuscript in preparation.

Kuhl, J., & Kazén, M. (1994). Self-discrimination and memory: State orientation and false self-ascription of assigned activities. *Journal of Personality and Social Psychology, 66,* 1103–1115.

Luciano, M., Wainwright, M. A., Wright, M. J., & Martin, N. G. (2006). The heritability of conscientiousness facets and their relationship to IQ and academic achievement. *Personality and Individual Differences, 40,* 1189–1199.

Lustman, P. J., Frank, B. L., & McGill, J. B. (1991). Relationship of personality characteristics to glucose regulation in adults with diabetes. *Psychosomatic Medicine, 53,* 305–312.

Mischel, W., Ebbesen, E. B., & Zeiss, A. R.

(1972). Cognitive and attentional mechanisms in delay of gratification. *Journal of Personality and Social Psychology, 21,* 204–218.

Mischel, W., Shoda, Y., & Peake, P. (1988). The nature of adolescent competencies predicted by preschool delay of gratification. *Journal of Personality and Social Psychology, 54,* 687–696.

Muraven, M., Baumeister, R. F., & Tice, D. M. (1999). Longitudinal improvement of self-regulation through practice: Building self-control through repeated exercise. *Journal of Social Psychology, 139,* 446–457.

Muraven, M., Collins, R. L., & Nienhaus, K. (2002). Self-control and alcohol restraint: An initial application of the self-control strength model. *Psychology of Addictive Behaviors, 16,* 113–120.

Muraven, M., Collins, L. R., Shiffman, S., & Paty, J. A. (2005). Daily fluctuations in self-control demands and alcohol intake. *Psychology of Addictive Behaviors, 19,* 140–147.

Muraven, M., Shmeuli, D., & Burkely, E. (in press). Conserving self-control strength. *Journal of Personality and Social Psychology.*

Muraven, M., & Slessareva, E. (2003). Mechanism of self-control failure: Motivation and limited resources. *Personality and Social Psychology Bulletin, 29,* 894–906.

Oaten, M., & Cheng, K. (2004). *Longitudinal gains in self-control following a money management program.* Manuscript under review.

Oaten, M., & Cheng, K. (2006a). Improved self-control: The benefits of a regular program of academic study. *Basic and Applied Social Psychology, 28,* 1–16.

Oaten, M., & Cheng, K. (2006b). Longitudinal gains in self-regulation from regular physical exercise. *British Journal of Health Psychology, 11,* 717–733.

Paulhus, D. L., & Levitt, K. (1987). Desirable responding triggered by affect: Automatic egotism? *Journal of Personality and Social Psychology, 52,* 245–259.

Plant, E. A., & Devine, P. G. (1998). Internal and external motivation to respond without prejudice. *Journal of Personality and Social Psychology, 75,* 811–832.

Powers, W. T. (1973). *Behavior: The control of perception.* Chicago: Aldine.

Pratt, T. C., & Cullen, F. T. (2000). The empirical status of Gottfredson and Hirschi's general theory of crime: A meta-analysis. *Criminology, 38,* 931–964.

Richeson, J. A., Baird, A. A., Gordon, H. L., Heatherton, T. F., Wyland, C. L., Trawalter, S., et al. (2003). An fMRI investigation of the impact of interracial contact on executive function. *Nature Neuroscience, 6,* 1323–1328.

Richeson, J. A., & Shelton, J. N. (2003). When prejudice does not pay: Effects of interracial contact on executive function. *Psychological Science, 14,* 287–290.

Rosen, C. L., Storfer-Isser, A., Taylor, H. G., Kirchner, H. L., Emancipator, J. L., & Redline, S. R. (2004). Breathing increased behavioral morbidity in school-aged children with sleep-disordered breathing. *Pediatrics, 114,* 1640–1648.

Rothbaum, F., Weisz, J. R., & Snyder, S. S. (1982). Changing the world and changing the self: A two-process model of perceived control. *Journal of Personality and Social Psychology, 42,* 5–37.

Schmeichel, B. J., Demaree, H. A., Robinson, J. L., & Pu, J. (2006). Ego depletion by response exaggeration. *Journal of Experimental Social Psychology, 42,* 95–102.

Schmeichel, B. J., Gailliot, M. T., & Baumeister, R. F. (2005). *Ego depletion undermines the benefits of the active self to memory.* Manuscript submitted for publication.

Schmeichel, B. J., Vohs, K. D., & Baumeister, R. F. (2003). Intellectual performance and ego depletion: Role of the self in logical reasoning and other information processing. *Journal of Personality and Social Psychology, 85,* 33–46.

Schmeichel, B. J., Vohs, K. D., & Baumeister, R. F. (2005). *Self-affirmation and the self's executive function.* Manuscript in preparation.

Schoenthaler, S., Amos, S., Doraz, W., Kelly, M. A., Muedeking, G., & Wakefield, J. (1997). The effect of randomized vitamin–mineral supplementation on violent and non-violent antisocial behavior among incarcerated juveniles. *Journal of Nutritional and Environmental Medicine, 7,* 343–352.

Shah, J., Higgins, E. T., & Friedman, R. S. (1998). Performance incentives and means: How regulatory focus influences goal attainment. *Journal of Personality and Social Psychology, 74,* 285–293.

Shoda, Y., Mischel, W., & Peake, P. K. (1990). Predicting adolescent cognitive and self-regulatory competencies from preschool delay of gratification: Identifying diagnostic conditions. *Developmental Psychology, 26,* 978–986.

Simpson, G. C., Cox, T., & Rothschild, D. R. (1974). The effects of noise stress on blood glucose level and skilled performance. *Ergonomics, 17,* 481–487.

Smith, R. W. (2002). Effects of relaxation on self-regulatory depletion. *Dissertation Abstracts International, 63*(5-B), 2605.

Sonnentag, S. (2003). Recovery, work engagement, and proactive behavior: A new look at the interface between nonwork and work. *Journal of Applied Psychology, 88,* 518–528.

Sonnentag, S., & Jelden (2005). *The recovery paradox: Why we don't exercise after stressful days.* Poster presented at the SIOP conference, Los Angeles.

Steele, C. M. (1988). The psychology of self-affirmation: Sustaining the integrity of the self. In L. Berkowitz (Ed.), *Advances in experimental social psychology* (Vol. 21, pp. 261–302). New York: Academic Press.

Tangney, J. P., Baumeister, R. F., & Boone, A. L. (2004). High self-control predicts good adjustment, less pathology, better grades, and interpersonal success. *Journal of Personality, 72,* 271–322.

Tice, D. M., Baumeister, R. F., Shmueli, D., & Muraven, M. (2007). Restoring the self: Positive affect helps improve self-regulation following ego depletion. *Journal of Experimental Social Psychology, 43,* 379–384.

Tice, D. M., Butler, J. L., Muraven, M. B., & Stillwell, A. M. (1995). When modesty prevails: Differential favorability of self-presentation to friends and strangers. *Journal of Personality and Social Psychology, 69,* 1120–1138.

Tice, D. M., Muraven, M., Slessareva, L., & Baumeister, R. F. (in press). Replenishing the self: Effects of positive affect on performance and persistence following ego depletion. *Journal of Experimental Social Psychology.*

Van Cauter, E., Polonsky, K. S., & Scheen, A. J. (1997). Roles of circadian and rhythmicity and sleep in human glucose regulation. *Endocrine Reviews, 18,* 716–738.

Virkkunen, M., & Huttunen, M. O. (1982). Evidence for abnormal glucose tolerance test among violent offenders. *Neuropsychobiology, 8,* 30–34.

Vohs, K. D., & Baumeister, R.F. (2006). *Depletion of self-regulatory resources makes people selfish.* Unpublished manuscript, University of Minnesota.

Vohs, K. D., Baumeister, R. F., & Ciarocco, N. J. (2005). Self-regulation and self-presentation: Regulatory resource depletion impairs impression management and effortful self-presentation depletes regulatory resources. *Journal of Personality and Social Psychology, 88,* 632–657.

Vohs, K. D., Gailliot, M. T., & Baumeister, R. F. (2006). *Self-control depletion increases passivity.* Manuscript in preparation.

Vohs, K. D., & Heatherton, T. F. (2000). Self-regulatory failure: A resourtce–depletion approach. *Psychological Science, 11,* 249–254.

Vohs, K. D., & Mead, N. L. (2006). *Self-regulatory resource depletion makes people more extreme in their impulses, urges, and judgments: A possible mechanism for ego depletion.* Manuscript in preparation.

Webb, T. L., & Sheeran, P. (2002). Can implementation intentions help to overcome ego-depletion? *Journal of Experimental Social Psychology, 39,* 279–286.

Weiland, P. E., Lassiter, G. D., Daniels, L., & Fisher, A. (2004, January). *Can nonconscious goals moderate self-regulatory failure?* Paper presented at the annual meeting of the Society for Personality and Social Psychology, Austin, TX.

West, R. (2001). Glucose for smoking cessation: Does it have a role? *CNS Drugs, 15,* 261–265.

CHAPTER 19

Self-Presentation of Personality

An Agency–Communion Framework

Delroy L. Paulhus
Paul D. Trapnell

OVERVIEW OF SELF-PRESENTATION

In its most general sense, all of human personality may be seen as self-presentational (Goffman, 1959; Sullivan, 1953t). That is, each human action communicates information about the actor. To most personality psychologists, the term also implies a degree of inauthenticity: Some actions are designed to convey a desired image rather than an accurate representation of one's personality. We follow suit here in using the term *self-presentation* to refer to motivated inaccuracy in self-portrayals. Because human motivation is so rich and diverse, self-presentation is no less so.

Indisputably, self-presentation is responsive to situational demands. When requested to do so, people can tailor their self-presentations exquisitely (e.g., Godfrey, Jones, & Lord, 1986; Holden & Evoy, 2005; Paulhus, Bruce, & Trapnell, 1995). They can also embellish their representations in important real-world encounters. Job applicants, for example, present themselves more favorably during interviews than they do after they have been hired (Rosse, Stecher, Miller, & Levin, 1998). People tend to self-promote more with potential dating partners than

they do in interactions with friends (Rowatt, Cunningham, & Druen, 1998; Tice, Butler, Muraven, & Stillwell, 1995). Proctored questionnaire administrations draw more socially desirable responding than do anonymous Internet studies (Richman, Weisband, Kiesler, & Drasgow, 1999). As a rule, people present themselves more favorably to public audiences than they do in private situations where the only audience is the self. Indeed, Baumeister (1982) viewed this discrepancy as the ultimate operationalization of self-presentation.

In this chapter, however, we are more concerned with chronic individual differences in self-presentation. We argue that such dispositions constitute strong and pervasive aspects of personality. People differ in the degree to which they are attuned to self-presentation demands, are motivated to self-present, and in the nature of the image they tend to present.

Both the process and individual differences literatures are immense. For book-length treatments, see Schlenker (1980), Rosenfeld, Giacalone, and Riordan (1995), or M. R. Leary (1995). Because our mandate here is to reframe rather than exhaust the literature, our coverage is necessarily selective. Our reframing is guided by an audience distinction (public vs. private) and a content distinction (agentic vs. communal image). As detailed below, an *agentic* image involves "getting ahead" whereas a *communal* image involves "getting along" (Bakan, 1966; Hogan, 1983). Our generic two-level framework is previewed in Figure 19.1. Throughout the chapter, we argue that the resulting four subtypes of self-presentation must be treated separately.

As noted already, our emphasis is on individual differences in self-presentation rather than the psychological processes maintaining these differences. However, the process literature has begun to fertilize the individual-differences literatures. Therefore, a brief review of the former is in order.

The Process of Self-Presentation

What psychological processes unfold during an episode of self-presentation? The answer is as complex as personality itself, and only a handful of researchers (e.g., Baumeister, Leary, Schlenker) have devoted sustained attention to the topic. Even fewer have focused on implications for assessment (e.g., Holden & Fekken, 1995; Rogers, 1974). The process most certainly involves the determination of whether or not one's behavior will be pub-

lic (i.e., observed by important others) and, if so, deciding on the appropriate image to present to that audience (Leary & Kowalski, 1990).

It is well known that awareness of an audience alters people's behavior in a variety of ways (Buss, 1980; Duval & Wicklund, 1972). But the production of an effective public self-presentation may require significant effort and attention. This process of regulating public self-presentations is often called *impression management*. If the context is private, there is no need for impression management, and people are often frank with themselves—even about issues that arouse shame and guilt. If the affective consequences are too severe, however, internal defensive processes such as *self-deception* are activated. Note that process researchers with a social-psychological bent tend to play down the inaccuracy implications. Instead, they emphasize that people are simply trying to establish and (to a large extent) live up to a chosen identity (Leary, 1995; Schlenker, Britt, & Pennington, 1996).

The contrast between impression management and self-deception corresponds roughly to the psychoanalytic distinction between conscious processes (e.g., suppression) and unconscious processes (e.g., repression). Within that tradition, the assumption is that

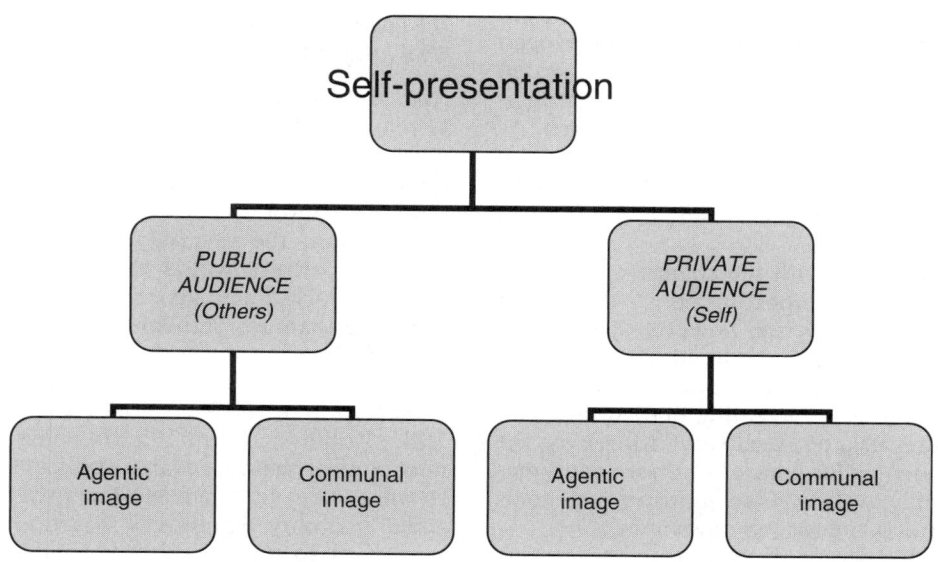

FIGURE 19.1. Hierarchy of self-presentation.

defensive processes can (in fact, must) operate outside of conscious awareness (Weinberger & Silverman, 1979; Westen, Gabbard, & Ortigo, Chapter 3, this volume). Confirmation of such self-deceptive processes in the laboratory has been constrained by prohibitions against inducing a serious psychological threat. One advance was the tightly controlled experiment conducted by Gur and Sackeim (1979): They demonstrated a motivated discrepancy between people's conscious and unconscious recognition of their own voices. Only a handful of other controlled experiments have verified the operation of an unconscious self-presentation process (Baumeister, Dale, & Sommer, 1998; Paulhus, Nathanson, & Lau, 2006; Quattrone & Tversky, 1984).

Those working within the information-processing tradition have characterized this distinction in terms such as in the language of *automatic* versus *controlled* self-presentation (Gilbert, Pelham, & Krull, 1988; M. R. Leary, 1995; Paulhus, 1995; Schlenker, 1980). For example, Paulhus and his colleagues showed clear evidence for an automatic component of self-presentation (e.g., Paulhus, 1995; Paulhus & Levitt, 1987). A key finding was that self-descriptions are more positive under a high cognitive load, for example, when respondents are speeded or engaged in a distracting task (Paulhus, Graf, & Van Selst, 1989).

Another research team provided a detailed account of the transformation of public to private self-presentation: Robert Hogan and John Johnson explained that repeated public self-presentations become automatized so that effort is no longer required. As a result, people's frank self-descriptions are eventually equivalent to their habitual self-presentations (Hogan, 1983; J. A. Johnson & Hogan, 1981).

Consistent with the cognitive tradition, such models attempt to minimize the role of motivation; implicitly, however, it pervades such models. For example, the choice among controlled behaviors is directed largely by motivation (e.g., recreating one's dating persona after negative feedback). Moreover, the conditions under which behavior is automatized may well involve motivational goals (e.g., practicing for job interviews).

In a welcome development, the process of self-presentation is now being studied at the physiological level. The self-regulation approach, for example, links psychological resources to physical resources. The fact that psychological resources are finite is evidenced by the demonstration that people show a measurable depletion in energy and performance after self-presentation episodes (Vohs, Baumeister, & Ciarocco, 2005). Moreover, those psychological resources can be renewed with a boost in glucose (Gailliot et al., 2007). Exciting new brain imaging research has begun to address self-presentation at the neuroscience level. For example, self-enhancement was reduced by activating the medial prefrontal cortex with transcranial magnetic stimulation (Kwan et al., 2007). This physiological work is especially important because it points to possible mechanisms for explaining deleterious effects of self-presentation (M. R. Leary, Tchividjian, & Kraxberger, 1999; Shepperd & Kwavnick, 1999).

In sum, public contexts tend to activate impression management processes tailored to the current audience. Although the result is typically a favorably biased self-portrayal, the key elements are flexibility and appropriateness. In private contexts, where the only audience is the self, personality descriptions may still be biased because of self-deception or habitualized impression management. In Figure 19.1, then, the private audience side subsumes self-deception as well as automatic self-presentation.

The Content of Self-Presentation: What Images Are Presented?

Are self-presentations infinite in number? Given the complexities of our social and work lives, do we really attempt to fine-tune the content of our images to suit each context? As Cantor and Kihlstrom (1987) have pointed out, the everyday management of such a repertoire would require a comprehensive "social intelligence" more elaborate in nature than any standard notions of "g." Instead, theorists suggest that people default to one of a finite number of standard self-presentation roles (e.g., Jones & Pittman, 1982; Robins & John, 1997b). Some people may confine themselves in a stylistic fashion to only one role, whereas others may show some flexibility (Paulhus & Martin, 1988). According to the early interactional framework of Timothy Leary (1957), people may show flexibility in undemanding situations but revert to their predominant role under stress.

To date, the most influential taxonomy of images is the quintet proposed by Jones and Pittman (1982): People can present themselves to embody intimidation, supplication, ingratiation, self-promotion, or exemplification. Research confirms that these five are indeed among the most common in everyday interactions (Bolino & Turnley, 1999).

Other research groups have been able to isolate a variety of self-presentation images (Holden & Evoy, 2005; M. R. Leary et al., 1999). Most comprehensive is the set of 12 self-presentational tactics isolated and measured by Lee, Quigley, Nesler, Corbet, and Tedeschi (1999). Interestingly, recent research using those same taxonomies suggests that the apparently varied measures can be summarized within two overarching themes (Trapnell & Paulhus, in press; Carey & Paulhus, 2008). The two default self-portrayals are (1) agentic (strong, competent, clever) and (2) communal (cooperative, warm, dutiful).

Such research helped convince us of the value of the agency–communion framework for organizing the content of self-presentations. Instead of enumerating the infinite variety of images that people are capable of displaying, we argue that the "Big Two" provide an efficient and coherent summary.

Individual Differences in Self-Presentation Attunement and Motivation

As previewed earlier, our focus in this chapter is on individual differences, rather than context effects, in self-presentation. At least three categories of individual differences have been given substantial attention: (1) attunement or attention to self-presentation, (2) motivation to engage in self-presentation, and (3) the amount of distortion involved in the self-presentation.

Attunement

Some individuals are more responsive to self-presentation issues than others. At least two personality concepts have generated substantial research by pairing an intuitively appealing concept with a solid research instrument.

Mark Snyder's (1974) conception of self-monitoring was that some people, more than others, attend to the social demands of their current situation and adjust their behavior to act in an appropriate fashion. His argument that people can self-report on these tendencies led to the development of his Self-Monitoring Scale (Snyder, 1974). The measure has seen wide usage, especially by social psychologists and, more recently, organizational psychologists. High scorers tend to show a variety of laboratory and real-world manifestations of their behavioral flexibility (e.g., Gangestad & Snyder, 2000).

Other researchers have reframed the concept of self-monitoring. For example, the claim for incremental validity of self-monitoring above and beyond extraversion has been questioned by John, Cheek, and Klohnen (1996). To make a similar point, Briggs and Cheek (1988) separated the extraversion component from the other-directedness factor with distinct subscales and showed distinctive correlates. Along with a revision to the concept, Lennox and Wolfe (1984) developed a revised instrument that partitioned ability and sensitivity subscales. Nonetheless, Snyder's scale continues to be the most popular choice in the research literature.

The other influential individual-difference construct addressing attunement is that of public self-consciousness (Buss, 1980). The idea is that some individuals are especially vigilant and reactive to public attention to their behavior. The standard instrument for measuring public self-consciousness is one of three subscales of the Public and Private Self-Consciousness scale: It also includes measures of private self-consciousness and social anxiety (Fenigstein, Scheier, & Buss, 1975).

Motivation

A variety of relevant personality constructs have arisen out of different assumptions about motivation. One assumption is that people differ in selfishness. Machiavellians, for example, are assumed to misrepresent themselves as part of a general pattern of instrumentally driven behavior (Christie & Geis, 1970). Other constructs based on the same assumption include subclinical psychopathy (Paulhus & Williams, 2002) and unmitigated agency (Helgeson & Fritz, 1999). In all these cases, exploitative self-presentation stems from a more general ego-centric personality.

On the other hand, chronic self-presentation may stem from chronic insecurity. Such was the basis for Crowne and Marlowe's (1964) concept of need for approval: Crowne (1979) concluded that the motive was more defensive than promotional. A similar notion underlay Watson and Friend's (1969) concept of fear of negative evaluation and some current conceptions of subclinical narcissism (e.g., Morf & Rhodewalt, 2001). A deep insecurity may also be the source of perfectionistic self-presentation (Sherry, Hewitt, Flett, Lee-Baggley, & Hall, 2007). Such defensive motivations are directly contrasted with the acquisitive motivations in Arkin's (1981) two-factor model: People may chronically self-present for either self-promotion or self-protection (see also, Lee et al., 1999; Millham, 1974).

Several research groups have offered taxonomies of possible motivations for self-presentation. Swann and colleagues have emphasized two: self-enhancement and self-verification (e.g., Swann, 1990). Others have suggested that people are motivated at various times to self-enhance, self-verify, or be accurate (M. R. Leary, 2007; Sedikides & Strube, 1997).

An even broader taxonomy of self-presentational motives was provided by Robins and John (1997b), who offered intuitively compelling labels to capture four reasons why people's self-perceptions might depart from reality. The egoist is motivated by self-enhancement; the politician, by popularity; the consistency-seeker, by consistency. Only the fourth type, the scientist, is motivated by accuracy. To date, there are no specific measures of these four tendencies, but the labels do ring true as capturing the primary motives for self-presentations.

Degree of Inaccuracy

The remainder of our chapter focuses on measuring the degree of distortion in an individual's self-presentation. Although the possible motives are numerous, the typical content of self-presentation tends to resonate with images of agency and communion. The crossing of those images with the public-versus-private audience distinction—as depicted in Figure 19.1—forms the basis for the third and fourth sections of this chapter.

AGENCY AND COMMUNION AS CONCEPTUAL COORDINATES FOR PERSONALITY

Here we elaborate on the two most common images in self-presentation efforts. The prominence of these two images, we argue, ensues from the centrality of two human metavalues: agency and communion.

Before we make that case directly, we provide the reader with a brief overview of the literature on that topic. These two images, as we show, are not arbitrarily picked from a cherry tree of options. In fact, they derive from the single most powerful framework for organizing the field of human personality. The agency–communion framework helps link values to motives, and motives to goals, traits, and biases (Paulhus & John, 1998). Ultimately, we argue, their influence extends to the content of self-presentation. Whether the audience is self or others, people organize the content of their self-portrayals in terms of these broad themes.

The Organizational Sweep of Agency and Communion

Originating with Bakan's (1966) book, the superordinate labels of *agency* and *communion* have helped frame key issues in personality psychology, social psychology, and psychotherapy. The theoretical impact of the agency–communion distinction was reviewed and extended in an influential chapter by Wiggins (1991). He pointed out parallel distinctions in the literatures on evolutionary theory, gender roles, language, and religion.

Applications of the agency–communion framework have not subsided in recent years. The two constructs have played central roles in recent work on interpersonal behavior measurement (Moskowitz & Zuroff, 2004), interpersonal measurement techniques (Pincus, Gurtman, & Ruiz, 1998), narrative interpretation (McAdams, Hoffman, Mansfield, & Day, 1996), social psychology (Abel & Wojiscke, 2007; Judd, James-Hawkins, Yzerbyt, & Kashima, 2005), and interpersonal psychotherapy (Kiesler & Auerbach, 2003; McMullen & Conway, 1997). Most recently, Len Horowitz and colleagues (2006) have reworked several ingredients of the earlier theoretical positions on agency and communion. As noted below, the agency–communion framework is especially useful in organizing literatures with broad evaluative implications.

The Interpersonal Axes

Even earlier than Bakan, a group of clinical researchers in the San Francisco Bay Area developed a similar two-factor conception of personality (Laforge, Leary, Naboisek, Coffey, & Freedman, 1954). Their work was elaborated in the influential book written by Timothy Leary (1957). They went beyond the two-axis framework to flesh in the intermediate angles and create what was later dubbed the interpersonal circumplex (Carson, 1969). Especially influential were Leary's labels for the trait-level concepts, namely, dominance and nurturance.

Central to their writings was the Sullivanian notion that personality emerges from interpersonal engagement. That notion is also a key element in most theories of self-presentation: Both an actor and an audience are indispensible to the concept.

Picking up from these earlier writers, Jerry Wiggins put the measurement of interpersonal traits on a solid footing. His extensive research program yielded the Interpersonal Adjective Scales, which remains the standard instrument for measuring both the interpersonal axes and the intermediate traits around the interpersonal circle (Wiggins, 1979). Later, McCrae and Costa (1989) linked the interpersonal circle tradition to the five-factor model by showing that dominance and nurturance axes of the interpersonal circumplex were associated with extraversion and agreeableness, respectively (see also Trapnell & Wiggins, 1990). Wiggins and Trapnell (1996) went further to identify agency and communion elements within each of the Big Five factors.

Agency and communion also came to play a key role in the contributions of Robert Hogan: The two axes helped frame his socioanalytic theory (Hogan, 1983). His characterization of agency and communion as "getting along and getting ahead" captured in felicitous fashion the two primary human motives. Along with John Johnson, Hogan

went further to argue that the nature of personality is essentially self-presentational (J. A. Johnson & Hogan, 1981). Their work is a key antecedent to our position that self-presentations of an agentic and/or communal nature are fundamental to personality.

Alternative Labels for the "Big Two" Factors

In recent years a number of other researchers have pointed to the value of a two-dimensional representation of personality (DeYoung, Peterson, & Higgins, 2002; Digman 1997; Judd et al., 2005; Saucier & Goldberg, 2001). Needless to say, all these models stand in stark contrast to the currently dominant five-factor organization (e.g., Costa & McCrae, 1992; John & Srivastava, 1999).

These alternative two-factor models have rather different theoretical histories, and none of the three applies the venerable agency–communion distinction. Digman's (1997) labels were *growth* and *socialization*, whereas Saucier and Goldberg (2001) suggested *dynamism* and *social propriety*. DeYoung and colleagues (2002) preferred the terms *plasticity* and *stability*.

Despite the disparate labels, a closer examination of the items and scale correlates reveals that those three models are remarkably similar in structure and content to the agency–communion model. Accordingly, we believe that our arguments about the content of self-presentation apply to all these two-factor models of personality content.

Note that, in all of these systems, the Big Two dimensions of personality are both positive: That is, society evaluates them both favorably. However, the nature of those two forms of positivity is dramatically different. Indeed, they implicate totally different value systems.

Agentic and Communal Values

The reigning structural model of values is undoubtedly that of Schwartz (1992). His model is a quasi-circumplex in which the relative compatibility or incompatibility of 10 value categories (e.g., power, benevolence, tradition) is represented by their relative distances around a circumplex. By dint of his methodology, Schwartz induced an inherent antagonism between agentic and communal values: They are contrasted on one bipolar dimension, *self-enhancement* (agency) versus *self-transcendence* (communion). The bipolarity of that axis was recently adduced as evidence that U.S. market capitalism promotes values inherently destructive to communion (Kasser, Cohn, Kanner, & Ryan, 2006).

Recently, however, research has indicated that orthogonal agency and communion dimensions can be identified both in Schwartz's value taxonomy and in comprehensive analyses of life goals (e.g., De Raad & Van Oudenhoven, 2008; Hinz, Brähter, Schmidt, & Albani, 2005; Roberts & Robins, 2000). Others have gone further to develop orthogonal measures of agentic and communal values (Locke, 2000; Trapnell & Paulhus, 2008).

Of key importance for this chapter is the notion that these two value systems culminate in rather different self-presentation styles (Paulhus & John, 1998). The style associated with agentic traits (egoism) involves exaggerated achievement striving and self-importance. In contrast, the style associated with communal traits (moralism) involves excessive adherence to group norms and minimization of social deviance.

Other Evaluative Domains

The need to distinguish two evaluative systems has become especially evident in three domains of psychological research: gender roles, dimensions of morality, and cultural values. Social scientists have long noted the strong historical and conceptual parallel between male versus female gender roles and agentic versus communal social roles. In the 1970s this parallel culminated in a new approach to assessing gender roles: Bem (1974) overturned the traditional bipolar notion by constructing independent measures of masculinity and femininity. However, Wiggins and Holzmuller (1978) showed that Bem's two dimensions are psychometrically indistinguishable from the orthogonal interpersonal circumplex dimensions of dominance and nurturance (cf. Spence, 1984).

A related controversy arose in the field of moral development. Gilligan (1982) argued that men and women need to be evaluated on different moral dimensions. Men should be evaluated with respect to instrumental (i.e., agentic) values; women, with regard to relationship (i.e., communal) values. Here again, we see the association of agency and communion with gender-based value systems.

A two-factor conception of self-presentation helps unify these literatures. Most societies make a clear distinction between what is desirable for men and what is desirable for women. From childhood, girls are encouraged to present themselves as "sugar, spice, and everything nice" and boys as "snips, snails, and puppy-dog tails." Even modern societies see no contradiction in honoring and encouraging both images.

Such complementary value systems are also evident in the new generation of research on cultural influences. Triandis's (1989) system led to the placement of countries and cultures within a two-factor system of individualistic and collectivistic values. Markus and Kitayama (1991) carried this distinction into the social psychological literature by contrasting *independent* self-concepts with *interdependent* self-concepts. The parallel between these cultural dimensions and the agency–communion coordinates is evident. In more recent writings, the issues are now specifically framed in terms of the agency and communion labels (Markus & Kitayama, 2003; Phalet & Poppe, 1997).

In sum, the dual values of agency and communion inevitably emerge when value systems are partitioned. Certainly they are implicit in the evaluation of morality, sex roles, and culture.

Links between Values, Motives, Traits, and Self-Presentation

Implicit in our discussion so far is a developmental sequence culminating in the agentic and communal images most typical in the content of self-presentation. In this section we spell out the sequence more explicitly.

Although differing in the details, most personality psychologists assume an interplay between traits, motives, values, and life goals (Roberts & Robins, 2000; Winter, John, Stewart, Klohnen, & Duncan, 2005; Woike, Gershkovich, Piorkowski, & Polo, 1999; see also Pervin, 1994, and the follow-up commentaries). Basic traits may partly determine values and goals (Bauer & McAdams, 2004; McCrae, 1994), may in part be goal-derived social categories (Borkenau, 1990; Read, Jones, & Miller, 1990), and may be inherently evaluative as well as descriptive (Peabody, 1984).

Paulhus and John (1998) have offered a developmental path sequence that applies specifically to the agency–communion model of personality. They argued that ontogeny of personality structure begins with (relatively orthogonal) genetic contributions from the Big Five traits (e.g., McCrae, Jang, Livesley, Riemann, & Angleitner, 2001). Gradually superimposed is the influence of socialization in the form of two preeminent values: agency and communion. Forces that inculcate one agentic trait will tend to inculcate the others (e.g., parents encouraging achievement); the same generalization holds for communal traits (e.g., religious training). Over the course of child development, then, this dual socialization process induces systematic correlations among the Big Five traits. Hence, the two-factor influence appears in higher-order factor analyses of the Big Five factors.

Interestingly, agency and communion also seem to have immediate impact on self-conceptions under conditions of acute evaluative load. For example, if respondents are hurried or forced to co-attend to a concurrent task, the five-factor structure reduces to a two-factor structure (Paulhus, 2002). In some respects, then, our two-factor self-conceptions are more "automatic" than our five-factor self-conceptions. As noted earlier, those automatic self-conceptions tend to emphasize agency or communion. Because automatic responses are socialized via repetition of controlled responses (Paulhus & John, 1998), the two-factor structure of agency and communion can ultimately be traced to society's two predominant socialized values.

Paulhus and John (1998) went further to argue that the two fundamental motives ensuing from two fundamental values are also responsible for the two-factor nature of biased responding. Individuals are rewarded for nurturing and maintaining the perception that they are agentic and/or communal. Accordingly, they err on the side of a biased presentation in those domains. This argument applies equally to socially desirable responding (see the third section) and private self-enhancement (see the fourth section).

SOCIALLY DESIRABLE RESPONDING

Socially desirable responding (SDR) is the term applied to self-presentation on self-report questionnaires (for a review, see Paulhus, 1991). When asked to rate their own personalities, people tend to bias their ratings in the favorable direction (Edwards, 1970). When measured as a stable individual difference, this tendency is often called a *social desirability response style*[1] (Jackson & Messick, 1962). As a local, context-driven behavior, it is known as an SD *response set*. The rationale behind measuring SDR is the diagnosis of dissimulation: High scores on an SDR measure raise concern about a respondent's answers on other questionnaires.

This concern extends to response tendencies beyond a simple positivity bias. People may purposely fabricate a unfavorable image, for example, by misrepresenting themselves as mentally ill (Baer, Rinaldo, & Berry, 2003) or incompetent (Furnham & Henderson, 1982).

A variety of SDR scales have been developed over the years. Attempts to determine the underlying dimensionality have utilized a variety of methods (e.g., Holden & Evoy, 2005; Messick, 1960; Paulhus, 1984) and have yielded a variety of answers. Here we focus on measures of favorable self-presentation and argue for two relatively orthogonal factors corresponding to the agency and communion axes introduced in the previous section.

We begin with a brief historical review of the construct *socially desirable responding*. That history led us ultimately to the view that the agency-versus-communion content distinction and public-versus-private context distinction could help organize and clarify the field. Figure 19.2 shows how these two distinctions map onto the generic framework provided earlier in Figure 19.1.

A History of Competing Operationalizations

Personality psychologists have interpreted SDR in (at least) three different ways. To some, SDR is an idiosyncratic behavior unique to questionnaire responses; to others, it is a personality construct that generalizes to other self-presentation contexts; still others see it as an accurate report of a desirable personality.

Such diversity in interpretations has led to a diversity of operationalizations. Unfortunately, this same diversity led to a singular lack of empirical convergence among SDR measures (Holden & Fekken, 1989; Jackson & Messick, 1962; Paulhus, 1984).

Minimalist Constructs

Some SDR scales are based on a compilation of the total amount of desirable responding in an individual's answers. One standard approach entails (1) collecting SD ratings of a large variety of items, and (2) assembling an SDR measure comprising those items with the most extreme desirability ratings (e.g., Edwards, 1970; Jackson & Messick, 1962; Saucier, 1994). The rationale is that individuals who claim the high-desirability items and disclaim the low-desirability items are likely to be responding on the basis of an item's desirability rather than its accuracy. This operationalization of SDR (e.g., Edwards's SD scale) was open to a serious criticism: Some people actually do have an abundance of desirable qualities and may just be telling the truth (e.g., Block, 1965).

An alternative operationalization of SDR has been labeled *role playing* (Wiggins, 1959). In this case, some participants are asked to "fake good," that is, respond to a wide array of items as if they were trying to appear socially desirable. Other participants are asked for a "straight take": that is, an accurate description of themselves. The items that best discriminate the two groups' responses are selected for the SDR measure. This approach led to the construction of the Minnesota Multiphasic Personality Inventory (MMPI) Malingering scale and Wiggins's Sd scale, which is still proving useful after 30 years (see Baer, Wetter, & Berry, 1992).

Although both operationalizations of social desirability seemed reasonable, representative measures (e.g., Edwards's SD-scale and Wiggins's Sd-scale) showed notoriously low intercorrelations (e.g., Jackson & Messick, 1962; Holden & Fekken, 1989; Paulhus, 1984; Wiggins, 1959). A critical difference in the two-item sets is that the endorsement rates of SD items were relatively high (e.g., "I usually expect to succeed in the things I do"), whereas the endorsement rates

for Sd items (e.g., "I never worry about my looks") were relatively low. To obtain a high score on the Sd scale, one must claim many rare but desirable traits. Thus the Sd scale (and similarly derived measures) indirectly incorporated the notion of exaggeration.

Conceptually Elaborate Constructs

Other attempts to develop SDR measures employed the rational method of test construction. Here, item composition involved specific hypotheses regarding the underlying construct (e.g., Eysenck & Eysenck, 1964; Crowne & Marlowe, 1964; Sackeim & Gur, 1978). The items were designed to trigger different responses in honest responders than in respondents motivated to appear socially desirable. In this respect, the notion of exaggerated positivity was incorporated in the item creation.

Such measures were available as far back as Hartshorne and May (1928). Most influential was the MMPI Lie scale, written to identify individuals deliberately dissembling their clinical symptoms (Hathaway & McKinley, 1951). Eysenck and Eysenck (1964) followed a similar rational procedure in developing the Lie scale of the Eysenck Personality Inventory.

Undoubtedly, the most comprehensive program of construct validity was that carried out by Crowne and Marlowe (1964) in developing their SDR measure. As with the other measures, the items concerned improbable virtues and common human frailties. In contrast to the purely empirical methods, high scores were accumulated by self-descriptions that were not just positive but *improbably* positive.

Crowne and Marlowe (1964) elaborated the character of high scorers by studying their behavioral correlates in great detail. Such research led the authors to a personality interpretation for the underlying construct, namely, *need for approval*. As a result, the Marlowe–Crowne scale, as it came to be called, served two roles in the subsequent personality literature: (1) as an indicator of dissimulation on questionnaires, and (2) as a measure of a personality construct in its own right. The two roles were linked: High scorers dissimulate on the Marlowe–Crowne scale because they fear disapproval from others (Crowne, 1979).

Accuracy Constructs

Other writers never accepted the dissimulation interpretation of SDR measures, maintaining instead that they measure known personality traits. High scorers are to be taken at their word and actually do enjoy a socially desirable character (Block, 1965; McCrae & Costa, 1983; Milholland, 1964). To support the accuracy position, these researchers provided evidence that the self-reports on SDR instruments correlate with reports by knowledgeable informants.

Historically, the most influential example is the vigorous set of arguments set out in Block's (1965) book, the *Challenge of Response Sets*. His view was that high scores on Edwards's SD scale (as well as the first factor of the MMPI) represented a desirable personality syndrome called ego resiliency. His evidence included the confirmation by knowledgeable observers (e.g., spouses) of many of the desirable qualities that were self-ascribed on the SD scale.

McCrae and Costa (1983) developed a similar argument for the accuracy of self-descriptions on the Marlowe–Crowne and EPQ Lie scales. Because high scores were largely sustained by spouses, McCrae and Costa suggested that they reflect good social adjustment instead of SDR.

An Integrative Perspective

Few personality assessors are willing to completely accept the accuracy position. An obvious case where respondents cannot be taken at their word is with the assessment of narcissism. A spate of studies has demonstrated that the favorable claims of narcissists (e.g., "People admire me") are rarely substantiated by the facts (e.g., Paulhus et al., 2003; Robins & John, 1997a). Instead, the data indicate that narcissists are better characterized by their insecurity and inaccuracy (Morf & Rhodewalt, 2001).

A reconciliation between the distortion and accuracy positions can be drawn from work by Millham and Jacobson (1978). They showed that high Marlowe–Crowne scorers would lie and cheat to impress experimenters of their good character. Such ironic distortion along with the accuracy demonstrated by other researchers can be explained under the umbrella construct of *need for approval*.

High scorers realize that carrying out socially conventional behavior is usually the best way to gain approval; they also realize that deceit works better in a number of situations where detection is very unlikely.

A related idea points to the effort to project an identity. To ensure that others accurately view one as well adjusted, there are times when one may have to deny certain "misleading" facts; to ensure that others view one accurately as autonomous, one may have to exaggerate the supportive evidence (Schlenker & Weigold, 1990).

In sum, the available unidimensional measures of SDR appear to tap some unclear combination of distortion and reality. The distortion component is implicated when respondents describe themselves in unrealistic terms across a variety of trait dimensions.

Two-Factor Models of SDR

Alpha and Gamma

The notion that SDR appears in two distinct forms was recognized by a number of early researchers (e.g., Jackson & Messick, 1962). Factor analyses consistently revealed two independent clusters of SDR measures noncommittally labeled *Alpha* and *Gamma*[2] by Wiggins (1964).

The Alpha factor was most clearly marked by Edwards's (1970) SD scale, the MMPI K-scale (Hathaway & McKinley, 1951), Byrne's (1961) Repression–Sensitization scale, and Sackeim and Gur's (1978) Self-Deception Questionnaire. Measures falling directly on the Gamma factor included Wiggins's (1959) Sd scale. Others loading strongly included Eysenck's Lie scale (Eysenk & Eysenck, 1964), the Marlowe–Crowne scale, the Good Impression scale (Gough, 1957), the MMPI Lie scale (Hathaway & McKinley, 1951), and Sackeim and Gur's (1978) Other-Deception Questionnaire. For many years, researchers debated how to interpret the Alpha and Gamma factors of SDR. Ultimately, Paulhus (1984) settled on the labels *Self Deception* and *Impression Management*.

A Two-Factor Measure

After several preliminary versions, Paulhus (1986) offered measures of these two factors with scales labeled *Self-Deceptive Enhancement* (SDE) and *Impression Management* (IM). Together, the scales formed early versions of the widely distributed Balanced Inventory of Desirable Responding— Version 6 (BIDR-6; Paulhus, 1991, 1998b). Sample items include SDE ("My first impressions about people are always right") and IM ("I always pick up my litter"). The BIDR is now as widely used as the Marlowe–Crowne scale.

The SDE and IM scales yielded a useful combination of response style measures in that they captured the two major SDR dimensions with only a small to moderate intercorrelation. Their utility was demonstrated in several studies of self-presentation in a job applicant context. Paulhus and colleagues (1995) showed that the IM scale, but not SDE, was extremely sensitive to faking instructions requesting various degrees of self-presentation. In some studies, IM has been shown to moderate the validity of personality scales (Holden, 2007). In an actual applicant setting, the IM scale showed a special sensitivity to self-presentation (Rosse et al., 1998).

In other studies, the SDE scale, but not the IM, predicted various kinds of self-promotional distortions. These include tendencies toward overclaiming (Paulhus et al., 2003), narcissism (Paulhus, 1998a) and hindsight bias (Hoorens, 1995). High-SDE individuals also exhibit a discordance with reality, as indicated by a discrepancy in self-ratings of agency relative to ratings by group consensus (Paulhus, 1998a). More recently, SDE has also shown utility in moderating the validity of other self-report scales (Berry, Page, & Sackett, 2007; Otter & Egan, 2007). More than 40 other studies, the majority from other laboratories, have helped elaborate the construct validity of the SDE and IM scales. For an extensive list, readers are invited to view the following website (*www.psych.ubc.ca/~dpaulhus/research/BIDR*).

The adjustment correlates of these response style measures correspond to the adjustment correlates of agency and communion. In general, SDE, but not IM, is positively related to self-perceptions of mental health (e.g., Bonanno, Field, Kovacevic, & Kaltman, 2002; Brown, 1998; Nichols & Greene, 1997; Paulhus, 1998b; Paulhus &

Reid, 1991). High SDE also has a positive association with task performance in certain circumstances (E. A. Johnson, 1995). In a study of discussion groups, however, high SDE scorers were perceived negatively after several meetings (Paulhus, 1998a). Those results bear directly on the debate about whether positive illusions are adaptive (see the fourth section).

Untangling Image Content and Audience

The labels *self-deception* and *impression management* turned out to be, at best, incomplete characterizations of Alpha and Gamma. The problem was uncovered by a series of studies that varied the self-presentation instructions (Paulhus, 2002). The Impression Management label for Gamma measures was originally justified by their sensitivity to instructional manipulations, such as "Respond in a socially desirable way" (e.g., Paulhus, 1984; Wiggins, 1964). Further research indicated that respondents interpreted such instructions to mean "Respond as if you are a 'nice person,' 'well socialized,' or 'good citizen.'" In retrospect, the instructions were tantamount to "Act communal."

With more agentic instructions (e.g., "Respond as if you are strong and competent"), Alpha measures were actually more responsive than Gamma measures (Paulhus, Tanchuk, & Wehr, 1999). In short, Alpha-related measures may be no more self-deceptive than are Gamma measures.

What, then, are we to make of the Alpha and Gamma factors of SDR? It appears that current measures of these factors confound content with manipulability. Both forms of distortion appear under anonymous conditions, suggesting a self-deceptive quality. Yet, with appropriate faking instructions, both are subject to impression management.

According to Paulhus (2002), the solution was to discard Alpha and Gamma and distinguish the content of SDR measures (agentic vs. communal) from their responsiveness to an audience manipulation (public vs. private). That distinction is represented by the two levels in Figure 19.2. Dissimulation to a public audience involves impression management of either agentic or communal forms. Dissimulation to a private audience (i.e., the self) involves self-deception via asset exaggeration and/or deviance denial.

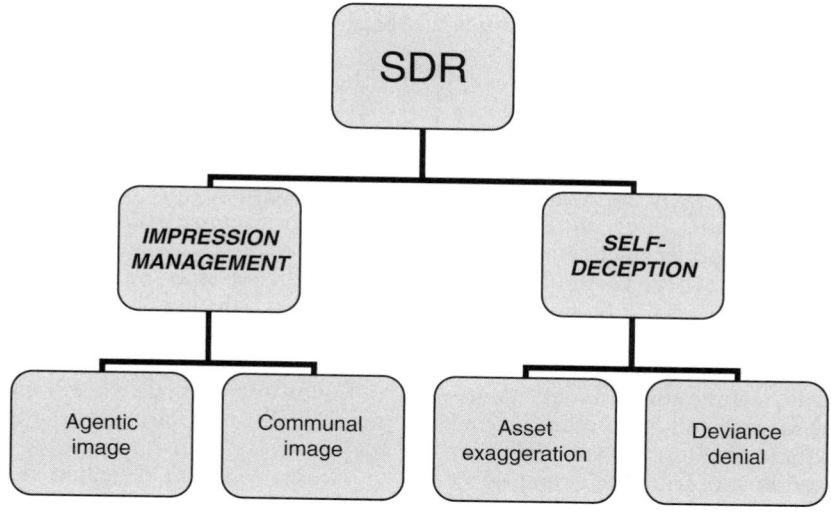

FIGURE 19.2. Hierarchy of socially desirable responding.

The content difference in SDR measures maps onto the agentic and communal values elucidated in the second section of this chapter. Excessive pressure from agentic values induces a tendency to exaggerate one's assets. This tendency leads to unrealistically positive self-perceptions on such personality traits as dominance, fearlessness, emotional stability, intellect, creativity, and even one's attractiveness. Self-perceptions of high scorers have a narcissistic, "superhero" quality. This self-deceptive distortion was summarized using the term *egoistic bias* (Paulhus & John, 1998). Similarly, excessive adherence to communal values induces a self-deceptive tendency to deny socially deviant impulses and claim sanctimonious, "saint-like" attributes. The tendency is played out in overly positive self-perceptions on such traits as agreeableness, dutifulness, and restraint. This version was labeled *moralistic bias* (Paulhus & John, 1998).

Responsiveness to audiences, that is, impression management, must also be distinguished in terms of content. People may be motivated to deliberately exaggerate their standing on agency or communion. The usual two clusters of traits are involved but the exaggeration is more deliberate. *Agency Management*, that is, asset-promotion or bragging, occurs on attributes such as competence, fearlessness, and creativity. Such behavior is most commonly seen in job ap-

plicants or in males attempting to impress a dating partner. Dissimulation on communal attributes is termed *Communion Management* and involves excuse making and damage control of various sorts. Such deliberate minimization of faults is likely in religious settings, in employees who are trying to exemplify integrity, or legal defendants trying to avoid punishment.

Measures of all four types of SDR measures are now available (Paulhus, 2005). Indeed, two of the four have been available for some time as subscales in the BIDR-6. Asset exaggeration can be measured with the SDE scale, now renamed Self-Deceptive Exaggeration to avoid confusion with the term *self-enhancement* in the fourth section. The Impression Management scale also remains useful but was renamed Communion Management to better indicate the scale's content.

Two new measures were developed to tap the unmeasured cells in Figure 19.2. The concept of self-deception on communal traits involves the denial of socially deviant thoughts and behaviors: They are incompatible with the preservation of one's social groups. The new subscale, *Self-Deceptive Denial* (SDD), includes such sample items as "I have never been cruel to anyone" and "I have never hated my parents." The fourth measure, *Agentic Management*, consists of items related to agency content but with low endorsement rates in straight-take administrations. The low endorsement rates for such items permit room for manipulators to deliberately enhance impressions of their agency. Examples are "I am very brave" and "No one is more talented than I." Such items tend not to be claimed, even by narcissists, under anonymous conditions. But the endorsement rate is higher under agency-motivated conditions than under anonymous conditions (Lonnqvist, Verkasalo, & Bezmenova, 2007).

The impression management scales—Agentic and Communal Management—appear to be most useful in tapping response sets rather than response styles. They perform very well in capturing the degree of situational press to appear agentic or communal (Carey & Paulhus, 2008). Because scores are influenced strongly by context subtleties, these scales are not especially useful as individual difference measures. In private administrations, much of the individual-difference variance represents actual content differences in positive qualities.

Summary

The traditional concern in the social desirability literature is with self-presentation on questionnaires. Such concern led to the development of numerous SDR scales measuring the degree to which respondents exaggerate their assets or minimize their social deviance. The assumption is that high scores indicate dissimulation not only on the SDR scale, but on all other questionnaires in the same package.

A 50-year history of structural analyses of SDR scales repeatedly confirmed that multiple underlying concepts were being tapped. We have argued here that a clearer understanding of this extensive literature emerges from our two-level framework: audience (public vs. private) and personality image (agency vs. communal).

The SDR approach has been of special interest to personality psychologists because of their continuing reliance on self-report questionnaires (Paulhus & Vazire, 2007; Tracy & Robins, this volume). Nonetheless, there remains some difficulty with confirming the degree to which SDR scales tap exaggeration, that is, departure from reality.

SELF-ENHANCEMENT

Although the concept of self-enhancement overlaps conceptually with SDR, its historical origins are quite distinct. It began with an early study suggesting that positive self-biases are maladaptive (Frenkel-Brunswik, 1939). Forty years later, two methodologically superior papers provided evidence that positive self-biases may be more adaptive than accurate self-evaluations (Alloy & Abramson, 1979; Lewinsohn, Mischel, Chaplin, & Barton, 1980). Those studies contributed to Taylor and Brown's (1988) assertion that positive illusions are both common and adaptive.

Rather than SDR scales, this literature employs measures such as social comparison (e.g., better than average) or self-criterion discrepancies. Because a normative comparison is involved, such measures promised to do a better job than do SDR scales in distinguishing distortion from truth.

Most writers follow Taylor and Brown (1988) in defining self-enhancement as an overly positive self-evaluation. The qualification—*overly positive*—is of central importance, given our requirement of inaccuracy in defining self-presentation. There is little dispute about the fact that some people harbor overly positive self-evaluations, whereas others are more accurate. To date, minimal attention has been paid to underestimated evaluations (but see Zuckerman & Knee, 1996).[3]

Self-enhancement can be demonstrated even on anonymous self-descriptions (Baumeister, 1982; Brown, 1998). As such, the phenomenon corresponds to the private-audience version of SDR. Because of its association with illusions rather than purposeful dissimulation, little attention has been directed at the public-audience version of self-enhancement (see Figure 19.3). Because self-reports vary with degree and nature of the audience, scores on self-enhancement measures should vary to the same degree as do SDR measures (Carey & Paulhus, 2008). Nonetheless, that issue has attracted less interest, and the following focus is on distortion in private self-beliefs.

Three issues have dominated the self-enhancement literature: One is how to measure self-enhancement; a second addresses

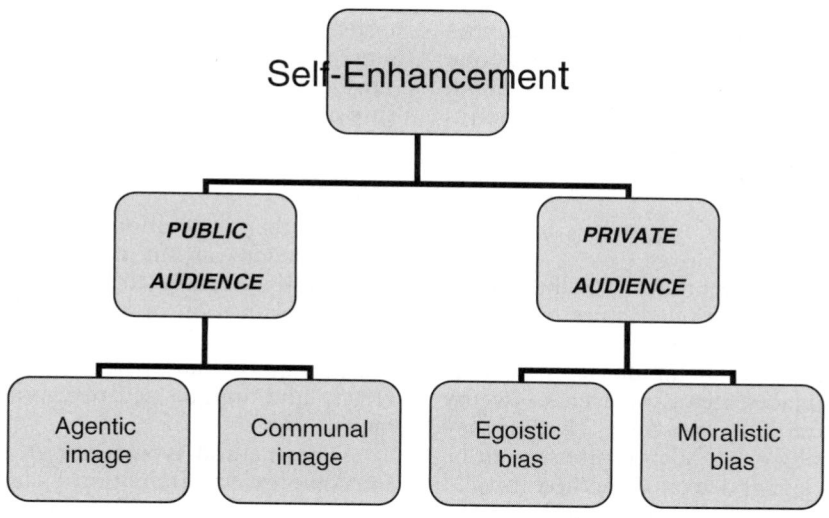

FIGURE 19.3. Hierarchy of self-enhancement.

the adaptiveness of self-enhancement; the third concerns the breadth and structure of self-enhancement.

Operationalizing Self-Enhancement

Although the concept might seem straightforward, much controversy has arisen over the choice of operationalization. Here we consider five types of operationalization that warrant special attention.

Social Comparison

The most popular choice has been to index self-enhancement as the tendency to view oneself more positively than one views others. Following Kwan, John, Kenny, Bond, and Robins (2004), we refer to this operationalization as *social comparison*. A well-replicated body of research indicates that a majority of people tend to rate themselves as above average on lists of evaluative traits (e.g., Alicke, 1985). If pervasive, this tendency certainly implies an illusion: After all, it is not possible for a large majority of people to actually be better than average.[4]

To index a general tendency, self-enhancement scores are typically aggregated across a wide set of evaluative traits. Respondents may be asked for separate ratings of self and others or, alternatively, a direct

comparison of themselves relative to the average other. A number of studies have confirmed that individuals scoring high on such indexes of self-enhancement tend to be well adjusted (Brown, 1986; Campbell, Rudich, & Sedikides, 2002; Kurt & Paulhus, 2008; Taylor, Lerner, Sherman, Sage, & McDowell, 2003).

Note, however, that this operationalization makes it difficult to distinguish self-enhancement from true differences in positive traits (Klar & Giladi, 1999; Robins & John, 1997b). After all, many people are actually above average, even across a large set of traits (Block & Colvin, 1994). In short, the social comparison operationalization lacks a reality criterion against which the validity of the self-descriptions can be evaluated.

Criterion Discrepancy

This limitation led a number of other researchers to operationalize self-enhancement as a *criterion discrepancy*, that is, the overestimation of one's positivity relative to a credible criterion. This category of measures includes both difference scores and residual scores. Rather than absolute values, higher numbers indicate the degree to which respondents' self-ratings exceed their criterion scores. Almost invariably, discrepancy measures of self-enhancement have shown negative associations with long-term adjustment outcomes (e.g., Colvin, Block, & Funder, 1995; John & Robins, 1994; Kwan, John, Kenny, Bond, & Robins, 2004; Paulhus, 1998a; Robins & Beer, 2001; Shedler, Mayman, & Manis, 1993: but see Bonanno et al., 2002).

Overclaiming Technique

The overclaiming technique (Paulhus et al., 2003) also emphasizes departure from reality, but in a different fashion. Respondents are asked to rate their familiarity with a set of persons, places, items, or events. Twenty percent of the items are foils: That is, they do not actually exist. Such responses can be scored via a signal detection method to yield both accuracy and bias scores for each respondent.

Of great practical advantage is the fact that the departure-from-reality aspect is included in the questionnaire along with the self-ratings. It is represented here by the answer key distinguishing real ones from foils: That is, a familiarity rating is accurate to the extent that real items are claimed and foils are disclaimed.

The original overclaiming questionnaire comprised academic items such as philosophy, history, literature, and science. On these items, the accuracy index correlated substantially with IQ scores, whereas the bias index correlated moderately with trait self-enhancement measures such as narcissism (Paulhus et al., 2003). When the items concerned lay topics such as sports, music, films, etc., the bias link was subtler. Correlations with narcissism were significant only for topics that the respondent valued.

Krueger's Method

This method might be called the idiosyncratic weighting method (Krueger, 1998; Sinha & Krueger, 1998). Each participant's self-ratings are correlated with his or her desirability ratings of the same items. Effectively, the method weights each rating by the desirability as judged by the rater. Other methods assume implicitly that the social consensus regarding the social desirability of each item within a test is shared by all respondents.

The method also has the advantage of adaptability because the weights can be adjusted to address context differences. For example, judgments of social desirability differ substantially across home, school, and leisure contexts.

Kwan's Method

Three other operationalizations of self-enhancement warrant mention here. Kwan's method (Kwan et al., 2004) utilizes the statistical sophistication of Kenny's (1994) social relations model. The technique decomposes self-perception into perceiver effect, target effect, and unique self-perception components.

The method is superior in controlling for complex contamination factors inherent in its competitors. The downside of this technique is that it can be applied only to round-robin ratings: That is, all participants have to rate each other.

Adaptiveness of Self-Enhancement

Taylor and Brown's (1988) claim for the adaptiveness of self-enhancement ("positive illusions") was supported by research such as the Brown (1986) study: He showed that individuals who claimed to be above average across a wide variety of traits also scored high on a standard self-esteem scale. A number of subsequent studies have shown the same pattern of adaptive outcomes (e.g., Campbell et al., 2002; Sedikides, Rudich, Gregg, Kumashiro, & Rusbult, 2004).

The Taylor–Brown proposition conflicted directly with traditional conceptions of mental health that emphasize the importance of perceiving oneself accurately (e.g., Allport, 1960; Jahoda, 1958). Critics of Taylor and Brown have tended to side with the more traditional view. In their comprehensive rebuttal, for example, Colvin and Block (1994) disputed both the logic and evidence presented for the adaptive value of self-enhancement. They acknowledged that positive illusions might be helpful in mood regulation and, therefore, might provide temporary relief from negative affect. Unacceptable to these critics was the notion that self-enhancement had sustained benefits.

To dispute the putative evidence, critics cited several specific faults with many of the studies cited by Taylor and Brown (1988). First was their use of the social comparison operationalization, which lacks a reality criterion against which the validity of the self-descriptions can be evaluated (Robins & John, 1997b).

Critics also pointed to the problem of using self-report outcomes when studying self-report predictors. If individual differences in self-favorability bias contaminate both the predictor and outcome, this common method variance would induce an artifactual positive correlation (Colvin & Block, 1994). For that reason, many critics have insisted that adaptiveness criteria be independent external measures, such as peer-rated adjustment (Paulhus, 1998a), expert ratings of adjustment (Colvin et al., 1995; Robins & John, 1997b), or school grades (Gramzow, Elliot, Asher, & McGregor, 2003; Robins & Beer, 2001).

Finally, a combination of the above two problems introduces an artifactual association even when hard outcome measures are used. If self-enhancement is operationalized by self-report (e.g., the social comparison index), then high scores represent a composite of true positive traits. But positive traits are known to yield objectively better life outcomes, including good adjustment (Block, 2002; Colvin & Block, 1994).

Such criticism led many researchers to turn to the criterion-discrepancy operationalization of self-enhancement.[5] When external criteria were used to evaluate outcomes, discrepancy measures of self-enhancement showed long-term maladaptive outcomes (e.g., Colvin et al., 1995; John & Robins, 1994; Paulhus, 1998a; Robins & Beer, 2001; Shedler et al., 1993). It is worth reviewing the key studies reported by critics.

Key Studies

The first empirical response to Taylor and Brown (1988) was the John and Robins (1994) study of performance in a group task. Each participant's self-rated performance was compared against two criterion measures: (1) others' ratings of the target's performance and (2) a concrete measure of success (money earned in the group exercise). The discrepancy between self-ratings and the two criterion measures provided

concrete indicators of self-enhancement. Results showed that higher scores on both indicators were negatively associated with ratings of adjustment by 11 trained psychologists.

Colvin and colleagues (1995) went further to conduct two longitudinal studies and a laboratory study. They assessed self-enhancement by comparing participants' self-evaluations with trained examiners' assessments of their personalities. Self-enhancement scores were then correlated with evaluations of adjustment from another set of trained observers. Results of their longitudinal studies showed that self-enhancement was associated with poor social skills and psychological maladjustment 5 years before and 5 years after the assessment of self-enhancement. The laboratory study showed that, in a confrontational situation, self-enhancers were rated negatively by both expert raters and peers.

Even with the discrepancy operationalization, however, the outcomes of self-enhancement are not uniformly negative. For example, Paulhus (1998a) investigated reactions to self-enhancers in two longitudinal studies where small groups met weekly for a total of 7 weeks. Results showed that, although high self-enhancers were initially perceived favorably, those perceptions became more and more negative over time. Paulhus concluded that self-enhancing tendencies were a "mixed blessing" (p. 1207).

This mixed blessing was also evident in later research reported by Robins and Beer (2001). In two studies, they showed that self-enhancing tendencies had short-term affective benefits. However, long-term damage was wrought to self-esteem and academic engagement as disconfirmation of overly positive self-assessments became evident. On objective indicators of academic performance, self-enhancement failed to predict higher academic performance or higher graduation rates. Gramzow and colleagues (2002) also used college grades as the outcome criterion. In two studies, higher discrepancies between reported and actual grade-point average (GPA) predicted poorer grades in the current course. Even with concrete behavioral criteria, then, the research seems to dispute claims that self-enhancement has any long-term adaptive outcomes.

Further Developments

Taylor and Brown (1994) responded to the critiques while holding fast to the original claim that self-enhancement is adaptive. Taylor and Armor (1996), however, clarified that position in two important ways. First, they explained that self-enhancement should be viewed not as a trait but as an adaptive strategy to be applied when needed. They also disputed the critique of using self-report self-esteem scales as criteria for adjustment: They argued that self-esteem is an inherent component of good psychological adjustment. Moreover, feeling good about oneself can only be measured via self-report.

In their most recent response, Taylor and her colleagues presented data indicating that (even) trait self-enhancement is adaptive (Taylor et al., 2003). That study was impressive in its breadth of operationalizations of self-enhancement—including the method favored by many critics, that is, self-criterion discrepancy. The criteria for adaptiveness included peer- and clinician-rated mental health. In support of the Taylor–Brown proposition, even the discrepancy operationalization seemed to show adaptive external correlates.

However, details of their method and results suggest that their conclusion should be regarded with some caution. Their discrepancy measure, for example, showed no significant associations with independently measured outcomes (e.g., clinician ratings and peer-judged mental health): All significant correlates were contaminated with self-report method variance. Moreover, the self-peer discrepancy measure employed a single peer rating, which is unlikely to be reliable. Other studies have used three or more raters (e.g., Colvin & Block, 1995; John & Robins, 1994; Paulhus, 1998a). In short, the measure that Taylor and colleagues treated as a discrepancy measure was ultimately another self-report of positive traits. Predictably, it showed adaptive external correlates—even when the latter were measured by valid external criteria.

However, support for the Taylor–Brown proposition can be found in research from other sources. In a field study of Bosnian war refugees, Bonanno and colleagues (2002) were able to measure discrepancy self-enhancement as well as clinician ratings of adjustment. Self-enhancers were rated as better adjusted. The extreme adversity of the situation makes this study unique among those using a discrepancy measure of self-enhancement.

Direct Competition

Only two studies have provided a head-to-head comparison of the adaptive value of self-enhancement operationalizations. Kwan and her colleagues compared three operationalizations (Kwan et al., 2004). In addition to the social comparison and discrepancy methods, they used their new technique described earlier. Results indicated that both the discrepancy measure and their novel measure were negatively related to task performance—the only objective outcome included in the study. The social comparison measure failed to predict the outcome.

Another head-to-head comparison of the social comparison and criterion-discrepancy methods expanded the outcomes to include four different measures of psychological adjustment (Kurt & Paulhus, 2008). Results showed that, in the same sample, social comparison had positive associations, and discrepancy measures had negative associations with externally evaluated adjustment—except self-rated self-esteem.

In sum, the literature indicates that the criterion-discrepancy measure is more valid than the social comparison method for tapping chronic self-enhancement. Based on research with the more valid measure, we conclude that chronic self-enhancement is linked to maladaptive attributes. The jury is still out on the direction of causation.

Three exceptions are noteworthy. One is that chronic self-enhancement may promote intrapsychic forms of adjustment, for example, self-esteem and happiness. Second is that self-enhancement may promote short-term interpersonal adjustment in the sense of engagement with strangers. Third, self-enhancement may pay off in traumatized samples (e.g., refugee victims), where formidable self-confidence is required for psychological survival.

In sum, no simple conclusion can be drawn regarding the Taylor–Brown claim for the adaptiveness of self-enhancement. In retrospect, this complexity is not surprising: It simply reaffirms the inherent difficulty of defining psychological adjustment (Asendorpf & Ostendorf, 1998; Paulhus, Fridhandler, & Hayes, 1997; Scott, 1968).

The Structure of Self-Enhancement

Although typically unspoken, the assumption in most research on self-enhancement is that the tendency generalizes across domains. It is assumed that respondents who self-enhance in one domain (e.g., their competence) also self-enhance in other domains. Paulhus and John (1998) challenged that assumption by asking "How many types of self-enhancement are there?"

Based on the evidence favoring the criterion-discrepancy method, Paulhus and John (1998) chose it as the unit of bias measurement. For each personality variable, a comparison was made between self-ratings and a more objective criterion, namely, ratings by knowledgeable peers (i.e., friends, family). In the case of intelligence, IQ scores were used as a criterion. Each self-rating was regressed on its corresponding peer rating to create a residual score representing the departure of the self-rating from reality. Factor analysis of a comprehensive set of personality variables was used to uncover the structure of self-enhancement.

Using the Big Five dimensions of personality plus intelligence to represent personality space, our factor analyses of residuals revealed a dimensionality smaller than the 5-D of either self- or peer ratings. The first two factors appeared as in Figure 19.4. Factor 1 was marked by the Extraversion and Openness residuals whereas Factor 2 was marked

by the Agreeableness and Dutifulness residuals.[6] Clearly, the structure of bias bears little resemblance to the standard Big Five structure. Instead, self-enhancement is organized in terms of agency and communion.

Several replication studies have helped to clarify the meaning of the bias factors through the addition of a wide variety of marker measures. These included traditional measures of SDR (BIDR, Marlowe–Crowne scale) as well as related measures of self-enhancement (e.g., Narcissistic Personality Inventory). The additions allowed us to project a variety of bias and personality measures onto the two bias factors.

Results showed a striking match with the SDR factors detailed in the third section of this chapter. SDE and narcissism projected onto the Agentic factor. Projections onto the Communal factor were strong for the Impression Management and Denial scales but weaker for Eysenck's Lie scale, the MMPI Lie scale, and the Marlowe–Crowne scale (Paulhus, 2002).

Another correspondence is informative: Positive Valence and Negative Valence (Benet-Martínez & Waller, 1997). Specifically, Positive Valence projected most clearly onto the Agentic factor, whereas Negative Valence projected onto the Communal factor. This correspondence adds to the construct validity of these two self-enhancement factors. Agentic self-enhancement concerns positive assets: People individuate by promoting their achievements. Communal self-enhancement concerns negative attributes: People submerge themselves in their groups by minimizing their social deviance.

Summary

Once again, our two-level framework has proved fruitful. The same Agentic and Communal self-presentation factors found in SDR have been recapitulated via the novel residual factoring method. This finding is noteworthy because the latter technique requires only personality content measures. In fact, there is no overlap whatsoever in the two methodologies. The convergence of results across the two techniques adds substantial credibility to both methods of factoring self-presentation. The interpretation of the self-enhancement factors becomes clearer,[7] and SDR factors gain more credibility as in-

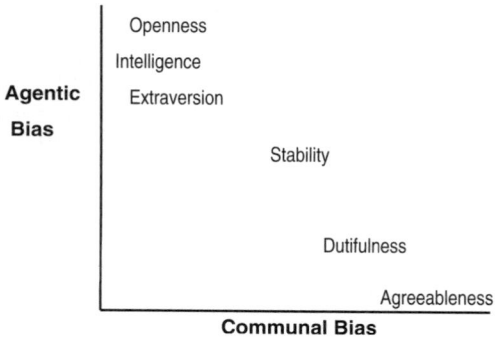

FIGURE 19.4. Structure of personality residuals.

dicators of departure from reality. That is, high scores on both factors involve overly positive self-descriptions.

Since publication of the Paulhus and John (1998) paper, attention to agentic and communal aspects of self-presentation has burgeoned. For example, Campbell and colleaguest (2002) utilized the distinction to clarify the difference between self-esteem and narcissism. Others have applied it to examining cultural differences in the structure of self-enhancement (Church et al., 2006; Kurman, 2001; Yik, Bond, & Paulhus, 1998). In search of a mechanism, Dijikic, Peterson, and Zelano (2005) found that memory distortion is greater for agentic than for communal self-enhancers. A variety of other self-enhancement behaviors have been shown to depend on the agency–communion distinction (Lonnqvist et al., 2007; Pauls & Stemmler, 2003).

FINAL CONCLUSIONS

The vast research on self-presentation is scattered across the literatures on social, clinical, and industrial-organizational psychology as well as personality, per se. Even within the latter, the literature is enormous and disconnected. In this chapter, we have tried to integrate the disconnected units within a two-level model. The first facet turns on the nature of the audience: public versus private. The second facet concerns the content of the image presented: People tend to offer images consistent with some combination of agentic qualities (strong, competent, clever) and communal qualities (cooperative, warm, dutiful).

That two-level model allowed us to organize three domains of research on self-presentation: socially desirable responding, self-enhancement, and, to a lesser extent, underlying cognitive processes. Resonating throughout the chapter is the historical failure of researchers to recognize the complex nature of positivity. Individuals motivated to self-present do not all behave the same way because the definition of positivity has (at least) two interpretations, and different audiences may differentially value those two forms of positivity.

NOTES

1. Abbreviating the term further to "social desirability" leads to misleading characterizations such as "high in social desirability." That terminology should be reserved for labeling individuals who possess desirable attributes.
2. Unfortunately confusion has ensured from the fact that Digman (1997) referred to similar factors as Alpha and Beta.
3. Part of the problem is where to draw the line. The same self-evaluation can be viewed as overestimated, underestimated, or accurate, depending on the choice of observer (Campbell & Fehr, 1990).
4. Although impossible if everyone were referring to the same dimension, individuals tend to define evaluative traits (e.g., intelligence) in idiosyncratic fashion to ensure that they score high (Dunning, 2005). In that sense, everyone can legitimately report being above average.
5. We use the term "discrepancy" to subsume difference scores and residual scores. Rather than an absolute values, we refer to directional values, with higher numbers indicating a self-rating greater than the criterion rating.
6. This result emerged when Conscientiousness was measured as Dutifulness rather than Ambition (Jackson, Paunonen, Fraboni, & Goffin, 1996). Dutifulness is most faithful, conceptually and empirically, to the Communal factor (Wiggins & Trapnell, 1990).
7. This convergence also helps to address allegations that discrepancy methods may be entirely misguided (Griffin, Murray, & Gonzalez, 1999; Zuckerman & Knee, 1996).

REFERENCES

Abel, A. E., & Wojiscke, B. (2007). Agency and communion from the perspective of self versus others. *Journal of Personality and Social Psychology, 93,* 751–763.

Alicke, M. D. (1985). Global self-evaluation as determined by the desirability and controllability of trait adjectives. *Journal of Personality and Social Psychology, 49,* 1621–1630.

Alloy, L. B., & Abramson, L. Y. (1979). Judgment of contingency in depressed and nondepressed students: Sadder but wiser? *Journal of Experimental Psychology: General, 108,* 441–485.

Allport, G. W. (1960). *Personality and social encounter.* Boston: Beacon Press.

Arkin, R. M. (1981). Self-presentational styles. In J. T. Tedeschi (Ed.), *Impression management theory and social psychological research* (pp. 311–333). New York: Academic Press.

Asendorpf, J. B., & Ostendorf, F. (1998). Is self-enhancement healthy?: Conceptual, psychometric, and empirical analysis. *Journal of Personality and Social Psychology, 74,* 955–966.

Baer, R. A., Rinaldo, J. C., & Berry, D. T. R. (2003). Response distortions in self-report assessment. In Rocío Fernández-Ballesteros (Ed.), *Encyclopedia of psychological assessment* (pp. 319–321). Thousand Oaks, CA: Sage.

Baer, R. A., Wetter, M. W., & Berry, D. T. (1992). Detection of underreporting of psychopathology on the MMPI: A meta-analysis. *Clinical Psychology Review, 12,* 509–525.

Bakan, D. (1966). *The duality of human existence: Isolation and communion in Western man.* Boston: Beacon Press.

Bauer, J. J., & McAdams, D. P. (2004). Personal growth in adults' stories of life transitions. *Journal of Personality, 72,* 573–602.

Baumeister, R. F. (1982). A self-presentational view of social phenomena. *Psychological Bulletin, 91,* 3–26.

Baumeister, R. F., Dale, K., & Sommer, K. L. (1998). Freudian defense mechanisms and empirical findings in modern social psychology: Reaction formation, projection, displacement, undoing, isolation, sublimation, and denial. *Journal of Personality, 66,* 1081–1124.

Bem, S. L. (1974). The measurement of psychological androgyny. *Journal of Consulting and Clinical Psychology, 42,* 165–172.

Benet-Martínez, V., & Waller, N. G. (1997). Further evidence for the cross-cultural generality of the "Big Seven" model: Imported and indigenous Spanish personality constructs. *Journal of Personality, 65,* 567–598.

Berry, C. M., Page, R. C., & Sackett, P. R. (2007). Effects of self-deceptive enhancement on personality-job performance relationships. *International Journal of Selection and Assessment, 15,* 94–109.

Block, J. (1965). *The challenge of response sets.* New York: Century.

Block, J. (2002). *Personality as an affect-processing system: Toward an integrative theory.* Mahwah, NJ: Erlbaum.

Block, J., & Colvin, R. D. (1994). Do positive illusions foster mental health?: Separating fiction from fact. *Psychological Bulletin, 116,* 28.

Bolino, M. C., & Turnley, W. H. (1999). Measuring impression management in organizations: A scale development based on the Jones and Pittman taxonomy. *Organizational Research Methods, 2,* 187–206.

Bonanno, G. A., Field, N. P., Kovacevic, A., & Kaltman, S. (2002). Self-enhancement as a buffer against extreme adversity: Civil war in Bosnia and traumatic loss in the United States. *Personality and Social Psychology Bulletin, 28,* 184–196.

Borkenau, P. (1990). Traits as ideal-based and goal-derived social categories. *Journal of Personality and Social Psychology, 58,* 381–396.

Briggs, S. R., & Cheek, J. M. (1988). On the nature of self-monitoring: Problems with assessment, problems with validity. *Journal of Personality and Social Psychology, 54,* 663–678.

Brown, J. D. (1986). Evaluations of self and others: Self-enhancement biases in social judgments. *Social Cognition, 4,* 353–376.

Brown, J. D. (1998). *The self.* Boston: McGraw-Hill.

Buss, A. H. (1980). *Self-consciousness and social anxiety.* San Francisco: Freeman.

Byrne, D. (1961). The Repression–Sensitization Scale: Rationale, reliability. and validity. *Journal of Personality, 29,* 334–349.

Campbell, K. W., Rudich, E. A., & Sedikides, C. (2002). Narcissism, self-esteem, and the positivity of self-views: Two portraits of self-love. *Personality and Social Psychology Bulletin, 28,* 358–365.

Campbell, J. D., & Fehr, B. A. (1990). Self-esteem and perceptions of conveyed impressions: Is negative affectivity associated with greater realism? *Journal of Personality and Social Psychology, 58,* 122–133.

Cantor, N., & Kihlstrom, J. F. (1987). *Personality and social intelligence.* Englewood Cliffs, NJ: Prentice Hall.

Carey, J., & Paulhus, D. L. (2008, August). *The structure of self-presentation scales.* Paper presented at the annual meeting of the American Psychological Association, Boston.

Carson, R. C. (1969). *Interaction concepts of personality.* Chicago: Aldine.

Christie, R., & Geis, F. L. (1970). *Studies in Machiavellianism.* New York: Academic Press.

Church, A. T., Katigbak, M. S., del Prado, A. M., Valdez-Medina, J. L., Miramontes, L. G., & Ortiz, F. A. (2006). A cross-cultural study of trait self-enhancement, explanatory variables, and adjustment. *Journal of Research in Personality, 40,* 1169–1201.

Colvin, C. R., & Block, J. (1994). Do positive illusions foster mental health? An examination of the Taylor and Brown formulation. *Psychological Bulletin, 116,* 3–20.

Colvin, C. R., Block, J., & Funder, D. C. (1995). Overly positive self-evaluations and personality: Negative implications for mental health. *Journal of Personality and Social Psychology, 68,* 1152–1162.

Costa, P. T., Jr., & McCrae, R. R. (1989). *Manual for the NEO Personality Inventory: Five Factor Inventory/ NEO-FFI.* Odessa, FL: PAR.

Costa, P. T., Jr., & McCrae, R. R. (1992). Four ways five factors are basic. *Personality and Individual Differences, 13,* 653–665.

Crowne, D. P. (1979). *The experimental study of personality.* Hillsdale, NJ: Erlbaum.

Crowne, D. P., & Marlowe, D. (1964). *The approval motive.* New York: Wiley.

De Raad, B., & Van Oudenhoven, J.P. (2008). Factors of values in the Dutch Language and their relationship to factors of personality. *European Journal of Personality, 22,* 81–108.

DeYoung, C. G., Peterson, Jordan B., & Higgins, D. M. (2002). Higher-order factors of the Big Five predict conformity: Are there neuroses of health? *Personality and Individual Differences, 33,* 533–552.

Digman, J. M. (1997). Higher-order factors of the Big Five. *Journal of Personality and Social Psychology, 73,* 1246–1256.

Djikic, M., Peterson, J. B., & Zelazo, P. D. (2005). Attentional biases and memory distortions in self-enhancers. *Personality and Individual Differences, 38,* 559–568.

Dunning, D. (2005). *Self-insight: Roadblocks and detours on the road to knowing thyself.* New York: Psychology Press.

Duval, T. S., & Wicklund, R. A. (1972). *A theory of objective self-awareness.* New York: Academic Press.

Edwards, A. L. (1957). *The social desirability variable in personality assessment and research.* Fort Worth, TX: Dryden Press.

Edwards, A. L. (1970). *The measurement of personality traits by scales and inventories.* New York: Holt, Rinehart & Winston.

Eysenck, S. B. G., & Eysenck, H. J. (1964). *Manual of the Eysenck Personality Inventory.* London: Stodder & Hougton.

Fenigstein, A., Scheier, M. F., & Buss, A. H. (1975). Public and private self-consciousness: Assessment and theory. *Journal of Consulting and Clinical Psychology, 43,* 522–527.

Frenkel-Brunswik, E. (1939). Mechanisms of self-deception. *Journal of Social Psychology, 10,* 409–420.

Furnham, A., & Henderson, M. (1982). The good, the bad, and the mad: Response bias in self-report measures. *Personality and Individual Differences, 3,* 311–320.

Gailliot, M. T., Baumeister, R. F., de Waal, C. N., Maner, J. K., Plant, E. A., Tice, D. M., et al. (2007). Self-control relies on glucose as a limited energy source: Willpower is more than a metaphor. *Journal of Personality and Social Psychology, 92,* 325–336.

Gangestad, S. W., & Snyder, M. (2000). Self-monitoring: Appraisal and reappraisal. *Psychological Bulletin, 126,* 530–555.

Gilbert, D. T., Pelham, B. W., & Krull, D. S. (1988). On cognitive busyness: When person perceivers meet persons perceived. *Journal of Personality and Social Psychology, 54,* 733–739.

Gilligan, C. (1982). *In a different voice: Psychological theory and women's development.* Cambridge, MA: Harvard University Press.

Godfrey, D., Jones, E. E., & Lord, C. G. (1986). Self-promotion is not ingratiating. *Journal of Personality and Social Psychology, 50,* 106–115.

Goffman, E. (1959). *The presentation of self in everyday life.* New York: Doubleday.

Gough, H. G. (1957). *Manual for the California Psychological Inventory.* Palo Alto, CA: Consulting Psychologists Press.

Gramzow, R. H., Elliot, A. J., Asher, E., & McGregor, H. A. (2002). Self-evaluation bias and academic performance: Some ways and some reasons why. *Journal of Research in Personality, 37,* 41–61.

Griffin, D., Murray, S., & Gonzalez, R. (1999). Difference score correlations in relationship research: A conceptual primer. *Personal Relationships, 6,* 505–518.

Gur, R. C., & Sackeim, H. A. (1979). Self-deception: A concept in search of a phenomenon. *Journal of Personality and Social Psychology, 37,* 147–169.

Hartshorne, H., & May, M. A. (1928). *Studies in deceit.* New York: Macmillan.

Hathaway, S. R., & McKinley, J. C. (1951). *MMPI manual.* New York: Psychological Corporation.

Helgeson, V. S., & Fritz, H. L. (1999). Unmitigated agency and unmitigated communion: Distinctions from agency and communion. *Journal of Research in Personality, 33,* 131–158.

Hinz, A., Brähler, E., Schmidt, P., & Albani, C. (2005). Investigating the circumplex structure of the Portrait Values Questionnaire (PVQ). *Journal of Individual Differences, 26,* 185–193.

Hogan, R. (1983). A socioanalytic theory of personality. In M. M. Page (Ed.), *Nebraska Symposium on Motivation* (Vol. 30, pp. 55–89). Lincoln: University of Nebraska Press.

Holden, R. R. (2007). Socially desirable responding does moderate personality scale validity both in experimental and nonexperimental contexts. *Canadian Journal of Behavioural Science, 39,* 184–201.

Holden, R. R., & Evoy, R. A. (2005). Personality inventory faking: A four-dimensional simulation of dissimulation. *Personality and Individual Differences, 39,* 1307–1318.

Holden, R. R., & Fekken, G. C. (1989). Three common social desirability scales: Friends, acquaintances, or strangers? *Journal of Research in Personality, 23,* 180–191.

Hoorens, V. (1995). Self-favoring biases, self-presentation, and the self–other asymmetry in social comparison. *Journal of Personality, 63,* 793–817.

Horowitz, L. M., Wilson, K. R., Turan, B., Zolotsev, P., Constantino, M. J., & Henderson, L. (2006). How interpersonal motives clarify the meaning of interpersonal behavior: A revised circumplex model. *Personality and Social Psychology Review, 10*, 67–86.

Jackson, D. N., & Messick, S. (1962). Response styles and the measurement of psychopathology. *Psychological Bulletin, 55*, 243–252.

Jackson, D. N., Paunonen, S. V., Fraboni, M., & Goffin, R. D. (1996). A five-factor versus six-factor model of personality structure. *Personality and Individual Differences, 20*, 33–45.

Jahoda, M. (1958). *Current concepts of positive mental health.* Oxford, UK: Basic Books.

John, O. P., Cheek, J. M., & Klohnen, E. C. (1996). On the nature of self-monitoring: Construct explication with Q-sort ratings. *Journal of Personality and Social Psychology, 71*, 763–776.

John, O. P., & Robins, R. W. (1994). Accuracy and bias in self-perception: Individual differences in self-enhancement and the role of narcissism. *Journal of Personality and Social Psychology, 66*, 206–219.

John, O. P., & Srivastava, S. (1999). The Big Five trait taxonomy: History, measurement, and theoretical perspectives. In L. A. Pervin & O. P. John (Eds.), *Handbook of personality psychology* (pp. 102–139). New York: Guilford Press.

Johnson, E. A. (1995). Self-deceptive responses to threat: Adaptive only in ambiguous circumstances. *Journal of Personality, 63*, 759–791.

Johnson, J. A., & Hogan, R. (1981). Moral judgments and self-presentations. *Journal of Research in Personality, 15*, 57–63.

Jones, E. E., & Pittman, T. S. (1982). Toward a theory of strategic self-presentation. In J. Suls (Ed.), *Psychological perspectives on the self* (pp. 231–262). Hillsdale, NJ: Erlbaum.

Judd, C. M., James-Hawkins, L., Yzerbyt, V., & Kashima, Y. (2005). Fundamental dimensions of social judgment: Understanding the relations between judgments of competence and warmth. *Journal of Personality and Social Psychology, 89*, 988–913.

Kasser, T., Cohn, S., Kanner, A. D., & Ryan, R. M. (2007). Some costs of American corporate capitalism: A psychological exploration of value and goal conflicts. *Psychological Inquiry, 18*, 1–22.

Kenny, D. A. (1994). *Interpersonal perception: A social relations analysis.* New York: Guilford Press.

Kiesler, D. J., & Auerbach, S. M. (2003). Integrating measurement of control and affiliation in studies of physician–patient interaction: The interpersonal circumplex. *Social Science and Medicine, 57*(9), 1707–1722.

Klar, Y., & Giladi, E. E. (1997). "No one in my group can be below the group's average": A robust positivity bias in favor of anonymous peers. *Journal of Personality and Social Psychology, 73*, 885–901.

Krueger, J. (1998). Enhancement bias in descriptions of self and others. *Personality and Social Psychology Bulletin, 24*, 505–516.

Kurman, J. (2001). Self-enhancement: Is it restricted to individualistic cultures? *Personality and Social Psychology Bulletin, 27*, 1705–1716.

Kurt, A., & Paulhus, D. L. (2008). Moderators of the adaptive value of self-enhancement: Operationalization, motivational domain, adjustment type , and evaluator. *Journal of Research in Personality.*

Kwan, V. S. Y., Barrios, V., Ganis, G., Gorman, J., Lange, C., Kumar, M., et al. (2007). Assessing the neural correlates of self-enhancement bias: A transcranial magnetic stimulation study. *Experimental Brain Research, 182*, 379–385.

Kwan, V. S. Y., John, O. P., Kenny, D. A., Bond, M. H., & Robins, R. W. (2004). Reconceptualizing individual differences in self-enhancement bias: An interpersonal approach. *Psychological Review, 111*, 94–110.

Laforge, R., Leary, T. F., Naboisek, H., Coffey, H. S., & Freedman, M. B. (1954). The interpersonal dimension of personality: II. An objective study of repression. *Journal of Personality, 23*, 129–153.

Leary, M. R. (1995). *Self-presentation: Impression management and interpersonal behavior.* Madison, WI: Brown & Benchmark.

Leary, M. R. (2007). Motivational and emotional aspects of the self. *Annual Review, 58*, 317–344.

Leary, M. R., & Kowalski, R. M. (1990). Impression management: A literature review and two-component model. *Psychological Bulletin, 107*, 34–47.

Leary, M. R., Tchividjian, L. R., & Kraxberger, B. E. (1999). Self-presentation can be hazardous to your health: Impression management and health risk. In R. F. Baumeister (Ed.), *The self in social psychology* (pp. 182–194). New York: Psychology Press.

Leary, T. (1957). *Interpersonal diagnosis of personality: A functional theory and methodology for personality evaluation.* Oxford, UK: Ronald Press.

Lee, S.-J., Quigley, B. M., Nesler, M. S., Corbet, A. B., & Tedeschi, J. T. (1999). Development of a self-presentation tactics scale. *Personality and Individual Differences, 26*, 701–722.

Lennox, R. D., & Wolfe, R. N. (1984). Revision of the self-monitoring scale. *Journal of Personality and Social Psychology, 46*, 1349–1364.

Lewinsohn, P. M., Mischel, W., Chaplin, W., & Barton, R. (1980). Social competence and depression: The role of illusory self-perceptions. *Journal of Abnormal Psychology*, *89*, 201–212.

Locke, K. D. (2000). Circumplex scales of interpersonal values: Reliability, validity, and applicability to interpersonal problems and personality disorders. *Journal of Personality Assessment*, *75*, 249–267.

Lonnqvist, J. E., Verkasalo, M., & Bezmenova, I. (2007). Agentic and communal bias in socially desirable responding. *European Journal of Personality*, *21*, 853–868.

Markus, H. R., & Kitayama, S. (1991). Culture and the self: Implications for cognition, emotion, and motivation. *Psychological Review*, *98*, 224–253.

Markus, H. R., & Kitayama, S. (2003). Culture, self, and the reality of the social. *Psychological Inquiry*, *14*, 277–283.

McAdams, D. P., Hoffman, B. J., Mansfield, E. D., & Day, R. (1996). Themes of agency and communion in significant autobiographical scenes. *Journal of Personality*, *64*, 339–377.

McCrae, R. R. (1994). New goals for trait psychology. *Psychological Inquiry*, *5*, 48–153.

McCrae, R. R., & Costa, P. T., Jr. (1983). Social desirability scales: More substance than style. *Journal of Consulting and Clinical Psychology*, *51*, 882–888.

McCrae, R. R., Jang, K. L., Livesley, W. J., Riemann, R., & Angleitner, A. (2001). Sources of structure: Genetic, environmental, and artifactual influences on the covariation of personality traits. *Journal of Personality*, *69*, 511–535.

McMullen, L. M., & Conway, J. B. (1997). Dominance and nurturance in the narratives told by clients in psychotherapy. *Psychotherapy Research*, *7*, 83–99.

Messick, S. (1960). Dimensions of social desirability. *Journal of Consulting Psychology*, *24*, 279–287.

Milholland, J. E. (1964). Theory and techniques of assessment. *Annual Review of Psychology*, *15*, 311–346.

Millham, J. (1974). Two components of need for approval score and their relationship to cheating following success and failure. *Journal of Research in Personality*, *8*, 378–392.

Millham, J., & Jacobson, L. I. (1978). The need for approval. In H. London & J. E. Exner (Eds.), *Dimensions of personality* (pp. 365–390). New York: Wiley.

Morf, C. C., & Rhodewalt, F. (2001). Unraveling the paradoxes of narcissism: A dynamic self-regulatory processing model. *Psychological Inquiry*, *12*, 177–196.

Moskowitz, D. S., & Zuroff, D. C. (2004). Flux, pulse, and spin: Dynamic additions to the personality lexicon. *Journal of Personality and Social Psychology*, *86*, 880–893.

Nichols, D. S., & Greene, R. L. (1997). Dimensions of deception in personality assessment: The example of the MMPI-2. *Journal of Personality Assessment*, *68*, 251–266.

Otter, Z., & Egan, V. (2007). The evolutionary role of self-deceptive enhancement as a protective factor against antisocial cognitions. *Personality and Individual Differences*, *43*, 2258–2269.

Paulhus, D. L. (1984). Two-component models of socially desirable responding. *Journal of Personality and Social Psychology*, *46*, 598–609.

Paulhus, D. L. (1986). Self-deception and impression management in test responses. In A. Angleitner & J. S. Wiggins (Eds.), *Personality assessment via questionnaire* (pp. 143–165). New York: Springer-Verlag.

Paulhus, D. L. (1991). Measurement and control of response bias. In J. P. Robinson, P. R. Shaver, & L. S. Wrightsman (Eds.), *Measures of personality and social psychological attitudes* (pp. 17–60). San Diego, CA: Academic Press.

Paulhus, D. L. (1994, August). *The multiplicity of meanings of social desirability.* Paper presented at the annual meeting of the American Psychological Association, Los Angeles.

Paulhus, D. L. (1995). Bypassing the will: The automatization of affirmations. In D. W. Wegner & J. W. Pennebaker (Eds.), *Handbook of mental control* (pp. 573–587). Hillsdale, NJ: Erlbaum.

Paulhus, D. L. (1998a). Interpersonal and intrapsychic adaptiveness of trait self-enhancement: A mixed blessing? *Journal of Personality and Social Psychology*, *74*, 1197–1208.

Paulhus, D. L. (1998b). *Manual for Balanced Inventory of Desirable Responding* (BIDR-7). Toronto: Multi-Health Systems.

Paulhus, D. L. (2002). Socially desirable responding: The evolution of a construct. In H. Braun, D. N. Jackson, & D. E. Wiley (Eds.), *The role of constructs in psychological and educational measurement* (pp. 67–88). Hillsdale, NJ: Erlbaum.

Paulhus, D. L. (2005, August). *The Comprehensive Inventory of Desirable Responding.* Paper presented at the meeting of the Society for Personality and Social Psychology, Memphis, TN.

Paulhus, D. L., Bruce, M. N., & Trapnell, P. D. (1995). Effects of self-presentation strategies on personality profiles and structure. *Personality and Social Psychology Bulletin*, *21*, 100–108.

Paulhus, D. L., Fridhandler, B., & Hayes, S. (1997). Psychological defense: Contemporary theory and research. In R. Hogan, J. A. Johnson, & S. R. Briggs (Eds.), *Handbook of personality psychology* (pp. 543–579). San Diego, CA: Academic Press.

Paulhus, D. L., Graf, P., & Van Selst, M. (1989). Attentional load increases the positivity of self-presentation. *Social Cognition, 7,* 389–400.

Paulhus, D. L., Harms, P. D., Bruce, M. N., & Lysy, D. C. (2003). The over-claiming technique: Measuring self-enhancement independent of ability. *Journal of Personality and Social Psychology, 84,* 681–693.

Paulhus, D. L., & John, O. P. (1998). Egoistic and moralistic biases in self-perception: The interplay of self-deceptive styles with basic traits and motives. *Journal of Personality, 66,* 1025–1060.

Paulhus, D. L., & Levitt, K. (1987). Desirable responding triggered by affect: Automatic egotism? *Journal of Personality and Social Psychology, 52,* 245–259.

Paulhus, D. L., & Martin, C. L. (1988). Functional flexibility: A new conception of interpersonal flexibility. *Journal of Personality and Social Psychology, 55,* 88–101.

Paulhus, D. L., Nathanson, C., & Lau, K. (2006). *Cheating on practice tests: A matter of self-deception?* Manuscript submitted for publication.

Paulhus, D. L., & Reid, D. B. (1991). Enhancement and denial in social desirable responding. *Journal of Personality and Social Psychology, 60,* 307–317.

Paulhus, D. L., Tanchuk, T., & Wehr, P. (1999, August). *Value-based faking on personality questionnaires: Agency and communion rule.* Paper presented at the annual meeting of the American Psychological Association, Boston.

Paulhus, D. L., & Vazire, S. (2007). The self-report method. In R. W. Robins, R. C. Fraley, & R. F. Krueger (Eds.), *Handbook of research methods in personality psychology* (pp. 224–239). New York: Guilford Press.

Paulhus, D. L., & Williams, K. M. (2002). The dark triad of personality: Narcissism, Machiavellianism, and psychopathy. *Journal of Research in Personality, 36,* 556–563.

Pauls, C. A., & Stemmler, G. (2003). Substance and bias in social desirability responding. *Personality and Individual Differences, 35,* 263–275.

Peabody, D. (1984). Personality dimensions through trait inferences. *Journal of Personality and Social Psychology, 46,* 384–403.

Pervin, L. A. (1994). A critical analysis of current trait theory. *Psychological Inquiry, 5,* 103–113.

Phalet, K., & Poppe, E. (1997). Competence and morality dimensions of national and ethnic stereotypes: A study in six Eastern-European countries. *European Journal of Social Psychology, 27,* 703–723.

Pincus, A. L., Gurtman, M. B., & Ruiz, M. A. (1998). Structural analysis of social behavior (SASB): Circumplex analyses and structural relations with the interpersonal circle and the five-factor model of personality. *Journal of Personality and Social Psychology, 74,* 1629–1645.

Quattrone, G. A., & Tversky, A. (1984). Causal versus diagnostic contingencies: On self-deception and on the voter's illusion. *Journal of Personality and Social Psychology, 46*(2), 237–248.

Read, S. J., Jones, D. K., & Miller, L. C. (1990). Traits as goal-based categories: The importance of goals in the coherence of dispositional categories. *Journal of Personality and Social Psychology, 58,* 1048–1061.

Richman, W. L., Weisband, S., Kiesler, S., & Drasgow, F. (1999). A meta-analytic study of social desirability response distortion in computer-administered and traditional questionnaires and interviews. *Journal of Applied Psychology, 84,* 754–775.

Roberts, B. W., & Robins, R. W. (2000). Broad dispositions, broad aspirations: The intersection of personality traits and life goals. *Personality and Social Psychology Bulletin, 26,* 1284–1296.

Robins, R. W., & Beer, J. S. (2001). Positive illusions about the self: Short-term benefits and long-term costs. *Journal of Personality and Social Psychology, 80,* 340–352.

Robins, R. W., & John, O. P. (1997a). Effects of visual perspective and narcissism on self-perception: Is seeing believing? *Psychological Science, 8,* 37–42.

Robins, R. W., & John, O. P. (1997b). The quest for self-insight: Theory and research on the accuracy of self-perceptions. In R. Hogan, J. Johnson, & S. R. Briggs (Eds.), *Handbook of personality psychology* (pp. 649–679). San Diego, CA: Academic Press.

Rogers, T. B. (1974). An analysis of two central stages underlying responding to personality items: The self-referent decision and response selection. *Journal of Research in Personality, 8,* 128–138.

Rosenfeld, P., Giacalone, R. A., & Riordan, C. A. (1995). *Impression management in organizations: Theory, measurement, practice.* London: Routledge.

Rosse, J. G., Stecher, M. D., Miller, J. L., & Levin, R. A. (1998). The impact of response distortion on preemployment personality testing and hiring decisions. *Journal of Applied Psychology, 83,* 634–644.

Rowatt, W. C., Cunningham, M. R., & Druen, P. B. (1998). Deception to get a date. *Personality and Social Psychology Bulletin, 24,* 1228–1242.

Sackeim, H. A., & Gur, R. C. (1978). Self-deception, self-confrontation, and consciousness. In G. E. Schwartz & D. Shapiro (Eds.), *Consciousness and self-regulation: Advances in research* (Vol. 2, pp. 139–197). New York: Plenum Press.

Saucier, G. (1994). Separating description and evaluation in the structure of personality attributes. *Journal of Personality and Social Psychology, 66,* 141–154.

Saucier, G., & Goldberg, L. R. (2001). Lexical studies of indigenous personality factors: Premises, products, and prospects. *Journal of Personality, 69,* 847–879.

Schlenker, B. R. (1980). *Impression management: The self-concept, social identity, and interpersonal relationships.* Monterey, CA: Brooks-Cole.

Schlenker, B. R., Britt, T. W., & Pennington, J. W. (1996). Impression regulation and management: A theory of self-identification. In R. M. Sorrentino & E. T. Higgins (Eds.), *Handbook of motivation and cognition: Vol. 3. The interpersonal context* (pp. 118–147). New York: Guilford Press.

Schlenker, B. R., & Weigold, M. F. (1990). Self-consciousness and self-presentation: Being autonomous versus appearing autonomous. *Journal of Personality and Social Psychology, 59,* 820–828.

Schwartz, S. H. (1992). Universals in the content and structure of values: Theoretical advances and empirical tests in 20 countries. In M. P. Zanna (Ed.), *Advances in experimental social psychology* (Vol. 25, pp. 1–66). San Diego, CA: Academic Press.

Scott, W. A. (1968). Concepts of normality. In E. F. Borgatta & W. W. Lambert (Eds.), *Handbook of personality: Theory and research.* Chicago: Rand-McNally.

Sedikides, C., Rudich, E. A., Gregg, A. P., Kumashiro, M., & Rusbult, C. (2004). Are normal narcissists psychologically healthy?: Self-esteem matters. *Journal of Personality and Social Psychology, 87,* 400–416.

Sedikides, C., & Strube, M. J. (1997). Self-evaluation: To thine own self be good, to thine own self be sure, to thine own self be true, and to thine own self be better. In M. P. Zanna (Ed.), *Advances in experimental social psychology* (Vol. 29, pp. 209–269). New York: Academic Press.

Shedler, J., Mayman, M., & Manis, M. (1993). The illusion of mental health. *American Psychologist, 48,* 1117–1131.

Shepperd, J. A., & Kwavnick, K. D. (1999). Maladaptive image maintenance. In R. M. Kowalski & M. R. Leary (Eds.), *The social psychology of emotional and behavioral problems: Interfaces of social and clinical psychology* (pp. 249–277). Washington, DC: American Psychological Association.

Sherry, S. B., Hewitt, P. L., Flett, G. L., Lee-Baggley, D. L., & Hall, P. A. (2007). Trait perfectionism and perfectionistic self-presentation in personality pathology. *Personality and Individual Differences, 42,* 477–490.

Sinha, R. R., & Krueger, J. (1998). Idiographic self-evaluation and bias. *Journal of Research in Personality, 32,* 131–155.

Snyder, M. (1974). Self-monitoring of expressive behavior. *Journal of Personality and Social Psychology, 30,* 526–537.

Spence, J. T. (1984). Masculinity, feminity, and gender-related traits: A conceptual analysis and critique of current research. *Progress in Experimental Personality Research, 13,* 1–97.

Sullivan, H. S. (1953). *The interpersonal theory of psychiatry.* New York: Norton.

Swann, W. B. J. (1990). To be adored or to be known? The interplay of self-enhancement and self-verification. In E. T. Higgins & R. M. Sorrentino (Eds.), *Handbook of motivation and cognition: Foundations of social behavior* (Vol. 2, pp. 408–448). New York: Guilford Press.

Taylor, S. E., & Armor, D. A. (1996). Positive illusions and coping with adversity. *Journal of Personality, 64,* 873–898.

Taylor, S. E., & Brown, J. D. (1988). Illusion and well-being: A social psychological perspective on mental health. *Psychological Bulletin, 103,* 193–210.

Taylor, S. E., & Brown, J. D. (1994). Positive illusions and well-being revisited: Separating fact from fiction. *Psychological Bulletin, 116,* 21–27.

Taylor, S. E., Lerner, J. S., Sherman, D. K., Sage, R. M., & McDowell, N. K. (2003). Portrait of the self-enhancer: Well adjusted and well liked or maladjusted and friendless? *Journal of Personality and Social Psychology, 84,* 165–176.

Tice, D. M., Butler, J. L., Muraven, M. B., & Stillwell, A. M. (1995). When modesty prevails: Differential favorability of self-presentation to friends and stranger. *Journal of Personality and Social Psychology, 69,* 1120–1138.

Trapnell, P. D., & Paulhus, D. L. (in press). Agentic and communal values: Their scope and measurement. *Journal of Personality Assessment.*

Trapnell, P. D., & Wiggins, J. S. (1990). Extension of the Interpersonal Adjective Scales to include the Big Five dimensions of personality. *Journal of Personality and Social Psychology, 59,* 781–790.

Triandis, H. C. (1989). The self and social behavior in differing cultural contexts. *Psychological Review, 96,* 506–520.

Vazire, S. (2006). Informant reports: A cheap, fast, and easy method for personality assessment. *Journal of Research in Personality, 40,* 472–481.

Vohs, K. D., Baumeister, R. F., & Ciarocco, N. J. (2005). Self-regulation and self-presentation: Regulatory resource depletion impairs impression management and effortful self-presentation depletes regulatory resources. *Journal of Personality and Social Psychology, 88*, 632–657.

Watson, D., & Friend, R. (1969). Measurement of social-evaluative anxiety. *Journal of Consulting and Clinical Psychology, 33*, 448–457.

Weinberger, J., & Silverman, L. H. (1990). Testability and empirical verification of psychoanalytic dynamic propositions through subliminal activation. *Psychoanalytic Psychology, 7*, 299–339.

Wiggins, J. S. (1959). Interrelationships among MMPI measures of dissimulation under standard and social desirability instructions. *Journal of Consulting Psychology, 23*, 419–427.

Wiggins, J. S. (1964). Convergence among stylistic response measures from objective personality tests. *Educational and Psychological Measurement, 24*, 551–562.

Wiggins, J. S. (1991). Agency and communion as conceptual coordinates for the understanding and measurement of interpersonal behavior. In D. Cicchetti & W. M. Grove (Eds.), *Thinking clearly about psychology: Essays in honor of Paul E. Meehl, Vol. 2. Personality and psychopathology* (pp. 89–113). Minneapolis: University of Minnesota Press.

Wiggins, J. S., & Holzmuller, A. (1978). Psychological androgyny and interpersonal behavior. *Journal of Consulting and Clinical Psychology, 46*, 40–52.

Wiggins, J. S., & Trapnell, P. D. (1996). A dyadic-interactional perspective on the five-factor model. In J.S. Wiggins (Ed.), *The five-factor model of personality* (pp. 88–162). New York: Guilford Press.

Winter, D. G., John, O. P., Stewart, A. J., Klohnen, E. C., & Duncan, L. E. (1998). Traits and motives: Toward an integration of two traditions in personality research. *Psychological Review, 105*, 230–250.

Woike, B. A., Gershkovich, I., Piorkowski, R., & Polo, M. (1999). The role of motives in the content and structure of autobiographical memory. *Journal of Personality and Social Psychology, 76*, 600–612.

Yik, M. S. M., Bond, M. H., & Paulhus, D. L. (1998). Do Chinese self-enhance or self-efface? It's a matter of domain. *Personality and Social Psychology Bulletin, 24*, 399–406.

Zuckerman, M., & Knee, C. R. (1996). A comment on Colvin, Block, and Funder (1995). *Journal of Personality and Social Psychology, 70*, 1250–1251.

CHAPTER 20

Attachment Theory and Its Place in Contemporary Personality Theory and Research

R. Chris Fraley
Phillip R. Shaver

While working in a home for maladjusted and delinquent boys in the 1930s, John Bowlby was struck by the boys' difficulty in forming close emotional bonds with others. After studying the family histories of the children, he learned that a disproportionate number of the boys had experienced severe disruptions in their early home lives. His observations led him to conclude that early parent–child relationships serve an important organizing role in human development and that disruptions in these relationships can have profound consequences on behavior, not only in the short term, but in the long term as well (Bowlby, 1944).

To better understand the significance of early relationships and how they shape human development, Bowlby turned to a variety of literatures, including those pertaining to psychodynamic theory (Freud, 1933/1965, 1940), the emerging ethological models of the 1950s and 1960s (e.g., Hinde, 1966), cognitive developmental psychology (e.g., Piaget, 1953), and the principles of control systems (e.g., Craik, 1943; Young, 1964). Over the next few decades he integrated ideas from each of these domains to forge a theoretical perspective now known as "attachment theory" (Bowlby, 1969/1982, 1973, 1980).

Bowlby's attachment theory has had an enormous impact on psychological science, in large part because it speaks to many of the enduring subjects that psychologists wish to understand (e.g., emotions, relationships, love and loss, personality, nature and nurture, development, psychological defense); and importantly, it does so in a way that has multidisciplinary appeal, bringing together ideas and observations from social psychology, developmental psychology, behavioral neuroscience and psychobiology, animal behavior, and clinical psychology. Indeed, by many standards, attachment theory is a strong candidate for being considered a "Grand Theory" in contemporary psychology. Nonetheless, the theory has never been fully embraced by contemporary personality psychologists, despite the fact that it was created to explain, in part, individual differences, personality organization and dynamics, and individual development.

One of the objectives of this chapter is to make the case that attachment theory should play a *central* role in contemporary personality theory and research. The theory offers conceptually rich "units of analysis" that are relevant for understanding much of personality functioning, a framework for modeling the structure of individual differences, and several testable hypotheses regarding the origin of individual differences and how those differences shape interpersonal development. But perhaps a more important reason why attachment theory warrants a more central role in contemporary personality psychology is that attachment theorists have struggled with many of the same conceptual issues with which personality psychologists have struggled over the past few decades (e.g., the person–situation debate, the stability of individual differences). As a result, attachment theory provides a rich and fertile testing ground for general models of personality processes, such as those that attempt to make sense of consistency and inconsistency in behavior (e.g., Mischel & Shoda, 1998), personality in context (Roberts, 2007), and patterns of stability and change in human experience (e.g., McCrae & Costa, 2006). Moreover, because attachment researchers have confronted many of the same conceptual issues that personality psychologists have, there may be common solutions to these problems.

We begin with a brief overview of attachment theory, highlighting some of the major topics studied by researchers over the years. We describe ways in which attachment theory and research have addressed core issues in personality theory, including units of analysis, the structure and origin of individual differences, and development. Finally, we discuss key challenges faced by attachment researchers, how those challenges mirror ones faced in personality research more generally, and how various ideas and findings in each area might be able to inform the other.

A BRIEF OVERVIEW OF ATTACHMENT THEORY

Bowlby developed attachment theory to explain the intense distress expressed by infants who are separated from their parents. He observed that separated infants go to extraordinary lengths (e.g., crying, clinging, frantically searching) either to prevent separation from, or reestablish proximity to, a missing parent. At the time of Bowlby's first writings, psychoanalytic theorists held that such emotional outbursts were manifestations of immature dependency, and many behaviorists thought that they were signs of dysfunctional parental reinforcements of dependency. Bowlby noted that such expressions are common to a wide variety of mammalian species, suggesting that they serve an evolutionary function.

Drawing on ethological theory, Bowlby postulated that *attachment behaviors*, such as crying and searching, are adaptive responses to separation from a primary attachment figure—someone who has a history of providing support, protection, and care to the child. Because human infants, like other mammalian infants, cannot feed or protect themselves, they are highly dependent on the care and protection of "older and wiser" adults. Bowlby argued that, over the course of evolutionary history, infants who were able to attract the attention of, and maintain proximity to, an attachment figure (i.e., by looking cute or by engaging in attachment behaviors) would be more likely to survive to a reproductive age. According to Bowlby, a motivational control system, which he called the "attachment behavioral system," was gradually "designed" by natural selection to do just that.

The attachment behavioral system is an important concept in attachment theory because it provides the conceptual bridge between ethological models of human development (e.g., Hinde, 1966) and modern theories of emotion regulation and personality (e.g., John & Gross, 2007). According to Bowlby, the attachment system essentially "asks" the following question: Is the attachment figure nearby, accessible, and attentive? If the child perceives the answer to be "yes," he or she feels loved, secure, and confident, and, behaviorally, is likely to explore his or her environment, play with others, and be sociable. If, however, the child perceives the answer to be "no," he or she experiences anxiety and, behaviorally, is likely to exhibit attachment behaviors ranging from simple visual searching to active following and vocal signaling (see Figure 20.1). These behaviors continue until either the child is able to reestablish a desirable level of physical or psychological proximity to the attachment figure, or the child wears down, as may happen in the context of a prolonged separation or loss.

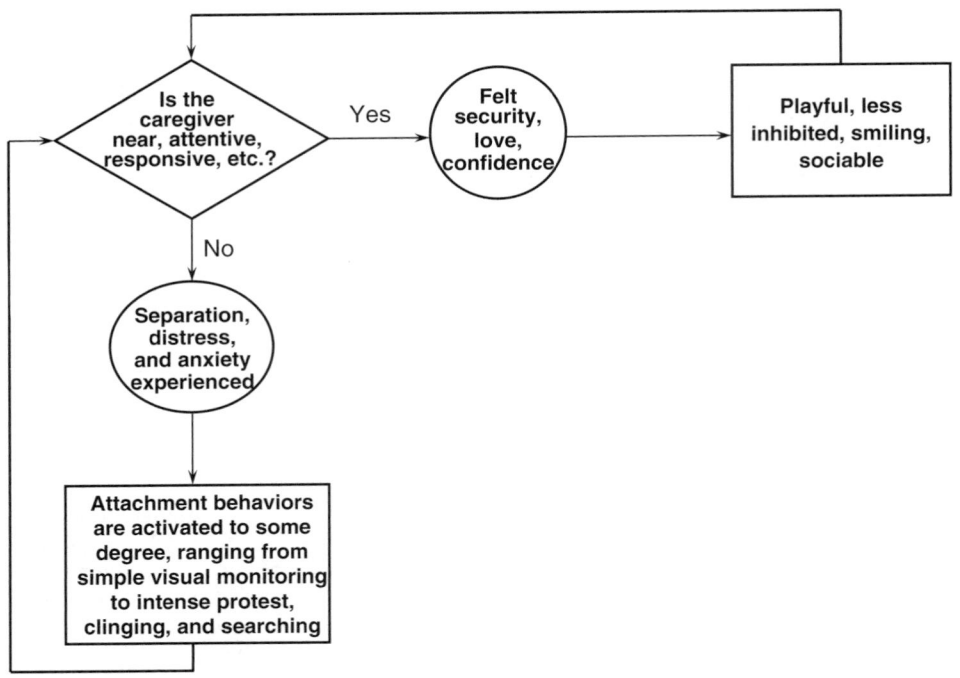

FIGURE 20.1. An illustration of the basic control mechanisms underlying Bowlby's conceptualization of the attachment behavioral system.

Bowlby believed that such experiences lead to despair and depression and have the potential to shape the expectations a child develops regarding self-worth and availability and accessibility of all significant others.

Individual Differences in Infant Attachment Patterns

Although Bowlby believed that the basic processes we have just described capture the normative dynamics of the attachment behavioral system, he recognized that there are individual differences in the way children appraise the accessibility of their attachment figures and regulate their attachment behavior in response to a threat. However, it was not until his colleague, Mary Ainsworth, began to study infant–parent separations systematically that a more complete and empirically informed understanding of these individual differences was established. Ainsworth and her students (Ainsworth, Blehar, Waters, & Wall, 1978) developed a technique called the "Strange Situation" to study infant–parent attachment. In the Strange Situation,

12-month-old infants and their parents are brought to the laboratory and systematically separated and reunited in a series of 3-minute scripted episodes. Most children (i.e., about 60%) behave in the way implied by Bowlby's normative theory. That is, they become upset when their parent leaves the room, but when he or she returns, they actively seek the parent and are easily comforted. Children who exhibit this pattern of behavior are often called "secure."

Other children (about 20% or less) are ill at ease initially, and upon separation become extremely distressed. Of great importance theoretically, when reunited with their parents they have difficulty being soothed and often exhibit conflicting behaviors that suggest that they want to be comforted but also want to "punish" their parent for leaving. These children are often called "anxious–resistant." The third pattern of attachment (shown by around 20% of children) is called *avoidant*. Avoidant children do not appear to be overly distressed by the separation, and upon reunion they actively avoid seeking contact with their parent, sometimes turning their attention, somewhat rigidly, to toys on the laboratory floor.

Ainsworth's research was important for at least three reasons. First, she provided one of the early empirical demonstrations of the ways in which attachment behavior is patterned in both safe and novel or threatening contexts. Second, she provided the first empirical taxonomy of individual differences in infant attachment patterns. According to her research, at least three "types" of children exist: those who are secure in their relationship with their parents, those who are anxious–resistant, and those who are anxious–avoidant. These individual differences have become the focus of most empirical research conducted on attachment. We discuss the relative merits of this particular taxonomy later, but for now we wish to highlight the fact that it was an important first step in delineating and studying individual differences in attachment.

Finally, and most importantly, Ainsworth demonstrated that these individual differences were predicted by infant–parent interactions in the home during the first year of life (i.e., before the Strange Situation assessments were made). Children who were classified as secure in the Strange Situation, for example, tended to have parents who were responsive to their needs. Children who were classified as insecure (i.e., as anxious–resistant or avoidant) often had parents who were insensitive to their needs or inconsistent or rejecting in their care. These data provided crucial support for some of Bowlby and Ainsworth's hypotheses about why some children develop secure relations with their caregivers, whereas other children develop insecure patterns.

A great deal of research since Ainsworth's has empirically tested some of her and Bowlby's claims about the origins of security and insecurity. Several longitudinal studies have documented associations between early maternal sensitivity and a child's attachment classification in the Strange Situation. For example, Grossmann and colleagues (K. Grossmann, Grossmann, Spangler, Suess, & Unzer, 1985) studied interactions between infants and their parents at home, and then later, when the infants were approximately a year old, brought them and their parents into the laboratory to participate in the Strange Situation. Children whose parents were rat-

ed as sensitive and responsive to their needs were more likely than other children to be classified as secure in the Strange Situation (see also Bates, Maslin, & Frankel, 1985; Isabella, 1993; Kiser, Bates, Maslin, & Bayles, 1986; see DeWolff & van IJzendoorn, 1997, for a review).

The association between infant–parent interactions and security has also been established experimentally. In one particularly interesting experiment, Anisfeld, Casper, Nozyce, and Cunningham (1990) randomly assigned parents who were participating in a parenting class to receive either a cozy, strap-on baby carrier or a plastic infant seat with a safety belt (which had the consequence of keeping the baby at a distance from the parents' bodies). Children whose parents had been assigned to the close-contact carrier condition were later more likely to be classified as secure in the Strange Situation than children whose parents received a plastic infant seat. Many experimental studies of nonhuman primates also demonstrate associations between maternal sensitivity and infant security and adaptation (Suomi, 1999), further suggesting that the infant–mother relationship can have effects on the way the child organizes his or her attachment behavior and regulates emotions.

Over the years there have been debates regarding the extent to which the attachment classifications are "merely" reflections of child temperament instead of capturing something about the way in which children organize their emotions and behavior in relation to a specific attachment figure—an organization based on the history of interactions with that figure. As some scholars have noted, there is only a modest overlap between attachment classifications when children are tested separately with their mothers and with their fathers (Fox, Kimmerly, & Schafer, 1991), suggesting that, to a large extent, the classifications are relationship-specific. This finding is difficult to explain if the attachment classifications are simply alternative ways of indexing a child's temperament. Moreover, most studies that have examined measures of temperament and attachment classifications have found weak or inconsistent associations between them (see Vaughn, Bost, & van IJzendoorn, 2008, for a review). This is not to say that temperament and parental relationships do not interact to affect a child's attachment classification (see, e.g., Mangelsdorf, Gunnar, Kestenbaum, Lang, & Andreas, 1990), but the findings we review here indicate that attachment classifications are not simply an alternative way of measuring temperament.

DEVELOPMENTAL PATHWAYS AND THE LEGACY OF EARLY EXPERIENCES

Over the past few decades there has been a great deal of research on the developmental implications of early attachment experiences (e.g., Grossmann, Grossmann, & Waters, 2005; Weinfield, Sroufe, Egeland, & Carlson, 2008). Most of this research has focused on the association between attachment classifications at 1 year of age and various later outcomes of developmental significance, such as ego resiliency, the ability to get along well and cooperate with peers, the ability to solve problems effectively, and psychopathology in adolescence (e.g., Carlson, 1998). Although there are exceptions, the majority of published studies demonstrate that early attachment status is related to many outcomes of interest to psychologists, not just in early childhood, but in later adolescence and young adulthood as well (e.g., Roisman, Madsen, Hennighausen, Sroufe, & Collins, 2001). Of course, there are varying perspectives on what those associations mean. The most common interpretation is the *organizational* perspective (Sroufe, 1979) that was inspired by Bowlby's discussion of developmental pathways.

In his 1973 volume, *Separation*, Bowlby analyzed the concept of developmental pathways by exploring the metaphor of a complex railway system. If a traveler were to begin his or her journey by selecting the main route, he or she would eventually reach a point at which the railroad branches into a number of distinct tracks. Some of these tracks would lead to distant, unfamiliar lands; others, although deviating from the main route, would run more or less parallel to it. As the traveler's journey progressed, he or she would be faced with new choices at each juncture. The choices the traveler made would have important implications for his or her journey and its ultimate destination.

Bowlby believed that the railway metaphor was a good way to characterize personality development. Early in life, there are many pathways along which a person might develop, and a variety of "destinations" at which the person might arrive (Sroufe & Jacobvitz, 1989). Some of these destinations involve high-functioning relationships with family members, peers, and romantic or marital partners; some do not. As people navigate alternative pathways, many get further away from their common origins, making their life trajectory increasingly difficult to transform. One of Bowlby's goals was to understand the pathways by which people develop and, importantly, to elucidate the processes that either keep them on a particular developmental course or allow them to deviate from routes previously established.

Bowlby's railway metaphor was inspired by C. H. Waddington's (1957) discussion of the cybernetics of cell development. Waddington, a developmental embryologist writing in the middle of the 20th century, was attempting to understand how a cell maintains a particular developmental trajectory in the face of external disturbances. He and others had observed that, once a cell begins to assume specific functions (e.g., becomes integrated into a structure that is destined to become the visual system), weak experimental interventions are unlikely to alter the cell's developmental trajectory. Although early in development a cell has the potential to assume many different fates, once a developmental trajectory becomes established, it becomes "canalized" or buffered, to some degree, making it less and less likely that the cell will deviate from that developmental course.

To illustrate these dynamics more concretely, Waddington compared them to the behavior of a marble rolling down a hill. In this analogy, the marble represents a cell, and the various troughs at the end of the landscape represent alternative developmental functions or "fates" the cell can assume. Waddington considered the specific shape of the landscape to be controlled by complex interactions among genes and between genes and the environment, leading Waddington to refer to it as the "epigenetic landscape."

After the marble begins its descent, it settles into one of several pathways defined by the valley floors of the epigenetic landscape. A slight push may force the marble away from its course, but the marble will eventually reestablish its trajectory. As the marble continues along the basin of a specific valley, it becomes increasingly unlikely that external forces will cause it to jump from one valley to the next. Certain features of the marble, such as its smoothness and momentum, help to keep it moving along the established path. Features intrinsic to the landscape itself also help to maintain the marble on its original pathway. The steepness and curvature of the hills, for example, serve to cradle the marble and buffer it from external forces.

Waddington considered the tendency for the marble to maintain its initial course in the face of external pressures to be an analogue to a fundamental self-regulatory process in cell development, "homeorhesis." Homeorhesis refers to the tendency of a system to maintain a specific developmental trajectory—or a course toward a specific developmental outcome—despite external perturbations. Waddington argued that the specific pathways available to the cell early in development are determined by the way the genes interact to initiate and control biochemical reactions. Moreover, he believed that these reactions operate in a manner that leads the valleys of the epigenetic landscape to become more entrenched over time. Thus, once a cell settles into one of several available pathways, it becomes increasingly likely to follow that pathway.

The concept "degree of canalization" was important to Bowlby, and he often wrote of "environmentally labile" traits to refer to properties that were less subject to canalization. In his 1969/1982 volume, *Attachment*, for example, he argued that the development of the attachment behavioral system is highly canalized, in the sense that the rudimentary set of control mechanisms and behavior programs needed to allow a child to regulate proximity to a caregiver emerges despite a diverse range of environmental circumstances. Bowlby believed, however, that the *specific way* in which a child comes to regulate his or her attachment behavior is influenced by interpersonal experiences, and if the system is to function appropriately in a specific caregiving environment, it needs to be calibrated, more or less, to that environment. Bowlby thought that early experiences within the family—especially those concerned with separation or threats of loss—were particularly influential in shaping the way a child's attach-

ment system becomes organized. According to his railway metaphor, early experiences in the family help to determine which of many possible routes an individual will travel.

In the context of personality development, Bowlby believed that once an initial pathway is established, there are a number of homeorhetic processes that keep a person on that pathway. He separated these homeorhetic processes into two broad categories. The first is the *caregiving environment*. To the extent that an individual's caregiving environment is stable, he or she is unlikely to experience interactions that challenge his or her representations of the world. Bowlby (1973) noted that a child is typically born into a family in which he or she has the same parents, same community, and the same broad ecology for long periods of time. Thus, it is during unusual periods of transition (e.g., parental divorce, relocating to a new town, being abused by an adult) that a person is most likely to be forced from one developmental track onto another. (This idea has been well supported in a 20-year longitudinal study by Waters, Merrick, Treboux, Crowell, & Albersheim, 2000).

Bowlby (1973) also discussed homeorhetic *intraindividual* or *psychodynamic* processes that can promote continuity. He noted that people often select their environments in ways that maximize the overlap between the psychological qualities of the situations and the people's experience-based expectations and preferences. Moreover, Bowlby argued, the mind generally assimilates new information into existing schemas rather than accommodating to it (an idea Bowlby borrowed from Piaget, whom he knew personally; see Collins & Read, 1994, for a discussion of this issue as it arises in the study of adult attachment and social cognition). Consistent with these ideas, empirical research has shown that people's working models influence the kinds of reactions they elicit from others (Arend, Gove, & Sroufe, 1979; Troy & Sroufe, 1987; Waters, Wippman, & Sroufe, 1979) and the kinds of inferences they make about people's intentions in experimental contexts (Brumbaugh & Fraley, 2006; Collins, 1996; Pierce, Sarason, & Sarason, 1992; Pietromonaco & Carnelley, 1994). Such dynamics allow working models to shape the kinds of interactions a person experiences, and in concert, help to maintain the individual's already partially canalized pathway through development. To the extent that an individual diverges from such a pathway, the changed route seems likely to be fairly close to its predecessor.

The important point is that Bowlby's theory offered a means (1) to understand how variation in an early caregiving environment can influence a child's development and (2) to acknowledge that it is not only the child who is affected by these experiences, but the subsequent developmental context and pathway as well. These processes are highly dynamic because, not only is the caregiving environment shaping the child's expectations about the world, but those expectations, in turn, influence the way people in the social world relate to the child. As a result, there is likely to be a detectable coherence over time in the way the child functions, and although the specific behaviors observed over time may change, the underlying themes that characterize the child's behavior may be relatively stable. One of the objectives of empirical research on attachment is to understand how caregiving environments affect children, how children's working models influence their environments in turn, and how the interplay between these two factors shapes children's developmental paths. Whereas certain kinds of experiences have the potential to alter a person's life course, the homeorhetic dynamics of the attachment system promote continuity and coherence over time.

ATTACHMENT IN ADULTS

Although Bowlby was primarily concerned with understanding the infant–caregiver relationship, he believed that attachment characterizes human experience from "the cradle to the grave." It was not until the mid-1980s, however, that researchers began to take seriously the possibility that attachment processes play out in adulthood in ways that go beyond what is predicted from infancy or childhood. Ideas about adult attachment were explored and developed in slightly different ways within different research traditions. Among developmental psychologists, researchers began to refine methods, such as the Adult Attachment Interview (AAI) (e.g., Main, Kaplan, & Cassidy, 1985; see review

by Hesse, in press), for understanding how young adults represent their early attachment experiences with parents. By studying transcripts based on an hour-long interview, Main and her colleagues developed a means of predicting which parents would have secure children and which would have insecure children, as assessed in the Strange Situation.

Their studies indicated that parents who are able to recall and describe their early experiences in a coherent fashion are more likely than others to have infants classified as "secure" in the Strange Situation. Such parents, called "secure and autonomous with respect to attachment," or just "secure," are able to collaborate effectively with the interviewer and provide accounts that are internally consistent. Other parents provide less coherent narratives. Some, for example, provide inconsistent information (e.g., describing their early relationships with parents as being "warm," yet narrating specific episodes in which they felt neglected or unappreciated by their parents). Some adults tend to minimize the relevance of their parents, whereas others appear to be overly enmeshed in these relationships. Many studies (reviewed by Crowell, Fraley, & Shaver, 2008) now confirm that adults' AAI classifications predict their children's attachment classifications (suggesting a degree of intergenerational transmission of attachment dynamics), their behavior toward their children, and their behavior toward their spouses or romantic partners (Roisman et al., 2007).

Among social and personality psychologists, the attachment dynamics and individual differences that Bowlby and Ainsworth discussed were examined in the context of close adult relationships, often of the romantic-sexual variety. Hazan and Shaver (1987) were two of the first researchers to explore Bowlby's ideas in this context. This research indicated that the emotional bond that develops between adult romantic partners is partly a function of the same motivational system—the attachment behavioral system—that gives rise to the emotional bond between infants and their caregivers. Further research revealed that adult romantic partners, like infants in relation to their caregivers, share the following features: (1) both infants and adults feel safer when their attachment figure is nearby and responsive; (2) both engage in close, intimate, bodily contact; (3) both feel insecure when their attachment figure is separated from them and inaccessible; (4) both share discoveries with each other; (5) both engage in mutual eye contact, touch each other's faces gently or playfully, snuggle and embrace, and seem fascinated and preoccupied with each other; and (6) both tend to use a special kind of communication, called "motherese" in the infant–parent relationship and "baby talk" in romantic relationships (Shaver, Hazan, & Bradshaw, 1988). On the basis of these parallels, it was argued that many adult romantic relationships, like infant–caregiver relationships, are *attachments*, and that romantic love is a property of the attachment behavioral system, as well as the somewhat distinct motivational systems that give rise to caregiving and sexuality (Hazan & Shaver, 1987; Shaver et al., 1988).

The idea that romantic relationships may be attachment relationships has had a profound influence on modern research in social and personality psychology. There are at least three important implications of this idea. First, if adult romantic relationships are attachment relationships, then we should observe the same kinds of individual differences in adult relationships that Ainsworth observed in infant–caregiver relationships. We may expect some adults, for example, to be secure in their relationships—to feel confident that their partners will be there for them, when needed, and feel open to depending on others and having others depend on them. We should expect other adults to be insecure in their relationships. For example, some insecure adults may be anxious–resistant: They worry that others do not love them sufficiently, and they are easily frustrated or angered when their attachment needs go unmet. Others may be avoidant: They may appear not to care much about close relationships and may prefer not to depend on other people or have others be dependent on them.

Second, if adult romantic relationships are attachment relationships, then the way in which adult relationships function should be similar to the way infant–caregiver relationships function. In other words, the same factors that facilitate exploration in children (i.e., having a responsive caregiver and the knowledge that he or she is available, if needed) should facilitate exploration in adults (i.e., having a responsive partner and knowing that he or she is available, when needed). The qualities that make an attachment figure "desirable" to an infant (i.e., being available, responsive, supportive) should also be desirable qualities in an adult romantic partner. Importantly, individual differences in attachment should influence relational and personal functioning in adulthood in the same ways they affect childhood behavior.

Third, whether an adult is secure or insecure in his or her adult relationships may be a partial reflection of his or her attachment experiences in childhood. As discussed previously, Bowlby believed that the mental representations or "working models" (i.e., expectations, beliefs, "rules" or "scripts" for behaving and thinking) that a child holds regarding relationships are a function of his or her experiences with caregivers. For example, a secure child tends to believe that others will be there for him or her because previous experiences have led to this conclusion. Once a child has developed such expectations, he or she will tend to seek out relational experiences consistent with those expectations and perceive others in ways colored by those beliefs. According to Bowlby, this kind of homeorhetic process should promote continuity in attachment patterns over the life course, although it is possible that a person's attachment pattern will change if his or her relational experiences are inconsistent with expectations. In short, if we assume that adult relationships are attachment relationships, it is possible that children who are secure as children will become adults who are secure in their romantic relationships.

In the following sections we briefly address some of these implications in light of early and contemporary research on adult attachment. This is not meant to be a comprehensive review (for a more comprehensive one, see Mikulincer & Shaver, 2007a); rather, it is designed to convey some of the major themes that have occupied attachment researchers over the past two decades while illustrating some of the ways in which the primary "units of analysis" in attachment research are studied.

DO WE OBSERVE THE SAME KINDS OF ATTACHMENT PATTERNS IN ADULTS THAT WE OBSERVE IN CHILDREN?

The earliest research on adult attachment examined associations between individual differences in adult attachment and the way people think about their romantic relationships and recall their childhood relationships with their parents. My colleague (P. R. S.) and I developed a simple questionnaire to measure these individual differences (which have been given different names by different investigators: "attachment styles," "attachment patterns," "attachment orientations," or "differences in the organization of the attachment system") (Hazan & Shaver, 1987). We asked research subjects to read the three paragraphs below and indicate which one best characterized the way they think, feel, and behave in close relationships (Hazan & Shaver, 1987):

> A. I am somewhat uncomfortable being close to others; I find it difficult to trust them completely, difficult to allow myself to depend on them. I am nervous when anyone gets too close, and often, others want me to be more intimate than I feel comfortable being.
> B. I find it relatively easy to get close to others and am comfortable depending on them and having them depend on me. I don't worry about being abandoned or about someone getting too close to me.
> C. I find that others are reluctant to get as close as I would like. I often worry that my partner doesn't really love me or won't want to stay with me. I want to get very close to my partner, and this sometimes scares people away.

Based on this three-category measure, we found that the frequencies of endorsing the different categories was similar to the frequencies observed in middle-class samples of infants in the Strange Situation: About 60% of adults classified themselves as secure (paragraph B), about 20% as avoidant (paragraph A), and about 20% as anxious–resistant (paragraph C) (Hazan & Shaver, 1987).

Although this measure was useful for documenting the association between attachment styles and relationship functioning, it did not allow a full test of the hypothesis that the same kinds of individual differences observed in infants might also be evident in adults. (For the most part, our measure assumed this to be true; it did not provide a means for testing the hypothesis.) We have explored this hypothesis in a variety of ways in subsequent research. For example, Brennan, Clark, and Shaver (1998) collected a large number of statements conceptually related to attachment (e.g., "I believe that others will be there for me when I need them"), correlated people's responses on them, and determined their underlying structure using factor analysis. Our findings indicated that there are two major attachment-style dimensions (see Figure 20.2). One of them was labeled "attachment-related anxiety." People with high scores on this dimension tend to worry whether their relationship partner is available, attentive, and responsive. People who score low on this dimension are more secure with respect to their partner's responsiveness. The other dimension is called "attachment-related avoidance." People who score high on this dimension prefer not to rely on others or open up emotionally to them. People who score low are more comfortable being intimate with others and relying on them for comfort and support. A prototypically secure adult scores low on both dimensions.

Recent analyses of the statistical patterning of infant behavior in the Strange Situation have revealed two conceptually similar dimensions, one indexing an infant's anxiety and resistance and the other indexing the child's willingness to use a parent as a safe haven and secure base (see Fraley & Spieker, 2003a, 2003b). These dimensions were also evident in a discriminant analysis included in Ainsworth and colleagues' (1978) book, but subsequent investigators tended to use attachment categories instead of the two continuous dimensions. Taken together, studies of the structure of measures of attachment orientation at different ages suggest that two major individual-difference dimensions exist at different points in the lifespan.

In light of Brennan and colleagues' findings, as well as taxometric research by Fraley and Waller (1998), most researchers currently conceptualize and measure attachment patterns dimensionally rather than categorically. The most popular measures of adult attachment style are Brennan and colleagues' Experiences in Close Relationships (1998) (ECR) and Fraley, Waller, and Brennan's (2000) Ex-

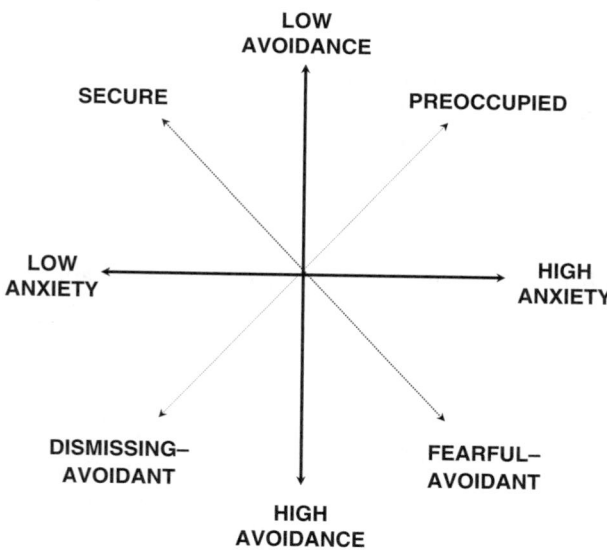

FIGURE 20.2. The two-dimensional model that is commonly used in contemporary social-personality research to conceptualize and partition individual differences in adult attachment. The cardinal lines represent the dimensions of attachment-related anxiety and avoidance, as described by Brennan et al. (1998). The diagonal lines capture the four prototypes described by Bartholomew and Horowitz (1991).

periences in Close Relationships—Revised (ECR-R), a slightly revised version of the ECR, based on item-response theory. Both self-report instruments provide scores on the two continuous dimensions: attachment-related anxiety and avoidance.

Although contemporary attachment researchers tend to focus on the two attachment dimensions of anxiety and avoidance in their research, it is important to note that this two-dimensional space covers many of the distinctions that have been made by other attachment researchers. For example, Hazan and Shaver's (1987) description of security refers to a combination of elements involving low anxiety and low avoidance, whereas their description of avoidance refers to someone who is high in avoidance and moderately high in attachment anxiety as well. Similarly, Bartholomew and Horowitz's (1991) four prototypes of security, preoccupation, fearful avoidance, and dismissing avoidance can be located in the two-dimensional space by rotating the anxiety and avoidance axes by 45 degrees, as show in Figure 20.2 (also see Griffin & Bartholomew, 1994). The prototypical dismissing individual, for example, is

high on the avoidance dimension and low on the anxiety dimension.

For the purposes of this chapter, most of the work that we review does not focus on distinguishing the two dimensions. We focus primarily on the way in which individual differences in security are related to other variables, while not always specifying whether security was measured using an older categorical measure or a linear combination of anxiety and avoidance, or whether only one of the two attachment dimensions was related to the outcome. These distinctions are sometimes important in attachment research, but a simplified discussion is sufficient here. We encourage interested readers to follow up these matters by reading the original publications.

DO ADULT ROMANTIC RELATIONSHIPS "WORK" THE SAME WAY AS INFANT–CAREGIVER RELATIONSHIPS?

There is now a large and heterogeneous body of research showing that adult romantic relationships do function in psychologically similar ways as infant–caregiver relationships, with some noteworthy exceptions, of course. Naturalistic research on adults separating from their partners at an airport demonstrated that behaviors indicative of attachment-related protest and caregiving occurred, and that regulation of these behaviors was associated with attachment style (Fraley & Shaver, 1998). For example, whereas couples who were about to separate (because one of them was leaving on an outbound flight) generally showed more attachment behavior (e.g., touching, watching, holding) than nonseparating couples, more avoidant adults displayed much less attachment behavior than less avoidant adults. In the sections below we discuss other parallels between infant–caregiver relationships and adult romantic relationships.

Partner Selection

Cross-cultural studies find that the secure pattern of attachment in infancy is universally considered the most desirable pattern by mothers (van IJzendoorn & Sagi-Schwartz, 2008). For obvious reasons, there is no similar study asking infants if they would prefer a security-inducing attachment figure. Adults seeking long-term relationships identify responsive caregiving qualities, such as attentiveness, warmth, and sensitivity, as most "attractive" in potential dating partners (Zeifman & Hazan, 1997). Despite the attractiveness of secure qualities, however, not all adults are paired with secure partners. Some evidence suggests that people end up in relationships with partners who confirm their existing beliefs about attachment relationships (Frazier, Byer, Fischer, Wright, & DeBord, 1997).

Secure-Base and Safe-Haven Behavior

In infancy, secure infants tend to be the most socially adjusted, in the sense that they are relatively resilient, get along well with their peers, and are well liked. Similar kinds of patterns are notable in research on adult attachment. Overall, secure adults tend to be more satisfied in their relationships than insecure adults. Their relationships are characterized by greater longevity, trust, commitment, and interdependence (e.g., Feeney, Noller, & Callan, 1994), and secure individuals are more likely to use romantic partners as a secure base from which to explore the world (e.g., Fraley & Davis, 1997).

Much of the research on adult attachment has been devoted to uncovering the behavioral and psychological mechanisms that promote security and secure-base behavior in adults. There have been two major discoveries thus far. First, and in accordance with attachment theory, secure adults are more likely than insecure adults to seek support from their partners when distressed (see Mikulincer & Shaver, 2007a, for a review). Moreover, they are more likely to provide support to their distressed partners (e.g., Simpson, Rholes, & Nelligan, 1992). Second, the attributions that insecure individuals make concerning their partner's behavior during and following relational conflicts exacerbate, rather than alleviate, their insecurities (e.g., Simpson, Rholes, & Phillips, 1996).

Avoidant Attachment and Defense Mechanisms

According to attachment theory, children differ in the kinds of strategies they adopt to regulate attachment-related anxiety. As mentioned earlier, following a separation and reunion between an infant and his or her parent, some insecure children approach the parents, but with ambivalence and resistance, whereas others withdraw from the parent, apparently minimizing attachment-related negative feelings and behavior. One of the big questions in the study of infant attachment is whether children who withdraw from their parents—avoidant children—are truly less distressed or whether their defensive behavior is a cover-up for their true feelings of vulnerability. Research that has measured the attentional capacity of children, heart rate, or stress hormone levels suggests that avoidant children are distressed by the separation, despite looking cool and unconcerned (e.g., Sroufe & Waters, 1977).

Recent research on adult attachment has revealed some interesting complexities concerning the relationships between avoidance and defense. Although some avoidant adults—the ones Bartholomew and Horowitz (1991) called fearfully avoidant—are poorly adjusted despite their defensive nature, others—the dismissingly avoidant—are able to use defensive strategies in an adaptive way. For example, in an experimental task in which adults were instructed to discuss losing their partner, we found that dismissing individuals (i.e., those who scored high on attachment-related avoidance but low on attachment-related anxiety) were just as physiologically distressed (as assessed by skin conductance measures) as other individuals (Fraley & Shaver, 1997). When instructed to suppress their thoughts and feelings, however, dismissing individuals were able to do so effectively. That is, they could deactivate their physiological arousal, to some degree, and minimize the occurrence of attachment-related thoughts. Fearfully avoidant individuals were not as successful in suppressing their emotions. This finding was replicated, but it was also discovered that avoidant adults were less proficient at inhibiting attachment-relevant thoughts and feelings when their attentional resources were depleted by a cognitively engaging task (Mikulincer, Dolev, & Shaver, 2004). This and other more naturalistic studies (e.g., Berant, Mikulincer, & Shaver, 2008) suggest that avoidant individuals' ability to suppress thoughts and feelings related to negative attachment experiences, as well as negative thoughts about themselves, is successful much of the time, perhaps partly because these thoughts can be avoided by not engaging in social interactions in which they would become salient. Under stress, however, the avoidant defenses may fail, leaving a generally cool and collected individual vulnerable to painful experiences.

ATTACHMENT THEORY AND CONTEMPORARY PERSONALITY RESEARCH

One of the objectives of this chapter is to make the case that attachment theory has the potential to play an important role in contemporary personality research. Up to this point we have discussed some of the basic ideas in attachment theory, highlighting the core units of analysis, the developmental aspects of the theory, and the role of individual differences in attachment research. In the following sections we expand upon this theme by discussing conceptual challenges or debates that have arisen both in attachment theory and in personality research more generally. Our intent is to highlight the ways in which these issues have been handled in both areas and to suggest that some of the ideas, models, and solutions that have been developed in personality research could be useful for better understanding attachment processes. We also contend that some of the ideas developed by attachment researchers have the potential to inform personality research more generally.

Consistency across Situations

Attachment researchers have tended to conceptualize attachment-related working models (cognitive–affective schemas) as generalized representations—representations that capture the broad, as opposed to the specific, relational themes common to diverse interpersonal experiences. This approach, which has sometimes been referred to as a "trait" or "individual-centered" approach (Kobak, 1994; Lewis, 1994), has obvious parallels to the trait concept in personality research and has been popular for a number of reasons. For one, if early childhood experiences with caregivers result in the formation of cognitive structures that are relatively general and stable, then these structures could be the basis for the continuity and coherence people display in their many close relationships. Although there are undoubtedly variations from one relationship to another in how a person relates to significant others, a trait perspective implies that there is likely to be a common thread tying together the individual's thoughts, feelings, and behavior across the different relationships and contexts.

Despite its appeal, the trait approach to attachment has been criticized on at least two grounds. First, researchers have observed that people exhibit different attachment patterns across different relationships. Baldwin, Keelan, Fehr, Ennis, and Koh-Rangarajoo (1996), for example, demonstrated that there is considerable within-person variability in the expectations and beliefs that people hold about different significant others. A man may consider his spouse to be warm, affectionate, and responsive while simultaneously viewing his mother as cold, rejecting, and aloof. The fact that substantial within-person variation (i.e., "inconsistency") exists in the way in which people relate to others raises a number of questions about how working models should be conceptualized in attachment theory.

This problem will be familiar to most personality researchers. Over 40 years ago

Walter Mischel published *Personality and Assessment*, a review of the field that is now best remembered for its critique of trait models of personality (Mischel, 1968). According to Mischel's interpretation of the evidence, the correlations among measures of behavior from one situation to the next were lower than expected, leading him to question the usefulness of the trait concept (see Ahadi & Diener, 1989, however, for alternative interpretations).

Attachment researchers have offered several potential solutions to the *inconsistency issue* in the study of attachment. One popular proposal has been that people hold different working models of different relationships, and that different models can exist at different levels of abstraction or generalization (e.g., Collins, Guichard, Ford, & Feeney, 2004; Overall, Fletcher, & Friesen, 2003). For example, people may hold relatively global representations of their "parents," but they also hold relationship-specific representations of their mothers and fathers. Thus, it is possible for the same person to exhibit varying degrees of security in relationships with two parents, assuming that there is a different history of security and support in the two relationships.

From this point of view, the challenge for attachment researchers is not to explain why people experience different degrees of security in their various relationships, but why there is some degree of consistency across relationships when each relationship has its own unique aspects. Collins and her colleagues (2004) suggested that, in addition to forming relationship-specific representations, people develop a more abstract, global representation that captures some kind of "average" of their experiences. Indeed, theoretical work on this possibility, using connectionist simulations, suggests that mental systems easily extract the "gist" or themes that are common to many different experiences and that these more abstract representations can be used to guide the model's response to new and ambiguous targets (Fraley, 2007). As a result, behavior in any one context can be driven both by global or abstract representations and by ones that are more specific to the relationship in question. The global representation is part of what creates similarity in a person's thoughts and feelings across relationships (and thus acts as a la-

tent factor, in a psychometric sense), whereas the relationship-specific representation captures knowledge and strategies for managing specific relationships (and thus explains relationship-specific variance).

Another explanation for the presence of some consistency across relationship partners is developmental in nature. If a relationship-specific representation is forged partly on the basis of those that already exist, we would expect a modest degree of association in security across different relationships. For example, if one relationship-specific representation (pertaining to Mother, say) was constructed before another (i.e., pertaining to one's romantic relationship partner), and if the former played a role in shaping the latter, then the two sets of relational experiences would be similar (and, thus, correlated across targets; see Figure 20.3). In this scenario, there is no global model or "trait," per se (although there is no reason why there could not be); the associations among the security levels of representations of different relationships is explained by existing models playing a causal (but incomplete) role in shaping the development of new models. The association is imperfect because the new relationships are unique in many respects.

Social-cognitive research on transference suggests that these kinds of dynamics occur and can be set in motion relatively easily with simple laboratory stimuli (e.g., Andersen & Chen, 2002). For example, when asked to rate how secure people feel with potential mates described in personal ads, participants are more likely to feel secure with

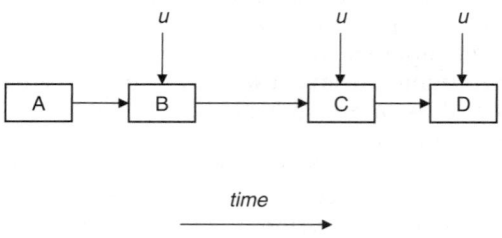

FIGURE 20.3. An illustration of one way in which attachment representations in different relationships could become correlated with one another in a manner that would suggest, in a factor analysis, that there is a "global" or latent factor when there really is not.

the people described in the ads when those ads have been constructed, unbeknownst to the research subjects, to resemble a former attachment figure (Brumbaugh & Fraley, 2006). This finding indicates that existing working models can be used to guide the interpretation of new experiences, thereby creating a degree of consistency.

These ideas bear on the consistency debate in personality psychology. In mainstream personality psychology, most of the initial responses to Mischel's arguments were "defensive" in nature—attempts to explain why Mischel was wrong or misrepresenting the facts rather than attempts to understand how it is that people can exhibit coherence in their thoughts, feelings, and behavior without necessarily behaving in similar ways across situations. Some proposals, for example, focused on the fact that the expected correlation between two "samples" of behavior should be relatively small, as expected from the psychometric principles of classical test theory, but that such correlations will increase as more and more instances are aggregated (Epstein, 1979, 1980). Other proposals focused on the idiosyncratic meaning of trait terms and how some traits might be relevant to some people while being irrelevant to others (thereby making their behavior less consistent across situations; see Bem & Allen, 1974; see also Baumeister & Tice, 1988, for a discussion).

One of the more recent rapprochements has come from Mischel himself. Mischel and Shoda's (1995; Chapter 7, this volume) cognitive–affective processing system (i.e., CAPS) model assumes that an important aspect of personality is the "if–then" associations people hold. A person can behave in a way that appears inconsistent if a researcher simply aggregates measures of honesty across situations, but the person may in fact be behaving in a way that is perfectly consistent with the way in which his or her associations are organized. For example, a person may be relatively sociable and outgoing among friends and family ("If with family, then feel free to express self"), but less talkative and shier when interacting with strangers ("If the situation and the other person's preferences are unknown, then refrain from sociable outbursts for the time being"). If we were to aggregate measures of sociable behavior across the two contexts, it might seem that

the person is "inconsistent," but the person's behavior might be quite lawful and coherent once the governing "ifs" and "thens" were taken into account.

The CAPS framework is similar to ones that have been adopted in the study of attachment, although the attachment approach incorporates traditional trait-like concepts (e.g., attachment styles, general working models) with more contextually specific factors, rather than removing trait-like constructs entirely. Indeed, theoretical simulations demonstrate that a connectionist cognitive system can construct both global representations and if–then representations in parallel, and that both kinds of representations can be used to guide behavior in new situations (Fraley, 2007). It should therefore be possible for personality researchers to consider models that enable traits and more dynamic and situation-specific aspects of personality to exist simultaneously.

Although additional solutions to the person–situation debate have been put forward (Fleeson's [2001] framework, e.g., strikes us as promising), the CAPS model is particularly worth discussing because in many ways it resembles ideas advanced by Bowlby (1969/1982, 1973, 1980) years before in his discussion of how working models are constructed and shape human experience. Moreover, some attachment researchers have explicitly embraced the CAPS framework as a means of understanding attachment dynamics in adult relationships (e.g., Zayas, Shoda, & Ayduk, 2002). Zayas and her colleagues provided a valuable discussion of how a close relationship can be viewed as a result of the interplay of two initially independent cognitive–affective systems (i.e., the two relationship partners) that eventually interlock and configure themselves in relation to each other. Such processes allow people to have preexisting working models that are initially used to make sense of partners as new relationships form, but also allow the working models to be reconfigured (and for new models to develop) as people continue their relationships. Ultimately, the way in which each person thinks, feels, and behaves in the relationship can be understood as lawful, but some of the classic concepts and measures used to study personality (e.g., measures of cross-situational consistency) may not always provide the best means of doing so.

Stability and Change: How Stable Are Attachment Patterns across Time?

One of the core themes in attachment research is that individual differences are relatively stable across time, but there have been heated debates about the extent to which attachment patterns are stable over the life course. Some scholars have highlighted the relative lack of stability in measures of attachment (e.g., Baldwin & Fehr, 1995; Kagan, 1996; Lewis, Feiring, & Rosenthal, 2000), whereas others have emphasized their stability (e.g., Waters et al., 2000). One reason these debates have been difficult to resolve is that test–retest correlation coefficients—the primary means of documenting and studying stability and change—can be difficult to interpret in a developmental context. If one were to assess a construct on two separate occasions and find a test–retest correlation of .30, some researchers might interpret it as

"small," whereas others might interpret it as "substantial."

It can be argued that test–retest coefficients across two time points are inadequate for determining whether a construct is stable (Fraley & Brumbaugh, 2004). To illustrate, consider the data shown in Figure 20.4. The solid curve illustrates a scenario in which the test–retest correlation between two measures of a construct is relatively high at the beginning of the life course (e.g., between ages 1 and 2), but gradually gets smaller as the test–retest interval increases. In fact, as the test–retest interval increases, the expected value of the test–retest correlation approaches zero. Now consider the dashed curve. In this scenario the stability correlations are relatively high across the early years and, although they drop to some extent, they approach a nonzero asymptote. The test–retest correlations between two measures of the construct are the same from age 1 to age 5 and from age 1 to age 35.

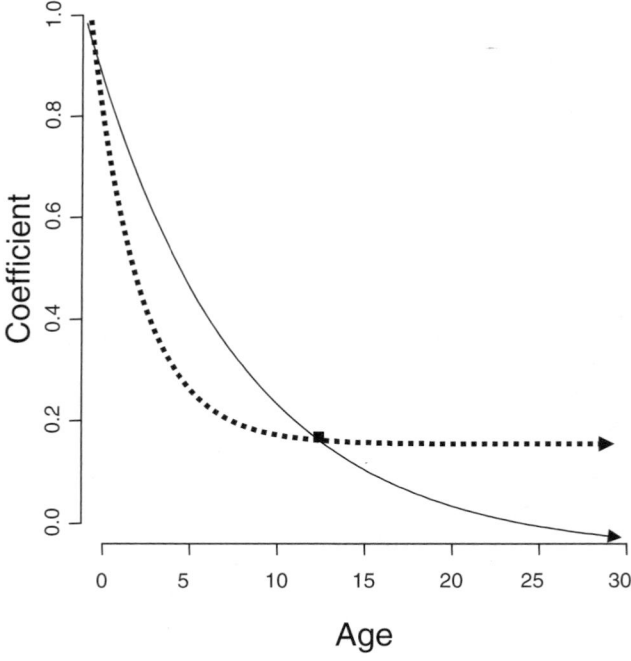

FIGURE 20.4. An illustration of the ambiguity of single test–retest correlation coefficients for understanding the stability of individual differences. In this diagram, a single correlation is compatible with two developmental predictions. One assumes that stability gradually decays over time, approaching zero in the limit (see the solid line). The other assumes that, although stability is not high, it does not continue to diminish as the test–retest interval increases (see the dashed line).

There are two important points to take away from this diagram. First, any test–retest coefficient (the bread and butter of longitudinal research on both personality and attachment) is compatible with two mutually exclusive scenarios: one in which there is a "stable degree of (in)stability" over time and one in which instability eventually "wins" and the long-run stability approaches zero. Most studies based on single test–retest coefficients are unable to address the original question: How stable are individual differences over long stretches of time? The second point is that questions about stability can be answered well only by studying test–retest correlations across multiple time points and estimating the asymptotic value of those correlations. It is the *pattern* of test–retest correlations over time that provides evidence of stability or instability, not the specific value of any one correlation, which has no clear meaning on its own (Fraley & Roberts, 2005).

Fraley (2002) initially discussed some of these issues in the context of attachment and formalized preliminary models that led to different predictions about the patterns of stability and change that should be observed in empirical studies. Based on a meta-analysis of the data that existed at the time, I concluded that attachment patterns were relatively stable from infancy to adulthood and that the asymptotic value of attachment stability was between .30 and .40. In other words, between age 1 and age 2, the expected stability is about .35, as it is between age 1 and age 25. The test–retest correlations tend to be higher in intervals across the adult years, which Fraley and Brumbaugh (2004) explained as being due to the accumulation of correlated variance across a person's environments.

These ideas were later adapted and elaborated to apply to similar debates in the study of personality traits (Fraley & Roberts, 2005). As in the domain of attachment research, debates have raged in trait research about the extent to which commonly studied personality traits are stable. Some researchers have argued that measures of personality are not highly stable over time (e.g., Lewis, 1999, 2001), whereas others have argued that they are (e.g., Caspi & Roberts, 2001; McCrae et al., 2000). Indeed, some researchers have argued that personality traits do

not change much at all past the age of 30, and that observed instability is largely due to measurement error (e.g., Costa & McCrae, 1994; but see Srivastava, John, Gosling, & Potter, 2003).

Fraley and Roberts (2005) formalized some of the ideas discussed in the literature on personality stability and change and illustrated the differential implications of those ideas for the patterns of stability that should be observed empirically over time. They reanalyzed meta-analytic data on the test–retest stability of personality measures and demonstrated that, as with attachment, the data on personality are compatible with the idea that there is a "stable degree of (in)stability" in personality. In short, the stability of individual differences from early childhood to later childhood and adulthood is relatively low, but it does not get lower as the test–retest interval increases. Moreover, the test–retest correlations in later life follow the same pattern but are higher than those seen in childhood, probably again due to the accumulation of correlated variance over time.

In summary, there is value in integrating the study of attachment and the study of personality. Both areas of study have struggled with the same issues, and in this case a solution that was developed in one area (i.e., the study of attachment) was able to affect the way in which personality researchers conceptualize and study stability and change.

What Is the Relation between Attachment and Trait Constructs?

One pressing issue for researchers working at the interface of attachment and personality is the association, both conceptual and empirical, between individual differences in attachment and personality traits, such as the Big Five dimensions (e.g., John & Srivastava, 1999). Theoretically, the issue is not as clear-cut as some might wish. As we discussed previously, Bowlby (1973) conceptualized attachment and development in a manner that was inspired by Waddington's (1957) discussion of cell development. As a result, Bowlby explicitly argued that a child's preexisting dispositions play a role in his or her responses to the environment; in some respects, they are responsible for the shape of the epigenetic stage upon which attachment relationships play out (e.g., Bowlby, 1973,

p. 369). But he also argued that the history of interactions between a child and his or her attachment figures is the more proximate and crucial determinant of the thoughts, feelings, and behaviors that the child experiences in close relationships, regardless of the preexisting dispositions upon which they are layered.

In the lingo of contemporary personality psychology, it is unclear from Bowlby's writings whether he considered basic personality traits to be independent predictors of interpersonal behavior, the starting point in a mediated casual chain, a potential moderator of the relations between attachment and interpersonal behavior, or some combination of the above. Regardless of this ambiguity, it is certain that he did not conceptualize individual differences in security as being "nothing more" than preexisting personality traits. In that spirit, it is worth noting that there has been a great deal of research over the past decade examining the way in which individual differences in security predict various outcomes, after statistically controlling for individuals' scores on measures of basic personality traits, such as neuroticism. For example, there is robust evidence that secure individuals tend to maintain stabler romantic relationships than insecure people (either anxious or avoidant) and report higher levels of relationship satisfaction and adjustment (see Mikulincer & Shaver, 2007a, for a review). This pattern has been consistently obtained in studies of both dating and married couples and cannot be explained by other personality factors, such as the Big Five personality traits or self-esteem (Noftle & Shaver, 2006). Moreover, research on seemingly basic affective responses reveals that measures of attachment predict emotional reactions even when basic personality traits are controlled (e.g., Erez, Mikulincer, van IJzendoorn, & Kroonenberg, 2008; Mikulincer, Gillath, & Shaver, 2002).

Despite the fact that individual differences in attachment are related to a variety of outcomes when basic personality traits are controlled, it is important to note that attachment and personality traits *are* related to one another in meaningful ways. Attachment anxiety, not surprisingly, is substantially correlated with neuroticism (r's in the .40–.50 range), and avoidant attachment is often negatively correlated (e.g., r's around –.20) with

agreeableness and extraversion (see Noftle & Shaver, 2006, for a detailed review). As a result, the core individual differences in attachment can be located in the well-known five-dimensional space advocated in much contemporary personality research. It seems unlikely, however, based on the evidence reviewed above, that these relations exist because the attachment dimensions are simply manifestations of the Big Five personality traits. In light of the previous discussion of the ways in which people can experience different levels of security with different significant others in their lives, it would be interesting for future research to examine the way relationship-specific measures of attachment relate to measures of basic personality traits and see if basic personality traits are able to explain part of what is common across varying relationships.

Adjustment and Psychopathology

Many "Grand Theories" of personality have something to say about disorders of personality—ways in which the functioning of the system can break down. Attachment theory is similar to Freudian and other psychoanalytic theories in focusing on defenses and pathology, but it also includes ideas about the paths to "optimal functioning" that have much in common with classic humanistic and self-actualization theories of personality (e.g., Maslow, 1968; Rogers, 1961) and with contemporary perspectives on subjective well-being and "positive psychology" (Aspinwall & Staudinger, 2003; Peterson, 2006). Attachment theory emphasizes not only fears and defenses related to attachment insecurities, but also the ways in which good relationships can build psychological resources and broaden perspectives and skills associated with a sense of security. Research consistently confirms that the sense of attachment security is associated with positive mental representations of others, a stable sense of self-efficacy and self-esteem, and reliance on constructive ways of coping, which in turn facilitate mental health and psychological functioning even in times of stress (see Mikulincer & Shaver, 2003, 2007a, for reviews). Moreover, securely attached people tend to feel generally safe and protected, and they can interact with others in a confident and open manner without being driven by a defensive need to protect a fragile or false self-concept (Mikulincer & Shaver, 2005).

There is extensive evidence that secure individuals are more likely than their insecure counterparts to possess personality characteristics and virtues emphasized in "positive psychology," such as resilience, optimism, hope, positive affectivity, curiosity and exploration, healthy autonomy, a capacity for love and forgiveness, feelings of interconnectedness and belongingness, tolerance, and kindness (see Lopez & Brennan, 2000; Mikulincer & Shaver, 2003, 2007a). Moreover, there are similarities between the way attachment security evolves from repeated episodes of attachment-figure availability and support and ideas discussed by classic humanistic psychologists about the parenting style that facilitates self-actualization (e.g., Maslow's [1968] concept of B-perception; Rogers's [1961] concept of "unconditional positive regard"). The common idea that recurs across different "positive" or humanistic theoretical frameworks is that experiences of being loved, accepted, and supported by others constitute the most important form of personal protection and provide a foundation for confronting adversity and maintaining equanimity and effective functioning in times of stress without interrupting natural processes of growth and self-actualization.

Recently, Mikulincer and Shaver (2005) reviewed extensive data showing that the sense of attachment security attenuates a wide array of defensive motives, such as the need for self-enhancement, needs for consensus and uniqueness, intergroup biases, defense of knowledge structures, and defense of cultural worldviews. Adult attachment research has consistently shown that a sense of attachment security acts as an inner resource that may supercede defensive needs and render defensive maneuvers less necessary. These defensive maneuvers and the resulting biases in the appraisals of self and others tend to be more characteristic of insecurely attached individuals. Mikulincer and Shaver noted that that these defensive needs indicate that a person has been forced by social experiences to face the world without adequate mental representations of attachment security and has had to struggle for a sense of self-worth.

According to Bowlby (1969/1982), the unavailability of security-providing attachment figures inhibits or blocks the activation of other behavioral systems, because a person who feels unprotected in the face of threats tends to be so focused on attachment needs that he or she lacks the attention and resources necessary to engage in other activities. This focus on attachment needs causes insecure people to be less tolerant of outgroup members (Mikulincer & Shaver, 2001), less humane in their values (Mikulincer et al., 2003), and less compassionate and altruistic (Mikulincer, Shaver, Gillath, & Nitzberg, 2005). Only when a sense of attachment security is restored can a person devote full attention and energy to other behavioral systems, such as exploration and caregiving. Interestingly, experimental induction of security causes beneficial short-term changes in people's attitudes, values, and altruistic behaviors (Mikulincer & Shaver, 2007b, 2007c), suggesting that the forces we have outlined here as childhood contributors to "positive" and "negative" personality tendencies can be applied even in adulthood, with therapeutic and ethical consequences.

Research supports the claim that secure individuals are more likely than insecure ones to exhibit all of Rogers's (1961) defining features of the "fully functioning person": openness to experience, existential living, organismic trust, experiential freedom, and creativity. Secure people are able to experience their thoughts and feelings deeply and to openly disclose these feelings to significant others, even if the thoughts and feelings are threatening and painful (e.g., Collins & Read, 1990; Mallinckrodt, Porter, & Kivlighan, 2005; Mikulincer & Orbach, 1995). Attachment security also facilitates cognitive openness and adaptive revision of knowledge structures, without arousing much fear of disapproval, criticism, or rejection (e.g., Green & Campbell, 2000; Mikulincer, 1997). Attachment security facilitates the savoring of good times and capitalizing on positive emotions, as evident in diary studies documenting secure people's enjoyment of daily activities and social interactions (e.g., Tidwell, Reis, & Shaver, 1996), as well as cognitive expansion following inductions of positive affect (e.g., Mikulincer & Sheffi, 2000). Securely attached people are able to engage in creative exploration and participate fully in the wider world while remaining sensitive and responsive to others' needs (e.g., Kunce & Shaver, 1994; Mikulincer, 1997). They are more likely than their avoidant peers to volunteer in their communities and have humanistic motives for so doing (Gillath, Bunge, Shaver, Wendelken, & Mikulincer, 2005).

In short, attachment theory offers a means to conceptualize a number of the qualities that have been emphasized in classical and contemporary research on personal adjustment and self-actualization. The theory does so within the same framework that is used to understand potential disorders of personality, thereby allowing the functional and dysfunctional aspects of personality functioning to be understood with a single set of concepts.

CONCLUDING COMMENTS

Attachment theory arose from the psychoanalytic stream of personality theorizing, but because Bowlby was unusually open to emerging cognitive and ethological approaches to human and nonhuman primate behavior, and because he and Ainsworth were both very empirically as well as theoretically oriented, the theory has remained open to other approaches and to subsequent theoretical and methodological developments. The theory naturally spans several usually separate areas of psychology: personality, social, developmental, clinical, and comparative. It is as congenial to "negative psychology" (i.e., focusing on psychopathology and dysfunction) as it is to "positive psychology" (prosocial behavior, self-actualization). The theory was cognitive in certain respects from the start, but it has become more sophisticated cognitively as researchers have used methods ranging from discourse analysis (in the AAI) to social cognition constructs and research paradigms. Although we have not stressed its connections with learning or behaviorist approaches to personality development, the ways in which parental behavior influence the attachment patterns of infants could easily, and perhaps productively, be conceptualized in learning theory terms. (We say this despite the fact that there was once considerable tension between attachment theorists and social learning theorists because of the behaviorist taboo on psychodynamic approaches.)

Attachment theory explains how social "situations" (i.e., interactions with regular caregivers) build personality (i.e., attach-

ment patterns) and how the resulting personality patterns then influence a person's choices among, and behavior in, social situations (especially close relationships). Most of the classic issues, debates, and conundrums in personality psychology have played themselves out within the field of attachment research, with largely productive results. We have not had space to say much about genetic influences or contemporary neuroscience methods, but there is already some interesting genetic and neuroscience research within the attachment domain (see, e.g., Coan, 2008; Gillath, Bunge, et al., 2005). Attachment theory and research provide a model of integration across what were once separate and ferociously defended fiefdoms within personality psychology. We look forward with great interest to the field's further development, diversification, and integration.

REFERENCES

Ahadi, S., & Diener, E. (1989). Multiple determinants and effect size. *Journal of Personality and Social Psychology, 56,* 398–406.

Ainsworth, M. D. S., Blehar, M. C., Waters, E., & Wall, S. (1978). *Patterns of attachment.* Hillsdale, NJ: Erlbaum.

Andersen, S. M., & Chen, S. (2002). The relational self: An interpersonal social-cognitive theory. *Psychological Review, 109,* 619–645.

Anisfeld, E., Casper, V., Nozyce, M., & Cunningham, N. (1990). Does infant carrying promote attachment? An experimental study of the effects of increased physical contact on the development of attachment. *Child Development, 61,* 1617–1627.

Arend, R., Gove, F. L., & Sroufe, L. A. (1979). Continuity of individual adaptation from infancy to kindergarten: A predictive study of ego-resiliency and curiosity in preschoolers. *Child Development, 50,* 950–959.

Aspinwall, L. G., & Staudinger, U. M. (Eds.). (2003). *A psychology of human strengths: Fundamental questions and future directions for a positive psychology.* Washington, DC: American Psychological Association.

Baldwin, M. W., & Fehr, B. (1995). On the instability of attachment style ratings. *Personal Relationships, 2,* 247–261.

Baldwin, M. W., Keelan, J. P. R., Fehr, B., Enns, V., & Koh-Rangarajoo, E. (1996). Social cognitive conceptualization of attachment working models: Availability and accessibility effects. *Journal of Personality and Social Psychology, 71,* 94–104.

Bartholomew, K., & Horowitz, L. (1991). Attachment styles among young adults: A test of the four-category model. *Journal of Personality and Social Psychology, 61,* 226–245.

Bates, J., Maslin, C., & Frankel, K. (1985). Attachment security, mother–child interactions, and temperament as predictors of behavior problem ratings at age three years. In I. Bretherton & W. Waters (Eds.), Growing points of attachment theory and research. *Monographs of the Society for Research in Child Development, 50*(1–2, Serial No. 209), 167–193.

Baumeister, R. F., & Tice, D. M. (1988). Metatraits. *Journal of Personality, 56,* 571–598.

Bem, D. J., & Allen, A. (1974). On predicting some of the people some of the time: The search for cross-situational consistencies in behavior. *Psychological Review, 81,* 506–520.

Berant, E., Mikulincer, M., & Shaver, P. R. (2008). Mothers' attachment style, their mental health, and their children's emotional vulnerabilities: A 7-year study of mothers of children with congenital heart disease. *Journal of Personality, 76,* 31–65.

Bowlby, J. (1944). Forty-four juvenile thieves: Their characters and home life. *International Journal of Psycho-Analysis, 25,* 19–52, 107–127.

Bowlby, J. (1973). *Attachment and loss: Vol. 2. Separation: Anxiety and anger.* New York: Basic Books.

Bowlby, J. (1980). *Attachment and loss: Vol. 3. Loss: Sadness and depression.* New York: Basic Books.

Bowlby, J. (1982). *Attachment and loss: Vol. 1. Attachment* (2nd ed.). New York: Basic Books. (Original work published 1969)

Brennan, K. A., Clark, C. L., & Shaver, P. R. (1998). Self-report measurement of adult attachment: An integrative overview. In J. A. Simpson & W. S. Rholes (Eds.), *Attachment theory and close relationships* (pp. 46–76). New York: Guilford Press.

Brumbaugh, C. C., & Fraley, R. C. (2006). Transference and attachment: How do attachment patterns get carried forward from one relationship to the next? *Personality and Social Psychology Bulletin, 32,* 552–560.

Carlson, E. A. (1998). A prospective longitudinal study of attachment disorganization/disorientation. *Child Development, 69,* 1107–1128.

Caspi, A., & Roberts, B. W. (2001). Personality development across the life course: The argument for change and continuity. *Psychological Inquiry, 12,* 49–66.

Coan, J. (in press). Toward a neuroscience of attachment. In J. Cassidy & P. R. Shaver (Eds.), *Handbook of attachment: Theory, research, and clinical applications* (2nd ed.). New York: Guilford Press.

Collins, N. L. (1996). Working models of attachment: Implications for explanation, emotion, and behavior. *Journal of Personality and Social Psychology, 71,* 810–832.

Collins, N. L., Guichard, A. C., Ford, M. B., & Feeney, B. C. (2004). Working models of attachment: New developments and emerging themes. In W. S. Rholes & J. A. Simpson (Eds.), *Adult attachment: Theory, research, and clinical implications* (pp. 196–239). New York: Guilford Press.

Collins, N. L., & Read, S. J. (1994). Cognitive representations of attachment: The structure and function of working models. In K. Bartholomew & D. Perlman (Eds.), *Advances in personal relationships: Vol. 5. Attachment processes in adulthood* (pp. 53–90). London: Jessica Kingsley.

Costa, P. T., Jr., & McCrae, R. R. (1994). Stability and change in personality from adolescence through adulthood. In C. F. Halverson, Jr., G. A. Kohnstamm, & R. P. Martin (Eds.), *The developing structure of temperament and personality from infancy to adulthood* (pp. 139–148). Hillsdale, NJ: Erlbaum.

Craik, K. (1943). *The nature of explanation.* Cambridge, UK: Cambridge University Press.

Crowell, J. A., & Fraley, R. C. (in press). Measures of individual differences in adolescent and adult attachment. In J. Cassidy & P. R. Shaver (Eds.), *Handbook of attachment: Theory, research, and clinical applications* (2nd ed.). New York: Guilford Press.

DeWolff, M., & van IJzendoorn, M. (1997). Sensitivity and attachment: A meta-analysis on parental antecedents of infant attachment. *Child Development, 68,* 571–591.

Epstein, S. (1979). The stability of behavior: I. On predicting most of the people most of the time. *Journal of Personality and Social Psychology, 37,* 1097–1126.

Epstein, S. (1980). The stability of behavior: II. Implications for psychological research. *American Psychologist, 35,* 790–806.

Erez, A., Mikulincer, M., van IJzendoorn, M. H., & Kroonenberg, P. M. (2008). Attachment, personality, and volunteering: Placing volunteerism in an attachment-theoretical framework. *Personality and Individual Differences, 44,* 64–74.

Feeney, J. A., Noller, P., & Callan, V. J. (1994). Attachment style, communication and satisfaction in the early years of marriage. In K. Bartholomew & D. Perlman (Eds.), *Advances in personal relationships: Vol. 5. Attachment processes in adulthood* (pp. 269–308). London: Jessica Kingsley.

Fleeson, W. (2001). Toward a structure- and process-integrated view of personality: Traits as density distributions of states. *Journal of Personality and Social Psychology, 80,* 1011–1027.

Fox, N. A., Kimmerly, N. L., & Schafer, W. D. (1991). Attachment to mother/attachment to father: A meta-analysis. *Child Development, 62,* 210–225.

Fraley, R. C. (2002). Attachment stability from infancy to adulthood: Meta-analysis and dynamic modeling of developmental mechanisms. *Personality and Social Psychology Review, 6,* 123–151.

Fraley, R. C. (2007). A connectionist approach to the organization and continuity of working models of attachment. *Journal of Personality, 75,* 1157–1180.

Fraley, R. C., & Brumbaugh, C. C. (2004). A dynamical systems approach to conceptualizing and studying stability and change in attachment security. In W. S. Rholes & J. A. Simpson (Eds.), *Adult attachment: Theory, research, and clinical implications* (pp. 86–132). New York: Guilford Press.

Fraley, R. C., & Davis, K. E. (1997). Attachment formation and transfer in young adults' close friendships and romantic relationships. *Personal Relationships, 4,* 131–144.

Fraley, R. C., & Roberts, B. W. (2005). Patterns of continuity: A dynamic model for conceptualizing the stability of individual differences in psychological constructs across the life course. *Psychological Review, 112,* 60–74.

Fraley, R. C., & Shaver, P. R. (1997). Adult attachment and the suppression of unwanted thoughts. *Journal of Personality and Social Psychology, 73,* 1080–1091.

Fraley, R. C., & Shaver, P. R. (1998). Airport separations: A naturalistic study of adult attachment dynamics in separating couples. *Journal of Personality and Social Psychology, 75,* 1198–1212.

Fraley, R. C., & Spieker, S. J. (2003a). Are infant attachment patterns continuously or categorically distributed? A taxometric analysis of strange situation behavior. *Developmental Psychology, 39,* 387–404.

Fraley, R. C., & Spieker, S. J. (2003b). What are the differences between dimensional and categorical models of individual differences in attachment?: Reply to Cassidy (2003), Cummings (2003), Sroufe (2003), and Waters and Beauchaine (2003). *Developmental Psychology, 39,* 423–429.

Fraley, R. C., & Waller, N. G. (1998). Adult attachment patterns: A test of the typological model. In J. A. Simpson & W. S. Rholes (Eds.), *Attachment theory and close relationships* (pp. 77–114). New York: Guilford Press.

Fraley, R. C., Waller, N. G., & Brennan, K. A. (2000). An item response theory analysis of self-report measures of adult attachment. *Journal of Personality and Social Psychology, 78,* 350–365.

Frazier, P. A., Byer, A. L., Fischer, A. R., Wright, D. M., & DeBord, K. A. (1996). Adult attachment style and partner choice: Correlational and experimental findings. *Personal Relationships, 3,* 117–136.

Freud, S. (1940). *An outline of psychoanalysis* (L. Strachey, Trans.). New York: Norton.

Freud, S. (1965). *New introductory lectures on psychoanalysis* (L. Strachey, Trans.). New York: Norton. (Original work published 1933)

Gillath, O., Bunge, S. A., Shaver, P. R., Wendelken, C., & Mikulincer, M. (2005). Attachment-style differences and ability to suppress negative thoughts: Exploring the neural correlates. *NeuroImage, 28,* 835–847.

Green, J. D., & Campbell, W. (2000). Attachment and exploration in adults: Chronic and contextual accessibility. *Personality and Social Psychology Bulletin, 26,* 452–461.

Griffin, D., & Bartholomew, K. (1994). Models of the self and other: Fundamental dimensions underlying measures of adult attachment. *Journal of Personality and Social Psychology, 67,* 430–445.

Grossmann, K., Grossmann, K. E., Spangler, G., Suess, G., & Unzer, L. (1985). Maternal sensitivity and newborn orienting responses as related to quality of attachment in northern Germany. In I. Bretherton & W. Waters (Eds.), Growing points of attachment theory and research. *Monographs of the Society for Research in Child Development, 50*(1–2, Serial No. 209), 233–256.

Grossmann, K. E., Grossmann, K., & Waters, E. (Eds.). (2005). *Attachment from infancy to adulthood: The major longitudinal studies.* New York: Guilford Pres.

Hazan, C., & Shaver, P. R. (1987). Romantic love conceptualized as an attachment process. *Journal of Personality and Social Psychology, 52,* 511–524.

Hesse, E. (2008). The Adult Attachment Interview: Historical and current perspectives. In J. Cassidy & P. R. Shaver (Eds.), *The handbook of attachment: Theory, research, and clinical applications* (2nd ed.). New York: Guilford Press.

Hinde, R. A. (1966). *Animal behavior: A synthesis of ethology and comparative psychology.* New York: McGraw-Hill.

Isabella, R. (1993). Origins of attachment: Maternal interactive behavior across the first year. *Child Development, 64,* 605–621.

John, O. P., & Gross, J. J. (2007). Individual differences in emotion regulation. In J. J. Gross (Ed.), *Handbook of emotion regulation* (pp. 351–372). New York: Guilford Press.

John, O. P., & Srivastava, S. (1999). The Big Five

trait taxonomy: History, measurement, and theoretical perspectives. In L. A. Pervin & O. P. John (Eds.), *Handbook of personality: Theory and research* (2nd ed., pp. 102–138). New York: Guilford Press.

Kagan, J. (1996). Three pleasing ideas. *American Psychologist, 51,* 901–908.

Kiser, L., Bates, J., Maslin, C., & Bayles, K. (1986). Mother–infant play at six months as a predictor of attachment security at thirteen months. *Journal of the American Academy of Child Psychiatry, 25,* 68–75.

Kobak, R. (1994). Adult attachment: A personality or relationship construct? *Psychological Inquiry, 5,* 42–44.

Kunce, L. J., & Shaver, P. R. (1994). An attachment-theoretical approach to caregiving in romantic relationships. In K. Bartholomew & D. Perlman (Eds.), *Advances in personal relationships: Vol. 5. Attachment processes in adulthood* (pp. 205–237). London: Jessica Kingsley.

Lewis, M. (1994). Does attachment imply a relationship or multiple relationships? *Psychological Inquiry, 5,* 47–51.

Lewis, M. (1999). On the development of personality. In L. A. Pervin & O. P. John (Eds.), *Handbook of personality: Theory and research* (2nd ed., pp. 327–346). New York: Guilford Press.

Lewis, M. (2001). Issues in the study of personality development. *Psychological Inquiry, 12,* 67–83.

Lewis, M., Feiring, C., & Rosenthal, S. (2000). Attachment over time. *Child Development, 71,* 707–720.

Lopez, F. G., & Brennan, K. A. (2000). Dynamic processes underlying adult attachment organization: Toward an attachment theoretical perspective on the healthy and effective self: Attachment and counseling psychology. *Journal of Counseling Psychology, 47,* 283–300.

Main, M., Kaplan, N., & Cassidy, J. (1985). Security in infancy, childhood, and adulthood: A move to the level of representation. *Monographs of the Society for Research in Child Development, 50*(1–2), 66–104.

Mallinckrodt, B., Porter, M. J., & Kivlighan, D. M., Jr. (2005). Client attachment to therapist, depth of in-session exploration, and object relations in brief psychotherapy. *Psychotherapy, 42,* 85–100.

Mangelsdorf, S., Gunnar, M., Kestenbaum, R., Lang, S., & Andreas, D. (1990). Infant proneness-to-distress temperament, maternal personality, and mother–infant attachment: Associations and goodness of fit. *Child Development, 61,* 820–831.

Maslow, A. H. (1968). *Toward a psychology of being* (2nd ed.). New York: Van Nostrand.

McCrae, R. R., & Costa, P. T., Jr. (2006). Cross-cultural perspectives on adult personality trait development. In D. K. Mroczek & T. D. Little (Eds.), *Handbook of personality development* (pp. 129–145). Mahwah, NJ: Erlbaum.

McCrae, R. R., Costa, P. T., Jr., Ostendorf, F., Angleitner, A., Hrebickova, M., Avia, M. D., et al. (2000). Nature over nurture: Temperament, personality, and life span development. *Journal of Personality and Social Psychology, 78,* 173–186.

Mikulincer, M. (1997). Adult attachment style and information processing: Individual differences in curiosity and cognitive closure. *Journal of Personality and Social Psychology, 72,* 1217–1230.

Mikulincer, M., Dolev, T., & Shaver, P. R. (2004). Attachment-related strategies during thought-suppression: Ironic rebounds and vulnerable self-representations. *Journal of Personality and Social Psychology, 87,* 940–956.

Mikulincer, M., Gillath, O., Sapir-Lavid, Y., Yaakobi, E., Arias, K., Tal-Aloni, L., et al. (2003). Attachment theory and concern for others' welfare: Evidence that activation of the sense of secure base promotes endorsement of self-transcendence values. *Basic and Applied Social Psychology, 25,* 299–312.

Mikulincer, M., Gillath, O., & Shaver, P. R. (2002). Activation of the attachment system in adulthood: Threat-related primes increase the accessibility of mental representations of attachment figures. *Journal of Personality and Social Psychology, 83,* 881–895.

Mikulincer, M., & Orbach, I. (1995). Attachment styles and repressive defensiveness: The accessibility and architecture of affective memories. *Journal of Personality and Social Psychology, 68,* 917–925.

Mikulincer, M., & Shaver, P. R. (2001). Attachment theory and intergroup bias: Evidence that priming the secure base schema attenuates negative reactions to out-groups. *Journal of Personality and Social Psychology, 81,* 97–115.

Mikulincer, M., & Shaver, P. R. (2003). The attachment behavioral system in adulthood: Activation, psychodynamics, and interpersonal processes. In M. P. Zanna (Ed.), *Advances in experimental social psychology* (Vol. 35, pp. 53–152). New York: Academic Press.

Mikulincer, M., & Shaver, P. R. (2005). Mental representations of attachment security: Theoretical foundation for a positive social psychology. In M. W. Baldwin (Ed.), *Interpersonal cognition* (pp. 233–266). New York: Guilford Press.

Mikulincer, M., & Shaver, P. R. (2007a). *Attachment in adulthood: Structure, dynamics, and change.* New York: Guilford Press.

Mikulincer, M., & Shaver, P. R. (2007b). Boosting

attachment security to promote mental health, prosocial values, and inter-group tolerance. *Psychological Inquiry, 18,* 139–156.

Mikulincer, M., & Shaver, P. R. (2007c). Reflections on security dynamics: Core constructs, psychological mechanisms, relational contexts, and the need for an integrative theory. *Psychological Inquiry, 18,* 197–209.

Mikulincer, M., Shaver, P. R., Gillath, O., & Nitzberg, R. A. (2005). Attachment, caregiving, and altruism: Boosting attachment security increases compassion and helping. *Journal of Personality and Social Psychology, 89,* 817–839.

Mikulincer, M., & Sheffi, E. (2000). Adult attachment style and cognitive reactions to positive affect: A test of mental categorization and creative problem solving. *Motivation and Emotion, 24,* 149–174.

Mischel, W. (1968). *Personality and assessment.* New York: Wiley.

Mischel, W., & Shoda, Y. (1995). A cognitive–affective system theory of personality: Reconceptualizing situations, dispositions, dynamics, and invariance in personality structure. *Psychological Review, 102,* 246–268.

Mischel, W., & Shoda, Y. (1998). Reconciling processing dynamics and personality dispositions. *Annual Review of Psychology, 49,* 229–258.

Noftle, E. E., & Shaver, P. R. (2006). Attachment dimensions and the Big Five personality traits: Associations and comparative ability to predict relationship quality. *Journal of Research in Personality, 40,* 179–208.

Overall, N. C., Fletcher, G. J. O., & Friesen, M. D. (2003). Mapping the intimate relationship mind: Comparisons between three models of attachment representations. *Personality and Social Psychology Bulletin, 29,* 1479–1493.

Peterson, C. (2006). *A primer in positive psychology.* New York: Oxford University Press.

Piaget, J. (1953). *Origins of intelligence in the child.* London: Routledge.

Pierce, G. R., Sarason, B. R., & Sarason, I. G. (1992). General and specific support expectations and stress as predictors of perceived supportiveness: An experimental study. *Journal of Personality and Social Psychology, 63,* 297–307.

Pietromonaco, P. R., & Carnelley, K. B. (1994). Gender and working models of attachment: Consequences for perceptions of self and romantic relationships. *Personal Relationships, 1,* 63–82.

Roberts, B. W. (2007). Contextualizing personality psychology. *Journal of Personality, 75,* 1071–1082.

Rogers, C. R. (1961). *On becoming a person.* Boston: Houghton Mifflin.

Roisman, G. I., Fraley, R. C., Holland, A., For-

tuna, K., Clausell, E., & Clarke, A. (2007). The Adult Attachment Interview and self-reports of attachment style: An empirical rapprochement. *Journal of Personality and Social Psychology, 92,* 678–697.

Roisman, G. I., Madsen, S. D., Hennighausen, K. H., Sroufe, L. A., & Collins, W. A. (2001). The coherence of dyadic behavior across parent–child and romantic relationships as mediated by the internalized representation of experience. *Attachment and Human Development, 3,* 156–172.

Shaver, P. R., Hazan, C., & Bradshaw, D. (1988). Love as attachment: The integration of three behavioral systems. In R. J. Sternberg & M. L. Barnes (Eds.), *The psychology of love* (pp. 68–99). New Haven, CT: Yale University Press.

Simpson, J. A., Rholes, W. S., & Nelligan, J. S. (1992). Support seeking and support giving within couples in an anxiety-provoking situation. *Journal of Personality and Social Psychology, 62,* 434–446.

Simpson, J. A., Rholes, W. S., & Phillips, D. (1996). Conflict in close relationships: An attachment perspective. *Journal of Personality and Social Psychology, 71,* 899–914.

Srivastava, S., John, O. P., Gosling, S. D., & Potter, J. (2003). Development of personality in early and middle adulthood: Set like plaster or persistent change? *Journal of Personality and Social Psychology, 84,* 1041–1053.

Sroufe, L. A. (1979). The coherence of individual development: Early care, attachment, and subsequent developmental issues. *American Psychologist, 34,* 834–841.

Sroufe, L. A., & Jacobvitz, D. (1989). Diverging pathways, developmental transformations, multiple etiologies and the problem of continuity in development. *Human Development, 32,* 196–204.

Sroufe, L. A., & Waters, E. (1977). Heart rate as a convergent measure in clinical and developmental research. *Merrill–Palmer Quarterly, 23,* 3–27.

Suomi, S. (1999). Attachment in rhesus monkeys. In J. Cassidy & P. R. Shaver (Eds.), *Handbook of attachment: Theory, research, and clinical applications* (pp. 181–197). New York: Guilford Press.

Tidwell, M. C. O., Reis, H. T., & Shaver, P. R. (1996). Attachment, attractiveness, and social interaction: A diary study. *Journal of Personality and Social Psychology, 71,* 729–745.

Troy, M., & Sroufe, L. A. (1987). Victimization among preschoolers: Role of attachment relationship history. *Journal of American Academy of Child and Adolescent Psychiatry, 26,* 166–172.

van IJzendoorn, M. H., & Sagi-Schwartz, A. (in press). Cross-cultural patterns of attachment: Universal and contextual dimensions. In J. Cassidy & P. R. Shaver (Eds.), *Handbook of attachment: Theory, research, and clinical applications* (2nd ed.). New York: Guilford Press.

Vaughn, B. E., Bost, K. K., & van IJzendoorn, M. H. (in press). Attachment and temperament: Additive and interactive influences on behavior, affect, and cognition during infancy and childhood. In J. Cassidy & P. R. Shaver (Eds.), *Handbook of attachment: Theory, research, and clinical applications* (2nd ed.). New York: Guilford Press.

Waddington, C. H. (1957). *The strategy of the genes: A discussion of some aspects of theoretical biology.* London: Allen & Unwin.

Waters, E., Merrick, S., Treboux, D., Crowell, J., & Albersheim, L. (2000). Attachment security in infancy and early adulthood: A twenty-year longitudinal study. *Child Development, 71,* 684–689.

Waters, E., Wippman, J., & Sroufe, L. A. (1979). Attachment, positive affect, and competence in the peer group: Two studies in construct validation. *Child Development, 50,* 821–829.

Weinfield, N. S., Sroufe, L. A., Egeland, B., & Carlson, E. A. (2008). Individual differences in infant–caregiver attachment: Conceptual and empirical aspects of security. In J. Cassidy & P. R. Shaver (Eds.), *Handbook of attachment: Theory, research, and clinical applications* (2nd ed., pp. 78–101). New York: Guilford Press.

Young, J. Z. (1964). *A model for the brain.* London: Oxford University Press.

Zayas, V., Shoda, Y., & Ayduk, O. N. (2002). Personality in context: An interpersonal systems perspective. *Journal of Personality, 70,* 851–898.

Zeifman, D., & Hazan, C. (1997). Attachment: The bond in pair-bonds. In J. A. Simpson & D. T. Kenrick (Eds.), *Evolutionary social psychology* (pp. 237–263). Mahwah, NJ: Erlbaum.

CHAPTER 21

Culture and Personality

Verónica Benet-Martínez
Shigehiro Oishi

I am *Homo sapiens*, I am American.
—Rozin (2003, p. 281)

Personality is shaped by both genetic and environmental factors; among the most important of the latter are cultural influences (Kluckhohn & Murray, 1948). Culture consists of shared meaning systems that provide the standards for perceiving, believing, evaluating, communicating, and acting among those who share a language, a historic period, and a geographic location (Triandis, 1996). More recently Chiu and Hong (2007) have defined culture as a network of knowledge that is both procedural (learned sequence of responses to particular cues) and declarative (representations of people, events, and norms) and is produced, distributed, and reproduced among a collection of interconnected people.

Culture is different from ethnicity in that *ethnicity* refers to a common background or social origins, shared culture and traditions that are distinctive, maintained between generations, and result in a sense of identity and group membership, and shared language or religious tradition (Senior & Bhopal, 1994). Culture is a broader construct than ethnicity because it encompasses macro-level processes and deals specifically with the values and norms that govern and organize a group of people (e.g., capitalistic culture), defining characteristics and behaviors that are deemed appropriate or inappropriate for an organized group (e.g., American business customs). Culture also specifies the context and environment (i.e., a specific place, time, and stimuli) in which ethnicity exists. Obviously, not all individuals sharing a common "cultural space" (e.g., the United States) have the same ethnicity (e.g., Hispanic, Asian American, African American). In addition, culture and ethnicity are different from race, in that *race* refers to a shared genetic heritage, expressed by common external physical characteristics such as facial features, skin color, and hair texture (e.g., Hispanic individuals can be white, such as Spaniards or Argentineans; black, such as individuals from Cuba or the Dominican Republic; or Native American, such as many Mexicans and Guatemalans).

Culture is transmitted through language, media messages, cultural practices and institutions, values and artifacts, and through the modeling of behavior (Cohen, 1996; Markus & Kitayama, 1994). Social scientists have recognized for decades that these influences have substantial psychological effects on individuals. However, culture does not have a deterministic influence on individuals' behavior. Rather, its influence is probabilistic (e.g., Allport, 1961; Stryker & Burke, 2000). Rohner's (1984) metaphor that compares culture to a game (with various rules) and people to its players clearly illustrates this point. Players can pick from different strategies and options, and sometimes even violate or modify the rules if they think they can get away with it. In other words, the degree to which players follow the rules differs across individuals, depending on their personal preferences, moods, and specific situations. This variation results in a great deal of within-culture heterogeneity and individual differences in the degree to which people endorse, internalize, and utilize particular rules (or norms; see Oishi, 2004, for a similar view).

Cultural influences on personhood were a prevalent concern in early personality psychology (e.g., Allport, 1961; Kluckhohn & Murray, 1948; McClelland, 1961), but, for reasons we discuss later, largely ignored in modern personality theory and research until the early 1990s. However, many cultural studies conducted during the last decade on issues such as self-processes, emotion, and personality traits have firmly established the following: Culture is a key determinant of what it means to be a person (see reviews by Church, 2000; Diener, Oishi, & Lucas, 2003; Markus & Kitayama, 1998; Triandis & Suh, 2002).[1]

In this chapter we review (1) key theories and studies dealing with cultural differences in levels and processes of various personality constructs (e.g., emotion, traits, identity) and (2) important conceptual issues personality researchers need to consider when conducting cultural research (see Benet-Martínez, 2007, for a review of cross-cultural methodological issues). With this review, we also hope to persuade personality researchers that cultural research offers exciting and interesting benefits and opportunities not available with traditional research approaches (Matsumoto, 2000). Cultural personality studies help elucidate how macro-contextual factors mediate and moderate personality outcomes (e.g., Schimmack, Radhakrishnan, Oishi, Dzokoto, & Ahadi, 2002), help dispel shaky cultural stereotypes (e.g., Terracciano, Mc-

Crae, Brant, & Costa, 2005), and test the generalizability of our theories (e.g., Benet-Martínez & John, 1998). Cultural studies, which often rely on multiple languages and samples, also offer personality researchers a way of dealing with classic methodological issues regarding construct validity and generalizability (e.g., need to control for possible confounding variables such as socioeconomic status [SES] or language proficiency; use of multisample, multitrait, multimethod designs; Benet-Martínez, 2007). The cultural perspective, in fact, may make us better at "seeing" personality. In other words, by understanding the cultural backdrop of a particular construct, behavior, or script, culturally informed personality researchers may correctly see individual differences and patterns of personality consistency and coherence where other researchers would only see extraneous or random variability.

HISTORICAL ANALYSIS

Most personality psychologists agree that the systematic study of how culture influences social and intrapersonality behavior should be an essential part of our discipline. Yet, cultural studies continue to be somewhat underrepresented in personality psychology (compared to social psychology, for instance). Why is this? One reason may be historical. Because of the serious methodological, theoretical, and ethical limitations of some of the studies on culture and personality conducted in the first half of the 20th century, some psychologists may still view cultural work on personality with skepticism.

The field of "culture and personality" (Benedict, 1934; Dubois, 1944; Kardiner, 1939) emerged in the first half of the 20th century driven mainly by psychoanalytically oriented anthropologists, psychologists, and psychiatrists. This movement thrived in the 1930s and 1940s and was considered by many an exciting and influential paradigm in the social sciences. According to recent reviews (e.g., Church & Ortiz, 2005; LeVine, 2001), the core propositions of this field were the following: (1) Each culture has a distinctive ethos, and all participants in that culture have internalized that ethos and developed a corresponding personality structure that is common to all them (the uniformity assumption); (2) childhood experiences, which are heavily culturally shaped, can be linked to predictable adult personality patterns (the continuity assumption); (3) adult personality characteristics prevalent in a nation directly impact its culture, institutions, historical and social trends, and psychopathology. Later, Sapir (1956), Wallace (1970), and others emphasized within-culture individual variations in personality and argued for the concept of "modal personality," which acknowledged the existence of both central tendencies (i.e., prevalent personality types in each culture) and individual variability.[2]

Unfortunately, during and after World War II, "culture and personality" tenets (e.g., the continuity and uniformity assumptions) and methods (e.g., projective techniques) were used to put forward the problematic notion of "national character," where whole nations such as Russia, Japan, and Germany were described in terms of a basic set of usually negative personality dispositions (e.g., fanaticism and restraint for the Japanese, rigidity and authoritarianism for the Germans). Because of the severe criticisms the national character studies received, the culture and personality field was stigmatized, and by the 1960s it had clearly "fallen from grace." Although a number of personality psychologists continued to show interest in personality from a cross-cultural perspective (e.g., McClelland, 1961), by the 1970s and 1980s, interest on the topic had vanished.

Cultural studies in personality resurged in the 1990s. Church (2001) notes some of the factors that led to this comeback: (1) a refinement of the concept of personality and its ability to predict behavior across situations (Kenrick & Funder, 1988); (2) the acceptance of the five-factor model (FFM) as an adequate taxonomy of personality differences; (3) the emergence of individualism and collectivism (I-C) as dimension that may link ecology, culture, and personality; (4) the multicultural movement in the United States; (5) the refinement of statistical methodology to address cross-cultural conceptual, linguistic, and measurement equivalence issues; and (6), the internationalization of scientific activity, which makes cross-cultural collaboration easier. Currently, the study of culture and personality is prosperous and being approached from a variety of theoretical perspectives.

CURRENT THEORETICAL MODELS

Broadly speaking, current research examining the role of culture in personality and social behavior can be seen as falling within either the cultural or cross-cultural approach. These two approaches have relatively distinct conceptual, methodological, and historical elements (Greenfield, 2000), although at times the differences between these two camps have been overemphasized.

The cultural psychology view endorses *relativist* and *constructivist* notions of personality and tends to favor emic (i.e., indigenous) over imposed-etic (i.e., imported) approaches to theory and instrument development. Specifically, it posits that personality—the affective, motivational, and cognitive dispositions that influence our evaluations and reactions to the environment—cannot be separated from the broad social and cultural context in which it develops and is expressed (Markus & Kitayama, 1998; Miller, 1997). As eloquently stated by Markus and Kitayama (1998), "A cultural psychological perspective implies that *there is no personality without culture*; there is only a biological entity" (p. 67, emphasis added). Thus, culture provides the context in which personality develops, is observed, and acquires meaning (for both the individual and the observer), and as a result, the existence of universal personality traits is questioned. In his recent review of the cultural and cross-cultural traditions, Church (2001) notes that the cultural approach is often characterized by (1) a concern with psychological processes (vs. individual differences); (2) a focus on highly contextual descriptions of psychological phenomenon in one or more cultures, with little expectation of finding cultural universals; and (3) an emphasis on experimental methodology, coupled with qualitative or interpretive approaches (Church, 2001). Most studies examining cultural influences on self-processes (e.g., self-enhancement, self-concept) and social behavior (e.g., attribution, dissonance) fit within the cultural perspective. Cultural psychology also speaks to the socially constructed nature of the construct of personality (e.g., how the notions of traits and personality consistency are particularly meaningful in the West).

The cross-cultural approach, on the other hand, treats culture and personality as relatively distinct entities and sees culture as an independent variable "outside" the individual (e.g., ecology, economic structure, value system) that influences personality and behavior (Triandis, 1996). Implicit in the cross-cultural approach is an ecocultural model with a causal sequence from ecology (e.g., the physical environment) to culture to socialization patterns (e.g., childrearing practices) to personality (Triandis & Suh, 2002). Church (2001) notes that the cross-cultural approach is characterized by (1) a focus on individual differences (e.g., in values, beliefs, etc., but particularly personality traits); (2) comparisons of multiple cultures in the search for cultural universals, or culture-specifics along with universals; (3) use of traditional, standardized psychometric questionnaires to measure both personality and culture; and (4) concern with the cross-cultural equivalence of constructs and measures. The majority of studies examining cultural influences on personality traits fit within the cross-cultural perspective.

A key differentiation within the cross-cultural approach is the distinction between the genotypic and phenotypic views, which have quite diverging stands about the meaning of personality traits and their cultural and biological basis. The *genotypic* view (McCrae & Costa, 1996) deems personality traits as endogenous and inherited basic tendencies that are largely independent from culture. In this approach, McCrae and Costa distinguish between "basic tendencies"—inherited, biologically based traits captured by their FFM—and "characteristic adaptations"—habits, values, beliefs, goals, and identities that develop from the interaction of basic tendencies and experience. Note that in this model only characteristic adaptations can be shaped by culture; thus, dispositions to be anxious, talkative, creative, accommodating, or disciplined (i.e., FFM traits) are culture-free. Two conclusions derive from this model: First, because basic personality tendencies (i.e., FFM traits) are biologically based, they should be universal; second, cultural differences on FFM levels should be taken as indicative of genetic differences between the cultural groups under study. Notice that this model also implies that responses to instruments such as the NEO Personality Inventory—Revised (NEO-PI-R; Costa & McCrae, 1992) reflect one's standing on the basic, biologically based tendencies, rather than characteristic adaptations.

Proponents of the *phenotypic* view (Saucier & Goldberg, 1996), on the other hand, conceptualize personality traits as observable behavioral regularities that reflect both genetic dispositions and characteristic adaptations to the sociocultural context. This view emphasizes the sociocognitive and linguistic basis of personality traits. It posits that lexically derived personality taxonomies such as the FFM reflect dispositions that have been encoded in the language because they represent attributes that are particularly significant for the society speaking that language. This approach views culture as an independent variable that may impact the level, expression, and correlates of traits *and* the underlying structure or dimensions of personality. According to this model, then, the basic personality constructs captured in personality taxonomies as well as individuals' responses to most trait inventories reflect observable (i.e., phenotypic) expressions, and thus no a priori assumptions about their genetic versus cultural basis can be made (only behavioral genetic studies can answer the last issue).

The boundaries between cultural and cross-cultural approaches are becoming less significant as the old debates between social and personality psychology about the meaning and status of the construct of personality finally die out, as new generations of cultural researchers are trained in multiple methods (psychometric, experimental, and interpretive), as the processes by which culture influences behavior become better understood, and as new data-analytic techniques (e.g., multigroup latent class analysis and multilevel analysis) become more readily available. Indeed, there are new models of culture and personality that attempt to integrate the cultural with cross-cultural perspectives. For instance, Church (2000) theorized that (1) traits exist in all cultures but explain behavior less in collectivist than in individualist cultures; (2) situational predictors of behavior are important universally, but more so in collectivist than in individualist cultures; and (3) cognitive and behavioral consistency exists universally but is less important in collectivist than in individualist cultures. Many empirical studies are also starting to combine features from both approaches, focusing on individual differences while supporting a view of culture and personality as mutually constituted, acknowledging bidirectional effects between culture and personality, and combining emic and imposed-etic methodology (e.g., Aaker, Benet-Martínez, & Garolera, 2000; Benet-Martínez, 1999; Benet-Martínez & Karakitapoglu-Aygun, 2003; Oishi & Diener, 2001). These approaches see personality variables (e.g., self- and other-ascribed traits, self-concept, well-being, goals) as often inseparable from cultural processes, in that the ways that situations are framed and experienced and the factors a person brings to a situation (e.g., expectations, values) are cultural products themselves.

TRAITS

Are there cultural differences in personality traits such as extraversion or emotional stability? This is often the type of question that comes to mind when thinking about the issue of cultural influences in personality. However, as our chapter attests, personality traits are only one of the several types of personality constructs and processes influenced by cultural forces. Furthermore, answering questions regarding possible cultural differences in personality traits requires first addressing more basic questions regarding the cross-cultural status of (1) the very notion of traits and traitedness (i.e., behavioral consistency), (2) the dimensional structures identified to organize trait variance (e.g., the FFM), and (3) the specific meanings and behaviors associated with broad and narrow personality traits (e.g., extraversion, assertiveness).

Some cultural psychologists have argued that the very notion of personality traits implies a belief in behavioral individuality, situational consistency, and temporal stability that is culture-specific (Markus & Kitayama, 1998). An impressive program of research on this issue by Church and his colleagues (e.g., 2003, 2006) provides some answers. For instance, in a large-scale study that included two individualistic cultures (United States and Australia) and four collectivistic cultures (Mexico, Philippines, Malaysia, Japan), Church and his colleagues (2006) found that implicit trait beliefs are endorsed in all cultural groups, although these beliefs are stronger in individualistic cultures. Furthermore, across the six cultures, trait beliefs seemed to be endorsed as much or more than contextual beliefs. Self-perceptions of one's own level of traitedness (i.e., behavioral consistency) seem to be more culturally dependent, however, and were lower in the collectivistic countries (except for Mexico).

The issue of whether the Big Five personality trait dimensions are cross-culturally robust and whether different, fewer, or more personality dimensions are needed in some cultures depends on the approach (imposed-etic or emic) taken to explore this issue. A comprehensive review of the many cross-cultural studies relying on translated versions of well-established personality questionnaires—that is, imposed-etic personality studies—goes beyond the scope of this chapter (see Church & Ortiz, 2005, or Triandis & Suh, 2002, for excellent reviews), so we will only summarize key studies and findings. Studies using translations of Anglo-based Big Five measures have reliably replicated the same five-factor structure across many different cultures and languages (McCrae & Costa, 1996). Additional support for the cross-cultural robustness of the Big Five dimensions comes from cross-cultural studies using translated versions of personality scales that do not measure the Big Five, per se, such as the Personality Research Form and the Nonverbal Personality Questionnaire (Paunonen & Ashton, 1998). Additionally, self- and peer ratings of the NEO-PI-R seem to converge in other cultures as much as they do in U.S. samples (Smith, Spillane, & Annus, 2006), and the same five factors emerge when the factor analyses are done at the nation level (Allik & McCrae, 2004). Lastly, Big Five scores correlate with various criteria (e.g., self- and relational esteem, self-construals, life satisfaction) quite consistently in Western and Asian samples (Benet-Martínez & Karakitapoglu-Aygun, 2003; Kwan, Bond, & Singelis, 1997). In conclusion, the cross-cultural evidence for the stability of the Anglo-based Big Five across cultures and languages is very impressive. This means that researchers can confidently and reliably measure these five personality dispositions (as defined in the Anglo-Saxon world) in other cultures. However, the psychometric applicability of the Anglo Big Five measures in other cultures does not speak to the validity of the Big Five to capture the local meaning and structure of personality traits in those other cultures (Benet-Martínez, 2007). In fact, it should be noted that translated versions of instruments tapping personality models different from the Big Five (e.g., Minnesota Multiphasic Personality Inventory [MMPI], Eysenck Personality Inventory, California Psychological Inventory, Big Seven model) also replicate quite well cross-culturally (Church, 2000; Smith et al., 2006). Only studies relying on emic or combined etic–emic approaches can directly address the issue of which personality dimensions are more robust cross-culturally (i.e., universal).

A comprehensive review of all the emic personality studies conducted in other languages and cultures also goes beyond the scope of this chapter. However, Cheung's programmatic work mapping the indigenous Chinese personality domain is worth mentioning (Cheung et al., 1996). Using combined emic–etic designs, Cheung and her colleagues (1996) identified four indigenous Chinese personality factors: Dependability, Interpersonal Relatedness, Social Potency, and Individualism. Joint-factor analyses of these indigenous scales and the Chinese-translated NEO-PI-R indicated that the Interpersonal Relatedness dimension is not represented in the Big Five personality space, and that the Openness to Experience domain is not represented in the Chinese personality space (Cheung et al., 2001). Not surprisingly, the Interpersonal Relatedness dimension taps personality dispositions that are uniquely central to Chinese relationships (but not encouraged in Anglo-Saxon cultures): strong orientation toward instrumental relationships, propriety in role and action, avoidance of internal and interpersonal conflict, and support of norms and traditions. Similarly, the dispositions tapped by Openness (imaginativeness, liberal thinking, and novelty seeking) seem to support Western cultures' emphasis on affective and intellectual freedom, expressiveness, and uniqueness.

Saucier and Goldberg (2001) carefully organized and meticulously compared lexical personality studies conducted in English and 12 other languages and concluded that, with the exception of Openness to Experience, most of these studies identified variants of four of the five factors (Neuroticism, Extraversion, Conscientiousness, and Agree-

ableness). Most emic studies that found more than five factors included additional dimensions representing culture-specific forms of Extraversion or Agreeableness subcomponents (e.g., face, interpersonal harmony, social reciprocity) or dimensions denoting social evaluation with regard to power, morality, or attractiveness. Saucier and Goldberg also conclude that the Anglo-based Big Five model replicates most predictably in emic personality studies when all of the following conditions are present: (1) the culture is of Northern European origin, (2) the personality descriptor pool contains only terms denoting trait dispositions (i.e., excludes evaluative terms), and (3) the factor analyses are done on ipsatized self-ratings.

In sum, even though the Anglo-based Big-Five structure is incompletely supported by some emic studies, dimensions resembling (i.e., cultural variants of) Extraversion, Agreeableness, Conscientiousness, and Neuroticism appear in most of these studies. All in all, these findings suggest that, whereas Openness to Experience may be a personality dimension unique to Anglo-based cultures, the other four dimensions have both universal and culture-specific components. Note that these results would seem to validate the phenotypic perspective of personality, which views taxonomic personality dimensions as reflecting both genetic dispositions and characteristic adaptations to the sociocultural context.

A neglected issue in the literature is the question of whether indigenous personality constructs have better predictive power than the Anglo-based Big Five traits. Katigbak, Church, Guanzon-Lapena, Carlota, and del Pilar (2002) found that Filipino indigenous inventories added modest incremental validity beyond the FFM in predicting common health, risk-related, and religious behaviors (i.e., smoking, drinking, gambling, accident proneness, and praying). Bond (2000), however, reports several studies with Chinese participants where indigenous dimensions predicted specific culture-bound behaviors, such as filial piety or gentle persuasion, well beyond the FFM. It should be noted that the use of both imported and indigenous personality scales (i.e., a combined emic–etic approach) is ideal in exploratory lexical and validational studies. However, this design may prove too expensive and lengthy in cultural studies simply interested in examining the link between personality and specific behavioral outcomes. As a compromising solution, Benet-Martínez and John (2000) have proposed the use of *quasi-indigenous* personality dimensions. This approach involves first identifying psychometrically a manageable set of indigenous personality descriptors that reliably measure the Big Five using local, culturally relevant terms, and then using these dimensions to predict the outcomes of interest.

Finally, recent research by McCrae and colleagues (Allik & McCrae, 2004; McCrae, Terracciano, et al., 2005) reports country-level scores on the FFM for 51 different cultures. The standing of particular countries on the Big Five traits was summarized in Table 2 in McCrae, Terracciano, et al., 2005; or Figures 1 and 2 in Allik & McCrae, 2004). These studies also report meaningful correlations between nation-level scores on the Big Five personality traits and nation-level scores on cultural values (individualism vs. collectivism, masculinity vs. femininity, power distance, and uncertainty avoidance) and socioeconomic indicators (e.g., gross domestic product [GDP]). These later results are particularly useful in that they provide a theoretical basis for interpreting the country-level mean personality differences. More recently, the research by this research group (Terracciano et al., 2005) has shed light on an important issue with profound social implications: the accuracy of cultural (self) stereotypes regarding personality (e.g., "the somber Scandinavian" or the "hot-tempered Mediterranean"). Almost 4,000 respondents in 49 cultures were asked to describe the personality of typical members of their own culture, and these scores were then compared with the actual personality scores of culture members (as assessed by self- and observer ratings). Results indicated that people's perceptions of the "stereotypical personality" of their native culture are very consistent but do not reflect individuals' actual personality traits.

AFFECT

The patterns of feeling, along with thinking and behaving, are signatures of one's personality (McCrae & Costa, 1999). As in the re-

search on personality traits, the first step for cross-cultural research in this area is to examine the degree of cross-cultural invariance in structure. Russell (1983) used similarity judgments and multidimensional scaling and found that Chinese, Japanese, Croatian, and Gujarati similarity judgments resulted in the circular structure of moods (pleasure–displeasure and arousal–sleepiness dimensions) similar to Canadians. Watson, Clark, and Tellegen (1984) conducted one of the first daily diary studies in Japan and investigated cross-cultural comparability in within-person structure of moods. It was also one of the longest daily diary studies to date (90 days!). Watson and colleagues obtained the two-factor structure (positive and negative mood factors) and factor loadings similar to the one previously found among Americans. The only major difference concerned the term "sleepy" (or *nemui*). In the United States, *sleepy* had a negative loading to the positive mood factor, whereas in Japan it did not load on the positive factor. This suggests that Americans were *not* sleepy when they were feeling positive moods, whereas Japanese were feeling sleepy sometimes when they were in positive moods. These differences might have come from cultural differences in general preference for high-activation versus low-activation positive moods: Americans typically prefer high-activation positive mood (e.g., excited) to low-activation positive mood (e.g., calm), whereas East Asians value low-activation positive mood as much as high-activation positive mood (Tsai, Knuston, & Fung, 2006). Individuals who value the experience of high-activation positive mood are likely to devalue that of low-activation mood such as sleepy.

Whereas Russell (1983) and Watson and colleagues (1984) found remarkable similarities in the structure of affect across cultures, recent research found systematic cultural variations as well. For instance, using the experience sampling method, Scollon, Diener, Oishi, and Biswas-Diener (2005) found that the factor loading of pride was quite different across cultures. Whereas pride loaded on the positive mood factor only among European Americans and Hispanic Americans, pride loaded on both positive and negative moods among Asian Americans, Japanese, and Indians (see also Oishi, 2007, in difference between Americans and Chinese on pride using item response theory). Likewise, Kitayama, Markus, and Kurosawa (2000) found that general happiness was strongly associated with interpersonally disengaging positive emotions (e.g., pride) among Americans, whereas it was strongly associated with interpersonally engaging positive emotions (e.g., *fureai*) among Japanese. The notable cultural difference involving pride observed above is also consistent with the cross-cultural literature on self-esteem and self-enhancement (Heine & Hamamura, 2007).

Besides the structural issues, researchers have investigated facial recognition and appraisal dimensions of emotions across cultures for decades. For instance, Ekman and colleagues (Ekman & Friesen, 1971; Ekman et al., 1987) showed that people from one culture can recognize emotion expressed by members of another culture with a great deal of accuracy (see also Haidt & Keltner, 1999; Tracy & Robins, in press). Following Darwin (1872/1965), Ekman and colleagues argued that facial expression and recognition are biologically determined and therefore universal. It should be noted, however, that there were also some cultural differences in Ekman et al.'s study. For instance, only 60–67% of Japanese participants correctly recognized disgust, fear, and anger, in comparison to 81–86% of American participants (see also Russell, 1994). The lower accuracy among Japanese might be due to their tendency to project the perspective of generalized others to the presented face (e.g., seeing "fear" in an "angry" face; Cohen & Gunz, 2002), and their tendency to attend to the target's eyes, which are less distinct across emotions than the mouth (e.g., Yuki, Maddux, & Masuda, 2007). In a comprehensive meta-analysis, Elfenbein and Ambady (2002) also showed that although many emotions are accurately recognized at above-chance levels universally, there is a sizable ingroup advantage in facial recognition (e.g., Chinese recognize Chinese facial expressions better than they recognize American facial expressions).

Whereas the majority of facial recognition studies used a single face to represent a single emotion, Masuda and colleagues (in press) devised a paradigm in which the focal face was presented with multiple other faces in the background. Given that our facial recognition in daily life takes place in the presence of other individuals, this paradigm has a greater degree of ecological validity than the still pictures often used in this literature. Using this new paradigm, these researchers showed that Japanese participants' facial recognition was affected by surrounding faces to a greater extent than Americans'. Using an eye-tracking method, these researchers further demonstrated that this cultural difference was explained by the perceptual attention given to the focal versus nonfocal objects in the visual field: Japanese gaze moved back and forth between the focal and background faces, whereas American gaze fixated at the focal face very quickly. These results indicate that, whereas there are a great deal of cultural similarities in facial recognition *outcomes* (final categorization), there are cultural differences in facial recognition *processes*.

In terms of appraisal dimensions, the majority of studies found more cross-cultural similarities than differences (see Mesquita & Frijda, 1992, for review). For example, Mauro, Sato, and Tucker (1992) found that the relevance of "primitive" dimensions such as pleasantness, attentional activity, certainty, coping potential, and goal/need conduciveness to 14 emotions was very similar in the United States, Japan, China, and Hong Kong. In contrast, the relevance of "complex" dimensions such as control, responsibility, and anticipated effort were quite different across cultures. Scherer (1997) also reported findings from 37 countries, showing that the relevance of eight appraisal dimensions for seven emotions was largely similar across cultures. One notable exception was the immorality dimension for disgust. Whereas the experience of disgust was strongly associated with immorality in the United States, New Zealand and Australia, it was unrelated in Latin American countries.

Although there is a remarkable degree of comparability across cultures in the structure, facial recognition, and appraisal of emotions, there are many other aspects of affect that differ. One of the most fundamental differences lies in the labeling of feeling states. Russell (1991) reviewed this literature and identified cultures that do not have the corresponding words for the so-called basic emotions. For instance, there is no word for *disgust* in Polish, Ifaluk, and Chewong. There is no word for *sadness* in Tahitian and Chewong, no word for *fear* in Ifaluk, Utku, and Pintupi, and no word for *surprise* in Fore, Dani, Malay, and Ifaluk. Even when there is the corresponding word, the conceptual comparability does not always exist. For example, there is a great deal of agreement that the most appropriate Japanese translation of depression is *yuutsu (憂鬱)*, and clearly there is a phenomenon labeled "depression" in Japan. Yet, Tanaka-Matsumi and Marsella (1976) found that the free associations given by English speakers were very different from those given by Japanese speakers, suggesting that the observable symptoms of depressions as well as how it feels to be "depressed" are different between Japanese and Americans. Because labeling is an important aspect of conscious awareness of feeling states, these linguistic differences should result in predictable cultural differences in the frequency and intensity of these affective states. In addition, connotative differences of emotions might give rise to different co-occurrence patterns of emotions across cultures.

There are also well-replicated cultural differences in the desirability of various emotions. Diener, Suh, Smith, and Shao (1995) found that Americans viewed the experience and expression of positive emotions more desirable and appropriate than Chinese. Using latent-class analysis, Eid and Diener (2001) also identified a culture-specific "class" among Chinese who viewed positive emotions as neither desirable nor undesirable. This class did not exist among Americans, Australians, or Taiwanese. A more recent study showed that people in Latin America value positive emotion and devalue negative emotion, even more than North Americans (Diener, Scollon, Oishi, Dzokoto, & Suh, 2000). Thus, the largest cultural difference in desirability of emotions lies not between East Asians and North Americans, but between East Asians and Latin Americans. It is also interesting that the frequency with which people feel any given emotion is different across cultures. Using a time-contingent recording method (i.e., reporting their emotions at a predetermined time, such as noon, 3:00 P.M., 6:00 P.M., and 9:00 P.M. for 8 tconsecutive days), Mesquita and Karasawa (2002) found that Japanese participants reported feeling "no emotion" more often than did Americans. If emotions are not experienced as often, it is then not surprising that the frequency of emotion itself is not as strong

a predictor of life satisfaction in collectivist nations as in individualist nations (Suh, Diener, Oishi, & Triandis, 1998). These findings suggest that desirability of emotion differs systematically across cultures, and these differences influence the role emotions play in people's daily life.

AFFECTIVE TRAITS

The aforementioned section focused on affective experiences. Next, we review cross-cultural research on affective traits. Many personality researchers theorize that extraversion and neuroticism are affective traits. Watson and Clark (1997), for instance, argue that divergent facets of extraversion (e.g., sensation seeking, dominance, sociability) could be "glued" by the latent construct of positive affectivity (PA). Lucas, Diener, Grob, Such, and Shao (2000) tested this idea across cultures and found that the correlation between PA and extraversion was significant in all 39 countries. Schimmack and colleagues (2002a) further demonstrated that the latent link between extraversion and hedonic balance (negative affectivity [NA]; PA–NA) was positive, and the link between neuroticism and hedonic balance was negative in the United States, Germany, Mexico, Japan, and Ghana. Interestingly, however, they found that the latent association between hedonic balance and life satisfaction was larger among Americans and Germans than among Mexicans, Japanese, and Ghanaians.

Some cultural psychologists (e.g., Markus & Kitayama, 1998; Shweder, 1991) questioned whether the factor-analytic results were really evidence for the existence of traits, arguing that the factor structure tells us more about semantic associations between items than behavioral co-occurrence. Cross-situational consistency provides a stronger piece of evidence than factor analysis for the existence of traits. To this end, Oishi, Diener, Scollon, and Biswas-Diener (2004) examined cross-situational consistency of affective experiences across cultures, using an experience sampling method. Replicating Diener and Larsen's (1984) earlier findings in the United States, Oishi and colleagues found a great deal of cross-cultural similarities in cross-situational consistency of affect at the between-person level in India, Japan, and the

United States ($r = .52$ for positive affect [e.g., happy persons alone were also happier with friends], and .51 for negative affect). Simultaneously, however, they discovered substantial cultural differences in the degree to which specific interpersonal contexts influenced their moods. For instance, Japanese moods varied more greatly between alone situations and with-friend situations than Americans. Based on these findings, Oishi and colleagues theorized that interindividual differences in affective experiences (e.g., Who is happy? Who is sad?) are determined largely by individuals' temperaments and biological constituents (see Ando et al., 2002; Yamagata et al., 2006), whereas within-individual variation in affective experiences (e.g., when does one feel happy or sad?) are largely driven by cultural factors. In other words, the mean levels of affect are thought to be influenced largely by genetic and biological factors, whereas the if–then patterns of affect (Mischel & Shoda, 1995) are thought to be influenced largely by cultural factors.

THINKING AND BEHAVING

Along with the patterns of feeling, patterns of thinking and action are integral to the definition of personality (McCrae & Costa, 1999). Thinking style also plays an important role in individual differences in well-being; for example, internal attribution of a negative event (Peterson & Seligman, 1984) and rumination (Lyubomirsky & Nolen-Hoeksema, 1993) are linked to depression, whereas optimism is associated with self-esteem and life satisfaction (Lucas, Diener, & Suh, 1996). A number of studies showed that North Americans are more optimistic than East Asians (e.g., Heine & Lehman, 1995). Nisbett and his colleagues have identified several important cultural differences on thinking styles between North Americans and East Asians (see Nisbett, 2004, for review). Confucian thinking common in East Asia tolerates contradiction, whereas the Western tradition, starting with Greek philosophy, is sensitive to contradiction. Confucian thinking is also known to be holistic and dialectical (e.g., paying attention to the whole), whereas Western thinking is known to be analytical (e.g., abstracting the essence). These different thinking styles have a profound implication for the way individu-

als evaluate their emotional experiences and themselves. Consistent with this idea, for instance, Schimmack, Oishi, and Diener (2002) found that the relation between the frequency of positive emotions and negative emotions was significantly more negative among North Americans and Western Europeans than among East Asians. In other words, in traditionally Confucian nations, the experience of positive and negative emotions was more independent than in Western nations, with their tradition of analytical thinking. Likewise, Spencer-Rodgers, Peng, Wang, and Hou (2004) found that East Asians endorsed both positive and negative aspects of the self, whereas European Americans endorsed either positive or negative aspects of the self. Furthermore, this cultural group difference was mediated by dialectical thinking style scores, indicating that dialectical thinking style explains between-culture differences and within-culture individual differences (*analytical* East Asians endorse either positive or negative self-statements, whereas *dialectical* European Americans endorse both positive and negative self-statements). In addition, Koo and Choi (2005) showed that holistic thinking is learned through education. Students of Oriental medicine were more holistic than students in other disciplines, and older students in Oriental medicine were more holistic than younger students in Oriental medicine. Besides the distinction between holistic and analytical styles, Kim (2002) found an interesting cultural difference in the role of speaking in thinking: Speaking helps North Americans think well, whereas it hinders East Asians' thinking. These findings suggest that cultural heritages affect how individuals think about themselves and others.

Levine, Norenzayan, and Philbrick (2001) conducted one of the few cross-cultural studies on behaviors and found that people living in Brazil, Costa Rica, and other Latin countries (cultures of *simpatia*) showed a greater degree of helping behaviors toward a stranger (the confederate) than people in other countries. Investigating the U.S. Southern culture of honor, Cohen, Nisbett, Bowdle, and Schwarz (1996) found that Southerners have a greater propensity to show physical aggression than Northerners in reaction to an insult. Southern laws were also more tolerant of violence when damaged honor was involved than Northern laws (Cohen, 1996).

Furthermore, Southern companies were more receptive to a fake applicant who had a violent past in reaction to the honor violation than were Northern companies (Cohen & Nisbett, 1997). These findings provide evidence that culture provides an important context in which personality traits such as empathy and aggression are expressed.

SELF-CONCEPT

In McCrae and Costa's (1999) schematic model of personality, self-concepts are the conscious aspects of personality that reflect not only temperaments but also characteristic patterns of adaptation. Given that characteristic adaptations are influenced by culture, it is expected that the ways in which individuals view themselves are, at least in part, culturally constructed. The content analysis of free self-descriptions revealed systematic cultural differences. For instance, participants from two traditional tribes in Kenya, the Samburu and the Masai, described themselves primarily in terms of social categories such as roles and group membership (over 80%) and rarely used personality traits (less than 2%; Ma & Schoeneman, 1997). In contrast, Kenyan college students in Nairobi as well as U.S. college students used personality traits and abilities much more than social categories in self-descriptions. Similarly, Americans used personality traits more often than did Japanese (Cousins, 1989). Interestingly, however, when specific contexts were given (e.g., at home), Japanese used personality traits as frequently as Americans. Thus, it is not that Japanese do not use personality traits in self-descriptions. Rather, Japanese use of personality traits in self-descriptions is much more context specific (see Kanagawa, Cross, & Markus, 2001, for situational variation in the Twenty Statements Test; also del Prado et al., 2007, for a review of this literature).

There is a large body of literature on self-esteem. In a recent international study, Schimmit and Allik (2005) found that (1) the mean self-esteem score was above neutral in all 53 nations, but (2) East Asian participants scored lower than the rest (especially Japanese, who scored the lowest). There is some evidence for an acculturation effect on self-esteem. For example, Japanese born and

raised in Canada reported higher self-esteem than Japanese who grew up in Japan but currently lived in Canada (Heine & Lehman, 2004; see similar acculturation findings on extraversion by McCrae, Yik, Trapnell, Bond, & Paulhus, 1998). Moreover, Japanese currently living in Canada reported higher self-esteem than Japanese living in Japan. In an extensive meta-analysis, Twenge and Crocker (2002) showed that Asian Americans also report lower self-esteem than European Americans (see, however, Robins, Trzesniewski, Tracy, Gosling, & Potter, 2002, for the null results). Interestingly, Asian Americans had slightly higher self-esteem than European Americans in the elementary school samples. But the advantage of Asian Americans no longer exists in middle school samples. In high school samples, European Americans report higher self-esteem than Asian Americans. Finally, in college samples, the difference is even larger. This meta-analysis sheds light on the developmental shift in degree of cultural differences in self-esteem.

Although self-esteem measured by explicit scales (e.g., Rosenberg Self-Esteem Scale) showed considerable mean differences between North Americans and Japanese, self-esteem measure by implicit methods, such as the name–letter preference (Kitayama & Karasawa, 1997) and implicit association test (Kobayashi & Greenwald, 2003; Yamaguchi et al., 2007), often yielded no cultural differences. This research suggests that cultural differences in explicit self-esteem might be due to cultural differences in desirability of pride and self-esteem. Namely, there is the possibility that Japanese and other East Asians report lower levels of explicit self-esteem than North Americans because of modesty (Kurman, 2003). Indeed, Akimoto and Sanbonmatsu (1999) designed a clever experiment with a public versus private self-evaluation condition and demonstrated that Japanese Americans evaluated their task performance less positively than European Americans only in the public condition. However, other findings cannot be explained by the modesty account. Kitayama, Markus, Matsumoto, and Norasakkunkit (1997), for instance, found that Japanese listed more negative self-descriptions than Americans across various anonymous conditions. False-feedback studies also found repeatedly that Japanese more readily accepted negative feedback than positive (Heine, Takata, & Lehman, 2000). In addition, Japanese reported that proud and embarrassing events felt equally far away, whereas North Americans reported that proud events felt closer in time than embarrassing events in an anonymous open-ended self-description task (Ross, Heine, Wilson, & Sugimori, 2005). In short, although there is a great deal of agreement on the sizable East–West difference in explicit measures of self-esteem, consensus has not yet emerged on why the magnitude of cultural difference on implicit measures of self-esteem is much smaller than that of explicit self-esteem.

Similar to the explicit self-esteem findings, many cross-cultural studies found that East Asians showed less self-enhancement than European Americans (see Heine & Hamamura, 2007, for a comprehensive meta-analysis). For instance, whereas the "better-than-average" effect is powerful among North Americans (College Board, 1976–1977), Japanese did not show the better-than-average effect (Markus & Kitayama, 1991). Recently, Sedikides, Gaertner, and Toguchi (2003) found that Japanese participants reported having collectivist traits more than the average other, suggesting that people universally self-enhance on the traits that are personally and culturally important to them (see also Sedikides, Gaertner, & Vevea, 2005). These results, however, directly contradict Heine and Renshaw's (2002) findings that Japanese showed more self-*effacement* on personally important traits. Because the self-enhancement studies using the average or typical others as a reference group have serious methodological problems (for one thing, it is impossible to disentangle their self-view and the view of "average other"; see Kenny, 1994), it is difficult to discern how much participants' self-reports are distorted. Thus, it is critical in the future to control for raters' bias via the social relations analysis (Kenny, 1994; Kwan, John, Kenny, Bond, & Robbins, 2004) and other methods in cultural research on self-enhancement (see, e.g., Su & Oishi, 2006).

Finally, several researchers have identified notable cultural differences in self-concept clarity and consistency. For example, Canadians reported having a clearer sense of who they are than Japanese (Campbell et al., 1996). In addition, Koreans' self-evaluation changed to a larger extent than Americans', depending on the question asked (e.g., "How extraverted versus how introverted are you?"; Choi & Choi, 2002). In a related vein, Suh (2002) showed that Americans' self-descriptions are more consistent across different roles than Koreans.' Moreover, replicating Donahue, Robins, Roberts, and John (1993), self-concept consistency was positively associated with well-being among European Americans. Furthermore, consistent persons were better liked by their peers among Americans. However, self-concept consistency was not associated with well-being among Koreans or likability ratings by their peers. Suh's findings are relevant to the most fundamental question about personality, namely, whether "persona" is a mask (the role one plays) or the actor him- or herself. Allport (1937) persuasively argued that personality should be the actor, or the true self. We agree with Allport's argument, in general, that the actor's unique way of adjusting to the environment should be a main target of personality research. Yet, Suh's findings illuminate that (1) role expectations are stronger in Korea than in the United States; (2) the degree to which the actor can exert an influence on the script is more restricted in Korea than in the United States; and (3) therefore, the opportunities to observe the expression of personality might be limited and the link between personality and behavior might be weaker in Korea than in the United States.

VALUES AND MOTIVATION

In empirical personality research, traits have been a central focus. Yet values and other related motivational constructs are just as important in understanding human personality. Vernon and Allport (1931), for instance, maintained that values are at the core of one's philosophy of life and provide a picture into the "total personality" (p. 231). Allport (1937, 1961) later argued that personality traits can be construed as the fully developed version of one's biological natural tendencies, or temperaments, whereas values reflect not only individuals' innate preferences but also ideal lifestyles. In order to understand how an individual uniquely adjusts to his or her environment (an important part of Allport's definition of personality), personality researchers need to understand not only a person's typical behavioral tendencies but also his or her unified philosophy of life.

Kluckhohn and Strodtbeck (1961) developed a value scale using a scenario method and consisting of five dimensions deemed important in the anthropological literature: human–nature orientation, time orientation, activity orientation, relational orientation, and nature of human. Using this scale, they conducted one of the first cross-cultural studies on values and found that Navaho preferred present time orientation to past or future time orientation and harmony with nature to mastery, compared to Mormons, Texans, and Spanish Americans. Although these efforts to measure values produced interesting findings, there was a great deal of concern about the comprehensiveness of earlier value scales. Rokeach (1973) developed his widely used value scale to address this limitation. He measured 18 instrumental values and 18 terminal values, using the ranking method. Shalom Schwartz and colleagues (e.g., Schwarz & Sagiv, 1995) extended the 36-item Rokeach Value Survey into a 54-item value survey, using a Likert scale. Schwartz and colleagues conducted a series of large-scale cross-cultural studies of values and validated the hierarchical structure of values. For example, in nationally representative samples Schwartz and Bardi (2002) showed that benevolence, self-direction, and universalism values were most important; power, tradition, and stimulation values were least important; and security, conformity, achievement, and hedonism values were in-between in many nations.

Along with Hofstede's (1980) work on individualism–collectivism and Schwartz's work on universal values, Ronald Inglehart's World Value Surveys (WVS) should be recognized as one of the most important contributions to culture and value research to date (Inglehart & Baker, 2000). Inglehart and Baker (2000) collected data on various values from all over the world, using a nationally representative sampling method in 1981–1982, 1990–1991, and 1995–1998. Their value items resulted in two major factors: self-expression versus survival orientations and tradition versus secular–rational orientations. Consistent with Hofstede and Schwartz's results, English-speaking and Protestant European nations were high on self-expression (similar to individualism), whereas former Communist nations, African nations, and South Asian nations were low on this dimension. In contrast, Protestant European nations, ex-Communist nations, and Japan were very high on secularism, whereas the United States was quite low on secularism, replicating well-known differences between the United States and Western Europe in religiosity and church attendance. Most interestingly, although Japanese responses in 1995 were more individualistic (high on self-expression) than in 1981, so were other nations (e.g., United States, Australia). Thus, the magnitude of cultural differences between Japan and other Western developed nations in 1995 was surprisingly similar to that in 1981 (Inglehart & Baker, 2000). These results have an important implication for the effect of globalization and Westernization on value orientations. Although many naive observers of culture often assume that developing nations will be Westernized and that globalization will quickly homogenize value orientations over time, so far, the WVS data suggest that globalization has not wiped out historical differences. Although value orientations do change over time (Rokeach & Ball-Rokeach, 1989), they change slowly. It seems fair to say that the cultural force for continuity seems to be more powerful than previously believed.

Despite these important discoveries in the 1990s and early 2000s, the landscape of culture and value research has shifted drastically from exuberant optimism to pessimism with the publication of Oyserman, Coon, and Kemmelmeier's (2002) meta-analysis. These researchers concluded that cultural differences in individualism and collectivism "were neither as large nor as systematic as often perceived" (p. 40). Their main criticism was that Hofstede's (1980) results were not replicated when various kinds of individualism–collectivism scales were used. Indeed, according to their meta-analysis, Americans were slightly *higher* on collectivism than Japanese (see also Takano & Osaka, 1999, for an earlier critique on the Japan–U.S. comparisons). It should be noted, however, that most studies reviewed by Oyserman and colleagues and Takano and Osaka were conducted in the 1980s and the 1990s and used raw means on a Likert scale. Unlike earlier cross-cultural studies (e.g.,

Klukhohn & Strodtbeck, 1961), therefore, these studies were susceptible to response styles. Indeed, when Schimmack, Oishi, and Diener (2005) statistically controlled for response styles (i.e., partialing out the mean of all value items), Hofstede's results converged quite well with Oyserman and colleagues' meta-analysis ($r = .50$, $p < .01$, as opposed to $r = .17$, *n.s.* without controlling for response styles). That is, nations deemed individualist in Hofstede indeed scored high on individualism in Oyserman and colleagues' meta-analysis, once response styles were statistically controlled. These findings underscore the importance of addressing response-style issues in cross-cultural research (see also, Bond, 1988; Heine, Lehman, Peng, & Greenholtz, 2002; Oishi et al., 2005, for other solutions).

In short, although culture and value research is currently in crisis, this should not prevent cross-cultural researchers from investigating this important topic. Chinese translation of "crisis" consists of two characters: 危機. The first character means "danger," but the second character means "opportunity." In the spirit of the Chinese interpretation, therefore, despite the current crisis, we believe that there is a great opportunity for cross-cultural research on values, now that the problems with previous research are clearly understood and that the simple solutions are provided. With the use of multiple methods, future research on culture and value is likely to generate important knowledge about the "total personality" across cultures, and should continue to be an integral part of culture and personality research.

In addition to explicit values, personality researchers have been interested in implicit motives since Murray (1938). In the late 1950s and early 1960s, Walter Mischel conducted one of the first cross-cultural studies on delay of gratification in the West Indies (e.g., Mischel, 1958, 1961). He found that African Trinidadian children chose the immediate reward more often than did East Indian Trinidadians and that this group difference could be explained by the proportion of absent fathers. McClelland (1961) was another pioneer in culture and motivation research. He used creative methodologies to measure need for achievement, ranging from content coding of folklore, children's stories, and literatures to vase designs, in various cultures over historical periods. For instance, he showed the positive correlation between achievement imagery in folk tales and the level of entrepreneurial activity in over 40 small-scale preliterate societies (e.g., Yoruba, Masai, Apache, Navaho). In addition, McClelland demonstrated that need for achievement seen in children's readers in 1925 predicted economic growth in 1950 among modern societies (e.g., Sweden, United States, Mexico, Russia). McClelland's cross-cultural research preceded the renewed interest in culture among leading economists and political scientists today (Harrison & Huntington, 2000) by 40 years.

Whereas the leading comparative economists and political scientists focus on stable values of various nations (Lipset & Lenz, 2000), McClelland (1961) was deeply interested in within-culture changes in motives as well. Most impressive, he demonstrated that the economic spur of Ancient Greece, 16th-century Spain, and 18th-century England was preceded by high levels of need for achievement seen in their respective literature. Furthermore, a subsequent decline in each culture was also predicted by lower need for achievement seen during the rapid economic growth. These historical analyses reveal that (1) dominant motives change over time within the same society, and (2) these changes are associated with systematic changes in economic activities later in time. In sum, McClelland's work demonstrates that need for achievement is not a stable "national character," but instead a dynamic motive that changes over time, depending on local and historical contexts. What seems like cultural differences in national character at any given time may simply be different phases of the same cycle. Whereas the cross-societal comparisons might evoke the "national character" and the notion of "cultural developmentalism," the cross-temporal comparisons clearly demonstrate that McClelland's work goes well beyond the traditional critique of national character and cultural developmentalism. Although David McClelland is not known for his cross-cultural work, his contribution to the culture and personality literature is worthy of the fullest recognition.

More recently, self-determination theorists (e.g., Richard Ryan, Kennon Sheldon, Valery Chirkov, and colleagues) conducted several cross-cultural studies on the needs for autonomy, relatedness, and competence. Whereas several researchers have questioned the centrality of need for autonomy in collectivist societies (e.g., Iyengar & Lepper, 1999; Oishi & Diener, 2001), self-determination researchers have gathered evidence in support of the universality of needs for autonomy, relatedness, and competence in various nations (e.g., Chirkov, Ryan, Kim, & Kaplan, 2003; Sheldon et al., 2004). The debate on universal versus culture-specific need for autonomy emerged in part as a result of diverging definitions of "autonomy." The self-determination theorists define autonomy by the degree of psychological internalization (e.g., personal importance), not by independence, per se (Chirkov et al., 2003), whereas several cultural psychologists define autonomy in terms of an individual's degree of freedom and choice (e.g., Iyengar & Lepper, 1999; Oishi & Diener, 2001). For example, Rudy, Sheldon, Awong, and Tan (2007) found that Chinese Canadian college students high in subjective well-being are those who report studying "because in my family, we want to know if our ideas are correct" and "because in my family, we enjoy doing our work well," whereas European Canadians high in subjective well-being are those who report studying "because I want to know if my ideas are correct" and "because I enjoy doing my school work well." According to self-determination theorists, both instances are a reflection of autonomy (the Chinese version is called "inclusive" autonomy) and indicate that the need for autonomy is universal.

In addition to the needs for autonomy, relatedness, and competence, various cultural differences in motivation have been reported. For instance, Russians, Koreans, and Asian Americans are more avoidance-oriented (e.g., they try to avoid failure) than European Americans (e.g., Elliot, Chirkov, Kim, & Sheldon, 2001). Similarly, Americans are more promotion-oriented (e.g., interested in success) than Italians, Chinese, Australians, Indians, and Japanese, whereas Italians, Spaniards, Americans, Indians, and Israelis are more locomotion-oriented (e.g., need to keep moving, get going) than Poles, Koreans, and Japanese (Higgins, Pierro, & Kruglanski, in press). Likewise, past success motivates European Americans to work harder, whereas past failure motivates Japanese to work harder (Heine et al., 2001).

These findings indicate that although most of the basic psychological needs (e.g., need for relatedness), if not all, seem to be present in every human being in every culture, what propels individuals can vary systematically across their local cultural contexts.

PSYCHOPATHOLOGY

There is a venerable research tradition on psychopathology in anthropology (e.g., La Barre, 1947). Kleinman (1977) revitalized this research topic by creating an interdisciplinary research area entitled "new cross-cultural psychiatry," later developed into the journal *Culture, Medicine, and Psychiatry*. In cross-cultural psychiatry researchers have tackled culture-specific illness, such as *taijin kyofu sho* in Japan (an extreme form of interpersonal anxiety), *ataque de nervios* among Latinos from the Caribbean (a form of anxiety and mood disorder whose symptoms include trembling and uncontrollable crying and verbal/physical aggression), and *anorexia nervosa* in the United States, as well as epidemiological issues such as prevalence and diagnosis across cultures (see Draguns & Tanaka-Matsumi, 2003; Lopez & Guarnaccia, 2000, for reviews).

In recent years there has been a concerted effort to create culturally sensitive diagnostic criteria such as the *Diagnostic and Statistical Manual of Mental Disorders* (4th ed., DSM-IV; Mezzich et al., 1999), reflecting the acceptance of the cross-cultural psychiatry approach in mainstream psychiatry (Kleinman and other influential cross-cultural psychiatrists were involved in the DSM-IV task force). Popular diagnostic scales such as the MMPI and MMPI-2 have been carefully translated and validated in many languages (e.g., 32 versions of the MMPI-2 were published by 1996; Butcher, 1996) and used extensively in numerous nations in diverse settings, ranging from clinics to military screening. Most important, research using the MMPI-2 has found many cross-cultural similarities in the profile types of various psychiatric patients (see Butcher, 2004, for review). In addition, large-scale cross-national epidemiological studies using the standardized diagnostic criteria have provided important information regarding similarities as well as differences across cultures in various psychopathologies (e.g., Jablensky et al., 1992). For instance, according to the study among Canadians, Iranians, Japanese, and Swiss conducted by the World Health Organization (1983), more than 76% of depressed patients in these nations reported a common pattern of depressive symptoms, including sadness, absence of joy, reduced concentration, and lack of energy. However, Draguns and Tanaka-Matsumi (2003) point out other findings: Guilt feelings are major symptoms of depression among North Americans, whereas guilt is not a common symptom of depression in Japan, China, India, Indonesia, or Africa.

Even when there are a great deal of commonalities in symptoms of a particular psychiatric category across cultures, the likelihood of this particular category being used in a diagnosis can vary across cultures. For example, Weisz, Chaiyasit, Weiss, Eastman, and Jackson (1995) showed that Thai teachers identified more externalizing problems in Thai children than did American teachers, even though objective raters identified more externalizing problems among American students than Thai. In other words, Thai teachers had a lower threshold for recognizing externalizing behaviors than American teachers, presumably because Thai students are, on average, more well-behaved than American students. These findings demonstrate the existence of the reference group effect in culture and psychopathology research (Heine et al., 2002). This is a significant issue in cross-cultural psychopathology research because, for example, the cultural difference in teachers' perceptions of students' behaviors will likely lead to the cultural difference in the number of students referred to mental health services, and then to the prevalence rate of a particular psychopathology. Furthermore, the similar cultural difference must exist among mental health professionals' perceptions of patients' behaviors as well as patients' self-evaluations, which directly affect the prevalence data across cultures. Indeed, Mexican-born Mexican Americans reported substantially lower prevalence rates of various psychological disorders than U.S.-born Mexican Americans (Burnam, Hough, Karno, Escobar, & Telles, 1987). Interestingly, Mexican-born Mexican Americans' prevalence rate was comparable to Mexicans living in Mexico city (Vega et al., 1998), so-

lidifying the idea that culture plays a role in the conception of psychopathologies and labeling of psychiatric categories. Thus, the prevalence data across cultures should be interpreted with these issues in mind.

Although the studies mentioned in this section emphasize cultural differences in psychopathology, behavioral genetic research has shown that many psychopathologies are heritable, ranging from the heritability coefficient of .80 for schizophrenia, to .50–.60 for alcoholism, .40–.50 for antisocial behavior, .40 for depression, and .30 for generalized anxiety disorder (Bouchard, 2004). There is no question that various psychopathologies are affected by genes. However, genes do not seem to work in a simple deterministic manner. Rather, the link between genes and observable behaviors is by no means direct, because environmental stimulations influence the likelihood that genes get activated (Marcus, 2004). To put these two lines of research together, then, psychopathologies clearly have biological foundations that are likely to be common among the human species. At the same time, however, situational antecedents (e.g., onset episodes) and the behavioral and affective manifestations of psychopathologies are likely to vary, depending on local, cultural, and historical contexts (e.g., hysteria in Freud's Victorian Austria, anorexia on college campuses in the United States in the 1990s and 2000s). In the end, epidemiological and behavioral genetics research on psychopathology should be supplemented by cultural psychological "thick" descriptions of these circumstantial and phenomenological aspects of psychopathology.

WITHIN-CULTURE CHANGES IN PERSONALITY

As the rates of Victorian-era hysteria and modern-day anorexia on U.S. college campuses indicate, the prevalence of a particular psychopathology changes over time, sometimes drastically, within the same culture. Given that genetic pools have not changed quickly within any given society, these changes must be instigated by sociocultural changes. One of the most exciting developments in culture and personality research, in our opinion, is the quantitative analysis of within-culture change in personality. Recent research on within-culture change in personality is similar to McClelland's (1961) work in spirit but different in terms of methodologies. Based on the longitudinal data from the Mills study, Roberts and Helson (1997), for instance, found that female participants became increasingly higher on self-focus and lower on norm adherence from 1958 to 1989, during which time American society is believed to have become more individualistic. This finding could be explained by personality maturation processes from ages 20 to 50. However, using a cross-temporal meta-analysis, Twenge and Campbell (2001) found that scores on the Rosenberg Self-Esteem Scale increased steadily from 1968 to 1994 in the United States, despite the steady decline in test scores, rise in divorce, and increasing crime rate during this period. Twenge and Campbell's data indicate that self-esteem of college students in the 1990s was higher than the self-esteem of college students in the 1960s. Thus, the maturation explanation does not apply to Twenge and Campbell's results. Together, then, these findings suggest that American college students, on average, became more self-focused and had increased self-esteem between the 1960s and 1990s (see, however, Trzesniewski, Donnellan, & Robins, in press, for the evidence of no change in narcissism).

Similarly, Twenge (2001a) found that American college students' scores on extraversion increased between 1966 and 1993. Twenge (2001b) also found that American women reported being more assertive and dominant from 1931 to 1945, then less assertive and dominant from 1946 to 1967, then again more assertive and dominant from 1968 to 1993. It is interesting to note that while self-esteem, extraversion, and assertiveness increased from the 1960s to the early 1990s, Americans' anxiety scores also increased during the same period of time (Twenge, 2000; see, however, Terracciano et al., 2005, for a counter-example among older adults). Although it is difficult to discern whether within-cultural changes in these personality scores reflect behavioral changes or changes in judgment criteria, these findings seem to capture an American cultural change toward greater individualism (self-focus, self-initiated social interaction) and competition (and the anxiety associated with it). The studies reviewed in this section, along with WVS data (Inglehart & Baker, 2000), pres-

ent a promising future direction for culture and personality research that explores the important issue of cultural change and persistence.

NEW DEVELOPMENTS AND FUTURE DIRECTIONS

The future of cultural personality studies is exciting. Personality researchers interested in how cultural factors influence personality-relevant processes and structures can profit from some new promising theoretical and methodological developments in the field, such as the integration of cultural and evolutionary approaches (Norenzayan & Heine, 2005; Rozin, 2003), the growing interest in the psychology of globalization and multiculturalism (Hong, Morris, Chiu, & Benet-Martínez, 2000), the application of brain imaging techniques to the understanding of cultural phenomenon such as race and identity (Eberhardt, 2005), and the availability of multilevel modeling statistical techniques to compare and link findings at the individual and cultural levels (Bryk & Raudenbush, 1992).

Some cultural researchers, informed by evolutionary theory, have proposed that many cross-cultural differences are, in fact, manifestations of deeper (universal and evolutionarily adaptive) psychological similarities in motivation and cognition (Higgins et al., in press; Norenzayan & Heine, 2005). The need for both cultural and cross-cultural psychology to respond to the theoretical and methodological questions posed by the growing phenomenon of multiculturalism cannot be overestimated. In their sampling and design choices, cultural researchers have often implicitly assumed that culture is a stable, uniform influence, and that nations and individuals are culturally homogeneous. But rapid globalization, continued massive migration, and the resulting demographic changes have resulted in social spaces (e.g., schools, homes, work settings) that are culturally diverse, and in a growing number of individuals who identify with, and live in more than, one culture (Hermans & Kempen, 1998; Hong et al., 2000). Current and future cultural studies need to move beyond traditional between-group cultural comparisons and develop theoretical models and methodologies that capture the multiplicity and malleability of cultural meaning *within* individuals. Some recent studies have taken this approach in examining the interplay between personality dispositions and psychosocial processes such as acculturation (Ryder, Alden, & Paulhus, 2000), multicultural attitudes (Van der Zee & Van Oudenhoven, 2001), bicultural identity structure (Benet-Martínez & Haritatos, 2005), and bilingualism (Chen, Benet-Martínez, & Bond, in press; Ramirez-Esparza, Gosling, Benet-Martínez, Potter, & Pennebaker, 2006).

Future cultural research can also benefit from exciting methodological advances. For instance, recent brain imaging studies show that individuals' preexisting social representations of race deeply affect their visual perception and neural processing of human faces and everyday objects (Eberhardt, 2005). Furthermore, because cultural and personality processes operating at the individual level may not replicate at the cultural level, and vice versa (Leung & Bond, 1989; see Tables 3 and 4 in Benet-Martínez, 2007), researchers can use multilevel modeling and latent-class techniques to deal with these complexities (e.g., Eid & Diener, 2001; Johnson, Kulesa, Cho, & Shavit, 2005; Oishi, Diener, Choi, Kim-Prieto, & Choi, 2007). These underused techniques have the potential of fostering a fruitful synergy between the field of personality—which has provided a wealth of information regarding individual-level psychological characteristics (e.g., traits and values)—and the fields of anthropology and sociology, which are very informative regarding culture-level phenomena (e.g., economy, religion, and many other key demographic factors).

Finally, although many studies have established that cultural forces influence the expression of personality (i.e., culture → personality effects; Benet-Martínez & Karakitapoglu-Aygun, 2003), almost no attention has been given to the processes by which personality may in turn influence culture (personality→culture effects; McCrae, 2004). Evidence from recent studies shows that our personalities shape the cultural contexts in which we live by influencing both micro-level (e.g., personal spaces, music preferences, content and style of personal webpages; Gosling, Ko, Mannarelli, & Morris, 2002; Rentfrow & Gosling, 2003; Vazire & Gosling, 2004) and macro-level (e.g., political orientation, social activism; Jost, Gla-ser, Kruglanski, & Sulloway, 2003) cultural elements. McCrae (2004) theorizes that aggregate levels of certain traits may lead to features of cultures, such as individualism versus collectivism. From the motivation science perspective, Higgins and colleagues (in press) theorize that universal motives (e.g., promotion, prevention) give rise to different manifestations of traits across cultures, depending on the strength of each motive. They hypothesize, for instance, that in cultures with strong promotion and locomotion motives, cultural traits that are conducive to and sustain these motives (e.g., extraversion) are likely to emerge. We believe that future cultural work in personality will benefit from using designs in which researchers also explore personality effects on culture.

CONCLUSION

The history of cultural research in personality reminds us of a story of an athletic star. It appeared in an academic scene out of "nowhere," and in a short period of time became the queen of the social and behavioral sciences. Like so many athletic stars, however, the enormous potentials of cultural personality research were never fulfilled due to a series of unfortunate events. Unlike athletic stars whose careers are cut short, the intellectual field of culture and personality has survived several injuries and has again become an important part of personality research. As shown above, the contribution of culture and personality research is substantial, ranging from elucidating links between individual and ecological influences on personality, to dispelling cultural stereotypes and national characters, to testing theory generalizability. Furthermore, cultural personality studies bring about tangible societal benefits by offering scientists, managers, policymakers, and the public ways to understand, manage, and benefit from the omnipresent cultural diversity that characterizes our society (Fowers & Richardson, 1996).

Now, again, the excitement for research on culture and personality is palpable. The grand ambition of early culture and personality researchers (e.g., Kluckhohn & Murray, 1948) can be realized with more measurement precision and more sophisticated data-analytic techniques than ever before. In a way, culture and personality research has finally begun to fulfill the century-old promise and to cultivate new and exciting horizons beyond the traditional research agendas.

ACKNOWLEDGMENTS

The two authors contributed equally and are listed in alphabetic order. We thank the following individuals for their valuable comments: Jesse Graham, Janetta Lun, and Felicity Miao.

NOTES

1. The terms "cross-cultural psychology" and "cultural psychology" refer to two different research traditions with somewhat distinct theoretical approaches, goals, and methodologies. However, for the sake of simplicity, throughout the chapter we often use the broader term "cultural" (e.g., cultural research, cultural studies) to refer to both kinds of traditions and their theories and methodologies.
2. Interestingly, as pointed out by LeVine (2001), several psychological studies of the relationship between personhood and society done at that time (e.g., Allport, 1961; Kluckhohn & Murray, 1948; McClelland, 1961) were, in fact, quite rigorous and sophisticated in their conceptualizations of both culture and personality.

REFERENCES

Aaker, J., Benet-Martínez, V., & Garolera, J. (2001). Consumption symbols as carriers of culture: A study of Japanese and Spanish brand personality constructs. *Journal of Personality and Social Psychology, 81*, 249–264.

Akimoto, S., & Sanbonmatsu, D. M. (1999). Differences in self-effacing behavior between European and Japanese Americans: Effect on competence evaluation. *Journal of Cross-Cultural Psychology, 30*, 159–177.

Allik, J., & McCrae, R. R. (2004). Toward a geography of personality traits: Patterns of profiles across 36 cultures. *Journal of Cross-Cultural Psychology, 35*, 13–28.

Allport, G. W. (1937). *Personality: A psychological interpretation*. New York: Holt.

Allport, G. W. (1961). *Patterns and growth in personality*. New York: Holt, Rinehart & Winston.

Ando, J., Ono, Y., Yoshimura, K., Onoda, N., Shimohara, M., Kanba, S., et al. (2002). The genetic structure of Cloninger's seven-factor model of temperament and character in a Japanese sample. *Journal of Personality, 70*, 583–610.

Benedict, R. (1934). *Patterns of culture*. Boston: Houghton Mifflin.

Benet-Martínez, V. (1999). Exploring indigenous Spanish personality constructs with a combined emic–etic approach. In J. C. Lasry, J. G. Adair, & K. L. Dion (Eds.), *Latest contributions to cross-cultural psychology* (pp. 151–175). Lisse, Netherlands: Swets & Zeitlinge.

Benet-Martínez, V. (2007). Cross-cultural personality research: Conceptual and methodological issues. In R. W. Robins, R. C. Fraley, & R. Krueger (Eds.), *Handbook of research methods in personality psychology* (pp. 170–190). New York: Guilford Press.

Benet-Martínez, V., & Haritatos, J. (2005). Bicultural Identity Integration (BII): Components and socio-personality antecedents. *Journal of Personality, 73*, 1015–1049.

Benet-Martínez, V., & John, O. (1998). *Los Cinco Grandes* across cultures and ethnic groups: Multitrait multimethod analyses of the Big Five in Spanish and English. *Journal of Personality and Social Psychology, 75*, 729–750.

Benet-Martínez, V., & John, O. P. (2000). Towards the development of quasi-indigenous personality constructs. *American Behavioral Scientist, 44*, 141–157.

Benet-Martínez, V., & Karakitapoglu-Aygun, Z. (2003). The interplay of cultural values and personality in predicting life-satisfaction: Comparing Asian- and European-Americans. *Journal of Cross-Cultural Psychology, 34*, 38–61.

Bond, M. H. (1988). Finding universal dimensions of individual variation in multicultural studies of values: The Rokeach and Chinese value surveys. *Journal of Personality and Social Psychology, 55*, 1009–1015.

Bond, M. H. (2000). Localizing the imperial outreach. *American Behavioral Scientist, 44*, 63–72.

Bouchard, T. J., Jr. (2004). Genetic influence on human psychological traits. *Current Directions in Psychological Science, 13*, 148–151.

Bryk, A. S., & Raudenbush, S. W. (1992). *Hierarchical linear models: Applications and data analysis methods*. Thousand Oaks, CA: Sage.

Burnam, A., Hough, R. L., Karno, M., Escobar, J. I., & Telles, C. (1987). Acculturation and lifetime prevalence of psychiatric disorders among Mexican Americans in Los Angeles. *Journal of Health and Social Behaviors, 28*, 89–102.

Butcher, J. N. (1996). *International adaptations of the MMPI-W: Research and clinical applications*. Minneapolis: University of Minnesota Press.

Butcher, J. N. (2004). Personality assessment without borders: Adaptations of the MMPI-2 across cultures. *Journal of Personality Assessment, 83,* 90–104.

Campbell, J. D., Trapnell, P. D., Heine, S. J., Katz, I. M., Lavallee, L. F., & Lehman, D. R. (1996). Self-concept clarity: Measurement, personality correlates, and cultural boundaries. *Journal of Personality and Social Psychology, 70,* 141–156.

Chen, S., Benet-Martínez, V., & Bond, M. H. (in press). Bicultural identity, bilingualism, and psychological adjustment in multicultural societies. *Journal of Personality.*

Cheung, F. M., Leung, K., Zhang, J. X., Sun, H. F., Gan, Y. G., Song, W. Z., et al. (2001). Indigenous Chinese personality constructs: Is the five-factor model complete? *Journal of Cross-Cultural Psychology, 32,* 407–433.

Chirkov, V., Ryan, R. M., Kim, Y., & Kaplan, U. (2003). Differentiating autonomy from individualism and independence: A self-determination theory perspective on internalization of cultural orientations and well-being. *Journal of Personality and Social Psychology, 84,* 97–109.

Chiu, C.-Y., & Hong, Y.-Y. (2007). Cultural processes: Basic principles. In A. W. Kruglanski & E. T. Higgins (Eds.), *Social psychology: Handbook of basic principles* (2nd ed., pp. 785–804). New York: Guilford Press.

Choi, I., & Choi, Y. (2002). Culture and self-concept flexibility. *Personality and Social Psychology Bulletin, 28,* 1508–1517.

Church, A. T. (2000). Culture and personality: Toward an integrated cultural trait psychology. *Journal of Personality, 68,* 651–703.

Church, A. T. (2001). Personality measurement in cross-cultural perspective. *Journal of Personality, 69,* 979–1006.

Church, A. T., Katigbak, M. S., Del Prado, A. M., Ortiz, F. A., Mastor, K. A., Harumi, Y., et al. (2006). Implicit theories and self-perceptions of traitedness across cultures: Toward integration of cultural and trait psychology perspectives. *Journal of Cross-Cultural Psychology, 37,* 694–716.

Church, A. T., & Ortiz, F. A. (2005). *Culture and personality.* In V. J. Derlaga, B. A. Winstead, & W. H. Jones (Eds.), *Personality: Contemporary theory and research* (3rd ed., pp. 420–456). Belmont, CA: Wadsworth.

Church, A. T., Ortiz, F. A., Katigbak, M. S., Avdeyeva, T. V., Emerson, A. M., Vargas-Flores, J. D., et al. (2003). Measuring individual and cultural differences in implicit trait theories. *Journal of Personality and Social Psychology, 85,* 332–347.

Cirkov, V., Ryan, R. M., Kim, Y., & Kaplan, U. (2003). Differentiating autonomy from individualism and independence: A self-determination theory perspective on internalization of cultural

orientation and well-being. *Journal of Personality and Social Psychology, 84,* 97–110.

Cohen, D. (1996). Law, social policy, and violence. *Journal of Personality and Social Psychology, 70,* 961–978.

Cohen, D., & Gunz, A. (2002). As seen by others ... : Perspectives on the self and the memories and emotional perceptions of Easterners and Westerners. *Psychological Science, 13,* 55–59.

Cohen, D., & Nisbett, R. E. (1997). Field experiments examining the culture of honor: The role of institutions in perpetuating norms about violence. *Personality and Social Psychology Bulletin, 23,* 1188–1199.

Cohen, D., Nisbett, R. E., Bowdle, B., & Schwarz, N. (1996). Insult, aggression, and the Southern culture of honor. *Journal of Personality and Social Psychology, 70,* 945–960.

College Board. (1976–1977). *Student descriptive questionnaire.* Princeton, NJ: Educational Testing Service.

Costa, P. T., & McCrae, R. R. (1992). *NEO PI-R professional manual.* Odessa, FL: Psychological Assessment Resources.

Cousins, S. D. (1989). Culture and self-perception in Japan and the United States. *Journal of Personality and Social Psychology, 56,* 124–131.

Darwin, C. (1965). *The expression of the emotions in man and animals.* Chicago: University of Chicago Press. (Original work published in 1872)

del Prado, A. M., Church, A. T., Katigbak, M. S., Miramontes, L. G., Whitty, M., Curtis, G. J., et al. (2007). Culture, method, and the content of self-concepts: Testing trait, individual-self-primacy, and cultural psychology perspectives. *Journal of Research in Personality, 41,* 1119–1160.

Diener, E., & Larsen, R. J. (1984). Temporal stability and cross-situational consistency of affective, behavioral, and cognitive responses. *Journal of Personality and Social Psychology, 47,* 871–883.

Diener, E., Oishi, S., & Lucas, R. E. (2003). Personality, culture, and subjective well-being: Emotional and cognitive evaluations of life. *Annual Review of Psychology, 54,* 403–425.

Diener, E., Scollon, C. K. N., Oishi, S., Dzokoto, V., & Suh, E. M. (2000). Positivity and the construction of life satisfaction judgments: Global happiness is not the sum of its part. *Journal of Happiness Studies, 1,* 159–176.

Diener, E., Suh, E. M., Smith, H., & Shao, L. (1995). National differences in reported subjective well-being: Why do they occur? *Social Indicators Research, 34,* 7–32.

Donahue, E. M., Robins, R. W., Roberts, B. W., & John, O. P. (1993). The divided self: Concurrent and longitudinal effects of psychological adjustment and social roles of self-concept differentiation. *Journal of Personality and Social Psychology, 64,* 834–846.

Draguns, J. G., & Tanaka-Matsumi, J. (2003). Assessment of psychopathology across and within cultures: Issues and findings. *Behaviour Research and Therapy, 41,* 755–776.

DuBois, C. (1944). *The people of Alor.* Minneapolis: University of Minnesota Press.

Eberhardt, J. L. (2005). Imaging race. *American Psychologist, 60,* 181–190.

Eid, M., & Diener, E. (2001). Norms for experiencing emotions in different cultures: Inter- and intranational differences. *Journal of Personality and Social Psychology, 81,* 869–885.

Ekman, P., & Friesen, W. V. (1971). Constants across cultures in the face and emotion. *Journal of Personality and Social Psychology, 17,* 124–129.

Ekman, P., Friesen, W. V., O'Sullivan, M., Chan, A., Diacoyanni-Tarlatzis, I., Heider, K., et al. (1987). Universals and cultural differences in the judgments of facial expressions of emotion. *Journal of Personality and Social Psychology, 53,* 712–717.

Elfenbein, H. A., & Ambady, N. (2002). On the universality and cultural specificity of emotion recognition: A meta-analysis. *Psychological Bulletin, 128,* 203–235.

Elliot, A. J., Chirkov, V. I., Kim, Y., & Sheldon, K. M. (2001). A cross-cultural analysis of avoidance (relative to approach) personal goals. *Psychological Science, 12,* 505–510.

Fowers, B. J., & Richardson, F. C. (1996). Why is multiculturalism good? *American Psychologist, 51,* 609–621.

Gosling, S. D., Ko, S. J., Mannarelli, T., & Morris, M. E. (2002). A room with a cue: Judgments of personality based on offices and bedrooms. *Journal of Personality and Social Psychology, 82,* 379–398.

Greenfield, P. M. (2000). Three approaches to the psychology of culture: Where do they come from? Where can they go? *Asian Journal of Social Psychology, 3,* 223–240.

Haidt, J., & Keltner, D. (1999). Culture and facial expression: Open-ended methods find more expressions and a gradient of recognition. *Cognition and Emotion, 13,* 225–266.

Harrison, L. E., & Huntington, S. P. (2000). *Culture matters: How values shape human progress.* New York: Basic Books.

Heine, S. J., & Hamamura, T. (2007). In search of East Asian self-enhancement. *Personality and Social Psychology Review, 11,* 4–27.

Heine, S. J., Kitayama, S., Lehman, D. R., Takata, T., Ide, E., Leung, C., et al. (2001). Divergent consequence of success and failure in Japan and North America: An investigation of self-improving motivations and malleable selves. *Journal of Personality and Social Psychology, 81,* 599–615.

Heine, S. J., & Lehman, D. R. (1995). Cultural variation in unrealistic optimism: Does the West feel more vulnerable than the East? *Journal of Personality and Social Psychology, 68,* 595–607.

Heine, S. J., & Lehman, D. R. (2004). Move the body, change the self: Acculturative effects of the self-concept. In M. Schaller & C. S. Crandall (Eds.), *The psychological foundations of culture* (pp. 305–331). Mahwah, NJ: Erlbaum.

Heine, S. J., Lehman, D. R., Peng, K., & Greenholtz, J. (2002). What's wrong with cross-cultural comparisons of subjective Likert scales?: The reference-group effect. *Journal of Personality and Social Psychology, 82,* 903–918.

Heine, S. J., & Renshaw, K. (2002). Interjudge agreement, self-enhancement, and liking: Cross-cultural divergences. *Personality and Social Psychology Bulletin, 28,* 442–451.

Heine, S. J., Takata, T., & Lehman, D. R. (2000). Beyond self-presentation: Evidence for self-criticism among Japanese. *Personality and Social Psychology Bulletin, 26,* 71–78.

Hermans, H., & Kempen, H. (1998). Moving cultures: The perilous problem of cultural dichotomies in a globalizing society. *American Psychologist, 53,* 1111–1120.

Higgins, E. T., Pierro, A., & Kruglanski, A. W. (in press). Rethinking culture and personality: How self-regulatory universals create cross-cultural differences. In R. M. Sorrentino (Ed.), *Handbook of motivation and cognition within and across cultures.* New York: Guilford Press.

Hofstede, G. (1980). *Culture's consequences.* Beverly Hills: Sage.

Hong, Y. Y., Morris, M., Chiu, C. Y., & Benet-Martínez, V. (2000). Multicultural minds: A dynamic constructivist approach to culture and cognition. *American Psychologist, 55,* 709–720.

Inglehart, R., & Baker, W. E. (2000). Modernization, cultural change, and the persistence of traditional values. *American Sociological Review, 65,* 19–51.

Iyengar, S. S., & Lepper, M. R. (1999). Rethinking the value of choice: A cultural perspective on intrinsic motivation. *Journal of Personality and Social Psychology, 76,* 349–366.

Jablensky, A., Sartorius, N., Ernberg, G., Anker, M., Korten, A., Cooper, J. E., et al. (1992). *Schizophrenia: Manifestations, incidence, and course in different cultures: A World Health Organization ten country study.* (Psychological Medicine Monograph Supplement 20). Cambridge, UK: Cambridge University Press.

Johnson, T., Kulesa, P., Cho, Y., & Shavit, S. (2005). The relation between culture and response styles: Evidence from 19 countries. *Journal of Cross-Cultural Psychology, 36,* 264–277.

Jost, J. T., Glaser, J., Kruglanski, A. W., & Sulloway, F. (2003). Political conservatism as motivated social cognition. *Psychological Bulletin, 129,* 339–375.

Kanagawa, C., Cross, S. E., & Markus, H. R. (2001). "Who am I?": The cultural psychology of the conceptual self. *Personality and Social Psychology Bulletin, 27,* 90–103.

Kardiner, A. (1939). *The individual and his society: The psychodynamics of primitive social organization.* New York: Columbia University Press.

Katigbak, M. S., Church, A. T., Guanzon-Lapena, M. A., Carlota, A. J., & del Pilar, G. H. (2002). Are indigenous personality dimensions culture specific?: Philippine inventories and the five-factor model. *Journal of Personality and Social Psychology, 82,* 89–101.

Kendrick, D. T., & Funder, D. C. (1988). Profiting from controversy: Lessons from the person–situation debate. *American Psychologist, 43,* 23–34.

Kenny, D. A. (1994). *Interpersonal perceptions: A social relations analysis.* New York: Guilford Press.

Kim, H. S. (2002). We talk, therefore we think?: A cultural analysis of the effect of talking on thinking. *Journal of Personality and Social Psychology, 83,* 828–842.

Kitayama, S., & Karasawa, M. (1997). Implicit self-esteem in Japan: Name letters and birthday numbers. *Personality and Social Psychology Bulletin, 23,* 736–742.

Kitayama, S., Markus, H. R., & Kurosawa, M. (2000). Culture, emotion, and well-being: Good feelings in Japan and the United States. *Cognition and Emotion, 14,* 93–124.

Kitayama, S., Markus, H. R., Matsumoto, H., & Norasakkunkit, V. (1997). Individual and collective processes in the construction of the self: Self-enhancement in the United States and self-criticism in Japan. *Journal of Personality and Social Psychology, 72,* 1245–1267.

Kleinman, A. (1977). Depression, somatization, and the "new cross-cultural psychiatry." *Social Science and Medicine, 11,* 3–9.

Kluckhohn, C., & Murray, H. E. (1948). *Personality in nature, society, and culture.* New York: Knopf.

Kluckhohn, F. R., & Strodtbeck, F. L. (1961). *Variations in value orientations.* Westport, CT: Greenwood Press.

Kobayashi, C., & Greenwald, A. G. (2003). Implicit–explicit differences in self-enhancement for Americans and Japanese. *Journal of Cross-Cultural Psychology, 34,* 522–541.

Koo, M., & Choi, I. (2005). Becoming a holistic thinker: Training effect of Oriental medicine on reasoning. *Personality and Social Psychology Bulletin, 31,* 1264–1272.

Kurman, J. (2003). Why is self-enhancement low in certain collectivist cultures? An investigation of two competing explanations. *Journal of Cross-Cultural Psychology, 34,* 496–510.

Kwan, V. S. Y., Bond, M. H., & Singelis, T. M. (1997). Pancultural explanations for life-satisfaction: Adding relationship harmony to self-esteem. *Journal of Personality and Social Psychology, 73,* 1038–1051.

Kwan, V. S. Y., John, O. P., Kenny, D. A., Bond, M. H., & Robbins, R. W. (2004). Reconceptualizing individual differences in self-enhancement bias: An interpersonal approach. *Psychological Review, 111,* 94–110.

La Barre, W. (1947). Primitive psychotherapy in Native American cultures: Peyotism and confession. *Journal of Abnormal and Social Psychology, 24,* 294–309.

Leung, K., & Bond, M. H. (1989). On the empirical identification of dimensions for cross-cultural comparisons. *Journal of Cross-Cultural Psychology, 20,* 133–151.

LeVine, R. A. (2001). Culture and personality studies, 1918–1960: Myth and history. *Journal of Personality, 69,* 803–818.

Levine, R. V., Norenzayan, A., & Philbrick, K. (2001). Cross-cultural differences in helping strangers. *Journal of Cross-Cultural Psychology, 32,* 543–560.

Lipset, S. M., & Lenz, G. S. (2000). Corruption, culture, and markets. In L. E. Harrison & S. P. Huntington (Eds.), *Culture matters: How values shape human progress* (pp. 112–124). New York: Basic Books.

Lopez, S. R., & Guarnaccia, P. J. J. (2000). Cultural psychopathology: Uncovering the social world of mental illness. *Annual Review of Psychology, 51,* 571–598.

Lucas, R. E., Diener, E., Grob, A., Suh, E. M., & Shao, L. (2000). Cross-cultural evidence for the fundamental features of extraversion. *Journal of Personality and Social Psychology, 79,* 452–468.

Lucas, R. E., Diener, E., & Suh, E. (1996). Discriminant validity of well-being measures. *Journal of Personality and Social Psychology, 71,* 616–628.

Lyubomirsky, S., & Nolen-Hoeksema, S. (1993). Self-perpetuating properties of dysphoric rumination. *Journal of Personality and Social Psychology, 65,* 339–349.

Ma, V., & Schoeneman, T. J. (1997). Individualism versus collectivism: A comparison of Kenyan and American self-concepts. *Basic and Applied Social Psychology, 19,* 261–273.

Marcus, G. (2004). *The birth of the mind.* New York: Basic Books.

Markus, H. R., & Kitayama, S. (1991). Culture and the self: Implications for cognition, emotion, and motivation. *Psychological Review, 98,* 224–253.

Markus, H. R., & Kitayama, S. (1998). The cultural psychology of personality. *Journal of Cross-Cultural Psychology, 29,* 63–87.

Masuda, T., Ellsworth, P., Mesquita, B., Leu, J., Tanida, S., & Veerdonk, E. (in press). Placing the face in context: Cultural differences in the perception of facial emotion. *Journal of Personality and Social Psychology.*

Matsumoto, D. R. (2000). *Culture and psychology: People around the world.* Delmar, CA: Wadsworth Thomson Learning.

Mauro, R., Sato, K., & Tucker, J. (1992). The role of appraisal in human emotions: A cross-cultural study. *Journal of Personality and Social Psychology, 62,* 301–317.

McClelland, D. C. (1961). *The achieving society.* New York: Van Nostrand.

McCrae, R. R. (2004). Human nature and culture: A trait perspective. *Journal of Research in Personality, 38,* 3–14.

McCrae, R. R., & Costa, P. T., Jr. (1996). Toward a new generation of personality theories: Theoretical contexts for the five-factor model. In J. S. Wiggins (Ed.), *The five-factor model of personality* (pp. 51–87). New York: Guilford Press.

McCrae, R. R., & Costa, P. T., Jr. (1999). A five-factor theory of personality. In L. A. Pervin & O. P. John (Eds.), *Handbook of personality* (2nd ed., pp. 139–153). New York: Guilford Press.

McCrae, R. R., Terracciano, A., & 79 members of the Personality Profiles of Cultures Project. (2005). Universal features of personality traits from the observer's perspective: Data from 50 cultures. *Journal of Personality and Social Psychology, 88,* 547–561.

McCrae, R. R., Yik, M. S. M., Trapnell, P. D., Bond, M. H., & Paulhus, D. L. (1998). Interpreting personality profiles across cultures: Bilingual, acculturation, and peer rating studies of Chinese undergraduates. *Journal of Personality and Social Psychology, 74,* 1041–1055.

Mesquita, B., & Frijda, N. H. (1992). Cultural variations in emotions: A review. *Psychological Bulletin, 112,* 179–204.

Mesquita, B., & Karasawa, M. (2002). Different emotional lives. *Cognition and Emotion, 16,* 127–141.

Mezzich, J. E., Kirmayer, L. J., Kleinman, A., Fabrega, H., Jr., Parron D. L., Good, B. J., et al. (1999). The place of culture in DSM-IV. *Journal of Nervous and Mental Disorders, 187,* 457–464.

Miller, J. G. (1997). Theoretical issues in cultural psychology. In J. W. Berry, Y. H. Poortinga, & J. Pandey (Eds.), *Handbook of cross-cultural psychology* (Vol. 1, 2nd ed., pp. 85–128). Boston: Allyn & Bacon.

Mischel, W. (1958). Preference for delayed reinforcement: An experimental study of a cultural observation. *Journal of Abnormal and Social Psychology, 56,* 57–61.

Mischel, W. (1961). Father-absence and delay of gratification: Cross-cultural comparisons. *Journal of Abnormal and Social Psychology, 63,* 116–124.

Mischel, W., & Shoda, Y. (1995). A cognitive–affective system theory of personality: Reconceptualizing situations, dispositions, dynamics, and invariance in personality structure. *Psychological Review, 102,* 246–268.

Murray, H. A. (1938). *Explorations in personality: A clinical and experimental study of fifty men of college age.* New York: Oxford University Press.

Nisbett, R. E. (2004). *The geography of thought: How Asians and Westerners think differently . . . and why.* New York: Free Press.

Norenzayan, A., & Heine, S. J. (2005). Psychological universals: What are they and how can we know? *Psychological Bulletin, 131,* 763–784.

Oishi, S. (2004). Personality in culture: A neo-Allportian view. *Journal of Research in Personality, 38,* 68–74.

Oishi, S. (2007). The application of structural equation modeling and item response theory to cross-cultural positive psychology research. In A. Ong & M. van Dulmen (Eds.), *Handbook of methods in positive psychology* (pp. 126–138). New York: Oxford University Press.

Oishi, S., & Diener, E. (2001). Goals, culture, and subjective well-being. *Personality and Social Psychology Bulletin, 27,* 1674–1682.

Oishi, S., Diener, E., Choi, D. W., Kim-Prieto, C., & Choi, I. (2007). The dynamics of daily events and well-being across cultures: When less is more. *Journal of Personality and Social Psychology, 93,* 685–698.

Oishi, S., Diener, E., Scollon, C. N., & Biswas-Diener, R. (2004). Cross-situational consistency of affective experiences across cultures. *Journal of Personality and Social Psychology, 86,* 460–472.

Oishi, S., Hahn, J., Schimmack, U., Radhakrishan, P., Dzokoto, V., & Ahadi, S. (2005). The measurement of values across cultures: A pairwise comparison approach. *Journal of Research in Personality, 39,* 299–305.

Oyserman, D., Coon, H. M., & Kemmelmeier, M. (2002). Rethinking individualism and collectivism: Evaluation of theoretical assumptions and meta-analyses. *Psychological Bulletin, 128,* 3–72.

Paunonen, S. V., & Ashton, M. C. (1998). The structured assessment of personality across cultures. *Journal of Cross-Cultural Psychology, 29,* 150–170.

Peterson, C., & Seligman, M. E. (1984). Causal explanations as a risk factor for depression: Theory and evidence. *Psychological Review, 91,* 347–374.

Ramirez-Esparza, N., Gosling, S., Benet-Martínez, V., Potter, J., & Pennebaker, J. (2006). Do bilinguals have two personalities? A special case of cultural frame-switching. *Journal of Research in Personality, 40,* 99–120.

Rentfrow, P. J., & Gosling, S. D. (2003). The do re mi's of everyday life: The structure and personality correlates of music preferences. *Journal of Personality and Social Psychology, 84,* 1236–1256.

Roberts, B. W., & Helson, R. (1997). Changes in culture, changes in personality: The influence of individualism in a longitudinal study of women. *Journal of Personality and Social Psychology, 72,* 641–651.

Robins, R. W., Trzesniewski, K. H., Tracy, J. L., Gosling, S. D., & Potter, J. (2002). Global self-esteem across the life span. *Psychology and Aging, 17,* 423–434.

Rohner, R. (1984). Toward a conception of culture for cross-cultural psychology. *Journal of Cross-Cultural Psychology, 15,* 111–138.

Rokeach, M. (1973). *The nature of human values.* New York: Free Press.

Rokeach, M., & Ball-Rokeach, S. J. (1989). Stability and change in American value priorities. *American Psychologist, 44,* 775–784.

Ross, M., Heine, S. J., Wilson, A. E., & Sugimori, S. (2005). Cross-cultural discrepancies in self-appraisals. *Personality and Social Psychology Bulletin, 31,* 1175–1188.

Rozin, P. (2003). Five potential principles for understanding cultural differences in relation to individual differences. *Journal of Research in Personality, 37,* 273–283.

Rudy, D., Sheldon, K. M., Awong, T., & Tan, H. H. (2007). Autonomy, culture, and well-being: The benefits of inclusive autonomy. *Journal of Research in Personality, 41,* 983–1007.

Russell, J. A. (1983). Pancultural aspects of the human conceptual organization of emotions. *Journal of Personality and Social Psychology, 45,* 1281–1288.

Russell, J. A. (1991). Culture and the categorization of emotion. *Psychological Bulletin, 110,* 426–450.

Russell, J. A. (1994). Is there universal recognition of emotion from facial expression? A review of the cross-cultural studies. *Psychological Bulletin, 115,* 102–141.

Ryder, A., Alden, L., & Paulhus, D. (2000). Is acculturation unidimensional or bidimensional?

A head-to-head comparison in the prediction of personality, self-identity, and adjustment. *Journal of Personality and Social Psychology, 79,* 49–65.

Sapir, E. (1956). *Culture, language, and personality.* Berkeley: University of California Press.

Saucier, G., & Goldberg, L. R. (1996). The language of personality: Lexical perspectives on the five-factor model. In J. S. Wiggins (Ed.), *The five-factor model of personality* (pp. 21–50). New York: Guilford Press.

Saucier, G., & Goldberg, L. R. (2001). Lexical studies of indigenous personality factors: Premises, products, and prospects. *Journal of Personality, 69,* 847–879.

Scherer, K. R. (1997). Profiles of emotion-antecedent appraisal: Testing theoretical predictions across cultures. *Cognition and Emotion, 11,* 113–150.

Schimmack, U., Oishi, S., & Diener, E. (2002). Cultural influences on the relation between pleasant emotions and unpleasant emotions: Asian dialectic philosophies or individualism–collectivism? *Cognition and Emotion, 16,* 705–719.

Schimmack, U., Oishi, S., & Diener, E. (2005). Individualism: A valid and important dimension of cultural differences between nations. *Personality and Social Psychology Review, 9,* 17–31.

Schimmack, U., Radhakrishnan, P., Oishi, S., Dzokoto, V., & Ahadi, S. (2002). Culture, personality, and subjective well-being: Integrating process models of life satisfaction. *Journal of Personality and Social Psychology, 82,* 582–593.

Schmitt, D. P., & Allik, J. (2005). Simultaneous administration of the Rosenberg Self-Esteem Scale in 53 nations: Exploring the universal and culture-specific features of global self-esteem. *Journal of Personality and Social Psychology, 89,* 623–642.

Schwartz, S. H., & Bardi, A. (2001). Value hierarchies across cultures: Taking a similarities perspective. *Journal of Cross-Cultural Psychology, 32,* 268–290.

Schwartz, S. H., & Sagiv, L. (1995). Identifying culture-specifics in the content and structure of values. *Journal of Cross-Cultural Psychology, 26,* 92–116.

Scollon, C. N., Diener, E., Oishi, S., & Biswas-Diener, R. (2005). An experience sampling and cross-cultural investigation of the relation between pleasant and unpleasant affect. *Cognition and Emotion, 19,* 27–52.

Sedikides, C., Gaertner, L., & Toguchi, Y. (2003). Pancultural self-enhancement. *Journal of Personality and Social Psychology, 84,* 60–79.

Sedikides, C., Gaertner, L., & Vevea, J. (2005). Pancultural self-enhancement reloaded: A meta-analytic reply to Heine. *Journal of Personality and Social Psychology, 89,* 539–551.

Senior, P. A., & Bhopal, R. (1994). Ethnicity as a variable in epidemiological research. *British Medical Journal, 309,* 327–330.

Sheldon, K. M., Elliot, A. J., Ryan, R. M., Chirkov, V., Kim, Y., Wu, C., et al. (2004). Self-concordance and subjective well-being in four cultures. *Journal of Cross-Cultural Psychology, 35,* 209–223.

Shweder, R. A. (1991). *Thinking through cultures.* Cambridge, MA: Harvard University Press.

Smith, G. T., Spillane, N. S., & Annus, A. M. (2006). Implications of an emerging integration of universal and culturally specific psychologies. *Perspectives on Psychological Science, 1,* 211–233.

Spencer-Rodgers, J., Peng, K., Wang, L., & Hou, Y. (2004). Dialectical self-esteem and East–West differences in psychological well-being. *Personality and Social Psychology Bulletin, 30,* 1416–1432.

Stryker, S., & Burke, P. J. (2000). The past, present, and future of an identity theory. *Social Psychology Quarterly, 63,* 284–297.

Su, J. C., & Oishi, S. (2006). *Culture and self-enhancement: A social relations analysis.* Manuscript submitted for publication.

Suh, E. M. (2002). Culture, identity consistency, and subjective well-being. *Journal of Personality and Social Psychology, 83,* 1378–1391.

Suh, E. M., Diener, E., Oishi, S., & Triandis, H. C. (1998). The shifting basis of life satisfaction judgments across cultures: Emotions versus norms. *Journal of Personality and Social Psychology, 74,* 482–493.

Takano, Y., & Osaka, E. (1999). An unsupported common view: Comparing Japan and the U.S. on individualism/collectivism. *Asian Journal of Social Psychology, 2,* 311–341.

Tanaka-Matsumi, J., & Marsella, A. J. (1976). Cross-cultural variations in the phenomenological experience of depression: I. Word association studies. *Journal of Cross-Cultural Psychology, 7,* 379–396.

Terracciano, A., Abdel-Khalek, A. M., Ádám, N., Adamovová, L., Ahn, C. K., Ahn, H. N., et al. (2005). National character does not reflect mean personality trait levels in 49 cultures. *Science, 310,* 96–100.

Terracciano, A., McCrae, R. R., Brant, L. J., & Costa, P. T., Jr. (2005). Hierarchical linear modeling analysis of the NEO-PI-R scales in the Baltimore Longitudinal Study of Aging. *Psychology and Aging, 20,* 493–506.

Tracy, J. L., & Robins, R. W. (2008). The nonverbal expression of pride: Evidence for cross-cultural recognition. *Journal of Personality and Social Psychology, 94,* 516–530.

Triandis, H. C. (1995). *Individualism and collectivism.* Boulder, CO: Westview.

Triandis, H. C. (1996). The psychological measurement of cultural syndromes. *American Psychologist, 51,* 407–415.

Triandis, H. C., & Suh, E. M. (2002). Cultural influences on personality. *Annual Review of Psychology, 53,* 133–160.

Trzesniewski, K. H., Donnellan, M. B., & Robins, R. W. (in press). Do today's young people really think they are so extraordinary?: An examination of secular changes in narcissism and self-enhancement. *Psychological Science.*

Tsai, J. L., Knutson, B., & Fung, H. H. (2006). Cultural variation in affect valuation. *Journal of Personality and Social Psychology, 90,* 288–307.

Twenge, J. M. (2000). The age of anxiety?: Birth cohort change in anxiety and neuroticism, 1952–1993. *Journal of Personality and Social Psychology, 79,* 1007–1021.

Twenge, J. M. (2001a). Birth cohort changes in extraversion: A cross-temporal meta-analysis, 1966–1993. *Personality and Individual Differences, 30,* 735–748.

Twenge, J. M. (2001b). Changes in women's assertiveness in response to status and roles: A cross-temporal meta-analysis, 1931–1993. *Journal of Personality and Social Psychology, 81,* 133–145.

Twenge, J. M., & Campbell, W. K. (2001). Age and birth cohort differences in self-esteem: A cross-temporal meta-analysis. *Personality and Social Psychology Review, 5,* 321–344.

Twenge, J. M., & Crocker, J. (2002). Race and self-esteem: Meta-analyses comparing whites, blacks, Hispanics, Asians, and American Indians and comment on Gray-Little and Hafdahl (2002). *Psychological Bulletin, 128,* 371–408.

Van der Zee, K. I., & Van Oudenhoven, J. P. (2001). The Multicultural Personality Questionnaire: Reliability and validity of self and other ratings of multicultural effectiveness. *Journal of Research in Personality, 35,* 278–288.

Vazire, S., & Gosling, S. D. (2004). E-perceptions: Personality impressions based on personal websites. *Journal of Personality and Social Psychology, 87,* 123–132.

Vega, W. A., Kolody, B., Aguilar-Gaxiola, S., Aldrete, E., Catalano, R., & Caraveo-Anduaga, J. (1998). Lifetime prevalence of DSM-III-R psychiatric disorders among urban and rural Mexican Americans in California. *Archive of General Psychiatry, 55,* 771–778.

Vernon, P. E., & Allport, G. W. (1931). A test for personal values. *Journal of Abnormal and Social Psychology, 26,* 231–248.

Wallace, A. F. C. (1970). *Culture and personality.* New York: Random House.

Watson, D., & Clark, L. A. (1997). Extraversion and its positive emotional core. In R. Hogan, J. Johnson, & S. Briggs (Eds.), *Handbook of personality psychology* (pp. 767–793). San Diego, CA: Academic Press.

Watson, D., Clark, L. A., & Tellegen, A. (1984). Cross-cultural convergence in the structure of mood: A Japanese replication and a comparison with U.S. findings. *Journal of Personality and Social Psychology, 47,* 127–144.

Weisz, J. R., Chaiyasit, W., Weiss, B., Eastman, K. L., & Jackson, E. W. (1995). A multimethod study of problem behavior among Thai and American children in school: Teacher reports versus direct observation. *Child Development, 66,* 402–412.

World Health Organization. (1983). *Depressive disorders in different cultures: Report of the WHO collaborative study of standardized assessment of depressive disorders.* Geneva: Author.

Yamagata, S., Suzuki, A., Ando, J., Ono, Y., Kijima, N., Yoshimura, K., et al. (2006). Is the genetic structure of human personality universal?: A cross-cultural twin study from North America, Europe, and Asia. *Journal of Personality and Social Psychology, 90,* 987–998.

Yamaguchi, S., Greenwald, A. G., Banaji, M. R., Murakami, F., Chen, D., Shiomura, K., et al. (2007). Apparent universality of positive implicit self-esteem. *Psychological Science, 18,* 498–500.

Yuki, M., Maddux, W. W., & Masuda, T. (2007). Are the windows to the soul the same in the East and West?: Cultural differences in using the eyes and mouth as cues to recognize emotions in Japan and the United States. *Journal of Experimental Social Psychology, 43,* 303–311.

CHAPTER 22

Persons, Situations, and Person–Situation Interactions

David C. Funder

A small scientific meeting of personality psychologists convened at a rustic lodge in the woods of Washington State. The purpose was to discuss the influence of dispositions and situations on behavior. Some participants were eminent researchers on the origins and implications of personality traits, whereas others believed that behavioral consistency had traditionally been overrated and that behavior was largely a function of the ever-changing situation. The attendees included Dr. X., a famous proponent of this latter point of view, who had recently published an influential book.

Gathered by the radio one night, the attendees heard a news bulletin: A notorious serial killer had escaped from a nearby prison. Pandemonium ensued. Particularly upset was Dr. X., who began plans to nail all windows shut and post a 24-hour guard. One of the more traditionally oriented personality psychologists patted him reassuringly on the back: "Relax, Dr. X.," he said, adding (sarcastically), "If the killer does show up, what he does next will depend on the situation!"[1]

What people do depends both on who they are—their dispositions such as personality traits—and the situation they are in. The obviousness of this statement only highlights how odd it is that each side of this equation

has fans. As the possibly-true anecdote above illustrates, and as the decades-long "person–situation debate" continues to prove (Funder, 2001; Kenrick & Funder, 1988), a surprising number of psychologists appear to be personally as well as professionally invested in believing that either situations or persons have stronger effects on behavior.

Why? Part of the reason may be sheer self-interest; a psychologist who has invested a lifetime learning the art of personality assessment will be understandably less than thrilled by arguments that personality variables don't really matter; on the other side, more than one career has been made by a willingness to point out that the correlations between personality and behavior are considerably lower than 1.0 and to argue that this implies that situations are what really matter.

But that is a cynical explanation, and I suspect that the more important reason why persons and situations both have fans—and why the rivalry between the two teams continues even now—is that each view of behavioral causation implies a different set of deeply held, if implicit, values. A belief that the situation is important may appear to remove limits on human potential because it implies that anybody—perhaps even the escaped killer referenced above—can cast off the burden of a past self and change his or her behavior at any moment, given the right set of circumstances. It is not uncommon to see the situational causation of behavior linked, usually implicitly but also sometimes explicitly, with virtues such as equality, adaptability, and even free will. On the other side, I suspect that some psychologists are disturbed—again, perhaps subconsciously—by a view of people as helplessly tossed about by the situational winds. Instead, it is possible to view psychological health as grounded in the development of a consistent self that is appropriate to a wide range of circumstances, and to view freedom as residing in the ability to forge a behavioral course independent of, or even resistant to, the situation. The famous protester in Tiananmen Square in 1989 who stood firm in the face of an oncoming tank was obviously not responding in the normative way to the situational forces that were present—that's why we admire him. Presumably, the determination of his behavior came from someplace deep inside.

Personal values such as these are deeply held and raise the stakes in the psychological debate over whether situations or persons are more important (Funder, 2006; Johnson, 1999). One purpose of the present chapter is to attempt to lower the stakes. My argument is that data and psychological analysis cannot resolve the underlying ideological question of whether it is better to be true to one's consistent sense of self or to respond flexibly to every situation as it comes along, or whether one of these approaches is more consistent with human nature than the other. Research cannot even resolve whether personal or situational influences on behavior are more powerful because these factors do not—except in rare and extreme circumstances—compete with each other in some kind of zero-sum game. As we shall see, each determinant of behavior can be strong at the same time, and neither gains its strength by taking it from the other. Furthermore, situations and persons *interact* in a way that goes beyond the statistical sense of this term. Exactly like genes and environments, neither can have any impact on the world at all without the contributions of both.

This chapter surveys how the main effects of persons and situations on behavior are generally assessed and sometimes compared and considers some of the pitfalls in that comparison. Then it summarizes how

person–situation interactions have been and could be studied, including some surprising implications of conceptualizations that focus on within-person variance and "*if–then*" profiles. The chapter describes how this research has been handicapped by the failure of psychologists to develop variables for the description of situations that are comparable in usefulness for the many variables available for describing personality dispositions, then it offers some suggestions for how a new generation of research—moving at last beyond a competition between persons and situations—may be able to illuminate what people do, when they do it, and why.

ASSESSING DISPOSITIONAL AND SITUATIONAL EFFECTS ON BEHAVIOR

The empirical assessment of dispositional and situational influences on behavior can be straightforward. To assess a dispositional effect, the researcher should measure a person's behavior in each of several situations and take the average. This average can be correlated (via the familiar Pearson r) with an average of the same individual's behavior across several *different* situations, or with his or her score on a personality trait measurement such as a test score. The first correlation is an index of the person's behavioral consistency and the second is a measure of the association between behavior and a specifically identified aspect of his or her personality. Either way, the correlation reflects dispositional influence on behavior. This is a standard method of research in personality psychology.

To assess a situational effect, the methodology is reversed. Instead of averaging across situations, the researcher averages across persons. A sample of people is placed (or found) in two (or more) different situations, and the behavior of the people in each situation is averaged. (Typically this situation is an experimental condition.) These averages can then be compared with each other, usually with a simple statistic such as a t-test. The difference in the means across the two situations reflects a situational influence on behavior. This is a standard method of research in social psychology.

These two methods share a number of properties. One is that the data analysis in each method is based on the same underlying statistical model. Traditionally, studies of dispositional variables use the correlation coefficient (Pearson's r), whereas experimental studies of situational effects use a t-test (in complex designs the analysis of variance), but these two numbers can be algebraically converted from one to the other. When this conversion is done—and it still is done too rarely—it turns out that some of the major effects of situations on behavior discovered by social psychology are of roughly the same size—generating r's in the range from about .30 to .40—as is typical of stronger effect sizes in the realm of personality (Funder & Ozer, 1983).

Another common property is that the larger the N—of individuals or of situations—across which the relevant average is computed, the more sensitively a researcher can detect a situational or dispositional effect on behavior. The typical social psychological experiment averages across a number of participants. A quick glance at the research literature (e.g., any issue of the *Journal of Experimental Social Psychology*) will verify that, in practice, this number is—at minimum—about 30 per condition. In contrast, a personality psychology study, if it measures any behaviors at all (as opposed to correlating questionnaires with each other), may only measure a single behavior per participant, rarely as many as two or three. As a result, the usual research design is much more sensitive to situational than to dispositional effects.

The reason for this discrepancy is to some degree pragmatic and to some degree traditional. Pragmatically, a researcher will find it is much more difficult and expensive to directly observe an individual research participant's behavior in, say, 30 different situations, than it is to place 30 participants into the same situation. As a result, the research tradition that developed over the decades within personality psychology sometimes seems to have almost forgotten that ideally one would wish to measure many behaviors for each participant. When Seymour Epstein made exactly this point in a series of articles in the 1970s and 1980s (Epstein, 1979, 1980), it was received by many as a new insight rather than an elementary principle (even though Epstein himself described

it as the latter), but subsequent standard research practice changed little.

Perhaps the most important shared aspect of the two methods is that because each is based on an average, both methods, in effect, blind themselves to the complementary behavioral influence. A paradigmatic study of dispositions, as described above, cannot detect the effect of the situation because it averages *across* situations in order to highlight individual differences. Similarly, a paradigmatic study of situations cannot detect the effect of dispositions because it averages across individuals to strike the mean for each experimental condition.[2] Still, these means, even by themselves, can be useful and informative.

Assessing Dispositional Effects

The mean scores people obtain on personality measures have generated a venerable research tradition. The foundation of this tradition is an effort to identify the important individual difference variables—personality traits—that are associated with the average behaviors of individuals, calculated across situations. Many candidates are available, ranging from the 100 items of the California Q-set (e.g., Block, 2008) to the widely used Big Five (e.g., McCrae & Costa, 1987, 1999). Some of these variables are highly specific; others are very general and the range of available content is vast. Allport and Odbert (1936) identified 17,953 trait terms in the dictionary, and there may be almost that many instruments available in the literature for measuring individual difference variables.

Once the relevant variables are identified, research can go in two directions. One direction is to go back in time and seek the origins of personality dispositions. A particularly exciting and lively recent line of research is outlining the origins of personality dispositions in patterns of early experience as they interact with genetic predispositions (e.g., Caspi et al., 2002, 2003). The other direction goes forward in time to assess (and perhaps predict) the life outcomes that eventually are associated with personality dispositions, which range from criminal behavior to success in occupations and relationships to—literally—the length of one's life (Ozer

& Benet-Martínez, 2006; Roberts, Kuncel, Shiner, Caspi, & Goldberg, 2007).

Assessing Situational Effects

The mean scores calculated by research on situations are used rather differently. Sometimes they are employed as parts of research programs intended to test broad theories of social behavior and cognition, such as, to name a couple of classic examples, self-perception theory and cognitive dissonance theory. Even more often, they are used to support mini-theories of effects of particular variables on behavior, such as (to name another classic example) the number of bystanders on the propensity to help in an emergency (Darley & Latané, 1968).

Overall, the research literature concerning the effects of situations is much less organized than that concerning the effects of dispositions. Whereas personality psychologists have offered numerous dispositional variables—arguably, too many—and have more-or-less achieved consensus on a small set of key variables (the Big Five), the situational variables examined in published research are almost completely ad hoc. One study may manipulate incentive, another will manipulate the content of a communication, and another may manipulate the number of bystanders present—and each of these situational variables will be studied in the context of assessing its effect on a different behavior, such as performance, compliance, or helping. As studies accumulate, they are generally organized implicitly or explicitly (e.g., in literature reviews) around the mini-theories the studies were designed to test, not in terms of the situational variables employed or their behavioral results. As a result, although the literature of experimental social psychology contains, latently, an enormous range of information about how situations affect behavior, it is not organized in such a way as to yield insights about what aspects of situations are important for determining which behaviors, or how they do it. Instead, as a general conclusion, we are left with little more than the oft-repeated observation that situations matter (e.g., Ross & Nisbett, 1991).

Many important psychologists have observed that the affect of a situation depends on the person who apprehends it. For example, Mischel (1977, p. 253) commented that "any given, objective stimulus condition may have a variety of effects, depending on how the individual construes and transforms it"; Bem and Allen (1974, p. 518) wrote that "the classification of situations ... will have to be in terms of the individual's phenomenology, not the investigator's"; and Allport (1937, p. 283) noted that "similarity is *personal*" (see Funder, 2006, p. 27).

However, the reasonableness and even obviousness of this "eye of the beholder" interpretation can mask some hidden pitfalls in thinking of situations this way. The eye-of-the-beholder argument implies that any aspect of a situation—say, a room full of people at a party—might be interpreted and experienced differently by different individuals, and it is this interpretation and experience that determine what they will do, not any concrete aspect of the situation itself. For example, an extravert might perceive the presence of other people as exciting, whereas a shy person might perceive the presence of the very same people, doing the very same things, as threatening.

Although this analysis is correct to the degree that people can react differently to the same stimulus, unless used with care it can inhibit rather than promote understanding the effect of situations on behavior, for two reasons. First, a moment's thought will reveal that such analysis subtly but effectively shifts the locus of causation from the situation back to the personal disposition. An *extravert* responds to the situation one way, and a *shy person* responds to the same situation in a different way. This is exactly the kind of individual difference mechanism that is the longstanding province of personality research, as shown, for example, in Gordon Allport's famous observation that

> for some the world is a hostile place where men are evil and dangerous; for others it is a stage for fun and frolic. It may appear as a place to do one's duty grimly; or a pasture for cultivating friendship and love. (1961, p. 266)

Allport was clear that the basis of these differences in perception was personality traits, which have "the capacity to render many stimuli functionally equivalent" (1961, p. 347). Thus, an analysis of how people perceive situations differently leads us right back to the traits that are the origins of these differences in perception and absorbs the analysis of situations into the analysis of dispositions.

A second shortcoming of the subjective analysis of situational effects is that it can come very close to complete circularity. A psychologist who wants to understand how situations—not dispositions—affect behavior will have to fall back on concluding that the first person is excited because she perceives the situation as exciting, whereas the second person feels threatened because he perceives the situation as threatening. Thus, psychological analysis requires information about what a situation actually is, as well as and separately from, how individuals perceive it. The difference is between what the classic personality psychologist Henry Murray (1938) called *alpha press*, the objective situation, and *beta press*, the subjective one. The difference is important. Indeed, an individual who manifests too large of a discrepancy may be fairly said to suffer from a delusion.

Fortunately, subjective and objective conceptualizations of situational effects may not be as much at odds as is sometimes presumed. In a pair of recent studies, we examined the similarity between pairs of situations using both subjective and objective methods (Furr & Funder, 2004). In the first study, we asked participants to rate the degree to which two experimental situations they had actually experienced seemed (subjectively) similar, tapping what Murray might have called *beta press*. In the second study, we assessed the relative pairwise similarity of six experimental situations in terms of two aspects of objective similarity (task and participants), tapping *alpha press*. Actual behavior, using the Riverside Behavioral Q-sort (RBQ; Funder, Furr, & Colvin, 2000), was coded from videotapes in both studies. The first study found that participants who saw the two experimental situations as more similar tended to be more consistent in their behavior across them. The second study found that participants were more consistent in their behavior across situations that were more objectively similar. These results demonstrate the importance of both alpha and beta press—the objective and subjective aspects of a situation—by showing that be-

havior is more consistent across situations to the degree that those situations are similar in either sense.

Our study (Furr & Funder, 2004) measured objective similarity in terms of a couple of elements that our experimental conditions did and did not share. What is needed for a more widely useful objective description of situations is a set of general variables that are independent of how any particular person experiences them or responds to the situation, analogous to the dispositional variables long used for the description of persons.

One effort currently in progress is the development of the Riverside Situational Q-sort (RSQ, pronounced "risqué"; Wagerman & Funder, 2006). The instrument is based on two theoretical principles. The first is that it seeks to describe situations at the middle or basic level likely to be most easily communicated and most useful for behavioral prediction and understanding. The items are written generally enough to be psychologically meaningful and behaviorally relevant, but specific enough to be rated with adequate reliability.

The second principle is that the items seek to describe situational variables that are directly relevant to the expression of personality, in a manner that is as comprehensive as possible. To accomplish this, the RSQ draws from a previously developed instrument for personality assessment, which has been widely acclaimed for its broad range: the California Adult Q-sort (CAQ; Bem & Funder, 1978; Block, 2008; McCrae, Costa, & Busch, 1986). Earlier, our lab developed the RBQ (Funder et al., 2000) on the same basis. We formulated descriptions of behaviors that would exemplify manifestations of each of the personality characteristics included in the CAQ. For example, the RBQ item "expresses criticism or skepticism" was written to describe behavior relevant to the CAQ item "is critical, skeptical, not easily impressed." We believe the early success of the RBQ is largely due to its foundation in the CAQ and the prior efforts at psychological comprehensiveness that went into the original instrument. Thus, we are following a similar strategy in developing items for the RSQ, writing items to describe characteristics of situations that afford the opportunity for expression of each of the personality characteristics included in the CAQ. For example, the CAQ item "is critical, skeptical, not easily impressed" yields the RSQ item "Someone is trying to impress someone or convince someone of something." The assumption is that in a situation that is accurately described by this property, a skeptical and critical person has an excellent opportunity to act accordingly, whereas the opposite sort of person may reveal his or her gullibility.

Development of the RSQ is in its early stages and much remains to be done, including using it to assess the relations between situational variables and behavior in a wide range of contexts, seeking to reduce the large number of items (currently 81) to an essential few analogous to the Big Five and mapping the items onto theoretical conceptualizations of situations.[3] Other researchers have also made a variety of different kinds of efforts to identify important, general variables for the description of situations (see, e.g., Kelly et al., 2003; Ten Berge & De Raad, 2002; Van Heck, Perugini, Caprara, & Froeger, 1994; Yang, Read, & Miller, 2006). The overall point of the present discussion goes beyond any particular instrument. Situations are important. However, it is one thing to say this—and it has been said, many times—and quite another to specify just what aspects of situations are important, and how. For this end to be achieved, it will be necessary to describe the psychologically relevant aspects of situations using a well-formulated set of variables with a wide range of applicability.

PERSON–SITUATION INTERACTIONS

So far the discussion has focused on the main effects of dispositional and situational variables, examined independently. But, of course, the two variables interact with each other. Psychologists have sometimes— often—viewed this interaction as competitive, as we saw in the anecdote that began this chapter. However, sometimes the analysis of the interaction between dispositional and situational variables views it as more cooperative.

Competitive Person–Situation Interactions

When viewed as competing, dispositions are implicitly conceptualized as forces that push on behavior from different directions: Dis-

positions, which are properties of individual persons, push from the inside (the "meaty side" of the dermis, in Gilbert's [1998, p. 21] memorable phrase), whereas situations push from the ("sunny") outside. This view of dispositions and situations as competing forces has a strong, almost irresistible intuitive appeal, and, as has already been observed, in this competition, many psychologists have already chosen a side to root for—generally personality psychologists support dispositions, whereas social psychologists cheer for the situation.

The comparison is tempting not just on the grounds of intuition and team spirit, but because a fundamental analytic tool in psychology, the analysis of variance, seems like it was almost specifically designed to allow situational and dispositional effects on behavior to be directly compared—and in a zero-sum manner, at that. The individual differences in behavior (or a dispositional variable associated with those differences) and the differences across experimental conditions (the manipulated situational variable that makes one condition different from another) yield main effects that can be easily calculated and compared with each other. Decades ago, Endler, Hunt, and Rosenstein (1962) used this basic procedure,[4] as, more recently (and in a more complex way), did Kenny, Mohr, and Levesque (2001). This seemingly straightforward approach turns out to have a number of complications, however.

One complication is that the estimate of the situational effect and of the dispositional effect only has implications beyond the bounds of the research study if the nature and range of the situational variables and of the dispositional variables are fairly representative of each type. If only a limited range of situations is included—and what experiment is not forced to severely restrict the range of situations it includes, compared to those that exist in the world?—and if only a limited range of individuals is included—and what study manages to include a sample of people truly representative of the population of the earth?—then the comparison between the two effects has little wider meaning.

Another complication is that even though the ANOVA conceptualization appears to imply that situational forces gain power over behavior only at the cost of dispositional sources, and vice versa, empirically this conclusion seems highly questionable. In one study we measured the cross-situational consistency of each of 62 behaviors (in a laboratory study using an early version of the RBQ), as well as the degree to which each behavior changed, on average (across participants), between the same two situations (Funder & Colvin, 1991). Across the behaviors, the correlation between consistency and change was –.01. Only in extreme cases, therefore—where a situation is so strong that everyone acts the same, or a personality disposition (or disorder?) is so strong that someone behaves without regard to the situation he or she is in—do situations and dispositions gain power at the expense of the other. In more ordinary and common circumstances, there is plenty of behavioral variance to go around.

The most important, conceptual objection to viewing dispositions and situations as competing forces is that, in order for either of them to have an effect on behavior, each *needs* the other (Johnson, 1997). Persons (and their dispositions) cannot exist outside of some sort of situation, and in a situation without people in it, no behavior will happen at all. This recognition has led writers such as Gilbert (1998), among others, to conclude that attribution theory's traditional way of distinguishing between dispositional attributions (ascribing behavioral causality to aspects of the person) and situational attributions (ascribing it to the situation) is fundamentally incoherent. Gilbert argues that, instead, dispositional attributions should be made only for an individual's behavior that is unusual; that is, different from what most other people do. Thus, if everybody puts on a coat on a cold day, the cause of any one person's behavior can be safely said to be the cold weather situation. The odd person (perhaps literally) who fails to wear a coat is doing so, presumably, because of something distinctive about him- or herself (e.g., an unusual immunity to, or eccentric liking for, cold).

This is a compelling analysis in most respects, but it leads to some surprising conclusions. For example, the classic studies of obedience by Milgram (1974) are almost universally described as demonstrating how the power of the situation to affect behavior, relative to the influence of personal dispositions, is much greater than anyone would

have expected (e.g., Ross & Nisbett, 1991). However, if we employ Gilbert's analysis, the direction of the violation of expectations is reversed. In a famous aspect of his research program, Milgram asked a panel of psychiatrists to estimate what percentage of his participants would obey a command to harm an innocent, protesting victim. They predicted almost nobody would. In Gilbert's analysis, this amounts to a prediction of a strong *situational* effect on behavior, because nearly everyone is predicted to act the same way. In fact, closer to 50% of the participants obeyed,[5] which amounts to an almost perfect demonstration of a strong *dispositional* effect on behavior.

From this perspective, it would be possible to conclude that the real take-home message from the Milgram research is that dispositions are much more important, relative to situations, than anyone ever thought! But really, what the analysis shows is that the fundamental dispositional–situational dichotomy, pitting one against the other, is poorly framed to begin with. Instead, the Milgram results can reasonably be read either of two ways: (1) The situational forces toward obedience (such as the experimenter saying "The experiment requires that you continue") was (perhaps surprisingly) stronger than the situational forces toward disobedience (such as the victim's protests). Or, (2) the dispositional forces toward obedience were (again, perhaps surprisingly) stronger than the dispositional forces toward empathy and disobedience.[6] On close examination, these interpretations are revealed to be equivalent. Notice, too, that neither of these equally valid interpretations pits the power of dispositions *against* the power of situations.

Cooperative Person–Situation Interactions

The study of person–situation interactions needs to move beyond frameworks that, like the analysis of variance or conventional attribution theory, cast them as competitors. A couple of possibilities can be suggested. Years ago, Buss (1979), among others, pointed out that persons and situations interact in at least three ways (see also Scarr & McCartney, 1983). One is the widely studied analysis of variance model, discussed above, which treats persons and situations as separate and independent contributors to behavior. The other two kinds of interaction are more cooperative: situational *selection* and situational *evocation*.

Situational selection is important because it addresses the fact that individuals do not just passively find themselves in the situations of their lives; they often actively seek and choose them. Thus, while a certain kind of bar may tend to generate a situation that creates fights around closing time, only a certain kind of person will choose to go to that kind of bar in the first place. Even if everybody at the bar ends up involved in the fight, therefore, the psychological excuse that "the situation made me do it" is less than completely persuasive. Instead, attributes of the person and the situation he or she chose have worked in tandem.

Situational evocation refers to the ways in which an individual's actions or even mere presence in a situation can change its dynamics. An aggressive person walking into a quiet discussion may change the situation dramatically for everyone there; a female walking into an all-male meeting, or vice versa, may change the situational dynamics by her or his mere presence. Again, notice how in these cases the attributes of a person are not competing with the attributes of the situation for control of behavior; they work together to produce the final result.

Buss pointed out, and it remains true, that both of these latter kinds of person–situation interaction are woefully understudied. In part this is because of the difficulty in empirically capturing dynamic processes such as the ways in which situations change during interactions as a function of what people do during them (see, e.g., Gottman & Bakeman, 1986). An even more important consideration, already mentioned, is the lack of general variables for describing the psychologically important elements of situations. Such variables will be necessary before research can study how situations are chosen and the ways in which they may change over time.

PERSON–SITUATION BEHAVIORAL PROFILES

A rather different approach to the person–situation interaction, suggested in recent years, is to turn research attention to variations of behavior *within* rather than across persons (e.g., Cervone, 2005; Fleeson, 2004; Mischel & Shoda, 1995). The idea is that every person varies his or her behavior across the situations of life, and that for each person this pattern of variation may be both consistent and idiosyncratic. Mischel and Shoda (1995) vividly labeled this approach the *if–then* conceptualization of personality: An individual is described in terms of his or her behavioral reactions to particular situations—for example: *if* at a party *then* the person is boisterous, whereas *if* in a seminar *then* the person is studious. It is the collection of such patterns that characterizes his or her personality.

Gordon Allport (1937) noted that every individual's pattern of behavior across contexts is unique and that, for this reason, all descriptions of individuals in terms of personality traits—which tend to assume a more-or-less common if–then pattern among the people they characterize—are at least a little bit misleading. For example, someone who is high on the trait of friendliness might initiate conversation when encountering a stranger. Although this might be true of friendly people, in general, a particular otherwise friendly person might hesitate to approach someone who reminds him of a previous, unpleasant encounter—a reaction that might be completely idiosyncratic to him and his personal history.

Going back even further, the classic pre-Skinnerian behaviorist John Watson (e.g., 1930) espoused a stimulus–response, or S–R, conceptualization of personality, in which a person's behavioral repertoire was described in terms of how he or she responds to the various situations—stimuli—that he or she encounters. This pattern of response was held to be a function of his or her unique learning history, and therefore was not presumed to have any general patterning or consistency across situations.

While it is eminently true that individuals vary their behavior across situations, and it is apparently true that each individual's pattern of variation is distinctive, to at least some degree, a personality psychology that decided to focus primarily on within-individual variation at the expense of between-individual variation would be forced to choose between a pair of less than completely attractive options.

One option is a return to old-fashioned Watsonian behaviorism, or a variant thereof. Watson believed that each individual could be understood only in terms of his or her unique learning history, and that his or her personality was manifested in an idiosyncratic pattern of S–R pairings. Watson's analysis has a couple of major disadvantages. One, noticed long ago by B. F. Skinner (1938), and others, is that people do more than respond passively to the stimuli that impinge on them; they initiate what Skinner called "operant" behaviors to actively create advantageous circumstances and advance their goals. Although it would be cumbersome, it might be possible to translate if–then conceptualizations into a more flexible Skinnerian rather than Watsonian version. A more fundamental problem with this kind of behavioristic approach, however, stems from its primary virtue, which is that it is completely idiographic. That is, there are as many S–R or if–then patterns as there are people on earth, each of which was generated by a unique learning history. While this may well be true, it is analytically daunting.

A second option for reconceptualizing personality in an if–then framework, and a way out of this dilemma, might be to gather groupings of patterns that resemble each other and classify people with those patterns as similar in some way. For example, the syndrome of rejection sensitivity (e.g., Downey & Feldman, 1996) has been described as characterizing a person who manifests the pattern of being kind and supportive in the early stages of a relationship, but insecure and demanding in the latter stages. Perhaps other kinds of if–then patterns could be identified that are shared by substantial numbers of individuals, which would allow individual differences to be conceptualized in a way that takes account of within-person behavioral variance.

Notice where this path has led us, however: right past personality dispositions, or traits, straight to the door of personality *types*. The idea of personality types has a long and controversial history (Mendelsohn, Weiss, & Feimer, 1982). This is not the place for a detailed account, but it can be noted that the idea of types goes back as far as Theophrastus (e.g., the penurious type), through Carl Jung (archetypes), to modern revivals such as a reconceptualization of the trait of self-monitoring as a type variable (Gangestad & Snyder, 1985) and a flurry of recent interest in three very general types characterized as overcontrolled, undercontrolled, and well adjusted (e.g., Caspi, 1998; Robins, John, Caspi, Moffitt, & Stouthamer-Loeber, 1996).

Personality types have a definite intuitive appeal. They have appeared to be useful tools for thinking about people in domains ranging from advertising (e.g., the suburban soccer mom) to the descriptions of personality disorders in the DSM-IV (e.g., the individual with histrionic personality disorder). Empirically and psychometrically, however, types have fared less well. The typological conception of psychological disorder appears to be yielding, slowly but surely, to a more dimensional—trait-like—approach (e.g., Clark, 2007). More generally, a number of recent studies—including those in a special issue of the *European Journal of Personality*—have converged on one robust conclusion: If the goal is the prediction of behavior—and that is the only way psychologists can empirically test whether their conceptualizations are correct—then types add little or nothing to what can be accomplished from traits alone (see Asendorpf, 2002; Costa, Herbst, McCrae, Samuels, & Ozer, 2002).

So where does that leave us? Gordon Allport followed his frank discussion of the way in which every person's pattern of behavior is unique with an admission that for psychological analysis some kind of simplification was going to be necessary, and that was all right because "some basic modes of adjustment ... from individual to individual are *approximately* the same" (Allport, 1937, p. 298). Maybe one person's extraversion is different from another's in minor respects, he said in effect, but they are still similar enough that it is useful and maybe even necessary to treat them as if they were the same. At least some of the within-person behavioral variance is idiosyncratic even to the person who displays it; in other words, it is error variance, which may be why robust person–situation interactions have proven so elusive (Chaplin, 1991). Even though Allport is remembered by some as a proponent of idiographic assessment, the bottom line for him was that patterns of behavior are common *enough* across individuals to be worth thinking of them, and assessing them, and then aggregating them, to produce measures of dispositions. Allport called them *traits*.

CONCLUSION:
BEYOND THE PERSON–SITUATION INTERACTION

It is easy, and probably too easy, to think of situational and dispositional causes of behavior as locked in opposition to each other. Except in extreme cases, they are not. Dispositions and situations both have important, robust, main effects. The only difference is that whereas many variables are available for describing dispositions, a psychologist wishing to describe a situation has very few options available at present. The time is past, one hopes, when it was sufficient to argue that situations are important on the basis of findings that dispositions do not account for all of the behavioral variance. The next generation of research needs to formulate variables to describe situations that are analogous, and function similarly, to the variables that describe dispositions.

Putting dispositions and situations together, many psychologists have acknowledged that it is the person–situation *interaction* that needs to be understood, not poorly framed questions concerning which is more important. The last four decades or so of research in personality have proven that this is easier said than done. The familiarity of the analysis of variance has tempted investigators into trying to apportion variance instead of understanding psychological dynamics. Attempts to focus attention on within-person behavioral variance appear to lead, in the end, either to a retreat to an outmoded form of behaviorism or to an almost equally outmoded typological approach. Yet again, we come to the need for good variables for describing situations as well as persons.

Dispositions and situations interact to determine what people do. Which dispositions and *which* aspects of situations (specifically) affect which behaviors? The search for specific answers to this seemingly straightforward question lays out a formidable research agenda. This agenda goes beyond the study of person–situation interactions to the three interactions derived from the *personality triad* of persons, situations, and behaviors, in which any element of the triad can be conceptualized in terms of the other two (Funder,

2006; see also Bandura, 1978). Behavior can be thought of as a function of the person and the situation, as has been discussed in this chapter. In addition, a person can be thought of in terms of the behaviors he or she performs in all the situations of his or her life (cf. Mischel & Shoda, 1995), and a situation, psychologically, can be conceptualized in terms of the behaviors that different people perform in it (cf. Bem & Funder, 1978). Another way to summarize these points is in the classic terms used by Lewin (1951): It is true, as he observed, that behavior is a function of the person and the situation, or $B = f(P, S)$. But it is also the case that $P = f(B, S)$ and $S = f(P, B)$. Pursuing the research implied by this conception moves personality psychology far beyond the competitive tug between person and situation that began this chapter and offers the potential to yield important theoretical insights and major contributions to the goals of psychology: to understand the bases of behavior and to promote human welfare.

ACKNOWLEDGMENTS

I am grateful for helpful comments from John A. Johnson and Richard Robins, but errors and omissions that remain are my sole responsibility.

NOTES

1. This story was told to me, years ago, by an eminent personality psychologist who claimed it really happened. It might not have, though, which is why I have concealed Dr. X.'s real name. In the words of Ken Kesey, "But it's the truth even if it didn't happen" (1962/1999, p. 7).
2. Actually, each method does pick up the complementary effect as part of the within-person or within-condition error variance, respectively. But this term does not separate the effect of the situation (in a traditional personality psychology study) or the effect of individual differences (in a traditional social psychology experiment) from measurement error. In practice, therefore, this term generally is treated as error variance that is useful for calculating statistical significance but otherwise ignored.
3. For a complete list of the items of the current version of the RSQ as well as the RBQ, and other relevant information, please visit our laboratory's website at *www.rap.ucr.edu*.
4. These investigators and most others doing similar research actually measured hypothetical

behaviors measured via questionnaire, rather than directly observed actual behaviors, but I shall pass over that important matter for now (Baumeister, Vohs, & Funder, 2006; Furr & Funder, 2007).

5. In the two most famous conditions, where the experimenter was present and the victim could be heard but not seen, the obedience rates were 63% (at Yale) and 48% (at "Research Associates of Bridgeport"). Across all conditions the average rate was 37.5% (Milgram, 1974, Tables, 2, 3, 4, and 5). See also Krueger and Funder (2004).

6. The traditional interpretation, of course, is that the situational forces toward obedience (e.g., the experimenter's orders) were stronger than dispositional forces toward disobedience (e.g., the participants' tendencies to be empathic to the victim). However, it would be precisely as valid—and equivalently misguided—to conclude that the dispositional forces toward obedience (e.g., the participants' conformist personalities) were generally stronger than situational forces toward disobedience (e.g., the victim's protests).

REFERENCES

Allport, G. W. (1937). *Personality: A psychological interpretation.* New York: Holt, Rinehart & Winston.

Allport, G. W. (1961). *Pattern and growth in personality.* New York: Holt, Rinehart & Winston.

Allport, G. W., & Odbert, H. S. (1936). Traitnames: A psycho-lexical study. *Psychological Monographs: General and Applied, 47,* 171–200.

Asendorpf, J. B. (2002). Editorial: The puzzle of personality types. *European Journal of Personality, 16,* 51–55.

Bandura, A. (1978). The self system in reciprocal determinism. *American Psychologist, 33,* 344–358.

Baumeister, R. F., Vohs, K. D., & Funder, D. C. (2007). Psychology as the science of self-reports and finger movements: Whatever happened to actual behavior? *Perspectives on Psychological Science, 2,* 396–403.

Bem, D. J., & Allen, A. (1974). On predicting some of the people some of the time: The search for cross-situational consistencies in behavior. *Psychological Review, 81,* 506–520.

Bem, D. J., & Funder, D. C. (1978). Predicting more of the people more of the time: Assessing the personality of situations. *Psychological Review, 85,* 485–501.

Block, J. (2008). *The Q-sort in character apprais-al: Encoding subjective impressions of persons quantitatively.* Washington, DC: American Psychological Association.

Buss, A. R. (1979). The trait–situation controversy and the concept of interaction. *Personality and Social Psychology Bulletin, 5,* 191–195.

Caspi, A. (1998). Personality development across the life course. In N. Eisenberg (Ed.), *Handbook of child psychology: Volume 3. Social, emotional, and personality development* (pp. 311–388). New York: Wiley.

Caspi, A., McClay, J., Moffitt, T. E., Mill, J., Martin, J., Craig, I. W., et al. (2002). Role of genotype in the cycle of violence in maltreated children. *Science, 297,* 851–854.

Caspi, A., Sugden, K., Moffitt, T. E., Taylor, A., Craig, I. W., Harrington, H., et al. (2003). Influence of life stress on depression: Moderation by a polymorphism in the 5-HTT gene. *Science, 301,* 386–389.

Cervone, D. (2005). Personality architecture: Within-person structures and processes. *Annual Review of Psychology, 56,* 423–452.

Chaplin, W. F. (1991). The next generation of moderator research in personality psychology. *Journal of Personality, 59,* 143–178.

Clark, L. A. (2007). Assessment and diagnosis of personality disorder: Perennial issues and an emerging reconceptualization. *Annual Review of Psychology, 58,* 227–257.

Costa, P. T., Jr., Herbst, J. H., McCrae, R. R., Samuels, J., & Ozer, D. J. (2002). The replicability and utility of three personality types. *European Journal of Personality, 16,* 573–588.

Darley, J. M., & Latané, B. (1968). Bystander intervention in emergencies: Diffusion of responsibility. *Journal of Personality and Social Psychology, 28,* 377–383.

Downey, G., & Feldman, S. I. (1996). Implications of rejection sensitivity for intimate relationships. *Journal of Personality and Social Psychology, 70,* 1327–1343.

Endler, N. S., Hunt, J. M., & Rosenstein, A. J. (1962). An S-R inventory of anxiousness. *Psychological Monographs, 76*(17), 1–33.

Epstein, S. (1979). The stability of behavior: I. On predicting most of the people much of the time. *Journal of Personality and Social Psychology, 37,* 1097–1126.

Epstein, S. (1980). The stability of behavior: II. Implications for psychological research. *American Psychologist, 35,* 790–806.

Fleeson, W. (2004). Moving personality beyond the person–situation debate: The challenge and opportunity of within-person variability. *Current Directions in Psychological Science, 13,* 83–87.

Funder, D. C. (2001). Personality. *Annual Review of Psychology, 52,* 197–221.

Funder, D. C. (2006). Towards a resolution of the personality triad: Persons, situations and behaviors. *Journal of Research in Personality, 40*, 21–34.

Funder, D. C., & Colvin, C. R. (1991). Explorations in behavioral consistency: Properties of persons, situations, and behaviors. *Journal of Personality and Social Psychology, 52*, 773–794.

Funder, D. C., Furr, R. M., & Colvin, C. R. (2000). The Riverside Behavioral Q-Sort: A tool for the description of social behavior. *Journal of Personality, 68*, 450–489.

Funder, D. C., & Ozer, D. J. (1983). Behavior as a function of the situation. *Journal of Personality and Social Psychology, 44*, 107–112.

Furr, R. M., & Funder, D. C. (2004). Situational similarity and behavioral consistency: Subjective, objective, variable-centered, and person-centered approaches. *Journal of Research in Personality, 38*, 421–447.

Furr, R. M., & Funder, D. C. (2007). Behavioral observation. In R. W. Robins, R. C. Fraley, & R. F. Krueger (Eds.), *Handbook of research methods in personality psychology* (pp. 273–291). New York: Guilford Press.

Gangestad, S. W., & Snyder, M. (1985). "To carve nature at its joints": On the existence of discrete classes in personality. *Psychological Review, 92*, 317–349.

Gilbert, D. T. (1998). Ordinary personology. In D. T. Gilbert, S. T. Fiske, & G. Lindzey (Eds.), *Handbook of social psychology* (Vol. 2, pp. 89–150). New York: McGraw-Hill.

Gottman, J. M., & Bakeman, R. (1986). *Observing interaction: An introduction to sequential analysis.* New York: Cambridge University Press.

Johnson, J. A. (1997). Units of analysis for description and explanation in psychology. In R. Hogan, J. A. Johnson, & S. R. Briggs (Eds.), *Handbook of personality psychology* (pp. 73–93). San Diego, CA: Academic Press.

Johnson, J. A. (1999, July). *Some hypotheses concerning attempts to separate situations from personality dispositions.* Paper presented at the sixth European Congress of Psychology, Rome. Available at *www.personal.psu.edu/~j5j/papers/rome.html*

Kelly, H. H., Holmes, J. G., Kerr, N. L., Reis, H. T., Rusbult, C. E., & Van Lange, P. A. (2003). *An atlas of interpersonal situations.* New York: Cambridge University Press.

Kenny, D. A., Mohr, C. D., & Levesque, M. J. (2001). A social relations variance partitioning of dyadic behavior. *Psychological Bulletin, 127*, 128–141.

Kenrick, D. T., & Funder, D. C. (1988). Profiting from controversy: Lessons from the person–situation debate. *American Psychologist, 43*, 23–34.

Kesey, K. (1999). *One flew over the cuckoo's nest.* New York: Penguin Books. (Original work published 1962)

Krueger, J. I., & Funder, D. C. (2004). Towards a balanced social psychology: Causes, consequences and cures for the problem-seeking approach to social behavior and cognition. *Behavioral and Brain Sciences, 27*, 313–327.

Lewin, K. (1951). *Field theory in social science.* New York: Harper.

McCrae, R. R., & Costa, P. T., Jr. (1987). Validation of the five-factor model of personality across instruments and observers. *Journal of Personality and Social Psychology, 52*, 307–317.

McCrae, R. R., & Costa, P. T., Jr. (1999). A five-factor theory of personality. In L. A. Pervin & O. P. John (Eds.), *Handbook of personality: Theory and research* (pp. 139–153). New York: Guilford Press.

McCrae, R. R., Costa, P. T., Jr., & Busch, C. M. (1986). Evaluating comprehensiveness in personality systems: The California Q-set and the five-factor model. *Journal of Personality, 54*, 430–446.

Mendelsohn, G. A., Weiss, D. S., & Feimer, N. R. (1982). Conceptual and empirical analysis of the typological implications of patterns of socialization and femininity. *Journal of Personality and Social Psychology, 42*, 1157–1170.

Milgram, S. (1974). *Obedience to authority: An experimental view.* New York: Harper & Row.

Mischel, W. (1977). On the future of personality measurement. *American Psychologist, 32*, 246–254.

Mischel, W., & Shoda, Y. (1995). A cognitive–affective system theory of personality: Reconceptualizing situations, dispositions, dynamics, and invariance in personality structure. *Psychological Review, 102*, 246–268.

Murray, H. A. (1938). *Explorations in personality.* New York: Oxford University Press.

Ozer, D. J., & Benet-Martínez, V. (2006). Personality and the prediction of consequential outcomes. *Annual Review of Psychology, 57*, 401–421.

Roberts, B. W., Kuncel, N. R., Shiner, R., Caspi, A., & Goldberg, L. R. (2007). The power of personality: The comparative validity of personality traits, socioeconomic status, and cognitive ability for predicting important life outcomes. *Perspectives on Psychological Science, 2*, 313–345.

Robins, R. W., John, O. P., Caspi, A., Moffitt, T. E., & Stouthamer-Loeber, M. (1996). Resilient, overcontrolled and undercontrolled boys:

Three personality types in early adolescence. *Journal of Personality and Social Psychology, 70,* 157–171.

Ross, L., & Nisbett, R. E. (1991). *The person and the situation: Perspectives of social psychology.* New York: McGraw-Hill.

Scarr, S., & McCartney, K. (1983). How people make their own environments: A theory of genotype → environment effects. *Child Development, 54,* 424–435.

Skinner, B. F. (1938). *The behavior of organisms: An experimental analysis.* New York: Appleton-Century.

Ten Berge, M. A., & De Raad, B. (2002). The structure of situations from a personality perspective. *European Journal of Personality, 16,* 81–102.

Van Heck, G. L., Perugini, M., Caprara, G. V., & Froeger, J. (1994). The Big Five as tendencies in situations. *Personality and Individual Differences, 16,* 715–731.

Wagerman, S. A., & Funder, D. C. (2006, January). *The Riverside Situational Q-Sort: A tool for understanding the psychological properties of situations.* Paper presented at the meeting of the Society for Personality and Social Psychology, Palm Springs, CA.

Watson, J. B. (1930). *Behaviorism* (rev. ed.). New York: Norton.

Yang, Y., Read, S. J., & Miller, L. C. (2006). A taxonomy of situations from Chinese idioms: Goal processes as a central organizing principle. *Journal of Research in Personality, 40,* 750–778.

PART VI

Cognitive and Motivational Processes

CHAPTER 23

The Psychological Unconscious

John F. Kihlstrom

Consciousness has two aspects: By virtue of *conscious awareness*, we gain introspective access to the mental states—the cognitions, emotions, and motives—that cause us to behave the way we do; and by virtue of *conscious control*, we gain voluntary control over the mental processes that generate those states—and, as a consequence, our behavior as well. The idea of the psychological unconscious is that at least some of the mental states and processes underlying behavior are either temporarily inaccessible or permanently unavailable to either conscious awareness or conscious control (Kihlstrom, 2007). Since the time of Freud, the psychological unconscious has been one of the most provocative aspects of personality theory—and it is also one of the most problematic and controversial.

HISTORICAL PERSPECTIVES

The unconscious mind is sometimes considered to be the intellectual property of psychodynamic approaches to personality and psychopathology whose evolution began in the 19th century (Ellenberger, 1970; Macmillan, 1991/1997), and especially the psychoanalytic tradition initiated by Sigmund Freud. Based on his observations of hysterical patients and his analysis of such phenomena as dreams, errors, and jokes, Freud initially proposed a topographical division of the mind into three mental compartments, or "systems," which he called *Cs*, *Pcs*, and *Ucs* (Freud, 1900/1953). The system *Cs*, or conscious mind, contains those thoughts, feelings, motives, and actions of which we are phenomenally aware at the moment. Consciousness is explicitly likened to a sensory organ capable of perceiving other mental contents. The system *Pcs*, by contrast, contains preconscious mental contents not currently in conscious awareness, but which are available to consciousness and which can be accessed and brought into awareness under certain conditions. Finally, the system *Ucs* contains unconscious mental contents that are unavailable to consciousness—that cannot enter awareness under any circumstances. According to Freud (1900/1953), contents are exchanged between the systems *Pcs* and *Cs* by virtue of *cathexis*—by having attention paid to, or withdrawn from, them; contents residing in the system *Ucs* are kept out of (or expelled from) the system *Pcs* by means of repression. As others (Erdelyi, 1985) have noted, this topographical model, with its spatial metaphors, may be read as an anticipation of modern multistore models of human information processing.

Freud maintained this account of the vicissitudes of consciousness for approximately two decades, but then introduced a wholesale revision of his view, shifting from a topographical to a functional analysis of the mind (Freud, 1923/1961). Although it might seem natural to graft the topographical model onto the functional one, such a connection proved untenable. The id is strictly unconscious, and except in cases of psychosis, can be known only through inference. By the same token, consciousness is necessarily a quality of the ego—after all, the ego functions expressly to permit us to become aware of external reality. At the same time, however, the defense mechanisms are also part of the ego, and their operations are not accessible to consciousness; and since the ego cannot be conscious of all of external reality at once, some of its contents (and, correspondingly, of the superego) must necessarily be preconscious.

The problem of reconciling the two different divisions of the mind, topographic and functional, was not solved by Freud before he died. Nevertheless, his assignment of some nonconscious mental functions to the ego, in both its defensive and nondefensive spheres, initiated an important research tradition within post-Freudian psychoanalysis. Beginning with the work of Anna Freud, and especially in the hands of Heinz Hartmann, David Rapaport, and George Klein, psychoanalytic ego psychology focused on the nondefensive, reality-oriented tasks of the ego. The research of the ego psychologists dealt with conventional topics of perception, memory, and thinking, and in many respects it resembled that being performed elsewhere in academic laboratories. In other respects, however, their work was quite different: It favored prose over nonsense syllables as stimulus materials, for example, took images and dreams seriously, and emphasized the interplay of emotional, motivational, and cognitive processes. The tradition of psychoanalytic ego psychology was linked most closely with mainstream experimental psychology by the work of Bruner, Klein, and others on the "New Look" in perception and attendant research on such topics as subliminal perception, perceptual defense and vigilance, and repression–sensitization (Bruner & Klein, 1960). In the present context, the most important feature of psychoanalytic ego psychology is that it took seriously the question of the psychological unconscious, and of the relations between conscious and nonconscious mental processes, at a time when most academic psychologists had difficulty taking even the notion of consciousness seriously.

Whereas Freud described the mechanism of the dynamic unconscious as one of repression, his intellectual rival, Pierre Janet, described it in terms of dissociation (actually, his term was *desaggregation*). Janet's work on hysteria was overshadowed by Freud's, and his magnum opus, *Psychological Automatisms*, unfortunately remains untranslated. For these reasons, Janet's theoretical ideas are known primarily through secondary sources (Ellenberger, 1970; Hilgard, 1977). These ideas were predicated on Claude Bernard's paradigm of analysis followed by synthesis: the study of elementary psychological functions taken separately, and then the reconstruction of the whole mind based on knowledge of these parts. The elementary mental functions were labeled psychological automatisms: complex intelligent acts that adjust to their circumstances and are accompanied by a rudimentary consciousness. Each automatism unites cognition, emotion, and motivation with action. Thus, automatisms resemble what some contemporary theorists would call productions (or production systems): condition–action units that are executed in response to appropriate contextual cues.

Janet (Ellenberger, 1970) held that under normal circumstances, all psychological automatisms are bound together into a single stream of consciousness: each accessible to introspection, and each susceptible to voluntary control. However, the occurrence of mental trauma, especially in a vulnerable individual, could result in the splitting off of one or more psychological automatisms from conscious monitoring and control. Under these circumstances, there would exist two or more streams of mental functioning (consciousness in James's broad sense), each processing inputs and outputs, but only one of which is accessible to phenomenal awareness and voluntary control. The dissociated automatisms constitute fixed ideas (*idee fixe*), which possess some degree of autonomy with respect to their development and effects on ongoing experience, thought, and action. The operation of these dissociated (as opposed to integrated or synthesized) psychological automatisms provides the mechanism for the major symptoms of hysteria: They produce the ideas, images, and behaviors that intrude, unbidden, on the stream of conscious thought and action; and their capacity to process information is responsible for the paradoxical ability of the hysterically blind or deaf to negotiate their environments successfully. Janet described these dissociated automatisms as *sub*conscious as opposed to *un*conscious, and considered repression as just one possible mechanism for dissociation.

Janet's ideas were championed by the American psychologist Morton Prince, and more recently by Ernest R. Hilgard (1977), who proposed a "neodissociation" theory of divided consciousness. Whether in its original or updated forms, dissociation theory provides a rather different view of nonconscious mental functioning than psychoanalytic theory. In the first place, dissociation theory holds that nonconscious mental contents are not necessarily restricted to primitive sexual and aggressive ideas and impulses, nor are they necessarily irrational, imagistic, or in any other way qualitatively different from conscious ones; they are simply not consciously accessible. In the second place, dissociation theory holds that the restriction of awareness need not be motivated by purposes of defense, nor need it necessarily have the effect of reducing conflict and anxiety; rather, it can occur simply as a consequence of particular psychological operations.

Within 19th-century academic psychology, perhaps the most forceful advocate of nonconscious mental life was William James. Following the onslaught of radical behaviorism, empirical interest in unconscious mental life declined precipitously in the years after World War I. Serious theoretical interest in nonconscious mental life had to wait the triumph of the cognitive revolution (Hilgard, 1980a), with its interest in attention, short-term memory, and even mental imagery. However, by implicitly identifying consciousness with "higher" mental processes, the classic multistore model left little or no room for the *psychological unconscious*—complex mental structures and processes that influence experience, thought, and action, but which are nevertheless inaccessible to phe-

nomenal awareness. The giant step—to the idea that mental states and processes could dynamically influence experience, thought, and action despite being inaccessible to phenomenal awareness and voluntary control—required a wholesale revision of our concepts of attention and memory.

THE COGNITIVE UNCONSCIOUS

The rediscovery of the unconscious by modern scientific psychology began with comparisons between automatic and effortful mental processes and between explicit and implicit memory. Since then, it has continued with the extension of the explicit–implicit distinction into the domains of perception, learning, and thought. Taken together, this literature describes the *cognitive unconscious* (Kihlstrom, 1987).

Automaticity and Unconscious Processing

The earliest information-processing theories of attention were based, to one degree or another, on the metaphor of the filter. Information that makes it past the filter is available for "higher" information-processing activities, whereas information that does not make it past the filter is not. This same attentional filter was also seen as the threshold that had to be crossed for information to be represented in phenomenal awareness. The filter theories of attention, in turn, raised questions about how permeable the attentional filter was, and how much information processing could occur preattentively. In part to solve these problems, the notion of an attentional filter was replaced by the notion of attentional capacity. Whereas the filter models conceived of information processing as serial in nature, the capacity models implied that several tasks could be carried out simultaneously, so long as their attentional requirements did not exceed available resources.

The capacity view, in turn, led to a distinction between *automatic* and *controlled* processes (LaBerge & Samuels, 1974; Posner & Snyder, 1975; Schneider & Shiffrin, 1977). Automatic processes are inevitably evoked by the presentation of specific stimulus inputs, regardless of any intention on the part of the subject. Once evoked, they are incorrigibly executed, in a ballistic fashion.

Automatic processes are effortless, in that they consume little or no attentional capacity. And they are efficient, in that they do not interfere with other ongoing mental activities. But in any case, automatic processes are unconscious in the strict sense that they are inaccessible to phenomenal awareness under any circumstances.

Challenges to capacity theory, from which the earliest ideas about automaticity emerged, have led to alternative theoretical conceptualizations of automaticity in terms of memory rather than attention. Nevertheless, the concept of automaticity has gained a firm foothold in the literature of cognitive psychology, and investigators have sought to develop methods to distinguish between the automatic and controlled contributions to task performance (Jacoby, 1991).

Implicit Memory

While automatic processes may be considered to be unconscious, the mental contents on which they operate, and which they in turn generate, are ordinarily thought to be available to conscious awareness. The further possibility, that cognitive processes can operate on mental states—percepts, memories, and the like—that are not themselves accessible to conscious awareness, was first raised in modern psychology in response to observations of priming in neurological patients with the *amnesic syndrome* resulting from bilateral damage to the medial temporal lobe, including the hippocampus. These patients cannot remember words that they have just studied, but nevertheless show normal levels of priming on tasks such as word-fragment completion and stem completion. On the basis of results such as these, Schacter (1987) drew a distinction between explicit memory, which involves the conscious recollection of some past event, and implicit memory, which is revealed by any change in task performance that is attributable to that event. Following Schacter, we may define implicit memory formally as *the effect of a past event on the subject's ongoing experience, thought, and action, in the absence of, or independent of, conscious recollection of that event.* Implicit memory is, in these terms, unconscious memory.

Priming has also been observed in various other forms of amnesia, including the anterograde and retrograde amnesia secondary to electroconvulsive therapy for depression; the anterograde amnesia produced by general anesthesia administered to surgical patients, as well as that associated with conscious sedation in outpatient surgery; memory disorders observed in dementia, including Alzheimer's disease, as well as those encountered in normal aging; hypnotic and posthypnotic amnesia following appropriate suggestions to hypnotizable subjects; and the "functional" or "psychogenic" amnesias encountered in genuine cases of dissociative disorder, including dissociative amnesia, dissociative fugue, and the interpersonality amnesia of dissociative identity disorder (also known as multiple personality disorder).

In each of these cases, the memory disorder primarily impairs explicit memory and spares implicit memory, which is either wholly or relatively intact. It is in this sense that implicit memory persists in the absence of explicit memory. However, implicit memory can be observed in individuals with normal memory functions as well. For example, normal subjects show significant savings in relearning for items that they can neither recall nor recognize. And although elaboration is an important determinant of explicit memory, "depth of processing" has relatively little impact on many priming effects. In nonamnesic individuals implicit memory may be said to be independent of explicit memory, in that priming does not depend on whether the prime is consciously remembered. Although some theoretical controversy surrounds the nature of implicit memory, the essential concept, including its dissociation from explicit memory, is now widely accepted.

Implicit Learning

Closely related to implicit memory is *implicit learning*. In Reber's (1967) classic experiments on artificial grammar learning, which introduced this term to psychological discourse, subjects were first asked to study a set of letter strings generated by an artificial grammar. Later, they were able to identify new grammatical letter strings at better than chance levels; however, they were unable to specify the grammatical rule that they had clearly induced from the study set. Apparently, they had acquired new knowledge (about the rules governing grammatical letter strings) through experience, but were unable to gain conscious access to this knowledge. In a paradigm somewhat similar to artificial grammar learning, subjects have learned to identify instances of novel concepts, such as patterns of dots that vary around a prototype, without being able to describe the defining or characteristic features of the concepts themselves; subjects can also detect the covariation between two features, such as hair length and personality, even though they cannot identify the basis for their predictions; they can learn the sequence in which certain stimuli will occur, without being able to specify the sequence itself; and they can learn to control the output of a complex system by manipulating an input variable, without being able to specify the relationship between the two.

Following the model of implicit memory, implicit learning may be defined as *a relatively permanent change in knowledge, resulting from experience, in the absence of conscious awareness of what has been learned* (Kihlstrom, 1996). Demonstrations that amnesic patients can acquire new procedural and declarative knowledge through experience, even though they do not remember the learning experiences themselves, have led some theorists to construe implicit learning as a variant on implicit memory. However, there is an important distinction between the two concepts: implicit memory is a feature of episodic knowledge, in which subjects lack conscious memory for a specific event in their lives. By contrast, in implicit learning subjects lack conscious access to certain pieces of semantic and procedural knowledge acquired through a learning experience. Implicit learning should be distinguished from merely *incidental* learning, in which new knowledge is acquired in the absence of instructions or intention to learn, but the subject retains conscious access to that knowledge. Incidental learning is unintended, whereas implicit learning is unconscious.

Nevertheless, the interpretation of implicit learning in terms of the acquisition of unconscious knowledge remains somewhat controversial. In the artificial grammar experiments, for example, the mere fact that subjects cannot articulate the Markov process by which grammatical strings were generated does not mean that they are unaware of what they have learned. Above-chance classification performance could well result from partial knowledge that is consciously accessible. The best that can be said, for now, is that the subjects in artificial grammar and sequence learning experiments often experience themselves as behaving randomly, without an awareness of what they are doing. However, this assumption rests on relatively informal evidence. A major item on the agenda in the study of implicit learning is to carry out more detailed analyses of subjects' experiences in implicit learning situations, to make sure that they are really unconscious of what they evidently know.

Implicit Perception

Effects analogous to implicit memory can be observed in perception: Just as there are palpable effects on experience, thought, and action of *past events that cannot be consciously remembered*, so there appear to be similar effects of *events in the current stimulus environment that cannot be consciously perceived*. At least in principle: A variety of methodological critiques have sought to demonstrate that events cannot be analyzed for meaning unless they have been consciously identified and attended to. However, beginning with the now-classic studies of Marcel (1983a, 1983b) and the work of Merikle and his associates (Cheesman & Merikle, 1984, 1986; Merikle & Reingold, 1990), an increasing body of literature has demonstrated unconscious perception in a manner that satisfies all but the most determined critics (Draine & Greenwald, 1998; Greenwald, Draine, & Abrams, 1996; Greenwald, Klinger, & Liu, 1989).

In traditional studies of subliminal perception, the stimulus is of extremely low intensity; otherwise, the stimulus is degraded by means of brief tachistoscopic presentation, or by a masking stimulus, as in Marcel's (1983a) studies. However, in other cases of implicit perception, the stimulus in question is not strictly subliminal. For example, Weiskrantz (1986) and his colleagues reported a patient who suffered extensive damage to the striate cortex of the occipital lobes. Although the patient reported an inability to see, he was nonetheless able to respond appropriately to some visual stimuli—a phenomenon called "blindsight." Similarly, patients with bilateral lesions to the mesial portions of the occipital and temporal cortex are unable to consciously recognize previously encountered faces as familiar—a condition known as prosopagnosia. Nevertheless, prosopagnosic patients show differential behavioral responses to old and new faces—a dissociation similar to the implicit memory seen in the amnesic syndrome. Similar phenomena have been observed in visual neglect syndromes resulting from damage to the temporoparietal areas of the cerebral cortex. In the domain of the "functional" disorders of perception, priming and related effects have been observed in cases of visual and auditory conversion disorder (also known as "hysterical" blindness and deafness), and in analogous phenomena of hypnosis, such as hypnotic blindness and deafness.

Finally, priming and similar effects have been observed in subjects whose attention has been deflected from the stimulus, so that it is processed outside conscious awareness. For example, a supraliminal stimulus may be presented in parafoveal segments of the visual field, or over the unattended channel in dichotic listening experiments. However, there are other circumstances where perception without awareness occurs even though the environmental stimulus is not degraded in any sense. Priming has also been observed in the attentional phenomena of *inattentional blindness*, *repetition blindness*, and the *attentional blink*—although to date there have been no demonstrations of priming in another attentional anomaly, known as *change blindness*.

Because perception without awareness extends to cases beyond stimuli that are subliminal or unattended, it seems more appropriate to make a broader distinction between explicit and implicit expressions of perception, paralleling the distinction between explicit and implicit memory (Kihlstrom, 1996; Kihlstrom, Barnhardt, & Tataryn, 1992). Explicit perception entails the subject's conscious perception of some object in the current environment, or the environment of the very recent past, as reflected in his or her ability to report the presence, location, form, identity, and/or activity of that object. Implicit perception refers to any change in the person's experience, thought, or action that is attributable to such an event, in the absence of (or independent of) conscious perception of that event. The term "implicit perception" captures a broader domain than is covered by the term "subliminal perception" because it covers the processing, outside of conscious awareness, of stimulus events that are normally perceptible in terms of intensity, duration, and other characteristics.

As with implicit learning, implicit perception effects are sometimes discussed under the rubric of implicit memory. However, it seems important to maintain the distinction between the two phenomena. In implicit memory, the subject was perceptually aware of the event at the time it occurred, but the memory of that event has been lost to conscious recollection. In implicit perception, the subjects were unaware of the event at the time it occurred; thus, it is the perception itself that is unconscious. The distinction can be illustrated by preserved priming in general anesthesia: Because the test takes place some time after the primes were presented, the priming might count as an instance of implicit memory; but because the patients were not aware of the primes at the time they were presented, the same phenomenon also counts as an instance of implicit perception.

Implicit Thought

Implicit memory, learning, and perception do not exhaust the domain of the psychological unconscious: It appears we can also have unconscious thoughts. Unconscious thought has been interpreted in terms of automaticity (Hassin, Uleman, & Bargh, 2005; Uleman & Bargh, 1989). However, there is some tantalizing evidence that thoughts themselves, and not just thinking, can be unconscious. For example, Bowers and his associates (Bowers, Regehr, Balthazard, & Parker, 1990) found that subjects could distinguish between soluble and insoluble word problems, without knowing what the solution to the soluble problem was. Employing similar materials, Shames (1994) showed that lexical decision judgments could be primed by the solution to a soluble word problem, even when subjects were unaware of the solution itself, an effect conceptually replicated by Jung-Beeman and Bowden (2000). Similarly, Bechara, Damasio, Tranel, and Damasio (1997) found that subjects showed anticipatory skin-conductance responses when making risky choices, even though they could not consciously discriminate between choices that were risky and those that were safe.

In each of these cases, the subjects seemed to be responding to a "feeling of knowing" analogous to that observed in metamemory tasks. Their choices are clearly being guided by something that is neither a percept (because the solution is not currently being presented to them) or a memory (because the solution has not been presented in the past). But by analogy to implicit perception and memory, we defined *implicit thought* as a mental representation—an idea or an image, for example—that influences ongoing experience, thought, and action in the absence of conscious awareness of that thought (Dorfman, Shames, & Kihlstrom, 1996; Kihlstrom, Shames, & Dorfman, 1996).

Implicit thought may underlie the phenomena of intuition, incubation, and insight in problem solving. Thus, intuition occurs when the thought is unconscious, insight occurs when the unconscious thought emerges into consciousness, and incubation may be thought of as the process by which the transformation from unconscious influence to conscious access takes place. Although intuition has acquired a negative reputation as a source of error in human judgment, more recent work on problem solving has been more open to the idea of unconscious influences (Bowden, Jung-Beeman, Fleck, & Kounios, 2006; Siegler, 2000). Although it is possible to "trick" intuitive judgment by taking advantage of priming effects, Bowers and his colleagues argued that intuitions represent our tendency, as intelligent problem solvers, to go beyond the information given by a problem or a retrieval cue (Bowers, Farvolden, & Mermigis, 1995). As the way out of the closed cognitive loop of induction and deduction, intuitions are important elements in the creative process—gut feelings that we are correct, without knowing why, or even whether, we are right. Viewed in this way, intuitions may have motivational value, keeping the problem solver at the problem, in the belief that a solution will be found.

What Does All This Have to Do with Personality?

The cognitive unconscious—cognitive processes that operate automatically and unconsciously, and percepts, memories, knowledge, and thoughts that are inaccessible to phenomenal awareness—is, naturally, of greatest interest to cognitive psychologists. But they are also relevant to personality psychologists. Allport (1937) defined a trait as "a generalized and localized neuropsychic system ... with the capacity to render many stimuli functionally equivalent, and to initiate and guide consistent (equivalent) forms of adaptive and expressive behavior" (p. 295). Setting aside the question of neural representation, the trait of friendliness, for example, can be construed as a cognitive disposition to perceive other people as friendly and to interpret behaviors as friendly (thus rendering "many stimuli functionally equivalent") and to behave toward others in a friendly manner (thus initiating and guiding "consistent forms of adaptive and expressive behavior." To the extent that these perceptions, interpretations, and behaviors occur automatically, then they will be perceived as "natural" aspects of the individual's personality ("That's just the way he is"), and they will also be perceived as "natural" by the person him- or herself ("That's just the way I am").

The cognitive unconscious is also relevant to cognitive social learning approaches to personality. Neither the original neobehaviorist formulations of social learning theory nor the more cognitively flavored versions offered subsequently made any particular reference to consciousness, but it is easy to see the potential relevance of unconscious processes to this view of personality. Imitation, a major form of social learning discussed by both Miller and Dollard (1941) and by Bandura (1977), may occur automatically. If percepts, memories, and thoughts can be represented outside of conscious awareness, Rotter's (1954) expectancies may be implicit as well as explicit. Kelly's (1955) personal construct theory allowed for preverbal, essentially unconscious, personal constructs as well as those that were consciously verbalizable. All of Mischel's (1973) social-cognitive learning person variables, including the cognitive-behavioral construction competencies, encoding strategies, and self-regulatory systems and plans, can operate unconsciously and automatically. More recently, Metcalfe and Mischel (1999) have distinguished between a "hot" social-cognitive system that operates automatically and unconsciously, and a "cool" one that operates consciously and deliberately. Although Bandura's (1986) social learning by precept (sponsored teaching) would seem to require consciousness on the part of the teacher, if not the learner, social learning by example may well occur implicitly as well as explicitly.

In the "social intelligence" interpretation of personality offered by Cantor and Kihlstrom (1987; Kihlstrom & Cantor, 2000), the individual's repertoire of procedural social knowledge, like all procedural knowledge, operates automatically and thus unconsciously; declarative social knowledge, represented in episodic and semantic memory, may be either explicit or implicit. Viewed from a cognitive perspective, the self may be viewed as one's mental representation of one's own personality, stored in memory just like any other knowledge structure (Kihlstrom, Beer, & Klein, 2002; Kihlstrom & Cantor, 1984; Kihlstrom et al., 1988; Kihlstrom & Klein, 1994, 1997; Kihlstrom, Marchese-Foster, & Klein, 1997). This self-knowledge structure is generally accessible to conscious awareness, which is why people—even amnesics, who have no conscious access to their recent autobiographical memories (S. B. Klein, Cosmides, & Costabile, 2003; S. B. Klein, Loftus, & Kihlstrom, 1996, 2002; Tulving, 1993)—are able to describe themselves and identify which aspects of their appearance, personality, and social relations are particularly important to their self-concepts. However, this self-knowledge is stored in memory, and we already know that memories can be implicit as well as explicit. Therefore, we have to concede that, in principle, some aspects of the self can be unconscious—as seems to be the case in multiple personality disorder, where the interpersonality amnesia appears to cover not just the actions and experiences of the patient's alter ego(s), but the self-concept(s) as well (Kihlstrom, 2001, 2005).

Now that the concept of unconscious mental life has been liberated from the death-grip of Freudian psychoanalysis, modern personality psychology seems to be more willing to think about unconscious processes (e.g., Asendorpf, 2007; Robinson, 2007; L. A. Rudman & Spencer, 2007). This is particularly the case for the concept of automaticity (Hassin et al., 2005; Uleman & Bargh, 1989). However, personality psychologists who wish to embrace the concept of unconscious life must beware of William James's warning that "the distinction between *the unconscious and the conscious being of the mental state* is the sovereign means for believing what one likes in psychology, and of turning what might become a science into a tumbling-ground for whimsies" (James, 1890/1980, p. 163, original emphasis). One of the dangers in psychology is the "psychologist's fallacy" (James, 1890/1980, p. 196) that his or her explanation of a subject's behavior is better than the subject's own. The dangers of the psychologist's fallacy are multiplied when the psychologist can resort to attributions of the subject's *unconscious* mental states. Fortunately, the literature on the cognitive unconscious has established fairly clear criteria for distinguishing between automatic and controlled processes, and for establishing dissociations between explicit and implicit perception and memory, that will prove useful as these concepts are increasingly embraced by personality psychologists.

BEYOND THE COGNITIVE UNCONSCIOUS

Implicit perception, learning, memory, and thought comprise the domain of the cognitive unconscious. But cognition is not the whole of mental life: the "trilogy of mind" includes emotion and motivation as well (Hilgard, 1980b). If we are going to accept the concepts of unconscious perception and memory as empirically valid, why shouldn't we extend the explicit–implicit distinction to emotion and motivation as well? We probably should—and when we do we come even closer to the traditional concerns of personality psychology.

Of course, feelings and goals can be activated automatically. Just as hunger and thirst arise from homeostatic mechanisms that respond automatically to changing levels of cell fluids and blood sugar, so it may well be that certain basic emotions, at least, are generated automatically in response to certain stimulus inputs, in the absence of conscious cognitive activity. In fact, the assertion that affect is independent of (conscious) cognition was the signal event in what might be called an *affective counterrevolution* in psychology (Zajonc, 1980, 1984), leading directly to the establishment of an affective science, or affective neuroscience, developing in parallel to, but largely independent of, cognitive science and cognitive neuroscience. But in these cases, although the generating process is unconscious, the resulting affective or conative state is presumably represented in conscious awareness. I feel hungry even if I am not aware of my blood-sugar levels, or how the hypothalamus processes them, and that feeling is conscious.

Similarly, subliminal exposure can influence my preferences, even if I am not aware of the exposures (Bornstein, 1989; Kunst-Wilson & Zajonc, 1980), and amnesic patients can acquire affective preferences without being able to remember any encounters with the objects of their affection (Johnson & Multhaup, 1992). But in both cases, the resulting preference itself is conscious. Emotional responses can serve as expressions of implicit perception and memory, but it is something else again for the emotional responses themselves to be unconscious. The question at issue is whether affective and conative states can be unconscious, in the same way that cognitive states such as percepts and memories can be.

The Motivational Unconscious

Paralleling the definitions of explicit and implicit memory, we can define explicit motivation as the conscious representation of a conative state, or the desire to engage in some particular activity, as represented by craving for food, yearning for love, and the like. By contrast, implicit motivation refers to changes in experience, thought, or action that are attributable to a person's motivational state independent of his or her conscious awareness of that state. In terms of measurement, explicit motivation tasks require the subject to reflect on, and report, his or her conscious desires; implicit motivation tasks do not. Of course, the existence of unconscious sexual and aggressive motives, inferred from symbolic representations such as symptoms and dream imagery, were the key to Freudian psychoanalysis. In the laboratory, implicit motivation might be exemplified by posthypnotic suggestion, in which the subject engages in suggested behavior without any awareness of the suggestion or even of any intention to act.

In the recent history of psychology, the concept of implicit motivation was first articulated by McClelland, Koestner, and Weinberger (1989)—interestingly, without any reference to the already-emerging concept of explicit memory. For McClelland et al., explicit motives are self-attributed: The person is aware of the motive, can reflect on it and report it in interviews or on personality questionnaires. Implicit motives, by contrast, are inferred from the person's performance on such exercises as the Thematic Apperception Test (TAT). As such, the distinction between explicit and implicit motives is an extension of McClelland's (1980) earlier distinction between respondent and operant motive measures. However, in this later formulation, McClelland and colleagues went beyond issues of measurement to postulate two dissociable motive systems, one explicit and the other implicit. One of these motive systems is accessible to conscious awareness; the other is not, and it influences the individual's experience, thought, and action unconsciously. By virtue of implicit motives, people engage in goal-oriented behavior without being aware of what their motives or goals are.

Or, at least, that is the hypothesis. McClelland and colleagues (1989) offered two types of evidence for the dissociation between explicit and implicit motives. First, the correlation between motive scores assessed through instruments such as the TAT and corresponding scores assessed through self-report questionnaires such as the Personality Research Form is notoriously low, averaging $r = .09$ in one meta-analysis (Spangler, 1992; Thrash & Elliot, 2002). Second, the two types of measurements predict different performance criteria (Bornstein, 1998; Woike, Mcleod, & Goggin, 2003). However, both types of evidence are ambiguous with respect to the distinction between conscious and unconscious motives. The low correlations between questionnaire and TAT measures may simply be a reflection of method variance, whereas the differential correlates of explicit and implicit motives may be due to the fact that the motives being measured are subtly different, despite their similar names. Most critically, in the present context, while the low correlations between TAT and questionnaire measures provide prima facie evidence of a dissociation between explicit and implicit motivation, the literature on implicit motivation does not yet contain carefully controlled comparisons that show that implicit motives are, indeed, inaccessible to conscious awareness (Schultheiss & Pang, 2007).

A rather different perspective on the motivational unconscious is offered by Bargh, as part of his general promotion of the concept of automaticity (Bargh, 1990; Bargh & Barndollar, 1996; Bargh, Gollwitzer, LeeChai, Barndollar, & Trotschel, 2001). According to the traditional folk-psychological model of motivation, the person consciously selects some intended behavior in order to achieve some goal, and then deliberately executes that behavior. Although it is commonly accepted that some skilled goal-directed behaviors are executed automatically and unconsciously, much like a concert pianist plays an arpeggio, Bargh also automates the process of goal selection—the selection of the music, not just the touch of fingers to keys. According to this *auto-motive* model, by virtue of having been frequently and consistently chosen in a particular situation, goals and motives themselves can be automatically and unconsciously invoked by environmental events. Once activated, then, goal-oriented behaviors can be executed outside of awareness as well.

It should be noted, however, that whereas the implicit motives discussed by McClelland and colleagues (1989) are themselves inaccessible to conscious awareness (at least on hypothesis), Bargh's (1997) auto-motive model asserts only that the person's motives are selected automatically, in the absence of conscious intention or choice. It does not necessarily follow that the person is not aware of the motives themselves. Thus, it may very well be that achievement or affiliation goals may be primed by events in the current or past environment, but these automatically elicited goals themselves may well be represented in the person's conscious awareness. In the absence of evidence that the motives themselves are inaccessible to phenomenal awareness, the automatically activated motives envisioned by Bargh are probably better construed as motivational expressions of implicit perception or memory, rather than as implicit motives.

The Emotional Unconscious

The idea of an emotional unconscious, too, has its roots in Freud's notion that repres-
sion and the other defense mechanisms were designed to render us unaware of our true emotional states—especially the anxiety elicited by the conflict between our instinctual urges and the demands of external physical and social realities. On the other hand, many modern authorities appear to consider the idea of unconscious emotion a contradiction in terms. According to conventional formulations, both the stimuli that elicit emotions and the processes that generate them may be unconscious, but the emotional feeling state must be conscious almost by definition. But, if we accept the James–Lange formulation that emotions are the perceptions of bodily responses to stimuli, and we have already agreed that percepts can be unconscious, then it does not seem unreasonable to argue that emotions, too, might be inaccessible to conscious awareness under some circumstances. Accordingly, and again following the model of implicit memory, we may define explicit emotion as the conscious awareness of a feeling state, such as fear or joy; and implicit emotion as any change in a person's experience, thought, or action that is attributable to an emotional state, in the absence of (or independent of) conscious awareness of that feeling state (Kihlstrom, Mulvaney, Tobias, & Tobis, 2000).

This non-Freudian view of the emotional unconscious has its roots in Lang's multiple-system theory of emotion (Lang, 1968). We usually think of the subjective, behavioral, and physiological components of emotion as covarying together: When people feel afraid, their heart rates go up and they avoid the fear stimulus. When their fear is reduced, heart rate and avoidance decrease as well. However, Lang proposed that these three systems are partially independent, so that under some conditions they can move in quite different directions. Rachman and Hodgson (1974) picked up on Lang's theme and applied the term *desynchrony* to cases where one component of emotional response is dissociated from the others (Zinbarg, 1998). The emotional unconscious represents a desynchrony in cases in which the subjective component of an emotion, the conscious feeling state, is absent, while the behavioral and/or physiological components persist outside of phenomenal awareness.

The emotional unconscious is anticipated in the neuropsychological model of fear offered by LeDoux (1996) and has begun to attract interest among personality and social psychologists (Feldman-Barrett, Niedenthal, & Winkielman, 2005; Lambie & Marcel, 2002). Nevertheless, it must be admitted that empirical evidence for unconscious emotion has been hard to find. Unconscious emotion is implicated in a variety of individual-difference constructs relating to emotional experience and expression, such as repressive coping style, alexithymia, and even anhedonia. For example, Lane and his colleagues proposed that emotional awareness proceeds through five stages of development, in the lowest two of which people are aware of bodily sensations and actions, but not of emotions, per se (Lane & Schwartz, 1987).

Still, very little if any of this research has used paradigms modeled on the study of implicit perception and memory to document dissociations between conscious and unconscious emotion—if, for no other reason than that the subjects in question were rarely actually asked what they are feeling. In the pioneering study of D. A. Weinberger, Schwartz, and Davidson (1979), for example, subjects identified as "repressors" showed patterns of physiological response to sexual and aggressive verbal phrases that were similar to those of highly anxious, but nondefensive, subjects. The implication is that individuals displaying a repressive coping style have a talent for desynchrony: They may not experience high levels of stress, even though their physiology is churning away anxiously. Unfortunately, however, Weinberger and colleagues did not ask the subjects to rate their distress while reading the stimuli; so, we do not actually know what they were feeling at the time the measurements were made.

This problem was corrected in more recent studies by Berridge and Winkielman (Berridge & Winkielman, 2003; Winkielman, Berridge, & Wilbarger, 2005), in which subliminal (masked) presentation of happy and sad faces led to changes in consummatory behavior on the part of the subjects. Here, the change in behavior counts as an index of implicit perception, but because subjects' self-reported feelings showed no differences between groups, it counts as an index of implicit emotion as well. The change in consummatory behavior is arguably a consequence of changed emotional state, even though the subjects were unaware of this change.

Perhaps the best evidence for the increasing acceptance of the possibility of unconscious emotion has been the widespread interest, among social psychologists, in the concept of implicit attitudes (Greenwald & Banaji, 1995; Greenwald et al., 2002; Wittenbrink & Schwarz, 2007), and especially in the popularity of the Implicit Association Test (IAT) as a means of measuring them (Greenwald & Farnham, 2000; Greenwald, Nosek, & Banaji, 2003; Nosek, Greenwald, & Banaji, 2005; Rudman, Greenwald, Mellott, & Schwartz, 1999). Attitudes are, of course, an aspect of emotion, as the pro–anti dimension of evaluation implies an "affect for or against a psychological object" (Thurstone, 1931). Attitudes, like emotions, are generally construed as conscious mental dispositions, which is why they are typically measured by self-report questionnaires and rating scales. But Greenwald and Banaji argued that people could also possess positive and negative attitudes about themselves and other people that affect ongoing social cognition and behavior outside of conscious awareness.

Implicit attitudes can be revealed by traditional priming methodologies, as when white subjects are faster to endorse positive traits as characteristic of whites and negative traits as characteristic of blacks (Dovidio, Evans, & Tler, 1986), or when words such as *doctor* and *nurse* affect response latencies when subjects classify first names as male or female (Blair & Banaji, 1996). But these and other early studies did not always include an assessment of subjects' explicit, conscious attitudes. In fact, a study by Wittenbrink, Park, and Judd (1997) showed that the magnitude of race-specific priming was correlated with scores on a questionnaire measure of racial prejudice. It is one thing for priming to serve as an unobtrusive measure (Webb, Campbell, Schwartz, & Sechrest, 1966) of attitudes that subjects are unwilling to disclose; it is quite another for priming to serve as an implicit measure of attitudes that subjects are unaware they have (Kihlstrom, 2004).

Thus, the construct of an implicit attitude confronts the investigator with two problems. First is to ensure that subjects are telling the truth about their consciously accessible attitudes—which is to say that any explicit measure must not be contaminated by such factors as social desirability and other aspects of impression management. The explicit measure must be as good an assessment of the subject's conscious attitudes as we can find. Second is to show that the implicit attitude is dissociated from the explicit attitude. This requires more than a straightforward comparison of scores on the explicit and implicit measures. In the comparison of explicit and implicit memory, for example, the cues presented to the subject—the first three letters of a target word, for example—are held constant across tests. In the explicit test, the subject is asked to recall a list item that began with the step; in the implicit test, the subject is asked to report the first word that comes to mind. When a priming measure of attitude is compared with an attitude questionnaire, or an attitude thermometer, any differences between the two may be due to method variance, not to any dissociation between conscious and unconscious attitudes (Kihlstrom, 2004).

Similar problems crop up with the IAT—which, despite its initial capitalization, is more of a general-purpose method than a formal psychological instrument. In a version of the IAT designed to assess implicit self-esteem (Greenwald & Farnham, 2000), subjects might classify items (such as *John* and *Horseheads*) as self-relevant or not, and then make "good–bad" judgments about words known to have a positive or negative valence (e.g., *diamond* and *poison*), or positive or negative trait labels. When the two concept sets are combined, subjects will make faster responses when connotatively similar concepts share a response. In this way, faster response latencies that occur when a subject has to make the same response to self-relevant items and positive words, compared to non-self-relevant items and negative words, are interpreted as indicating high self-esteem. The IAT has become enormously popular; a quick PsycInfo search yielded 261 papers from its introduction, in 1998, through the end of 2006—but its interpretation is fraught with unresolved difficulties (Arkes & Tetlock, 2004; Blanton, Jaccard, Gonzales, & Christie, 2006; Brendl, Markman, & Messner, 2001). For example, the IAT is essentially a forced-choice measure, in which any advantage in response latency counts as evidence of a corresponding attitude. Thus, an individual who is positively disposed toward both whites and blacks, but who simply favors whites more (for whatever reason), will be regarded as equally prejudiced as an individual who actually favors whites and disfavors blacks. More critically, perhaps, differences in response latency can be produced by differences in both target difficulty and task difficulty. Thus, an individual who does not know many blacks, or much about blacks, may seem to be prejudiced, when in fact he or she is simply ignorant. Greenwald, Banaji, and others involved in what has come to be known as "Project Implicit" (*projectimplicit.net*) have tried to address these and other problems—sometimes with rhetoric (Banaji, Nosek, & Greenwald, 2004), but more often with data (Greenwald, Nosek, Banaji, & Klauer, 2005; Greenwald, Nosek, & Sriram, 2006). As a result, the psychometric properties of the IAT have improved as its scope has broadened.

One critical issue, however, remains unclear: whether the IAT actually measures unconscious attitudes, or whether it is an unobtrusive measure of conscious attitudes. In two surveys, the average correlation between the IAT and self-report measures of the same attitude (the latter typically by means of a "thermometer"-type rating scale) were $r = .25$ (Greenwald, McGhee, & Schwartz, 1998), $r = .43$ (Greenwald et al., 2003). A recent comprehensive survey of explicit–implicit correlations across 56 different domains yielded median rs (depending on the details of the calculation) of .37–.48. These correlations, although relatively low compared to those obtained between two explicit measures of the same construct (Cunningham, Preacher, & Banaji, 2001), are far from trivial; they are, for example, far above the correlations reported between TAT and questionnaire scores of human motives (Spangler, 1992). They are higher than Mischel's (1968) "personality coefficient" of .30, and about at the upper limit of what one would expect from correlations between questionnaire scores and measures of human performance. Given that the correlations between IAT and self-report measures are of at least "medium" strength by Cohen's (1988) standards, it appears that the IAT is best construed as an unobtrusive measure of conscious attitudes, rather than as a measure of unconscious attitudes. The impression that the IAT is *intended* to be an unobtrusive measure of conscious attitudes is strengthened by the fact that much of the evidence for improvements in the IAT (Greenwald et al., 2003) comes in the form of *increased* correlations with self-report measures.

THIS IS NOT
YOUR PSYCHOANALYST'S UNCONSCIOUS

Freud did not discover the psychological unconscious (Ellenberger, 1970; D. B. Klein, 1977; Whyte, 1960), but he did popularize the idea of unconscious mental life. Accordingly, there has been some tendency to claim that findings such as those summarized here prove that Freud was right after all (Bornstein & Masling, 1998; Erdelyi, 1985, 1996, 2006; Shevrin, Bond, Brakel, Hertel, & Williams, 1996; J. Weinberger & Westen, 2001; Westen, 1998a, 1998b, 1999). For example, Westen (1998b), after performing a review not unlike the present one, concluded that "the notion of unconscious processes is not psychoanalytic voodoo, and it is not the fantasy of muddle-headed clinicians. It is not only clinically indispensable, but it is good science" (p. 35).

True enough, so far as it goes, but Westen ignores the fact that none of the literature he has reviewed bears on the particular view of unconscious mental life offered by Freud. The fact that amnesic patients show priming effects on word-stem completion tasks and can acquire positive and negative emotional responses to other people, without having any conscious recollection of the experiences responsible for these effects, cannot be offered in support of a theory that attributes conscious behavior to repressed sexual and aggressive urges. None of the experiments reviewed involve sexual or aggressive contents, none of their results imply defensive acts of repression, and none of their results support hermeneutic methods of interpreting manifest contents in terms of latent contents. To say that this body of research supports psychoanalytic theory is to make what the philosopher Gilbert Ryle called a category mistake.

Rapaport (1960) importantly distinguished among four levels of psychoanalytic theorizing. At the highest, "metapsychological" level are broad, and frankly untestable, assumptions such as "the crucial determinants of behaviors are unconscious" (p. 46); nestled under that is a hierarchy of general,

specific, and empirical propositions that are increasingly testable. And it is at these levels where psychoanalytic theory crashes on the shoals of reality. For example, nothing in the evidence reviewed here even remotely suggests that the unconscious is a repository of primitive sexual and aggressive instincts. Nor is there any evidence for the idea that mental contents are rendered unconscious by means of a defensive process of repression. Nor is there any evidence that psychological trauma instigates amnesia via repression, or that the recovery of repressed memories is critical to the success of psychotherapy, or that neurotic symptoms are really implicit, if symbolic, memories of trauma (Kihlstrom, 2006; McNally, 2003; Pope, Oliva, & Hudson, 2000). All that really survives is Freud's distinction between conscious, preconscious, and unconscious mental life. In the modern usage, "unconscious" refers to those that are inaccessible to conscious awareness in principle, under any circumstances, whereas "preconscious" refers to mental contents that could be accessible to conscious awareness, if conditions were right. While preconscious percepts and memories are typically degraded, as in subliminal perception, "subconscious" mental contents are more fully analyzed. But even here, the modern definition of unconscious processes and preconscious contents owes nothing to Freud.

One response to this state of affairs is to argue that psychoanalytic theory itself has evolved since Freud, and that it is therefore unfair to bind psychoanalysis so tightly to the Freudian vision of repressed infantile sexual and aggressive urges, symbolically represented in dreams, errors, and symptoms, and revealed on the couch through free association. Westen (1998b) himself attempted this gambit, arguing that critics of psychoanalysis attack an archaic, obsolete version of psychodynamic theory and ignore more recent developments such as ego psychology and object relations theory. But, to borrow the language of the Vietnam war, this perspective destroys the village in order to save it. Culturally, the 20th century was the century of Sigmund Freud, not the century of Heinz Kohut or Melanie Klein. Freud's legacy is not to be assessed in terms of ideas that emerged since Freud died, but rather in terms of the ideas propounded by Freud himself through the 24 volumes of his *Col-*

lected Works. Chief among these is a particular view of unconscious mental life—a view that, to date, has found little or no support in empirical science. And, it must be said, the modern psychological laboratory offers little or nothing to support the theories of Kohut or Klein, either.

THE DENIAL OF CONSCIOUSNESS

One place where Freud's influence can be felt, however remotely, is in the contemporary enthusiasm, among many personality and social psychologists, for the concept of automaticity—a trend that I have come to call the *automaticity juggernaut* (Kihlstrom, 2008). Certainly, the concept of automaticity has come to play a powerful role in personality and social psychology (Bargh, 1984; Chaiken & Trope, 1999; Wegner & Bargh, 1998). The general argument is that some of the processes involved in social cognition, and some of the processes by which social cognitions are translated into social behavior, are executed automatically. Thus, it is generally accepted that attitudes, impressions, and other social judgments, as well as aggression, compliance, prejudice, and other social behaviors, are often mediated by automatic processes that operate outside phenomenal awareness and voluntary control.

Beyond that, however, some personality and social psychologists have argued that social cognition and behavior are dominated by unconscious, automatic processes, to the virtual exclusion of conscious, controlled ones (Bargh, 1997; Bargh & Chartrand, 1999; Bargh & Uleman, 1989; Langer, 1978). Similarly, Wegner concluded that automatic processes typically dominate controlled ones (Wegner & Schneider, 1989), and more recently asserted that conscious will is an illusion, and that the real causes of human action are unconscious, automatic processes (Kihlstrom, 2004c; Wegner, 2002). And Wilson, while initially proposing a dual-process model of attitudes, both controlled and automatic (Wilson, Lindsey, & Schooler, 2000), has more recently concluded that "Freud's view of the unconscious was far too limited. When he said ... that consciousness is the tip of the mental iceberg ... it may be more the size of a snowball on top of that iceberg"

(Kihlstrom, 2004b, 2004c; Wilson, 2002). Both Bargh (1997) and Wegner (Wegner & Smart, 1997) have expressly replaced Freud's view of unconscious determination with the more modern concept of automaticity.

To some extent, the widespread embrace of automaticity is a reaction to an earlier view of social interaction that seemed to inappropriately emphasize conscious, rational, cognitive processes at the expense of the unconscious, irrational, emotive, and conative. But the embrace of automaticity also represents a reverting to earlier situationist views within social psychology (Berkowitz & Devine, 1995; Ross & Nisbett, 1991). This regressive situation has been clearly articulated by Bargh (1997), who noted that "as Skinner argued so pointedly, the more we know about the situational causes of psychological phenomena, the less need we have for postulating internal conscious mediating processes to explain those phenomena" (p. 1). In fact, Bargh has concluded that automaticity solves the problem of Skinnerian radical behaviorism by showing how environmental stimuli are connected to organismal responses by a web of intervening processes that unfold automatically (Bargh & Ferguson, 2000). Bargh's position is not classically Skinnerian, because he shares the central dogma of cognitive social psychology: that social behavior is caused by the actor's internal mental representation of the situation, rather than the situation as it might be described objectively. But by asserting that this internal mental representation is itself constructed automatically and perhaps influences behavior preconsciously, he maintains a superficial allegiance to cognitivism while at the same time harkening back to radical situationism. If the cognitive processes underlying social cognition and social behavior are largely automatic, then not too much thought has gone into them.

The irony in the popularity of automaticity is that there is no empirical evidence to support the proposition that social behavior is exclusively, or even predominantly, determined by automatic processes. Most studies of automaticity in personality and social psychology simply do not include a control condition invoking controlled processes. And in the few studies where the power of automatic and controlled processes has been directly compared, as with Jacoby's (1991) process-dissociation procedure, controlled processes almost always prove to be stronger (Payne, 2005; Uleman, Blader, & Todorov, 2005). The automaticity juggernaut, far from representing an evidence-based conclusion about the nature of human social cognition and behavior, seems rather to reflect a kind of "shyness" about consciousness (Flanagan, 1992)—at best, a stance of conscious inessentialism, which holds that consciousness is necessary for adaptive action; and at worst, a stance of epiphenomenalism, which holds that consciousness has no causal function at all. One who has spent the better part of his professional career trying to get his colleagues to take a non-Freudian view of unconscious mental life seriously is reminded of Aesop's fable of King Midas (or is it The Frogs Asking for a King?): Be careful what you wish for.

CONSCIOUSNESS, THE PSYCHOLOGICAL UNCONSCIOUS, AND THE SELF

More positively, experimental studies of the psychological unconscious shed light on the nature of consciousness itself. At a psychological level of analysis, it seems that conscious awareness requires that a mental representation of an event be connected with some mental representation of the self as agent or experiencer of that event (Kihlstrom, 1993, 1997). Of course, the idea that consciousness and self are deeply intertwined is not new. In his discussion of the stream of consciousness, James (1890/1980) wrote that "the first fact for ... psychologists is that thinking of some sort goes on" (p. 219). He also wrote, immediately thereafter, that "thought tends to personal form" (p. 220)—that is, every thought (by which James meant every conscious mental state) is part of a personal consciousness:

> The only states of consciousness that we naturally deal with are found in personal consciousnesses, minds, selves, concrete particular I's and you's [sic]. ... It seems as if the elementary psychic fact were not *thought* or *this thought* or *that thought*, but *my thought*, every thought being owned. ... On these terms the personal self rather than the thought might be treated as the immediate datum for psychology. The universal conscious fact is not "feelings exist" or "thoughts exist" but "*I* think" and "*I* feel." (p. 221, original emphasis)

In other words, an episode of ongoing experience, thought, and action becomes conscious if, and only if, a link is made between the mental representation of the event itself and some mental representation of the self (Kihlstrom et al., 2002; Kihlstrom & Cantor, 1984; Kihlstrom & Klein, 1997) as the agent or experiencer of that event. Janet (1907) put it so well:

> The complete consciousness which is expressed by the words, "I see, I feel a movement" ... contains a new term, the word "I," which designates ... the idea of personality, of my whole person. ... There are then in the "I feel," two things in presence of each other: a small, new, psychological fact, a little flame lighting up— "feel"—and an enormous mass of thoughts already constituted into a system—"I." These two things mingle, combine: and to say "I feel" is to say that the already enormous personality has seized upon and absorbed that little, new sensation which has just been produced.

It is precisely this mental representation of self that is missing in cases of unconscious influence. As Claparede (1911/1951) put it, when describing the implicit memory of an amnesic patient: "If one examines the behavior of such a patient, one finds that everything happens as though the various events of life, however well associated with each other in the mind, were incapable of integration with *the me* itself" (p. 71).

What unites the various phenomena of the psychological unconscious—implicit perception, memory, learning, and thought; implicit motivation and emotion as well—is the loss of the link between whatever is going through the person's mind at the moment and a mental representation of the self currently active in working memory. In this way, the study of unconscious mental life, by shedding light on the importance of the self for consciousness, suggests how James's two candidates for the "datum of psychology"—thought and self—fit into a single, unified whole. The psychological unconscious, which might have remained the province of cognitive psychology, returns to the domain of personality psychology in modern form, without the excess baggage of Freudian psychodynamics.

REFERENCES

Many relevant references have been eliminated in the interest of space. For a more complete list of references, see *socrates.berkeley.edu/~kihlstrm/ Pervin3.htm.*

Allport, G. W. (1937). *Personality: A psychological interpretation.* New York: Holt, Rinehart & Winston.

Arkes, H. R., & Tetlock, P. E. (2004). Attributions of implicit prejudice, or "Would Jesse Jackson 'fail' the Implicit Association Test?". *Psychological Inquiry, 15,* 257–321.

Asendorpf, J. B. (2007). Implicit representations and personality. *International Journal of Psychology, 42,* 145–148.

Banaji, M. R., Nosek, B. A., & Greenwald, A. G. (2004). No place for nostalgia in science: A response to Arkes and Tetlock. *Psychological Inquiry, 15,* 279–289.

Bandura, A. (1977). *Social learning theory.* Englewood Cliffs, NJ: Prentice-Hall.

Bandura, A. (1986). *Social foundations of thought and action: A social cognitive theory.* Englewood Cliffs, NJ: Prentice-Hall.

Bargh, J. A. (1984). Automatic and conscious processing of social information. In R. S. Wyer & T. K. Srull (Eds.), *Handbook of social cognition* (pp. 1–43). Hillsdale, NJ: Erlbaum.

Bargh, J. A. (1990). Auto-motives: Preconscious determinants of social interaction. In E. T. Higgins & R. M. Sorrentino (Eds.), *Handbook of motivation and cognition* (pp. 93–130). New York: Guilford Press.

Bargh, J. A. (1997). The automaticity of everyday life. In R. S. Wyer (Ed.), *Advances in social cognition* (Vol. 10, pp. 1–61). Mahwah, NJ: Erlbaum.

Bargh, J. A., & Barndollar, K. (1996). Automaticity in action: The unconscious as repository of chronic goals and motives. In P. M. Gollwitzer & J. A. Bargh (Eds.), *The psychology of action: Linking cognition and motivation to behavior* (pp. 457–481). New York: Guilford Press.

Bargh, J. A., & Chartrand, T. L. (1999). The unbearable automaticity of being. *American Psychologist, 54*(7), 462–479.

Bargh, J. A., & Ferguson, M. J. (2000). Beyond behaviorism: On the automaticity of higher mental processes. *Psychological Bulletin, 126*(6), 925–945.

Bargh, J. A., Gollwitzer, P. M., LeeChai, A., Barndollar, K., & Trotschel, R. (2001). The automated will: Nonconscious activation and pursuit of behavioral goals. *Journal of Personality and Social Psychology, 81*(6), 1014–1027.

Bargh, J. A., & Uleman, J. S. (1989). Introduction. In J. S. Uleman & J. A. Bargh (Eds.), *Unintended thought: Causes and consequences for judgment, emotion, and behavior* (pp. 3–51). New York: Guilford Press.

Bechara, A., Damasio, H., Tranel, D., & Damasio, A. R. (1997). Deciding advantageously before knowing the advantageous strategy. *Science, 275,* 1293–1295.

Berkowitz, L., & Devine, P. G. (1995). Has social psychology always been cognitive? What is "cognitive" anyhow? *Personality and Social Psychology Bulletin, 21*(7), 696–703.

Berridge, K. C., & Winkielman, P. (2003). What is an unconscious emotion? (The case for unconscious "liking"). *Cognition and Emotion, 17,* 181–211.

Blair, I. V., & Banaji, M. R. (1996). Automatic and controlled processes in stereotype priming. *Journal of Personality and Social Psychology, 70,* 1142–1163.

Blanton, H., Jaccard, J., Gonzales, P. M., & Christie, C. (2006). Decoding the Implicit Association Test: Implications for criterion prediction. *Journal of Experimental Social Psychology, 42*(2), 192–212.

Bornstein, R. F. (1989). Exposure and affect: Overview and meta-analysis of research, 1968–1987. *Psychological Bulletin, 106,* 265–289.

Bornstein, R. F., & Masling, J. M. (Eds.). (1998). *Empirical perspectives on the psychoanalytic unconscious.* Washington, DC: American Psychological Association.

Bowden, E. M., Jung-Beeman, M., Fleck, J., & Kounios, J. (2006). New approaches to demystifying insight. *Trends in Cognitive Sciences, 9,* 322–328.

Bowers, K. S., Farvolden, P., & Mermigis, L. (1995). Intuitive antecedents of insight. In S. M. Smith, T. M. Ward, & R. A. Finke (Eds.), *The creative cognition approach* (pp. 27–51). Cambridge, MA: MIT Press.

Bowers, K. S., Regehr, G., Balthazard, C., & Parker, K. (1990). Intuition in the context of discovery. *Cognitive Psychology, 22,* 72–110.

Brendl, C. M., Markman, A. B., & Messner, C. (2001). How do indirect measures of evaluation work?: Evaluating the inference of prejudice in the Implicit Association Test. *Journal of Personality and Social Psychology, 81*(5), 760–773.

Bruner, J., & Klein, G. S. (1960). The functions of perceiving: New Look retrospect. In B. Kaplan & S. Wapner (Eds.), *Perspectives in psychological theory* (pp. 61–77). New York: International Universities Press.

Cantor, N., & Kihlstrom, J. F. (1987). *Personality and social intelligence.* Englewood Cliffs, NJ: Prentice-Hall.

Chaiken, S., & Trope, Y. (Eds.). (1999). *Dual-process theories in social psychology.* New York: Guilford Press.

Cheesman, J., & Merikle, P. M. (1986). Distinguishing conscious from unconscious perceptual processes. *Canadian Journal of Psychology, 40,* 343–367.

Claparede, E. (1951). [Recognition and me-ness]. In D. Rapaport (Ed.), *Organization and pathology of thought: Selected sources* (pp. 58–75). New York: Columbia University Press. (Original work published 1911)

Cohen, J. (1988). *Statistical power analysis for the behavioral sciences* (2nd ed.). Hillsdale, NJ: Erlbaum.

Cunningham, W. A., Preacher, K. J., & Banaji, M. (2001). Implicit attitude measures: Consistency, stability, and convergent validity. *Psychological Science, 12,* 163–170.

Dorfman, J., Shames, V. A., & Kihlstrom, J. F. (1996). Intuition, incubation, and insight: Implicit cognition in problem solving. In G. Underwood (Ed.), *Implicit cognition* (pp. 257–296). Oxford, UK: Oxford University Press.

Dovidio, J. F., Evans, N., & Tler, R. B. (1986). Racial stereotypes: The contents of their cognitive representations. *Journal of Experimental and Social Psychology, 22,* 22–37.

Draine, S. C., & Greenwald, A. G. (1998). Replicable unconscious semantic priming. *Journal of Experimental Psychology: General, 127*(3), 286–303.

Ellenberger, H. F. (1970). *The discovery of the unconscious: The history and evolution of dynamic psychiatry.* New York: Basic Books.

Erdelyi, M. H. (1985). *Psychoanalysis: Freud's cognitive psychology.* New York: Freeman.

Erdelyi, M. H. (1996). *The recovery of unconscious memories: Hypermnesia and reminiscence.* Chicago: University of Chicago Press.

Erdelyi, M. H. (2006). The unified theory of repression. *Behavioral and Brain Sciences, 29,* 499–551.

Feldman-Barrett, L., Niedenthal, P. M., & Winkielman, P. (Eds.). (2005). *Emotion and consciousness.* New York: Guilford Press.

Freud, S. (1953). The interpretation of dreams. In J. Strachey (Ed.), *The standard edition of the complete psychological works of Sigmund Freud* (Vols. 4–5). London: Hogarth Press. (Original work published 1990)

Freud, S. (1961). The ego and the id. In J. Strachey (Ed.), *The standard edition of the complete psychological works of Sigmund Freud* (Vol. 19). London: Hogarth Press. (Original work published 1923)

Flanagan, O. (1992). *Conscousness reconsidered.* Cambridge, MA: MIT Press.

Greenwald, A. G., & Banaji, M. R. (1995). Implicit social cognition: Attitudes, self-esteem, and stereotypes. *Psychological Review, 102,* 4–27.

Greenwald, A. G., Banaji, M. R., Rudman, L. A., Farnham, S. D., Nosek, B. A., & Mellott, D. S.

(2002). A unified theory of implicit attitudes, stereotypes, self-esteem, and self-concept. *Psychological Review, 109*(1), 3–25.

Greenwald, A. G., Draine, S. C., & Abrams, R. L. (1996). Three cognitive markers of unconscious semantic activation. *Science, 273,* 1699–1702.

Greenwald, A. G., & Farnham, S. D. (2000). Using the Implicit Association Test to measure self-esteem and self-concept. *Journal of Personality and Social Psychology, 79*(6), 1022–1038.

Greenwald, A. G., Klinger, M. R., & Liu, T. J. (1989). Unconscious processing of dichotically masked words. *Memory and Cognition, 17,* 35–47.

Greenwald, A. G., McGhee, D. E., & Schwartz, J. L. K. (1998). Measuring individual differences in implicit cognition: The Implicit Association Test. *Journal of Personality and Social Psychology, 74,* 1464–1480.

Greenwald, A. G., Nosek, B. A., & Banaji, M. R. (2003). Understanding and using the Implicit Association Test: I. An improved scoring algorithm. *Journal of Personality and Social Psychology, 85,* 197–216.

Greenwald, A. G., Nosek, B. A., Banaji, M. R., & Klauer, K. C. (2005). Validity of the salience asymmetry interpretation of the Implicit Association Test: Comment on Rothermund and Wentura (2004). *Journal of Experimental Psychology: General, 134,* 420–425.

Greenwald, A. G., Nosek, B. A., & Sriram, N. (2006). Consequential validity of the Implicit Association Test: Comment on Blanton and Jaccard (2006). *American Psychologist, 61,* 56–61.

Hassin, R. R., Uleman, J. S., & Bargh, J. A. (Eds.). (2005). *The new unconscious.* New York: Oxford University Press.

Hilgard, E. R. (1977). *Divided consciousness: Multiple controls in human thought and action.* New York: Wiley.

Hilgard, E. R. (1980a). Consciousness in contemporary psychology. *Annual Review of Psychology, 31,* 1–26.

Hilgard, E. R. (1980b). The trilogy of mind: Cognition, affection, and conation. *Journal for the History of the Behavioral Sciences, 16,* 107–117.

Jacoby, L. L. (1991). A process dissociation framework: Separating automatic from intentional uses of memory. *Journal of Memory and Language, 13,* 513–541.

James, W. (1980). *Principles of psychology.* Cambridge, MA: Harvard University Press. (Original work published 1890)

Janet, P. (1907). *The major symptoms of hysteria.* New York: Macmillan.

Johnson, M. K., & Multhaup, K. S. (1992). Emotion and MEM. In S.-A. Christianson

(Ed.), *Handbook of emotion and memory* (pp. 33–66). Hillsdale, NJ: Erlbaum.

Jung-Beeman, M., & Bowden, E. M. (2000). The right hemisphere maintains solution-related activation for yet-to-be solved insight problems. *Memory and Cognition, 28,* 1231–1241.

Kelly, G. (1955). *The psychology of personal constructs.* New York: Norton.

Kihlstrom, J. F. (1987). The cognitive unconscious. *Science, 237,* 1445–1452.

Kihlstrom, J. F. (1993). The psychological unconscious and the self. *Ciba Foundation Symposium, 174,* 147–167.

Kihlstrom, J. F. (1996). Perception without awareness of what is perceived, learning without awareness of what is learned. In M. Velmans (Ed.), *The science of consciousness: Psychological, neuropsychological and clinical reviews* (pp. 23–46). London: Routledge.

Kihlstrom, J. F. (1997). Consciousness and me-ness. In J. D. Cohen & J. W. Schooler (Eds.), *Scientific approaches to consciousness* (pp. 451–468). Mahwah, NJ: Erlbaum.

Kihlstrom, J. F. (2001). Dissociative disorders. In P. B. Sutker & H. E. Adams (Eds.), *Comprehensive handbook of psychopathology* (3rd ed., pp. 259–276). New York: Plenum Press.

Kihlstrom, J. F. (2004a). Implicit methods in social psychology. In C. Sansone, C. C. Morf, & A. T. Panter (Eds.), *The Sage handbook of methods in social psychology* (pp. 195–212). Thousand Oaks, CA: Sage.

Kihlstrom, J. F. (2004b). An unwarrantable impertinence [Commentary on *The Illusion of Conscious Will* by D. M. Wegner]. *Behavioral and Brain Sciences, 27,* 666–667.

Kihlstrom, J. F. (2005). Dissociative disorders. *Annual Review of Clinical Psychology, 1,* 277–253.

Kihlstrom, J. F. (2006). Trauma and memory revisited. In B. Uttl, N. Ohta, & A. L. Siegenthaler (Eds.), *Memory and emotions: Interdisciplinary perspectives* (pp. 259–291). New York: Blackwell.

Kihlstrom, J. F. (2008). The automaticity juggernaut. In J. Baer, J. C. Kaufman, & R. F. Baumeister (Eds.), *Psychology and free will* (pp. 155–180). New York: Oxford University Press.

Kihlstrom, J. F., Barnhardt, T. M., & Tataryn, D. J. (1992). Implicit perception. In R. F. Bornstein & T. S. Pittman (Eds.), *Perception without awareness: Cognitive, clinical, and social perspectives* (pp. 17–54). New York: Guilford Press.

Kihlstrom, J. F., Beer, J. S., & Klein, S. B. (2002). Self and identity as memory. In M. R. Leary & J. Tangney (Eds.), *Handbook of self and identity* (pp. 68–90). New York: Guilford Press.

Kihlstrom, J. F., & Cantor, N. (1984). Mental representations of the self. In L. Berkowitz (Ed.), *Advances in experimental social psychology* (Vol. 17, pp. 1–47). New York: Academic Press.

Kihlstrom, J. F., & Cantor, N. (2000). Social intelligence. In R. J. Sternberg (Ed.), *Handbook of intelligence* (pp. 359–379). New York: Cambridge University Press.

Kihlstrom, J. F., Cantor, N., Albright, J. S., Chew, B. R., Klein, S. B., & Niedenthal, P. M. (1988). Information processing and the study of the self. In L. Berkowitz (Ed.), *Advances in experimental social psychology: Vol. 21. Social psychological studies of the self: Perspectives and programs* (pp. 145–178). San Diego, CA: Academic Press.

Kihlstrom, J. F., & Klein, S. B. (1994). The self as a knowledge structure. In R. S. Wyer & T. K. Srull (Eds.), *Handbook of social cognition: Vol. 1. Basic processes* (pp. 153–208). Hillsdale, NJ: Erlbaum.

Kihlstrom, J. F., & Klein, S. B. (1997). Self-knowledge and self-awareness. In J. G. Snodgrass & R. L. Thompson (Eds.), *The self across psychology: Self-recognition, self-awareness, and the self concept* (pp. 5–17). New York: New York Academy of Sciences.

Kihlstrom, J. F., Marchese-Foster, L. A., & Klein, S. B. (1997). Situating the self in interpersonal space. In U. Neisser & D. A. Jopling (Eds.), *The conceptual self in context: Culture, experience, self-understanding* (pp. 154–175). New York: Cambridge University Press.

Kihlstrom, J. F., Mulvaney, S., Tobias, B. A., & Tobis, I. P. (2000). The emotional unconscious. In E. Eich, J. F. Kihlstrom, G. H. Bower, J. P. Forgas, & P. M. Niedenthl (Eds.), *Cognition and emotion* (pp. 30–86). New York: Oxford University Press.

Kihlstrom, J. F., Shames, V. A., & Dorfman, J. (1996). Intimations of memory and thought. In L. M. Reder (Ed.), *Implicit memory and metacognition* (pp. 1–23). Mahwah, NJ: Erlbaum.

Klein, D. B. (1977). *The unconscious: Invention or discovery?* Santa Monica, CA: Goodyear.

Klein, S. B., Cosmides, L., & Costabile, K. A. (2003). Preserved knowledge of self in a case of Alzheimer's dementia. *Social Cognition, 21*(2), 157–165.

Klein, S. B., Loftus, J., & Kihlstrom, J. F. (1996). Self-knowledge of an amnesic patient: Toward a neuropsychology of personality and social psychology. *Journal of Experimental Psychology: General, 125*(3), 250–260.

Klein, S. B., Loftus, J., & Kihlstrom, J. F. (2002). Memory and temporal experience: The effects of episodic memory loss on an amnesic patient's ability to remember the past and imagine the future. *Social Cognition, 20,* 353–379.

Kunst-Wilson, W. R., & Zajonc, R. B. (1980). Affective discrimination of stimuli that cannot be recognized. *Science, 207,* 557–558.

LaBerge, D., & Samuels, S. J. (1974). Toward a theory of automatic information processing in reading. *Cognitive Psychology, 6*(2), 293–323.

Lambie, J. A., & Marcel, A. J. (2002). Consciousness and the varieties of emotion experience: A theoretical framework. *Psychological Review, 109*(2), 219–259.

Lane, R. D., & Schwartz, G. E. (1987). Levels of emotional awareness: A cognitive-developmental theory and its application to psychopathology. *American Journal of Psychiatry, 144,* 133–143.

Lang, P. J. (1968). Fear reduction and fear behavior: Problems in treating a construct. In J. M. Schlein (Ed.), *Research in psychotherapy* (Vol. 3, pp. 90–103). Washington, DC: American Psychological Association.

Langer, E. J. (1978). Rethinking the role of thought in social interaction. In J. H. Harvey, W. J. Ickes, & R. F. Kidd (Eds.), *New directions in attribution research* (Vol. 2, pp. 35–58). Potomac, MD: Erlbaum.

LeDoux, J. E. (1996). *The emotional brain: The mysterious underpinnings of emotional life.* New York: Simon & Schuster.

Macmillan, M. (1991/1997). *Freud evaluated: The completed arc.* Cambridge, MA: MIT Press.

Marcel, A. J. (1983a). Conscious and unconscious perception: An approach to the relations between phenomenal experience and perceptual processes. *Cognitive Psychology, 15,* 238–300.

Marcel, A. J. (1983b). Conscious and unconscious perception: Experiments on visual masking and word recognition. *Cognitive Psychology, 15,* 197–237.

McClelland, D. C. (1980). Motive dispositions: The merits of operant and respondent measures. *Review of Personality and Social Psychology, 1,* 10–41.

McClelland, D. C., Koestner, R., & Weinberger, J. (1989). How do self-attributed and implicit motives differ? *Psychological Review, 96,* 690–702.

McNally, R. J. (2003). *Remembering trauma.* Cambridge, MA: Harvard University Press.

Merikle, P. M., & Reingold, E. M. (1990). Recognition and lexical decision without detection: Unconscious perception? *Journal of Experimental Psychology: Human Perception and Performance, 16,* 574–583.

Metcalfe, J., & Mischel, W. (1999). A hot/cool system analysis of delay of gratification: Dynamics of willpower. *Psychological Review, 106,* 3–19.

Miller, N. E., & Dollard, J. (1941). *Social learning and imitation.* New Haven, CT: Yale University Press.

Mischel, W. (1968). *Personality and assessment.* New York: Wiley.

Mischel, W. (1973). Toward a cognitive social learning reconceptualization of personality. *Psychological Review, 80*(4), 252–253.

Nosek, B. A., Greenwald, A. G., & Banaji, M. R. (2005). Understanding and using the Implicit Association Test: II. Method variables and construct validity. *Personality and Social Psychology Bulletin, 31,* 166–180.

Payne, B. K. (2005). Conceptualizing control in social cognition: How executive functioning modulates the expression of automatic stereotyping. *Journal of Personality and Social Psychology, 89,* 489–503.

Pope, H. G., Oliva, P. S., & Hudson, J. I. (2000). Repressed memories: B. Scientific status. In D. L. Faigman, D. H. Kaye, M. J. Saks, & J. Sanders (Eds.), *Modern scientific evidence: The law and science of expert testimony* (Vol. 1, pp. 154–195). St. Paul, MN: West.

Posner, M. I., & Snyder, C. R. R. (1975). Attention and cognitive control. In R. L. Solso (Ed.), *Information processing and cognition: The Loyola Symposium* (pp. 55–85). New York: Wiley.

Rachman, S., & Hodgson, R. E. (1974). Synchrony and desynchrony in measures of fear. *Behaviour Research and Therapy, 12,* 311–318.

Rapaport, D. (1960). The structure of psychoanalytic theory: A systematizing attempt. *Psychological Issues, 2*(2), Whole No. 6.

Reber, A. S. (1967). Implicit learning of artificial grammars. *Journal of Verbal Learning and Verbal Behavior, 6,* 855–863.

Robinson, M. D. (2007). Lives lived in milliseconds: Using cognitive methods in personality research. In R. W. Robins, R. C. Fraley, & R. F. Krueger (Eds.), *Handbook of research methods in personality psychology* (pp. 345–359). New York: Guilford Press.

Ross, L., & Nisbett, R. E. (1991). *The person and the situation: Perspectives of social psychology.* Philadelphia: Temple University Press.

Rotter, J. B. (1954). *Social learning and clinical psychology.* Englewood Cliffs, NJ: Prentice-Hall.

Rudman, L. A., Greenwald, A. G., Mellott, D. S., & Schwartz, J. L. K. (1999). Measuring the automatic components of prejudice: Flexibility and generality of the Implicit Association Test. *Social Cognition, 17*(4), 437–465.

Rudman, L. A., & Spencer, S. J. (2007). The implicit self. *Self and Identity, 6,* 97–100.

Schacter, D. L. (1987). Implicit memory: History and current status. *Journal of Experimental Psychology: Learning, Memory, and Cognition, 13,* 501–518.

Schneider, W., & Shiffrin, R. M. (1977). Controlled and automatic human information processing: I. Detection, search, and attention. *Psychological Review, 84*(1), 1–66.

Schultheiss, O. C., & Pang, J. S. (2007). Measuring implicit motives. In R. W. Robins, R. C. Fraley, & R. F. Krueger (Eds.), *Handbook of research methods in personality psychology* (pp. 322–344). New York: Guilford Press.

Shames, V. A. (1994). *Is there such a thing as implicit problem-solving?* Unpublished doctoral dissertation, University of Arizona, Tucson.

Shevrin, H., Bond, J. A., Brakel, L. A. W., Hertel, R. K., & Williams, W. J. (1996). *Conscious and unconscious processes: Psychodynamic, cognitive, and neurophysiological convergences.* New York: Guilford Press.

Siegler, R. S. (2000). Unconscious insights. *Current Directions in Psychological Science, 9*(3), 79–83.

Spangler, W. D. (1992). Validity of questionnaire and TAT measures of need for achievement: Two meta-analyses. *Psychological Bulletin, 112,* 140–154.

Thrash, T. M., & Elliot, A. J. (2002). Implicit and self-attributed achievement motives: Concordance and predictive validity. *Journal of Personality, 70*(5), 729–755.

Thurstone, L. L. (1931). The measurement of attitudes. *Journal of Abnormal and Social Psychology, 4,* 25–29.

Tulving, E. (1993). Self-knowledge of an amnesic individual is represented abstractly. In T. K. Srull & R. S. Wyer (Eds.), *Advances in social cognition* (Vol. 5, pp. 147–156). Hillsdale, NJ: Erlbaum.

Uleman, J. S., & Bargh, J. A. (Eds.). (1989). *Unintended thought.* New York: Guilford Press.

Uleman, J. S., Blader, S. L., & Todorov, A. (2005). Implicit impressions. In R. R. Hassin, J. S. Uleman, & J. A. Bargh (Eds.), *The new unconscious* (pp. 362–392). New York: Oxford University Press.

Webb, E. J., Campbell, D. T., Schwartz, R. D., & Sechrest, L. (1966). *Unobtrusive measures: Nonreactive research in the social sciences.* Chicago: Rand McNally.

Wegner, D. M. (2002). *The illusion of conscious will.* Cambridge, MA: MIT Press.

Wegner, D. M., & Bargh, J. A. (1998). Control and automaticity in social life. In D. Gilbert, S. T. Fiske, & G. Lindzey (Eds.), *Handbook of social psychology* (Vol. 1, pp. 446–496). Boston: McGraw-Hill.

Wegner, D. M., & Schneider, D. J. (1989). Mental control: The war of the ghosts in the machine. In J. S. Uleman & J. A. Bargh (Eds.), *Unintended thought* (pp. 287–305). New York: Guilford Press.

Wegner, D. M., & Smart, L. (1997). Deep cognitive activation: A new approach to the unconscious. *Journal of Consulting and Clinical Psychology, 65,* 984–995.

Weinberger, D. A., Schwartz, G. E., & Davidson, R. J. (1979). Low-anxious, high-anxious, and repressive coping styles: Psychometric patterns and behavioral and physiological responses to stress. *Journal of Abnormal Psychology, 88,* 369–380.

Weinberger, J., & Westen, D. (2001). Science and psychodynamics: From arguments about Freud to data. *Psychological Inquiry, 12*(3), 129–132.

Weiskrantz, L. (1986). *Blindsight: A case study and implications.* Oxford, UK: Oxford University Press.

Westen, D. (1998a). The scientific legacy of Sigmund Freud: Toward a psychodynamically informed psychological science. *Psychological Bulletin, 124,* 333–371.

Westen, D. (1998b). Unconscious thought, feeling, and motivation: The end of a century-long debate. In R. F. Bornstein & J. M. Masling (Eds.), *Empirical perspectives on the psychoanalytic unconscious* (pp. 1–44). Washington, DC: American Psychological Association.

Westen, D. (1999). The scientific status of unconscious processes: Is Freud really dead? *Journal of the American Psychoanalytic Association, 47*(4), 1061–1106.

Whyte, L. L. (1960). *The unconscious before Freud.* New York: Basic Books.

Wilson, T. D. (2002). *Strangers to ourselves: Discovering the adaptive unconscious.* Cambridge, MA: Belknap Press of Harvard University Press.

Wilson, T. D., Lindsey, S., & Schooler, T. Y. (2000). A model of dual attitudes. *Psychological Review, 107*(1), 101–126.

Winkielman, P., Berridge, K. C., & Wilbarger, J. L. (2005). Unconscious affective reactions to masked happy versus angry faces influence consumption behavior and judgments of value. *Personality and Social Psychology Bulletin, 31,* 121–135.

Wittenbrink, B., Judd, C. M., & Park, B. (1997). Evidence for racial prejudice at the implicit level and its relationship with questionnaire measures. *Journal of Personality and Social Psychology, 72,* 262–274.

Wittenbrink, B., & Schwarz, N. (Eds.). (2007). *Implicit measures of attitudes.* New York: Guilford Press.

Woike, B., Mcleod, S., & Goggin, M. (2003). Implicit and explicit motives influence accessibility to different autobiographical knowledge. *Personality and Social Psychology Bulletin, 29,* 1046–1055.

Zajonc, R. B. (1980). Feeling and thinking: Preferences need no inferences. *American Psychologist, 35,* 151–175.

Zajonc, R. B. (1984). On the primacy of affect. *American Psychologist, 39,* 117–123.

Zinbarg, R. E. (1998). Concordance and synchrony in measures of anxiety and panic reconsidered: A hierarchical model of anxiety and panic. *Behavior Therapy, 29,* 301–323.

CHAPTER 24

Implicit Motives

Oliver C. Schultheiss

Implicit motives are motivational dispositions that operate outside of a person's conscious awareness and are aimed at the attainment of specific classes of incentives and the
avoidance of specific classes of disincentives.
In this chapter, I review the affective, cognitive, physiological, and behavioral functions
of implicit motives; the assessment of motive
dispositions; and the role of implicit motives
in political, economic, and societal phenomena. I also outline a conceptual model to account for some key differences between implicit motives and conscious modes of goal
striving.

PROFILES OF IMPLICIT MOTIVES

Over the past 50 years, most implicit motive
research has focused on achievement, affiliation, and power motives. Individuals with
a strong achievement motive get a kick out
of doing something well or improving on
a task; individuals with a strong affiliation
motive experience close, harmonious contact
with other people as satisfying; and individuals with a strong power motive derive pleasure from having an impact on and dominat-
ing others (e.g., McClelland, 1987; Winter,
1996). In the following sections, I provide
short profiles of these three motives and dis-

cuss the hope and fear aspects of implicit motives. A systematic overview of these motives
and their correlates is given in Table 24.1.

The Achievement Motive

The psychological kernel of the achievement
motive is the *capacity to derive satisfaction
from the autonomous mastery of challenging
tasks* (McClelland, Atkinson, Clark, & Lowell, 1953; Schultheiss & Brunstein, 2005).
Achievement-motivated individuals prefer to
work on tasks of medium difficulty, on which
the chances of success are neither too high
nor too low and that demand their full concentration and effort (McClelland, 1987). If
they cannot choose and solve such tasks on
their own terms, but are given explicit advice and direction on how to do it, they are
likely to leave the field and invest no effort
in the task (Spangler, 1992). Individuals low
in achievement, in contrast, typically avoid
medium-difficulty tasks, because they require
effort, and success is neither likely to come
quickly nor guaranteed in the first place. So
why do achievement-motivated people like
to solve challenging tasks and why are they
so fiercely independent-minded about it?
 A look at the developmental precursors of achievement motivation, identified
in longitudinal and observational studies,

TABLE 24.1. Incentives and Correlates of Major Implicit Motives

| | Motive | | |
	Achievement	Affiliation	Power
Incentive	Autonomous mastery of challenging tasks	Social closeness with others	Having impact on others; dominating others
Disincentive	Failure to master a challenging task on one's own	Discord, rejection, loneliness	Defeat; another's dominance
Physiological correlates	Release of arginine-vasopressin (?)	Release of progesterone, oxytocin (?); enhanced immune system function	Sympathetic nervous system activation, release of testosterone (impact) and cortisol (defeat), compromised immune system function, cardiovascular activation/disease
Socialization origins	Early, age-appropriate demands for independence	Moderate lack of parental responsiveness to infant	Parental permissiveness for sex and aggression
Behavioral correlates	Entrepreneurial success, innovativeness	More liking of and agreement with similar others, but also more disliking of dissimilar others	Managerial and career success; sex and aggression; seeks visibility and prestige
Societal, economic, and historical correlates	Economic growth, innovation; civil war, ineffective leadership	Peace, disarmament; political scandal	War, arms increase; effective leadership

provides some important clues. Parents of high-achievement children are more likely to reward their children warmly for independent mastery of developmental hurdles such as toilet training, but are also more likely to punish them for not mastering challenging tasks on their own, and generally set their demands slightly above what the child is already able to master (Heckhausen & Heckhausen, in press; McClelland & Pilon, 1983; Rosen & D'Andrade, 1959; Winterbottom, 1958). In other words, children who later have a strong achievement motive have been trained to associate the encounter of challenges and the effort their mastery requires with a positive feeling that occurs after they have surmounted the challenge. They have also learned that lack of independent mastery is associated with negative consequences—hence their preference for solving challenges independently (Schultheiss & Brunstein, 2005).

Later in life, achievement-motivated individuals not only prefer moderately chal-

lenging tasks that they are allowed to master on their own terms, they also prefer tasks and work settings in which they can obtain frequent feedback on how well they are currently doing in order to optimize their performance (e.g., Brunstein & Schmitt, 2004). But not any kind of feedback will do. As recent studies by Brunstein and Hoyer (2002) and Brunstein and Maier (2005) have documented, achievement-motivated individuals prefer feedback with reference to an individual norm that tells them how well they are doing now relative to how well they did previously. They remain generally uninterested in how well they are doing relative to a social norm, that is, relative to other people's performance, except under very specific circumstances (cf. Brunstein & Meier, 2005; see also Veroff, 1969).

The developmental precursors and core characteristics of achievement motivation help explain why high-achievement individuals excel at some tasks in life but fail in others. High levels of achievement motivation are an asset in job contexts in which people can have full control over goal setting and implementation and also have access to frequent feedback on how they are doing. For this reason, high-achievement individuals succeed in business and many kinds of entrepreneurial activity, as long as they have full control over how the business is run and can see how well it is doing by, for instance, checking the daily cash flow (McClelland, 1961, 1965; McClelland & Franz, 1992; Wainer & Rubin, 1969). Achievement-motivated individuals' performance fizzles, however, when they work in jobs that require managerial or "people" skills (Andrews, 1967; Jacobs & McClelland, 1994; McClelland & Boyatzis, 1982). The focus in such jobs is no longer on what the achievement-motivated person may perceive as the best possible goal, the best possible way to achieve it, and having full control over the process. Rather, managerial positions require the delegation of work to others, finding compromises between conflicting views and interests, and making personnel decisions—none of which has any strong appeal for achievement-motivated individuals.

This may also explain why achievement-motivated individuals perform so dismally at the very highest levels of "management." Among U.S. presidents, as Winter (1991) has shown by content-coding presidential inauguration speeches, high levels of achievement motivation are associated with a strong sense of idealism but also with what historians judge to be an active-negative leadership style—that is, a flurry of political activity that fails to deliver (e.g., Presidents Wilson, Hoover, Nixon, and Carter). According to Winter (1996), achievement-motivated presidents start out with idealistic, "best-possible-outcome" goals. But because in politics they have to compromise and negotiate and cannot retain full control over goal setting and implementation, they soon become frustrated. They may also try to compensate by rigidly clinging to their idealistic goals and, unwilling to compromise, achieve comparatively little in the end.

The Affiliation Motive

At the core of the affiliation motive is a *capacity to derive satisfaction from establishing, maintaining, and restoring positive re-* *lationships with others* (Atkinson, Heyns, & Veroff, 1958). Individuals high in this need respond with approach behavior to nonverbal signals of affiliation, such as facial expressions of joy, and with vigilance and avoidance behavior to nonverbal signals of rejection and hostility, such as facial expressions of anger (e.g., Schultheiss & Hale, 2007; Schultheiss, Pang, Torges, Wirth, & Treynor, 2005). In other words, they want to be with individuals who are friendly and accepting and distance themselves from people who are not.

In their interpersonal behavior affiliation-motivated individuals are prone to engage in warm, friendly behavior toward those they like (cf. Winter, 1996). For instance, high-affiliation individuals, relative to low-affiliation individuals, interact more with others whom they perceive to be friendly or similar to themselves (e.g., Lansing & Heyns, 1959); like others more who express opinions similar to their own (e.g., Byrne, 1962); are more willing to make concessions to others whose goodwill is important to them (e.g., Langner & Winter, 2001); make more eye contact with others in noncompetitive situations (e.g., Exline, 1963); and are more willing to take others' needs into consideration in their own actions (e.g., Hardy, 1957).

Because individuals high in affiliation motivation cannot bear discord with others, however, they are also prone to distancing themselves from those they perceive as rejecting. Relative to low-affiliation individuals, they dislike others more who express disagreeing opinions (e.g., Byrne, 1961); they further augment such differences by changing their own opinions away from disagreeing others (Burdick & Burnes, 1958); they avoid eye contact with others whom they perceive to be antagonistic (e.g., Exline, 1963); and they are less likely to accept as a work partner someone whose opinions are too dissimilar to their own (Byrne, 1961).

Comparatively little is known about the developmental precursors of the affiliation motive. In a longitudinal study, high levels of affiliation motivation in adulthood could be traced back to more parental use of praise as a socialization technique, but also to the mother's being less responsive to the child's crying (McClelland & Pilon, 1983; see also Lundy & Potts, 1987). These findings suggest that the affiliation motive may be rooted at least partly in early separation anxiety or an avoidant attachment, but unfortunately the link between affiliation motivation and patterns of early attachment is largely unexplored.

Outside of the laboratory, high-affiliation individuals are more likely than low-affiliation individuals to experience high emotional and physical well-being, particularly if they are high in intimacy motivation, a facet of affiliation motivation that is oriented toward love and transcendence (e.g., McAdams & Vaillant, 1982; McClelland, 1989; Zeldow, Daugherty, & McAdams, 1988). In achievement contexts, affiliation-motivated individuals excel at tasks that require cooperation with other individuals (Atkinson & O'Connor, 1966; French, 1958) or bring them social approval (Atkinson & O'Connor, 1966), but show inferior performance on competitive tasks (Koestner & McClelland, 1992). Although high-affiliation individuals rarely make it to management positions in strongly hierarchical business organizations, presumably because their need for harmonious relationships with others clashes with the ruthless kind of leadership expected of top managers (McClelland, 1987), they shine as managers in companies with "flat" hierarchies, in which managers are expected to aid the integration of task groups (e.g., Litwin & Siebrecht, 1967).

Among U.S. presidents a strong need for affiliation is associated with a greater likelihood of scandal and the resignation of a member of the cabinet or the White House staff as a consequence. Winter (1991) speculates that high-affiliation presidents, such as George W. Bush, are more likely than others to be influenced by the suggestions of close friends, who may not always be the best advisors. On the positive side, affiliation-motivated presidents are more likely to sign arms limitation treaties and thus to contribute to peaceful relationships with other nations. Similar peace-promoting effects of affiliation motivation have also been found in motivational analyses of Soviet Politburo members (Hermann, 1980).

The Power Motive

Individuals high in power motivation have a *capacity to derive pleasure from having physical, mental, or emotional impact on other in-*

dividuals or groups of individuals and to experience the impact of others on themselves as aversive (Schultheiss, Wirth, et al., 2005; Veroff & Veroff, 1972; Winter, 1973). This double-faced aspect of the power motive is aptly illustrated in Figure 24.1, which shows that power-motivated individuals are quick to pick up and retain behaviors that helped them dominate others, but equally quick to inhibit behaviors that, in the past, have been associated with their being defeated by others. Note also that although the ultimate goal of the power motive may be dominance over others, the canonical definition of the power motive focuses on an intermediate step toward dominance, namely, having *impact* on others, which is *not* synonymous with being dominant.

This is an important distinction, because it is often assumed that the drive for power manifests itself as an in-your-face kind of aggressive and domineering behavior. Yet, among many mammalian species, particularly primates (cf. de Waal, 1998), this type of behavior is rarely a successful strategy to attain dominance, and it is not what typically characterizes individuals high in power motivation. Although they can be aggressive

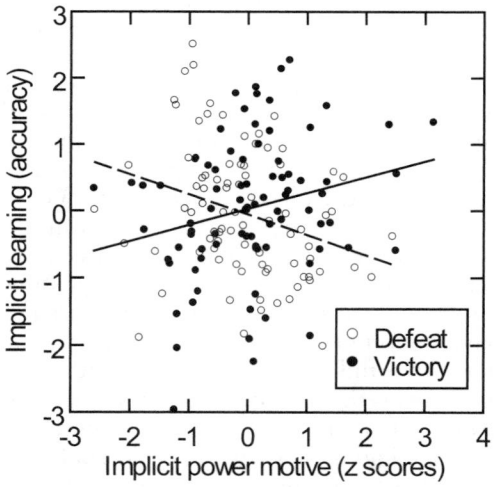

FIGURE 24.1. Effects of victory and defeat in a dominance contest and implicit power motivation on implicit learning of instrumental behavior (visuomotor sequences). Solid line, victory condition; dashed line, defeat condition. Based on Schultheiss, Wirth, et al. (2005).

and irresponsible (cf. Dutton & Strachan, 1987; Winter, 1988), more often they have been found to be very clever and intelligent in their quest for impact experiences (McClelland, 1975, 1987). For instance, in one study (Schultheiss & Brunstein, 2002), participants were videotaped while they presented their view on the ethics of experimentation with animals to another person. When judges later viewed the videotapes they did not rate participants who were high in implicit power motivation as more assertive or less friendly than other participants. But they did rate them as more persuasive and competent. The impression of higher competence in power-motivated individuals was not mediated by what participants actually said, but by how they said it: Compared to low-power individuals, high-power participants used more gesturing, were more likely to raise their eyebrows to emphasize the importance of what they said, and spoke more fluently. Thus, power-motivated individuals often employ behavioral strategies that allow them to have lasting and socially acceptable impact on others (e.g., by influencing their beliefs and opinions), rather than resorting to directly aggressive and coercive behaviors that are likely to backfire in many social contexts and relationships (e.g., Ridgeway, 1987).

Perhaps as a consequence of their considerable interpersonal intelligence, power-motivated individuals are more likely to ascend to the highest levels of management in hierarchically organized corporations (McClelland & Boyatzis, 1982; McClelland & Burnham, 1976) and, more generally, to have productive and successful careers (McClelland & Franz, 1992; Peterson & Stewart, 1993). However, when working in leadership positions, power-motivated individuals become vulnerable to ingratiating behavior by subordinates (Fodor & Farrow, 1979) and favor an autocratic style of decision making that leaves little room for subordinates' input (Fodor & Smith, 1982). Another way for power-motivated individuals to have impact is to "make a splash," to do something that will increase their social visibility by attracting others' attention. For instance, high-power individuals are more likely than low-power individuals to make risky bets in gambling to get attention (McClelland & Teague, 1975; McClelland &

Watson, 1973). For the same reason, they are also more likely to purchase extravagant cars and consumer goods (Winter, 1973). Finally, the implicit power motive is also involved in various forms of generativity (e.g., Peterson & Stewart, 1996). For instance, McClelland (1975) found the power motive to be positively correlated with sharing and giving in mature individuals, and power-motivated individuals are attracted to jobs that allow them to teach others (Winter, 1973). In women, high levels of power motivation are correlated with having more children and being more involved in parenting (Peterson & Stewart, 1993).

In the political arena, high levels of power motivation are associated with the proactive initiation of armed conflicts, as has been observed in U.S. presidents and South African leaders during the apartheid regime (Winter, 1980, 1991). U.S. presidents high in the need for power have a higher risk of being assassinated (e.g., Kennedy, Lincoln), but are also held in greater esteem by historians than low-power presidents (Winter, 1991).

In many studies (e.g., McClelland & Boyatzis, 1982; Schultheiss & Brunstein, 2002), the effects of power motivation on behavior depend on individuals' level of activity inhibition—a measure of their propensity to engage right-hemispheric functions under stressful and challenging conditions (Schultheiss, Riebel, & Jones, 2006). In general, high-power individuals show more sophisticated power behavior when they are high in activity inhibition and blunter and more aggressive manifestations of their need for impact when they are low in this variable.

Developmentally, the power motive may be rooted in parental permissiveness for sexual and aggressive behavior before the age of 5 (McClelland & Pilon, 1983), which may explain why some high-power adults express their need for impact in the form of aggression, drinking, and frequent sex, often with changing partners (e.g., McClelland, 1975; McClelland, Davis, Kalin, & Wanner, 1972; Schultheiss, Dargel, & Rohde, 2003b; Winter, 1988). However, growing up with younger siblings appears to transform the power motive into more responsible forms of impact seeking, such as holding office or becoming politically active (Winter, 1988). Also, the presence and involvement of a father in the child's parenting appears to facilitate the development of a "socially intelligent" power motive (McClelland, 1987; McClelland & Pilon, 1983).

Hope and Fear Components of Implicit Motives

Almost from the start of implicit motive research more than 50 years ago, researchers realized that a given motive may not be a unitary construct, but represent two complementary motivational orientations, one directed toward attaining a motive-specific incentive (approach or hope motivation) and one directed toward avoiding a motive-specific disincentive (avoidance or fear motivation) (e.g., McClelland et al., 1953). In each motivational domain, these orientations may give rise to similar types of behaviors, despite their different aims. For instance, in the domain of achievement motivation, Heckhausen (1963) differentiates a hope for success from a fear of failure motive. Individuals predominantly high in hope for success want to do well on tasks because they associate pleasure with successful mastery of challenges, whereas individuals predominantly high in fear of failure want to do well on tasks to avoid the negative outcomes associated with the failure to master challenges independently (e.g., parental punishment). Similarly, Veroff and Veroff (1972) argued that the power motive bifurcates into a hope of power and a fear of weakness component, with individuals high in hope of power seeking to have impact for the pleasure of the impact experience, and individuals high in fear of weakness seeking to have impact to avoid becoming someone else's target of impact. Finally, Boyatzis (1973) pointed out that in many empirical studies the affiliation motive seems to be characterized by a strong fear of rejection component, which propels individuals to seek contact with others to avoid loneliness and isolation. He suggested that this fear component of affiliation motivation is complemented by a hope-for-closeness component, a motivational orientation toward the positive incentive of love. This idea later gave rise, in part, to the development of a measure of implicit intimacy motivation, which aimed to capture the love aspect of affiliation motivation (McAdams, 1992).

The issue became even more complex when some scholars suggested that some-times people may actually *fear* the very incentive at the core of a given motive, thereby adding a third variant to the manifestations of some motives. Thus, Horner (1972) argued for the existence of a fear-of-success motive, and noted that people characterized by it avoid doing well on achievement tasks because they fear the social repercussions of standing out academically. In support of this notion, subsequent research showed that individuals high in fear of success scored low on measures of the implicit achievement motive (Karabenick, 1977). And Winter (1973) suggested that some people are uncomfortable with having power or impact over others and therefore avoid it. This idea has gained considerable support recently with the discovery that individuals very low in implicit power motivation do not seem to be indifferent to the impact incentive, but actually respond to impact experiences as if they were aversive and stressful for them (cf. Schultheiss, Wirth, et al., 2005; Wirth, Welsh, & Schultheiss, 2006; see also Figure 24.1). It also seems plausible that individuals with very low affiliation motivation scores may avoid closeness to others, similar to individuals with an avoidant attachment style, but to date there is little evidence to support this claim (cf. McAdams, Lester, Brand, McNamara, & Lensky, 1988).

In their discussion of the hope and fear components of achievement motivation, Schultheiss and Brunstein (2005) presented a framework derived from basic instrumental learning principles, which is extended here to provide an integrated account of the various hope and fear components of all three major implicit motives studied so far (see Table 24.2). The framework distinguishes between whether instrumental behavior to attain an incentive is executed or not and whether incentive attainment is associated with reward or punishment, derived either from the incentive itself or from its social consequences. This 2 × 2 framework describes three fundamental modes of motivation based on predominant learning experiences:

1. In the *active approach*, instrumental behavior aimed at incentive attainment has been rewarded, thus increasing the likelihood of future occurrences of the behavior for the sake of gaining pleasure. Hope of success, hope of power, and hope of intimacy are the

TABLE 24.2. A 2 × 2 Framework for the Description of Hope and Fear Aspects of the Implicit Needs for Power, Achievement, and Affiliation

	Reward follows	Punishment follows
Behavior is executed	Active approach (hope) motive Hope of power Hope of success Hope of intimacy	Passive avoidance (anti-) motive Fear of power Fear of success Fear of intimacy
Behavior is not executed	—	Active avoidance (fear) motive Fear of weakness Fear of failure Fear of rejection

components associated with this motivational mode in the motive domains of achievement, power, and affiliation, respectively.

2. In the *active avoidance* mode, lack of (effective) instrumental behavior is punished, which also leads to an increase of instrumental behavior in the future, although primarily for the sake of gaining relief. Fear of failure, fear of weakness, and fear of rejection represent the manifestations of this motivational focus for the three motive domains, respectively.

3. In contrast to the active approach and active avoidance modes, which are both associated with high levels of motivated behavior and can therefore coexist in a person, the *passive avoidance* mode represents an anti-motive, because here active attainment of the incentive is followed by punishment, which leads to the inhibition of behavior aimed at the incentive. As a consequence, the person with a strong fear of success shows a conspicuous absence of achievement-related behavior, particularly in the presence of achievement cues, which now act as a warning sign for the punishment associated with incentive attainment. Similarly, the person with a strong fear-of-power motive suppresses behavioral impulses aimed at impact, because having impact has become associated with punishment; and the person with a fear-of-intimacy motive avoids getting too involved with others, because intimate closeness has had aversive consequences in this person's learning history.

Whereas active approach and active avoidance components of a given implicit motive are not mutually exclusive and can actually co-occur within the same person (cf. Heckhausen, 1963; Winter, 1973), the relationship between these active motivational modes and the passive-avoidance anti-motive is an inverse one by functional necessity. This may also explain why, as previously described, individuals scoring very low on measures of implicit motives show signs of behavioral inhibition and avoidance in response to motive-specific incentives.

The 2 × 2 framework also yields a fourth mode, termed here "passive approach." Because the very lack of active, instrumental effort is being rewarded here (akin to learned helplessness induced by reward that is not contingent on performance; cf. Eisenberger & Cameron, 1996), this mode is not assumed to play a role in motivation proper and is not discussed further.

Other Motives

While the implicit needs for achievement, power, and affiliation have each generated voluminous bodies of research, other implicit motives have also been proposed and examined. A study on the measurement of implicit hunger motivation (Atkinson & McClelland, 1948), in fact, represents the opening salvo to McClelland and Atkinson's large-scale research programs on implicit motives. In addition, implicit motive measures have been developed for the assessment of curiosity (e.g., Maddi, Propst, & Feldinger, 1965), sexual motivation (Clark, 1952), and fear (Walker et al., 1958). Although these motives represent fundamental needs with distinct and well-described physiological substrates (e.g., Panksepp, 1998), implicit motive research has so far failed to systematically explore them. Implicit motive measures for aggression have also been developed (Feshbach, 1955; Kornadt, 1987), but they overlap substantially with implicit power motivation. Moreover, the status of aggression as a motivational need in its own right is debatable (cf. Panksepp, 1998; Schultheiss & Wirth, in press).

MEASUREMENT OF IMPLICIT MOTIVES

We recently provided a detailed discussion of the measurement of implicit motives in the *Handbook of Research Methods in Personality Psychology* (Schultheiss & Pang, 2007). In brief, the most frequently used method of assessing implicit motives is the picture story exercise (PSE; McClelland, Koestner, & Weinberger, 1989). The PSE requires research participants to write imaginative stories about four to eight photographs or drawings showing people in various social situations (e.g., a captain talking to a passenger, two women working in a laboratory). These stories are then scored with empirically derived and validated content-coding systems (cf. Schultheiss & Pang, 2007, for further details). Higher scores resulting from the coding of PSE stories for a given motive are seen as a reflection of a stronger motivational need disposition.

Coding systems for the assessment of power, affiliation, and achievement motivation from PSE stories have been revised and refined considerably over time, and a compilation of most existing coding systems for implicit motives was most recently published by Smith (1992). Winter (1991, 1994) developed an integrated coding system that allows researchers to code all three major motives simultaneously and can be applied to PSE stories as well as other types of verbal material (e.g., political speeches, diaries).

Reliability of PSE-based implicit motive measures is sufficient for research purposes. Interrater reliability between two independent coders scoring the same stories is typically higher than 80%, reflecting a high degree of objectivity of the coding rules. We reported the following meta-analytically derived retest stability coefficients: .71 after 1 day, .60 after 1 week, .52 after 1 month, and .37 after 1 year (Schultheiss & Pang, 2007). Internal consistency estimates (e.g., Cronbach's alpha) are not suitable for the assessment of the PSE's reliability (for discussions of this issue, see Atkinson, 1981; Reuman, 1982; Schultheiss & Pang, 2007).

Recent years have seen a resurgence of interest in the assessment of implicit motives that has led to new or revised content coding measures (e.g., Pang, 2006; Siegel & Weinberger, 1997), a better description of the picture cues used in the PSE (Pang & Schultheiss, 2005; Schultheiss & Brunstein, 2001), more rigorous evaluations of the suitability of various picture cues for motive measurement (Blankenship et al., 2006; Hofer & Chasiotis, 2004), and the introduction of computer-based PSE administration (Blankenship & Zoota, 1998; Pang & Schultheiss, 2005). Renewed interest has also led to attempts to measure implicit motives by means other than the PSE, such as the Operant Motive Test (OMT; Kuhl, Scheffer, & Eichstaedt, 2003), the Multi-Motive Grid (MMG; Sokolowski, Schmalt, Langens, & Puca, 2000; see also Johnston, 1957), and an adaptation of the Implicit Association Test (IAT; Brunstein & Schmitt, 2004). However, convergent measurement validity (i.e., does the new measure correlate with the PSE?) and convergent criterion validity (i.e., does the new measure predict the same criteria as the PSE?) of these new instruments with existing PSE motive measures still need to be clearly established.

HOW IMPLICIT MOTIVES DIFFER FROM SELF-ATTRIBUTED NEEDS AND GOALS

One of the most striking and pervasive findings emerging from more than 50 years of research on implicit motives is the observation that the correlation between PSE measures and self-reports of need strength in a given motivational domain is typically close to zero. For instance, correlations between PSE and questionnaire measures of achievement motivation were .06 in a study with 195 German students (Schultheiss & Brunstein, 2001) and .02 in a sample of 323 American college students (Pang & Schultheiss, 2005). Similarly, a meta-analysis reported by Spangler (1992) yielded an average variance overlap of less than 1% between PSE and questionnaire measures of achievement motivation. Negligibly low correlations between the PSE and questionnaires are not unique to the domain of achievement, but have also been consistently reported for the domains of power and affiliation (e.g., King, 1995; Pang & Schultheiss, 2005; Schroth, 1985). The lack of variance overlap between PSE and self-report measures of motivation extends even to the goals people choose and pursue in their daily lives. For instance, individuals high in implicit affiliation motivation are not more or less committed to affiliation and relationship goals than individuals low in implicit affiliation motivation (King, 1995; Schultheiss, Jones, Davis, & Kley, 2006). What the stubborn lack of substantial between-measures correlations suggests, then, is that, in general, *people do not have conscious access to the strength of their motives, as assessed with the PSE, and that the motivational needs and goals they ascribe to themselves cannot be interpreted as valid indicators of their underlying motive dispositions.* For this reason, McClelland and colleagues (1989) labeled motivational constructs assessed with the PSE *implicit motives* and motivational constructs assessed through self-report methods *self-attributed* or *explicit motives.*

Implicit and Explicit Motives Predict Different Types of Behavior

Perhaps even more important than the finding that implicit and explicit motives do not overlap is the observation that the two types of constructs respond to different types of stimuli and predict different kinds of validity criteria. In an early study of the differences between implicit and explicit achievement motivation, deCharms, Morrison, Reitman, and McClelland (1955) found that high scores on an achievement motive questionnaire, but not high scores on the achievement motive PSE, predicted research participants' likelihood of adjusting their judgments of artwork to those of a proclaimed expert and also to rate a target person described as unsuccessful in more negative terms. On the other hand, high scores on the PSE achievement motive measure, but not high scores on the achievement motive questionnaire, predicted good recall of facts from a story and superior performance on a scrambled-word test. Consistent with these early observations, Biernat (1989) found that implicit achievement motivation (PSE) predicted

good performance on an arithmetic task, but not the likelihood of volunteering for a task group leadership position, whereas explicit achievement motivation did not predict arithmetic task performance but did predict participants' inclination to be task group leader. Similarly, Brunstein and Hoyer (2002; see also Brunstein & Maier, 2005) reported that the implicit achievement motive predicts good performance on an attention task, particularly after negative individual-norm feedback, but not participants' choice of whether to continue with the task or do something else, whereas a measure of explicit achievement motivation positively predicted the choice to continue, particularly after participants were led to believe that they had done worse than others, but not the actual performance on the task.

Such differences between implicit and explicit measures of motivation have also been reported for other motives (e.g., J. A. Craig, Koestner, & Zuroff, 1994; Koestner, Weinberger, & McClelland, 1991). For instance, we found that the implicit power motive, but not the explicit need for dominance, predicted performance on a computer game that allowed players to enter a high-score ranking list and thereby obliterate the entries of previous players (Schultheiss & Brunstein, 1999). Notably, in the same study, the explicit need for dominance, but not the implicit power motive, was a positive predictor of participants' stated commitment to reach the highest rank on the high-score list ($r = .30$, $p < .05$; Schultheiss, 1996). However, the explicit need for dominance did not predict actual performance in the game.

Taken together, these studies suggest a double dissociation between implicit and explicit motives and their behavioral correlates, such that implicit motives are more likely to predict performance measures than choices and judgments, and explicit motives are more likely to predict choices and judgments than performance (cf. Bornstein, 2002). This characterization of the differences in predictive validity between implicit and explicit motives is probably too coarse to apply across the board (see, e.g., Brunstein & Maier, 2005, for an illustration of specific circumstances under which implicit and explicit achievement motives conjointly influence performance). But it is consistent with meta-analytic findings (Spangler, 1992) and can serve as a useful heuristic for predicting which type of measure will perform well for which types of outcomes in the laboratory and in the field.

Implicit and Explicit Motives Respond to Different Types of Cues

Whereas the distinction between measures of performance and measures of judgments and choices characterizes critical differences between implicit and explicit motives at the behavioral-output end, the two types of motives also respond to different types of information at the input stage of information processing. Specifically, a growing body of evidence suggests that implicit motives are more likely to become engaged by nonverbal cues than by verbal cues. Klinger (1967) observed that individuals responded to watching an affiliation-oriented or achievement-oriented experimenter, even when they could not hear his verbal instructions, with increases in affiliation or achievement motivation expressed in the PSE. We demonstrated that experimenters who verbally described a power-related goal to their participants failed to arouse participants' power motive (Schultheiss & Brunstein, 1999, 2002). Only after participants had had an opportunity to translate the assigned goal into an experiential format through a goal imagery exercise did their power motive predict goal commitment and task performance. Finally, our recent research indicates that facial expressions of emotion are particularly salient nonverbal cues for implicit motives. Facial signals of friendliness and hostility interact with individuals' implicit affiliation motive, and facial signals of dominance and submission interact with individuals' implicit power motive to shape attentional orienting and instrumental learning (Schultheiss & Hale, 2007; Schultheiss, Pang, et al., 2005).

Explicit motives, in contrast, respond preferentially to verbal cues. The aforementioned findings by deCharms and colleagues (1955) provide a good illustration of this point. Individuals high in explicit achievement motivation were sensitive to an alleged expert's verbal judgments about works of art and over time changed their own judgments toward the expert's position. But they were not influenced by the cues inherent in the achievement tasks (story recall, scrambled-word test) to which individuals with a strong implicit motive responded. In his meta-analysis of the range and conditions of predictive validity of implicit and explicit achievement motives measures, Spangler (1992) also found strong support for the notion that explicit motives respond to different cues than implicit motives. Across studies, high scores on questionnaire measures of achievement predict achievement-related behaviors particularly well in the presence of achievement-focused instructions (e.g., "Today you are going to play a ring toss game. ... We want to see how good you are at this"; Atkinson & Litwin, 1960, p. 54). But they did not predict behavior well in the absence of such verbal cues or in the presence of strong task-intrinsic cues, such as task-based feedback about one's performance increases or decreases.

An Information-Processing Model of Implicit and Explicit Motives

I have presented an information-processing account of implicit and explicit motives (Schultheiss, 2001; see also Schultheiss, 2007b; Schultheiss & Pang, 2007) that draws on these sets of findings as well as on earlier conceptual work on the differences between implicit and explicit motives (Cantor & Blanton, 1996; McClelland, 1980; McClelland et al., 1989; Weinberger & McClelland, 1990) and on distinctions between implicit and explicit aspects of cognition and emotion proposed by social, cognitive, and biopsychologists (e.g., Gazzaniga, 1985; LeDoux, 2002; Nisbett & Wilson, 1977; Paivio, 1986; Rolls, 1999; Squire & Zola, 1996; T. D. Wilson, 2002; Zajonc, 1980). A schematic overview of the model is presented in Figure 24.2.

According to this model, implicit motives preferentially respond to *nonverbal cues and incentives* and, after arousal, are particularly likely to have an impact on *nondeclarative measures of motivation*, that is, measures of behaviors and processes that are not accessible to, or controlled by, a person's self-concept or verbally represented intentions. Nondeclarative measures include physiological responses aimed at promoting biologically rooted needs (e.g., changes in blood pressure and heart rate, hormone release, muscle tone), acquisition of new stimulus–stimulus associations and goal-directed behaviors through processes of Pavlovian and

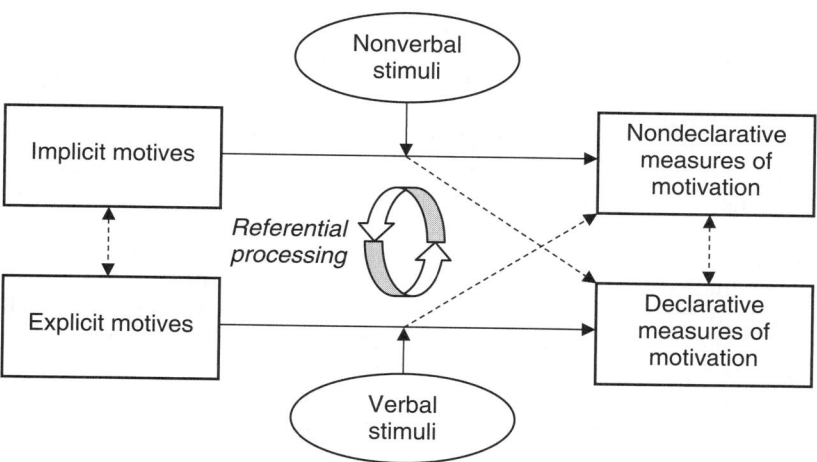

FIGURE 24.2. Information-processing model of implicit and explicit motivation. Solid lines indicate significant influence or correlation, whereas dashed lines indicate lack of significant influence or correlation. Based on Schultheiss (2001, 2007b) Schultheiss and Brunstein (2005), and Schultheiss and Pang (2007).

instrumental learning, and utilization of such learned stimulus connections and behaviors in the appropriate contexts. Explicit motives, on the other hand, preferentially respond to *verbal–symbolic cues* and influence *declarative measures of motivation*, that is, measures that tap into a person's verbally represented sense of self and the attitudes, judgments, decisions, and goals associated with it. Valence judgments, choice behavior, assessments of self-regulatory control, and personal goal listings are all examples of declarative measures of motivation (cf. Schultheiss, 2007b, for further discussion of the significance of the declarative–nondeclarative distinction for the conceptualization and assessment of personality).

A key aspect of the information-processing model of motivation, as sketched out in Figure 24.2 is the proposition of a mechanism by which verbal cues can interact with implicit motives to influence both declarative and nondeclarative measures of motivation. The mechanism is *referential processing*, the process through which verbal labels are retrieved and assigned to nonverbal percepts, and, conversely, mental images are generated in response to words (Paivio, 1986). Referential processing represents an active effort to connect the verbal and nonverbal domains of experience: It takes additional time and effort, however slight, to name an object as opposed to only perceive

it; likewise, a word is more quickly read than the object to which it refers is conjured up as a mental image. Based on work by Bucci (1984, 1985, 1997), Weinberger and McClelland (1990) speculated that implicit and explicit motivational systems can become better aligned through referential processing. We recently obtained evidence in support of this notion (Schultheiss & Brunstein, 1999, 2002). In a series of studies, participants were assigned power- or affiliation-related goals and then either had an opportunity to translate these verbally represented goals into an experiential, nonverbal format through guided goal imagery procedures (goal imagery group) or not (control group). We found that declarative (e.g., goal commitment, self-reported activation) and nondeclarative (e.g., task performance, expressive behavior) measures of motivation were contingent on participants' implicit motives (assessed with a PSE) in the goal imagery groups, but were independent of their implicit motives in the control groups. These findings indicate that an active effort to translate verbal goal representations into nonverbal representations allows implicit motives to "understand" and respond to verbal stimuli, which would otherwise be incapable of engaging them.

Whereas alignment between implicit and explicit motivation may often depend on having the opportunity in a given situation to engage in referential processing, as in our studies (Schultheiss & Brunstein, 1999, 2002), implicit–explicit alignment may also be the result of stable interindividual differences in people's referential processing ability; that is, it may reflect the degree of their general *referential competence*. In support of this idea, we found that in individuals with high referential competence, as measured by their response speed on a color-naming task (cf. Bucci, 1984), higher levels of implicit affiliation motivation significantly predicted more negative ratings of words expressing hostile emotions (e.g., *furious*, *mad*, *angry*), whereas the affiliation motive did not predict such ratings among individuals low in referential competence (Schultheiss & Schad, 2006). Taken together, these findings suggest that referential processing can help make individuals' self-attributed needs and explicit goals more similar to, and perhaps also more integrated with, their implicit motives in the long run.

Other moderators of the relationship between implicit and explicit motives have also been proposed. These include methodological factors in the assessment of motives (Thrash, Elliot, & Schultheiss, 2007), self-determination (Thrash & Elliot, 2002), the ability to quickly down-regulate negative affect (Baumann, Kaschel, & Kuhl, 2005; Brunstein, 2001), and private body consciousness, self-monitoring, and preference for consistency (Thrash et al., 2007). More research is needed to determine whether these moderators reliably influence the alignment between implicit and explicit motives and how they relate to each other as well as to the referential processing mechanism I proposed (Schultheiss, 2001).

PHYSIOLOGICAL AND HEALTH CORRELATES OF IMPLICIT MOTIVES

It does not take much to recognize in the implicit needs for affiliation and power the human manifestations of fundamental motivational systems present in nearly all mammals and many nonmammalian species, too. Most social animals are propelled by the need to form durable attachments to their parents, offspring, or kin to ensure safety and protection (affiliation) and by the need to rise in the social hierarchy to secure and control scarce resources (dominance; cf. E. O.

Wilson, 1980). As a consequence, mammalian and nonmammalian species share many physiological and brain systems that facilitate affiliative and dominant behaviors (cf. Schultheiss & Wirth, in press). For instance, the gonadal steroid hormone testosterone promotes dominant behavior across various species (Monaghan & Glickman, 1992), and the same is true of the peptide hormone oxytocin in the context of affiliation and attachment (Insel & Young, 2001). The case for a universal motivational need for achievement is harder to make, and perhaps this motive is either a species-specific adaptation in humans or represents a secondary, derived motive that is rooted in a need to maintain an intact relationship with one's caregivers (cf. Elliot & Thrash, 2004; Rosen & D'Andrade, 1959). On the other hand, some primates and other mammals are also known to take an interest in, and perhaps derive pleasure from, exploring and mastering their nonsocial environment (e.g., Boesch-Achermann & Boesch, 1993; McClelland, 1987), which may point to the existence of phylogenetic roots of the achievement motive.

In the following sections, I review evidence for the involvement of specific endocrine and physiological systems in implicit power, affiliation, and achievement motivation and also highlight some of the health correlates associated with implicit motivational needs.

Physiological and Health Correlates of the Power Motive

Arousal of power motivation in laboratory and field experiments leads to clear-cut increases in sympathetic nervous system activation, and this effect is more pronounced in individuals with a strong dispositional power motive (McClelland, 1982). Power-motivated individuals respond to power arousal or dominance challenges with increases in saliva and urine levels of the sympathetic catecholamines epinephrine, norepinephrine, and their metabolites (McClelland, Davidson, & Saron, 1985; McClelland, Floor, Davidson, & Saron, 1980; McClelland, Ross, & Patel, 1985; Steele, 1973, as cited in McClelland, 1987), increased blood pressure (Fontana, Rosenberg, Marcus, & Kerns, 1987), and increased muscle tone (Fodor, 1985). Perhaps as an outcome of frequent or stressful power arousal experiences, power-motivated individuals are more likely to have chronically elevated blood pressure (McClelland, 1979). It should be noted that many of these findings emerge more strongly if high levels of power motivation co-occur with high levels of activity inhibition, an index of relative right-hemispheric activation during stress (Schultheiss, Riebel, & Jones, 2006; the right hemisphere controls sympathetic activation and stress responses, cf. Wittling, 1995).

Implicit power motivation has also been linked to salivary testosterone levels. Across several studies, slight positive correlations between basal testosterone levels and implicit power motive scores have been observed in men (e.g., Dabbs, Hopper, & Jurkovic, 1990; Schultheiss, Campbell, & McClelland, 1999; Schultheiss, Wirth, et al., 2005). More importantly, anticipation of a successful outcome of a dominance challenge (Schultheiss et al., 1999) and actual success in one-on-one dominance contests leads to transient testosterone increases in power-motivated men (Schultheiss et al., 1999; Schultheiss & Rohde, 2002; Schultheiss, Wirth, et al., 2005), which appear to have reinforcing effects on instrumental behavior (Schultheiss & Rohde, 2002; Schultheiss, Wirth, et al., 2005). In power-motivated women, dominance contests lead to a general transient testosterone increase, regardless of contest outcome, and testosterone does not appear to be related to instrumental learning (Schultheiss, Wirth, et al., 2005). Some evidence also suggests that power-motivated women respond with sustained estradiol increases to a dominance success and estradiol reductions to a defeat (Stanton & Schultheiss, 2007). Defeat during a dominance contest leads to increases of the stress hormone cortisol in both men and women (Wirth et al., 2006) and to testosterone decreases in men (Schultheiss et al., 1999; Schultheiss & Rohde, 2002; Schultheiss, Wirth, et al., 2005).

The observed changes in sympathetic catecholamines, testosterone, and cortisol in response to power arousal and dominance outcomes in men represent the operation of a functionally integrated neuroendocrine mechanism that subserves male dominance motivation (Sapolsky, 1987; Schultheiss, 2007a). Sympathetic catecholamines are typically released in situations in which the individual can actively cope with a challenge, such as beating an opponent in a contest, and they have fast, stimulating effects on testosterone release from the gonads (Sapolsky, 1987). Testosterone further aids active coping with dominance challenges by increasing energy supply to the muscles and lowering the threshold for aggressive behavior through its actions on the brain. In contrast to challenges that are perceived to be manageable, cortisol is released in situations in which the individual is exposed to an uncontrollable stressor, such as being defeated and subjected to another's dominance. Cortisol inhibits testosterone release from the gonads (Sapolsky, 1987), thereby lowering the individual's inclination to engage in further, potentially costly and fruitless dominance battles. According to this model, testosterone increases in power-motivated male winners of a dominance contest represent the net effect of relatively greater sympathetic catecholamine release throughout the challenge, whereas testosterone decreases in male power-motivated losers represent the net effect of relatively greater cortisol release during and after the challenge. Although testosterone is known to facilitate dominant and aggressive behavior in females, too (e.g., Dabbs, Ruback, Frady, Hopper, & Sgoutas, 1988; van Honk et al., 2001), the exact causal mechanisms and functional roles of the fast, contest-induced testosterone increases and the differential estradiol changes observed in power-motivated women remain to be explored.

In several studies, stressed power motivation has also been linked to compromised immune system functioning and impaired health (Jemmott, 1987; McClelland, 1989). During exam periods, high-power students, relative to low-power students, showed elevated and prolonged sympathetic stress responses and suppressed levels of secretory immunoglobulin A (sIgA), the immune system's first line of defense against pathogens in the mucosal tissues of the body (Jemmott et al., 1983; McClelland, Alexander, & Marks, 1982; McClelland et al., 1985). Stressed power motivation is also associated with decreased natural killer cell activity (Jemmott et al., 1990). As a consequence of compromised immune system functions, high-power individuals who experience frequent or severe power stress are more likely than low-power individuals to become ill (McClelland & Jemmott, 1980; McClelland et al., 1980,

1982, 1985). Although it has not been explored in greater detail why stressed power motivation translates into impaired immune system functioning, the immunosuppressive effects of strongly or chronically elevated cortisol levels appear to be a plausible mechanism (cf. Wirth et al., 2006). Notably, high levels of power motivation in combination with low-power stress and success in power-related endeavors have been found to predict low levels of physical symptoms and overall good health (McClelland, 1989), which suggests that the implicit power motive is not a general vulnerability for impaired health.

Physiological and Health Correlates of the Affiliation Motive

High levels of implicit affiliation motivation are associated with indicators of parasympathetic nervous system (PNS) activity (Jemmott, 1987; McClelland, 1989). Compared to low-affiliation individuals, individuals high in affiliation at age 30 have lower blood pressure at age 50 (McClelland, 1979). They also maintain better immune system functioning during stress, as evidenced by enhanced release of sIgA during exam periods (Jemmott et al., 1983; McClelland, Ross, & Patel, 1985). In the absence of stressors, individuals with a strong implicit affiliation motive show better immunocompetence than individuals with a weak affiliation motive (Jemmott et al., 1990), and they also respond with greater sIgA increases to positive affiliation arousal (e.g., watching a documentary about Mother Teresa; McClelland & Kirshnit, 1988). Experimental arousal of affiliation motivation leads to increases in peripheral dopamine release (McClelland, Patel, Stier, & Brown, 1987), which is involved in blood pressure down-regulation and other PNS-related functions (e.g., Duncker et al., 1997). Likely as a consequence of enhanced PNS activity and the high level of immune system functioning associated with it, high-affiliation individuals are, overall, less likely to become ill than others (Jemmott, 1987; McClelland, 1989; McClelland & Jemmott, 1980), particularly if they experience low levels of stress or have low levels of activity inhibition, indicating left-hemispheric engagement during stress (Schultheiss, Riebel, & Jones, 2006; the left hemisphere is associated with PNS activation; cf. Wittling,

1995). The one blemish on the affiliation motive's "health record" is the finding that diabetics are more likely than nondiabetics to be characterized by high levels of affiliation motivation and low levels of activity inhibition (McClelland, Brown, Patel, & Kelner, 1988; cited in McClelland, 1989). Although a causal role of affiliation motivation in diabetes remains to be established, McClelland (1989) has speculated that the affiliation motive may predispose individuals for diabetes through greater food intake and higher blood sugar levels via the effects of peripheral dopamine on the liver.

Another line of research points to a link between implicit affiliation motivation and the steroid hormone progesterone. Women who take oral contraceptives (which contain progesterone) have higher levels of affiliation motivation than women not taking "the pill" or men (Schultheiss, Dargel, & Rohde, 2003a). Also, higher levels of affiliation motivation are preceded by greater increases of progesterone in the course of women's menstrual cycle (Schultheiss et al., 2003b), and a recent laboratory study found increases in progesterone to be associated with increases in affiliation motivation (Wirth & Schultheiss, 2006). Finally, we found that movie-induced arousal of affiliation motivation, but not of power motivation, leads to fast progesterone increases in both women and men (Schultheiss, Wirth, & Stanton, 2004). We (Schultheiss et al., 2004) speculated that the observed changes in progesterone may reflect the ovarian action of oxytocin, a hormone involved in affiliative behavior in animals and humans (Insel & Young, 2001). We also (Wirth & Schultheiss, 2006) offered an alternative explanation: Progesterone exerts anxiolytic effects in the brain and may thereby help down-regulate fight–flight stress responses and promote tend-and-befriend (Taylor et al., 2000) affiliative behavior. This interpretation is consistent with high-affiliation individuals' better stress resistance (McClelland, 1989) and with the observation that affiliative behavior increases during threat (Gump & Kulik, 1997; Schachter, 1959). Thus, we argue for a bidirectional relationship between affiliation motivation and progesterone, in which a strong affiliation motive leads to increased progesterone release, particularly during stress, and high levels of progesterone, in turn, facilitate affiliation motivation (Wirth & Schultheiss, 2006).

Physiological and Health Correlates of the Achievement Motive

The biological correlates of the achievement motive have received the least attention so far, despite the fact that intriguing clues to the existence of such correlates emerged almost from the beginning of achievement motivation research. For instance, Mücher and Heckhausen (1962) found, in a study with 33 male participants, that higher levels of achievement motivation correlated .65 with leg muscle tone during rest. Mueller and Beimann (1969; see also Mueller, Kasl, Brooks, & Cobb, 1970) reported that men with high levels of uric acid, a risk factor for gout, have higher levels of hope for success and lower levels of fear of failure than men with normal uric acid levels. Finally, Bäumler (1975; cf. Schultheiss & Brunstein, 2005) showed that administration of a drug that increases central dopaminergic transmission leads to increases in hope for success, whereas administration of a drug that decreases dopaminergic transmission leads to decreases in both hope for success and fear of failure. Unfortunately, none of these reported correlates of achievement motivation have been studied more systematically so far.

A more consistent picture emerged from research on achievement motivation and urine excretion. After observing, in two previous studies, that high implicit achievement motivation was associated with low-volume urine samples collected by research participants (as cited in McClelland, 1995; McClelland et al., 1980; McClelland, Maddocks, & McAdams, 1985). McClelland (1995) experimentally tested the notion that high levels of achievement motivation lead to low urine excretion. He found that participants' baseline implicit achievement motive predicted low urine sample volume after achievement arousal, but not in a neutral control condition. Moreover, in the arousal condition the achievement motive predicted better recall for achievement-related material on a memory test, and better recall was negatively correlated with urine-sample volume. McClelland attributed these effects to the release of the peptide hormone arginine-vasopressin (AVP), which promotes water retention in the body and episodic memory processes in the brain (cf. Beckwith, Petros, Bergloff, & Staebler, 1987; Stricker & Verbalis, 2002). However, the achievement motive–AVP hypothesis has not been tested directly yet.

CORE MOTIVATIONAL FUNCTIONS OF IMPLICIT MOTIVES

Most theories of motivation agree that motivation *directs* behavior, in time and space, towards desired goals (incentives) and away from aversive "anti-goals" (disincentives) and that it *energizes* behavior directed at such outcomes (e.g., Carver & Scheier, 1998; Pfaff, 1999; Toates, 1986). Because both the orientation of attention toward incentive cues and the selective learning of cues, contexts, and behaviors that are associated with goal attainment are seen as specific, critical aspects of motivation by many theorists (e.g., W. Craig, 1918; Epstein, 1982; Lang, Bradley, & Cuthbert, 1997; Teitelbaum, 1966), McClelland (1987) has differentiated the directing function of motivation into an orienting function and a selecting function. Ultimately, the orienting, selecting, and energizing functions of motivation follow from the central feature of motivated behavior, namely, that it is aimed at hedonically charged goals (e.g., Berridge & Robinson, 2003; Bindra, 1978; Cabanac, 1979; Epstein, 1982; Toates, 1986). Epstein (1982) argued that behavior is only then truly motivated if there is a hedonic response (behavioral, autonomic, or endocrine) to goal attainment. Similarly, Berridge (2004) has proposed that it is hedonic pleasure experienced in commerce with an object that makes the object desirable or wanted. Without this attribution of pleasure to an object (termed *incentive salience;* cf. Berridge & Robinson, 1998), the individual would not be motivated to approach it. In the following material I review the evidence for a role of implicit motives in hedonic responses to incentives, learning of cues, contexts, and behaviors associated with incentive attainment; orienting of attention toward incentive cues; and energizing of behavior aimed at incentive attainment. Figure 24.3 provides an overview of how these functions of implicit motives act in concert.

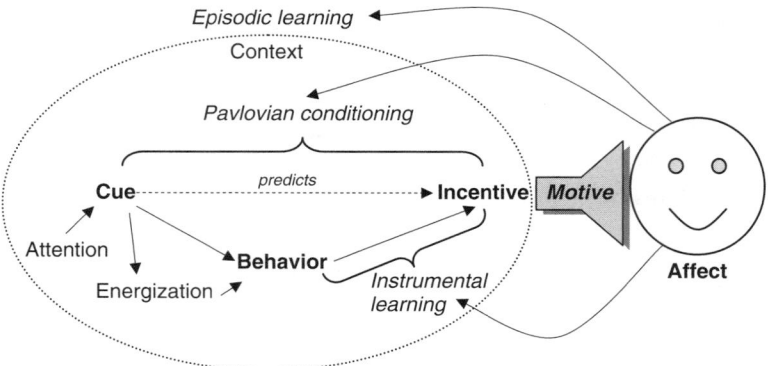

FIGURE 24.3. Schematic overview of implicit motive effects on affect, learning, attention, and behavioral energizing.

Motives Amplify Affective Responses to Incentives

Atkinson (1957) argued that a capacity to have a strong affective response to motive-specific incentives and disincentives is at the core of an implicit motive. In other words, motives act as *affect amplifiers*, making incentive attainment more rewarding, and encounters with disincentives more aversive. The reward- and punishment-augmenting effects of implicit motives have been documented most clearly in studies of affect and instrumental learning.

Evidence for an affect-amplifying function of implicit motives comes from studies of facial expressions, which in humans and other mammals represent a prime indicator of the hedonic impact of goal attainment (cf. Berridge, 2000). In humans, spontaneous smiles reflect a positive hedonic response, and frowns reflect a negative hedonic response, to a wide variety of stimuli and situations (Cacioppo, Petty, Losch, & Kim, 1986; Dimberg, 1997), and there is evidence that facial hedonic responses to motive-specific stimuli are more pronounced in high-motive as compared to low-motive individuals. For instance, relative to individuals low in power motivation, power-motivated people frown more intensively when faced with a dominant-acting person, but do not show this expression when encountering a submissive-acting person (Fodor, Wick, & Hartsen, 2006). Individuals with a strong affiliation motive respond with smiling to friendly encounters with other people (McAdams, Jackson, &

Kirshnit, 1984), but with frowns to an interaction partner whom they expect to oppose their views (Schultheiss, 1996). Individuals with a weak affiliation motive do not show these responses to affiliation incentives and disincentives.

The affect-amplifying function of motives can also be observed at the level of endocrine responses. As previously described, power-motivated winners of a dominance contest showed a postcontest increase in gonadal steroid hormones, which, through their actions on the brain, contribute to reinforcement, decreased anxiety, and increased aggression (Schultheiss, 2007a; Schultheiss, Wirth, et al., 2005). Power-motivated losers, on the other hand, registered a contest-induced decrease in gonadal steroid levels. These effects were not observed in winners and losers low in power motivation.

Research on the implicit achievement motive shows that motives also influence the expectation of affective reward associated with incentive attainment, another critical feature of motivational processes (cf. Berridge, 2004; Dickinson & Balleine, 1994; Epstein, 1982). Halisch and Heckhausen (1989) and Brunstein and Maier (2005) observed that high-achievement individuals expect to get more pleasure out of mastering a challenging task and less pleasure out of mastering an easy task than do low-achievement individuals.

Finally, the affect-augmenting function of motives can also manifest in subjective feeling states under specific circumstances (see Schultheiss, Wirth, et al., 2005, for further discussion of the boundary conditions of this effect). In an experience sampling study McAdams and Constantian (1983) observed that individuals high in implicit intimacy motivation, compared to those low in this variable, experienced more positive affect during interactions with others in their everyday lives. In two studies we found that success and failure in goal pursuits—such as getting a good grade, finding a romantic partner, or spending more time with one's friends—affect individuals' well-being only to the extent that such pursuits are backed up by strong implicit motives (Brunstein, Schultheiss, & Grässmann, 1998; Schultheiss, Jones, Davis, & Kley, in press). Participants whose goals were supported by strong implicit motives experienced feelings of happiness and an absence of depressive symptoms when they had success in their goal pursuits, but suffered from impaired mood and depressive symptoms when they encountered setbacks and failure en route to their goals. For goals that were not supported by strong implicit motives, on the other hand, variations in goal progress were not directly related to emotional well-being and depressive symptoms.

Motives Shape Incentive-Driven Learning Processes

Through their hedonic impact on the individual, rewards and punishments influence the learning, retention, and utilization of the stimuli and behaviors by which they were preceded and the contexts in which they occurred. Therefore, implicit motives, in interaction with the encounter of motive-specific incentives and disincentives, should scale the degree to which individuals show evidence of (1) Pavlovian conditioning in response to incentive cues, (2) learning of behavior that is instrumental for incentive attainment (including inhibition of behavior that precedes an encounter with a disincentive), and (3) memory for the episodic context in which an incentive (or disincentive) occurs. Research supports a role of implicit motives in learning on all three accounts.

Pavlovian conditioning mechanisms have been assumed to be at the core of implicit motives from the outset. McClelland and colleagues (1953) theorized that the implicit achievement motive is aroused by

cues that have become associated with, and thus predict, successful mastery of challenging tasks, similar to Ivan Pavlov's canine subjects, whose appetite was aroused by the sound of a metronome that predicted the arrival of food. Recent research shows that Pavlovian conditioning does, in fact, play a role in implicit motives. We found that power-motivated individuals show attentional avoidance of salient abstract cues that have been conditioned to high-dominance facial expressions of emotion (joy, anger) (Stanton, Wirth, & Schultheiss, 2006), a finding that parallels high-power individuals' attentional avoidance of high-dominance faces (Schultheiss & Hale, 2007; see below). Although research on the role of implicit motives in Pavlovian conditioning is still in the early stages, these findings corroborate a central assumption of McClelland and colleagues' account of motive arousal and are also consistent with research that shows Pavlovian conditioning to be at the core of many nondeclarative emotional and motivational processes (e.g., LeDoux, 2002).

Evidence for a role of instrumental learning in implicit motives has grown substantially over the past couple of years. Using implicit learning tasks developed by cognitive psychologists (e.g., Curran, 1997; Nissen & Bullemer, 1987), we found replicable evidence across several experimental studies that high-power individuals show superior performance on visuomotor sequences whose execution has become associated with winning a dominance contest, but impaired performance on sequences whose execution was followed by a defeat (cf. Figure 24.1; (Schultheiss & Rohde, 2002; Schultheiss, Wirth, et al., 2005).

In another line of research, we have shown that the implicit needs for power and affiliation influence instrumental learning in response to nonverbal dominance and affiliation signals (Schultheiss, Pang, et al., 2005). For instance, relative to individuals low in power motivation, high-power individuals showed enhanced learning of a visuomotor sequence whose execution was "rewarded" by the presentation of an emotional expression signaling the sender's low dominance.

More recently, Pang (2006) has provided evidence that implicit instrumental learning can also be shaped by the implicit achievement motive. Both hope-for-success and fear-of-failure components of this motive predicted generally enhanced performance on visuomotor sequences participants had worked on during an achievement arousal phase of the experiment. Hope for success was a particularly good predictor of sequence execution when participants had received intermittent positive or negative achievement feedback during the arousal phase, but not when feedback was given continuously.

Evidence for a role of implicit motives in episodic memory, including autobiographical memory, is strong. Research on the achievement motive uncovered early on that individuals high in achievement motivation have better recall of unfinished tasks than individuals low in achievement motivation, who in turn have better recall of completed tasks (Atkinson, 1953; Weiner, 1965; see also Kazen & Kuhl, 2005). Later, research on the relationship between the implicit needs for power and intimacy and autobiographical memory showed that power-motivated individuals were particularly likely to recall power-related peak experiences from their lives, whereas intimacy-motivated individuals had superior memory for intimacy-related peak experiences (McAdams, 1982; McAdams, Hoffmann, Mansfield, & Day, 1996). Similar findings emerged from research by Woike and colleagues, who studied the effects of agentic (achievement and power) and communal (affiliation and intimacy) motives on individuals' memory for agentic and communal episodes in their lives (Woike, 1994, 1995; Woike, Gershkovich, Piorkowski, & Polo, 1999; Woike & Polo, 2001). Across studies, participants high in agentic motivation recalled more agentic episodes, and participants high in communal motivation recalled more communal episodes. Woike (1995) and Woike, Mcleod, and Goggin (2003) further differentiated this motive-congruent memory effect by showing that it emerges only for emotional or specific, but not for nonemotional or generalized, autobiographical memories.

Another approach that has been used to study motive effects on memory involves the presentation of stories featuring vivid motive-related episodes. Studies based on this paradigm indicate that high levels of a given motive, measured before story presentation, predict better recall of motive-congruent story elements (e.g., deCharms et al., 1955;

McClelland, 1995; McClelland, Maddocks, & McAdams, 1985; see also McClelland, Scioli, & Weaver, 1998).

In summary, there is substantial evidence for a selecting function of implicit motives, and this selecting function is particularly strong in conjunction with emotionally arousing material—that is, encounters with motive-specific incentives and disincentives. Thus, high levels of an implicit motive influence (1) learning of cues that predict an emotionally charged motive-specific incentive or disincentive (Pavlovian conditioning), (2) behaviors that result in incentive consummation or frustration (instrumental conditioning), and (3) the unique spatial and temporal context in which the (dis-)incentive was encountered (episodic learning). From a neuropsychological perspective, an involvement of the amygdala in the selecting functions of motives appears very likely, since this brain structure plays a key role in the processing of emotional stimuli, is critically involved in Pavlovian conditioning, and provides emotional modulation of learning in other memory systems, such as implicit learning (striatum) and episodic memory (hippocampus; cf. Cahill, 2000; Eichenbaum & Cohen, 2001; LeDoux, 2002).

Motives Direct Attention toward Incentive Cues

According to McClelland (1987), implicit motives make a person sensitive to cues that predict motive-specific incentives and disincentives. Such cues represent particularly salient stimuli that automatically attract the person's attention. Early evidence for an attention-directing function of implicit motives came from a study of the effects of affiliation motivation on signal detection (Atkinson & Walker, 1958). When presented with slides that depicted social (human faces) and nonsocial (furniture) information in random locations, at low illumination, and in quick succession, high-affiliation individuals were more likely than low-affiliation individuals to detect the faces. More recently, we used a dot-probe task to assess effects of implicit motives on attentional orienting to facial expressions in two studies (Schultheiss & Hale, 2007). We predicted that the power motive should influence attentional orienting to faces signaling low or high dominance, and the affiliation motive should influence attentional orienting to faces signaling affiliation or rejection. In support of these predictions, we found that high-power individuals, compared to low-power individuals, oriented their attention toward surprised faces (low dominance) but away from happy or angry faces (both high dominance; cf. Hess, Blairy, & Kleck, 2000; Knutson, 1996). Individuals high in affiliation motivation, relative to those low in this motive, oriented their attention toward happy faces, a highly affiliative signal, but also toward hostile, angry faces, perhaps reflecting the heightened sensitivity for rejection signals observed in many earlier studies on affiliation motivation (cf. Boyatzis, 1973).

The studies by Atkinson and Walker (1958) and we (Schultheiss & Hale, 2007) provide evidence for the alerting and orienting aspects of attention, respectively (cf. Posner, 1995). It remains an open question whether implicit motive modulation of attention can also be documented for the executive control of attention, that is, for individuals' ability to focus attention on one task and ignore interfering information (e.g., motivational incentive cues).

Motives Energize Behavior Aimed at Incentive Attainment

After a motive has become aroused by the presence of cues signaling a possible encounter with an incentive or disincentive, behavior directed at attaining the incentive or avoiding the disincentive becomes highly energized, as reflected by the recruitment of physiological systems supporting behavioral engagement with the environment (e.g., sympathetic activation) and quicker onset as well as more effective (e.g., faster, more frequent, more forceful) execution of instrumental behavior (e.g., Ikemoto & Panksepp, 1999; McClelland, 1987; Wright & Brehm, 1989). Evidence for an energizing function has been obtained for all three major motives.

As already noted, high-achievement individuals were found to have higher muscle tone than low-achievement individuals, and this difference was particularly pronounced when participants were working on challenging tasks, compared to a rest condition (Mücher & Heckhausen, 1962). Another measure of sympathetic activation, galvanic skin response, is also increased in high-

achievement individuals in anticipation of a challenge, indicating greater energizing (Raphelson, 1957). Bäumler's (1975) previously mentioned finding that dopamine agonists increase, and antagonists decrease, achievement motivation expressed in the PSE suggests that this motivational need may engage the mesolimbic dopamine system, which is directly involved in response invigoration (Ikemoto & Panksepp, 1999).

Beyond these physiological indicators of an energizing function of the achievement motive, behavioral studies using simple measures of response speed, persistence, and performance output also strongly suggest that the achievement motive energizes behavior aimed at the mastery of challenges. In contrast to low-achievement individuals, high-achievement individuals show shorter response latencies on mental concentration tasks, particularly in response to negative feedback (Brunstein & Hoyer, 2002; Brunstein & Maier, 2005); persist longer on challenging anagram (Feather, 1966) and mental arithmetic tasks (Wendt, 1955); and solve more items on anagram (deCharms et al., 1955), arithmetic (Biernat, 1989; Schroth, 1987; Wendt, 1955), and digit–letter substitution tasks (French, 1958) in a fixed amount of time.

Similar to achievement-motivated individuals, people high in implicit power motivation also show signs of increased physiological preparedness for effort expenditure. In a study by Steele (1973; also described in McClelland, 1987), high-power individuals responded with increased physiological activation to power-arousing speeches, as reflected in strongly elevated urinary catecholamine metabolites after power arousal, compared to a neutral control condition and an achievement arousal condition. In another study, Steele (1977) found that power-arousing speeches also lead to greater subjective activation in high-power individuals as compared to low power-individuals or high-power individuals in a neutral speech control condition. We found similar results: Power-motivated individuals felt more activated while playing a computer game that allowed them to ascend in a high-score list (Schultheiss & Brunstein, 1999). This same study also provided evidence for power-motive-driven energizing of performance driven by the power motive: High-power individuals scored more points than low-power individuals, but only after their implicit power motive had been aroused properly (cf. section "Implicit and Explicit Motives Respond to Different Types of Cues").

Finally, individuals high in affiliation motivation also show signs that they more frequently or intensively engage in behaviors that allow them to connect to other people in positive, friendly ways. Individuals high in intimacy motivation, compared to individuals low in this motive, smile and laugh more and use more "we" references when interacting with others (McAdams et al., 1984; McAdams & Powers, 1981). They are also more likely to think about their friends and relatives and to talk to them during the course of the day (J. A. Craig et al., 1994; McAdams & Constantian, 1983). Similar findings have also been obtained for the original measure of implicit affiliation motivation (Lansing & Heyns, 1959; McAdams & Constantian, 1983). If the incentives are right, a direct effect of affiliation motivation on energizing, as reflected in performance on a simple achievement task can also be observed: In two separate studies designed to examine the effects of achievement motivation on performance, high-affiliation participants unexpectedly performed particularly well on a challenging digit–letter substitution task (Atkinson & O'Connor, 1966; French, 1958). These findings have been explained by the fact that in both studies all participants were male and were supervised by a female experimenter (French, 1958; McClelland, 1987).

THE BIGGER PICTURE: IMPLICIT MOTIVES IN ECONOMY, SOCIETY, AND HISTORY

One of the most remarkable aspects of the implicit motive construct is the fact that it can be used to predict an incredibly broad array of phenomena, ranging from basic physiological processes (such as hormone release) to fundamental cognitive functions (such as attention and learning) to long-term trends in individuals' everyday experience and behavior. But implicit motive measures can be taken even further and used to describe and explain political, economic, societal, and historical processes. In the following material, I illustrate this point with research on the role of achievement motivation in economic growth and the significance of power

and affiliation motivation in war and peace. Further examples and details can be found in McClelland (1975, 1987) and Winter (1996).

Achievement Motivation and Economic Growth

The first and perhaps most well-developed effort to link implicit motives to societal phenomena was made by McClelland (1961) in the book *The Achieving Society*. Drawing on Max Weber's (1905) influential ideas on the contribution of the Protestant work ethic to the rise of capitalism, McClelland argued that a Protestant upbringing is more likely than a non-Protestant upbringing to foster in children the independent mastery of challenges, thus sowing the seeds of a strong achievement motive. As adults, these children are more likely than others to engage in entrepreneurial activities and develop technological innovations, thereby contributing to a nation's economic welfare. In support of these ideas, McClelland (1961) reported evidence that schoolchildren from Protestant families had higher achievement motive scores on the PSE than children from Catholic families. The previously described research on the effects of parental demands for independent mastery of age-appropriate tasks on children's achievement motivation is also consistent with the idea that Protestant values of independent accomplishment provide the matrix for the development of a strong need for achievement (cf. McClelland & Pilon, 1983; Rosen & D'Andrade, 1959; Winterbottom, 1958).

McClelland (1961) also provided evidence that high-achievement individuals are more likely to engage in small-business and innovative enterprises, a frequently replicated finding (e.g., Langens, 2001; McClelland, 1965; Singh & Gupta, 1977; Wainer & Rubin, 1969). To support his claim that a societal concern with independent achievement has a causal effect on economic growth, McClelland scored children's readers and school books from different nations for achievement imagery at two different times (1925 and 1950) and related the scores to concurrent and subsequent levels of national energy consumption as a measure of economic output. Across both assessments, McClelland found evidence that collective levels of achievement motivation were independent of concurrent energy consumption, but positively predicted energy consumption increases in the subsequent 25-year time period. This finding suggests that high levels of endemic achievement motivation preceded, and perhaps caused, subsequent economic growth as a generation of children who had been reared to master challenges independently became adults and entered the workforce. Findings in support of McClelland's theory of achievement motivation and economic growth were also reported by others. deCharms and Moeller (1962) found that during a period from 1810 to 1950, increases of achievement imagery in American children's readers strongly predicted increases in the U.S. patent index, a measure of the nation's technological innovation rate and positively related to economic growth, with a time lag of 20 years. Bradburn and Berlew (1961) compared achievement motive imagery assessed in samples from English literary works written between 1550 and 1800 with energy consumption in London (gains in coal imports) across the same time span and found that increases in energy consumption closely followed increases in collective achievement motivation with a time lag of 30–50 years.

McClelland and Winter (1971) put the theory of achievement motivation and economic growth to the test by selecting two Indian cities with similar initial levels of employment and then training small business owners in one of them to think and behave like high-achievement individuals (e.g., set moderately challenging goals, take personal responsibility, seek feedback, write PSE stories with a high degree of achievement imagery). Two years after the training, employment in the city where the training had taken place had increased much more than in the "control" city, where no trainings had been conducted. However, the real test of the effectiveness of the achievement training came, quite unexpectedly, 1 year later, when an economic depression hit the country. Employment rates in both cities dropped, but they dropped more in the control city than in the "training" city. Three years after the depression, employment rates in the training city were on the rebound and actually exceeded predepression levels, whereas employment rates in the control city showed no sign of recovering. In combination with the previously described studies on energy consumption and patent index changes, McClel-

land and Winter's (1971) study thus provides considerable evidence for the validity of McClelland's (1961) model of achievement motivation and economic growth.

Power and Affiliation, War and Peace

Comparing the occurrence of war and peace in English and U.S. history with changes in power and affiliation motive levels, assessed by coding popular books, plays, and songs from both countries and across different historic periods, McClelland (1975) observed the following dynamic relationship between motivational variables and a country's belligerence versus peacefulness:

Stage 1: High levels of both affiliation and power precede the passing of social reforms, leading to a drop in collective affiliation motivation due to satisfaction of this need.

Stage 2: Power motivation continues to be high, but affiliation motivation is low; the nation becomes more aggressive and wages war against other countries.

Stage 3: As a consequence of the satisfaction of power needs through war, collective levels of power motivation drop, and in response to the threat caused by war, collective levels of affiliation motivation rise, triggering a period of peace. Power motivation levels subsequently rebound, thus bringing the pattern full circle to Stage 1.

Winter (1993) confirmed several key features of this model, providing three different lines of evidence. For a time span from 1603 to 1988 in British history, he compared motive patterns scored from the "Sovereign's Speeches," written by members of the government and presented by the king or queen of England at the beginning of each session of the Parliament, in years in which Britain went to war with motive patterns in years in which Britain did not go to war. In each case Winter also looked at motive patterns 1–5 years before the crucial comparison year. He found that, as predicted by the McClelland model, a clear predominance of power motivation over affiliation motivation preceded Britain's entry into war, with a lead time of 1 year. Conversely, power motive levels in the Sovereign's Speeches were significantly lower in years in which Britain ended a war than in years in which it was at war and did not end the war. Power motive levels also tended to decline further for a couple of years after a war ended.

In a second study, Winter (1993) analyzed motive patterns in British and German government-to-government communications before the outbreak of World War I. In the early phase of the crisis triggered by the assassination of Archduke Franz Ferdinand in Sarajevo, both governments used significantly more affiliation imagery than power imagery in their communications. However, this pattern reversed in the late phase of the crisis, with power imagery outweighing affiliation imagery, and the outcome of the escalation was the beginning of World War I.

In a third study, Winter (1993) demonstrated that a reduction in power motivation can also lead to the peaceful outcome of a crisis. Coding the government-to-government communications exchanged by the Kennedy administration and the Khrushchev Politburo during the Cuban missile crisis in 1962 for motive imagery, Winter observed that the dialogue between the two governments was initially characterized by a clear predominance of power motive imagery. However, in the late stage of the crisis, communications became more saturated with affiliation imagery, and power imagery decreased. The outcome of this shift from a concern with having impact on the other party to having friendly relationships with it was a peaceful resolution of the crisis.

In later studies, Winter (e.g., Langner & Winter, 2001) not only replicated the basic finding that a relative preponderance of power motivation over affiliation motivation in the communications between conflict parties precedes the beginning of an armed conflict. He also demonstrated, in archival analyses of real crises and in laboratory studies of conflict behavior, that one side's power motivation fuels the conflict through the endorsement of negative concessions (i.e., opposing the other side's concessions and suggestions for conflict solution; taking unilateral assertive action), thus escalating the conflict. In contrast, if one party is high in affiliation motivation, it is more likely to make positive concessions during negotiations (e.g., suggesting ways to facilitate dialogue and conflict resolution; accepting the other side's concessions), thus helping to deescalate the conflict.

One might wonder what motivational imagery scored from political documents or the popular literature actually represents. Is there any methodological or conceptual continuity with the implicit motives measured by the PSE in individuals? Methodologically, the same coding systems that have been developed for, and used with, the PSE can be used, without substantial modifications, with any other text document based on verbal or written language (e.g., McClelland, 1961, 1975; Winter, 1991). Thus, although the scored texts may originate from different intentions and contexts (writing imaginative stories in the case of the PSE; communicating with audiences or adversaries in the case of political texts; expressing current concerns, needs, and conflicts within a given culture and historical time in the case of popular literature), the same types of images that are coded in research participants' PSEs are also scored from political documents and popular literature. Commenting on the issue of conceptual continuity, McClelland (1987) argued that the behavioral correlates of motives measured at the collective level (e.g., from the popular literature) closely resemble those of motives assessed in the individual. For instance, much as individuals with a strong achievement motive are likely to be successful in business, societies with high collective achievement motivation levels tend to thrive economically. Similarly, individuals with a strong power motive tend to be assertive, and political entities and societies with high power motivation levels behave more assertively in the international arena, too. According to McClelland, these parallels suggest that collective motive levels represent, to some extent, the average motive levels of the individuals living in a particular society at a given historical time; they also support the idea that there is continuity in the construct validity of motives measured at individual and collective levels.

CONCLUSION

The study of implicit motives remains an active field of research in personality psychology. In recent years, interdisciplinary approaches to motive research have brought new discoveries and enhanced rigor to the field. This reinvigoration is partly due to methodological and conceptual advances in other disciplines and increased cross-talk between scientific disciplines. For instance, methods developed and fine-honed by cognitive psychologists and endocrinologists are now used to study the effects of motives on attention, implicit learning, episodic memory, and hormone changes. Advances in functional neuroimaging now even allow researchers to explore how implicit motives are "embrained" (Schultheiss, Wirth, et al., 2006). Today, dissociations between conscious and nonconscious forms of goal striving can be better understood conceptually on the basis of sophisticated models of information processing and learning (e.g., Paivio, 1986; Schultheiss, 2007b) and the interplay of brain systems in the generation and regulation of behavior (e.g., Rolls, 1999).

Another reason for the continuing interest in implicit motives may lie in this field's emphasis on the observation and measurement of actual behavioral phenomena rather than on self-report measures of personality and behavior. As personality psychology, and psychology in general, has grown more aware of the limits of humans' introspective access to the real causes of their behavior (e.g., Gazzaniga, 1985; Kagan, 1994, 2002; T. D. Wilson, 2002), many researchers now strive to develop measures that tap into the nonconscious reaches of the human mind. The rapidly growing number of personality measures based on the IAT is testament to this development. From the very start more than 50 years ago, research on implicit motives was based *exactly* on the premise that humans lack direct insight into many important wellsprings of their behavior (McClelland, 1984) and that therefore both the motivational needs that drive behavior as well as the effects of these dispositions on behavior need to be assessed with indirect methods (which, ironically, are often more direct than asking people what they *believe* they are doing, or what they believe causes their behavior). For a long time, this insistence on nondeclarative measurement of personality and motivation made implicit motive research the "odd one out" in personality psychology (cf. McClelland, 1996). But implicit motive researchers have used this relative separation from the mainstream of personality psychology to advance conceptual and empirical work on motives (cf. McClelland et al., 1989), to con-nect to other disciplines (e.g., endocrinology, immunology; cf. McClelland, 1989), and to build a strong case for the validity of implicit motives. As a consequence, the implicit motive construct today offers a well-developed, far-reaching, and fascinating approach for scholars who are interested in using methods that do not rely on self-reports to study personality, motivation, and behavior.

ACKNOWLEDGMENTS

I would like to thank Kent Berridge and Barbara Woike for their helpful comments on an earlier draft of this chapter. Parts of the research summarized in this chapter were supported by Deutsche Forschungsmeinschaft Grant Nos. SCHU 1210/1-2, 1-3, and 2-2; National Institute of Mental Health Grant No. 1 R03 MH63069-01; and National Science Foundation Grant No. BCS 0444301.

REFERENCES

Andrews, J. D. W. (1967). The achievement motive and advancement in two types of organization. *Journal of Personality and Social Psychology, 6,* 163–168.

Atkinson, J. W. (1953). The achievement motive and recall of interrupted and completed tasks. *Journal of Experimental Psychology, 46,* 381–390.

Atkinson, J. W. (1957). Motivational determinants of risk-taking behavior. *Psychological Review, 64,* 359–372.

Atkinson, J. W. (1981). Studying personality in the context of an advanced motivational psychology. *American Psychologist, 36,* 117–128.

Atkinson, J. W., Heyns, R. W., & Veroff, J. (1958). The effect of experimental arousal of the affiliation motive on thematic apperception. In J. W. Atkinson (Ed.), *Motives in fantasy, action, and society: A method of assessment and study* (pp. 95–104). Princeton, NJ: Van Nostrand.

Atkinson, J. W., & Litwin, G. H. (1960). Achievement motive and test anxiety conceived as motive to approach success and motive to avoid failure. *Journal of Abnormal and Social Psychology, 60,* 52–63.

Atkinson, J. W., & McClelland, D. C. (1948). The effects of different intensities of the hunger drive on thematic apperception. *Journal of Experimental Psychology, 28,* 643–658.

Atkinson, J. W., & O'Connor, P. (1966). Neglected factors in studies of achievement-oriented performance: Social approval as an incentive and performance decrement. In J. W. Atkinson &

N. T. Feather (Eds.), *A theory of achievement motivation* (pp. 299–326). New York: Wiley.

Atkinson, J. W., & Walker, E. L. (1958). The affiliation motive and perceptual sensitivity to faces. In J. W. Atkinson (Ed.), *Motives in fantasy, action, and society: A method of assessment and study* (pp. 360–366). Princeton, NJ: Van Nostrand.

Baumann, N., Kaschel, R., & Kuhl, J. (2005). Striving for unwanted goals: Stress-dependent discrepancies between explicit and implicit achievement motives reduce subjective well-being and increase psychosomatic symptoms. *Journal of Personality and Social Psychology, 89,* 781–799.

Bäumler, G. (1975). *Beeinflussung der Leistungsmotivation durch Psychopharmaka: I. Die 4 bildthematischen Hauptvariablen* [The effects of psychoactive drugs on achievement motivation: I. The four motivation scales]. *Zeitschrift für Experimentelle und Angewandte Psychologie, 22,* 1–14.

Beckwith, B. E., Petros, T. V., Bergloff, P. J., & Staebler, R. J. (1987). Vasopressin analogue (DDAVP) facilitates recall of narrative prose. *Behavioral Neuroscience, 101*(3), 429–432.

Berridge, K. C. (2000). Measuring hedonic impact in animals and infants: Microstructure of affective taste reactivity patterns. *Neuroscience and Biobehavioral Reviews, 24*(2), 173–198.

Berridge, K. C. (2004). Motivation concepts in behavioral neuroscience. *Physiology and Behavior, 81*(2), 179–209.

Berridge, K. C., & Robinson, T. E. (1998). What is the role of dopamine in reward: hedonic impact, reward learning, or incentive salience? *Brain Research Reviews, 28*(3), 309–369.

Berridge, K. C., & Robinson, T. E. (2003). Parsing reward. *Trends in Neuroscience, 26*(9), 507–513.

Biernat, M. (1989). Motives and values to achieve: Different constructs with different effects. *Journal of Personality, 57,* 69–95.

Bindra, D. (1978). How adaptive behavior is produced: A perceptual-motivational alternative to response-reinforcement. *Behavioral and Brain Sciences, 1,* 41–91.

Blankenship, V., Vega, C. M., Ramos, E., Romero, K., Warren, K., Keenan, K., et al. (2006). Using the multifaceted Rasch model to improve the TAT/PSE measure of need for achievement. *Journal of Personality Assessment, 86*(1), 100–114.

Blankenship, V., & Zoota, A. L. (1998). Comparing power imagery in TATs written by hand or on the computer. *Behavior Research Methods, Instruments, and Computers, 30,* 441–448.

Boesch-Achermann, H., & Boesch, C. (1993). Tool use in wild chimpanzees: New light from dark forests. *Current Directions in Psychological Science, 2,* 18–21.

Bornstein, R. F. (2002). A process dissociation approach to objective–projective test score interrelationships. *Journal of Personality Assessment, 78,* 47–68.

Boyatzis, R. E. (1973). Affiliation motivation. In D. C. McClelland & R. S. Steele (Eds.), *Human motivation: A book of readings* (pp. 252–276). Morristown, NJ: General Learning.

Bradburn, N. M., & Berlew, D. E. (1961). Need for achievement and English industrial growth. *Economic Development and Cultural Change, 10,* 8–20.

Brunstein, J. C. (2001). *Persönliche Ziele und Handlungs- versus Lageorientierung: Wer bindet sich an realistische und bedürfniskongruente Ziele?* [Personal goals and action versus state orientation: Who builds a commitment to realistic and need-congruent goals?]. *Zeitschrift für Differentielle und Diagnostische Psychologie, 22,* 1–12.

Brunstein, J. C., & Hoyer, S. (2002). *Implizites und explizites Leistungsstreben: Befunde zur Unabhängigkeit zweier Motivationssysteme* [Implicit and explicit achievement strivings: Empirical evidence of the independence of two motivational systems]. *Zeitschrift für Pädagogische Psychologie, 16,* 51–62.

Brunstein, J. C., & Maier, G. W. (2005). Implicit and self-attributed motives to achieve: Two separate but interacting needs. *Journal of Personality and Social Psychology, 89*(2), 205–222.

Brunstein, J. C., & Schmitt, C. H. (2004). Assessing individual differences in achievement motivation with the Implicit Association Test. *Journal of Research in Personality, 38*(6), 536–555.

Brunstein, J. C., Schultheiss, O. C., & Grässmann, R. (1998). Personal goals and emotional well-being: The moderating role of motive dispositions. *Journal of Personality and Social Psychology, 75*(2), 494–508.

Bucci, W. (1984). Linking words and things: Basic processes and individual variation. *Cognition, 17,* 137–153.

Bucci, W. (1985). Dual coding: A cognitive model for psychoanalytic research. *Journal of the American Psychoanalytic Association, 33,* 571–607.

Bucci, W. (1997). *Psychoanalysis and cognitive science: A multiple code theory.* New York: Guilford Press.

Burdick, H. A., & Burnes, A. J. (1958). A test of "strain toward symmetry" theories. *Journal of Abnormal and Social Psychology, 57,* 367–370.

Byrne, D. (1961). Interpersonal attraction as a function of affiliation need and attitude similarity. *Human Relations, 14,* 283–289.

Byrne, D. (1962). Response to attitude similarity-dissimilarity as a function of affiliation need. *Journal of Personality, 30,* 164–177.

Cabanac, M. (1979). Sensory pleasure. *Quarterly Review of Biology, 54*(1), 1–29.

Cacioppo, J. T., Petty, R. E., Losch, M. E., & Kim, H. S. (1986). Electromyographic activity over facial muscle regions can differentiate the valence and intensity of affective reactions. *Journal of Personality and Social Psychology, 50*(2), 260–268.

Cahill, L. (2000). Modulation of long-term memory in humans by emotional arousal: Adrenergic activation and the amygdala. In J. P. Aggleton (Ed.), *The amygdala: A functional analysis* (pp. 425–446). New York: Oxford University Press.

Cantor, N., & Blanton, H. (1996). Effortful pursuit of personal goals in daily life. In P. M. Gollwitzer & J. A. Bargh (Eds.), *The psychology of action: Linking cognition and motivation to behavior* (pp. 338–359). New York: Guilford Press.

Carver, C. S., & Scheier, M. F. (1998). *On the self-regulation of behavior.* New York: Cambridge University Press.

Clark, R. A. (1952). The projective measurement of experimentally induced levels of sexual motivation. *Journal of Experimental Psychology, 44*, 391–399.

Craig, J. A., Koestner, R., & Zuroff, D. C. (1994). Implicit and self-attributed intimacy motivation. *Journal of Social and Personal Relationships, 11*, 491–507.

Craig, W. (1918). Appetites and aversions as constituents of instincts. *Biological Bulletin of Woods Hole, 34*, 91–107.

Curran, T. (1997). Higher-order associative learning in amnesia: Evidence from the serial reaction time task. *Journal of Cognitive Neuroscience, 9*, 522–533.

Dabbs, J. M., Hopper, C. H., & Jurkovic, G. J. (1990). Testosterone and personality among college students and military veterans. *Personality and Individual Differences, 11*, 1263–1269.

Dabbs, J. M., Ruback, R. B., Frady, R. L., Hopper, C. H., & Sgoutas, D. S. (1988). Saliva testosterone and criminal violence among women. *Personality and Individual Differences, 9*, 269–275.

de Waal, F. B. (1998). *Chimpanzee politics: Power and sex among apes* (rev. ed.). Baltimore: Johns Hopkins University Press.

deCharms, R., & Moeller, G. H. (1962). Values expressed in American children's readers. *Journal of Abnormal and Social Psychology, 64*, 136–142.

deCharms, R., Morrison, H. W., Reitman, W., & McClelland, D. C. (1955). Behavioral correlates of directly and indirectly measured achievement motivation. In D. C. McClelland (Ed.), *Studies in motivation* (pp. 414–423). New York: Appleton-Century-Crofts.

Dickinson, A., & Balleine, B. (1994). Motiva-tional control of goal-directed action. *Animal Learning and Behavior, 22*, 1–18.

Dimberg, U. (1997). Psychophysiological reactions to facial expressions. In U. Segerstrale & P. Molnar (Eds.), *Nonverbal communication: Where nature meets culture* (pp. 47–60). Mahwah, NJ: Erlbaum.

Duncker, D. J., Haitsma, D. B., van der Geest, I. E., Stubenitsky, R., van Meegen, J. R., Man in't Veld, A. J., et al. (1997). Systemic, pulmonary and coronary haemodynamic actions of the novel dopamine receptor agonist in awake pigs at rest and during treadmill exercise. *British Journal of Pharmacology, 120*(6), 1101–1113.

Dutton, D. G., & Strachan, C. E. (1987). Motivational needs for power and spouse-specific assertiveness in assaultive and nonassaultive men. *Violence and Victims, 2*(3), 145–156.

Eichenbaum, H., & Cohen, N. J. (2001). *From conditioning to conscious recollection: Memory systems of the brain.* New York: Oxford University Press.

Eisenberger, R., & Cameron, J. (1996). Detrimental effects of reward: Reality or myth? *American Psychologist, 51*, 1153–1166.

Elliot, A. J., & Thrash, T. M. (2004). The intergenerational transmission of fear of failure. *Personality and Social Psychology Bulletin, 30*(8), 957–971.

Epstein, A. N. (1982). The physiology of thirst. In D. W. Pfaff (Ed.), *Physiological mechanisms of motivation* (pp. 25–55). New York: Springer.

Exline, R. V. (1963). Explorations in the process of person perception: Visual interaction in relation to competition, sex, and need for affiliation. *Journal of Personality, 31*, 1–20.

Feather, N. T. (1966). The relationship of persistence at a task to expectation of success and achievement-related motives. In J. W. Atkinson & N. T. Feather (Eds.), *A theory of achievement motivation* (pp. 117–133). New York: Wiley.

Feshbach, S. (1955). The drive-reducing function of fantasy behavior. *Journal of Abnormal and Social Psychology, 50*, 3–11.

Fodor, E. M. (1985). The power motive, group conflict, and physiological arousal. *Journal of Personality and Social Psychology, 49*, 1408–1415.

Fodor, E. M., & Farrow, D. L. (1979). The power motive as an influence on use of power. *Journal of Personality and Social Psychology, 37*(11), 2091–2097.

Fodor, E. M., & Smith, T. (1982). The power motive as an influence on group decision making. *Journal of Personality and Social Psychology, 42*, 178–185.

Fodor, E. M., Wick, D. P., & Hartsen, K. M. (2006). The power motive and affective response to assertiveness. *Journal of Research in Personality, 40*, 598–610.

Fontana, A. F., Rosenberg, R. L., Marcus, J. L., & Kerns, R. D. (1987). Type A behavior pattern, inhibited power motivation, and activity inhibition. *Journal of Personality and Social Psychology, 52,* 177–183.

French, E. G. (1958). Some characteristics of achievement motivation. In J. W. Atkinson (Ed.), *Motives in fantasy, action, and society* (pp. 270–277). Princeton, NJ: Van Nostrand.

Gazzaniga, M. S. (1985). *The social brain: Discovering the networks of the mind.* New York: Basic Books.

Gump, B. B., & Kulik, J. A. (1997). Stress, affiliation, and emotional contagion. *Journal of Personality and Social Psychology, 72*(2), 305–319.

Halisch, F., & Heckhausen, H. (1989). Motive-dependent versus ability-dependent valence functions for success and failure. In F. Halisch, J. H. L. van den Bercken, & S. Hazlett (Eds.), *International perspectives on achievement and task motivation* (pp. 51–67). Amsterdam: Swets & Zeitlinger.

Hardy, K. R. (1957). Determinants of conformity and attitude change. *Journal of Abnormal and Social Psychology, 54,* 289–294.

Heckhausen, H. (1963). *Hoffnung und Furcht in der Leistungsmotivation* [Hope and fear components of achievement motivation]. Meisenheim am Glan: Anton Hain.

Heckhausen, H., & Heckhausen, J. (in press). *Motivation and action* (2nd ed.). New York: Cambridge University Press.

Hermann, M. G. (1980). Assessing the personalities of Soviet Politburo members. *Personality and Social Psychology Bulletin, 6,* 332–352.

Hess, U., Blairy, S., & Kleck, R. E. (2000). The influence of facial emotion displays, gender, and ethnicity on judgments of dominance and affiliation. *Journal of Nonverbal Behavior, 24,* 265–283.

Hofer, J., & Chasiotis, A. (2004). Methodological considerations of applying a TAT-type picture-story test in cross-cultural research: A comparison of German and Zambian adolescents. *Journal of Cross-Cultural Psychology, 35*(2), 224–241.

Horner, M. S. (1972). Toward an understanding of achievement-related conflicts in women. *Journal of Social Issues, 28,* 157–175.

Ikemoto, S., & Panksepp, J. (1999). The role of nucleus accumbens dopamine in motivated behavior: A unifying interpretation with special reference to reward-seeking. *Brain Research Reviews, 31*(1), 6–41.

Insel, T. R., & Young, L. J. (2001). The neurobiology of attachment. *Nature Reviews: Neuroscience, 2*(2), 129–136.

Jacobs, R. L., & McClelland, D. C. (1994). Moving up the corporate ladder: A longitudinal study of the leadership motive pattern and managerial success in women and men. *Consulting Psychology Journal of Practice and Research, 46,* 32–41.

Jemmott, J. B. (1987). Social motives and susceptibility to disease: Stalking individual differences in health risks. *Journal of Personality, 55,* 267–298.

Jemmott, J. B., Borysenko, J. Z., Borysenko, M., McClelland, D. C., Chapman, R., Meyer, D., et al. (1983). Academic stress, power motivation, and decrease in secretion rate of salivary secretory immunoglobulin A. *Lancet, 8339,* 1400–1402.

Jemmott, J. B., Hellman, C., McClelland, D. C., Locke, S. E., Kraus, L., Williams, R. M., et al. (1990). Motivational syndromes associated with natural killer cell activity. *Journal of Behavioral Medicine, 13,* 53–73.

Johnston, R. A. (1957). A methodological analysis of several revised forms of the Iowa Picture Interpretation Test. *Journal of Personality, 25,* 283–293.

Kagan, J. (1994). *Galen's prophecy.* New York: Westview Press.

Kagan, J. (2002). *Surprise, uncertainty, and mental structures.* Cambridge, MA: Harvard University Press.

Karabenick, S. A. (1977). Fear of success, achievement and affiliation dispositions, and the performance of men and women under individual and competitive conditions. *Journal of Personality, 45,* 117–149.

Kazen, M., & Kuhl, J. (2005). Intention memory and achievement motivation: Volitional facilitation and inhibition as a function of affective contents of need-related stimuli. *Journal of Personality and Social Psychology, 89*(3), 426–448.

King, L. A. (1995). Wishes, motives, goals, and personal memories: Relations of measures of human motivation. *Journal of Personality, 63,* 985–1007.

Klinger, E. (1967). Modeling effects on achievement imagery. *Journal of Personality and Social Psychology, 7,* 49–62.

Knutson, B. (1996). Facial expressions of emotion influence interpersonal trait inferences. *Journal of Nonverbal Behavior, 20,* 165–182.

Koestner, R., & McClelland, D. C. (1992). The affiliation motive. In C. P. Smith (Ed.), *Motivation and personality: Handbook of thematic content analysis* (pp. 205–210). New York: Cambridge University Press.

Koestner, R., Weinberger, J., & McClelland, D. C. (1991). Task-intrinsic and social-extrinsic sources of arousal for motives assessed in fantasy and self-report. *Journal of Personality, 59,* 57–82.

Kornadt, H.-J. (1987). The aggression motive and

personality development: Japan and Germany. In F. Halisch & J. Kuhl (Eds.), *Motivation, intention and volition* (pp. 115–140). Berlin: Springer.

Kuhl, J., Scheffer, D., & Eichstaedt, J. (2003). *Der Operante Motiv-Test (OMT): Ein neuer Ansatz zur Messung impliziter Motive* [The Operant Motive Test (OMT): A new approach to implicit motive assessment]. In F. Rheinberg & J. Stiensmeier-Pelster (Eds.), *Diagnostik von Motivation und Selbstkonzept* [Assessment of motivation and self-concept] (pp. 129–150). Göttingen, Germany: Hogrefe.

Lang, P. J., Bradley, M. M., & Cuthbert, B. N. (1997). Motivated attention: Affect, activation, and action. In P. J. Lang, R. F. Simons, & M. T. Balaban (Eds.), *Attention and orienting: Sensory and motivational processes* (pp. 97–135). Mahwah, NJ: Erlbaum.

Langens, T. A. (2001). Predicting behavior change in Indian businessmen from a combination of need for achievement and self-discrepancy. *Journal of Research in Personality, 35,* 1–14.

Langner, C. A., & Winter, D. G. (2001). The motivational basis of concessions and compromise: Archival and laboratory studies. *Journal of Personality and Social Psychology, 81,* 711–727.

Lansing, J. B., & Heyns, R. W. (1959). Need affiliation and frequency of four types of communication. *Journal of Abnormal and Social Psychology, 58,* 365–372.

LeDoux, J. E. (2002). *The synaptic self.* New York: Viking.

Litwin, G. H., & Siebrecht, A. (1967). Integrators and entrepreneurs: Their motivation and effect on management. *Hospital Progress, 48*(9), 67–71.

Lundy, A., & Potts, T. (1987). Recollection of a transitional object and needs for intimacy and affiliation in adolescents. *Psychological Reports, 60,* 767–773.

Maddi, S. R., Propst, B. S., & Feldinger, I. (1965). Three expressions of the need for variety. *Journal of Personality, 33,* 82–98.

McAdams, D. P. (1982). Experiences of intimacy and power: Relationships between social motives and autobiographical memory. *Journal of Personality and Social Psychology, 42,* 292–302.

McAdams, D. P. (1992). The intimacy motive. In C. P. Smith (Ed.), *Motivation and personality: Handbook of thematic content analysis* (pp. 224–228). New York: Cambridge University Press.

McAdams, D. P., & Constantian, C. A. (1983). Intimacy and affiliation motives in daily living: An experience sampling analysis. *Journal of Personality and Social Psychology, 45,* 851–861.

McAdams, D. P., Hoffmann, B. J., Mansfield, E.

D., & Day, R. (1996). Themes of agency and communion in significant autobiographical scenes. *Journal of Personality, 64,* 339–377.

McAdams, D. P., Jackson, J., & Kirshnit, C. (1984). Looking, laughing, and smiling in dyads as a function of intimacy motivation and reciprocity. *Journal of Personality, 52,* 261–273.

McAdams, D. P., Lester, R. M., Brand, P. A., McNamara, W. J., & Lensky, D. B. (1988). Sex and the TAT: Are women more intimate than men? Do men fear intimacy? *Journal of Personality Assessment, 52,* 397–409.

McAdams, D. P., & Powers, J. (1981). Themes of intimacy in behavior and thought. *Journal of Personality and Social Psychology, 40,* 573–587.

McAdams, D. P., & Vaillant, G. E. (1982). Intimacy motivation and psychosocial adjustment: A longitudinal study. *Journal of Personality Assessment, 46,* 586–593.

McClelland, D. C. (1961). *The achieving society.* New York: Free Press.

McClelland, D. C. (1965). Achievement and entrepreneurship: A longitudinal study. *Journal of Personality and Social Psychology, 1,* 389–392.

McClelland, D. C. (1975). *Power: The inner experience.* New York: Irvington.

McClelland, D. C. (1979). Inhibited power motivation and high blood pressure in men. *Journal of Abnormal Psychology, 88,* 182–190.

McClelland, D. C. (1980). Motive dispositions: The merits of operant and respondent measures. In L. Wheeler (Ed.), *Review of personality and social psychology* (Vol. 1, pp. 10–41). Beverly Hills: Sage.

McClelland, D. C. (1982). The need for power, sympathetic activation, and illness. *Motivation and Emotion, 6,* 31–41.

McClelland, D. C. (1984). *Motives, personality, and society: Selected papers.* New York: Praeger.

McClelland, D. C. (1987). *Human motivation.* New York: Cambridge University Press.

McClelland, D. C. (1989). Motivational factors in health and disease. *American Psychologist, 44,* 675–683.

McClelland, D. C. (1995). Achievement motivation in relation to achievement-related recall, performance, and urine flow: A marker associated with release of vasopressin. *Motivation and Emotion, 19,* 59–76.

McClelland, D. C. (1996). Does the field of personality have a future? *Journal of Research in Personality, 30,* 429–434.

McClelland, D. C., Alexander, C., & Marks, E. (1982). The need for power, stress, immune function, and illness among male prisoners. *Journal of Abnormal Psychology, 91,* 61–70.

McClelland, D. C., Atkinson, J. W., Clark, R. A.,

& Lowell, E. L. (1953). *The achievement motive*. New York: Appleton-Century-Crofts.

McClelland, D. C., & Boyatzis, R. E. (1982). Leadership motive pattern and long-term success in management. *Journal of Applied Psychology, 67*, 737–743.

McClelland, D. C., Brown, D., Patel, V., & Kelner, S. P. (1988). *Affiliation motivation and eating behavior in adult insulin dependent diabetics*. Unpublished manuscript, Boston University, Department of Psychology, Boston.

McClelland, D. C., & Burnham, D. H. (1976). Power is the great motivator. *Harvard Business Review, 54*, 100–110.

McClelland, D. C., Davidson, R. J., & Saron, C. (1985). Stressed power motivation, sympathetic activation, immune function, and illness. *Advances, 2*, 42–52.

McClelland, D. C., Davis, W. N., Kalin, R., & Wanner, E. (1972). *The drinking man*. New York: Free Press.

McClelland, D. C., Floor, E., Davidson, R. J., & Saron, C. (1980). Stressed power motivation, sympathetic activation, immune function, and illness. *Journal of Human Stress, 6*, 11–19.

McClelland, D. C., & Franz, C. E. (1992). Motivational and other sources of work accomplishments in mid-life: A longitudinal study. *Journal of Personality, 60*, 679–707.

McClelland, D. C., & Jemmott, J. B. (1980). Power motivation, stress and physical illness. *Journal of Human Stress, 6*, 6–15.

McClelland, D. C., & Kirshnit, C. (1988). The effect of motivational arousal through films on salivary immunoglobulin A. *Psychology and Health, 2*, 31–52.

McClelland, D. C., Koestner, R., & Weinberger, J. (1989). How do self-attributed and implicit motives differ? *Psychological Review, 96*, 690–702.

McClelland, D. C., Maddocks, J. A., & McAdams, D. P. (1985). The need for power, brain norepinephrine turnover, and memory. *Motivation and Emotion, 9*, 1–9.

McClelland, D. C., Patel, V., Stier, D., & Brown, D. (1987). The relationship of affiliative arousal to dopamine release. *Motivation and Emotion, 11*, 51–66.

McClelland, D. C., & Pilon, D. A. (1983). Sources of adult motives in patterns of parent behavior in early childhood. *Journal of Personality and Social Psychology, 44*, 564–574.

McClelland, D. C., Ross, G., & Patel, V. (1985). The effect of an academic examination on salivary norepinephrine and immunoglobulin levels. *Journal of Human Stress, 11*, 52–59.

McClelland, D. C., Scioli, A., & Weaver, S. (1998). The effect of implicit and explicit motivation on recall among old and young adults. *International Journal of Aging and Human Development, 46*, 1–20.

McClelland, D. C., & Teague, G. (1975). Predicting risk preferences among power related tasks. *Journal of Personality, 43*, 266–285.

McClelland, D. C., & Watson, R. I. (1973). Power motivation and risk-taking behavior. *Journal of Personality, 41*, 121–139.

McClelland, D. C., & Winter, D. G. (1971). *Motivating economic achievement: Accelerating economic development through psychological training*. New York: Free Press.

Monaghan, E. P., & Glickman, S. E. (1992). Hormones and aggressive behavior. In J. B. Becker, S. M. Breedlove, & D. Crews (Eds.), *Behavioral endocrinology* (pp. 261–285). Cambridge, MA: MIT Press.

Mücher, H. P., & Heckhausen, H. (1962). Influence of mental activity and achievement motivation on skeletal muscle tonus. *Perceptual and Motor Skills, 14*, 217–218.

Mueller, E. F., & Beimann, M. (1969). *Die Beziehung der Harnsäure zu Testwerten der nach Heckhausen gemessenen Leistungsmotivation* [Relationship between uric acid and Heckhausen's measure of achievement motivation]. *Zeitschrift für Experimentelle und Angewandte Psychologie, 16*(2), 295–306.

Mueller, E. F., Kasl, S. V., Brooks, G. W., & Cobb, S. (1970). Psychosocial correlates of serum urate levels. *Psychological Bulletin, 73*(4), 238–257.

Nisbett, R. E., & Wilson, T. D. (1977). Telling more than we can know: Verbal reports on mental processes. *Psychological Review, 84*, 231–259.

Nissen, M. J., & Bullemer, P. (1987). Attentional requirements of learning: Evidence from performance measures. *Cognitive Psychology, 19*, 1–32.

Paivio, A. (1986). *Mental representations: A dual coding approach*. New York: Oxford University Press.

Pang, J. S. (2006). *Hope of success and fear of failure*. Unpublished doctoral dissertation, University of Michigan, Ann Arbor.

Pang, J. S., & Schultheiss, O. C. (2005). Assessing implicit motives in U.S. college students: Effects of picture type and position, gender and ethnicity, and cross-cultural comparisons. *Journal of Personality Assessment, 85*(3), 280–294.

Panksepp, J. (1998). *Affective neuroscience: The foundations of human and animal emotions*. New York: Oxford University Press.

Peterson, B. E., & Stewart, A. J. (1993). Generativity and social motives in young adults. *Journal of Personality and Social Psychology, 65*, 186–198.

Peterson, B. E., & Stewart, A. J. (1996). Antecedents and contexts of generativity motivation at midlife. *Psychology and Aging, 11*, 21–33.

Pfaff, D. W. (1999). *Drive: Neurobiological and molecular mechanisms of sexual motivation*. Cambridge, MA: MIT Press.

Posner, M. I. (1995). Attention in cognitive neuroscience: An overview. In M. S. Gazzaniga (Ed.), *The cognitive neurosciences* (pp. 615–624). Cambridge, MA: MIT Press.

Raphelson, A. C. (1957). The relationships among imaginative, direct verbal, and physiological measures of anxiety in an achievement situation. *Journal of Abnormal and Social Psychology, 54,* 13–18.

Reuman, D. A. (1982). Ipsative behavioral variability and the quality of thematic apperceptive measurement of the achievement motive. *Journal of Personality and Social Psychology, 43*(5), 1098–1110.

Ridgeway, C. L. (1987). Nonverbal behavior, dominance, and the basis of status in task groups. *American Sociological Review, 52,* 683–694.

Rolls, E. T. (1999). *The brain and emotion.* Oxford, UK: Oxford University Press.

Rosen, B. C., & D'Andrade, R. (1959). The psychological origins of the achievement motive. *Sociometry, 22,* 185–218.

Sapolsky, R. M. (1987). Stress, social status, and reproductive physiology in free-living baboons. In D. Crews (Ed.), *Psychobiology and reproductive behavior: An evolutionary perspective* (pp. 291–322). Englewood Cliffs, NJ: Prentice-Hall.

Schachter, S. (1959). *The psychology of affiliation.* Stanford, CA: Stanford University Press.

Schroth, M. L. (1985). The effect of differing measuring methods on the relationship of motives. *Journal of Psychology, 119,* 213–218.

Schroth, M. L. (1987). Relationships between achievement-related motives, extrinsic conditions, and task performance. *Journal of Social Psychology, 127,* 39–48.

Schultheiss, O. (1996). *Imagination, Motivation und Verhalten* [Imagination, motivation, and behavior]. Unpublished dissertation thesis, Friedrich-Alexander-Universität, Erlangen, Germany.

Schultheiss, O. C. (2001). An information processing account of implicit motive arousal. In M. L. Maehr & P. Pintrich (Eds.), *Advances in motivation and achievement: Vol. 12. New directions in measures and methods* (pp. 1–41). Greenwich, CT: JAI Press.

Schultheiss, O. C. (2007a). A biobehavioral model of implicit power motivation arousal, reward and frustration. In E. Harmon-Jones & P. Winkielman (Eds.), *Social neuroscience: Integrating biological and psychological explanations of social behavior* (pp. 176–196). New York: Guilford Press.

Schultheiss, O. C. (2007b). A memory-systems approach to the classification of personality tests: Comment on Meyer and Kurtz (2006). *Journal of Personality Assessment, 89*(2), 197–201.

Schultheiss, O. C., & Brunstein, J. C. (1999). Goal imagery: Bridging the gap between implicit motives and explicit goals. *Journal of Personality, 67,* 1–38.

Schultheiss, O. C., & Brunstein, J. C. (2001). Assessing implicit motives with a research version of the TAT: Picture profiles, gender differences, and relations to other personality measures. *Journal of Personality Assessment, 77*(1), 71–86.

Schultheiss, O. C., & Brunstein, J. C. (2002). Inhibited power motivation and persuasive communication: A lens model analysis. *Journal of Personality, 70,* 553–582.

Schultheiss, O. C., & Brunstein, J. C. (2005). An implicit motive perspective on competence. In A. J. Elliot & C. S. Dweck (Eds.), *Handbook of competence and motivation* (pp. 31–51). New York: Guilford Press.

Schultheiss, O. C., Campbell, K. L., & McClelland, D. C. (1999). Implicit power motivation moderates men's testosterone responses to imagined and real dominance success. *Hormones and Behavior, 36*(3), 234–241.

Schultheiss, O. C., Dargel, A., & Rohde, W. (2003a). Implicit motives and gonadal steroid hormones: Effects of menstrual cycle phase, oral contraceptive use, and relationship status. *Hormones and Behavior, 43,* 293–301.

Schultheiss, O. C., Dargel, A., & Rohde, W. (2003b). Implicit motives and sexual motivation and behavior. *Journal of Research in Personality, 37,* 224–230.

Schultheiss, O. C., & Hale, J. A. (2007). Implicit motives modulate attentional orienting to perceived facial expressions of emotion. *Motivation and Emotion, 31*(1), 13–24.

Schultheiss, O. C., Jones, N. M., Davis, A. Q., & Kley, C. (in press). The role of implicit motivation in hot and cold goal pursuit: Effects on goal progress, goal rumination, and depressive symptoms. *Journal of Research in Personality.*

Schultheiss, O. C., & Pang, J. S. (2007). Measuring implicit motives. In R. W. Robins, R. C. Fraley, & R. F. Krueger (Eds.), *Handbook of research methods in personality psychology* (pp. 322–344). New York: Guilford Press.

Schultheiss, O. C., Pang, J. S., Torges, C. M., Wirth, M. M., & Treynor, W. (2005). Perceived facial expressions of emotion as motivational incentives: Evidence from a differential implicit learning paradigm. *Emotion, 5*(1), 41–54.

Schultheiss, O. C., Riebel, K., & Jones, N. M. (2006). *Activity inhibition: A predictor of lateralized brain function during stress?* Manuscript submitted for publication.

Schultheiss, O. C., & Rohde, W. (2002). Implicit power motivation predicts men's testosterone changes and implicit learning in a contest situation. *Hormones and Behavior, 41,* 195–202.

Schultheiss, O. C., & Schad, D. (2006). [Referential competence as a moderator of the effects of implicit motives on declarative measures of emotion.] Unpublished raw data.

Schultheiss, O. C., & Wirth, M. M. (in press). Biopsychological aspects of motivation. In J. Heckhausen & H. Heckhausen (Eds.), *Motivation and action*. New York: Cambridge University Press.

Schultheiss, O. C., Wirth, M. M., & Stanton, S. J. (2004). Effects of affiliation and power motivation arousal on salivary progesterone and testosterone. *Hormones and Behavior, 46*(5), 592–599.

Schultheiss, O. C., Wirth, M. M., Torges, C. M., Pang, J. S., Villacorta, M. A., & Welsh, K. M. (2005). Effects of implicit power motivation on men's and women's implicit learning and testosterone changes after social victory or defeat. *Journal of Personality and Social Psychology, 88*(1), 174–188.

Schultheiss, O. C., Wirth, M. M., Waugh, C. E., Stanton, S., Meier, E., & Reuter-Lorenz, P. (2006). *Exploring the motivational brain: Effects of implicit power motivation on brain activation in response to facial expressions of emotion*. Manuscript submitted for publication.

Siegel, P., & Weinberger, J. (1997, August). *Capturing the MOMMY AND I ARE ONE merger fantasy: The oneness motive*. Paper presented at the 105th annual convention of the American Psychological Association, Chicago.

Singh, S., & Gupta, B. S. (1977). Motives and agricultural growth. *British Journal of Social and Clinical Psychology, 16*, 189–190.

Smith, C. P. (Ed.). (1992). *Motivation and personality: Handbook of thematic content analysis*. New York: Cambridge University Press.

Sokolowski, K., Schmalt, H. D., Langens, T. A., & Puca, R. M. (2000). Assessing achievement, affiliation, and power motives all at once: The multi-motive grid (MMG). *Journal of Personality Assessment, 74*(1), 126–145.

Spangler, W. D. (1992). Validity of questionnaire and TAT measures of need for achievement: Two meta-analyses. *Psychological Bulletin, 112*, 140–154.

Squire, L. R., & Zola, S. M. (1996). Structure and function of declarative and nondeclarative memory systems. *Proceedings of the National Academy of Sciences, 93*(24), 13515–13522.

Stanton, S. J., & Schultheiss, O. C. (2007). Basal and dynamic relationships between implicit power motivation and estradiol in women. *Hormones and Behavior, 52*(5), 571–580.

Stanton, S. J., Wirth, M. M., & Schultheiss, O. C. (2006, January). *Effects of perceivers' implicit power motivation on attentional orienting to Pavlovian-conditioned cues of anger and joy*. Paper presented at the annual meeting of the Society for Personality and Social Psychology, Palm Springs, CA.

Steele, R. S. (1973). *The physiological concomitants of psychogenic motive arousal in college males*. Unpublished doctoral dissertation, Harvard University, Boston.

Steele, R. S. (1977). Power motivation, activation, and inspirational speeches. *Journal of Personality, 45*, 53–64.

Stricker, E. M., & Verbalis, J. G. (2002). Hormones and ingestive behaviors. In J. B. Becker, S. M. Breedlove, & D. Crews (Eds.), *Behavioral endocrinology* (2nd ed., pp. 451–473). Cambridge, MA: MIT Press.

Taylor, S. E., Klein, L. C., Lewis, B. P., Gruenewald, T. L., Gurung, R. A., & Updegraff, J. A. (2000). Biobehavioral responses to stress in females: Tend-and-befriend, not fight-or-flight. *Psychological Review, 107*(3), 411–429.

Teitelbaum, P. (1966). The use of operant methods in the assessment and control of motivational states. In W. K. Honig (Ed.), *Operant behavior: Areas of research and application* (pp. 565–608). New York: Appleton-Century-Crofts.

Thrash, T. M., & Elliot, A. J. (2002). Implicit and self-attributed achievement motives: Concordance and predictive validity. *Journal of Personality, 70*, 729–756.

Thrash, T. M., Elliot, A. J., & Schultheiss, O. C. (2007). Methodological and dispositional predictors of congruence between implicit and explicit need for achievement. *Personality and Social Psychology Bulletin, 33*, 961–974.

Toates, F. (1986). *Motivational systems*. Cambridge, UK: Cambridge University Press.

van Honk, J., Tuiten, A., Hermans, E., Putman, P., Koppeschaar, H., Thijssen, J., et al. (2001). A single administration of testosterone induces cardiac accelerative responses to angry faces in healthy young women. *Behavioral Neuroscience, 115*(1), 238–242.

Veroff, J. (1969). Social comparison and the development of achievement motivation. In C. P. Smith (Ed.), *Achievement-related motives in children* (pp. 46–101). New York: Sage Foundation.

Veroff, J., & Veroff, J. B. (1972). Reconsideration of a measure of power motivation. *Psychological Bulletin, 78*, 279–291.

Wainer, H. A., & Rubin, I. M. (1969). Motivation of research and development entrepreneurs: Determinants of company success. *Journal of Applied Psychology, 53*, 178–184.

Walker, E. L., Atkinson, J. W., Veroff, J., Birney, R. C., Dember, W., & Moulton, R. W. (1958). The expression of fear-related motivation in thematic apperception as a function of the proximity to an atomic explosion. In J. W. Atkinson (Ed.), *Motives in fantasy, action, and society: A method of assessment and study* (pp. 143–159). Princeton, NJ: Van Nostrand.

Weber, M. (1905). *Die protestantische Ethik und der Geist des Kapitalismus: I. Das Problem* [The Protestant ethic and the spirit of capitalism: I. The problem]. *Archiv für Sozialwissenschaft und Sozialpolitik, 20,* 1–54.

Weinberger, J., & McClelland, D. C. (1990). Cognitive versus traditional motivational models: Irreconcilable or complementary? In E. T. Higgins & R. M. Sorrentino (Eds.), *Handbook of motivation and cognition: Foundations of social behavior* (Vol. 2, pp. 562–597). New York: Guilford Press.

Weiner, B. (1965). Need achievement and the resumption of incompleted tasks. *Journal of Personality and Social Psychology, 1,* 165–168.

Wendt, H.-W. (1955). Motivation, effort, and performance. In D. C. McClelland (Ed.), *Studies in motivation* (pp. 448–459). New York: Appleton-Century-Crofts.

Wilson, E. O. (1980). *Sociobiology: The abridged edition.* Cambridge, MA: Harvard University Press.

Wilson, T. D. (2002). *Strangers to ourselves: Discovering the adaptive unconscious.* Cambridge, MA: Harvard University Press.

Winter, D. G. (1973). *The power motive.* New York: Free Press.

Winter, D. G. (1980). An exploratory study of the motives of Southern African political leaders measured at a distance. *Political Psychology, 2,* 75–85.

Winter, D. G. (1988). The power motive in women—and men. *Journal of Personality and Social Psychology, 54,* 510–519.

Winter, D. G. (1991). Measuring personality at a distance: Development of an integrated system for scoring motives in running text. In D. J. Ozer, J. M. Healy, & A. J. Stewart (Eds.), *Perspectives in personality* (Vol. 3, pp. 59–89). London: Kingsley.

Winter, D. G. (1993). Power, affiliation, and war: Three tests of a motivational model. *Journal of Personality and Social Psychology, 65,* 532–545.

Winter, D. G. (1994). *Manual for scoring motive imagery in running text* (4th ed.). Unpublished manuscript, Department of Psychology, University of Michigan, Ann Arbor.

Winter, D. G. (1996). *Personality: Analysis and interpretation of lives.* New York: McGraw-Hill.

Winterbottom, M. R. (1958). The relation of need for achievement to learning experiences in independence and mastery. In J. W. Atkinson (Ed.), *Motives in fantasy, action, and society: A method of assessment and study* (pp. 453–478). Princeton, NJ: Van Nostrand.

Wirth, M. M., & Schultheiss, O. C. (2006). Effects of affiliation arousal (hope of closeness) and affiliation stress (fear of rejection) on progesterone and cortisol. *Hormones and Behavior, 50,* 786–795.

Wirth, M. M., Welsh, K. M., & Schultheiss, O. C. (2006). Salivary cortisol changes in humans after winning or losing a dominance contest depend on implicit power motivation. *Hormones and Behavior, 49*(3), 346–352.

Wittling, W. (1995). Brain asymmetry in the control of autonomic-physiologic activity. In R. J. Davidson & K. Hugdahl (Eds.), *Brain asymmetry* (pp. 305–357). Cambridge, MA: MIT Press.

Woike, B. A. (1994). Vivid recollection as a technique to arouse implicit motive-related affect. *Motivation and Emotion, 18,* 335–349.

Woike, B. A. (1995). Most-memorable experiences: Evidence for a link between implicit and explicit motives and social cognitive processes in everyday life. *Journal of Personality and Social Psychology, 68,* 1081–1091.

Woike, B. A., Gershkovich, I., Piorkowski, R., & Polo, M. (1999). The role of motives in the content and structure of autobiographical memory. *Journal of Personality and Social Psychology, 76*(4), 600–612.

Woike, B. A., McLeod, S., & Goggin, M. (2003). Implicit and explicit motives influence accessibility to different autobiographical knowledge. *Personality and Social Psychology Bulletin, 29*(8), 1046–1055.

Woike, B. A., & Polo, M. (2001). Motive-related memories: Content, structure, and affect. *Journal of Personality, 69*(3), 391–415.

Wright, R. A., & Brehm, J. W. (1989). Energization and goal attractiveness. In L. A. Pervin (Ed.), *Goal concepts in personality and social psychology* (pp. 169–210). Hillsdale, NJ: Erlbaum.

Zajonc, R. B. (1980). Feeling and thinking: Preferences need no inferences. *American Psychologist, 35,* 151–175.

Zeldow, P. B., Daugherty, S. R., & McAdams, D. P. (1988). Intimacy, power, and psychological well-being in medical students. *Journal of Nervous and Mental Disease, 176,* 182–187.

CHAPTER 25

Personality and the Capacity for Religious and Spiritual Experience

Robert A. Emmons
Justin L. Barrett
Sarah A. Schnitker

A chapter on the psychology of religion has never before appeared in a personality handbook. Religion has often been overlooked, neglected, minimized, and marginalized, despite the fact that religion was of great interest to the founding figures of the field, including Gordon Allport and Henry Murray. This neglect is striking in that one of the hallmarks of personality psychology that distinguishes it from other fields is its focus on a comprehensive understanding of the person. Accordingly, personality psychology should have a distinctive relationship with the psychology of religion. Personality psychology provides a natural home for the study of religion and spirituality in that a concern with the transcendent is an inherent part of what it means to be human (Emmons, 1999; Kirkpatrick, 1999). Spiritual or religious goals, beliefs, and practices are central to many people's lives and are powerful influences on cognition, affect, motivation, and behavior. Because spirituality and religiousness are profound aspects of people's lives, it would seem that in order to know about people (McAdams, 1995), personologists must know about the religious side of people's lives. Certainly personality psychology is not alone in its omission of the religious side of life; Rozin (2006) notes that the topic receives scant attention in introductory, social, and developmental textbooks.

Personality psychologists are said to "provide glimpses of what it's like to be human" (Carver, 1996, p. 331). Spiritual or religious goals, beliefs, and practices are not only a distinctive component of a person, for many *they are* the core of the personality. National polls repeatedly report that over 90% of Americans believe in God. In one survey, nearly three-quarters of those nationally polled reported that "my whole approach to life is based on my religion" (Bergin & Jensen, 1990, p. 4). Thus, for at least a substantial percentage of the population, an acute sense of spirituality is likely to be central to their self-concept, identity, and relationship to God and others. Today, between 3 and 4 billion people of the world's population are adherents of the major religions. Across the lifespan, spirituality and religion are important, perhaps central, dimensions of human experience. Even among groups thought to be unconcerned with spiritual matters, religious concern is active. Data from American adolescents show that 95% believe in God, and three-quarters try to follow the teachings of their religion; almost half of American youth say they frequently pray alone, and 36% are involved in church youth groups (Smith & Denton, 2005). About 40% of adults worship weekly, and, among the elderly, approximately 50% of persons age 65 and older attend religious services at least weekly (Barna, n.d.). In the United States alone, 82% of the population reportedly believes in life after death (Davis, Smith, & Marsden, 1998), and the majority (70%) of people believe in eternal judgment and hell (Winseman, 2004).

Data also indicate that people's religious commitments, behaviors, and identities change as they pass through adulthood. Longitudinal studies show that adults in the United States generally become more religious as they age. Religiousness is quite stable in a rank-order sense (test–retest correlations have ranged from .40 to .70 over 10-, 20-, 30-, and even 40-year intervals during adulthood; Idler & Kasl, 1997; Lubinski, Schmidt, & Benbow, 1996; Wink & Dillon, 2001), but many adults' absolute levels of religiousness change over the life course. Given that personality psychologists concern themselves with stability and change in personality, these shifts in religious commitments are interesting theoretically.

THE RELIGION AND PERSONALITY LANDSCAPE

Religion Defined

In order for progress to occur in a scientific discipline, there must be some consensus concerning the meaning of core constructs and their measurement. A lack of precision does hamper progress in the field. Religion is a "set of beliefs, symbols, and practices about the reality of superempirical orders that make claims to organize and guide human life" (Smith, 2003, p. 118). Other features of religion include a belief in a reality beyond ordinary existence, a distinction between the sacred and the secular, ritual or corporate worship, a moral code of ethical principles, a striving to attain levels of consciousness beyond normal experience, the use of sacred texts, a belief in an afterlife, and an emotional connection to the transcendent (Smart, 1996).

It has become fashionable, both culturally and in the scientific literature, to differentiate between the spiritual and the religious. The noun "spirit" and the adjective "spiritual" are being used to refer to an ever-increasing range of experiences rather than being reserved for those occasions of use that specifically imply the existence of nonmaterial forces or persons. The word "spirituality" comes from the Latin *spiritus*, meaning breath, or "the animating or vital principle of a person" (*Oxford English Dictionary*). In Christian theology, spirituality may most naturally be defined as the result of the work of the Holy Spirit in humans—more specifically, in humans' souls and in their activities. Because psychology must deal with natural rather than supernatural levels of description and explanation, however, spirituality has been defined in solely human terms as "a deep sense of belonging, of wholeness, of connectedness, and of openness to the infinite" as that which involves "ultimate and personal truths," and as "a way of being and experiencing that which comes about through awareness of a transcendent dimension and that is characterized by certain identifiable values in regard to self, others, nature, life and whatever one considers to be the Ultimate" (Elkins, 2005, p. 139). Spirituality—in contrast to religion—means something spontaneous, informal, creative, and universal; it means authentic inner experience, and it implies freedom of individual expression, of seeking, and even of religious experimenting (Elkins, 2005).

In contrast, religions are rooted in authoritative spiritual traditions that transcend the person and point to larger realities within which the person is embedded: "A religion is a unified set of beliefs and practices relative to sacred things, that is to say, things set apart and forbidden-beliefs and practices which unite into one single moral community, called a Church, all those who adhere to them" (Wilson, 2002, p. 222). Spiritualities *may* be contextualized within faith communities, though they need not be. Religions are sets of beliefs, symbols, and practices about the reality of superempirical orders that make claims to organize and guide human life. They include a covenant faith community with teachings and narratives that enhance the search for the sacred and encourage morality. The term "religiosity" refers to motivating commitments to supernatural beings, powers, and places, as well as dispositions to form these beliefs. Such supernatural objects are normally viewed as "gods." Whereas some have argued that the movement toward spirituality represents a movement away from traditional religion, others contend that the increased emphasis on spirituality indicates an increased respect for the inner, contemplative practices of traditional religious systems.

Religion and Personality Traits

Determining how religiousness is related to the major dimensions of human personality has been an important starting point for improving relations between personality psychology and the scientific study of religion. In the last decade, many researchers have investigated whether individual differences in religiousness are associated with personality traits.

Religion and the Five-Factor Model

The five-factor trait model (FFM) of personality offers a starting point for exploring the relationship between religiousness and personality functioning. Several recent studies have employed measures of the constructs in the Big Five, or five-factor personality taxonomy (these are: whether one is open to experience, conscientious, extraverted, agreeable, neurotic) (e.g., see John, Naumann, & Soto, Chapter 4, this volume; McCrae & Costa, Chapter 5, this volume), to examine the association of religiousness and personality. Kosek (1999), MacDonald (2000), and Taylor and MacDonald (1999) found that measures of Agreeableness and Conscientiousness were positively associated with measures of religious involvement and intrinsic religious orientation. MacDonald found somewhat different patterns of correlations across the Big Five, depending on the domain of spirituality examined. A factor labeled "Cognitive orientation toward spirituality" was associated with Extraversion, Agreeableness, Openness, and Conscientiousness, whereas an experiential form of spirituality was related to Extraversion and Openness only. A meta-analytic review (Saroglou, 2002) found that religiousness is consistently associated with high Agreeableness and Conscientiousness and low Psychoticism, whereas it is unrelated to the other Big Five traits.

Correlations between five-factor scales and religiosity are often significant but typically run in the low range. For example, intrinsic religiosity correlated with Agreeableness and Conscientiousness ($r = .25, .23$) in a large sample ($N = 1,129$) of Canadian undergraduates (Taylor & MacDonald, 1999), whereas extrinsic religiosity correlated negatively with Openness ($r = -.18$). One other generalization that appears warranted is that Openness tends to be negatively correlated with more fundamentalist measures of religiousness. McCrae and Costa's (1996) model of personality may prove useful for understanding how basic trait tendencies are channeled into characteristic adaptations that include culturally conditioned religious and spiritual goals and attitudes.

Explaining Links between the FFM and Religiousness

By understanding the Big Five personality traits as basic tendencies, religiousness can be conceptualized as a characteristic adaptation that some people in some cultural contexts adopt to "fulfill" or express basic personality tendencies (McCrae & Costa, 1996). For example, conscientious and/or agreeable people (in some cultural contexts) tend to fulfill their tendencies toward conformity, order, or prosociality by being religious. People high in Conscientiousness and Agreeableness both are motivated to conform to rules and laws, although for different reasons (Costa & McCrae, 1995). Conscientiousness motivates people to abide by rules and conventions. Formal religious practices often provide a clear, delineated value system that might appeal to conscientious people but that might cause less conscientious people to bristle. Psychologically, religion may also be considered as a way to enhance self-control. Historically, a major motive for religion is the need to reign in unacceptable impulses, especially those involving sex and aggression (Pargament, 1997). People desire to have things under control, to believe in their capacity to change a situation as well as in their capacity to change themselves in order to change reality. Furthermore, people gain a feeling of control by making sense out of what is happening (e.g., seeing misfortune as part of a large, cosmic plan) and being able to predict what will occur in the future. So, religion satisfies this need for control. Furthermore, religious individuals tend to be high in the personality trait of Conscientiousness or Planfulness (a broad factor in the FFM of personality) and low in impulsiveness.

Agreeableness also motivates people to abide by conventions, particularly out of concern for the feelings and rights of others. Therefore, Agreeableness might move people toward religiousness in adulthood in part out of concern for minimizing conflict and maintaining harmony with their families by remaining faithful to the family's religious systems. It is also possible that agreeable people are more amenable to maintaining a religious faith partly out of an earnest desire to maintain positive relations with God or to be involved in a value system that promotes kindness, altruism, forgiveness, and love. Although much of the theorizing regarding the dynamics of the personality–religiousness relationship has focused on how certain traits might influence people's religiousness, the causal direction of these relationships remains largely unexplored. Especially during early development, religious involvement could contribute to the formation of Conscientiousness or Agreeableness, or personality and religiosity could mutually reinforce one another.

Spiritual Transcendence

In addition to linking religiousness to the FFM, evidence is accruing that spirituality may represent a (previously unrecognized) sixth major dimension of personality (Mac-Donald, 2000; Piedmont, 1999). Other recent research has similarly noted that spirituality and religiousness are omitted from structural models of personality that are developed around the FFM (Saucier & Goldberg, 1998). Piedmont (1999) demonstrated the value of the FFM for advancing the scientific study of religion. He suggests that the FFM can provide an empirical reference point for evaluating the development of new measures of religiousness and for evaluating the meaning of existing measures. Ozer and Reise (1994) advise that personality researchers routinely correlate their particular measure with the FFM. Given the proliferation of measurement instruments in the psychology of religion, researchers would do well to heed this advice.

Spiritual transcendence is "the capacity of individuals to stand outside of their immediate sense of time and place and to view life from a larger, more objective perspective. This transcendent perspective is one in which a person sees a fundamental unity underlying the diverse strivings of nature" (Piedmont, 1999, p. 988). In developing the Spiritual Transcendence Scale (STS), a consortium of theological experts from diverse faith traditions, including Buddhism, Hinduism, Quakerism, Lutheranism, Catholicism, and Judaism, was assembled. This focus group identified aspects of spirituality that were common to all of these faiths. The resulting items were analyzed within the context of the FFM and were shown to constitute an independent individual-differences dimension. The STS manifested a single overall factor comprised of three "facet" scales: *Prayer Fulfillment*, a feeling of joy and contentment that results from personal encounters with a transcendent reality (e.g., "I find inner strength and/or peace from my prayers or meditations"); *Universality*, a belief in the unitive nature of life (e.g., "I feel that on a higher level all of us share a common bond"); and *Connectedness*, a belief that one is part of a larger human reality that cuts across generations and across groups (e.g., "I am concerned about those who will come after me in life").

The STS evidenced incremental validity by significantly predicting a number of relevant psychological outcomes (e.g., stress experience, social support, interpersonal style) even after the predictive effects of personality were removed (Piedmont, 1999). For the STS to be shown to capture a universal aspect of spirituality, it would be necessary to demonstrate that the instrument remains reliable and valid in culturally diverse, religiously heterogeneous samples. Piedmont and Leach (2002) have documented the utility of the STS in a sample of Muslims, Indian Hindus, and Christians. Support was found for two of the facet scales and the overall domain (Connectedness was not found to be reliable) in this sample. The STS was presented in English, a second language for these participants. This may have created difficulties in understanding the terminology or the exemplars used, as items lacked relevance in this culture. Nonetheless, these data highlight the value of cross-cultural research on spirituality and show the STS to reflect spiritual qualities relevant across very different religious traditions.

Ultimate Concerns

Yet another way to conceptualize personality and religion is in terms of goals or strivings, or what I (R. A. E.) and my colleagues have called "ultimate concerns" (Emmons, 1999; Emmons, Cheung, & Tehrani, 1998). Following Tillich (1957), among others, I (Emmons, 1999) argued that both religion and spirituality deal with ultimate concerns of people, and I developed a research program to identify ultimate concerns and their role in human personality and subjective well-being. A religious perspective can illuminate the origins of some of the most profound human strivings. Religions, as authoritative faith traditions, are systems of information that provide individuals with knowledge and resources for living a life of purpose and direction. Religion and goals are intertwined in human experience. One of the functions of a religious belief system and a religious worldview is to provide "an ultimate vision of what people should be striving for in their lives" (Pargament & Park, 1995, p. 15) and the strategies to reach those ends. Religions recommend the ultimate goal of binding with the sacred and prescribe rituals for its realization. It has been found that not only is it possible to reliably assess the search for the sacred in personal goals, but that individual differences in sacred goals predicted well-being more strongly than any other category of striving that has been studied, exceeding those for intimacy, power, or generativity goals (Emmons et al., 1998).

PERSONALITY AND RELIGION: EMPIRICAL POINTS OF CONTACT

Recent research on religion and spirituality as human phenomena is almost as vast and diverse as religious and spiritual life itself. A literature search using the PsychINFO database for the 10-year period 1997–2006 returned nearly 2,400 title citations for the terms "spirituality" and "spiritual" and over 1,700 for "religion" and "religiosity." This review, therefore, must be quite selective, of necessity.

Religion and Virtue

The study of virtue, at the intersection of the psychology of religion, personality psychology, moral philosophy, and the psychology of emotion, is making a comeback in psychology. Partly responsible for this resurgence is the positive psychology movement that has sought systematically to classify human strengths and virtues into a comprehensive taxonomy (Peterson & Seligman, 2004). Considerable research is addressing positive aspects of human functioning and variables that describe more uplifting features of human experience (e.g., optimism, hope, and altruism). Concepts such as forgiveness, love, hope, humility, gratitude, self-control, and wisdom appear as highly prized human dispositions in Jewish, Christian, Muslim, Buddhist, and Hindu thought and are affirmed universal principles in world philosophies and ethical systems.

Among the virtues, forgiveness has been an especially vigorous research area, and is a process that links readily to concerns in clinical, counseling, and health psychology. Inspired by (but not limited to) religious systems, research is answering fundamental questions about what forgiveness is and isn't, how it develops, what are its physiological correlates and physical effects, whether it is always beneficial, and how people—if they are so motivated—might be helped to forgive. Both researchers and applied psychologists have usually treated forgiveness as synonymous with forgivingness—as a characteristic of the individual (the offended party in a transaction) that is relatively consistent across relationships and across offenses within a given relationship. McCullough and Hoyt (2002) examined forgiveness ratings across a variety of transgressions in close relationships (with friends, parents, and romantic partners) and concluded that some people are dispositionally more willing to forgive than others. Specifically, between 22 and 44% of variance in respondents' willingness to forgive a specific transgression was attributable to stable individual differences in forgivingness. Personality factors that best predicted forgivingness in that study were Agreeableness (positively) and Neuroticism (negatively). With regard to the place of forgiveness in personality, Ashton and Lee (2001) recently posited that forgiveness/non-retaliation is one of three major traits that underlies prosocial tendencies and can account for individual differences in the major dimensions of agreeableness and emotional stability. Most religions place a premium on forgiveness, and accordingly, most religious individuals say that they value forgiveness. Interestingly, however, a recent study showed that religious people were actually more retaliatory (behaviorally) against a norm violator, even though they reported themselves to have been more forgiving (Greer, 2005).

Religion, Spirituality, and Well-Being

The growth in empirical research on religious and spiritual topics has quite likely been influenced by many factors, not the least of which is the growing body of research demonstrating that religious and spiritual variables affect human health and subjective well-being. Patients in health care settings generally welcome attention to spiritual aspects of their illness by their health providers. Work on the "faith factor" has been conducted by sociologists, epidemiologists, psychologists, and physicians and has explored the health impacts of religion on adherents. Religious practices and experiences have measurable effects on important psychosocial and health outcomes, and these effects seem to be independent of at least some plausible alternative mediators (including social support, age, and health status). An impressive research literature, though not uncontroversial, has documented that religious practices are associated with reduced morbidity and mortality across the lifespan. For example, religious practices, including participation in religious activities such as prayer and attending services, has been linked to better coping with stress, prevention of and recovery from illness, and even longevity. Proximal mechanisms for these links are being explored. Many religious rituals, ceremonies, and practices are biologically significant events. Ongoing research with participants engaged in meditation and trance demonstrate changes in brain-wave patterns, heart and pulse rate, skin conductance, and other autonomic functions.

A series of recent studies controlling for personality with five-factor personality measures has tested specifically the relationship between spirituality and most facets of subjective well-being. Considerable evidence now exists that the FFM accounts for considerable variance related to psychosocial outcomes but does not eliminate religiosity's predictive ability. Controlling for age, gender, marital status, and personality with Methodist ministers ($N = 320$), spirituality predicted less psychological exhaustion and more cognitive well-being (Golden, Piedmont, Ciarrocchi, & Rodgerson, in press). In a sample of Maltese undergraduates ($N = 312$), spiritual transcendence predicted both positive affect and cognitive well-being, over and above personality, but did not predict negative affect (Galea, 2003). A similar pattern emerged in a sample of male sex offenders ($N = 194$), with faith maturity predicting positive affect and cognitive well-being but not negative affect (Geary, 2003). Spiritual transcendence predicted cognitive well-being over personality but neither negative affect or positive affect (Walsh, 2001) in problem gamblers ($N = 100$). Finally, faith maturity predicted cognitive well-being over personality but was unrelated to negative emotionality in female patients with breast cancer (Ciarrocchi & Deneke, 2005). Ciarrocchi and Deneke (2005) found that measures of spirituality made a unique contribution in predicting subjective well-being by virtue of their relation to positive emotionality and life satisfaction. Spirituality, defined as perceived closeness to God, added an element to well-being that was not accounted for by age, gender, personality, or the social support provided in the religious setting. The role spirituality plays in its relationship with well-being varies according to the components of well-being. Religiosity also predicts hope and optimism over and above the FFM (Ciarrochi, Dy-Liacco, & Deneke, in press).

These results are notable in that, despite using a variety of instruments to measure both personality and well-being, the pattern of the outcomes is similar in most of the studies. Spirituality predicted the positive aspects of subjective well-being, but failed to predict negative emotionality, as first noted by Watson and Clark (1993). Overall these results render Fredrickson's (2002) theory plausible: that the major influence of religion on well-being may be its ability to enhance positive emotions. She hypothesized that positive emotion mediates the beneficial effects of religion through the "most reliable path" (2002, p. 211) of meaning. In other words, religion provides meaning, which creates positive emotions leading to the development of personal capacities that then ensure health and well-being.

Critics (e.g., Sloan, Bagiella, & Powell, 2001) have argued, however, that established relationships between religiousness and health are not robust and that more rigorous epidemiological studies are needed before the health benefits of spiritual practices can inform public policy. It is likely that future waves of research will incorporate increasingly sophisticated research designs and statistical analyses in order to disentangle linkages between religious activities and health outcomes.

Religious Conversion and Spiritual Transformation

Religious conversion has long been a topic of interest for researchers concerned with understanding personality and religion. The importance of spiritual transformation is stressed in an abundance of world religions. Ranging from the conversion of St. Paul to Christianity on the road to Damascus to the transformation of Siddhartha Guatama, religions have long highlighted and exemplified transformative spiritual experiences.

Examining the history of the personality field, religious conversion can be counted as one of the first psychological topics to be scientifically studied (Starbuck, 1899). Indeed, the underlying self-processes of conversion receive considerable exposition in James's (1902) seminal work, *The Varieties of Religious Experience*. Long-standing interest in the study of religious conversions and spiritual transformations is partly attributable to the unique opportunity afforded by these phenomena to observe the dynamics of personality change. Due to a variety of factors, including genetic and environmental influences, person–environment transactions, and crystallized self-perceptions, researchers have found that adult personality is moderately stable across the life course (Roberts, Wood, & Caspi, Chapter 14, this volume). Religious/spiritual transformation may be one of the few life events recognized to engender substantial and dramatic personality change.

However, spiritual transformation is not always dramatic and complete, as is often typified by classical conversion paradigms. The extravagant and dramatic transformation of the individual's entire meaning system, goals, and ultimate concerns, referred to as "quantum change" (Miller & C'deBaca, 1994, 2001) or "amazing conversions" (Altemeyer & Hunsberger, 1997), is distinguishable from other forms of conversions or spiritual transformations. Paloutzian (2005) identifies a bevy of changes in personality that may result from a spiritual transformation, ranging from an increase or decrease in adherence to the same religion, to a change in a specific element within a person's worldview, to a complete overhaul of ultimate concerns and life purpose. Other researchers have also illuminated the diversity of experiences that could be labeled spiritual transformations or religious conversions. Given the plethora of conceptualizations, what are the defining aspects of *spiritual transformation* and *religious conversion*? And, what factors distinguish between these two constructs?

First, conversion and transformation are both separable from learning, developmental, and maturational processes in that transformative experiences display a distinctiveness of change whereby the convert can identify a time before which he or she held a different array of spiritual beliefs and goals than those held after the transformative experience (Paloutzian, 2005). This is not to say that transformative experiences must be sudden or acute; they may actually take variable amounts of time, ranging from seconds to years. Instead, researchers highlight *distinctiveness* as a key identifying theme of spiritual transformation.

Paloutzian (2005) models spiritual transformation and religious conversion as a change in the meaning system. Paloutzian, Richardson, and Rambo (1999) maintain that spiritual transformation leads to changes in the second and third levels of McAdams's (Chapter 8, this volume; 1995) construction of personality. Essentially, McAdams proposes that personality can be conceptualized hierarchically, beginning with traits and temperament at Level 1; then goals, strivings, and characteristic adaptations at Level 2; and finally a person's life narrative at Level 3. Level 1 personality traits are fairly stable across adulthood and contain a large biological component (Costa & McCrae, 1994); therefore, it is not surprising that studies provide little evidence that a person's core personality traits (such as those represented by the Big Five) change as a result of religious conversion or spiritual transformation (Piedmont, 2005). However, researchers do find substantial changes in personality resulting from conversion at the level of the person's strivings and life narrative. For example, an atheist who becomes a Protestant may accumulate new strivings such as "obey God" or "read my Bible" (see Emmons, 1999, for examples of spiritual strivings), or he or she may change the strivings so that he or she no longer desires to become an actor but instead strives to become an evangelist. Similarly, a recent convert may reframe his or her life narrative, utilizing a redemption paradigm, to provide personal meaning. Thus, Paloutzian (2005) conceptualizes spiritual transformation as a reorganization of an individual's goals and meaning system. Other researchers would also add that spiritual transformation is not only a reorganization but also a reorientation of the individual toward the sacred (Mahoney & Pargament, 2004) and transcendent (Piedmont, 1999). Apparently, James (1902) was not far from modern conceptualizations when he described conversion as the movement of religious ideas from the periphery of one's consciousness to the "habitual center of energy."

Although the model of religious conversion and spiritual transformation as a change in the meaning system is well accepted by the majority of researchers in the field, greater dissension surrounds the question of the distinctions and relations between religious conversion and spiritual transformation. Paloutzian (2005) maintains that religious conversions are a subset of the larger category of spiritual transformations, and that religious conversion is specifically oriented toward a religious system whereas spiritual transformation may include a change relative to whatever is transcendent to the individual. Conversely, Zinnbauer and Pargament (1998) demarcate religious conversion as a higher-order category defined as a radical change in the self in response to internal or external stress; and they postulate spiritual conversion as a constituent process whereby the self becomes identified with a spiritual force. Notably, they remark that joining a new religious group is not tantamount to

religious conversion, as it may or may not involve a radical change in the self.

Researchers have produced a fair amount of empirical work examining spiritual transformations and religious conversions, although several methodological limitations have restricted interpretation of the data. Specifically, a large proportion of studies utilize retrospective reports of preconversion personality and measure the convert's perceived change instead of actual change. For example, in their study of religious change among college undergrads Zinnbauer and Pargament (1998) simply asked participants if they had experienced a conversion over the past 2 years and then asked them to retrospectively report their pre- and postconversion experiences. Although this is an acceptable launching point to commence inquiry into the topic, such retrospective reports pose serious limitations. It is unclear whether or not participants are able to accurately contrast their pre- and postconversion personality and experiences. Beckford (1978) comments that converts' retrospective reports are quite subjective and tend to overemphasize the negative past in contrast to the positive postconversion state, as they narrate their own life stories to fit "scripts" provided by their religious traditions. Retrospective reports may also be contaminated by stereotypical views of how spiritual conversions are "supposed" to change personality. Robins, Noftle, Trzesniewski, and Roberts (2005) found that college students perceived considerable change in the major dimensions of their personality, but analyses were unable to rule out the possibility that these perceived changes reflected stereotypes of how the college experience and the transition to adulthood are thought to influence personality development.

Therefore, it seems quite imperative for researchers to adopt more longitudinal methods that utilize multiple measures beyond self-perceived change, including informant reports as well as further measures of actual change. Researchers should especially aim to acquire true preconversion measurement by pretesting a large number of participants and then following up with those who actually experience a conversion over time compared to controls.

Even if such changes are made in study designs, researchers still must deal with response-shift bias: that is, changes in the participants' internal standards for measures (see Howard & Dailey, 1979, for further elucidation of response-shift bias). For example, participants' standards of morality may become more stringent following conversion, such that they may give themselves the same scale score on an evaluation of their moral behavior, despite the fact that they have demonstrated great increases in moral behavior by any objective standards. A possible solution is to use retrospective self-reports in conjunction with objective measures of change (Sprangers, 1989; Zinnbauer & Pargament, 1998).

Another solution to the problem of systematic biases in self-reports of change is to use observer or informant ratings of spirituality and morality. Research in the psychology of religion has underutilized observer ratings, especially as compared to how routinely they are used in personality research (Piedmont, McCrae, Riemann, & Angleitner, 2000). Demonstrating cross-observer convergence in religious and spiritual changes would be an important methodological advance in the study of the conversion experience. Beyond convergence, observer rating data are important sources of information in their own right, providing information on how a person has been perceived to have changed spiritually by others (Piedmont et. al, 2000). As an illustration, an outpatient drug rehabilitation program was found to produce significant shifts in most of the traits of the FFM in a sample of 30 adult clients—shifts that were noticeable by observers and that were not simply attributable to either self-reports or to symptom relief (Piedmont, 2001).

Despite the apparent limitations and difficulties of research in this area, scientists have garnered considerable insight concerning religious conversions and spiritual transformations. Pertaining to the precursors of spiritual transformations, researchers have amassed considerable support for the thesis that acute stress and a sense of personal inadequacy or disintegration often precede conversion (e.g., Galanter, 1982; Rosen & Nordquist, 1980; Ullman, 1989; Zinnbauer & Pargament, 1998). Moreover, chronic stressors are related to the occurrence of conversion. Ullman (1989) found that converts, as opposed to nonconverts, reported a greater

degree of emotional stress during childhood, higher incidence of an absent father, and more traumatic life events. Moreover, Kirkpatrick (1997, 1998) has shown that individuals who exhibit an insecure adult attachment style are more likely to report a new relationship with God in the 4 years following the initial measurement of adult attachment. Kirkpatrick's findings seem to support the hypothesis that conversion acts as compensation for secure attachment relationships with other people. However, it should be noted that conversion is not equivalent to spiritual maturity, as higher levels of spiritual growth are actually reported for those with secure attachment styles (Granqvist, 1998).

In addition to stress and a sense of personal inadequacy, a variety of other factors have been proposed as precursors of conversion. It seems likely that those individuals who already possess a religiously based orienting system would be more likely to experience spiritual transformation during stressful conditions (Pargament, 1997). Additionally, Rambo (1993) highlights the importance of broader cultural factors in providing individuals with access to religious symbols, myths, and rituals that may facilitate conversion. Finally, certain demographic groups report more conversions than others. For example, conversions are found to occur most often during adolescence, with females converting 1–2 years earlier than males, on average (Hood, Spilka, Hunsberger, & Gorsuch, 1996). This finding seems reasonable, as adolescence is a time of identity formation and a time when individuals challenge normative systems.

Regarding the consequences of religious conversions and spiritual transformations, researchers have demonstrated strong correlations between conversion and a multitude of positive outcomes. Paloutzian (1981) found that converts reported significantly higher purpose in life than nonconverts, and Zinnbauer and Pargament (1998) reported an increased sense of competency and adequacy in converts. Such findings support the idea of conversion as a process of transforming the self from a state of disintegration to one of integrity and wholeness. Additionally, converts to new religious groups, even those considered cults, demonstrate dramatic decreases in drug use, mitigation of neurotic distress, renewed vocational motivation, increased compassion, and decreased psychosomatic symptoms (Hood et al., 1996). However, due to the previously mentioned limitations of most conversion research (i.e., a lack of longitudinal designs), little is known regarding the sustainability of changes in personality brought about by conversion experiences. In Paloutzian's purpose-in-life study, he did find higher levels of purpose for those reporting a conversion more than 6 months previous, but the validity of this finding as a basis for drawing any definitive conclusions about the sustainability of changes is limited.

EXPLAINING RELIGION: EVOLUTION AND COGNITION

The field of personality deals not only with describing individual differences but also with the development of universal laws of human behavior. Thus the field of personality must grapple with the challenge of explaining the universality of religious beliefs and behaviors. The evolution of religion and its possible adaptive function have been the subject of considerable recent investigation by a wide array of researchers with diverse theoretical and methodological approaches. Cognitive scientists, evolutionary psychologists, and cultural anthropologists are prominent among these researchers. Rather than focus on institutions or group affiliation, these scholars have primarily studied elements typical of religious life, including beliefs in supernatural agents, transmission of religious concepts, ideas about the afterlife, and the role of cognition and affect in ritual. Primary debates in the area concern whether religious thought and behavior arise from capacities evolved for other selective advantages (e.g., Boyer, 2001), or whether religion itself confers selective advantage (e.g., Wilson, 2002). Also disputed is the relative importance of implicit, less culturally variable cognition versus explicit, more culturally variable cognition in explaining religious thought and behavior (e.g., White-house, 2004).

Cognitive–evolutionary approaches to religion come in three varieties: *neurotheology*, *group selection*, and *cognitive science of religion*. Though all possess some connections to evolutionary perspectives, the three schools take importantly different approaches to explaining religion.

Neurotheology is primarily concerned with identifying which components and dynamics of the brain underlie religious experiences and subsequent religious behavior. Neurotheology is the only one of the three varieties of cognitive-evolutionary approaches that emphasizes mystical experience of the sort William James regarded as central to religion (James, 1902). The aim of this area is to identify religious phenomena as the (perhaps accidental) output of evolved neural circuitry. Evolved brains have components that have arisen because of their usefulness to survival—components that happen to interact in such a way as to generate religious experiences. These experiences are shared and codified into common religious beliefs.

A recognized role for brain imaging in the study of human religious and spiritual phenomena has emerged. The capacity for spiritual and religious experience is inseparably connected to the architecture of the mind–brain. With rapid advances in the development of techniques to measure brain activity, neuroscientific approaches to the human spirit are receiving increasing attention. The hemodynamics of blood and oxygen flow or glucose metabolism in the brain, as revealed by positron emission tomography (PET) or functional magnetic resonance imaging (fMRI), suggest that spiritual practices such as meditation and prayer involve increased activity in frontal brain structures, as well as those other brain areas that form a system to regulate and focus attention (Azari, 2006). Specifically, meditation is associated with decreased activity in the superior parietal lobe, which is correlated with spatial and temporal orientation, thus contributing the sense of "oneness" or felt unity common in spiritual experiences. Perhaps unsurprisingly, there is also evidence that prayer involves increased activity in brain regions known to be involved in the production of language (Newberg & Newberg, 2005).

According to the *group selection hypothesis*, religious systems encourage prosocial behavior, and groups that exhibit prosocial behavior (cooperation, lack of cheating and stealing) will tend to out-survive and out-reproduce groups that do not exhibit these traits (Wilson, 2002). Because religious communities have stronger prosocial tendencies, they cooperate better. As they cooperate better, they survive and thrive better than competing communities. Hence, religious communities—and whatever genetic information accounts for their religiosity and prosociality—will tend to survive and expand at a greater rate than nonreligious communities. Over time, then, people with the biological disposition to be religious will increasingly outnumber nonreligious people. This selection process thereby accounts for the widespread existence of religious people. Group selection theory seeks to reconcile evolutionary biology with the frequently made paradoxical observation that many religious systems codify rules that appear to diminish reproductive fitness. Wilson's solution is to view natural selection as a multilevel process such that it plays an important explanatory role. Group selection theory appears to fit some empirical observations but has not gone unchallenged (Henig, 2007; Numbers & Numbers, 2003).

Evolutionary-minded social scientists have proposed that religious behaviors constitute costly signals that contribute to social cohesion. These behaviors publicize the message that an individual shares the same values as the group, and their costliness (in terms of time, effort, material resources, and sometimes pain) makes them hard to fake. These theorists situate religious ritual within a broader, nonhuman evolutionary continuum related to socially adaptive behaviors.

Research has verified that religious people seem to be inspired by these prosocial ideals, at least in the way they perceive themselves and desire to be. Invariably across cultures and religious contexts, religiosity is associated with the tendency to be agreeable, generous, warm (see the Agreeableness factor of the five-factor model), to be friendly and not distant (low psychoticism in the Eysenck's model of personality), to be ready to undertake altruistic actions if necessary, and to forgive and grant high importance to the value of benevolence. The evidence indicates that religious persons are prosocial because they are empathic and because it is important for them to be fair, honest, and show respect for prosocial norms. Religion may also encourage nonaggression, nonviolence, and nonconflict as a positive effect rather than prosocial, helping, altruistic behavior; for instance, in many religions the prohibition of killing is not applied only to the act of murder but is extended to the prohibition of killing the other through slanderous words and thoughts (at least with respect to the ingroup). Yet there is evidence for religion's ability to motivate aggression, especially when the religion is of the fundamentalist variety (McCullough & Willoughby, in press).

The most developed field identified with evolutionary accounts of religion is called the *cognitive science of religion* (Andresen, 2001; Barrett, 2004; Boyer, 2001; McCauley & Whitehouse, 2005; Tremlin, 2006). Cognitive scientists argue that religion is a constellation of human phenomena that is represented and communicated by naturally occurring cognitive processes. Numerous research programs in cognitive and developmental psychology have converged on the view that religious concepts heavily rely on implicit, essentially universal causal reasoning. This perspective, known as the "naturalness of religion thesis," posits that religious concepts, such as belief in god(s), the successful interpersonal transmission of these concepts, and the development of practices based on these concepts, rely on the use of mental tools operating in cross-culturally recurrent conditions (Barrett, 2000; Boyer, 1994). In other words, ordinary cognition plus exposure to ordinary environments accounts for religion. No special domain for religious thought need be postulated (Lawson & McCauley, 1990). More specifically, the cognitive science of religion starts with the following assumptions:

1. By virtue of a common human biology inhabiting a remarkably uniform natural world, core structures of mind develop similarly everywhere.
2. Human minds are not general-purpose information-processing devices but are highly specialized conglomerates of many functional subsystems that solve particular problems.
3. These subsystems importantly shape perception and cognition regarding the natural and social world.
4. These contours of human minds inform and constrain recurrent patterns of human thought and action, including religious (and other cultural) thought and action.
5. Hence, recurrent features of religious

thought and action (e.g., belief in gods) can be explained (or predicted) by appealing to requisite conceptual structures. Particular thoughts and actions will occur more frequently among humans than other possible thoughts and actions by virtue of their foundation in the dynamics of human minds.

For example, a number of cognitive scientists have noted that the *counterintuitive* concepts (ones that violate expectations) that characterize religious beliefs are both attention arresting and memorable (Barrett, 2000, 2004; Boyer, 1994, 2001; Sperber & Wilson, 1995). Experimental tests on four continents have validated these observations (Barrett & Nyhof, 2001; Boyer & Ramble, 2001). Furthermore, people have a built-in bias to detect human-like agency in their environment (Guthrie, 1993). This *hypersensitive agency detection device* (HADD; Barrett, 2004) might lead people to posit supernatural agents to account for unexplained events such as "miraculous" healings or signs. An example of an event that may trigger HADD is the following true story taken from Barrett (2004): Doug was in a grain silo when a propane explosion occurred. Surviving the first blast that buckled the doors and blasted out the windows, he resigned himself to die in the subsequent blast. Instead, he heard a voice say "not yet" and felt himself lifted up through a second story window and deposited on the ground outside. Moments later the silo and barn exploded into rubble. Given that his body moved in a way that was not readily explained by the nonreflective beliefs of his naive physics system, and his life-saving movement out of a window seemed goal-directed, Doug's HADD detected agency at play and registered the automatic belief that the event was caused by an unseen agent. Moving this automatic belief to a reflective one involving supernatural agents was perfectly natural, given the circumstances.

By virtue of their agentic attributes, gods are readily incorporated into numerous domains of social activity, including moral reasoning. Including gods in such reasoning increases their nonreflective plausibility by increasing the number of mental tools that accept and affirm their existence and activity. Why are gods so readily incorporated into domains of morality, fortune, and mis-

fortune? First, people are always searching the environment to explain events, and they have a tendency to evoke social or intentional causes when obvious mechanical or biological causes are absent or insufficient. Second, unusual fortune or misfortune happens. Intuitively, such unusual events as the sudden, tragic death of a loved one, or the winning of the lottery, demand an explanation. Probabilistic explanations ring hollow to people's intuitive mental tools that demand causal explanations. Gods enter the story because of the particular sorts of counterintuitive properties they possess. Not only do they have unusual powers that might enable them to perform acts resulting in great fortune or misfortune, but perhaps more importantly, their invisibility and super-knowledge gives them "strategic information" about what people do in private (Bering, 2006b; Boyer, 2001). People envision gods as possessing knowledge of socially strategic information—of having unlimited perceptual access to socially maligned behaviors that occur in private and therefore outside the perceptual boundaries of everyday human agents. Morally sensitive gods do and may reward or punish them. The notions of gods with strategic information and moral reasoning mutually reinforce each other's plausibility and cultural transmission.

Accumulating research further indicates that humans exhibit a developmental predisposition to believe in such socially infallible supernatural agents, appearing in early childhood (Barrett & Richert, 2003). Cross-cultural studies conducted with children between the ages of 3 and 12 indicate that young children may possess an "intuitive theism" that prompts them to see intentional purpose in the natural world that cannot be attributed to people but only to specially powerful supernatural agents (Kelemen, 2005). Therefore, mental tools predispose people to hold religious beliefs. In this sense, widespread belief in gods arises from the operation of natural processes of the human mind. In the views of cognitive scientists, belief in gods does not amount to anything strange or peculiar; on the contrary, such belief is nearly inevitable. In answering the questions of why would anyone believe in God, the answer from cognitive science is that the design of our minds leads us to believe (Barrett, 2004).

EXAMPLE: GRATITUDE AS A DISPOSITION AND RELIGIOUS EMOTION

Gratitude has been well established as a universal human attribute. Its presence is felt and expressed in different ways by virtually all peoples, of all cultures, worldwide (Emmons & McCullough, 2004). The fact that gratitude is universal across all cultures suggests that it is part of human nature. Gratitude is likewise a recurrent religious sentiment, often reflected in gift giving and other social exchange between humans and their gods (Burkert, 1996). Some of the most profound experiences of gratitude can be religiously based or associated with reverent wonder and an acknowledgment of the universe (Goodenough, 1998), including the perception that life itself is a gift. In the great monotheistic religions of the world, the concept of gratitude permeates texts, prayers, and teachings. Worship with gratitude to God for the many gifts and mercies are common themes, and believers are urged to develop this quality.

Gratitude from an Evolutionary Perspective

Like other emotional dispositions, gratitude can be considered at many levels of analysis. For example, from a biocultural or evolutionary perspective that emphasizes social–functional accounts of emotion (Keltner, 2003), gratitude helps individuals form and maintain relationships. As relationships are essential to the survival and well-being of individuals, groups, and societies, a biocultural approach to gratitude suggests that it, like other social emotions, evolved to solve certain recurring problems in the human social landscape.

Specifically, the emotion of gratitude has been hypothesized to have developed in order to solve problems of group governance. Sociologist Georg Simmel (1950) argued that gratitude was a cognitive–emotional supplement serving to sustain one's reciprocal obligations. Because formal social structures such as the law and social contracts are insufficient to regulate and ensure reciprocity in human interaction, people are socialized to have gratitude, which then serves to remind them of their need to reciprocate. Thus, during exchange of benefits, gratitude prompts one person (a beneficiary) to be bound to another (a benefactor), thereby reminding ben-

eficiaries of their reciprocity obligations. He referred to gratitude as "the moral memory of mankind. ... If every grateful action ... were suddenly eliminated, society (at least as we know it) would break apart" (1950, p. 388).

Gratitude also provides an emotional basis for reciprocal altruism. In his seminal article, Robert Trivers (1971) speculated on the evolutionary functions of gratitude. Trivers viewed gratitude as an evolutionary adaptation that regulates people's responses to altruistic acts. Gratitude for altruistic acts is a reward for adherence to the universal norm of reciprocity and is a mediating mechanism that links the receipt of a favor to the giving of a return favor. The effect of this emotion is to create a desire to reciprocate. From this perspective, gratitude serves as a mental mechanism that calibrates the extent of debt owed—the larger the debt, the larger the sense of gratitude. Recent research indicates that gratitude may be a psychological mechanism underlying reciprocal exchange in both human and nonhuman primates (Bonnie & de Waal, 2004). McCullough, Kilpatrick, Emmons, and Larson (2001) synthesized historical perspectives and recent research on gratitude in our theory of gratitude as a moral affect—that is, one with moral precursors and consequences. By experiencing gratitude, a person is motivated to carry out prosocial behavior, energized to sustain moral behaviors, and is inhibited from committing destructive interpersonal behaviors. Because of its specialized functions in the moral domain, McCullough and colleagues likened gratitude to empathy, sympathy, guilt, and shame, which all occupy a special place in the grammar of moral life. Whereas empathy and sympathy operate when people have the opportunity to respond to the plight of another person, and guilt and shame operate when people have failed to meet moral standards or obligations, gratitude operates typically when people acknowledge that they are the recipients of prosocial behavior. Specifically, McCullough and colleagues posited, first, that gratitude serves as a *moral barometer*, providing individuals with an affective readout that accompanies the perception that another person has treated them kindly or prosocially. Second, gratitude serves as a *moral motive*, stimulating people to behave prosocially after they have been the beneficiaries of other people's prosocial behavior. Recent empirical evidence does indeed suggest that gratitude can shape costly prosocial behavior (Bartlett & DeSteno, 2006). Third, gratitude serves as a *moral reinforcer*, encouraging prosocial behavior by reinforcing people for their previous prosocial behavior.

We have argued that gratitude is a human strength in that it enhances individuals' personal and relational well-being and is quite possibly beneficial for society as a whole. Results on the correlates of dispositional gratitude appear to bear out this formulation. As a disposition, gratitude is a generalized tendency to recognize and respond with positive emotions (appreciation, thankfulness) to the role of other individuals' (moral agents') kindness and benevolence in the positive experiences and outcomes experienced. Existing research suggests that gratitude is a typically pleasant experience that is linked to contentment, happiness, and hope.

Gratitude has also been scientifically examined at the level of a personality trait or disposition. As a trait, gratitude is the tendency to perceive benevolence on the part of others and to respond with thankful feelings and cognitions (e.g., perceptions of being "gifted" by another's actions) and a desire to reciprocate. Two trait measures of gratitude have been published: The Gratitude Questionnaire (GQ-6; McCullough, Emmons, & Tsang, 2002) and the Gratitude Resentment and Appreciation Test (GRAT; Watkins, Woodward, Stone, & Kolts, 2003). High scorers on the GQ report more frequent positive emotions, life satisfaction, vitality, and optimism and lower levels of depression and stress (McCullough et al., 2002). Similarly, scores on the GRAT correlate positively and moderately with positive states and traits such as internal locus of control, intrinsic religiosity, and life satisfaction; moreover, scores correlate negatively and moderately with negative states and traits such as depression, extrinsic religiosity, narcissism, and hostility. In one experiment, high scorers on the GRAT showed a positive memory bias: They recalled a greater number of positive memories when instructed to do so and even rated their memories of unpleasant experiences more positively over time, relative to the initial emotional impact of these negative events (Watkins, Grimm, & Kolts, 2004). Importantly, these data showing that gratitude is correlated with beneficial outcomes is not limited to self-reports. Notably, the family, friends, partners, and others that surround participants consistently report that people who practice gratitude seem measurably happier and are more pleasant to be around. Grateful people are rated by others as more helpful, more outgoing, more optimistic, and more trustworthy (McCullough et al., 2002).

Gratitude and Costly Signaling Theory

It is possible to draw a conceptual linkage between evolutionary and theological perspectives on gratitude by invoking the "costly signaling theory" (CST) of religious behavior (Bulbulia, 2004; Irons, 2001; Sosis, 2003). Recent developments in the scientific study of religion have applied this theory to explain religious belief and behavior. According to CST, both public and private religious behaviors (i.e., ritual activities such as fasting, prayer, worship, and tithing) can be regarded as "costly" in that they incur significant effort without prospect of immediate returns. In their roles as signaling devices these religious rituals and behaviors can become reliable indicators of commitment (of the person enacting them) to the religious community (see Rapaport, 1999, for a similar analysis). By engaging in these religious practices the religious adherent is saying, in effect, "Look, I would not be devoting so much time to these irrational and useless activities unless I was truly committed to the group." No free rider would be willing to consistently engage in apparently useless ritual activities; thus adherents can separate the sheep from the goats by looking at their willingness to comply with all of the group's ritual obligations. Identifying who is and is not in compliance with the rules facilitates group cohesion and cooperation because adherents can have confidence that they are not being exploited by free riders (Fehr & Rockenbach, 2004; Sosis, 2003). Furthermore, evolutionary models of sexual selection in humans suggest that both men and women use "strength of character" as a reliable, hard-to-fake signal or cue of fitness in a mate. Interestingly, surveys (see review in Steen, Kachorek, & Peterson, 2003) find that strength of character is considered to be sexy and highly attractive and involves such virtues as the capacity to love and be loved, honesty, humor, enthusiasm, kindness, gratitude, forgiveness, playfulness, self-control, and wisdom. These character strengths are consciously cultivated and highly prized by most, and perhaps all, of the major world religions.

Theologians have recognized the effectiveness of public expression of compliance with ritual forms. A public religious expression, such as a testimony of thanksgiving in response to answered prayer, can authenticate commitment to one's god and to one's faith community. This testimony, if it is repetitive and sincere, provides concrete evidence of the giver's commitment that not only reinforces and strengthens his or her faith but signals to other believers the person's level of the commitment to the group and to their shared ideology. For instance, a family ritual of saying grace before meals is a simple example of how thanksgiving practices can be inculcated within groups and lead to increased cohesiveness. Theologian Patrick D. Miller (1994) documented the communal character of praise and thanksgiving in Biblical theology. When an individual corporately testifies to God's gracious beneficence, the faith community becomes a "circle of thanksgiving to God" (p. 195), and the resultant effect is the enhancing and strengthening of communal ties and a powerful reminder to the individual that he or she is not autonomous and self-sufficient (P. D. Miller, 1994). Such public acts also increase the devotion of believers through dissonance reduction dynamics (Aronson, 1999), thus contributing to their efficacy and cultural staying power. Commitment is then strengthened through dissonance-reduction dynamics.

As mentioned above "costly signals" require strategic costs—that is, costs that extend beyond the baseline costs that all behavioral actions entail, and that are therefore hard to fake by individuals not truly committed to cooperative interchange. Cooperative relationships can greatly benefit participating individuals, but they are at risk of exploitation by "free riders"—individuals who want to take but not give. It is important to realize just how destructive a free rider can be to attempts to cooperate (de Quervain et al., 2004). If a group of people who are engaged in a common work begin to sense that one of their members is not putting anything into the work but is nevertheless still drawing salary or benefits, then every other individual in

the group begins to adjust his or her performance accordingly, until eventually all trust collapses among members of the group and they disband before accomplishing their purpose. Successful group cooperation requires reliable methods of identifying cheaters and free riders. The ability to identify genuine cooperators and fakes or free riders is crucial for those wishing to pursue cooperative exchanges. Interestingly, recent studies combining neuroimaging with behavioral game experiments have shown that neostriatal and limbic prefrontal dopaminergic networks are activated when cheaters/free riders are identified and punished (Fehr & Gächter, 2002; Fehr & Rockenbach, 2004; de Quervain et al., 2004). Fehr and Rockenbach interpret this finding as indicating that evolution has endowed humans with proximate mechanisms that render altruistic behavior as intrinsically rewarding.

While multiple institutional procedures have evolved to spot and punish free riders, we are interested here in how religious emotions might contribute to the process. It is clear how the common emotions contribute: You get angry, even enraged, when you are being exploited by a free rider, and you vow never to trust that person again. By contrast, after a successful bout of cooperation with a trustworthy individual, you increase your level of liking, comfort, and trust in that individual. But what about the religious versions of the emotions of trust, gratitude, forgiveness, and so forth?

We contend that religious emotions help us identify free riders and genuine cooperators because all of the religious emotions contribute to the *virtues* or "strengths of character." If a person has genuinely acquired the traditional religious virtues, then he or she is likely to be a trustworthy companion. The crucial distinction, we believe, is that *genuine cooperators will acquire a reputation for trustworthiness and integrity, whereas free riders will not be able to sustain the high costs of acting with integrity, consistency, and generosity.* The importance of trustworthiness and character is even more pronounced when social groups increase in size and number, such that adherents can no longer rely on reputation or repeated interactions with an individual. In large groups of people free riders find ways to escape identification in the crowd. Perceived strength of character or "trustworthiness" of an individual should, therefore, reliably indicate an individual's willingness to engage in cooperative enterprises. Thus, considerations derived from CST predict that a premium will be placed on the neurobehavioral ability to both perceive and signal trustworthiness. The religious emotions would facilitate the ability to both perceive and display traits of trustworthiness. If I am, for example, perceived as a grateful person, then it likely means that I have received an unmerited gift at some point in the recent past. If I have received an unmerited gift, then it is likely that some important person or group trusted me enough to cooperate with me and liked me enough to confer extraordinary benefits on me in the course of that cooperation. Thus, sustaining over time the behavioral disposition of "gratitude" could bring even more *benefits* to the grateful individual because it will mark the person as trustworthy. From this theoretical framework, then, it is easy to understand why people would believe that the good things that they have in life—those blessings for which they are grateful—were intentionally given to them for their benefit. Our mental tools support such an inferential process. It would be far more unnatural to see these "blessings" as randomly occurring, or attribute them to luck or fate. This being the case, gratitude is a nearly inevitable outcome of how our mind works. When the blessings that we have cannot be attributed to human benevolence, attributions to God's goodness become all the more likely. Therefore, people are more likely to sense a divine hand in cherished experiences that cannot easily be attributed to human effort—the birth of a child, a miraculous recovery from illness, the restoration of an estranged relationship—for which gratitude to God is the apt response.

While some of this discussion of the evolutionary basis of religion and virtue is admittedly speculative, it is our opinion that there is much to be gained by an increasing dialogue and collaboration between psychologists who specialize in the psychology of religion and our colleagues in evolutionary biology, neuroscience, philosophy, anthropology, and cognitive science, so that developments in the psychology of religion and personality take into account and build upon advances in these related scientific disciplines.

CONCLUSION

Over a half century ago, Gordon Allport stated "If we ask what psychology has contributed to our understanding of the religious nature of man, the answer is, 'Less than we might wish'" (Allport, 1955, p. 93). Over the past decade progress into understanding the role of religion and spirituality in personality has begun to accelerate. Much progress has been made at the interface of personality psychology and the psychology of religion, as personality researchers from diverse theoretical positions have begun to view religion as a fruitful topic for empirical study. Although personality psychology has made admirable advances since Allport's (1955) lament about our ignorance regarding religiousness, we still know considerably less about this domain of human functioning than we might wish. Dialogue and collaboration between personality psychologists who specialize in religion and our colleagues in evolutionary biology, neuroscience, philosophy, anthropology, and cognitive science has been rapidly expanding. The result of these collaborative efforts is that developments in the personality psychology of religion take into account and build upon advances in these related scientific disciplines. This collaboration represents significant progress toward pursuing Allport's vision of a psychology of personality that takes seriously the religious dimension of human functioning.

REFERENCES

Allport, G. W. (1955). *Becoming: Basic considerations for a psychology of personality*. New Haven, CT: Yale University Press.

Altemeyer, B., & Hunsberger, B. (1997). *Amazing conversions: Why some turn to faith and others abandon religion*. Amherst, NY: Prometheus Press.

Andresen, J. (2001). *Religion in mind: Cognitive perspectives on religious belief, ritual, and experience*. New York: Cambridge University Press.

Aronson, E. (1999). *The social animal* (8th ed.). New York: Worth.

Ashton, M. C., & Lee, K. (2001). A theoretical basis for the major dimensions of personality. *European Journal of Personality, 15,* 327–353.

Azari, N. P. (2006). Neuroimaging studies of religious experience: A critical review. In P. Mc-

Namara (Ed.), *Where science and God meet: How brain and evolutionary studies alter our understanding of religion* (Vol. 2, pp. 33–54.) Westport, CT: Praeger.

Barna Group Survey Reports. (n.d.). *Church attendance.* Retrieved October 20, 2006, from *www.barna.org/FlexPage. aspx?Page=Topic&TopicID=10.*

Barrett, J. L. (2000). Exploring the natural foundations of religion. *Trends in Cognitive Sciences, 4,* 29–34.

Barrett, J. L. (2004). *Why would anyone believe in God?* Walnut Creek, CA: Altamira Press.

Barrett, J. L., & Nyhof, M. A. (2001). Spreading non-natural concepts: The role of intuitive conceptual structures in memory and transmission of cultural materials. *Journal of Cognition and Culture, 1,* 69–100.

Barrett, J. L., & Richert, R. A. (2003). Anthropomorphism or preparedness? Exploring children's concept of God. *Review of Religious Research, 44,* 300–312.

Bartlett, M. Y., & DeSteno, D. (2006). Gratitude and prosocial behavior: Helping when it costs you. *Psychological Science, 17,* 319–325.

Beckford, J. A. (1978). Accounting for conversion. *British Journal of Sociology, 29,* 249–262.

Bergin, A. E., & Jensen, J. P. (1990). Religiosity of psychotherapists: A national survey. *Psychotherapy: Theory, Research, Practice, Training: Special issue on Psychotherapy and Religion, 27,* 3–7.

Bering, J. M. (2006). The folk psychology of souls. *Behavioral and Brain Sciences, 29,* 453–498.

Bonnie, K. E., & de Waal, F. B. M. (2004). Primate social reciprocity and the origin of gratitude.In R. A. Emmons & M. E. McCullough (Eds.), *The psychology of gratitude* (pp. 213–229). New York: Oxford University Press.

Boyer, P. (1994). *The naturalness of religious ideas: A cognitive theory of religion.* Berkeley, CA: University of California Press.

Boyer, P. (2001). *Religion explained.* New York: Basic Books.

Boyer, P., & Ramble, C. (2001). Cognitive templates for religious concepts: Cross-cultural evidence for recall of counter-intuitive representations. *Cognitive Science, 25,* 535–564.

Bulbulia, J. (2004). Religious costs as adaptations that signal altruistic intention. *Evolution and Cognition, 10,* 19–38.

Burkert, W. (1996). *Creation of the sacred: Tracks of biology in early religions.* Cambridge, MA: Harvard University Press.

Carver, C. S. (1996). Emergent integration in contemporary personality psychology. *Journal of Research in Personality: Special issue on the future of personality, 30,* 319–334.

Ciarrocchi, J. W., & Deneke, E. (2005). Happiness and the varieties of religious experience: Religious support, practices, and spirituality as predictors of well-being. *Research in the Social Scientific Study of Religion, 15,* 209–233.

Ciarrocchi, J. W., Dy-Liacco, G.S., & Deneke, E. (in press). Gods or rituals?: Relational faith, spiritual discontent, and religious practices as predictors of hope and optimism. *Journal of Positive Psychology.*

Costa, P. T., Jr., & McCrae, R. B. (1994). Set like plaster?: Evidence for the stability of adult personality. In T. F. Heatherton & J. L. Weinberger (Eds.), *Can personality change?* (pp. 21–40). Washington, DC: American Psychological Association.

Costa, P. T., Jr., & McCrae, R. R. (1995). Domains and facets: Hierarchical personality assessment using the revised NEO personality inventory. *Journal of Personality Assessment, 64,* 21–50.

Davis, J. A., Smith, T. W., & Marsden, P. V. (1998). *General social survey cumulative codebook, 1972–1998.* Storrs, CT: Roper Center.

de Quervain, D. J., Fischbacher, U., Treyer, V., Schellhammer, M., Schnyder, U., & Buck, A., et al. (2004). The neural basis of altruistic punishment. *Science, 305,* 1254–1258.

Elkins, D. N. (2005). A humanistic approach to spiritually-oriented psychotherapy. In L. Sperry & E. P. Shafranske (Eds.), *Spiritually-oriented psychotherapy* (pp. 131–152). Washington, DC: American Psychological Association.

Emmons, R. A. (1999). *The psychology of ultimate concerns: Motivation and spirituality in personality.* New York: Guilford Press.

Emmons, R. A., Cheung, C., & Tehrani, K. (1998). Assessing spirituality through personal goals: Implications for research on religion and subjective well-being. *Social Indicators Research, 45,* 391–422.

Emmons, R. A., & McCullough, M. E. (2004). *The psychology of gratitude.* New York: Oxford University Press.

Fehr, E., & Gächter, S. (2002). Altruistic punishment in humans. *Nature, 415,* 137–140.

Fehr, E., & Rockenbach, B. (2004). Human altruism: Economic, neural, and evolutionary perspectives. *Current Opinion in Neurobiology, 14,* 784–790.

Fredrickson, B. L. (2002). How does religion benefit health and well-being? Are positive emotions active ingredients? *Psychological Inquiry, 13,* 209–213.

Galanter, M. (1982). Charismatic religious sects and psychiatry: An overview. *American Journal of Psychiatry, 139,* 1539–1548.

Galea, M. (2003). The impact of child abuse on the psycho-spiritual status, religious behavior, and family dynamics of Maltese college students (Doctoral dissertation, ProQuest Information & Learning). *Dissertation Abstracts*

International: Section B: The Sciences and Engineering, 64, 1933.

Geary, B. (2003). The contribution of spirituality to well-being in sex offenders (Doctoral dissertation, ProQuest Information & Learning). *Dissertation Abstracts International: Section B: The Sciences and Engineering, 64,* 2431.

Golden, J. L. (2002). Spirituality as a predictor of burnout among united Methodist clergy: An incremental validity study (Doctoral dissertation, ProQuest Information & Learning). *Dissertation Abstracts International: Section B: The Sciences and Engineering, 63,* 576.

Golden, J., Piedmont, R. L., Ciarrocchi, J. W., & Rodgerson, T. (in press). Spirituality and burnout: An incremental validity study. *Journal of Psychology and Theology.*

Goodenough, U. (1998). *The sacred depths of nature.* New York: Oxford University Press.

Granqvist, P. (1998). Religiousness and perceived childhood attachment: On the question of compensation and correspondence. *Journal for the Scientific Study of Religion, 37,* 350–367.

Greer, T. (2005). "We are a religious people; we are a vengeful people." *Journal for the Scientific Study of Religion, 44,* 45–47.

Guthrie, S. E. (1993). *Faces in the clouds: A new theory of religion.* New York: Oxford University Press.

Henig, R. M. (2007). Darwin's God. *New York Times.* Retrieved March 5, 2007, from *www.nytimes.com/2007/03/04/magazine/04evolution.t.html?pagewanted=8&en=43cfb46824423cea&ei=5090&ex=1330664400.*

Hood, R. W., Jr., Spilka, B., Hunsberger, B., & Gorsuch, R. (1996). *The psychology of religion: An empirical approach* (2nd ed.). New York: Guilford Press.

Howard, G. S., & Dailey, P. R. (1979). Response-shift bias: A source of contamination of self-report measures. *Journal of Applied Psychology, 64,* 144–150.

Idler, E. L., & Kasl, S. V. (1997). Religion among disabled and nondisabled persons: II. Attendance at religious services as a predictor of the course of disability. *Journals of Gerontology: Series B: Psychological Sciences and Social Sciences, 52,* 306–316.

Irons, W. (2001). Religion as a hard-to-fake sign of commitment. In R. M. Nesse (Ed.), *Evolution and the capacity for commitment* (pp. 290–309). New York: Sage Foundation.

James, W. (1902). *The varieties of religious experience.* New York: Longmans.

Kelemen, D. (2005). Are children "intuitive theists"?: Reasoning about purpose and design in nature. *Psychological Science, 15,* 295–301.

Keltner, N. L. (2003). The ABCs of psychobiology. *Perspectives in Psychiatric Care, 39,* 123–126.

Kirkpatrick, L. A. (1997). A longitudinal study of changes in religious belief and behaviors as a function of individual differences in adult attachment style. *Journal for the Scientific Study of Religion, 36,* 207–217.

Kirkpatrick, L. A. (1998). God as a substitute attachment figure: A longitudinal study of adult attachment style and religious change in college students. *Personality and Social Psychology Bulletin, 24,* 961–973.

Kosek, R. B. (1999). Adaptation of the Big Five as a hermeneutic instrument for religious constructs. *Personality and Individual Differences, 27,* 229–237.

Lawson, E. T., & McCauley, R. N. (1990). *Rethinking religion: Connecting cognition and culture.* New York: Cambridge University Press.

Lubinski, D., Schmidt, D. B., & Benbow, C. P. (1996). A 20-year stability analysis of the study of values for intellectually gifted individuals from adolescence to adulthood. *Journal of Applied Psychology, 81,* 443–451.

MacDonald, D. A. (2000). Spirituality: Description, measurement, and relation to the five-factor model of personality. *Journal of Personality, 68,* 153–197.

Mahoney, A., & Pargament, K. I. (2004). Sacred changes: Spiritual conversion and transformation. *Journal of Clinical Psychology, 60,* 481–492.

McAdams, D. P. (1994). Can personality change? Levels of stability and growth in personality across the lifespan. In T. F. Heatherton & J. L. Weinberger (Eds.), *Can personality change?* (pp. 299–313). Washington, DC: American Psychological Association.

McAdams, D. P. (1995). What do we know when we know a person? *Journal of Personality, 63,* 365–396.

McCauley, R. N., & Whitehouse, H. (2005). Introduction: New frontiers in the cognitive science of religion. *Journal of Cognition and Culture* [Special issue], *5,* 1–13.

McCrae, R. R., & Costa, P. T., Jr. (1996). Toward a new generation of personality theories: Theoretical contexts for the five-factor model. In J. S. Wiggins (Ed.), *The five-factor model of personality* (pp. 51–87). New York: Guilford Press.

McCullough, M. E., Emmons, R. A., & Tsang, J. (2002). The grateful disposition: A conceptual and empirical topography. *Journal of Personality and Social Psychology, 82,* 112–127.

McCullough, M. E., & Hoyt, W. T. (2002). Transgression-related motivational dispositions: Personality substrates of forgiveness and their links to the Big Five. *Personality and Social Psychology Bulletin, 28,* 1556–1573.

McCullough, M. E., Kilpatrick, S. D., Emmons, R. A., & Larson, D. B. (2001). Is gratitude a moral affect? *Psychological Bulletin, 127*, 249–266.

McCullough, M. E., & Willoughby, B. L. B. (in press). Religion, self-regulation, and self-control. *Psychological Bulletin*.

Miller, P. D. (1994). *They cried to the Lord: The form and theology of Biblical prayer*. Minneapolis: Fortress Press.

Miller, W. R., & C'deBaca, J. (1994). Quantum change: Toward a psychology of transformation. In T. F. Heatherton & J. L. Weinberger (Eds.), *Can personality change?* (pp. 253–280). Washington, DC: American Psychological Association.

Miller, W. R., & C'deBaca, J. (2001). *Quantum change: When epiphanies and sudden insights transform ordinary lives*. New York: Guilford Press.

Newberg, A. B., & Newberg, S. K. (2005). The neuropsychology of religious and spiritual experience. In R. F. Paloutzian & C. L. Park (Eds.), *Handbook of the psychology of religion and spirituality* (pp. 199–215). New York: Guilford Press.

Numbers, R. L., & Numbers, K. S. (2003, March–April). Religion red in tooth and claw. *American Scientist Online*. Retrieved May 3, 2007, from *www.americanscientist.org/template/BookReviewTypeDetail/assetid/17182;jsessionid=baa9*.

Ozer, D. J., & Reise, S. P. (1994). Personality assessment. *Annual Review of Psychology, 45*, 357–388.

Paloutzian, R. F. (1981). Purpose in life and value changes following conversion. *Journal of Personality and Social Psychology, 41*, 1153–1160.

Paloutzian, R. F. (2005). Religious conversion and spiritual transformation: A meaning-system analysis. In R. F. Paloutzian & C. C. Park (Eds.), *Handbook of the psychology of religion and spirituality* (pp. 331–347). New York: Guilford Press.

Paloutzian, R. F., Richardson, J. T., & Rambo, L. R. (1999). Religious conversion and personality change. *Journal of Personality, 67*, 1047–1079.

Pargament, K. I. (1997). *The psychology of religious coping: Theory, research, practice*. New York: Guilford Press.

Pargament, K. I., & Park, C. L. (1995). Merely a defense?: The variety of religious means and ends. *Journal of Social Issues: Special issue on religious influences on personal and societal well-being, 51*, 13–32.

Peterson, C., & Seligman, M. E. P. (2004). *Character strengths and virtues: A handbook of classification*. Washington, DC: American Psychological Association.

Piedmont, R. L. (1999). Does spirituality represent the sixth factor of personality?: Spiritual transcendence and the five-factor model. *Journal of Personality, 67*, 985–1013.

Piedmont, R. L. (2001). Cracking the plaster cast: Big Five personality change during intensive outpatient counseling. *Journal of Research in Personality, 35*, 500–520.

Piedmont, R. L. (2005). The role of personality in understanding religious and spiritual constructs. In R. F. Paloutzian & C. C. Park (Eds.), *Handbook of the psychology of religion and spirituality* (pp. 253–273). New York: Guilford Press.

Piedmont, R. L., & Leach, M. M. (2002). Cross-cultural generalizability of the spiritual transcendence scale in India. *American Behavioral Scientist, 45*, 1888–1901.

Piedmont, R. L., McCrae, R. R., Riemann, R., & Angleitner, A. (2000). On the invalidity of validity scales: Evidence from self-reports and observer ratings in volunteer samples. *Journal of Personality and Social Psychology, 78*, 582–593.

Rambo, L. R. (1993). *Understanding religious conversion*. New Haven, CT: Yale University Press.

Rapaport, L. G. (1999). Provisioning of young in golden lion tamarins (callitrichidae, leontopithecus rosalia): A test of the information hypothesis. *Ethology, 105*, 619–636.

Robins, R. W., Noftle, E., Trzesniewski, K. H., & Roberts, B. W. (2005). Do people know how their personality has changed? Correlates of perceived and actual personality change in young adulthood. *Journal of Personality, 73*, 489–521.

Rosen, A. S., & Nordquist, T. A. (1980). Ego developmental level and values in a yogic community. *Journal of Personality and Social Psychology, 39*, 1152–1160.

Rozin, P. (2006). Domain denigration and process preference in academic psychology. *Perspectives on Psychological Science, 1*, 365–376.

Saroglou, V. (2002). Religion and the five factors of personality: A meta-analytic review. *Personality and Individual Differences, 32*, 15–25.

Saucier, G., & Goldberg, L. R. (1998). What is beyond the Big Five? *Journal of Personality, 66*, 495–524.

Simmel, G. (1950). *The sociology of Georg Simmel*. Glencoe, IL: Free Press.

Simpson, J. A., & Weiner, E. S. C. (1989). *The Oxford English dictionary* (2nd ed., Vols. 1–20). New York: Oxford University Press.

Sloan, R. P., Bagiella, E., & Powell, T. (2001). Without a prayer: Methodological problems, ethical challenges, and misrepresentations in the study of religion, spirituality, and medicine.

In T. G. Plante & A. C. Sherman (Eds.), *Faith and health: Psychological perspectives* (pp. 339–354). New York: Guilford Press.

Smart, N. (1996). *Dimensions of the sacred: An anatomy of the world's beliefs.* Berkeley: University of California Press.

Smith, C. (2003). *Moral, believing animals: Human personhood and culture.* New York: Oxford University Press.

Smith, C., & Denton, M. L. (2005). *Soul searching: The religious and spiritual lives of American teenagers.* Oxford: Oxford University Press.

Sosis, R. (2003). Why aren't we all Hutterites?: Costly signaling theory and religious behavior. *Human Nature, 14,* 91–127.

Sperber, D., & Wilson, D. (1995). *Relevance: Communication and cognition.* Oxford, UK: Blackwell.

Sprangers, M. (1989). Subject bias and the retrospective retest in retrospect. *Bulletin of the Psychonomic Society, 27,* 11–14.

Starbuck, E. D. (1899). *The psychology of religion.* London: Walter Scott.

Steen, T. A., Kachorek, L. V., & Peterson, C. (2003). Character strengths among youth. *Journal of Youth and Adolescence, 32,* 5–16.

Taylor, A., & MacDonald, D. A. (1999). Religion and the five factor model of personality: An exploratory investigation using a Canadian university sample. *Personality and Individual Differences, 27,* 1243–1259.

Tillich, P. (1957). *Dynamics of faith.* New York: Harper & Row.

Tremlin, T. (2006). *Minds and gods: The cognitive foundations of religion.* New York: Oxford University Press.

Trivers, R. L. (1971). The evolution of reciprocal altruism. *Quarterly Review of Biology, 46,* 35–57.

Ullman, C. (1989). *The transformed self: The psychology of religious conversion.* New York: Plenum Press.

Walsh, K. F. (2001). *Shed some light: Open the door. A descriptive study of the feeling of peak experience while listening to or performing music* (Doctoral dissertation, ProQuest Information & Learning). *Dissertation Abstracts International: Section B: The Sciences and Engineering, 61*(9), 5011.

Watkins, P. C., Grimm, D. L., & Kolts, R. (2004). Counting your blessings: Positive memories among grateful persons. *Current Psychology: Developmental, Learning, Personality, Social, 23,* 52–67.

Watkins, P. C., Woodward, K., Stone, T., & Kolts, R. L. (2003). Gratitude and happiness: Development of a measure of gratitude and relationships with subjective well-being. *Social Behavior and Personality, 31,* 431–452.

Watson, D., & Clark, L. A. (1993). Behavioral disinhibition versus constraint: A dispositional perspective. In D. M. Wegner & J. W. Pennebaker (Eds.), *Handbook of mental control* (pp. 506–527). Upper Saddle River, NJ: Prentice Hall.

Whitehouse, H. (2004). *Modes of religiosity: A cognitive theory of religious transmission.* Walnut Creek, CA: AltaMira Press.

Wilson, D. S. (2002). *Darwin's cathedral: Evolution, religion, and the nature of society.* Chicago: University of Chicago Press.

Wink, P., & Dillon, M. (2001). Religious involvement and health outcomes in late adulthood: Findings from a longitudinal study of women and men. In T. G. Plante & A. C. Sherman (Eds.), *Faith and health: Psychological perspectives* (pp. 75–106). New York: Guilford Press.

Winseman, A. L. (2004, May 25). Eternal destinations: Americans believe in Heaven, Hell. *Gallup Poll National Survey Commentary.* Retrieved May 3, 2007, from *www.galluppoll.com/content/?ci=11770&pg=1.*

Zinnbauer, B. J., & Pargament, K. I. (1998). Spiritual conversion: A study of religious change among college students. *Journal for the Scientific Study of Religion, 37,* 161–180.

CHAPTER 26

Self-Determination Theory and the Role of Basic Psychological Needs in Personality and the Organization of Behavior

Richard M. Ryan
Edward L. Deci

THE IMPORTANCE OF PSYCHOLOGICAL THEORY

Although it is not always reflected in the discourse of contemporary psychology, the most proximal determinants of human behavior lie in *experience*. It is the manner in which people interpret events and the perceived relations of those events to the actors' psychological needs that provide the *regnant causes* of intentional actions (Ryan & Deci, 2004).

Attesting to this point, consider that the most practical behavioral interventions are those that focus on changing a person's experience. Humans typically influence others through psychological (rather than physical) means: for example, facilitating insight or inspiration, engaging in persuasion, making salient subjectively relevant information or values, conveying regard or distain, or changing contingencies to specifically alter others' explicit motives and goals. Even when people attempt to engineer others' behavior by directly controlling their environments (as advocated by B. F. Skinner, 1953), how the recipients experience the controls mediates how they respond. Similarly, even

as neuroscience gains increasingly detailed knowledge concerning the material underpinnings of experience, intervening at the level of people's subjective experience will continue to be the most practical means of changing human behavior (Breckler, 2006). Thus, when people's *aim* is behavior change, altering others' experience is the most available means for achieving the desired effect.

The significance of human experience goes beyond the scientific enterprise. Existentially, what defines a person's life is the way in which it is experienced. Well-being, mental health, and a life well lived are all about experiencing love, freedom, efficacy, and meaningful goals and values (Bauer, McAdams & Sakaeda, 2005; Ryan, Huta, & Deci, 2008), all of which are psychological phenomena. Although there are outer signs of successful living, they are unreliable compared to people's true experiences of their lives. The rich can be depressed and the poor happy; the famous can be lonely and the introvert secure. Thus, within their "objective" circumstances, the most important feature in people's lives is their experience of living, so enhancing that experience, with its various consequences, is an important focus for psychological interventions.

In sum, it is typically people's feelings, beliefs, motives, and goals, and the *perceived* environment within which these feelings, beliefs, motives, and goals arise, that organize subsequent behavior. Yet oddly empirical psychology today still often finds suspect, or actively discounts, the importance of "subjective" phenomenon, when it is precisely subjective phenomenon that the discipline of psychology ought to lawfully explain.

SELF-DETERMINATION THEORY AND THE EMPIRICAL STUDY OF HUMAN EXPERIENCE

Self-determination theory (SDT; Deci & Ryan, 1985b; Ryan & Deci, 2000b) is unabashedly a psychological approach to human behavior, which means that it typically considers people's experience to be the proximal determinant of action. In other words, the theory focuses on the way people interpret internal or external stimulus inputs, which, we assert, gain meaning and power from their direct or indirect relation to people's basic psychological needs. It is in this nexus of stimulus events or contexts and people's psychological needs that their subjective or functional experiences arise. Thus, it is there that we find what we believe to be the most important concepts for predicting behavior and its consequences (Ryan & Deci, 2004).

Although experience is the proximal determinant of most behaviors, it is important not to equate psychological experience with *self-reports*. Self-reports are themselves behaviors and thus must be considered in terms of *their* determinants (Robins & John, 1997). Although they can be useful for studying people's experiences and behaviors, self-reports are also shaped in part by the motives operative in the perceived social context of self-reporting and the person's interpretation of what is being asked. Moreover, people's experiences are frequently richer than what they can say about them, which makes phenomenology, or the study of experience, different from a self-report psychology. Thus, a psychology of experience may make use of self-reports, but it can also make use of inferences about experience as hypothetical intervening constructs, a point that Tolman (1932) argued so persuasively decades ago.

SDT does use hypothetical constructs. In its empirical investigations of behaviors, along with their antecedents, correlates, and consequences, the theory uses both self-reports and observations to define key psychological constructs. For example *intrinsic motivation* is defined as behavior done for its inherent satisfactions, and it is assessed behaviorally in terms of freely pursued behaviors, and experientially by a perceived internal locus of causality and feelings of interest. SDT also includes constructs concerning basic psychological needs as they shape the implicit and explicit meanings, or *functional significance*, people give to contexts and life events. SDT thus stands in the tradition of Heider (1958), White (1959), and deCharms (1968) in formalizing the principles through which persons organize and explain their own and others' actions, and the relations of various types of motives, reasons, and intentions to subsequent behavior. Although behavior can be studied at multiple levels of analysis and is both underpinned by people's biology and encapsulated within their culture, psychological principles remain the primary focus of SDT, for they typically supply the regnant causes of actions. It is through psychological processes that the chain of microphysical events that "compose into" complex behaviors is organized (Ryan & Deci, 2004).

At the same time that SDT is a theory of personal experience, it is also a theory of human nature, for it maintains that understanding subjective experience requires that one specify the nature of the self and its integrative tendencies as well as the basic psychological needs that lend greater salience to some events than to others (Ryan, 1995). Within SDT, specification of these natural or inherent needs, which have gravitational weight in behavioral dynamics, emerged empirically from a series of investigations over many years. As we studied motivational processes in laboratory experiments and field research, we found that a deep and meaningful theoretical explanation of phenomena that were otherwise isolated required an assumption of a small set of basic psychological needs, namely, those for autonomy, competence, and relatedness. This has led, successively, to four sets of formal propositions that we refer to as *mini-theories*, each of which focuses on a different set of phenomena. The four mini-theories are connected and integrated by their relations to the core concept of basic psychological needs, and together they constitute SDT. Thus, the theoretical framework has grown in complexity over time, and it has also analyzed an increasing number of topics and moved into an increasing number of applied domains over the years.

SDT began as an exploration of the determinants of *intrinsic motivation*, of why people (and other organisms) often behave not so much for extrinsic incentive as for the satisfactions inherent in the behaving. This early work was formalized as *cognitive evaluation theory* (CET; Deci & Ryan, 1980) and concerned how social-contextual factors support, versus thwart, people's needs for autonomy and competence and thus impact their intrinsic motivation. Subsequently, SDT moved onto empirical work focused on *internalization*, that is, the question of how people acquire and integrate nonintrinsically motivated regulations and values. This second mini-theory, labeled *organismic integration theory* (OIT; Deci & Ryan, 1985b; Ryan & Connell, 1989), incorporates the idea of an assimilative, integrative, or synthetic tendency, which has been central to organismic theories of personality and development such as those of Freud (1923/1962), Piaget (1971), Goldstein (1939), and Rogers (1951). It attempts to explain what facilitates or forestalls that core integrative process and what results when the process is facilitated or forestalled to varying degrees (Ryan, 1995). The study of internalized, as well as intrinsic, motives led to a fuller consideration of the concept of relatedness as a basic psychological need, in addition to the needs for autonomy and competence that had proven essential in the formulation of CET.

Other research focused on individual differences in motivational orientations as predictors of behavior and other aspects of personality; and this work was formalized as *causality orientations theory* (COT; Deci & Ryan, 1985a, 1985b). Most recently, we outlined *basic psychological need theory* (BPNT; Deci & Ryan, 2000; Ryan & Deci, 2002), a fourth mini-theory that examines the extent to which personal and social events satisfy the postulated needs and thus promote, to varying degrees, healthy development and psychological well-being (Ryan & Deci,

2001, 2004). This mini-theory also provides the foundation for a theoretical formulation about how differing goal contents are associated with wellness (T. Kasser & Ryan, 1996; Vansteenkiste, Ryan, & Deci, in press). Subsequent theoretical formulations associated with SDT's four mini-theories have included how awareness functions to foster integration and need satisfaction (Brown & Ryan, 2003), how individual psychological processes flourish (or are derailed) at situational, domain, and even cultural levels of analysis (Chirkov, Ryan, Kim, & Kaplan, 2003; Vallerand, 1997), how vitality and energy are enhanced or depleted (e.g., Moller, Deci, & Ryan, 2006; Ryan & Frederick, 1997), and how basic psychological needs play a critical role in personal relationships (Deci, La Guardia, Moller, Scheiner, & Ryan, 2006; Ryan, La Guardia, Solky-Butzel, Chirkov, & Kim, 2005).

In this chapter, we address the concept of basic psychological needs, review the four mini-theories and some of the evidence supporting them, and briefly survey some new directions and applications of the theory. Our intention is to provide a comprehensive and coherent motivational framework for the empirical study of human personality in social contexts, as it develops and functions, affecting people's behavior and their psychological and physical health.

THE CONCEPT OF PSYCHOLOGICAL NEEDS: ITS HISTORY AND USAGE WITHIN SDT

SDT is built upon the assumption that there are specifiable psychological nutriments, which, when afforded by an individual's social context, facilitate personality growth, well-being, and integrity (Deci & Ryan, 2000; Ryan & Deci, 2000a). These nutriments for personality—that is, these *basic psychological needs*—describe the universal, cross-developmental supports upon which integrated functioning depends, and which, in an ultimate sense, determine both the mental health of individuals and the vitality of the communities within which they are embedded.

Historically, the concept of psychological needs has been employed by theorists in two distinct ways, only one of which we endorse and utilize. The first, and by far the most common, use defines needs as desires that people differentially hold and that motivate behavior across situations. From this perspective, the central concept is the strength of the needs, which are viewed as individual differences. Thus, need strength is said to be learned as a function of interactions with the social environment, and it is then used either as a direct or interactive predictor of other personality characteristics, behaviors, or psychological conditions. The second usage involves a more restrictive concept of needs as nutriments that are essential for an organism's development and wellness. This use of the term "needs" leads researchers to focus more on the degree to which they are satisfied versus thwarted rather than on their strength.

Needs as Wants or Desires

The best-known theorists to use the concept of psychological needs were Murray (1938) and McClelland (1985). They both used needs in the first sense—as individual differences in the strength of a person's motives or desires. Specifically, Murray defined a need as "a force which organizes perception, apperception, intellection, conation and action in such a way as to transform in a certain direction an existing, unsatisfying, situation" (Murray, 1938, p. 124). Based on this broad definition, he postulated an array of both psychological and physical needs, including not only quite obvious needs such as that for affiliation, but also more specific desires such as the need to dominate others, and its opposite, the need to defer and submit. Murray and McClelland, as well as the scholars who followed in their tradition, used this broad concept of needs to generate a rich and productive body of research assessing the strength of individuals' needs and using that to predict a range of outcomes (e.g., Koestner & McClelland, 1990; McAdams, 1989; Winter, 1973).

It is noteworthy that Murray's conception of needs could be applied to virtually any motivating force or impetus to behavior. People's desires, motives, wants, or strivings all represent "forces that organize perception and action." Thus, Murray's definition fits with equal appropriateness into phrases like a dehydrated man's utterance that "I

need water" (Murray's thirst need) and a billionaire's remark that "I need another sports car" (Murray's acquisitive need). Although both "needs" may organize and activate goals, cognitions, and behaviors, there is no differentiation between objective needs, or necessities for health and wellness, and mere personal desires. In fact, although all of the motives Murray identified in his lengthy list of so-called needs can be salient energizers of behavior, many of them might be the products of insults to the psyche (e.g., the need for abasement, see Ryan, 2005), and some may produce as much damage as good for psychological health (e.g., acquisitiveness, see T. Kasser & Ryan, 1996).

Needs as Essential Nutriments

SDT uses the alternative and more circumscribed definition of needs. Specifically, we denote a basic psychological need as a *nutriment essential for psychological growth, integrity, and wellness*. This formulation of the term "needs" thus parallels the role of physiological needs for physical growth and integrity, because both psychological needs and physiological needs concern the conditions and supports that are necessary for human beings to thrive. The concept of physiological needs, so defined, was central to Hull's (1943) drive theory of motivation and learning. Thus, our concept of need shares this defining element with Hull's but not Murray's concept of need, and it shares with Murray's (1938) but not Hull's concept the fact that the level of focus is psychological rather than physiological.

Because SDT defines needs as necessities for healthy development, the theory maintains that it is not necessary for people to be aware of, or to culturally value, basic psychological needs in order for their thwarting to have a negative functional impact on well-being. For example, a woman might say that she does not need relationships to be happy, but deprivation of the relatedness need will nonetheless be manifest as some type of decrement in both personal development and well-being. So viewed, needs are *objective* rather than subjective (Braybrooke, 1987; Plant, Lesser, & Taylor-Gooby, 1980); people require them whether or not they think they do, and failures of satisfaction will thus have specifiable negative consequences. In the same way that, without proper socialization, children may not learn to value or prefer foods that are nutritious, instead valuing high-fat foods that objectively harm them, in some social contexts children may be more influenced to regulate themselves in controlled rather than autonomous ways, or to be more oriented toward selfishness than relatedness, even though doing so will harm them psychologically. Additionally, when people have been routinely unable to satisfy basic needs, they may block awareness of these needs as a way of defensively not having to experience the state of deprivation. For example, a person who avoids opportunities for relatedness may do so as an attempt to subjectively cope with a painful interpersonal past, but nonetheless, failure to obtain relatedness would still objectively be connected to psychological degradation.

Regardless of whether an individual is explicitly aware of needs, SDT maintains that the human psyche innately seeks out these nutriments and gravitates to sources of their fulfillment, either by directly seeking their gratification, or indirectly seeking it through need substitutes or compensatory activities. Psychological needs are thus hypothesized to energize much of human behavior, and many subjective desires are derived from the dynamics of basic needs. For example, materialists, who strongly desire wealth and possessions, are frequently people whose developmental backgrounds are characterized by need deficits in autonomy and relatedness (see, e.g., T. Kasser, Ryan, Zax, & Sameroff, 1995). Basic need deprivation in turn leads to a psychological sense of insecurity, which the acquisition of material excess is intended to ameliorate. Thus, although materialists may focus on material acquisition as a source of self-esteem and feelings of worth, this acquisitive activity does not "pay off" in terms of wellness because acquisition does not satisfy needs for autonomy and relatedness (T. Kasser & Ryan, 1996). As such, in SDT's framework Murray's "need for acquisitiveness" is not a need at all but a derivative motive—something that can become particularly strong for an individual in reaction to something more basic that has been missing. This "dynamic" approach allows us to predict both the etiology of derivative motives and the reason they do not enhance

well-being, even when achieved (e.g., Niemiec, Ryan, & Deci, 2007).

Positing basic needs also has importance for understanding and predicting the impact of variations in cultural and social systems (Vansteenkiste et al., in press). SDT suggests that societies and cultures maintain stability only by meeting the fundamental needs of their individual members. As detailed within OIT, supports for basic needs facilitate people's internalization of familial and cultural values. In the absence of internalization, social values can be maintained only through coercion and pressure, which is more like duct tape than a social glue. That is, societies function most stably and optimally when they provide opportunities for needs, both physical *and* psychological, to be fulfilled (Chirkov, Ryan, & Willness, 2005).

Three Basic Psychological Needs

Because of the restrictiveness of our definition of needs, our list, unlike Murray's, is very short. We thus far posit only three basic and universal psychological needs: those for autonomy, competence, and relatedness. *Autonomy* concerns the self-organization and endorsement of one's behavior. It refers to the feeling that deCharms (1968) described as "being an origin." More generally, autonomy concerns feeling volitional and congruent with respect to what one does (Ryan & Connell, 1989; Ryan & Deci, 2004). The opposite of autonomy is not dependence but heteronomy, which means feeling controlled by forces, whether external or internal, that are alien to the self. *Competence* refers to feeling effective in one's actions—that is, experiencing opportunities to exercise, expand, and express one's capacities (Deci, 1975; E. Skinner, 1995; White, 1959). Feelings of competence are enhanced by engaging optimal challenges and receiving positive feedback; they are diminished by conditions that deprive one of control over outcomes, signify that one does not have the capacities necessary for the task at hand, or are too easy. *Relatedness* refers to feeling connected with others and having a sense of belonging within one's community (Deci & Ryan, 1991; Reis & Patrick, 1996). Relatedness satisfactions entail a sense that one is significant to others, which is often manifest in others' willingness to care for one or to receive the care one has to offer (Ryan et al., 2005).

The criterion for distinguishing a need from a motive, again, pertains to its necessity for growth, integrity, and wellness. As we show later in the chapter, SDT provides evidence that when any of the three basic psychological needs for autonomy, competence, and relatedness are frustrated or thwarted, the individual will exhibit diminished motivation and well-being. Conversely, it is largely only insofar as behaviors satisfy one or more of these basic needs that they foster positive experience and a sense of vitality and mental health. By using a restrictive and verifiable definition of needs, we avoid what has been historically perhaps the most common criticism of need-related theories; namely, that there is a potentially infinite list of needs that can be postulated. In fact, we have seen little evidence for any psychological needs beyond the three we have isolated (Ryan & Deci, 2000a). Moreover, the list allows us to examine various aspects of social environments, whether concrete events or boarder societal factors, and to make a clear set of hypotheses about how they will affect aspects of growth, integrity, or wellness.

The Universality of Basic Needs

Another significant implication of our definition of psychological needs is that they are natural and universal. Psychological needs are natural in the sense that they are an invariant, indeed foundational, aspect of the psychological architecture of the human organism, and they are universal in that they apply to all persons regardless of gender, upbringing, or culture. Stated simply, SDT maintains that the effects of need support versus deprivation will generalize across all individuals and cultural contexts. It does not imply, however, that all individuals or cultural groups will explicitly value or support these needs, or that the needs will be satisfied versus thwarted in the same ways in different cultures or developmental epochs. Basic psychological needs may be expressed differently, and the vehicles through which they are satisfied may differ in different societies or stages of life, but their necessity is unchanging. Although cultures differ, for example, with some espousing the primacy of the group over the individual and others

espousing the primacy of the individual over the group, this does not, for example, negate the underlying necessities of all people satisfying the needs for relatedness and autonomy, respectively.

Indeed, it is a fundamental tenet of SDT that the reason people have a developmental readiness to adopt and internalize ambient cultural values is that by doing so they satisfy basic psychological needs. By assimilating the values of their group, individuals become more connected and related, and more competent and effective. Furthermore, the tendency for the individuals to make ambient values their own—that is, to integrate them into their sense of self—allows them to experience enactment of these values as autonomous. Put differently, needs supply the underlying processes that explain how cultures become part of individual personality. These essentials are thus apparent across historical, cultural, political, and economic contexts.

On the other hand, economic and cultural contexts can be compared in terms of the degree to which they support versus thwart the fulfillment of basic needs. Put differently, not all cultures, contexts, or economic structures are equally "good" for humans. Some may be better at satisfying their members' basic psychological needs, and those cultures or economies will be expected to have members with a higher average well-being. This point differentiates SDT from the absolute cultural relativism that characterizes much of modern social science (see, e.g., Iyengar & DeVoe, 2003; Schweder, Mahapatra, & Miller, 1990) that views cultures as molding a fully malleable, if not empty, human nature. In contrast to that relativist view, which fails to provide an explanation for cultural transformation—that is, for people changing their cultures—the psychology of needs contained in SDT clarifies the limits of cultural imposition and specifies the means through which people seek changes in cultures (see Inghilleri, 1999). SDT also suggests directions for human betterment and thriving, which clearly some cultures and economic systems have been more adept at than others (Vansteenkiste et al., in press).

We turn now to a brief description of each of the four mini-theories that make up SDT, and then move on to a few recent advances in theoretical and applied work related to SDT.

COGNITIVE EVALUATION THEORY

As already noted, from the time of the earliest work leading to SDT, we have made a distinction between intrinsic and extrinsic motivation. When *intrinsically motivated* people engage in an activity because they find the activity itself interesting and personally satisfying. Intrinsic motivation is a spontaneous motivator of proactive growth-promoting behaviors and a critical element in healthy cognitive and personality development. *Extrinsic motivation* propels us to engage in an activity because it leads to some separable consequence, such as the attainment of a reward, the avoidance of a punishment, or the achievement of a valued instrumental outcome.

Early cognitive theories of motivation, most notably expectancy–value theories (e.g., Atkinson, 1964; Porter & Lawler, 1968; Vroom, 1964), implied or asserted that these two types of motivation were additive, yielding total motivation. The first studies of intrinsic motivation with humans tested that assertion. Specifically, Deci (1971) explored whether providing extrinsic rewards to people for doing a task they were intrinsically motivated to do would result in a total motivation equivalent to the addition of the two. Deci found that when extrinsic rewards were given to people for doing an intrinsically interesting task, they subsequently evidenced less intrinsic motivation than they had had before being rewarded. In other words, the extrinsic and intrinsic motivations were not additive; instead, the introduction of extrinsic incentives *decreased* intrinsic motivation for the activity. In contrast, positive competence feedback increased intrinsic motivation, suggesting that this type of input was positively associated with intrinsic motivation.

The undermining of intrinsic motivation by rewards was a very controversial finding (e.g., Calder & Staw, 1975; Scott, 1976) largely because of the centrality of operant behaviorism (B. F. Skinner, 1953) within psychology at that time. Indeed the finding has remained somewhat controversial in the years since (e.g., Eisenberger, Pierce, & Cameron, 1999). Nonetheless, there have been more than 100 published experiments examining the effects of extrinsic rewards on intrinsic motivation, and a definitive meta-analysis (Deci, Koestner, & Ryan, 1999) confirmed that tangible rewards are indeed, on average, detrimental to intrinsic motivation. However, within CET reward effects are more complex than this "on average" effect might indicate, and a consideration of how reward effects are experienced by their recipients will allow a more finely tuned understanding of these effects.

Functional Significance: Informational and Controlling

CET was originally formulated to explain reward effects and, more broadly, the effects of extrinsic factors (e.g., deadlines, imposed goals, competition, surveillance, and evaluations), on intrinsic motivation (Deci, 1975; Deci & Ryan, 1980). Stated specifically, CET posits that any motivating factor (e.g., a reward) has two functional aspects that affect people's intrinsic motivation—a *controlling aspect* and an *informational aspect*—and that it is the relative salience of the controlling and informational aspects of the factor that determines its effect on people's intrinsic motivation. The *controlling* aspect thwarts satisfaction of the need for autonomy, for it leads people to experience their behavior as having an *external perceived locus of causality* (deCharms, 1968). Whether or not the motivator coerces (as is the case with threats of punishment; Deci & Cascio, 1972) or seduces (as is the case with rewards; Deci, 1971), if the motivator is experienced as controlling, it will undermine people's sense of autonomy. The *informational* aspect, in contrast, satisfies the need for competence by signifying effective performance. Thus, the informational aspect enhances intrinsic motivation primarily through strengthening perceived competence.

Implicit in this theoretical proposition is the idea that it is the interpretation of situational factors by the person that affects the person's intrinsic motivation. In the terms of CET, rewards and other extrinsic motivators have a *functional significance* to people—that is, a psychological meaning as a function of the degree to which the informational or controlling aspects are salient. As such, this represents a concrete instance of how it is the person's phenomenology in the situation that determines the effects of the situational factor on his or her motivation. CET also specifies aspects of the social context that tend to conduce to a controlling or informational significance for an event, but experience remains the hypothetical variable that mediates the outcomes. Understanding the relation of events to experience thus helps one know how to structure and deliver rewards effectively, without compromising either people's positive experiences or subsequent interest in the activity.

Other External Events and Social Contexts

After the initial experiments on tangible and verbal rewards, other experiments examined the effects of other concrete events on intrinsic motivation. For example, results of the studies indicated that deadlines (Amabile, DeJong, & Lepper, 1976), competition (Deci, Betley, Kahle, Abrams, & Porac, 1981), surveillance (Lepper & Greene, 1975; Plant & Ryan, 1985), judgmental evaluations (even when positive) (Smith, 1975), and imposed goals (Mossholder, 1980) undermined intrinsic motivation. We interpret the findings as indicating that, on average, people experience these events as controlling, or, using the concept introduced by deCharms (1968), the events tend to shift the perceived locus of causality for the behavior from internal to external, thus diminishing people's sense of autonomy. In contrast, the events of offering people choice about what to do or how to do it (Zuckerman, Porac, Lathin, Smith, & Deci, 1978) and acknowledging people's feelings about a situation (Koestner, Ryan, Bernieri, & Holt, 1984) have been found to enhance intrinsic motivation because they tend to promote a more internal perceived locus of causality, thus satisfying people's need for autonomy.

Additional studies indicated that for positive feedback to have its enhancing effects on intrinsic motivation, it has to be given in a noncontrolling way so that people feel responsible for the performance that is being affirmed (Fisher, 1978; Ryan, 1982). Furthermore, studies showed that negative performance feedback tended to decrease intrinsic motivation because it signifies incompetence, thus thwarting the need for competence (Deci & Cascio, 1972; Vallerand & Reid, 1984). In many cases, negative feedback also decreases extrinsic motivation by conveying that people cannot attain desired outcomes. This message will leave them *amotivated*, or lacking in either intrinsic or extrinsic motivation for the relevant activities.

Considerable research on CET has examined the general ambience of situations—that is, whether the social context tends to be autonomy supportive or to be controlling and pressuring. Consistently, studies have found positive links between interpersonal contexts that are autonomy supportive and both intrinsic motivation and well-being (Deci, Schwartz, Sheinman, & Ryan, 1981; Ryan, 1982). Furthermore, experiments showed that offering rewards in an autonomy-supportive way tends to enhance intrinsic motivation relative to no rewards and no feedback, but it does lead to less intrinsic motivation than just positive feedback that is comparable to what is conveyed by the rewards. This finding indicates that positive competence information conveyed by these "performance-contingent" rewards can have a positive effect on intrinsic motivation, but that this is not due to the reward per se but rather the competence feedback it provides (Deci et al., 1999; Ryan, Mims, & Koester, 1983).

In sum, CET focuses primarily on the enhancement or undermining of intrinsic motivation and posits that factors that conduce to perceived autonomy and competence are essential for maintained and enhanced intrinsic motivation. From this formulation has come a number of field studies in classroom, work, sport, and game contexts, in which factors associated with autonomy and competence have impacted intrinsic motivation (Ryan & Deci, 2000b).

ORGANISMIC INTEGRATION THEORY

Much of the research encompassed by CET tended to show how extrinsic rewards and contingencies can undermine intrinsic motivation, which is a prototype of autonomous behavior, implying that extrinsically motivated behavior tends not to be autonomous. Indeed, there was a period in which many writers generally considered intrinsic and extrinsic motivation to be antagonistic, suggesting that the former is autonomous or self-determined, whereas the latter is not only not autonomous but is detrimental to it (see, e.g., deCharms, 1968). However, the SDT perspective has been that, although rewards and other extrinsic motivators do often undermine intrinsic motivation, extrinsically motivated behavior can be autonomous. We suggested (e.g., Ryan, Connell, & Deci, 1985) that extrinsic motivation can become autonomous via *internalization*, a process through which external values and regulations can be taken in and integrated, to varying degrees, with one's sense of self. OIT was formulated to explicate the phenomena associated with the process of internalization of extrinsic motivation (Deci & Ryan, 1985b).

OIT specifies four types of extrinsic motivation and distinguishes them on the basis of the degree to which the motivation has been fully internalized and transformed into self-determined motivation. More specifically, the four types of extrinsic motivation fall along a continuum of relative autonomy in terms of the degree to which the resulting behavior associated with the four types of motivation will be autonomous or self-determined. All four types of extrinsic motivation do represent types of motivation, so they stand in contrast to *amotivation*, which represents a lack of motivation. Furthermore, they differ from intrinsic motivation because the basis for even the most internalized type of extrinsic motivation is not interest in the activity per se but rather in the activity's instrumental importance. Thus the four types of extrinsic motivation lie on the relative autonomy continuum between amotivation, which is accompanied by the experience of lowest autonomy, and intrinsic motivation, which is characterized by a high level of autonomy.

The least autonomous type of extrinsic motivation is *external regulation*, which is the classic type of extrinsic motivation based in rewards and punishments. It is the type of extrinsic motivation that was investigated in many of the experiments discussed in the CET section, and it is the type that was central to operant behaviorism. When externally regulated, people act because of the external contingencies besetting them. The principle problem with external motivation is not that it isn't a powerful motivator, but rather that it does not *internally* motivate, so it has poor maintenance and transfer.

The next type of extrinsic motivation, moving along the relative autonomy continuum, is *introjected regulation*. This type of extrinsic regulation involves behavior being controlled by an internalized motivation, but it is not one that people have fully endorsed. Rather, it is as if the internalized regulation is controlling the person in whom it resides. With introjected regulation, people are internally controlled to do what they "have to do" to maintain self-esteem (e.g., to affirm their self-worth), to avoid feeling guilty, or to live up to their beliefs about what will lead to others' approval. Introjected regulation is a very interesting case because it is a type of internal motivation that is more controlled than autonomous.

Identified regulation is the third type of extrinsic motivation and is a relatively self-determined type of extrinsic motivation, for people have identified with the personal importance of the activity for their own self-selected goals, values, or aspirations. Thus, they have accepted the regulation as their own by transforming it into a personally endorsed type of regulation. Finally, *integrated regulation* is a highly self-determined type of extrinsic motivation. It occurs as people evaluate an identification and bring it into coherence with other aspects of themselves. Without integration, identifications would be important to people but might not be well coordinated with other aspects of the self— that is, with other values, goals, and needs. Integrated regulation approximates intrinsic motivation in its degree of self-determination, but whereas intrinsic motivation is the innate motivation that emerges spontaneously from interest, integrated regulation is based in the importance of an activity for the person's values and goals.

The relative autonomy continuum of motivation appears in Figure 26.1. Amotivation, the four types of extrinsic motivation, and intrinsic motivation are arranged in the figure from left to right, showing increasing amounts of the degree to which the types of motivation represent autonomy and an expression of one's true sense of self.

Facilitating versus Inhibiting Internalization

OIT proposes that people are naturally inclined to internalize attitudes, values, be-

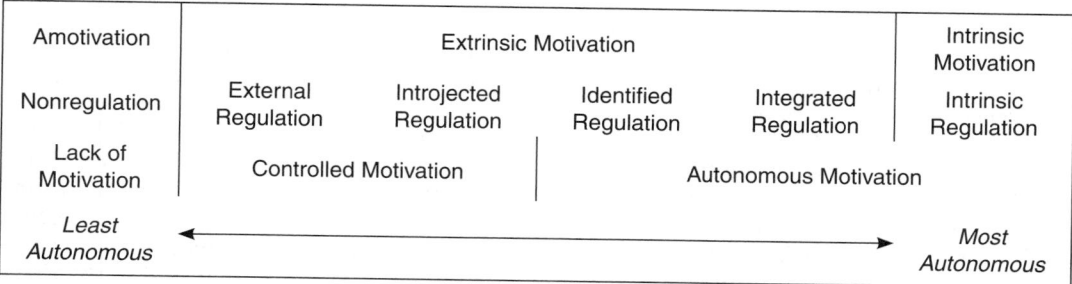

FIGURE 26.1. The types of motivation and regulation within self-determination theory as specified in organismic integration theory. The degree of relative autonomy for each type of motivation and regulation becomes greater within each row as it moves from left to right.

haviors, and mores that are ambient in their social environments and endorsed by others with whom they are (or wish to be) connected. Yet the theory further proposes that when the social environment allows satisfaction of the basic psychological needs, people will be most inclined to internalize and integrate aspects of the social world, including extrinsic motivations, but when the social environment thwarts need satisfaction, people will be less effective in their internalizations. Stated differently, when the social context is such that people can build their competencies, connect with others, and act in ways that are self-endorsed, they will be most inclined to integrate into the self the structures that are transmitted by the social world. However, when it is relatively controlling, people will be more resistant to taking in and integrating these structures. Moreover, OIT suggests that people are most inclined to internalize norms, values, and practices they can comprehend and competently perform. In short, internalization is impacted by all three basic needs.

Substantial research has supported the proposition that people internalize values and regulations more fully when the socializing context is more supportive of autonomy. For example, Deci, Eghrari, Patrick, and Leone (1994) did a laboratory experiment in which they found that three facilitating factors—(1) providing a rationale for a requested behavior, (2) acknowledging people's feeling about the behavior (e.g., that they might find it boring), and (3) highlighting choice rather than control—all contributed to making the context supportive of needs and thus to facili-

tating internalization. When the facilitating factors were present, greater internalization occurred. In contrast, when these facilitating factors were not present (e.g., when the context was controlling), the little internalization that did occur resulted in introjected regulation rather than integrated regulation. Other studies have also shown that internalization is most effective in autonomy-supportive interpersonal contexts. For example, Williams and Deci (1996) found that medical students internalized course values more fully when the learning context was more supportive of autonomy, and Grolnick and Ryan (1989) showed that parents who were rated by interviewers as more autonomy supportive had children who had more fully internalized the value of learning and were more self-regulated in their motivation for schoolwork.

Autonomous and Controlled Motivation

Research on the internalization of extrinsic motivation is important for many reasons, most notably because many activities that are central to our lives are not particularly interesting and thus not intrinsically motivating, but are done for instrumental or extrinsic reasons. Many behaviors entailed in work, school, sport, or the arts, for example, are not inherently interesting, even if they have a clear function or purpose. Yet it is possible to be autonomous in carrying out such extrinsically motivated activities. Accordingly, this research shifted primary attention from the distinction between intrinsic and extrinsic motivation, which was the basis for the development of CET, to the distinction between autonomous and controlled motivation.

Stated differently, SDT emphasizes the difference between autonomous motivation (including identified/integrated extrinsic motivation and intrinsic motivation) and controlled motivation (including extrinsic motivation that is regulated externally or by introjects), and much of the application of the theory focuses on promoting change from controlled forms of regulation to more autonomous forms of regulation.

Consequences and Correlates of Autonomous Motivation

Work that informed the development of CET and OIT has been important, in part, because research has made clear that there are strong positive relations between autonomous motivation and both effective performance and psychological health and well-being. Thus, by understanding how to maintain and enhance autonomous motivation, we are in a position to facilitate more adaptive behaviors and experiences. While enhancing autonomous motivation is a matter that can be argued to be of some importance in its own right, its value derives largely from the positive correlates and consequences associated with autonomous (versus controlled) motivation. Accordingly, a great deal of research, both laboratory experiments and field research, has examined this issue. The general hypothesis guiding the research states that both autonomous motivation in individuals and autonomy support in the social context will promote more effective performance and better psychological health and well-being.

The literature attesting to the veracity of this hypothesis is very large (Ryan & Deci, 2000b), so we provide just a few examples. Using a method developed by Ryan and Connell (1989) to assess autonomous motivation as a domain-specific individual difference, Ryan, Rigby, and King (1993) found that individuals' autonomous motivation for engaging in religious behaviors was positively related to their psychological well-being; morbidly obese patients whose motivation was more autonomous lost more weight and maintained the loss better (Williams, Grow, Freedman, Ryan, & Deci, 1996); individuals who were more autonomous in their moti-

vation toward the environment engaged in more proenvironment behaviors than those who were more controlled (Green-Demers, Pelletier, & Menard, 1997); and people who were more autonomous in following politics enjoyed learning about politics more and were more likely to vote than people whose motivation was more controlled (Koestner, Losier, Vallerand, & Carducci, 1996). These are but a few of the varied studies that have related the autonomous motivation of children and adults to positive consequences in many of life's domains.

Other studies have related autonomy support in the social context to various performance and well-being outcomes. For example, experiments have examined this issue with respect to learning, in each case distinguishing between superficial learning (i.e., rote memorization) and deeper learning (i.e., conceptual understanding). In an experiment done with college students learning about neurophysiology, Benware and Deci (1984) found that when the context supported more active engagement with the learning activity, students evidenced better conceptual understanding and comparable rote memorization compared to when the context was more pressuring and controlling. Comparable results were found for an experimental manipulation with fifth-grade students, and in addition, assessment of the children's motivation indicated that when they were more autonomously motivated they maintained their learning better over time (Grolnick & Ryan, 1987).

Still other studies have found that when people experience an interpersonal climate as more supportive of autonomy, they display greater well-being. For example, adult outpatients who experienced their physician as more autonomy supportive adhered to their medication prescriptions better than those who found their physicians more controlling (Williams, Rodin, Ryan, Grolnick, & Deci, 1998); working adults who experienced their supervisors as more autonomy supportive experienced greater need satisfaction at work and, in turn, displayed more engagement and better psychological health (Baard, Deci, & Ryan, 2004); and high-school students from Russia and the United States who experienced their teachers and parents as more autonomy supportive were also more engaged in their schoolwork and showed better psychological adjustment (Chirkov & Ryan, 2001).

CAUSALITY ORIENTATIONS THEORY

The various types of autonomous and controlled motivation discussed within OIT are considered to be types of regulation that represent behavior- or domain-specific individual difference. However, they are viewed as being only moderately stable, because we believe that social-contextual conditions will influence the strength of the various types of regulation, leading to changes in these more specific motivational orientations. Indeed, for example, several studies have been done to document the enhancement of autonomous motivation (i.e., identified, integrated, and intrinsic regulation) by autonomy-supportive social contexts (e.g., Williams, Freedman, & Deci, 1998).

Within SDT we also recognize that it is sometimes useful to characterize people's general or global motivational orientations. COT was formulated as a third mini-theory to explicate individual differences in general motivational orientations (Deci & Ryan, 1985a). The theory specifies three orientations: the autonomy orientation, the controlled orientation, and the impersonal orientation. The *autonomy orientation* indexes the degree to which people tend to interpret the social context as autonomy supportive and informational; tend to be aware of their own inner needs, interests, and values and use them as guides for their behavior, all of which conduce toward autonomous self-regulation. The *controlled orientation* reflects the degree to which people look for cues and controls in the environment or in their own introjects and let those regulate and determine their behavior. Thus, this orientation concerns people's behavior being directed by demands, rewards, threats, and self-esteem contingencies. The *impersonal orientation* represents the degree to which people tend to feel as if they have no control over desired outcomes in their lives and thus experience a general sense of loss and amotivation.

Causality orientations are viewed as developmental outcomes in which the interaction of the active organism with a social environment—which, to varying degrees, supports autonomy, controls behavior, and/or conveys incompetence over multiple situations and extended periods of time—result in a specifiable level of each orientation. Thus, people come to view themselves in relation to their environments as somewhat autonomous, somewhat controlled, and somewhat impersonal, and the three orientations can be used to predict various outcomes (Vallerand, 1997).

Research (Deci & Ryan, 1985a) has found the autonomy orientation to be associated with greater ego development (Loevinger, 1985), self-actualization, and self-esteem, as well as the tendency to support autonomy in others. The autonomy orientation has also predicted successfully maintaining weight loss in a low-calorie diet program (Williams et al., 1996) and being engaged and well adjusted in one's job or volunteer work (Gagné & Deci, 2005). Studies have found the controlled orientation to be linked to proneness to conformity, public self-consciousness, and the Type A coronary-prone behavior pattern. Williams and colleagues (1996) found the controlled orientation to predict less maintenance of positive behavior change. Finally, our research found the impersonal orientation to be positively associated with tendencies toward depression, self-derogation, external locus of control, and social anxiety, and negatively related to self-actualization and self-esteem (Deci & Ryan, 1985a).

A number of researchers have elaborated on the implications of COT. For example, Koestner and colleagues (1996) related the causality orientations to more effective emotional regulation, and Koestner, Bernieri, and Zuckerman (1992) showed that more controlled versus autonomy-oriented persons exhibit less consistency among attitudes, traits, and behaviors. Hodgins and Knee (2002) reviewed evidence that autonomous versus controlled persons are less defensive and more open interpersonally, thus enhancing capacities for relatedness and personal growth (e.g., Knee, Lonsbary, Canevello, & Patrick, 2005). Neighbors and Knee (2003) have shown how causality orientations predict proneness to peer pressure and conformity. These represent just a few studies bespeaking the importance of these individual differences in how persons orient to the world and motivate their own actions and interactions.

BASIC PSYCHOLOGICAL NEEDS THEORY

As already discussed, central to SDT is the proposition that there are three fundamental and universal psychological needs: the needs for competence, autonomy, and relatedness. These needs are a linchpin for all four of the SDT mini-theories. They are central to CET because they provide an account of how social-contextual factors affect intrinsic motivation and its corresponding outcomes. They are important for OIT because they provide an account of internalization and how the social context affects internalization and integration of extrinsic motivation and how that relates to healthy development. They are relevant to COT because they explain the development of the different motivational orientations and why they relate differently to other psychological constructs, as well as effective performance and psychological well-being.

As this research has developed, we found it increasingly necessary to formulate a fourth mini-theory, labeled basic psychological needs theory (BPNT; Ryan & Deci, 2002), that makes explicit our assumptions concerning needs and their relations, not just to motivational processes, but to wellness and vitality more generally. This is especially important for developing testable hypotheses about the varied effects of goals and aspirations on life outcomes, and for our cross-cultural perspective on the universal underpinnings of human psychological dynamics. The basic tenets of BPNT include the following:

1. Psychological needs define the necessary cross-developmental and cross-cultural nutriments for wellness and optimal functioning.
2. Various motives, aspirations, and goals can be evaluated with respect to their potential for satisfying or thwarting basic needs, and thus their impact on wellness will follow from these relations.
3. Within- and between-person variations in wellness are a function of need satisfaction, with all three needs demonstrating independent and interactive contributions.

Several studies have directly measured satisfaction of the needs for autonomy, competence, and relatedness in various settings to examine its relations to motivation, performance, and well-being. As examples, need satisfaction predicted both performance evaluations and psychological adjustment of employees in a banking firm (Baard et al., 2004); satisfaction of the basic needs predicted security of attachment at the between-person level and also to parents and peers at the within-person level (La Guardia, Ryan, Couchman, & Deci, 2000); all three needs were predictive of more optimal relationship functioning (Patrick, Knee, Canevello, & Lonsbary, 2007); college students' reports of well-being varied from day to day as a function of the variations in need satisfaction (Reis, Sheldon, Gable, Roscoe, & Ryan, 2000); and satisfaction of the basic needs in the daily lives of elderly residents in an institution for the aged were positively related to well-being and perceived health (V. M. Kasser & Ryan, 1999).

Need Satisfaction and the Big Five Traits

Needs are postulated to reflect inherent dimensions of organismic functioning by specifying those nutriments associated with thriving. As such, need satisfaction is not an enduring aspect of the personality, because it meaningfully fluctuates with changing environmental supports and the person's capacity to find satisfaction within them. In short, need satisfaction is not a trait. Traits, by contrast, reflect more enduring characteristics that differentiate between people (see John, Naumann, & Soto, Chapter 4, this volume; McCrae & Costa, Chapter 5, this volume); they have predictive value across situations, time, and domains. Yet traits also fluctuate at a within-person level. That is, people can be more or less extraverted than one another, but it is also true that each person is more extraverted in some situations and less so in others. In fact, there is evidence of substantial within-person variation in traits, but there had not been a systematic account of that variation.

According to SDT the variation in traits is quite systematic. Specifically, SDT predicts that people will express traits closer to their ideal trait profiles when in contexts that support autonomy, competence, and relatedness. Thus, recently researchers found that, at a within-person level, when people were with social partners who were more autonomy supportive, they were both more satisfied and vital, and expressed Big Five traits closer to their ideals, which in the context of relationships meant that they were more extraverted, open, and agreeable and were less neurotic than their general or average trait dispositions (Lynch, La Guardia, & Ryan, 2007). These results were similar to those obtained in another study (Sheldon, Ryan, Rawsthorne, & Ilardi, 1997), which found a similar pattern for different life domains in which people could be more versus less authentic.

Need Satisfaction across Cultures

Numerous studies have also examined need satisfaction across cultures. Insofar as SDT maintains that the basic needs are universal, it has been important to empirically test the effects of need satisfaction in a wide variety of cultures with different societal values and mores. Although few have disputed the significance of either relatedness or competence needs across cultures, the most controversial issues have concerned the need for autonomy. In our view this is because, in a number of theories (e.g., Markus & Kitayama, 1991), the issue of autonomy is conflated with the issue of independence and individualism, whereas in the SDT view autonomy concerns the *self-endorsement and valuing if one's own practices*, and thus it can accompany dependence or independence, individualism or collectivism, traditionalisms or modernisms. However, when any of these practices or values are imposed or introjected, the theory suggests, ill-being results.

A growing body of evidence is supporting the critical role played by all three needs across cultures. For example, in samples of employees in Bulgarian companies operating primarily by central planning principles and employees of a U.S. company operating by capitalist principles, employees' basic need satisfaction predicted both engagement at work and psychological health and well-being (Deci et al., 2001). Chirkov and colleagues (2003) studied the internalization of values in Korea, Russia, Turkey, and the United States, assessing the degree to which people in these cultures experienced autonomy with respect to ambient cultural practices. Results indicated that feeling greater autonomy (or fuller internalization) was associated with

well-being in all cultures. Chirkov and colleagues (2005) also examined Canadian and Brazilian students and found that in these cultures, both cultural fit and well being were associated with need satisfactions, which were facilitated by autonomy-supportive contexts. Sheldon, Elliot, Kim, and Kasser (2001) examined what makes events satisfying in Korean and U.S. samples and found that all three basic needs had explanatory salience in both cultures. In sum, these and numerous other studies have provided strong evidence that basic psychological needs, including autonomy, are universally important for well-being across cultures.

Aspirations and Life Goals

One of the central findings of SDT has been that if a goal is pursued for autonomous reasons, it will be associated with psychological health and well-being. Other SDT-related work has investigated the *content* of goals, suggesting that some goal contents are more aligned with well-being because they promote satisfaction of the basic psychological needs and thus will be associated with both greater happiness and personal growth (Bauer et al., 2005; Ryan, Sheldon, Kasser, & Deci, 1996).

Kasser and Ryan (1996) assessed the importance people place on the life goals of wealth, fame, and image, which are closely associated with the American Dream, as well as the life goals of personal growth, relationships, and community. They referred to the former group of goals (i.e., wealth, fame, and image) as *extrinsic aspirations*, indicating that their attainment does not promote inherent need satisfaction but rather is a means to an end and may in fact represent an attempt by people to get external validation of their personal worth as a substitute for not experiencing basic need satisfaction. Another set of goals (i.e., growth, relationships, and community) was labeled *intrinsic aspirations*, conveying that these goals are more directly linked to satisfaction of the basic psychological needs for autonomy, competence, and relatedness. They found first that intrinsic and extrinsic goal types were distinguishable in factor analyses. They also found that the relative importance an individual placed on extrinsic aspirations was negatively related to a wide array of well-being indicators, whereas the relative importance of intrinsic aspirations was positively related to well-being. This same phenomenon was demonstrated in both Russian and U.S. samples (Ryan et al., 1999). Indeed, subsequent research has replicated this basic finding in adults, school-age children, businesspersons, and the residents of numerous other nations. In fact, Grouzet and colleagues (2005) showed the reliability of the intrinsic versus extrinsic goal distinction across 15 varied cultures.

Goal Contents and Motives

Just as the finding about the undermining of intrinsic motivation by extrinsic rewards (especially monetary rewards) was controversial when it first appeared in the early 1970s, the finding that extrinsic goal contents (especially wealth) are associated with ill-being has also been controversial. For example, Carver and Baird (1998) and Srivastava, Locke, and Bartol (2001) have suggested that it is not the goal contents but the motives behind them that are detrimental. Because extrinsic goal contents and controlled regulations are correlated, Carver and Baird argued that it is likely the controlled motivation rather than the extrinsic goal that is problematic for well-being. In response, we and our colleagues did a set of three studies to examine this issue (Sheldon, Ryan, Deci, & Kasser, 2004). We assessed both the goal contents (extrinsic vs. intrinsic) and motives (controlled vs. autonomous) and found, as expected, that extrinsic aspirations did correlate significantly with controlled regulation of the goal pursuits. However, we entered both the goal contents and motives into simultaneous analyses and found that each variable contributed significant independent variance. In other words, the relative importance of extrinsic goals was negatively related to psychological ill-being even after the variance in ill-being explained by controlled regulation had been removed.

Goal Attainment

The above-mentioned studies of goal contents all assessed the importance people place on goals. The next issue considered in this field of research was the relation of goal attainment to well-being. The important question is, does the attainment of all valued goals yield positive well-being outcomes, or

might the content of the goals moderate the relation of the goal attainment to well-being? Goals theorists such as Locke and Latham (1990) have suggested that attainment of all valued goals is beneficial for people. SDT maintains, however, that goal attainments are associated with wellness as a function of their capacity to yield basic psychological need satisfactions. Examining this issue in the United States and Russia, it was found that the degree to which people attained extrinsic aspirations was not related to their well-being, after controlling for attainment of intrinsic aspirations; whereas their attainment of intrinsic aspirations was uniquely related to well-being after controlling for attainment of extrinsic aspirations (T. Kasser & Ryan, 2001; Ryan et al., 1999). More recently, we did a longitudinal study in which we considered change in well-being as a function of change in intrinsic and extrinsic goal attainment (Niemiec, Ryan, et al., 2007). We found that attainment of intrinsic goals led to increases in well-being and decreases in ill-being; however, attainment of extrinsic goals did not affect well-being and added to people's ill-being. Furthermore, the positive effect of intrinsic aspirations on well-being was mediated by satisfaction of the three basic psychological needs. In short, strong relative pursuit of extrinsic aspirations is associated with poorer psychological well-being, and attainment of extrinsic aspirations does not help well-being—in fact, it may contribute to people's ill-being. In contrast, both the pursuit and attainment of intrinsic goals is strongly related to psychological health.

Goal Framing

In the studies of goals reviewed so far, intrinsic and extrinsic goals were assessed as individual differences, and the relative strength of people's intrinsic versus extrinsic goals was used to predict outcomes. In other research, however, Vansteenkiste and his colleagues have conducted experiments in which the concepts of intrinsic and extrinsic goals were used to frame people's engagement with a task. In these experiments, participants were told that doing a particular activity would be instrumental to either an intrinsic or extrinsic goal, and then the behavior and experience of the two groups of participants were examined. Furthermore, many of the studies by

Vansteenkiste and colleagues on goal framing also investigated the effects of presenting the goals with an autonomy-supportive versus controlling communication style. For example, in one set of studies, learning situations were used in which (1) education students learned about recycling and reusing materials either to help save the environment (intrinsic goal) or to save money (extrinsic goal); (2) business students learned about approaches to communicating either for personal development (intrinsic) or to be more successful at work (extrinsic); and (3) younger students learned a physical activity either to be healthier (intrinsic) or to look better (extrinsic) (Vansteenkiste, Simons, Lens, Sheldon, & Deci, 2004). These conditions were crossed with communication style, and the outcomes were indicators of learning, performance, and persistence. All three studies yielded similar results: Persons given intrinsic goal framing subsequently learned the material more deeply, took additional opportunities to find out about the topics, and performed better when tested on what they had learned, compared with those given extrinsic goal framing. Furthermore, those who were given a goal induction with an autonomy-supportive style learned and performed better than those who were given it with a controlling style, as predicted on the basis of OIT. Finally, interactions revealed that the condition in which the intrinsic goal framing was given in an autonomy-supportive way not only led to the most positive outcomes, but these outcomes were more positive than would be expected from the two main effects.

In sum, studies of intrinsic versus extrinsic goals, whether done with individual differences in the importance of the goals or with the framing of tasks in terms of intrinsic versus extrinsic goals, indicate that holding intrinsic goals is associated with more positive learning, performance, and well-being outcomes than is the case for holding extrinsic goals.

SELECTED RECENT RESEARCH IN SDT

As a broad theory of motivation and psychological development, SDT has many applications and possible extensions. Recently SDT research has been very active in a number

of new areas that cannot be adequately reviewed herein. For example, Vallerand and his colleagues have differentiated two forms of passion, namely *harmonious passion* and *obsessive passion*. The former is characterized by greater internalization and integration of a person's passion into identity, whereas the latter is characterized by more controlled motives. Using this distinction Vallerand and colleagues (e.g., 2003) have shown important differences in both persistence and wellness as people pursue passions. Sheldon and his colleagues (e.g., Sheldon, Elliot, et al., 2004) have focused on the *self-concordance* of personal goals and strivings (Emmons, 1986), defined in terms of both more autonomous versus controlled motivation and greater linkages with basic needs, showing in both U.S. and international samples that greater self-concordance enhances both wellness and performance. SDT research has also focused on distinguishing hedonic from eudaimonic processes in well-being, examining both the antecedents and consequences of each (Ryan & Deci, 2001; Ryan et al., 2008). These strains of research on people's passions, the self-concordance of personal goals and strivings, and the pathways to wellness illustrate the ways in which the SDT framework is generative of new hypotheses and findings of applied significance.

In what follows we highlight, again for illustrative purposes, three of the other areas of recent interest: the role of awareness and mindfulness in behavior regulation, the importance of autonomy support in fostering enduring intimate relationships; and a theory of psychological energy or vitality.

Awareness and Mindfulness

Considerable research has now confirmed that social contexts have a substantial effect on the degree to which people are autonomously motivated, the degree to which they place greatest importance on intrinsic life goals, and, in turn, the degree to which they display greater human thriving. But self-determination is by no means just a function of social contexts. It is a personal characteristic, and people have the possibility of displaying more self-determination regardless of the social climate. That is, even in situations that are quite pressuring and demanding, people can still act with a relatively high level of autonomy. Furthermore, people who are quite strongly control oriented can take responsibility for becoming more autonomy oriented. The key to such a change is awareness.

Awareness, according to Perls (1973), is relaxed attention. Simply to attend to something is not enough for awareness; the attention must be interested, open-minded, and relaxed. Introjects, for example, can force one to attend to some internal or external stimulus, but that is not awareness because it is forced and has an underlying agenda. Awareness is about wondering what will emerge when you attend to something and take interest in whatever it is. Indeed, awareness is about letting true meanings emerge rather than imposing meanings on stimuli. By being more aware of their own internal conditions—of their needs, feelings, interests, values, desires, and introjects—people can make their own choices even when they are surrounded by pressures and criticisms, and they can move toward a regulation that is guided by choices more of the time. In short, people can, through awareness, turn controls into information to be used in making choices that are meaningful and right for them.

Although the relation of awareness to self-determination has long been a topic with SDT (Deci & Ryan, 1980, 1985b), SDT researchers have recently begun to examine the awareness issue using the concept of *mindfulness* (Brown & Ryan, 2003), which has been studied both as an experience at a particular time (i.e., a state) and as a more enduring tendency (i.e., an individual difference or trait). Acting in a self-regulating way is facilitated when one is openly in touch with what is actually occurring in the moment, as well as with one's personal interests and values; this is particularly so in situations that are not supportive of the person's need satisfaction. In the Brown and Ryan research both the disposition and state of being aware of and receptive to one's inner psychological experiences and values were found to be associated with more autonomous motivation, more positive affect, and greater well-being. Mindfulness has also been facilitated with brief inductions and with longer-term programs intended to bring people to a state of greater internal quiet and centeredness, and it has resulted in various positive outcomes

(Brown, Ryan, & Creswell, 2007). For example, using a brief induction, Broderick (2005) found that those participants in the mindfulness condition were more able to cope effectively with dysphoric moods. Using longer programs to induce mindfulness, Kabat-Zinn, Lipworth, and Burney (1985) found that it reduced psychological symptoms in pain patients, and Brown and Ryan (2003) found that mindfulness decreased fatigue, stress, and disturbed mood in cancer patients.

Our central premise is that, through mindfulness, people can take responsibility for becoming more autonomous, thus gradually ameliorating the negative effects that have resulted from their being controlled and amotivated in various past and present circumstances. For instance, Legault, Green-Demers, Grant, and Chung (2007) showed that persons with more autonomous motivation to regulate prejudice demonstrated both lower explicit and implicit prejudice. Niemiec, Brown, and Ryan (2007) recently showed in multiple experiments that people high in mindfulness did not show the defensive reactions involving prejudice and outgroup derogation that typically follow from the mortality salience inductions used within terror management theory (Greenberg, Solomon, & Pyszczynski, 1997). Mindfulness allows people to explore their inner psychic landscape and to gain insight into why, for example, they may be passive, controlled, apathetic, or alienated. With this increased insight they will be in a position to develop greater sensitivity to inner needs and outer realities, and the autonomy to act in ways that yield greater ongoing need satisfaction.

At the same time it is important to note that explicit awareness is not always a necessary condition for acting autonomously. Many behaviors in which we engage are habitual and automatic, and some are unconsciously primed (see Kilstrom, Chapter 23, this volume; Schultheiss, Chapter 24, this volume). In our view (see Deci & Ryan, 1980; Ryan & Deci, 2006), however, implicit processes can instigate either autonomous or controlled activities and goals. Often habitual and automatic behaviors serve purposes that would, when reflected upon, be fully self-endorsed (e.g., automatically shifting one's car into a higher gear as RPMs rise), whereas others are associated with behaviors that are not self-congruent (e.g., impulsive eating or aggression). In other words, the issue of implicit versus explicit processing is not isomorphic with that of autonomy versus control. Nonetheless having the capacity to reflectively access motives and goals, and being able to accept or reject potential actions on the basis of integrated interests and values are critical capacities for autonomous functioning.

Close Relationships

SDT maintains that healthy and satisfying close personal relationships require satisfaction of the basic psychological needs for autonomy and competence as well as for relatedness. Several recent SDT studies have tested this reasoning. For example, La Guardia and colleagues (2000) assessed students' security of attachment with their mothers, fathers, romantic partners, and best friends, in addition to their level of satisfaction of the needs for autonomy, competence, and relatedness within each of those relationships. The researchers reported that need satisfaction with a particular relational partner accounted for significant variance in attachment security with that partner. That is, there was substantial within-person variability in security of attachment with different partners, and basic need satisfaction within relationships explained that variability. Subsequent analyses considered the three needs separately, and it turned out that satisfaction of each of the separate needs within a relationship was a significant predictor of security of attachment in that relationship. In more recent research multiple relationships were examined within persons in diverse cultural samples drawn from China, Russia, and the United States (Lynch et al., 2007). Here, too, it was found that perceived autonomy accounted for within-person variations in relationship-specific satisfaction and vitality, an effect that was not moderated by cultural membership of the individual's style of self-construal.

Another example of the SDT studies of relationships examined mutuality of autonomy support as a predictor of need satisfaction, relationship quality, and well-being among close friends (Deci et al., 2006). Using a method developed by Griffin and Gonzales (1995) for analyzing dyad data, the researchers found that there tended to be mutuality

in the level of autonomy support provided by each partner in close friendships and that receiving autonomy support from one's close friend was associated with greater need satisfaction, relationship quality, and well-being. Further analyses indicated that giving support for autonomy to a close friend also was positively related to basic need satisfaction, relationship quality, and well-being for the giver, after controlling for the autonomy support received.

In short, both giving and receiving autonomy support in a close friendship are related to relationship quality and well-being. Interestingly, similar findings were reported by Knee and colleagues (2005) in the context of heterosexual couples, and Patrick and colleagues (2007) showed that need satisfaction was not only related to individual well-being but also relational wellness. Ryan and colleagues (2005) also showed that one's willingness to depend on another person is a function of perceived need supports. As the dynamics of relationships are studied in more detail, it is becoming ever clearer that the quality and depth of connections between people is a function of the degree to which satisfactions of all three basic needs is afforded in their relationship.

Psychological Energy and Self-Regulation: Vitality and Its Sources

The idea that the regulation of behavior has costs in terms of energy dates back at least to Breuer and Freud. The empirical study of psychological energy has, however, become more active over the last decade. SDT researchers have specifically focused on *energy dynamics* and how motives determine either vitalization or depletion. For example, Ryan and Frederick (1997) showed that activities and lifestyles associated with basic need satisfaction foster greater vitality and feelings of aliveness, whereas factors associated with thwarted autonomy, competence, and relatedness deplete energy. Nix, Ryan, Manly, and Deci (1999) also demonstrated that the same activity was less draining when it was either self- or autonomously directed, compared to being externally directed or controlled. More recently, Moller, Ryan, and colleagues (2006) showed that autonomous self-regulation based in true choice is not subject to the ego-depletion effect (e.g., Baumeister, 2002).

Thus, SDT offers some important caveats to Baumeister's (2002) ego-depletion model.

More specifically, the ego-depletion model suggests that the exercise of self-regulation or volition is generally depleting. SDT argues, however, that it is specifically controlling forms of self-regulation that deplete. In contrast, autonomy, or true volition, in which the self endorses and organizes the action, does not lead to depletion. Moreover, whereas ego-depletion models do not specify a psychological source of energy or revitalization, SDT specifically suggests that people gain regulatory energy through need fulfillment. Thus, events in which there are positive experiences of autonomy, competence, or relatedness strengthen the self and the subjective energy on which it draws.

APPLYING SDT IN LIFE'S DOMAINS

An enormous amount of research has examined basic SDT principles in a variety of real-world settings. For example, much work has been done in the realm of education, showing that when teachers are more autonomy supportive, students become more autonomously motivated, show better adjustment and well-being, and tend to learn better, especially at the conceptual level (Reeve, Deci, & Ryan, 2004). These studies have spanned from the elementary school level (e.g., Deci, Schwartz, et al., 1981; Ryan & Grolnick, 1986) to college level chemistry courses (Black & Deci, 2000). Studies of parents have similarly shown how controlling versus autonomy-supportive parenting techniques undermine interest, persistence, performance, and adjustment in the academic domain (see Grolnick, 2003; Grolnick & Ryan, 1989).

In the domain of work organizations, Deci, Connell, and Ryan (1989) found that the autonomy supportiveness of first-line managers in a Fortune 500 company predicted the levels of their employees' trust, felt security, and satisfaction with job characteristics. Furthermore, an intervention intended to teach managers to be more autonomy supportive did result in increased support of autonomy by managers, relative to a control group that did not get the intervention, and even more importantly the enhanced autonomy support of managers re-

sulted in increased trust and satisfaction in their employees. Other studies (e.g., Baard et al., 2004) have indicated that managers' autonomy support predicted the degree of need satisfaction experienced by their employees, even when controlling for the employees' autonomous causality orientation. In turn, the degree of need satisfaction predicted the employees' performance evaluations, and it negatively predicted their anxiety and somatic symptoms. In short, autonomy support in the workplace has been found to enhance autonomous motivation, need satisfaction, performance, and well-being in various studies in the United States and abroad (Gagné & Deci, 2005).

Another area where SDT has been applied to guide many studies, including randomized clinical trials, is medical encounters between practitioners and patients. Autonomy support provided by practitioners has been found to predict increases in perceived competence and autonomous motivation for engaging in a treatment regimen, and these in turn have predicted such outcomes as smoking cessation, glycemic control, lower LDL cholesterol, and adherence to medication (see Williams, Deci, & Ryan, 1998, for a review). Furthermore, an intensive autonomy-supportive intervention was developed for smoking cessation. Relative to usual care in the community, participants in the intervention group displayed increases in autonomous motivation, perceived competence, adherence to medications intended to facilitate cessation, as well as actual cessation at the end of 6 months (Williams, McGregor, Sharp, Levesque, et al., 2006). A follow-up study indicated that there was still significantly greater abstinence in the intervention group than the control group 18 months after the beginning of treatment (Williams, McGregor, Sharp, Kouides, et al., 2006).

The importance of autonomy support and basic need satisfaction have also been demonstrated in domains as diverse as sport (Gagné, Ryan, & Bargmann, 2003), politics (Koestner et al., 1996), aging (V. M. Kasser & Ryan, 1999), pro-environmental behavior (Green-Demers et al., 1997), video games (Ryan, Rigby, & Przybylski, 2006), and psychotherapy (Markland, Ryan, Tobin, & Rollnick, 2005), among others. A comprehensive review of such empirically grounded, real-world demonstrations and applications of SDT-derived principles is well beyond the scope of this review. Yet, the growing body of real-world findings based on SDT shows again how consideration of the psychological factors that proximally determine behavior provides the most practical approaches for changing social practices and improving human outcomes.

CONCLUSION

SDT has at its core the concept of basic, universal psychological needs for competence, autonomy, and relatedness. Unlike most other theories that use the concept of psychological needs to assess individual differences in motive strength, SDT proposes that these basic needs represent the necessary nutriments for healthy, full functioning. Thus, SDT specifies that these needs must be satisfied for individuals to experience optimal psychological development, performance, and well-being within any domain and across cultural contexts. As it has developed, SDT has used the concept of basic psychological needs to integrate a wide range of phenomena that have been encompassed by SDT's four mini-theories; namely, cognitive evaluation theory, organismic integration theory, causality orientations theory, and basic psychological needs theory. Moreover, the concept of basic psychological needs has been useful in extending SDT to a variety of new research areas, including subjective energy, mindfulness, and close relationships. Finally, the concept of needs has proven to be practically useful, as shown by SDT's applications in far-ranging domains: education, parenting, work, medicine, sport and exercise, politics, aging, and psychotherapy. SDT, in short, has aimed at providing a fuller understanding of what it is that people truly need for optimal living, and all that distracts from, or undermines, those needs being fulfilled.

Despite the growth of SDT as a framework of study, as an empirically based open theory SDT has much room for continued refinement and expansion of its propositions, as well as for improvements in the specification and implementation of theory-based interventions aimed at behavioral, organizational, and social change. As a psychologically focused theory, SDT will also need to continue to interface with both more molecular levels of analysis in the neurosciences (e.g., Ryan, Deci, Grolnick, & La Guardia, 2006) and more global analyses supplied by economic, cultural, and historical perspectives (Vansteenkiste et al., in press). Yet the primary focus of SDT will remain on human psychology, where all of these levels of analysis intersect in the determination of human experience, which not only gives rise to our behavior but also represents the substance of our living existence. SDT thus remains unabashedly psychological in its approach because, as we see it, it is at that level of analysis that hypotheses concerning the questions of central concern to humans can most readily be advanced. More importantly, a psychological level of analysis is the most pertinent to making a practical, real-world difference in how we behave and to shaping the values we internalize and embrace.

REFERENCES

Amabile, T. M., DeJong, W., & Lepper, M. (1976). Effects of externally imposed deadlines on subsequent intrinsic motivation. *Journal of Personality and Social Psychology, 34,* 92–98.

Atkinson, J. W. (1964). *An introduction to motivation.* Princeton, NJ: Van Nostrand.

Baard, P. P., Deci, E. L., & Ryan, R. M. (2004). Intrinsic need satisfaction: A motivational basis of performance and well-being in two work settings. *Journal of Applied Social Psychology, 34,* 2045–2068.

Bauer, J. J., McAdams, D. P., & Sakaeda, A. (2005). Interpreting the good life: How mature, happy people frame their autobiographical memories. *Journal of Personality and Social Psychology, 88,* 203–217.

Baumeister, R. F. (2002). Ego depletion and self-control failure: An energy model of the self's executive function. *Self and Identity, 1,* 129–136.

Benware, C., & Deci, E. L. (1984). Quality of learning with an active versus passive motivational set. *American Educational Research Journal, 21,* 755–765.

Black, A. E., & Deci, E. L. (2000). The effects of student self-regulation and instructor autonomy support on learning in a college-level natural science course: A self-determination theory perspective. *Science Education, 84,* 740–756.

Braybrooke, D. (1987). *Meeting needs.* Princeton, NJ: Princeton University Press.

Breckler, S. J. (2006). Science directions: The newest age of reductionism. *Monitor on Psychology, 37,* 23.

Broderick, P. C. (2005). Mindfulness and coping with dyscphoric mood: Contrasts with rumination and distraction. *Cognitive Therapy and Research, 29*(5), 501–510.

Brown, K. W., & Ryan, R. M. (2003). The benefits of being present: Mindfulness and its role in psychological well-being. *Journal of Personality and Social Psychology, 84,* 822–848.

Brown, K. W., Ryan, R. M., & Creswell, J. D. (2007). Mindfulness: Theoretical foundations and evidence for its salutary effects. *Psychological Inquiry, 18,* 177–182.

Calder, B. J., & Staw, B. M. (1975). The interaction of intrinsic and extrinsic motivation: Some methodological notes. *Journal of Personality and Social Psychology, 31,* 76–80.

Carver, C. S., & Baird, E. (1998). The American dream revisited: Is it what you want or why you want it that matters? *Psychological Science, 9,* 289–292.

Chirkov, V. I., & Ryan, R. M. (2001). Parent and teacher autonomy-support in Russian and U.S. adolescents: Common effects on well-being and academic motivation. *Journal of Cross-Cultural Psychology, 32,* 618–635.

Chirkov, V. I., Ryan, R. M., Kim, Y., & Kaplan, U. (2003). Differentiating autonomy from individualism and independence: A self-determination theory perspective on internalization of cultural orientations and well-being. *Journal of Personality and Social Psychology, 84,* 97–110.

Chirkov, V. I., Ryan, R. M., & Willness, C. (2005). Cultural context and psychological needs in Canada and Brazil: Testing a self-determination approach to the internalization of cultural practices, identity, and well-being. *Journal of Cross-Cultural Psychology, 36,* 423–443.

deCharms, R. (1968). *Personal causation: The internal affective determinants of behavior.* New York: Academic Press.

Deci, E. L. (1971). Effects of externally mediated rewards on intrinsic motivation. *Journal of Personality and Social Psychology, 18,* 105–115.

Deci, E. L. (1975). *Intrinsic motivation.* New York: Plenum Press.

Deci, E. L., Betley, G., Kahle, J., Abrams, L., & Porac, J. (1981). When trying to win: Competition and intrinsic motivation. *Personality and Social Psychology Bulletin, 7,* 79–83.

Deci, E. L., & Cascio, W. F. (1972, April). *Changes in intrinsic motivation as a function of negative feedback and threats.* Paper presented at the meeting of the Eastern Psychological Association, Boston.

Deci, E. L., Connell, J. P., & Ryan, R. M. (1989). Self-determination in a work organization. *Journal of Applied Psychology, 74,* 580–590.

Deci, E. L., Eghrari, H., Patrick, B. C., & Leone, D. R. (1994). Facilitating internalization: The self-determination theory perspective. *Journal of Personality, 62,* 119–142.

Deci, E. L., Koestner, R., & Ryan, R. M. (1999). A meta-analytic review of experiments examining the effects of extrinsic rewards on intrinsic motivation. *Psychological Bulletin, 125,* 627–668.

Deci, E. L., La Guardia, J. G., Moller, A. C., Scheiner, M. J., & Ryan, R. M. (2006). On the benefits of giving as well as receiving autonomy support: Mutuality in close friendships. *Personality and Social Psychology Bulletin, 32,* 313–327.

Deci, E. L., & Ryan, R. M. (1980). The empirical exploration of intrinsic motivational processes. In L. Berkowitz (Ed.), *Advances in experimental social psychology* (Vol. 13, pp. 39–80). New York: Academic Press.

Deci, E. L., & Ryan, R. M. (1985a). The General Causality Orientations Scale: Self-determination in personality. *Journal of Research in Personality, 19,* 109–134.

Deci, E. L., & Ryan, R. M. (1985b). *Intrinsic motivation and self-determination in human behavior.* New York: Plenum Press.

Deci, E. L., & Ryan, R. M. (1991). A motivational approach to self: Integration in personality. In R. Dienstbier (Ed.), *Nebraska Symposium on Motivation: Vol. 38. Perspectives on motivation* (pp. 237–288). Lincoln: University of Nebraska Press.

Deci, E. L., & Ryan, R. M. (2000). The "what" and "why" of goal pursuits: Human needs and the self-determination of behavior. *Psychological Inquiry, 11,* 227–268.

Deci, E. L., Ryan, R. M., Gagné, M., Leone, D. R., Usunov, J., & Kornazheva, B. P. (2001). Need satisfaction, motivation, and well-being in the work organizations of a former Eastern Bloc country. *Personality and Social Psychology Bulletin, 27,* 930–942.

Deci, E. L., Schwartz, A. J., Sheinman, L., & Ryan, R. M. (1981). An instrument to assess adults' orientations toward control versus autonomy with children: Reflections on intrinsic motivation and perceived competence. *Journal of Educational Psychology, 73,* 642–650.

Eisenberger, R., Pierce, W. D., & Cameron, J. (1999). Effects of reward on intrinsic motivation—negative, neutral, and positive: Comment on Deci, Koestner, and Ryan. *Psychological Bulletin, 125,* 677–691.

Emmons, R. A. (1986). Personal strivings: An approach to personality and subjective well-being. *Journal of Personality and Social Psychology, 51,* 1058–1068.

Fisher, C. D. (1978). The effects of personal control, competence, and extrinsic reward systems on intrinsic motivation. *Organizational Behavior and Human Performance, 21,* 273–288.

Freud, S. (1962). *The ego and the id.* New York: Norton. (Original work published 1923)

Gagné, M., & Deci, E. L. (2005). Self-determination theory and work motivation. *Journal of Organizational Behavior, 26,* 331–362.

Gagné, M., Ryan, R. M., & Bargmann, K. (2003). The effects of parent and coach autonomy support on need satisfaction and well-being of gymnasts. *Journal of Applied Sport Psychology, 15,* 372–390.

Goldstein, K. (1939). *The organism.* New York: American Book.

Green-Demers, I., Pelletier, L. G., & Menard, S. (1997). The impact of behavioral difficulty on the saliency of the association between self-determined motivation and environmental behaviors. *Canadian Journal of Behavioural Science, 29,* 157–166.

Greenberg, J., Solomon, S., & Pyszczynski, T. (1997). Terror management theory of self-esteem and social behavior: Empirical assessments and conceptual refinements. In M. P. Zanna (Ed.), *Advances in experimental social psychology* (Vol. 29, pp. 61–139). San Diego, CA: Academic Press.

Griffin, D., & Gonzales, R. (1995). Correlational analysis of dyad-level data in the exchangeable case. *Psychological Bulletin, 118,* 430–439.

Grolnick, W. S. (2003). *The psychology of parental control: How well-meant parenting backfires.* Hillsdale, NJ: Erlbaum.

Grolnick, W. S., & Ryan, R. M. (1987). Autonomy in children's learning: An experimental and individual difference investigation. *Journal of Personality and Social Psychology, 52,* 890–898.

Grolnick, W. S., & Ryan, R. M. (1989). Parent styles associated with children's self-regulation and competence in school. *Journal of Educational Psychology, 81,* 143–154.

Grouzet, F. M., Kasser, T., Ahuvia, A., Dols, J. M., Kim, Y. Lau, S., et al. (2005). The structure of goals across 15 cultures. *Journal of Personality and Social Psychology, 89,* 800–816.

Heider, F. (1958). *The psychology of interpersonal relations.* New York: Wiley.

Hodgins, H. S., & Knee, C. R. (2002). The integrating self and conscious experience. In E. L. Deci & R. M. Ryan (Eds.), *Handbook of self-determination research* (pp. 87–100). Rochester, NY: University of Rochester Press.

Hull, C. L. (1943). *Principles of behavior: An introduction to behavior theory.* New York: Appleton-Century-Crofts.

Inghilleri, P. (1999). *From subjective experience to cultural change.* New York: Cambridge University Press.

Iyengar, S. S., & DeVoe, S. E. (2003). Rethinking the value of choice: Considering cultural mediators of intrinsic motivation. In V. Murphy-Berman & J. J. Berman (Eds.), *Nebraska Symposium on Motivation: Cross-cultural differences in perspectives on self* (Vol. 49, pp. 129–174). Lincoln: University of Nebraska Press.

Kabat-Zinn, J., Lipworth, L., & Burney, R. (1985). The clinical use of mindfulness meditation for the self-regulation of chronic pain. *Journal of Behavioral Medicine, 8,* 162–190.

Kasser, T., & Ryan, R. M. (1996). Further examining the American dream: Differential correlates of intrinsic and extrinsic goals. *Personality and Social Psychology Bulletin, 22,* 80–87.

Kasser, T., & Ryan, R. M. (2001). Be careful what you wish for: Optimal functioning and the relative attainment of intrinsic and extrinsic goals. In P. Schmuck & K. M. Sheldon (Eds.), *Life goals and well-being: Towards a positive psychology of human striving* (pp. 115–129). Goettingen, Germany: Hogrefe & Huber.

Kasser, T., Ryan, R. M., Zax, M., & Sameroff, A. J. (1995). The relations of maternal and social environments to late adolescents' materialistic and prosocial values. *Developmental Psychology, 31,* 907–914.

Kasser, V. M., & Ryan, R. M. (1999). The relation of psychological needs for autonomy and relatedness to vitality, well-being, and mortality in a nursing home. *Journal of Applied Social Psychology, 29,* 935–954.

Knee, C. R., Lonsbary, C., Canevello, A., & Patrick, H. (2005). Self-determination and conflict in romantic relationships. *Journal of Personality and Social Psychology, 89*(6), 997–1009.

Koestner, R., Bernieri, F., & Zuckerman, M. (1992). Self-determination and consistency between attitudes, traits, and behaviors. *Personality and Social Psychology Bulletin, 18,* 52–59.

Koestner, R., Losier, G. F., Vallerand, R. J., & Carducci, D. (1996). Identified and introjected forms of political internalization: Extending self-determination theory. *Journal of Personality and Social Psychology, 70,* 1025–1036.

Koestner, R., & McClelland, D. (1990). Perspectives on competence motivation. In L. Pervin (Ed.), *Handbook of personality: Theory and research* (pp. 527–548). New York: Guilford Press.

Koestner, R., Ryan, R. M., Bernieri, F., & Holt, K. (1984). Setting limits on children's behavior: The differential effects of controlling versus informational styles on intrinsic motivation and creativity. *Journal of Personality, 52,* 233–248.

La Guardia, J. G., Ryan, R. M., Couchman, C. E., & Deci, E. L. (2000). Within-person variation in security of attachment: A self-determination theory perspective on attachment, need fulfillment, and well-being. *Journal of Personality and Social Psychology, 79,* 367–384.

Legault, L., Green-Demers, I., Grant, P., & Chung, J. (2007). On the self-regulation of implicit and explicit prejudice: A self-determination theory perspective. *Personality and Social Psychology Bulletin, 33,* 732–749.

Lepper, M. R., & Greene, D. (1975). Turning play into work: Effects of adult surveillance and extrinsic rewards on children's intrinsic motivation. *Journal of Personality and Social Psychology, 31,* 479–486.

Locke, E. A., & Latham, G. P. (1990). *A theory of goal setting and task performance.* Englewood Cliffs, NJ: Prentice-Hall.

Loevinger, J. (1985). Revision of the sentence completion test for ego development. *Journal of Personality and Social Psychology, 48,* 420–427.

Lynch, M. F., La Guardia, J. G., & Ryan, R. M. (2007). *On being yourself: Ideal, actual, and relationship-specific trait self-concept and the support of autonomy.* Manuscript submitted for publication.

Markland, D., Ryan, R. M., Tobin, V. J., & Rollnick, S. (2005). Motivational interviewing and self-determination theory. *Journal of Social and Clinical Psychology, 24,* 811–831.

Markus, H. R., & Kitayama, S. (1991). Culture and the self: Implications for cognition, emotion, and motivation. *Psychological Review, 92,* 224–253.

McAdams, D. P. (1989). *Intimacy: The need to be close.* New York: Doubleday.

McClelland, D. C. (1985). *Human motivation.* Glenview, IL: Scott, Foresman.

Moller, A. C., Deci, E. L., & Ryan, R. M. (2006). Choice and ego-depletion: The moderating role of autonomy. *Personality and Social Psychology Bulletin, 32,* 1024–1036.

Mossholder, K. W. (1980). Effects of externally mediated goal setting on intrinsic motivation: A laboratory experiment. *Journal of Applied Psychology, 65,* 202–210.

Murray, H. A. (1938). *Explorations in personality.* New York: Oxford University Press.

Neighbors, C., & Knee, C. R. (2003). Self-determination and the impact of social comparison information. *Journal of Research in Personality, 37*(6), 529–546.

Niemiec, C. P., Brown, K. W., & Ryan, R. M. (2007). *Being present when facing death: The role of mindfulness in terror management processes.* Manuscript submitted for publication.

Niemiec, C. P., Ryan, R. M., & Deci, E. L. (2007). The Path Taken: Consequences of attaining intrinsic and extrinsic aspirations in post-college life. Manuscript submitted for publication.

Nix, G., Ryan, R. M., Manly, J. B., & Deci, E. L. (1999). Revitalization through self-regulation:

The effects of autonomous versus controlled motivation on happiness and vitality. *Journal of Experimental Social Psychology, 35,* 266–284.

Patrick, H., Knee, C. R., Canevello, A., & Lonsbary, C. (2007). The role of need fulfillment in relationship functioning and well-being: A self-determination theory perspective. *Journal of Personality and Social Psychology, 92,* 434–457.

Perls, F. S. (1973). *The Gestalt approach and eyewitness to therapy.* Ben Lomond, CA: Science and Behavior Books.

Piaget, J. (1971). *Biology and knowledge.* Chicago: University of Chicago Press.

Plant, R., Lesser, H., & Taylor-Gooby, P. (1980). *Political philosophy and social welfare: Essays on the normative basis of welfare provision.* London: Routledge & Kegan Paul.

Plant, R., & Ryan, R. M. (1985). Intrinsic motivation and the effects of self-consciousness, self-awareness, and ego-involvement: An investigation of internally controlling styles. *Journal of Personality, 53,* 435–449.

Porter, L. W., & Lawler, E. E. (1968). *Managerial attitudes and performance.* Homewood, IL: Irwin-Dorsey.

Reeve, J., Deci, E. L., & Ryan, R. M. (2004). Self-determination theory: A dialectical framework for understanding sociocultural influences on student motivation. In D. M. McInerney & S. Van Etten (Eds.), *Big theories revisited* (pp. 31–60). Greenwich, CT: Information Age.

Reis, H. T., & Patrick, B. P. (1996). Attachment and intimacy: Component processes. In E. T. Higgins & A. W. Kruglanski (Eds.), *Social psychology: Handbook of basic principles* (pp. 523–563). New York: Guilford Press.

Reis, H. T., Sheldon, K. M., Gable, S. L., Roscoe, J., & Ryan, R. M. (2000). Daily well-being: The role of autonomy, competence, and relatedness. *Personality and Social Psychology Bulletin, 26,* 419–435.

Robins, R. W., & John, O. P. (1997). The quest for self-insight: Theory and research on accuracy and bias in self-perception. In R. T. Hogan, J. A. Johnson, & S. R. Briggs (Eds.), *Handbook of personality psychology* (pp. 649–679). New York: Academic Press.

Rogers, C. (1951). *Client centered therapy.* Boston: Houghton Mifflin.

Ryan, R. M. (1982). Control and information in the intrapersonal sphere: An extension of cognitive evaluation theory. *Journal of Personality and Social Psychology, 43,* 450–461.

Ryan, R. M. (1995). Psychological needs and the facilitation of integrative processes. *Journal of Personality, 63,* 397–427.

Ryan, R. M. (2005). The developmental line of autonomy in the etiology, dynamics and treatment of borderline personality disorders. *Development and Psychopathology, 17,* 987–1006.

Ryan, R. M., Chirkov, V. I., Little, T. D., Sheldon, K. M., Timoshina, E., & Deci, E. L. (1999). The American dream in Russia: Extrinsic aspirations in two cultures. *Personality and Social Psychology Bulletin, 25,* 1509–1524.

Ryan, R. M., & Connell, J. P. (1989). Perceived locus of causality and internalization: Examining reasons for acting in two domains. *Journal of Personality and Social Psychology, 57,* 749–761.

Ryan, R. M., Connell, J. P., & Deci, E. L. (1985). A motivational analysis of self-determination and self-regulation in education. In C. Ames & R. E. Ames (Eds.), *Research on motivation in education: The classroom milieu* (pp. 13–51). New York: Academic Press.

Ryan, R. M., & Deci, E. L. (2000a). The darker and brighter sides of human existence: Basic psychological needs as a unifying concept. *Psychological Inquiry, 11,* 319–338.

Ryan, R. M., & Deci, E. L. (2000b). Self-determination theory and the facilitation of intrinsic motivation, social development, and well-being. *American Psychologist, 55,* 68–78.

Ryan, R. M., & Deci, E. L. (2001). On happiness and human potentials: A review of research on hedonic and eudaimonic well-being. In S. Fiske (Ed.), *Annual review of psychology* (Vol. 52, pp. 141–166). Palo Alto, CA: Annual Reviews.

Ryan, R. M., & Deci, E. L. (2002). An overview of self-determination theory: An organismic–dialectical perspective. In E. L. Deci & R. M. Ryan (Eds.), *Handbook of self-determination research* (pp. 3–33). Rochester, NY: University of Rochester Press.

Ryan, R. M., & Deci, E. L. (2004). Autonomy is no illusion: Self-determination theory and the empirical study of authenticity, awareness, and will. In J. Greenberg, S. L. Koole, & T. Pyszczynski (Eds.), *Handbook of experimental existential psychology* (pp. 449–479). New York: Guilford Press.

Ryan, R. M., & Deci, E. L. (2006). Self-regulation and the problem of human autonomy: Does psychology need choice, self-determination, and will? *Journal of Personality, 74,* 1557–1585.

Ryan, R. M., Deci, E. L., Grolnick, W. S., & La Guardia, J. G. (2006). The significance of autonomy and autonomy support in psychological development and psychopathology. In D. Cicchetti & D. J. Cohen (Eds.), *Developmental psychopathology* (pp. 795–849). Hoboken, NJ: Wiley.

Ryan, R. M., & Frederick, C. M. (1997). On energy, personality and health: Subjective vitality as a dynamic reflection of well-being. *Journal of Personality, 65,* 529–565.

Ryan, R. M., & Grolnick, W. S. (1986). Origins and pawns in the classroom: Self-report and projective assessments of children's perceptions. *Journal of Personality and Social Psychology, 50,* 550–558.

Ryan, R. M., Huta, V., & Deci, E. L. (2008). Living well: A self-determination theory perspective on eudaimonia. *Journal of Happiness Studies, 9,* 139–170.

Ryan, R. M., La Guardia, J. G., Solky-Butzel, J., Chirkov, V., & Kim, Y. (2005). On the interpersonal regulation of emotions: Emotional reliance across gender, relationships, and cultures. *Personal Relationships, 12,* 145–163.

Ryan, R. M., Mims, V., & Koestner, R. (1983). Relation of reward contingency and interpersonal context to intrinsic motivation: A review and test using cognitive evaluation theory. *Journal of Personality and Social Psychology, 45,* 736–750.

Ryan, R. M., Rigby, C. S., & Przybylski, A. (2006). The motivational pull of video games: A self-determination theory approach. *Motivation and Emotion, 30,* 347–364.

Ryan, R. M., Rigby, S., & King, K. (1993). Two types of religious internalization and their relations to religious orientations and mental health. *Journal of Personality and Social Psychology, 65,* 586–596.

Ryan, R. M., Sheldon, K. M., Kasser, T., & Deci, E. L. (1996). All goals are not created equal: An organismic perspective on the nature of goals and their regulation. In P. M. Gollwitzer & J. A. Bargh (Eds.), *The psychology of action: Linking cognition and motivation to behavior* (pp. 7–26). New York: Guilford Press.

Schweder, R. A., Mahapatra, M., & Miller, J. G. (1990). Culture and moral development. In J. Stiger & G. Herdt (Eds.), *Cultural psychology: Essays on comparative human development* (pp. 130–204). Cambridge, UK: Cambridge University Press.

Scott, W. E., Jr. (1976). The effects of extrinsic rewards on "intrinsic motivation": A critique. *Organizational Behavior and Human Performance, 15,* 117–129.

Sheldon, K. M., Elliot, A. J., Kim, Y., & Kasser, T. (2001). What is satisfying about satisfying events? Testing 10 candidate psychological needs. *Journal of Personality and Social Psychology, 80,* 325–339.

Sheldon, K. M., Elliot, A. J., Ryan, R. M., Chirkov, V., Kim, Y., Wu, C., et al. (2004). Self-concordance and subjective well-being in four cultures. *Journal of Cross-Cultural Psychology, 35,* 209–223.

Sheldon, K. M., Ryan, R. M., Deci, E. L., & Kasser, T. (2004). The independent effects of goal contents and motives on well-being: It's both what you pursue and why you pursue it.

Personality and Social Psychology Bulletin, 30, 475–486.

Sheldon, K. M., Ryan, R. M., Rawsthorne, L. J., & Ilardi, B. (1997). "Trait" self and "true" self: Cross-role variation in the Big Five personality traits and its relations with psychological authenticity and subjective well-being. *Journal of Personality and Social Psychology, 73,* 1380–1393.

Skinner, B. F. (1953). *Science and human behavior.* New York: Macmillan.

Skinner, E. A. (1995). *Perceived control, motivation, and coping.* Thousand Oaks, CA: Sage.

Smith, W. E. (1975). *The effect of anticipated vs. unanticipated social reward on subsequent intrinsic motivation.* Unpublished doctoral dissertation, Cornell University, Ithaca, NY.

Srivastava, A., Locke, E. A., & Bartol, K. M. (2001). Money and subjective well-being: It's not the money, it's the motive. *Journal of Personality and Social Psychology, 80,* 959–971.

Tolman, E. C. (1932). *Purposive behavior in animals and men.* New York: Century.

Vallerand, R. J. (1997). Toward a hierarchical model of intrinsic and extrinsic motivation. In M. P. Zanna (Ed.), *Advances in experimental social psychology* (Vol. 29, pp. 271–360). San Diego, CA: Academic Press.

Vallerand, R. J., Blanchard, C., Mageau, G. A., Koestner, R., Ratelle, C., Léonard, M., et al. (2003). *Les passions de l'ame*: On obsessive and harmonious passion. *Journal of Personality and Social Psychology, 85,* 756–767.

Vallerand, R. J., & Reid, G. (1984). On the causal effects of perceived competence on intrinsic motivation: A test of cognitive evaluation theory. *Journal of Sport Psychology, 6,* 94–102.

Vansteenkiste, M., Ryan, R. M., & Deci, E. L. (in press). Self-determination theory and the explanatory role of psychological needs in human well-being. In L. Bruni, F. Comim, & M. Pugno (Eds.), *Capabilities and happiness.* Oxford, UK: Oxford University Press.

Vansteenkiste, M., Simons, J., Lens, W., Sheldon, K. M., & Deci, E. L. (2004). Motivating learning, performance, and persistence: The synergistic effects of intrinsic goal contents and autonomy-supportive contexts. *Journal of Personality and Social Psychology, 87,* 246–260.

Vroom, V. H. (1964). *Work and motivation.* New York: Wiley.

White, R. W. (1959). Motivation reconsidered: The concept of competence. *Psychological Review, 66,* 297–333.

Williams, G. C., & Deci, E. L. (1996). Internalization of biopsychosocial values by medical students: A test of self-determination theory. *Journal of Personality and Social Psychology, 70,* 767–779.

Williams, G. C., Deci, E. L., & Ryan, R. M. (1998). Building health-care partnerships by supporting autonomy: Promoting maintained behavior change and positive health outcomes. In A. L. Suchman, P. Hinton-Walker, & R. Botelho (Eds.), *Partnerships in healthcare: Transforming relational process* (pp. 67–87). Rochester, NY: University of Rochester Press.

Williams, G. C., Freedman, Z., & Deci, E. L. (1998). Supporting autonomy to motivate patients with diabetes for glucose control. *Diabetes Care, 21,* 1644–1651.

Williams, G. C., Grow, V. M., Freedman, Z., Ryan, R. M., & Deci, E. L. (1996). Motivational predictors of weight loss and weight-loss maintenance. *Journal of Personality and Social Psychology, 70,* 115–126.

Williams, G. C., McGregor, H. A., Sharp, D., Kouides, R. W., Levesque, C., Ryan, R. M., et al. (2006). A self-determination multiple risk intervention trial to improve smokers' health. *Journal of General Internal Medicine, 21,* 1288–1294.

Williams, G. C., McGregor, H. A., Sharp, D., Levesque, C., Kouides, R. W., Ryan, R. M., et al. (2006). Testing a self-determination theory intervention for motivating tobacco cessation: Supporting autonomy and competence in a clinical trial. *Health Psychology, 25,* 91–101.

Williams, G. C., Rodin, G. C., Ryan, R. M., Grolnick, W. S., & Deci, E. L. (1998). Autonomous regulation and long-term medication adherence in adult outpatients. *Health Psychology, 17,* 269–276.

Winter, D. G. (1973). *The power motive.* New York: Free Press.

Zuckerman, M., Porac, J., Lathin, D., Smith, R., & Deci, E. L. (1978). On the importance of self-determination for intrinsically motivated behavior. *Personality and Social Psychology Bulletin, 4,* 443–446.

CHAPTER 27

Creativity and Genius

Dean Keith Simonton

Creativity and genius are highly desirable but also rather elusive qualities. Employers in high-tech industries often wish that their workers were more creative, and so creativity workshops have proliferated that purport to attain that end. Parents are usually pleased to learn that they have given birth to a "budding genius," and will often fight hard to get their child enrolled in special programs for the gifted.

Although a person can exhibit creativity without being a genius, and be a genius without being creative, both characteristics can converge in a single personality. Indeed, the creative genius is often viewed as the highest or purest manifestation of both creativity and genius. Isaac Newton, René Descartes, Miguel de Cervantes, Leonardo da Vinci, and Ludwig van Beethoven offer clear-cut examples. Creative genius is so highly valued that special honors are devoted to its recognition—the Nobel Prize perhaps constituting the most conspicuous example. A more recent instance is the special grants awarded by the MacArthur Foundation, for which recipients the mass media have taken to confer the official title of "genius."

Of the two attributes, *genius* has the longer history as an individual-difference variable. The first scientific study was Galton's (1869) book on *Hereditary Genius*. Creativity, in contrast, did not come into its own as an independent research topic until nearly a century later. Often this latter development is taken as beginning with Guilford's (1950) presidential address before the American Psychological Association. Yet it was not until the 1960s that research on creativity really exploded. The *Journal of Creative Behavior*, for example, did not begin publication until 1962. Although creativity research got a late start, it quickly overtook research on genius as a topic in personality research. Despite something of a decline in interest in the 1980s, research on creativity has resurged. This increased activity is evident in the founding of the *Creativity Research Journal* in 1988, the recent publication of several edited volumes (e.g., Sternberg, 1999), including the *International Handbook of Creativity Research* (Kaufman & Sternberg, 2006), plus the publication of the two-volume *Encyclopedia of Creativity* (Runco & Pritzker, 1999). With this upsurge has come an increased interest in genius as well (e.g., Eysenck, 1995; Simonton, 1999a).

The main goal of this chapter is to provide an overview of the substantive findings and issues regarding individual differences in creativity and genius, with a special emphasis on the two combined. But before we can begin that task, I first must define the two key terms.

DEFINITIONS

What do we mean when we call someone "creative"? How do we know when a person can be considered a "genius"? Because creativity is perhaps the most difficult to define, I start with the first question.

Creativity

Creativity involves the generation of creative ideas. At least two prerequisites must be met for an idea to be deemed "creative." First, the idea must represent a relatively uncommon response—the criterion of *originality*. An idea that arose from only one person in the history of the human race is considered more original than an idea that emerged from many people. Of course, originality is not an absolute, all-or-none criterion. Instead, we can speak of degrees of originality. Second, to count as creative, an original idea must exhibit *adaptiveness*. That is, the idea must provide the solution to some significant problem or achieve some important goal. Without this second criterion it would be difficult to separate the rambling thoughts of a psychotic from the shocking innovations of an avant-garde artist. Notice that this condition may also admit of degrees. Some solutions may prove superior to others. In any event, a creative idea must simultaneously meet both stipulations. The higher the combined value of both originality and adaptiveness, the higher is the level of creativity.

Although most researchers would agree with this abstract conception of creativity, they often differ when they turn to the concrete study of the phenomenon. This divergence occurs because there is more than one way to investigate the emergence of creative ideas. These different ways essentially represent contrary levels of psychological analysis. Three viewpoints, in particular, are paramount (Simonton, 2003c):

1. Creativity can be viewed as a *mental process* (or collection of processes) that results in the production of ideas simultaneously original and adaptive. This is the per-

spective favored by cognitive psychologists who study problem solving and insight using either laboratory experiments or computer simulations.

2. Creativity can be seen as a characteristic of a *product*, such as a discovery, invention, poem, painting, or composition. A product is deemed creative if it satisfies the combined criteria of originality and adaptiveness. The former criterion might specifically entail novelty, surprise, and complexity, whereas the latter criterion might involve truth, beauty, elegance, and virtuosity, the specifics depending on the particular domain of creativity. The study of creative products is the primary occupation of psychologists in experimental aesthetics, albeit some psychologists have also attempted to comprehend better the nature of scientific products.

3. Creativity is a trait or personality profile that characterizes a *person*. That is, it is some quality or capacity that some individuals have more than others, and some may not have at all. For instance, creativity may consist of some special combination of such individual-difference factors as intelligence, ambition, determination, independence, openness, and originality. Needless to say, this is the perspective adopted by personality psychologists who wish to identify that set of personal attributes that distinguish creative individuals from people who display little, if any, creativity.

These are the process, product, and person definitions of creativity. These three definitions are not totally independent. At the very least, we might hope that creative products are generated by creative persons using creative processes. It is for this reason that investigators will often combine two or three perspectives in a single inquiry. For example, psychologists might examine cross-sectional variation in cognitive styles, the latter then determining the odds that a person will use the mental operations necessary for the generation of creative ideas (e.g., Sternberg & Lubart, 1995). Other researchers might gauge individual differences in creativity in terms of their comparative output of creative products, and then attempt to predict that variation using cognitive and personality variables (e.g., Feist, 1993; Helmreich, Spence, Beane, Lucker, & Matthews, 1980; Simonton, 1992). Nonetheless, most investigators tend to concentrate on just one of the three perspectives, the remaining two becoming secondary at best. This is true for the bulk of the personality research, which usually concentrates on the creative person, assigning noticeably less attention to the process and product aspects.

Genius

The term "genius" has a much longer history than that of "creativity." In fact, the word originates in the times of Ancient Rome, when each person was believed to be born with a kind of "guardian angel." This private genius looked out for the individual's fate. As time went on, genius became integrated with the person. First it was extended to encompass those qualities that made an individual unique. This usage is still common in some Romance languages, such as Spanish, in which genius (*genio*) can denote a person's temperament or disposition. Later still, the term acquired a more restrictive usage, namely, the distinctive abilities and attributes that enabled certain individuals to make major contributions to human culture. This signification still retained something of the idiosyncratic significance of the previous meanings, but with a more narrow application. Not everyone had genius.

Beginning with Galton's 1869 *Hereditary Genius*, the term found its way into the behavioral sciences. The word then began to accrue a more objective and quantitative meaning. Eventually, psychologists proposed two rather contrary operational definitions of the construct: the psychometric and the historiometric.

Psychometric Definition

Galton (1869) conceived of genius in terms of the normal distribution of what he called "natural ability." Those individuals whose natural ability placed them in the remote upper tail of the bell-shaped distribution were identified as geniuses. Unfortunately, although Galton (1883) attempted to devise instruments that would directly measure individual differences in natural ability, the resulting "anthropometric" methods failed miserably. However, the advent of the intelligence test placed Galton's conception on a much sounder basis. Although these tests were originally designed to help identify children who were below average in intellect, they soon were used to label children as intellectually gifted. Pioneers such as Lewis Terman (1925) and Leta Hollingworth (1942) helped to establish the practice of styling a child a "genius" if he or she scored above a certain set level on some standardized IQ test, such as the Stanford–Binet. Later, when adult intelligence tests emerged, this psychometric definition was carried over with minimal modification. A genius was simply a child or adult who scored above some predetermined level.

Often the cutoff was put at IQ 140, a hypothetical threshold that has found its way into many dictionaries and encyclopedias (e.g., *American Heritage*, 1992). Others would relax the criterion somewhat. For instance, the Mensa Society sets the figure at two standard deviations above the population mean, which results in a requirement of around 132 on many tests. Naturally, because scores on IQ tests can be considered interval variables, genius can be also conceived in a more continuous fashion. It is then possible to speak of relative degrees of genius. Indeed, this very practice has inspired the appearance of additional clubs of even more elite intellects. The Four Sigma Society requires its members to be four standard deviations above the mean (or around IQ 164), while the Mega Society stipulates an IQ only obtained by one in a million (or around IQ 176). The highest-grade genius, according to the *Guinness Book of Records* (McFarlan, 1989), is supposedly Marilyn Vos Savant, whose IQ is claimed to be 228.

The psychometric definition of genius has many assets. One important advantage is the impressive reliabilities of the best intelligence tests, which tend to be among the most reliable of all psychometric instruments. Another is the applicability of the definition to any population for which there exists an appropriate IQ test. Hence, the definition is as applicable to children as it is to adults. On the other hand, psychometric genius also encounters problem when it is extended to the domain of creative achievement. As is discussed later, the association between intelligence and creativity is very weak for both child and adult samples. In fact, the correlation tends to become negligible for populations that are above-average in intelligence

(Simonton, 1985). Although there is some debate exactly where the association begins to disappear, the figure of IQ 120 is often bandied about in the research literature (Barron & Harrington, 1981). Such a threshold implies that the various grades of intellectual genius do not necessarily correspond to the different grades of creative genius.

A concrete illustration of this lack of correspondence may be found in Terman's classic *Genetic Studies of Genius* (Terman, 1925). Having selected more than 1,500 children on the basis of exceptional IQ scores, Terman conducted a longitudinal study to determine whether these young geniuses would grow up to become highly accomplished adults (Terman & Oden, 1959). Although many attained considerable success, it is fair to say that none achieved the highest levels of acclaim. For example, there were no Nobel laureates among the group. The ironic fact eventually emerged that among those screened in the early 1920s were two children who grew up to earn Nobel prizes in physics, namely, William Shockley in 1956 and Luis Alvarez in 1968. Yet their childhood IQs were not high enough to get either one of them included in Terman's elite sample (Winner, 1996).

Historiometric Definition

When Galton wrote his *Hereditary Genius*, there existed no psychometric measures that could be used to define genius. Therefore, Galton introduced a rather different operational definition, the historiometric (Woods, 1911). According to this alternative, genius is defined in terms of an individual's contributions to a particular domain of human achievement. A genius is then a person whose effects on a domain are so numerous and so distinctive that the domain is appreciably transformed. The most prominent geniuses often make names for themselves by becoming eponyms for discoveries, movements, or events. Illustrations include the Copernican revolution, Newtonian physics, Darwinism, Pasteurization, and Freudian slips. Furthermore, as in the psychometric definition, historiometric assessment can be designed to gauge the relative magnitude of genius (Simonton, 1990). The greater is the degree of impact, the more prominent is the individual's reputation and hence the higher is the caliber of genius (see, e.g., J. M. Cattell,

1903; Ludwig, 1992b; Simonton, 1998a). Thus, according to their comparative impression on the classical repertoire, Mozart can be said to have displayed more genius than Salieri, just as Salieri can be styled a greater genius than Türk. Assertions such as this can be based on two distinct kinds of measurements: eminence and productivity.

1. *Eminence measures* gauge the total global impact an individual has made upon a given domain (Simonton, 1990). This impact may be defined according to the ratings of peers or experts (e.g., Helson & Crutchfield, 1970; Roe, 1953); the receipt of special honors or awards, such as the Nobel prize (e.g., Rothenberg, 1979, 1990); the frequency of performance, discussion, or citation (e.g., Feist, 1993; Martindale, 1995b; Simonton, 1991b, 1992); or the amount of space assigned the individual in encyclopedias, biographical dictionaries, history texts, anthologies, and other reference works (e.g., J. M. Cattell, 1903; Murray, 2003; Simonton, 1998a).

2. *Productivity measures* assess the number of concrete contributions an individual has made to a given domain (Albert, 1975). These most commonly consist of counts of books, articles, poems, paintings, inventions, compositions, and the like (e.g., Matthews, Helmreich, Beane, & Lucker, 1980; Simonton, 1977, 1997), although occasionally more refined units may be used, such as the number of melodies created by composers (e.g., Simonton, 1991b). These tabulations may include all works generated, regardless of impact, or they may include only those works that were influential, as determined by citation or performance frequencies, for example (Simonton, 1977, 1991a).

Fortunately, because productivity constitutes the single most prominent predictor of differential eminence, these two alternative definitions are, for all practical purposes, equivalent (Albert, 1975; Simonton, 1997). Beyond this convergence, historiometric definitions have other measurement virtues. First, historiometric measures have clear "face validity"; that is, they seem to correspond closely with what most people would consider indicative of creative achievement. If Beethoven, Michelangelo, Shakespeare, or Descartes are not accorded the status of creative genius, it is doubtful that the word could have any meaning whatsoever. Second, research indicates that such measures have highly respectable reliabilities, with multiple indicators of eminence or productivity usually displaying coefficient alphas in the upper .80s and .90s (Simonton, 1977, 1984, 1991a). Third, research has also shown that such measures display a high degree of cross-cultural invariance (e.g., Simonton, 1991c). For example, the most eminent figures according to the African American minority culture are also the most eminent figures according to the European American majority culture of the United States (Simonton, 1998a). Fourth, historiometric assessments enjoy a high degree of transhistorical stability (Simonton, 1991c). Despite the existence of occasional exceptions—such as Johann Sebastian Bach and Gregor Mendel—those who are most famous in their own time also tend to be the most eminent today (see also Farnsworth, 1969; Rosengren, 1985). This result is important because it suggests that whenever psychologists study distinguished contemporaries, it is highly likely that those luminaries will continue to have exceptional posthumous reputations (Simonton, 1998b).

One last feature of the historiometric definition is worth noting. The word "genius" was first used as a label for those persons who made outstanding creative contributions. However, it eventually became applicable to other forms of exceptional achievement. As a result, it is now acceptable to talk of political, military, religions, and entrepreneurial genius. Thus, the historiometric definition can apply to accomplishment in leadership domains as well as that in creativity domains (Simonton, 1990). To be sure, the products of a leader are not the same as those of a creator, and so the productivity definition cannot be used. Nonetheless, it is often possible to gauge both creators and leaders on a comparable scale of differential eminence, something first demonstrated by James McKeen Cattell back in 1903. This common denominator has permitted psychologists to examine the similarities and contrasts in the personality profiles of distinguished creators and leaders (e.g., Cox, 1926; Simonton, 1991d; Thorndike, 1950).

Although it is feasible to speak of genius in leadership domains as well as genius in creative domains, the current chapter concentrates on the latter. There are three reasons for this focus. First, the research literature on the personal characteristics of leaders is so immense that it would easily take up considerable space (Simonton, 1995). Second, individual-difference variables appear to play a much less conspicuous role in outstanding leadership than they do in exceptional creativity. Very often situational factors dominate over individual factors (Simonton, 1995). Even when personal attributes play some role, frequently their effects are moderated by contextual variables. Third, although leaders can clearly qualify as geniuses by the historiometric definition, they are rather less likely to do so under the psychometric definition. Not only do leaders often display lower levels of intellectual ability than do creators (Cox, 1926; Simonton, 1976), but in addition there is evidence that leadership effectiveness can actually be compromised by an excessively high intelligence (Simonton, 1995). Sometimes the relation between leadership and intelligence may be best described by a curvilinear, inverted-U function (Simonton, 1985). This nonmonotonic association contrasts greatly with what is observed for creativity.

Having defined the terms and delineated this chapter's scope, I next wish to provide a general personality sketch of the highly creative individual. After doing so, I turn to a discussion of some of the key issues in the study of the creative personality.

GENERAL PERSONALITY SKETCH

Since the onset of research on the creative personality, researchers have periodically published reviews of the central research findings (e.g., Barron & Harrington, 1981; Feist, 1998). These reviews show that the body of research seems to have reached a consensus regarding the factors associated with cross-sectional variation in creativity. That is, individuals who display high levels of creativity appear to differ from less creative individuals on numerous cognitive and dispositional characteristics. The most conspicuous overall feature of this distinctive profile is its complexity. The creative genius often has the appearance of being a bundle of highly variable and sometimes even contradictory attributes. To make this point, consider the following six clusters of findings:

1. Creative individuals are almost invariably more intelligent than average, at least by a standard deviation or more (Barron & Harrington, 1981; Haensly & Reynolds, 1989). Yet as pointed out earlier, intelligence appears to operate more as a threshold function (Simonton, 1994). Below a certain minimal intellect, it is improbable that a person can display culturally significant levels of creative behavior. But beyond this threshold level, further increases in intelligence may or may not translate into higher degrees of creative genius. Someone with IQ 200 may not be any more creative than someone with IQ 120, and may even be less so—albeit it is likely that the most creative person with the higher IQ will display more creativity than the most creative person with the lower IQ.

2. Complicating the picture all the more is the fact that intelligence is not a homogeneous construct but rather may consist of distinguishable intelligences (see, e.g., Gardner, 1983; Paulhus, Wehr, Harms, & Strasser, 2002; Sternberg, 2003). In Guilford's (1967) classic "structure of intellect model" intelligence is broken into 120 distinct types, only a subset of which has any direct involvement in creativity (Bachelor & Michael, 1997). Particularly crucial is the distinction between convergent and divergent processes. Convergent thought endeavors to identify the single correct response to a given problem situation, whereas divergent thought tries to generate many different responses. The latter concept has led to the emergence of a large number of divergent thinking tests that have had some success in predicting creativity (Simonton, 2003b). In a similar vein, some investigations suggest that creative individuals exhibit the capacity for generating many unusual associative linkages between otherwise diverse concepts or stimuli (Eysenck, 1995; Mednick, 1962; Rothenberg, 1979). The creative mind is thus cognitively rich, with complex semantic networks loosely interlinking various ideas (Martindale, 1995a).

3. Paralleling this cognitive richness is the creator's perceptual richness. Creative persons exhibit a tremendous amount of openness to diverse experiences and demonstrate exceptional tolerance of ambiguity (Harris, 2004; McCrae, 1987; Peterson & Carson, 2000). Indeed, they tend to actively seek out novelty and complexity (Barron, 1963; MacKinnon, 1978). Especially fascinating is the ability to engage in "defocused attention," which enables the creator to attend to more than one stimulus and/or cognition at the same time (Ansberg & Hill, 2003; Martindale, 1995a; Mendelsohn, 1976). Not surprisingly, given these results, creative personalities are more likely to display a wide range of interests and hobbies (e.g., Gough, 1979; Root-Bernstein, Bernstein, & Garnier, 1995). Consistent with this point is the tendency for creative individuals to be omnivorous readers (Chambers, 1964; Simonton, 1984). This breadth often takes the form of extraordinary versatility that enables creators to make contributions to more than one domain of achievement (Cassandro, 1998; Raskin, 1936; R. K. White, 1931).

4. Beyond these more cognitive aspects of the creative disposition are the motivational attributes. Creators deeply love what they do and thus show exceptional enthusiasm, energy, and commitment to their chosen domain of creative endeavor (e.g., Chambers, 1964; Roe, 1953). So strong is this emotional involvement that creators are often perceived by family and friends as "workaholics"—an attribution that is not without empirical justification (Helmreich, Spence, & Pred, 1988; Matthews et al., 1980). In any case, because of this characteristic, creators are extremely persistent in the face of obstacles and disappointments (e.g., Chambers, 1964; Cox, 1926; see also Duckworth, Peterson, Matthews, & Kelly, 2007). They do not give up easily. Yet at the same time, creative individuals tend to be highly flexible, altering strategies and tactics—and even problems—when repeated failure seems to recommend such action. This behavioral flexibility is facilitated by the tendency to work on multiple projects, each at various stages of development (Hargens, 1978; Root-Bernstein, Bernstein, & Garnier, 1993). Furthermore, these projects are interrelated in complex ways, forming what has been styled a "network of enterprises" (Gruber, 1989). As a consequence, the solution to one problem often provides the needed clue for getting around an impasse in the solution of another problem (Simonton, 2004).

5. The foregoing cognitive and motivational attributes are usually coupled with a characteristic social orientation. Creative individuals are far more likely to be introverted than extraverted (e.g., Eysenck, 1995; Roe, 1953). Indeed, this introversion can reach the level of being rather remote,

withdrawn, and even antisocial (R. B. Cattell, 1963; Eysenck, 1995). At the same time, creative persons are prone to exhibit a high degree of independence and autonomy, often displaying a pronounced rebellious streak in their categorical refusal to conform to conventional norms (e.g., Crutchfield, 1962; Eysenck, 1995; Roe, 1953).

6. Creative individuals, and especially creative geniuses, seem to show higher than average rates of psychopathology of various kinds (Jamison, 1993; Ludwig, 1995; Simonton, 2005). This tendency is indicated by disorders such as suicidal depression as well as alcoholism or other forms of substance abuse (Goertzel, Goertzel, & Goertzel, 1978; Ludwig, 1995; Post, 1996). In addition, highly creative personalities often produce elevated scores on psychometric instruments that are indicative of mental disorder or emotional instability, such as the psychoticism scale of the Eysenck Personality Questionnaire (Eysenck, 1995) or the clinical subscales of the Minnesota Multiphasic Personality Inventory (Barron, 1969; MacKinnon, 1978). Creativity is also negatively associated with the ability to filter out irrelevant information (Carson, Peterson, & Higgins, 2003). Although this characteristic is positively correlated with openness to experience (Carson et al., 2003; Peterson, Smith, & Carson, 2002), it is also positively associated with both psychoticism and psychosis (Eysenck, 1995; Stavridou & Furnham, 1996). Yet the surprising point is that creators appear to have unusual levels of ego strength or other psychological resources that enable them to hold these adverse forces in check (Barron, 1969; Carson et al., 2003; R. B. Cattell & Butcher, 1968).

I hasten to point out that the empirical and theoretical literature is by no means consistent regarding the above personality sketch. Many researchers would delete one or more of the listed attributes, and a few researchers would omit virtually all of them. The points raised in the next section will help us understand why.

SPECIFIC SUBSTANTIVE ISSUES

Seven critical questions complicate any attempt to understand the personality of the creative genius. These questions concern everyday versus exceptional achievements, childhood versus adulthood creativity, cognitive versus dispositional attributes, scientific versus artistic creativity, nature versus nurture in creative development, individual versus situational determinants of creativity, and empirical versus theoretical personality profiles. I discuss each issue in the following material (see Simonton, in press, for a more detailed discussion).

Everyday versus Exceptional Achievements

The primary focus of the personality sketch was to describe the creative genius. The implicit assumption is that the most eminent creators provide the most typical or characteristic profile of cognitive and dispositional traits. Yet many studies of creative behavior examine more mundane forms of the phenomenon, such as workers in industrial research and development units. Indeed, much research in creativity investigates student populations, including children. Therefore, to what extent are the personality profiles gathered from the examination of creative geniuses truly indicative of more everyday creators? There are two alternative responses.

On the one hand, we can argue that the creative genius differs only in degree from an individual whose creativity will never earn significant recognition beyond the confines of a rather circumscribed time and place. In other words, there exists some continuum linking the universally recognized genius with the average person on the street. On this continuum may be placed various intermediate grades of creators. All of the traits associated with creativity would then vary according to a person's placement on this latent continuum. Eysenck (1995), for example, argued that psychoticism represented just such a dimension. Low levels of psychoticism predict the absence of creativity, and increased psychoticism predicts ever elevated creativity. The genius emerges at the exalted level, near the dangerous borderline between creativity and madness.

One attractive feature of this continuity hypothesis is the fact that creative behavior itself displays some degree of continuity. This aspect of continuity is most obvious when creativity is gauged in terms of the output of creative products. Lifetime creative productivity forms a well-defined ratio scale on which people may vary. In the sciences, for instance, there are those who made no contribution, those who made two, those who made three, and so forth. Furthermore, there already exists ample evidence that the magnitude of creative output can display a monotonic relationship with certain personality traits (e.g., Eysenck, 1995). Hence, continuous variation in creative behavior may be grounded in an underlying variation in personality.

On the other hand, we can take the position that there are qualitative differences among the various forms that creativity may take. To appreciate this alternative, consider seven hypothetical levels of creative attainment:

1. *Those who have made a significant and enduring impact on their chosen domain of creative activity, and who have left a major imprint on general culture.* Besides producing contributions in their fields, these figures became virtual icons of popular culture. Their images grace T-shirts, their lives become the basis for plays and movies, and their works the subject of television documentaries.

2. *Those who have made a significant and enduring impact on their chosen domain of creative activity, but who have left virtually no imprint on general culture.* These figures will always have at least a modest place in the encyclopedias and biographical dictionaries, but will probably never become household names.

3. *Those who endeavored to make lasting contributions to their chosen domain of creative activity, but failed.* Such individuals enjoyed only a transient or local celebrity, but their "15 minutes of fame" have long since elapsed. Their works long forgotten, they have been reduced to footnotes in esoteric histories of their fields.

4. *Those who attempted to make a lasting contribution, but who never managed to make even the most minimal impression on their colleagues or on audiences or appreciators.* These are the scientists who publish journal articles that no one reads or cites, artists whose works appear in local galleries without success, and composers whose works get a one-time performance by an amateur orchestra.

5. *Those who never succeed in producing something that went beyond private consumption.* These are the inventors who tinker around in the garage but who never patent

anything; the Sunday afternoon artists who paint landscapes and seascapes; the amateur poets whom no one even knows write poetry in their spare time. If these silent creators do venture something for the appreciation of the larger world, it never makes it past the preliminary evaluation of a patent official, selection juror, or journal editor.

6. *Those who do not create anything of their own, but do display a profound appreciation of the creativity of others.* They may read scientific or literary magazines, attend concerts of new music, or regularly visit art galleries. If they have the resources, such persons may even become patrons of the arts, demonstrating their creativity in the elevated tastes they show in their commissions or purchases.

7. *Those who don't like new ideas or newfangled technologies, and who believe that art, music, and literature are for whimsy pseudo-intellectuals and nerds.* The height of their creative appreciation extends no higher than a boxing match or a war movie.

Now it could be that these seven levels are mere points on an underlying personality dimension that provides the basis for creativity. But it may be more likely that qualitative shifts appear at certain places. To begin with, there may be a profound contrast between producing creative ideas and appreciating those ideas. Why are some people satisfied with absorbing the novel ideas of others whereas others feel the compulsion to express themselves through some form of creative work? Even if we confine our attention to those who actively generate products for public evaluation, certain discontinuities are possible. For example, might there not be a difference between amateur and professional creators? And even among the professional creators, might there not be a contrast between the successful and unsuccessful ones? Finally, might those creators who attain universal acclaim depart in significant ways from those whose success is confined to a narrow discipline?

To address such questions, we must determine if it is necessary for distinct traits to "kick in" for a person to cross over from one level to the next. It may also be the case that some of the underlying personality effects are nonlinear or nonmonotonic. An interesting example is the relation between versatility and eminence in science (Sulloway, 1996).

Rather than discover a positive linear function, an intriguing J-curve was found. The most famous scientists are those who make contributions to many different domains of science, whereas the next most famous were those who specialized in a single circumscribed topic. The least eminent were those who were neither highly specialized nor highly versatile. To the extent that versatility reflects some deeper personality disposition, then this curvilinear function implies the existence a peculiar discontinuity in the etiology of creative genius.

Needless to say, if creativity falls into qualitatively distinct types, then there would have to exist more than one "typical" personality profile. Even creative geniuses might feature two or more different profiles.

Childhood versus Adulthood Creativity

So far we have been discussing creativity in adult samples. Yet studies of creativity, including many of the classic investigations in this field, often focus on children (e.g., Getzels & Jackson, 1962; Wallach & Kogan, 1965). Besides its theoretical interest, this issue can have significant practical consequences for the design and evaluation of programs for the education of gifted children (Colangelo & Davis, 2002). Nevertheless, these inquiries have a somewhat ambiguous status from the standpoint of understanding the personality basis of creativity and genius. There are two main difficulties.

First is the matter of identification. How does the researcher decide that a given child is creative? One common approach is to make this decision according to performance on some "creativity test," usually some measure of divergent thinking (Runco, 1992). Yet this approach somewhat begs the question. Such assessment is only as good as the instruments are valid. Unfortunately, the divergent and convergent validity of various creativity tests can sometimes be rather low (Simonton, 2003b; see, e.g., Carson, Peterson, & Higgins, 2005). An alternative approach is to identify creativity according to actual behavioral performance—the generation of genuine creative products. This method is especially useful in the case of children who display precocious talent, such as child prodigies in a particular domain of creativity. Nonetheless, this line of attack does not completely remove the validity problem. It is

extremely rare for children (and even adolescents) to generate products that satisfy adult standards of creativity (Winner, 1996). The products may reveal a precocious acquisition of specialized skills and a degree of virtuosity in the execution of those skills, but without displaying the originality and adaptiveness necessary to compete with the output of mature creators (Runco, 1989). Given these problems of identification, it is not always safe to assume that the personality profile characteristic of youthful creativity is the same as that for adulthood creativity (see, e.g., Parloff, Datta, Kleman, & Handlon, 1968). The selection procedures may not entail sufficiently overlapping criteria.

Second is the matter of continuity. Development from childhood through adolescence and even adulthood is fraught with a great variety of changes in cognitive makeup and personality structure. Besides progressive developmental differentiation of various functions, specific personality traits may wax and wane, with particularly dramatic effects taking place during puberty. Some of these transformations may be exogenous (environmental) and others endogenous (genetic), but in combination they signify the instability of youth's constitution during the course of their growth and maturation. At various points during the course of development, creativity may undergo spurts and slumps, and may even vanish altogether—for the remainder of a person's life (Albert, 1996; Runco & Charles, 1997). Even in adulthood, creativity may come and go, whether we assess it psychometrically (McCrae, Arenberg, & Costa, 1987) or historiometrically (Simonton, 1988, 1989, 1997). These developmental instabilities within individuals hold even though differences in creativity across individuals may be relatively stable over time.

It should be pointed out that these two difficulties are mitigated, if not entirely obliterated, when we revert to the psychometric definition of genius. That is, if genius is defined as an exceptionally high IQ, then the problem of identification disappears by definitional fiat. Furthermore, such IQ scores are highly stable across childhood, adolescence, and adulthood (Simonton, 1976; Terman & Oden, 1959). The main source in developmental instability would then probably be concentrated in the personality profiles that characterize highly intelligent persons. However, even if these latter profiles were highly stable across time, that stability would not contribute much to our understanding of the dispositional qualities of the exceptional creator. For both in youth and in maturity, the personality profiles of highly intelligent individuals differ markedly from those of highly creative individuals (Albert, 1994; Getzels & Jackson, 1962; Wallach & Kogan, 1965). The psychometric genius and the historiometric genius are different people from a dispositional perspective (Simonton, 1994).

Cognitive versus Dispositional Attributes

Research on individual differences in creativity may be said to have roots in two distinct psychological traditions. The first harks back to the Gestalt psychologists who were the pioneers in research on problem solving and insightful behavior. In line with this tradition, much research on creativity has focused more on the creative process than the person. Some investigators have even gone so far as to suggest that creativity is a mental operation accessible to all, and thus largely unrelated to general individual-difference dimensions (e.g., Weisberg, 1992). Creative geniuses are merely persons who have acquired the necessary expertise in a given domain, but otherwise they employ the same cognitive processes as the rest of us in problem-solving situations. In contrast, other researchers in this cognitive tradition maintain that the person is indeed important, because creative individuals are those who have superior access to certain special mental operations, such as the capacity for remote association (Mednick, 1962), divergent thought (Guilford, 1967), or some other process. Many older psychometric instruments were, in fact, predicated on the assumption that individual differences in creativity were grounded in certain cognitive abilities (e.g., Mednick, 1962). Also in this class of studies may be placed the work on how creativity relates to cognitive styles, or distinctive patterns of thinking (e.g., Sternberg & Lubart, 1995). Whatever the specifics, this tradition asserts that a complete understanding of the creator requires that we understand the cognitive process behind creativity. If individual differences exist in the capacity for creativity (besides those grounded in domain-specific expertise), then this variation has to do with creative cognition (Finke, Ward, & Smith, 1992).

The second research tradition may be said to have its source in personality and clinical assessment. Here researchers are fascinated with the richness of the human personality, with its complex domains of differentiating interests and values, emotions and motives, activities and reactions. For investigations in this tradition, the creative genius must have a highly distinctive profile of traits that enables him or her to exhibit creativity. Some investigators have even argued that this defining cluster of dispositional attributes is far more critical in a creative life than are any putative cognitive differences (e.g., Dellas & Gaier, 1970; cf. Feist & Barron, 2003). Of course, this second tradition implies a whole different manner of constructing "creativity tests." Rather than measure the intellectual capacity for certain cognitive operations, the tests may assess preferences, attitudes, and activities associated with creative behavior (e.g., Davis, 1975, 1989). Standard personality measures may even be used to identify the characteristic profile of the highly creative person (R. B. Cattell & Butcher, 1968; Gough, 1979, 1992; MacKinnon, 1978). In such circumstances, the assessment of creativity becomes a matter of scoring performance on a generic inventory rather than the application of a test specifically designed to tap the creative personality.

Although some researchers have taken extreme positions, advocating exclusively either cognitive or dispositional assessment, many recent investigators have argued for the involvement of both intellect and personality in the making of a creative individual (e.g., Eysenck, 1995; Simonton, 2004; Sternberg & Lubart, 1995). Creativity of the highest order, especially that of the creative genius, may require a special combination of cognitive and dispositional attributes. In fact, it may be the distinctiveness of that combination that renders exceptional creativity so rare. The vast majority of the population may be missing one or more essential components (Simonton, 1999b).

Scientific versus Artistic Creativity

Researchers often treat creativity as a single, relatively homogeneous phenomenon. Creativity is the result of some generic capacity for generating original and adaptive ideas without regard to the specific domain in which the creativity takes place. Although this simple view may have some justification when discussing everyday creativity or the creativity displayed by children, it becomes clearly invalid when extended to extraordinary creativity, especially when it attains the level of creative genius. The expected cognitive and dispositional profiles vary conspicuously according to the type of creative achievement. The disciplinary contrast that has attracted the most empirical documentation is that between scientific and artistic creativity (Feist, 1998). Expressed in general terms, creative scientists tend to exhibit traits that fall somewhere between those of the creative artist and those of the average human being (Simonton, 2004). For example, remote associations and divergent thinking are less prominent, and that which does occur is more restricted to concepts within the scientific specialty—in contrast to artists who seem to have wild ideas about almost everything. The scientific genius also tends to have a more conventional, predictable, and stable personality structure than does the artistic genius. Especially remarkable is the less conspicuous inclination toward psychopathology seen in great scientists, albeit even here this characteristic may still be more prominent than found in the general population (Ludwig, 1995; Raskin, 1936). The only major attribute on which scientists score more prominently than artists, relative to the normal baseline, is intelligence (Cox, 1926). On the average, the brightest creative geniuses are those who make major contributions to scientific disciplines. In Cox's (1926) study of 301 geniuses, for example, the estimated IQs for scientists were around a standard deviation higher than those for artists (see also Walberg, Rasher, & Hase, 1978). However, these mean differences may merely reflect the tendency of intelligence to be conceived in terms of the kinds of cognitive skills that are most suitable for exceptional performance in science.

I should point out that the foregoing differentiations represent only the "first cut" in laying out some typology of creative personality. Although scientists are broadly different from artists, neither scientific nor artistic creators form homogeneous groups. In the sciences, for instance, some personality differences separate contributors to the mathematical, physical, biological, and be-

havioral or social sciences (Chambers, 1964; Roe, 1953; Terman, 1954). Thus, social scientists, as a group, are more extraverted than are most natural scientists. Even within a particular scientific discipline, revolutionary scientists tend to be much more "artistic" in their disposition than are practitioners of what Kuhn (1970) styled "normal science" (Simonton, 2004). In the arts the variability in empirical profiles is even more remarkable (Cox, 1926; Ludwig, 1992a). This diversity is perhaps most apparent in Ludwig's (1995) recent study of psychopathology in eminent creators. The incidence rates for various disorders depends very much on the prevalent form of artistic expression. Poets tend to suffer from extremely high rates, for example, whereas architects are more similar to the scientists in their susceptibility to psychopathology (see also Kaufman, 2000–2001; Post, 1994).

It should now be evident that there are many types of creative personalities, not just one. This variability is reflected not just in their dispositions but in their backgrounds too. For instance, scientific creators, in contrast to artistic creators, hail from backgrounds that tend to favor more conformity, conventionality, and stability (Simonton, 2004). But this fact brings us naturally to the next substantive issue.

Nature versus Nurture in Creative Development

One of the oldest controversies in psychology is the relative importance of nature and nurture in human development. Interestingly, this issue was first raised—and christened—with respect to the study of creative genius. The debate began with Galton's 1869 *Hereditary Genius*, in which he attempted to show that genius of all kinds clustered into talented family pedigrees. Galton explicitly took the position that genius is born rather than made. It was the immediate consequence of the genetic inheritance of extraordinary intelligence, energy, and determination. This extreme stance was soon challenged, most notably by Candolle in 1873, who endeavored to show how the appearance of scientific creativity was contingent on a diverse array of climatological, political, and sociocultural factors. As a result, Galton conceded that that both factors may play a role in the emergence of creative genius. This concession was ably made in his 1874 book on *English Men of Science: Their Nature and Nurture.* The subtitle is significant, for it represents the first formal use of the terms "nature" and "nurture" to label the debate.

Unfortunately, later research on genius and creativity moved even further away from the position that development was a function of both biological endowment and environmental influences. This movement toward nurture accounts can be partly ascribed to the increased dominance of psychology in the United States, which tended to emphasize learning as the central factor in personality development. In addition, the eugenics movement founded by Galton—which attempted to improve the gene pool through direct intervention—seemed discredited by the genocidal programs of the Nazi regime during World War II. But perhaps most importantly, a great deal of research seemed to show that the development of creativity was contingent on a host of environmental factors (Simonton, 1987), including variables concerning birth order and family size; early traumatic experiences; the home intellectual environment; formal education and special training; geographic, ethnic, religious, or professional marginality; and the larger political, social, cultural, and economic milieu. This large inventory of developmental variables seemed to prove that nurture was supreme over nature in the appearance of creative talent and genius.

However, recently the tide has turned against this extreme environmentalist view—a turnaround due to the advent of modern behavioral genetics (Lykken, 1998), including the sophisticated analysis of monozygotic and dizygotic twins. It now appears rather likely that at least a portion of what it takes to display creativity, outstanding or otherwise, arises from our genes (Simonton, 1999b). In fact, research in behavioral genetics suggests that some so-called environmental factors might actually be genetic in their underlying causality (Plomin & Bergeman, 1991; Scarr & McCartney, 1983). There are two main ways in which genetics makes significant contributions:

1. Offspring obtain their genotypes from the parental genotypes. However, the *parental genotype is also associated with a particular parental phenotype, part of which may leave an imprint on the home environment.* For instance, highly intelligent parents will more likely have more intellectual and cultural hobbies and recreational activities. As a consequence, the home may be filled with books, magazines, art prints, and music recordings. This available stimulation may then be improperly given all of the credit for the appearance of a young genius. Yet the apparent connection may be partly or completely spurious from a causal standpoint. It is the shared genotype, not the home circumstances per se, that may be responsible for the bulk of the developmental effect.

2. Even more dramatically, we must recognize that *a person's genotype helps shape the environment in which the phenotype must emerge.* Children or adolescents are not passive receptacles (*tabula rasa*) on which events impinge; rather, these youth act upon their world, trying to make it conform more closely to their abilities and interests. They may ask their parents to provide them with music lessons, to purchase certain books or magazines, to visit science or art museums, and so forth. Indeed, there is ample anecdotal evidence that gifted children will often continue to pursue activities in the face of active parental discouragement. Blaise Pascal, who independently invented a large portion of Euclidean geometry, continued to study mathematics on his own even after his father deliberately hid books on that subject, believing that his son was slighting classical studies.

It is crucial to recognize the possibility that genes might affect the environment in a manner that sometimes is extremely subtle and therefore not easily deciphered. Take, for instance, the research suggesting that creative geniuses exhibit higher rates of orphanhood or parental loss in childhood or adolescence (e.g., Eisenstadt, 1978; Ludwig, 1995; Roe, 1953; Silverman, 1974; Walberg, Rasher, & Parkerson, 1980). This might be seen as an obvious case of a nurture effect, and this developmental influence is often so interpreted (e.g., Eisenstadt, Haynal, Rentchnick, & De Senarclens, 1989). Presumably such traumatic experiences can dramatically change the course of personality development. Nevertheless, it can be readily argued that this linkage represents a hidden genetic effect (Simonton, 1994). To provide but one such alternative interpretation, we know that the parents of geniuses tend to have gotten married later in life and to have had their offspring at later ages than is the norm (Bowerman, 1947; Ellis, 1926; Galton, 1874; Raskin, 1936). This may simply reflect the fact that highly intelligent and ambitious people tend to delay family responsibilities until they have fully established their careers. If so, then when all other factors are held constant, it could be that this phenomenon alone might account for the higher incidence of parental loss. The traumatic event itself has no developmental consequence. What does have an effect is that the young genius inherited those qualities that enable him or her to succeed in life, such as intelligence and drive.

Of course, at present we cannot say with any precision precisely the relative contributions of nature and nurture to creative development. Insofar as creativity depends on intellectual growth, then the genetic contribution should be substantial. After all, intelligence features among the highest heritability coefficients of all individual-difference variables (Plomin & Petrill, 1997). At the same time, the heritability coefficients for motives, dispositions, interests, and values are rather less prominent, genes at best accounting for only half as much variance as they account for in intellectual traits (Bouchard, 1994; Bouchard, Lykken, McGue, Segal, & Tellegen, 1990). Thus, the determination of the comparative impact of nature and nurture for creativity must depend on the determination of the relative importance of the diverse characteristics that enter into the profile of the creative person. If intelligence is the primary factor, then more than half of creativity may be ascribed to genetic influences. But if personality attributes provide the most critical components of the profile, then maybe less than a quarter of the observed individual differences may be attributed to genetic makeup.

Individual versus Situational Determinants of Creativity

Thus far we have assumed that creativity has its locus *inside* the person—that it is an individual characteristic or behavior. Not all researchers accept this viewpoint, however (e.g., Csikszentmihaly, 1990). Many sociologists and anthropologists have argued that creativity, even genius, is more a sociocultural than an individual phenomenon (e.g., White, 1949). There are two main arguments for this position, one general and the other specific.

The general argument ensues from the fact that creative genius is not evenly distributed across history and geography. Instead, exceptional creativity tends to cluster into what Kroeber (1944) called *cultural configurations*. Typically, there will exist long periods in the history of any civilization in which creative activity is virtually nil ("dark" ages), punctuated by other periods in which creativity reaches the greatest heights ("golden" and "silver" ages). The Classical Age of Greece or the Italian Renaissance are prime examples. Kroeber has documented the existence of these configurations in every civilization that has ever existed in the world, and so we cannot doubt that this is a very general phenomenon. Moreover, Kroeber and others argue from this secure fact that the creative genius is basically an epiphenomenon produced by the zeitgeist, or "spirit of the times." At best, the creators are mere spokespersons for the culture in which they live.

The specific argument concerns the curious phenomenon called *multiples* (Merton, 1961). These occur whenever two or more individuals independently, and often simultaneously, come up the exact same scientific discovery or technological invention. Classic examples include the creation of calculus by Newton and Leibnitz, the discovery of Neptune by Adams and Leverrier, the theory of evolution by natural selection by Darwin and Wallace, and the invention of the telephone by Bell and Gray. In fact, some have claimed that the number of such multiple discoveries and inventions easily runs into the hundreds, if not thousands (Merton, 1961). Furthermore, many social scientists have argued that the very occurrence of these events prove that creativity ensues from the sociocultural system, and not from the individual (e.g., Lamb & Easton, 1984). At a particular moment in the history of any creative domain, certain ideas become absolutely inevitable, and so it really makes no difference who actually makes the contribution. The new ideas are "in the air" to be picked by anyone. Indeed, some proponents of this social-deterministic account have actually argued that the discoverer or inventor does not even need to possess any special intellectual or dispositional attributes (e.g., L. White, 1949).

Needless to say, if these arguments are correct, then creativity and genius would no longer become the proper subject of psychological analysis, for creative genius would become a sociocultural process. Nonetheless, scrutiny of both arguments reveal several weaknesses that seriously undermine the thesis of sociocultural determinism (Simonton, 2004). In the case of cultural configurations, for instance, it has been shown that certain political, economic, cultural, social, and disciplinary circumstances play an important part in creative development, and thus the milieu is operating *through* creative individuals (Simonton, 2003b). An excellent example is the impact of role models on the early development of the creative genius. In the case of multiples, it is possible to construct theoretical models of the phenomenon that are based on how creativity operates within individual minds (Simonton, 2004). Not only can these psychological models explicate the same phenomenon, but in addition they lead to precise predictions that have so far withstood empirical tests. According to these alternative models, the contribution of the sociocultural milieu is limited to the provision of the necessary (but not sufficient) conditions for the emergence of certain ideas. The creative genius must do the rest.

Although recent research seems to undermine a strong form of sociocultural determinism, that is not tantamount to the claim that creativity and genius are located entirely in the individual. On the contrary, there exists ample empirical evidence that the creative person is open to all sorts of external influences that directly affect the amount and type of creativity displayed (Simonton, 2003a). Furthermore, to some extent, creativity operates as a state rather than trait variable, changing from moment to moment according to the circumstances, social and otherwise (Amabile, 1996; Paulus & Nijstad, 2003; Simonton, 2004). Indeed, this openness to extrinsic influences is what inspires many researchers to search for environmental stimuli that are the most conductive to the manifestation of creative behavior. Especially crucial are various disciplinary networks, such as collaborative and competitive relationships with colleagues in the same field (Simonton, 2004). In fact, it

is this social exchange that may be partly responsible for the clustering of creative genius into cultural configurations.

These data suggest that creativity is not just a cognitive, developmental, and personological phenomenon, but a social-psychological phenomenon as well (Simonton, 2000). Creative behavior is affected by a host of factors that reside outside the individual creator.

Empirical versus Theoretical Personality Profiles

Much of the research on the personality basis of creativity has been purely empirical in nature. Investigators have often been content with simply subjecting creative individuals to standard assessment techniques in order to determine the personality profiles that correspond with the syndrome. Nevertheless, five theoretical systems or orientations have been put forward as providing a personality basis for the phenomenon: psychoanalytic, humanistic, cognitive, economic, and evolutionary.

1. *Psychoanalytic theories.* Although far from Sigmund Freud's main focus, the founder of psychoanalysis had interests in both creativity and genius. These interests are evident in both his psychobiographical study of Leonardo da Vinci and his theory of creativity, which was rooted in primary-process thought (Freud, 1908/1959). Although Freud's ideas continue to leave an impression on scholarly inquiry, that impact now is more concentrated in the humanities than in psychological sciences (but see Gedo, 1997). Nonetheless, some modern psychologists continue to argue that the creative process depends partly on the operation of imagery akin to primary process (Martindale, 1995; Simonton, 2004; Suler, 1980). Even so, this imagery is more cognitive than psychodynamic in nature. In particular, modern thinkers do not evoke the intrusion of unconscious impulses from the "id."

2. *Humanistic theories.* Humanistic psychologists have often theorized about the significance of creativity in the constitution of the healthy human being. Creativity had a special place in Abraham Maslow's (1959, 1972) theory of the self-actualizing person, and several of the self-actualizers whom he studied were creative geniuses of

note (Maslow, 1970). However, with the minor exception of Carl Rogers's (1954) theory of creativity (see, e.g., Harrington, Block, & Block, 1987), these humanistic theories have inspired relatively little empirical research in mainstream psychology. Moreover, the proposed linkage between creativity and mental health seems to run counter to the connection between creative genius and psychopathology (but see Simonton, 2005).

3. *Cognitive theories.* For the most part, cognitive psychologists have tended to take little interest in personality factors, no matter what the phenomenon. Creativity, in particular, is often viewed as primarily, if not entirely, a matter of intellect rather than character (Weisberg, 1992). Nonetheless, researchers have greatly broadened the cognitive perspective, most notably Sternberg and Lubart (1995), who have linked creativity with both cognitive styles and various personality traits. In the reverse direction, personality researcher Eysenck (1995) has attempted to make a direct link between psychoticism and the cognitive processes underlying the creative process. Also worth note are attempts to examine creativity from the standpoint of attribution theory and social cognition (Kasof, 1995). To some undetermined extent, creativity may be more in the "eyes of the beholder," such that personality traits may lead to the attribution of creativity without participating directly in the creative process.

4. *Economic theories.* The work of Sternberg and Lubart (1995) is interesting for another reason than its integration of intellectual and dispositional variables: They have also cast their formulation in economic terms, calling it an investment theory of creativity (Sternberg & Lubart, 1991). Theirs is not the only attempt to comprehend the creative person in economic terms (e.g., Rubenson & Runco, 1992). Although these theories differ in details, economic interpretations tend to view the creative individual as someone who (a) invests in "human capital" pertaining to a particular enterprise, (b) takes exceptional risks to achieve exceptional goals, and (c) possesses the personal resources, including the optimal character, to make the risky investments pay off.

5. *Evolutionary theories.* Darwin's theory of evolution has left a major impression on the behavioral sciences, and research on creativity is no exception. In fact, the first psychologist to discuss the creative individual in Darwinian terms was William James (1880) well over a century ago. Evolutionary psychologists have used Darwinian theory to integrate the creative process with the creative person (Martindale, 1995a; Simonton, 1999a). In addition, some evolutionary psychologists have used the theory to embed both the creative individual and the creative product in the larger sociocultural context (Martindale, 1990; Simonton, 2004). One especially striking feature is that Darwinian theory has led to combinatorial models that yield precise, mathematically derived predictions (Simonton, 1997, 2004).

Although theorizing has been very active, we are still far from having in hand a universally accepted theory. Until we do, it will be impossible to know the precise causal connection between personality and creativity—or even whether a causal connection actually exits. In addition, it will always be precarious using personality inventories to assess the creative potential of individuals, until we can establish with some confidence that certain dispositional traits have a necessary empirical link with the creative process and the generation of creative products.

FUTURE PROSPECTS

It should be apparent from the foregoing discussion that research on creativity and genius has already produced an extremely rich, complex, and controversy-laden literature. It is certainly not a topic for those researchers who wish to investigate a subject where questions are easily posed and more easily answered. Indeed, it is possible that many psychologists are scared away from the field simply owing to the several methodological and theoretical difficulties it presents. Nonetheless, creativity and genius are human realities too practically important for psychologists to ignore (Sternberg & Lubart, 1996). Whether we are speaking of everyday creativity at home and work or the highly acclaimed accomplishments of creative genius, this is a phenomenon that has affected the lives of everyone and will probably continue to do so for the duration of human civilization. Therefore, it is hardly a topic that is going to languish into oblivion. That does not mean that research activity will not wax and wane as the field progresses. Such oscillations have happened in the past, and they will probably continue to do so in the future. Nevertheless, inquiries into creativity will be continually revived as new developments take place in other fields of psychological study.

I believe that this resurgence will be the case specifically in regard to research on the creative personality. Studies into the dispositional attributes of creators and geniuses have slackened considerably since their heyday in the 1970s (Feist & Runco, 1993). Nonetheless, much of this decline may merely reflect a more pervasive slump in personality research as a whole. Now that personality has recovered its vitality and mission as a substantial subdiscipline of psychology, I foresee increased attention to those personal qualities that enable individuals to exhibit creativity—even creativity that assumes the form of genius.

REFERENCES

Albert, R. S. (1975). Toward a behavioral definition of genius. *American Psychologist, 30*, 140–151.

Albert, R. S. (1994). The achievement of eminence: A longitudinal study of exceptionally gifted boys and their families. In R. F. Subotnik & K. D. Arnold (Eds.), *Beyond Terman: Contemporary longitudinal studies of giftedness and talent* (pp. 282–315). Norwood, NJ: Ablex.

Albert, R. S. (1996). Some reasons why childhood creativity often fails to make it past puberty into the real world. In M. A. Runco (Ed.), *Creativity from childhood through adulthood: The developmental issues* (pp. 43–56). San Francisco: Jossey-Bass.

Amabile, T. M. (1996). *Creativity in context.* Boulder, CO: Westview Press.

American Heritage Electronic Dictionary (3rd ed.). (1992). Boston: Houghton Mifflin.

Ansberg, P. I., & Hill, K. (2003). Creative and analytic thinkers differ in their use of attentional resources. *Personality and Individual Differences, 34*, 1141–1152.

Bachelor, P. A., & Michael, W. B. (1997). The structure-of-intellect model revisited. In M. A. Runco (Ed.), *The creativity research handbook* (Vol. 1, pp. 155–182). Cresskill, NJ: Hampton Press.

Barron, F. X. (1963). The needs for order and for disorder as motives in creative activity. In C. W. Taylor & F. X. Barron (Eds.), *Scientific creativity: Its recognition and development* (pp. 153–160). New York: Wiley.

Barron, F. X. (1969). *Creative person and creative process.* New York: Holt, Rinehart & Winston.

Barron, F. X., & Harrington, D. M. (1981). Creativity, intelligence, and personality. *Annual Review of Psychology, 32*, 439–476.

Bouchard, T. J., Jr. (1994). Genes, environment, and personality. *Science, 264*, 1700–1701.

Bouchard, T. J., Jr., Lykken, D. T., McGue, M., Segal, N. L., & Tellegen, A. (1990). Sources of human psychological differences: The Minnesota study of twins reared apart. *Science, 250*, 223–228.

Bowerman, W. G. (1947). *Studies in genius.* New York: Philosophical Library.

Carson, S., Peterson, J. B., & Higgins, D. M. (2003). Decreased latent inhibition is associated with increased creative achievement in high-functioning individuals. *Journal of Personality and Social Psychology, 85*, 499–506.

Carson, S., Peterson, J. B., & Higgins, D. M. (2005). Reliability, validity, and factor structure of the Creative Achievement Questionnaire. *Creativity Research Journal, 17*, 37–50.

Cassandro, V. J. (1998). Explaining premature mortality across fields of creative endeavor. *Journal of Personality, 66*, 805–833.

Cattell, J. M. (1903). A statistical study of eminent men. *Popular Science Monthly, 62*, 359–377.

Cattell, R. B. (1963). The personality and motivation of the researcher from measurements of contemporaries and from biography. In C. W. Taylor & F. Barron (Eds.), *Scientific creativity: Its recognition and development* (pp. 119–131). New York: Wiley.

Cattell, R. B., & Butcher, H. J. (1968). *The prediction of achievement and creativity.* Indianapolis, IN: Bobbs-Berrill.

Chambers, J. A. (1964). Relating personality and biographical factors to scientific creativity. *Psychological Monographs: General and Applied, 78*(Whole No. 584), 1–20.

Colangelo, N., & Davis, G. A. (Eds.). (2002). *Handbook of gifted education* (3rd ed.). Boston: Allyn & Bacon.

Cox, C. (1926). *The early mental traits of three hundred geniuses.* Stanford, CA: Stanford University Press.

Crutchfield, R. (1962). Conformity and creative thinking. In H. E. Gruber, G. Terrell, & M. Wertheimer (Eds.), *Contemporary approaches to creative thinking* (pp. 120–140). New York: Atherton Press.

Csikszentmihaly, M. (1990). The domain of creativity. In M. A. Runco & R. S. Albert (Eds.),

Theories of creativity (pp. 190–212). Newbury Park, CA: Sage.

Davis, G. A. (1975). In frumious pursuit of the creative person. *Journal of Creative Behavior, 9,* 75–87.

Davis, G. A. (1989). Testing for creative potential. *Contemporary Educational Psychology, 14,* 257–274.

de Candolle, A. de (1873). *Histoire des sciences et des savants depuis deux siecles* [History of the sciences and scientists in the last two centuries]. Geneva: Georg.

Dellas, M., & Gaier, E. L. (1970). Identification of creativity: The individual. *Psychological Bulletin, 73,* 55–73.

Duckworth, A. L., Peterson, C., Matthews, M. D., & Kelly, D. R. (2007). GRIT: Perseverance and passion for long-term goals. *Journal of Personality and Social Psychology, 92,* 1087–1101.

Eisenstadt, J. M. (1978). Parental loss and genius. *American Psychologist, 33,* 211–223.

Eisenstadt, J. M., Haynal, A., Rentchnick, P., & De Senarclens, P. (1989). *Parental loss and achievement.* Madison, CT: International Universities Press.

Ellis, H. (1926). *A study of British genius* (rev. ed.). Boston: Houghton Mifflin.

Eysenck, H. J. (1995). *Genius: The natural history of creativity.* Cambridge, UK: Cambridge University Press.

Farnsworth, P. R. (1969). *The social psychology of music* (2nd ed.). Ames: Iowa State University Press.

Feist, G. J. (1993). A structural model of scientific eminence. *Psychological Science, 4,* 366–371.

Feist, G. J. (1998). A meta-analysis of personality in scientific and artistic creativity. *Personality and Social Psychology Review, 2,* 290–309.

Feist, G. J., & Barron, F. X. (2003). Predicting creativity from early to late adulthood: Intellect, potential, and personality. *Journal of Research in Personality, 37,* 62–88.

Feist, G. J., & Runco, M. A. (1993). Trends in the creativity literature: An analysis of research in the *Journal of Creative Behavior* (1967–1989). *Creativity Research Journal, 6,* 271–286.

Finke, R. A., Ward, T. B., & Smith, S. M. (1992). *Creative cognition: Theory, research, applications.* Cambridge, MA: MIT Press.

Freud, S. (1959). Creative writers and daydreaming. In J. Strachey (Ed. & Trans.), *Standard edition of the complete psychological works of Sigmund Freud* (Vol. 9, pp. 141–153). London: Hogarth Press. (Original work published 1908)

Galton, F. (1869). *Hereditary genius: An inquiry into its laws and consequences.* London: Macmillan.

Galton, F. (1874). *English men of science: Their nature and nurture.* London: Macmillan.

Galton, F. (1883). *Inquiries into human faculty and its development.* London: Macmillan.

Gardner, H. (1983). *Frames of mind: A theory of multiple intelligences.* New York: Basic Books.

Gedo, J. E. (1997). Psychoanalytic theories of creativity. In M. A. Runco (Ed.), *The creativity research handbook* (Vol. 1, pp. 29–39). Cresskill, NJ: Hampton Press.

Getzels, J., & Jackson, P. W. (1962). *Creativity and intelligence: Explorations with gifted students.* New York: Wiley.

Goertzel, M. G., Goertzel, V., & Goertzel, T. G. (1978). *300 eminent personalities: A psychosocial analysis of the famous.* San Francisco: Jossey-Bass.

Gough, H. G. (1979). A creative personality scale for the adjective check list. *Journal of Personality and Social Psychology, 37,* 1398–1405.

Gough, H. G. (1992). Assessment of creative potential in psychology and the development of a creative temperament scale for the CPI. In J. C. Rosen & P. McReynolds (Eds.), *Advances in psychological assessment* (Vol. 8, pp. 225–257). New York: Plenum Press.

Gruber, H. E. (1989). The evolving systems approach to creative work. In D. B. Wallace & H. E. Gruber (Eds.), *Creative people at work: Twelve cognitive case studies* (pp. 3–24). New York: Oxford University Press.

Guilford, J. P. (1950). Creativity. *American Psychologist, 5,* 444–454.

Guilford, J. P. (1967). *The nature of human intelligence.* New York: McGraw-Hill.

Haensly, P. A., & Reynolds, C. R. (1989). Creativity and intelligence. In J. A. Glover, R. R. Ronning, & C. R. Reynolds (Eds.), *Handbook of creativity* (pp. 111–132). New York: Plenum Press.

Hargens, L. L. (1978). Relations between work habits, research technologies, and eminence in science. *Sociology of Work and Occupations, 5,* 97–112.

Harrington, D. M., Block, J. H., & Block, J. (1987). Testing aspects of Carl Rogers's theory of creative environments: Child-rearing antecedents of creative potential in young adolescents. *Journal of Personality and Social Psychology, 52,* 851–856.

Harris, J. A. (2004). Measured intelligence, achievement, openness to experience, and creativity. *Personality and Individual Differences, 36,* 913–929.

Helmreich, R. L., Spence, J. T., Beane, W. E., Lucker, G. W., & Matthews, K. A. (1980). Making it in academic psychology: Demographic and personality correlates of attainment. *Journal of Personality and Social Psychology, 39,* 896–908.

Helmreich, R. L., Spence, J. T., & Pred, R. S. (1988). Making it without losing it: Type A, achievement motivation, and scientific attainment revisited. *Personality and Social Psychology Bulletin, 14,* 495–504.

Helson, R., & Crutchfield, R. S. (1970). Mathematicians: The creative researcher and the average Ph.D. *Journal of Consulting and Clinical Psychology, 34,* 250–257.

Hollingworth, L. J. (1942). *Children beyond 180 IQ: Origin and development.* Yonkers-on-Hudson, NY: World Book.

James, W. (1880). Great men, great thoughts, and the environment. *Atlantic Monthly, 46,* 441–459.

Jamison, K. R. (1993). *Touched with fire: Manic–depressive illness and the artistic temperament.* New York: Free Press.

Kasof, J. (1995). Explaining creativity: The attributional perspective. *Creativity Research Journal, 8,* 311–366.

Kaufman, J. C. (2000–2001). Genius, lunatics and poets: Mental illness in prize-winning authors. *Imagination, Cognition, and Personality, 20,* 305–314.

Kaufman, J. C., & Sternberg, R. J. (2006). (Eds.). *International handbook of creativity research.* New York: Cambridge University Press.

Kroeber, A. L. (1944). *Configurations of culture growth.* Berkeley: University of California Press.

Kuhn, T. S. (1970). *The structure of scientific revolutions* (2nd ed.). Chicago: University of Chicago Press.

Lamb, D., & Easton, S. M. (1984). *Multiple discovery: The pattern of scientific progress.* Avebury, UK: Avebury.

Ludwig, A. M. (1992a). Creative achievement and psychopathology: Comparison among professions. *American Journal of Psychotherapy, 46,* 330–356.

Ludwig, A. M. (1992b). The Creative Achievement Scale. *Creativity Research Journal, 5,* 109–124.

Ludwig, A. M. (1995). *The price of greatness: Resolving the creativity and madness controversy.* New York: Guilford Press.

Lykken, D. T. (1998). The genetics of genius. In A. Steptoe (Ed.), *Genius and the mind: Studies of creativity and temperament in the historical record* (pp. 15–37). New York: Oxford University Press.

MacKinnon, D. W. (1978). *In search of human effectiveness.* Buffalo, NJ: Creative Education Foundation.

Martindale, C. (1990). *The clockwork muse: The predictability of artistic styles.* New York: Basic Books.

Martindale, C. (1995a). Creativity and connectionism. In S. M. Smith, T. B. Ward, & R. A. Finke (Eds.), *The creative cognition approach* (pp. 249–268). Cambridge, MA: MIT Press.

Martindale, C. (1995b). Fame more fickle than fortune: On the distribution of literary eminence. *Poetics, 23,* 219–234.

Maslow, A. H. (1959). Creativity in self-actualizing people. In H. H. Anderson (Ed.), *Creativity and its cultivation* (pp. 83–95). New York: Harper & Row.

Maslow, A. H. (1970). *Motivation and personality* (2nd ed.). New York: Harper & Row.

Maslow, A. H. (1972). A holistic approach to creativity. In C. W. Taylor (Ed.), *Climate for creativity* (pp. 287–293). New York: Pergamon Press.

Matthews, K. A., Helmreich, R. L., Beane, W. E., & Lucker, G. W. (1980). Pattern A, achievement striving, and scientific merit: Does Pattern A help or hinder? *Journal of Personality and Social Psychology, 39,* 962–967.

McCrae, R. R. (1987). Creativity, divergent thinking, and openness to experience. *Journal of Personality and Social Psychology, 52,* 1258–1265.

McCrae, R. R., Arenberg, D., & Costa, P. T., Jr. (1987). Declines in divergent thinking with age: Cross-sectional, longitudinal, and cross-sequential analyses. *Psychology and Aging, 2,* 130–136.

McFarlan, D. (Ed.). (1989). *Guinness book of world records.* New York: Bantam.

Mednick, S. A. (1962). The associative basis of the creative process. *Psychological Review, 69,* 220–232.

Mendelsohn, G. A. (1976). Associative and attentional processes in creative performance. *Journal of Personality, 44,* 341–369.

Merton, R. K. (1961). Singletons and multiples in scientific discovery: A chapter in the sociology of science. *Proceedings of the American Philosophical Society, 105,* 470–486.

Murray, C. (2003). *Human accomplishment: The pursuit of excellence in the arts and sciences, 800 b.c. to 1950.* New York: HarperCollins.

Parloff, M., Datta, L., Kleman, M., & Handlon, J. (1968). Personality characteristics which differentiate creative male adolescents and adults. *Journal of Personality, 36,* 528–552.

Paulhus, D. L., Wehr, P., Harms, P. D., & Strasser, D. I. (2002). Use of exemplar surveys to reveal implicit types of intelligence. *Personality and Social Psychology Bulletin, 28,* 1051–1062.

Paulus, P. B., & Nijstad, B. A. (Eds.). (2003). *Group creativity: Innovation through collaboration.* New York: Oxford University Press.

Peterson, J. B., & Carson, S. (2000). Latent inhibition and openness to experience in a high-achieving student population. *Personality and Individual Differences, 28,* 323–332.

Peterson, J. B., Smith, K. W., & Carson, S. (2002). Openness and extraversion are associated with reduced latent inhibition: Replication and commentary. *Personality and Individual Differences, 33,* 1137–1147.

Plomin, R., & Bergeman, C. S. (1991). The nature of nurture: Genetic influence on environmental measures. *Behavioral and Brain Sciences, 14,* 373–386.

Plomin, R., & Petrill, S. A. (1997). Genetics and intelligence: What's new? *Intelligence, 24,* 53–77.

Post, F. (1994). Creativity and psychopathology: A study of 291 world-famous men. *British Journal of Psychiatry, 165,* 22–34.

Post, F. (1996). Verbal creativity, depression and alcoholism: An investigation of one hundred American and British writers. *British Journal of Psychiatry, 168,* 545–555.

Raskin, E. A. (1936). Comparison of scientific and literary ability: A biographical study of eminent scientists and men of letters of the nineteenth century. *Journal of Abnormal and Social Psychology, 31,* 20–35.

Roe, A. (1953). *The making of a scientist.* New York: Dodd, Mead.

Rogers, C. R. (1954). Toward a theory of creativity. *ETC: A Review of General Semantics, 11,* 249–260.

Root-Bernstein, R. S., Bernstein, M., & Garnier, H. (1993). Identification of scientists making long-term, high-impact contributions, with notes on their methods of working. *Creativity Research Journal, 6,* 329–343.

Root-Bernstein, R. S., Bernstein, M., & Garnier, H. (1995). Correlations between avocations, scientific style, work habits, and professional impact of scientists. *Creativity Research Journal, 8,* 115–137.

Rosengren, K. E. (1985). Time and literary fame. *Poetics, 14,* 157–172.

Rothenberg, A. (1979). *The emerging goddess: The creative process in art, science, and other fields.* Chicago: University of Chicago Press.

Rubenson, D. L., & Runco, M. A. (1992). The psychoeconomic approach to creativity. *New Ideas in Psychology, 10,* 131–147.

Runco, M. A. (1989). The creativity of children's art. *Child Study Journal, 19,* 177–189.

Runco, M. A. (1992). Children's divergent thinking and creative ideation. *Developmental Review, 12,* 233–264.

Runco, M. A., & Charles, R. E. (1997). Developmental trends in creative potential and creative performance. In M. A. Runco (Ed.), *The creativity research handbook* (Vol. 1, pp. 115–152). Cresskill, NJ: Hampton Press.

Runco, M. A., & Pritzker, S. (Eds.). (1999). *Encyclopedia of creativity* (2 vols.). San Diego, CA: Academic Press.

Scarr, S., & McCartney, K. (1983). How people make their own environments: A theory of genotype → environmental effects. *Child Development, 54,* 424–435.

Silverman, S. M. (1974). Parental loss and scientists. *Science Studies, 4,* 259–264.

Simonton, D. K. (1976). Biographical determinants of achieved eminence: A multivariate approach to the Cox data. *Journal of Personality and Social Psychology, 33,* 218–226.

Simonton, D. K. (1977). Eminence, creativity, and geographic marginality: A recursive structural equation model. *Journal of Personality and Social Psychology, 35,* 805–816.

Simonton, D. K. (1984). *Genius, creativity, and leadership: Historiometric inquiries.* Cambridge, MA: Harvard University Press.

Simonton, D. K. (1985). Intelligence and personal influence in groups: Four nonlinear models. *Psychological Review, 92,* 532–547.

Simonton, D. K. (1987). Developmental antecedents of achieved eminence. *Annals of Child Development, 5,* 131–169.

Simonton, D. K. (1988). Age and outstanding achievement: What do we know after a century of research? *Psychological Bulletin, 104,* 251–267.

Simonton, D. K. (1989). The swan-song phenomenon: Last-works effects for 172 classical composers. *Psychology and Aging, 4,* 42–47.

Simonton, D. K. (1990). *Psychology, science, and history: An introduction to historiometry.* New Haven, CT: Yale University Press.

Simonton, D. K. (1991a). Career landmarks in science: Individual differences and interdisciplinary contrasts. *Developmental Psychology, 27,* 119–130.

Simonton, D. K. (1991b). Emergence and realization of genius: The lives and works of 120 classical composers. *Journal of Personality and Social Psychology, 61,* 829–840.

Simonton, D. K. (1991c). Latent-variable models of posthumous reputation: A quest for Galton's G. *Journal of Personality and Social Psychology, 60,* 607–619.

Simonton, D. K. (1991d). Personality correlates of exceptional personal influence: A note on Thorndike's (1950) creators and leaders. *Creativity Research Journal, 4,* 67–78.

Simonton, D. K. (1992). Leaders of American psychology, 1879–1967: Career development, creative output, and professional achievement. *Journal of Personality and Social Psychology, 62,* 5–17.

Simonton, D. K. (1994). *Greatness: Who makes history and why.* New York: Guilford Press.

Simonton, D. K. (1995). Personality and intellectual predictors of leadership. In D. H. Saklofske & M. Zeidner (Eds.), *International handbook of personality and intelligence* (pp. 739–757). New York: Plenum Press.

Simonton, D. K. (1997). Creative productivity: A predictive and explanatory model of career trajectories and landmarks. *Psychological Review, 104,* 66–89.

Simonton, D. K. (1998a). Achieved eminence in minority and majority cultures: Convergence versus divergence in the assessments of 294 African Americans. *Journal of Personality and Social Psychology, 74,* 804–817.

Simonton, D. K. (1998b). Fickle fashion versus immortal fame: Transhistorical assessments of creative products in the opera house. *Journal of Personality and Social Psychology, 75,* 198–210.

Simonton, D. K. (1999a). *Origins of genius: Darwinian perspectives on creativity.* New York: Oxford University Press.

Simonton, D. K. (1999b). Talent and its development: An emergenic and epigenetic model. *Psychological Review, 106,* 435–457.

Simonton, D. K. (2000). Creativity: Cognitive, developmental, personal, and social aspects. *American Psychologist, 55,* 151–158.

Simonton, D. K. (2003a). Creative cultures, nations, and civilizations: Strategies and results. In P. B. Paulus & B. A. Nijstad (Eds.), *Group creativity: Innovation through collaboration* (pp. 304–328). New York: Oxford University Press.

Simonton, D. K. (2003b). Creativity assessment. In R. Fernández-Ballesteros (Ed.), *Encyclopedia of psychological assessment* (Vol. 1, pp. 276–280). London: Sage.

Simonton, D. K. (2004). *Creativity in science: Chance, logic, genius, and zeitgeist.* Cambridge, UK: Cambridge University Press.

Simonton, D. K. (2005). Are genius and madness related?: Contemporary answers to an ancient question. *Psychiatric Times, 22*(7), 21–23.

Simonton, D. K. (in press). *Genius 101.* New York: Springer.

Stavridou, A., & Furnham, A. (1996). The relationship between psychoticism, trait-creativity, and the attentional mechanism of cognitive inhibition. *Personality and Individual Differences, 21,* 143–153.

Sternberg, R. J. (Ed.). (1999). *Handbook of creativity.* Cambridge, UK: Cambridge University Press.

Sternberg, R. J. (2003). *Wisdom, intelligence, and creativity synthesized.* New York: Cambridge University Press.

Sternberg, R. J., & Lubart, T. I. (1991). An investment theory of creativity and its development. *Human Development, 34,* 1–31.

Sternberg, R. J., & Lubart, T. I. (1995). *Defying the crowd: Cultivating creativity in a culture of conformity.* New York: Free Press.

Sternberg, R. J., & Lubart, T. I. (1996). Investing in creativity. *American Psychologist, 51,* 677–688.

Suler, J. R. (1980). Primary process thinking and creativity. *Psychological Bulletin, 88,* 144–165.

Sulloway, F. J. (1996). *Born to rebel: Birth order, family dynamics, and creative lives.* New York: Pantheon.

Terman, L. M. (1925). *Mental and physical traits of a thousand gifted children.* Stanford, CA: Stanford University Press.

Terman, L. M. (1954). Scientists and nonscientists in a group of 800 gifted men. *Psychological Monographs: General and Applied, 68*(Whole No. 378), 1–44.

Terman, L. M., & Oden, M. H. (1959). *The gifted group at mid-life.* Stanford, CA: Stanford University Press.

Thorndike, E. L. (1950). Traits of personality and their intercorrelations as shown in biography. *Journal of Educational Psychology, 41,* 193–216.

Walberg, H. J., Rasher, S. P., & Hase, K. (1978). Iq correlates with high eminence. *Gifted Child Quarterly, 22,* 196–200.

Walberg, H. J., Rasher, S. P., & Parkerson, J. (1980). Childhood and eminence. *Journal of Creative Behavior, 13,* 225–231.

Wallach, M. A., & Kogan, N. (1965). *Modes of thinking in young children.* New York: Holt, Rinehart & Winston.

Weisberg, R. W. (1992). *Creativity: Beyond the myth of genius.* New York: Freeman.

White, L. (1949). *The science of culture.* New York: Farrar, Straus.

White, R. K. (1931). The versatility of genius. *Journal of Social Psychology, 2,* 460–489.

Winner, E. (1996). *Gifted children: Myths and realities.* New York: Basic Books.

Woods, F. A. (1911). Historiometry as an exact science. *Science, 33,* 568–574.

PART VII
Emotion, Adjustment, and Health

CHAPTER 28

Emotion and Emotion Regulation

Personality Processes and Individual Differences

James J. Gross

William James argued that emotions are central to our psychological economy. Without emotions, he said, "No one portion of the universe would then have importance beyond another; and the whole character of its things and series of its events would be without significance, character, expression, or perspective" (1902, p. 150). What an empty life that would be! We'd feel no love when we saw our children; no sadness when we botched an important job interview; no amusement when a friend regaled us with stories of collegiate misdeeds; and no embarrassment when we used the wrong name in addressing a colleague. Our once-colorful world would be bleached a dull, lifeless gray. We'd drift along aimlessly, under slack sails, bereft of the impulses that motivate and direct our everyday pursuits.

In the past few decades, researchers from a variety of disciplines have begun to examine emotion and emotion-related processes in growing numbers (Gross, 1999). These disciplines include psychology, neuroscience, biology, ethology, anthropology, sociology, psychiatry, philosophy, computer science, economics, linguistics, and history. Findings have begun to accumulate: Each week brings journals with new findings on emotion, each month brings new books on emotion, and each year brings new journals focused primarily on emotion. It is now clearer than ever before that emotions are complex multicomponential processes, at once biologically based and socially constructed. Given the interdisciplinary nature of emotion research, however, relatively few psychologists have had formal training in the topic. Fewer still have the luxury of keeping abreast of the burgeoning literature on emotion.

What is needed is a basic framework for organizing the growing number of findings. My aim in this chapter is to provide such a framework. My particular goal is to provide a conceptual map and readable introduction useful to researchers interested in personality processes and individual differences. In the first section, I consider what emotion is and describe what I refer to as the "modal model" of emotion. In the second section, I use this model to organize my selective review of research on basic emotional processes and related individual differences. In the third section, I describe a process model of emotion regulation. In the fourth section, I use this process model to organize my selective review of research on personality processes and individual differences related to emotion regulation. Throughout this chapter, my strategy is to first focus on basic emotional processes and then to discuss individual differences in these emotional processes.

EMOTION

Approaches, Definitions, and the "Modal Model"

Approaches to Emotion

In his *Origin of Species*, Darwin (1859/1962) argued that "instincts are as important as corporeal structures for the welfare of each species, under its present conditions of life ... and if it can be shown that instincts do vary ever so little, then I can see no difficulty in natural selection preserving and continually accumulating variations of instinct to any extent that was profitable" (p. 245). Darwin's views powerfully influenced the earliest psychologists. William James (1884) wrote that "the nervous system of every living thing is but a bundle of predispositions to react in particular ways upon the contact of particular features of the environment." (p. 190). McDougal (1923) asserted that humans have 13 instincts (e.g., parenting, food seeking, repulsion, curiosity, gregariousness), and defined emotion as "a mode of experience which accompanies the working within us of instinctive impulses" (p. 128).

The vagueness of the notion of instinct and the absence of criteria with which to verify the correctness of statements concerning instincts soon made scientists worry. To combat "the erroneous belief that one can approach the problem of instinctive behavior patterns with non-inductive methods and pronounce upon 'instinct' without defined experiments," Lorenz (1937/1970, p. 259) and other early ethologists used careful observation and rigorous deprivation experiments. Rather than the murky concept of instinct, they spoke of *fixed action patterns* (FAPs). These patterns, as Eibl-Eibesfelt (1975) put it, refer to the fact that "in the behavioral repertoire of an animal one encounters recognizable and therefore 'form-constant' movements that do not have to be learned by the animal and provide, like morphological characteristics, distinguishing features of a species" (p. 16).

Psychologists who were impressed by the continuity between human and nonhu-man emotions—as Darwin had been—soon made use of the notion of FAPs. For example, Tomkins (1962) spoke of an "affect program." Plutchik (1962) saw emotions as biologically based adaptive behavior patterns. Ekman (1972) drew upon the notion of an FAP in his "facial affect program." At the same time, however, many took pains to emphasize that in the case of human emotion, the link between releaser and response was probabilistic, not certain. Scherer (1984) made this point when he described emotion as a "decoupled reflex." Most also distanced themselves from the stereotypy implied by the notion of an FAP. Frijda (1986) emphasized that "to the extent that action programs are fixed and rigid, the concept of action tendency loses much of its meaning. ... To the extent that the program is flexible, however, action tendency, and action readiness generally, become meaningful concepts. Flexible programs are those that are composed of alternative courses of action, that allow for variations in circumstances and for feedback from actions executed" (p. 83). Lazarus (1991a) similarly stressed response flexibility, arguing that "in more advanced species, especially humans, through evolution, hardwired affect programs have given way to a complex and flexible process" (p. 198).

Others distanced themselves considerably further from the early ethologists' notion of an FAP. Although such theorists acknowledged that emotions have biological (and evolutionary) bases, they saw emotions as arising more from social than from biological factors and were concerned with the functions emotions serve in a particular context (Averill, 1980). Some theorists of this ilk— the social constructivists—took a cultural perspective and focused on the processes by which particular cultures define and shape the emotions of its members (Armon-Jones, 1986; Harre, 1986; Markus & Kitayama, 1991; Mesquita & Albert, 2007). Others— psychological constructivists—emphasized how evolutionarily based biological responses (which they referred to as core affect, or feelings of goodness or badness and activation or quiescence) are translated in a given individual into specific emotional responses via the retrieval of semantic knowledge that links these changes in core affect to the particular features of the local environment (Barrett, 2006b; Russell, 2003). It should be noted that appearances (and rhetoric) notwithstanding, there is no inherent conflict between evolutionary accounts (which draw attention to biological bases and evolutionary functions) and constructivist accounts (which draw attention to cultural bases and social functions) (Sabini & Schulkin, 1994).

Defining Emotion

As we have seen, emotion theorists differ in their relative emphasis on biological givens versus culture- and individual-specific learning and practices. Despite these differences, many theorists share a conception of emotion in which three features are emphasized.[1]

The first feature has to do with *what gives rise to emotions*. Emotions arise when an individual attends to a situation and understands it as being relevant to his or her current goals (Armon-Jones, 1986; Clore & Ortony, 1998; Lazarus, 1991a). These goals may be biologically based (e.g., to expel a noxious substance) or culturally derived (e.g., to honor one's elders). Whatever the goal may be, and whatever the situation means to the individual, it is this meaning in relation to a goal that gives rise to emotion. As either the goal or the situation's meaning change over time, the emotion will also change.

The second feature has to do with *what makes up an emotion*. Emotions are multifaceted, embodied phenomena that involve loosely coupled changes in the domains of *subjective experience*, *behavior*, and *peripheral physiology* (Mauss, Levenson, McCarter, Wilhelm, & Gross, 2005). The experiential aspect of emotion refers to what it feels like from a first-person perspective as an emotion unfolds. The behavioral aspect refers to the fact that emotions often either increase or decrease the likelihood that we will do something (e.g., approach others or burst into tears) (Frijda, 1986). The peripheral physiological aspect refers to the fact that the impulses to act in certain ways (and not act in others) are associated with autonomic and neuroendocrine changes that both anticipate the associated behavioral responses (thereby providing metabolic support for the action) and follow it, often as a consequence of the motor activity associated with the emotional response. One crucial—and much debated—question is just how tightly coupled changes in various response modalities are (Barrett,

2006a). Unfortunately, evidence on response coherence is quite limited. What evidence is available to date suggests a rather modest degree of coupling among response systems (Mauss et al., 2005), but it is not yet well understood what contextual and personal factors moderate the level of response coherence.

The third feature has to do with the *malleability* of emotion. Emotions frequently interrupt what we are doing and lead us to think, feel, and behave differently than we otherwise might have (Frijda, 1986; Simon, 1967). However, emotions compete with other responses occasioned by our goals and the situations we are in, and do not automatically trump other possible responses. This means that emotions can be, and often are, modified as they arise and then play themselves out. The malleability of emotion has been emphasized since William James (1884), who viewed emotions as response tendencies that may be modulated in a large number of ways. It is this third aspect of emotion that forms the basis for our ability to regulate our emotions, to which we turn in the second half of this chapter.

The "Modal Model" of Emotion

These three features of emotion are emphasized in many different theories of emotion (e.g., Arnold, 1960; Buck, 1985; Ekman, 1972; Frijda, 1986; Izard, 1977; Lazarus, 1991a; Levenson, 1994; Plutchik, 1962; Scherer, 1984; Tomkins, 1962). I view them as constituting what might be called a consensual or "modal" model of emotion (Barrett, Ochsner, & Gross, 2006; Gross, 1998a; Gross & Thompson, 2007). According to this *modal model*, emotions arise in the context of a person–situation transaction that compels attention, has a particular meaning to the individual, and gives rise to a coordinated yet malleable multisystem response to the ongoing person–situation transaction.

In Figure 28.1, I present the situation–attention–appraisal–response sequence specified by the modal model. This sequence begins with a situation that is attended to in various ways, which gives rise to appraisals; that is, assessments (among other things) of the situation's familiarity, valence, and value relevance (Ellsworth & Scherer, 2003). These appraisals, in turn, give rise to emotion re-

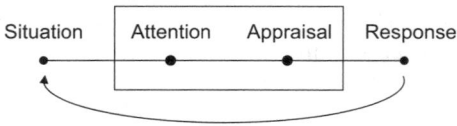

FIGURE 28.1. The "modal model" of emotion. From Gross and Thompson (2007). Copyright 2007 by The Guilford Press. Reprinted by permission.

sponse tendencies, ranging from tiny pangs of guilt, to full-scale outbursts of emotion rich with vivid emotion experience, behavioral displays, and a whole host of powerful physiological changes. Because these responses often change the situation that gave rise to the response in the first place, the model has an arrow to indicate the response feeding back to (and modifying) the situation.

Basic Processes and Individual Differences

Using the modal model as an organizing framework, in the following sections I selectively review the literature on basic emotional processes and related individual differences.

Situations

William James (1884) likened emotional responses to the turning of a key in a lock. This analogy implies that emotions are a direct— almost unmediated—response to certain events. Even today, this perspective still has currency. For example, Buck (1985) argued that internal and external emotion-eliciting stimuli impinge on the emotion system directly and without cognitive mediation. This "direct view" suggests that it should be possible to provide descriptions of the objective situations that lead to particular emotions. However, given the flexibility of input– output relations that characterizes human emotions, descriptions of antecedent conditions for specific emotions in everyday life have been largely anecdotal. Lists such as the one offered by Ellsworth (1994) are typical: "loss of support or sense of direction, separation from a mother, sudden intense noises, abrupt movements, caresses, and secondary sexual characteristics" (p. 151). As Ellsworth admits, "the actual research record is quite thin" (p. 151).

In one empirical study of emotion antecedents, Scherer, Summerfield, and Wallbott (1983) asked students to recall events that elicited joy, sadness, anger, and fear. Subjects then described these events, and raters coded subjects' descriptions of the antecedents of their emotions. General categories were derived inductively, including news (good or bad), relationships, success/self-esteem, experiences (pleasant or unpleasant), material objects (gain or loss), organic tissue (well or damaged), among others. News was important to none of the emotions, whereas success/self-esteem was important to all. Categories that discriminated among emotions included the relationship category (important to all emotions but fear), experiences (important to joy and fear but not sadness or anger), material objects (prominent in anger), and organic tissue (important to fear). When described at this level of abstraction, however, these antecedents are a far cry from the direct triggers called to mind by James's (1884) lock-and-key analogy.

Another approach to the study of emotion antecedents has been taken in the clinical domain. In these studies, researchers examine individual differences in emotion by focusing on the situations to which a person has been (or is being) exposed. This *life-events* tradition employs a semistructured interview such as the Life Events and Difficulties Schedule to rate the stressfulness of present or past situations (Brown, 2000). Research from this tradition is concerned with the likely meaning of a situation as rated not by the individual him- or herself, but rather by a set of knowledgeable raters. Although it is acknowledged that what a situation means to a particular person is crucial, these meanings are derived through an analysis of the environmental context itself, not via self-reports of internal states.

When assessing the impact of the environment, one complexity is captured by the notion of *evocative transactions*, which refers to the fact that individuals differ in the responses they evoke from others (Caspi & Roberts, 1999). That is, each individual is a stimulus to which others respond, and in that sense, each person brings an important part of the situation wherever he or she may go. In one study, for example, depressed women did not differ from nondepressed individuals in the levels of objective stress and adversity they encountered, but they did differ in the frequency of dependent interpersonal events—stressful interpersonal interactions that were created, at least in part, by the depressed individuals themselves (Hammen, 1991). In a similar vein, Bolger and Schilling (1991) used daily diaries to track stressors in a sample of married subjects. They found that subjects who scored higher in neuroticism had more arguments with spouses and others than subjects who scored low in neuroticism. Even within similar environments, then, evocative interaction patterns lead to importantly different emotion antecedents, and hence individual differences in emotional responding.

In recent years, exciting new developments have emerged in the study of how individual differences emerge as a function of the environments in which people are living. These developments have focused on person × environment interactions. Sometimes person variables are psychological, such as low self-esteem. In one such study, Brown and colleagues showed that severe life events were twice as likely to be followed by a depressive episode in individuals with low as compared to high self-esteem (Brown, Andrews, Harris, Adler, & Bridge, 1986). In other studies, the relevant person variables are biological. One example is provided by Caspi and colleagues (2003), who asked why stressful life experiences lead to psychopathology in some individuals but not in other individuals. To address this question, Caspi and colleagues used a prospective design to study individuals who differed in serotonin transporter genes and had either two short alleles, one short and one long allele, or two long alleles. They found that compared to individuals with two long alleles, individuals with one or two copies of the short allele showed more depressive symptoms, clinical cases of depression, and suicidality when they had experienced significant life stress (see also Canli, Chapter 11, this volume). Importantly, these genetic and environmental effects do not seem to be additive, but are rather interactive. As Kendler and Prescott (2006) put it, there seems to be genetic control over sensitivity to the stressful features of the environment, such that some individuals (those who have genetic diatheses) appear to suffer greater harm from stressful environments than those without such diatheses.

Attention

According to the modal model, *potentially* upsetting or delightful situations are only *actually* upsetting or delightful if attention is directed to relevant aspects of the situation. In this sense, attention is the gateway to emotion. However, this way of putting it misses half of the story because even as attention enables emotion, emotion in turn shapes attention. This bidirectional and mutually reinforcing interplay between emotion and attention is currently a major focus of investigation (Phelps, 2006).

Scherer (1994) has suggested that individuals continually scan their internal and external environments looking for "news," much as a radar operator in an air control tower might scan for incoming airplanes. This scanning process is well illustrated by the "cocktail party effect," in which an emotionally significant stimulus (e.g., a person's name) is registered and then attended to even though the person was initially otherwise engaged (Cherry, 1953). The finding that potentially significant aspects of the environment are automatically registered and then are attended to—as time permits—has been replicated in many different contexts. Although both negative and positive information may be "newsworthy" in this sense, researchers generally have focused on potentially threatening stimuli that are relevant to universal and highly valued goals such as individual survival (e.g., Ohman & Mineka, 2001).

Importantly, even as attention permits emotion to begin to unfold, emotion modulates the attentional focus on potentially significant aspects of the environment (Niedenthal & Kitayama, 1994). Thus, in the case of a potential threat, attention facilitates processing of information related to the threat, and this potentiates a negative emotional response. This negative emotional response, in turn, increases attentional focus toward the potential threat, leading to further enhancements in information processing, and hence to increased negative emotional responding. This interplay between attention and emotion may be understood in functional terms. When something important to the individual is at stake, attention is directed toward potentially significant aspects of the environment, and if these aspects of the environment are seen as relevant and important (leading emotion to arise), additional processing resources are dedicated to the environment as the individual works out what is happening and how to best respond. It appears that the amygdala may mediate this facilitation of attention by emotion (Phelps, 2006), and the links between attention and emotion have been cleverly captured in a number of laboratory studies. For example, A. K. Anderson and Phelps (2001) have shown that (1) healthy participants demonstrate enhanced attention for negatively valenced stimuli relative to neutral stimuli, but (2) individuals with left-amygdalar lesions do not show this attentional enhancement for negatively valenced material.

As soon as a potentially significant event is registered and attended to, the individual is likely to interrupt ongoing behavior (Simon, 1967) and begin to mount a response aimed at effectively managing the threat or opportunity presented by the situation. A number of early-appearing responses have been described, including orienting responses, startle responses, and defensive responses (Cook & Turpin, 1997). Historically, these early-appearing responses are seen as falling outside the realm of emotional responding per se (Ekman, Friesen, & Simons, 1985). Emotion researchers typically have focused on the later-appearing and more flexible response tendencies that support more generalized approach or withdrawal behavior (Lang, 1995). These behavioral tendencies may be indexed using electromyography (EMG; e.g., Cacioppo, Berntson, Larsen, Poehlmann, & Ito, 2000) or by electroencephalography (EEG; e.g., Harmon-Jones, 2003).

So far, I have considered features of the attention–emotion relationship that are thought to be widely shared. However, there is evidence that individual differences are both present and important in these processes. Studies of individual differences in attentional processes that have bearing on emotion have focused primarily on the role of attentional biases in mood and anxiety disorders. For example, individuals with high versus low levels of anxiety are quicker to direct their attention to threatening stimuli (MacLeod, Mathews, & Tata, 1986; Mogg & Bradley, 1999). This effect is clearest early in information processing (i.e., when stimuli

are presented very briefly; see Mogg & Bradley, 2006).

Appraisal

With respect to the appraisal step in the modal model, a number of appraisal theorists have offered lists of meaning dimensions (for a review, see Scherer, Schorr, & Johnstone, 2001). For example, Ellsworth (1994) reported six meaning dimensions: novelty (Is this relevant?), valence (Is this good or bad?), certainty (How sure can I be about novelty or valence?), control (Can I handle this?), agency (Who or what caused this?), and norm–self-concept compatibility (Does this meet my own or the group's goals?). The earliest of these appraisals refers to the initial steps of registration and attention described above, whereas the later appraisals involve more elaborated meaning analysis of the unfolding situation. The basic logic of this approach is captured by Frijda's (1988) Law of Apparent Reality: "Emotions are elicited by events appraised as real, and their intensity corresponds to the degree to which this is the case" (p. 352). Even situations that are patently artificial (e.g., a film or a play) can arouse emotions as long as the individual sees them as meaningful (see Frijda, 1989, for a discussion of aesthetic emotions; see Rottenberg, Ray, and Gross, 2007, for film clips that elicit discrete emotions).

Individual differences in interpretations of situations powerfully shape emotional responses. *Reactive transactions* refer to individual differences in how the same environment is interpreted and experienced (Caspi & Roberts, 1999). In Figure 28.1, this notion moves us from a consideration of objective stimuli to the evaluations we make of these stimuli. Cognitive therapists such as Ellis, Beck, and Seligman have long emphasized the role of such evaluations in creating individual differences in emotional responding. Although they have emphasized the extremes of anxiety and depression, the logic of their analysis applies with equal force to normal variation in emotion. For example, aggressive children frequently expect others to be aggressive, and may read hostile intent into neutral behaviors of others (Dodge, 1991). At the other extreme, optimists see good news in neutral or ambiguous situations (Scheier & Carver, 1985). These differences in evaluation matter. For example, Aspinwall and Taylor (1992) found that optimistic undergraduates had lower levels of distress during their freshman year than did less optimistic classmates. In a study of dating couples, Srivastava, McGonigal, Richards, Butler, and Gross (2006) found that both optimists and their partners indicated greater relationship satisfaction, and when discussing a conflict, optimists and their partners saw each other as engaging more constructively during the conflict, which in turn led both partners to feel that the conflict was better resolved 1 week later. In a 1-year follow-up, men's optimism predicted relationship status: 75% of couples with men at or above the median were still together at 1 year, contrasted with 54% of couples with men below the median.

Emotional Responses

Like many others before me, I find it useful to distinguish among three major response domains: emotion experience, emotion-expressive behavior, and emotion physiology.[2]

EMOTION EXPERIENCE

Despite its importance, surprisingly little is known about the psychological and biological underpinnings of emotion experience (Barrett, Mesquita, Ochsner, & Gross, 2007). In part, this gap is due to the field's suspicion regarding phenomenological accounts of mental processes. How, then, has research been done on emotion experience? Contemplating the awesome range of emotion experience, researchers generally have taken one of two approaches. The first approach is to examine specific categories of emotion experience. Proponents of this categorical approach give emotions such as sadness, fear, or anger their own chapter headings and describe the phenomenology of each (e.g., Lazarus, 1991a). The second approach is to examine broader dimensions of emotion experience that these categories share. Two dimensions emerge reliably, with emotions arrayed along the circle formed by these two dimensions, labeled variously as pleasantness and activation (Larsen & Diener, 1992; Russell, 1980; Russell & Barrett, 1999) or positive and negative activation (Cacioppo,

Gardner, & Bernston, 1999; Watson, Wiese, Vaidya, & Tellegen, 1999).

From a categorical perspective, a number of questionnaires assess individual differences in the experience of specific emotions such as anxiety (J. A. Taylor, 1953) and anger (Spielberger & Sydeman, 1994). There also are omnibus inventories designed to assess multiple emotions, such as the Differential Emotions Scale (Izard, Libero, Putnam, & Haynes, 1993), the Multiple Affect Adjective Checklist (Zuckerman & Lubin, 1985), the Positive and Negative Affect Schedule—Expanded Form (PANAS-X; Watson & Clark, 1994), and the Profile of Mood States (McNair, Lorr, & Droppleman, 1971). Researchers have used these measures to document stable individual differences in the experience of specific emotions. Another approach is to assess individual differences not in the experience of any particular emotion, but rather in the nature of emotion experience itself. For example, using the Levels of Emotional Awareness Scale, Lane and colleagues have measured individual differences in the complexity of emotion labels given to feelings associated with particular (hypothetical) situations (Lane, Quinlan, Schwartz, Walker, & Zeitlin, 1990). At the one extreme are alexithymics (G. J. Taylor, Bagby, & Parker, 1997), who experience negative affect but have little capacity to identify and describe their feelings. At the other extreme are individuals who show high levels of emotional awareness, as evidenced by their capacity to appreciate and describe complex blends of emotions.

From a dimensional perspective, Watson and colleagues' Positive and Negative Affect Schedule (PANAS; Watson, Clark, & Tellegen, 1988) assesses individual differences in positive and negative activated affect. Another approach is to examine the relative weight that individuals give to each dimension of emotion experience when describing their experience. Feldman (1995; Barrett 1998, 2004) has explored individual differences in the use of the dimensions of pleasantness and activation in describing emotion experience. Virtually all subjects used the pleasantness dimension, but they differed in the degree to which they used the activation dimension. For some individuals, emotion experience was essentially the difference between "good" and "bad" (a flattened circle).

Others made more fine-grained distinctions among their emotion experiences (a fully developed version of the emotion circumplex).

The dimensional perspective brings into focus the structural similarities between emotion and personality (Meyer & Shack, 1989). In particular, the dimensional perspective suggests a mapping between the dimension of negative emotion and neuroticism, and between the dimension of positive emotion and extraversion. These links have been born out in several studies (e.g., Emmons & Diener, 1985; Tellegen, 1985; Watson & Clark, 1984, 1992; Watson et al., 1999; for a discrete emotions perspective, see Gross, Sutton, & Ketelaar, 1998; Izard et al., 1993). For example, Costa and McCrae (1980) found that neuroticism predicted negative affect in everyday life, whereas extraversion predicted positive affect; these relations held over even a 10-year period. On the basis of these relations, McCrae and Costa (1991) have proposed that neuroticism and extraversion represent temperamental personality dimensions that predispose individuals to negative and positive emotions, respectively.

BEHAVIORAL RESPONSES

Behavioral responses in emotion can be verbal or nonverbal. Verbal behavior refers to what we say, for instance, when we are angry. Some of the speech content involves descriptions of feeling states (e.g., "I'm angry"). Other speech content taps into shared metaphors commonly used to describe emotional states (Lakoff, 1987), including heat (e.g., "I'm hot-headed") and explosions (e.g., "I'm so angry I could explode"). In addition to semantic content, verbal behavior also includes *how* we say what we say (e.g., loudly vs. softly). Research has shown that alterations in fundamental frequency—which relate to level of sympathetic activation—represent one dimension of vocal responding (Scherer, 1986); the voice also may contain information about specific emotions (Johnstone & Scherer, 2000; Scherer & Wallbott, 1994).

Emotional responses can also be nonverbal. One particularly salient form of nonverbal behavior is emotion-expressive facial behavior, which results from the contractions of facial muscles that move the overlying skin and connective tissue (Rinn, 1984). One point of debate has been whether dif-

ferent emotions are reliably associated with different facial expressions. To address this question, researchers have examined whether naive participants can reliably identify posed expressions thought to be associated with different emotions with greater than chance accuracy. There is evidence for greater than chance recognition for anger, disgust, fear, happiness, pride, sadness, and surprise (Ekman, 1994; Izard, 1994; Keltner & Ekman, 2000; Russell, 1994; Tracy & Robins, 2004). What is less clear, however, is whether everyday emotions are typically associated with distinct emotion-expressive behavior. Despite the commonsense appeal of this idea, the evidence for this proposition is surprisingly sparse.

Personality psychologists have long been concerned with individual differences in expressive behavior (Allport & Vernon, 1933). One approach to quantifying expressive behavior is to use global ratings, either of specific emotions (e.g., amusement, disgust) or broad dimensions (e.g., pleasantness, intensity). With a modest amount of training, coders reliably make such global judgments (e.g., Gross & Levenson, 1993; Kring, Smith, & Neale, 1994). To allow greater precision in describing facial expressive behavior, Ekman and Friesen (1978) developed the Facial Action Coding System (FACS). This anatomically based coding system specifies 44 distinct facial movements ("action units"), which are then combined (via a "code book") into inferences about emotional responses (for a review of studies using FACS, see Ekman & Rosenberg, 1997). A third approach is to measure facial behavior using facial electromyography (EMG; e.g., Cacioppo, Martzke, Petty, & Tassinary, 1988). This approach has the advantage of continuous measurement. EMG sensors also can register activity that is too weak to produce visible movements of facial muscles.

Self-report measures of emotional expressivity also have been developed. Initial measures were unidimensional (e.g., Friedman, Prince, Riggio, & DiMatteo, 1980; Kring et al., 1994), but more recent measures have emphasized the multifaceted nature of emotional expressivity (Gross & John, 1997, 1998). In our work, for example, we have found that three correlated facets consistently emerge in both self-reports and peer ratings of expressivity, namely Positive Expressivity,

Negative Expressivity, and Impulse Strength (conceptualized as the strength of the emotional impulses). These facets differentially predict criterion measures: Positive Expressivity predicts amusement expressions such as laughing (but not sadness expressions), and Negative Expressivity predicts sadness expressions such as crying (but not amusement expressions). These findings suggest the need for a hierarchical model, in which specific expressivity facets are subsumed under a more general expressivity factor (Gross & John, 1997).

PHYSIOLOGICAL RESPONSES

When we are emotional, our bodies respond: We sweat, our hearts pound, and we breathe more quickly. In William James's famous thought experiment regarding emotion, he suggested that "if we fancy some strong emotion, and then try to abstract from our consciousness of it all the feelings of its characteristic bodily symptoms, we find we have nothing left behind, no 'mind-stuff' out of which the emotion can be constituted, and that a cold and neutral state of intellectual perception is all that remains" (James, 1884, p. 193). James's view that different emotions are associated with different patterns of autonomic and somatic responses accords well with common sense. When we are angry, it seems quite clear that our body is reacting very differently from when we are happy, sad, or in a relatively neutral state (Levenson, 1994).

Surprisingly, empirical findings have not provided strong support for this commonsensical view. Levenson (1992) reported that despite decades of research, only a modest number of distinctions among emotions seemed well-supported, including (1) heart rate acceleration during anger, (2) heart rate acceleration during fear, (3) heart rate acceleration during sadness, (4) heart rate deceleration during disgust, and (5) greater peripheral vasoconstriction in fear than anger. Cacioppo and colleagues (2000) concluded that "the results are far from definitive regarding emotion-specific autonomic patterning" (p. 180) and presented a model in which afferent feedback was frequently undifferentiated and yet was perceived as being highly patterned. Although Cacioppo and colleagues did not rule out the existence

of specific autonomic responses in emotion, they found stronger evidence for general approach- or withdrawal-related physiological responses than for emotion-specific responses. Gray (1994) went further, arguing that the autonomic and endocrine systems were "the *wrong* places to look" for emotion specificity because these systems are concerned with housekeeping functions that bear no clear relation to specific emotions (p. 243).

If peripheral systems are the wrong place to look for evidence of emotion specificity, where should we look? The answer for many has been the brain. More than 60 years ago, Papez (1937) proposed that emotions arise in a circuit that involves the hypothalamus, anterior thalamus, cingulate, and hippocampus. Over the next few decades, MacLean (1949, 1975, 1990) added additional brain regions to the Papez model, including the amygdala, prefrontal cortex, and septal nuclei. MacLean called this phylogenetically old circuit the *limbic system*, and this term has gained wide popularity. However, because there are no clear criteria for deciding what is part of this system, the list of brain regions associated with the limbic system has continued to grow without an end in sight. This uncontrolled growth has led to the consensus that "the concept suffers from imprecision at both the structural and functional levels" (LeDoux, 1993, p. 109), and hence may have outlived its usefulness.

To increase precision in the analysis of brain regions subserving emotion, neuroscience tools developed for research on cognitive processes have been used to study emotion. This approach has led to the emergence of the field of affective neuroscience (Davidson & Sutton, 1995; Panksepp, 1991). Based largely on animal models, affective neuroscientists have argued that emotions arise not in one but in multiple neural circuits (e.g., Gray, 1994; Panksepp, 1998). For example, Panksepp (1991) has suggested that "the brain appears to contain a number of functionally and anatomically distinct emotional circuits" for emotions such as separation distress, fear, rage, curiosity, and play (p. 63).

The advent of noninvasive neuroimaging techniques in the past few decades has permitted affective neuroscientists to test these claims, and several meta-analyses of these studies have been conducted (Murphy, Nimmo-Smith, & Lawrence, 2003; Phan,

Wager, Taylor, & Liberzon, 2002). Results of these meta-analyses suggest that some brain regions are activated in virtually all emotions—for example, the medial prefrontal cortex. One likely possibility is that this section of the brain plays a general role in attention and appraisal related to emotion. Other brain regions, however, seem to be preferentially related to specific emotions. For example, fear is often associated with amygdalar activation, and sadness is often associated with activation of the cingulate cortex, just below the corpus callosum (although it should be noted that activation in these brain regions is by no means specific to these emotions; see Barrett & Wager, 2006). As with the peripheral findings, the evidence for discrete circuits at present is not strong.

Individual differences are evident in neural systems involved in emotional responding. Thus, extraversion has been associated with greater responsivity in a distributed set of dopaminergically innervated brain regions, including the nucleus accumbens and amygdala (Cohen, Young, Baek, Kessler, & Ranganath, 2005; Depue & Collins, 1999; Knutson & Bhanji, 2006). Work by Canli and colleagues also has implicated the amygdala: In a series of studies, these researchers found that extraverts responded more strongly in the amygdala to both smiling faces and positive pictures (Canli et al., 2001; Canli, Sivers, Whitfield, Gotlib, & Gabrieli, 2002).

One point of particular focus in research on individual differences in physiological responses in emotion has been the primarily subcortical amygdala-related circuits implicated in fear conditioning. Kagan and Snidman (1991) have championed the notion that individual differences in the amygdalar circuit give rise to individual differences in inhibition—which they operationalize as fear proneness and a hesitation to approach novel stimuli. As they put it: "One of our major assumptions is that inhibited children, and by inference high-motor-high-cry infants, have a low threshold of reactivity in the central nucleus of the amygdala and its projections to the hypothalamus, sympathetic chain, and cardiovascular system" (p. 859). Kagan and colleagues tested this hypothesis in a functional magnetic resonance imaging (fMRI) study of young adults who had been classified when they were infants as either inhibited or uninhibited (Schwartz, Wright, Shin,

Kagan, & Rauch, 2003). These participants viewed a series of familiar and unfamiliar faces. As Kagan had predicted, when the inhibited participants viewed unfamiliar faces, their amygdalas showed higher levels of activation than did the amygdalas of uninhibited participants. The two groups did not differ, however, when they were viewing familiar faces, suggesting that it was the newness of the faces that led the inhibited individuals' amygdalas to respond more strongly than did the uninhibited individuals

EMOTION REGULATION

Approaches, Definitions, and a Process Model

As we have seen, the modal model holds that emotions arise when a person attends to and evaluates a situation in ways that lead to a coordinated set of experiential, behavioral, and physiological responses. Because emotion-related attentional and appraisal processes typically operate outside of awareness, emotions seem to come and go of their own accord. However, on closer inspection, emotions are often actively managed (or mismanaged). The topic of emotion regulation is a relatively late addition to the field of emotion, but a concern with emotion regulation is anything but new. Indeed, emotion regulation has been a focus in the study of psychological defenses (Freud, 1926/1959), stress and coping (Lazarus, 1966), attachment (Bowlby, 1969), and self-regulation (Mischel, Shoda, & Rodriguez, 1989). What is new is the theoretical and empirical advances that have been made in recent years, thanks to a dramatic increase in attention to this topic (Gross, 2007). One sign of this increased attention is the over 150-fold increase in citations containing the phrase "emotion regulation" (from 4 to 651) from 1990 to 2005.

Approaches to Emotion Regulation

From an evolutionary perspective, emotions represent the "wisdom of the ages" (Lazarus, 1991b, p. 820), prompting us to respond in ways that have been proven advantageous over the millennia. One apparent embarrassment for this evolutionary perspective, however, is the degree to which emotions seem to be *unhelpful* in our everyday efforts to meet the challenges posed by the world around us.

With alarming regularity, it seems, we have to ignore or even override our emotions in order to perform well during a challenging test or avoid a nasty blowup with a colleague.

Evolutionary accounts address the need for emotion regulation by conceiving of emotions as "decoupled reflexes" (Scherer, 1984). On this view, one of the most important adaptive properties of emotions is the degree to which they are (usually) advisory rather than obligatory. This advisory property is thought to stem from the fact that we humans have inherited much of the subcortical emotion-generative machinery with which other mammals have been endowed. What distinguishes humans, on this view, is the degree to which emotions can be regulated by top-down influences from the neocortex. This conception has led to a concerted effort to discern the biological bases of emotion regulation (e.g., Ochsner & Gross, 2005), with a view to better understanding the mechanisms that permit emotions to be up- and down-regulated.

Other approaches to emotion regulation focus more directly on its social and cognitive aspects. Emotion regulation typically occurs in social contexts (Gross, Richards, & John, 2006), and these contexts are powerfully shaped by larger societal forces. Among other things, cultures differentially support different emotions (Mesquita & Albert, 2007; Plutchik, 1994). For example, in individualistic cultural contexts, people generally seek out high-arousal positive emotional states, whereas in collectivistic cultural contexts, people generally seek out low-arousal positive emotional states (Tsai, Knutson, & Fung, 2006). Even within a culture, however, there seem to be important differences in emotion regulatory behaviors. How can we explain such differences? One possibility is that people differ in their *beliefs* regarding emotion and emotion regulation, and these differences might, in turn, shape whether people try to regulate their emotions, and—when they do so—which emotion-regulatory strategies they employ.

To test this hypothesis, Tamir, John, Srivastava, and Gross (2007) modified items from the Implicit Theories of Intelligence Scale (Dweck, 1999) to refer to general beliefs about the extent to which emotions are malleable and incremental (e.g., "If they want to, people can change the emotions that they have") or fixed and uncontrollable (e.g., "The truth is, people have very little control over their emotions"). They then administered this measure to students facing a crucial life transition, namely the transition to college. Findings revealed that participants did differ in their beliefs about emotion, and participants with incremental as opposed to entity views of emotion reported greater self-efficacy in emotion regulation, and greater use of reappraisal. By the end of freshman year, participants with incremental views of emotion reported greater levels of positive emotions, lesser levels of negative emotions, higher levels of well-being, and lower levels of depression. Incremental participants also had higher levels of social adjustment and lower levels of loneliness. These findings indicate that participants' naive beliefs concerning their emotions—as either fixed or malleable—influenced how they regulated their emotions and how they fared in one important life transition, namely the transition to college.

Defining Emotion Regulation

Surveying the many ways in which individuals seek to influence their emotions, *emotion regulation* may be defined as the ways individuals influence which emotions they have, when they have them, and how they experience or express them (Gross, 1998b). Such regulation may be automatic or controlled, and may be unconscious or conscious (Mauss, Evers, Wilhelm & Gross, 2006). Because emotions are multicomponential processes that unfold over time, emotion regulation involves changes in the duration or intensity of behavioral, experiential, and/or physiological responses (Gross & Thompson, 2007). It's important to note that any given emotion regulation process may be used to make things either better or worse, depending on the context. For example, cognitive strategies that dampen negative emotions may help a medical professional operate efficiently in stressful circumstances, but also may neutralize negative emotions associated with empathy, thereby decreasing his or her helpfulness.

What are people hoping to accomplish when they regulate their emotions? Typically, people are trying to decrease the experiential and/or behavioral aspects of negative emotions such as anger, fear, and sadness (Gross et al., 2006). However, positive emotions are also down-regulated, such as when individuals try to look less amused than they feel by a child's inappropriate comment, or when they try to neutralize a positive mood in order to be able to properly attend to a friend's feelings of distress or to interact with a stranger (Erber, Wegner, & Therriault, 1996). Emotion regulation also may involve maintaining or increasing emotion, such as when we share good news with others, or, in the context of negative emotion, when bill collectors try to increase their anger to help collect delinquent accounts (Sutton, 1991); when people high on neuroticism cultivate negative emotions in order to maximize performance (Tamir, 2005); or when people who believe that being angry will help them in a performance context choose to engage in activities that will lead them to feel angry (Tamir, Mitchell, & Gross, 2008).

A Process Model of Emotion Regulation

A very large number of processes are involved in decreasing, maintaining, or increasing one or more aspects of emotion. Indeed, relevant processes range from changing one's job to calling one's mother to keeping a "stiff upper lip." How should we conceptualize the potentially overwhelming number of processes involved in regulating our own or others' emotions?

My strategy has been to undertake a conceptual analysis of the processes underlying diverse emotion regulatory acts. Using the modal model of emotion shown in Figure 28.1 as a starting point, I have argued that emotion regulatory acts may be seen as having their primary impact at different points in the emotion-generative process (Gross, 2001). In particular, I have suggested that each of the emotion-generative processes specified by the modal model is a potential target for regulation. In Figure 28.2, therefore, I have redrawn the modal model, highlighting five points at which individuals can regulate their emotions. These five points represent five families of emotion regulation processes: situation selection, situation modification, attentional deployment, cognitive change, and response modulation.

Basic Processes and Individual Differences

In the following sections, I use the process model of emotion regulation shown in Figure 28.2 as an organizing framework for a selective review of the literature on basic emotion regulation processes and individual differences. At the outset, it's worth noting that the distinctions made in this model are conceptual rather than empirical. What someone does in everyday life to regulate emotions—such as taking a walk on the beach after a stressful day at work—often involves multiple regulatory processes. Nonetheless, this process model provides a conceptual framework useful for understanding the causes, consequences, and mechanisms underlying basic emotion regulatory processes.

With respect to individual differences in emotion regulation, one could imagine (at least) three critical dimensions. The first has

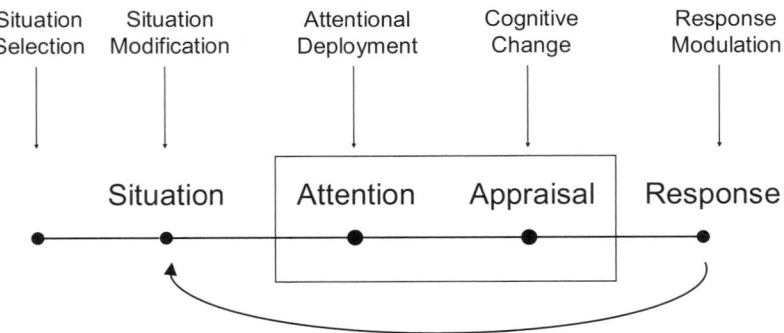

FIGURE 28.2. A process model of emotion regulation that highlights five families of emotion regulation strategies. From Gross and Thompson (2007). Copyright 2007 by The Guilford Press. Reprinted by permission.

to do with an individual's emotion regulatory goals. What does the individual believe constitutes appropriate emotion experience, expression, and physiological responding in a given situation? The second domain has to do with how frequently an individual attempts to regulate emotions in each of a variety of ways. How often does an individual use a particular strategy to achieve a given emotion regulatory goal? The third has to do with what an individual is capable of. How able is the individual to regulate emotions in a particular way if he or she is highly motivated to do so? Eventually, we need constructs that distinguish among these three individual-difference domains for each of the major forms of emotion regulation. At this point, unfortunately, we are far from that goal. In the sections that follow, I focus principally on the second dimension and consider how frequently individuals typically use particular forms of emotion regulation.

Situation Selection

The first type of emotion regulation is *situation selection*. This family of regulatory processes is placed at the left-most point in Figure 28.2 because it affects the situation to which a person is exposed, and thus shapes the emotion trajectory from the earliest possible point. Situation selection involves actions that make it more likely that we will be in a situation we expect will give rise to the emotions we'd like to have (or less likely that we'll be in a situation that will give rise to emotions we'd prefer not to have).

What distinguishes situation selection from the many other actions in which we engage everyday that—at least in part—are governed by a hedonic calculus? Situation selection refers to the subset of such actions, namely those taken with a view to how they will affect future emotional responses. Often, it is possible to guess the trajectory our emotions will have if we don't take steps to influence those emotions. This awareness motivates us to take steps to alter the default emotional trajectory via situation selection. Thus we may try hard to avoid situations we know will bring us face-to-face with a grumpy neighbor, or we may actively seek out situations that will provide us with contact with friends and loved ones.

Individuals seek out situations consistent with their dispositions (Caspi & Rob-

erts, 1999). Thus, extraverts seek out social situations that provide opportunities for fun and enjoyment, thereby influencing the emotions they experience (Clark & Watson, 1988). Individuals high in sensation seeking search out challenges and risky situations because they enjoy the thrill and excitement that these situations provide (Zuckerman, 1979). Individuals high in attachment avoidance avoid attachment-related contexts that are, for them, associated with high levels of anxiety (Shaver & Mikulincer, 2007). (Attachment avoidance in adult romantic relationships is assessed by items such as "I get uncomfortable when a romantic partner wants to be very close"; Brennan, Clark, & Shaver, 1998.)

From a Big Five perspective, one of the most relevant personality dimensions may be conscientiousness, which refers to socially prescribed impulse control such as thinking before acting, delaying gratification, and planning, organizing, and prioritizing tasks (John & Srivastava, 1999). These traits suggest that individuals high in conscientiousness should be more likely to engage in situation selection than individuals low in conscientiousness. Compared to the low-conscientiousness individuals, they should be able to avoid knowingly entering or getting trapped in situations that cause them negative emotions. For example, the highly conscientious college student who knows she will feel bad about not finishing her class paper on time will decline a social invitation before completing the paper. By carefully choosing situations that are consistent with their goals and plans, these individuals end up doing fewer things they later come to regret.

Situation Modification

Potentially emotion-eliciting situations— whether a flat tire on the way to an important appointment or loud music next door at 3:00 A.M.—do not necessarily call forth emotions. After all, we can convert a meeting into a phone conference or convince a neighbor to tone down a raucous party. Such efforts to directly modify the situation so as to alter its emotional impact constitute a second family of emotion regulatory processes, shown next in line in Figure 28.2. In the stress and coping tradition, this type of emotion regulation is referred to as problem-focused coping (Lazarus & Folkman, 1984).

Individual differences in situation modification largely have been studied in the context of problem-focused coping. Currently, the most commonly used coping measure is the COPE (Carver, Scheier, & Weintraub, 1989), which, among other things, assesses *active coping*. Individuals high on active coping say that they respond to difficult or stressful events by concentrating their efforts on doing something about the situation. From a Big Five perspective, extraversion—in particular, the facet of dominance or assertiveness—is especially relevant to situation modification (Costa & McCrae, 1992). Compared to more introverted individuals, extraverts forcefully pursue their goals, seeking out and achieving positions of leadership, and freely expressing both positive and negative emotions (e.g., C. Anderson, John, Keltner, & Kring, 2001; Gross & John, 1998). Instead of sitting at home and fuming at a loud party next door, the assertive individual knock's on the neighbor's door and asks him or her to turn the music down.

Attentional Deployment

The first two forms of emotion regulation—situation selection and situation modification—shape the situation to which an individual will be exposed. However, it is also possible to regulate emotions without actually changing the environment. Situations have many aspects; *attentional deployment* refers to influencing emotional responding by redirecting attention within a given situation. Attentional deployment is thus an internal version of situation selection, in that attention is used to select which of many possible "internal situations" are active for an individual at any point in time. In Figure 28.2, attentional deployment comes after situation modification in the emotion trajectory.

In one form or another, attentional deployment is used throughout the lifespan, particularly when it is not possible to change or modify the situation. Specific forms of attentional deployment include distraction, concentration, and rumination. In distraction an individual refocuses attention on nonemotional aspects of the situation or moves attention away from the immediate situation altogether. Through concentration, an individual can create a self-sustaining transcendent state that Csikszentmihalyi (1975) calls

"flow." Rumination involves attentional focus on feelings and their consequences. Rumination increases negative emotion (Bushman, 2002; Morrow & Nolen-Hoeksema, 1990; Ray, Wilhelm, & Gross, 2008), and is associated with increased and/or prolonged amygdalar activation in response to negative pictures and negative words (Ray et al., 2005; Siegle, Steinhauser, Thase, Stenger, & Carter, 2002).

Several individual-difference constructs involve attentional deployment. Repressive copers deflect attention away from potentially threatening stimuli (Boden & Baumeister, 1997; Krohne, 1996). Monitors turn attention toward threatening stimuli, whereas blunters turn away from threatening stimuli (Miller, 1987). Compared with those low in neuroticism, individuals high in neuroticism are less able to shift attention from motivationally relevant stimuli when doing so is desirable (Wallace & Newman, 1997). From a Big Five perspective, conscientiousness is particularly relevant: Being able to focus on a task and deploy attention to goal-relevant features of the environment is one of the defining features of conscientiousness (e.g., self-discipline, deliberation, and order; Costa & McCrae, 1992), and low levels of conscientiousness have been linked to the attentional deficits so common in attention-deficit/hyperactivity disorder (ADHD; Nigg et al., 2002).

Perhaps the most prominent individual-difference construct in the domain of attentional deployment is rumination. Individuals who tend to ruminate have higher levels of depression (Just & Alloy, 1997; Lyubomirsky & Nolen-Hoeksema, 1993). Chronic ruminators also have longer-lasting depressive symptoms (Nolen-Hoeksema, McBride, & Larson, 1997), and increased occurrences of depressive episodes (Nolen-Hoeksema, 2000; Spasojevic & Alloy, 2001).

Cognitive Change

Even after a potentially emotion-eliciting situation has arisen and been attended to, emotion need not follow. This is because emotion further requires that the individual imbue the situation with a certain kind of meaning. *Cognitive change* (shown fourth in line in Figure 28.2) refers to changing one or more of the appraisals one makes in a way that alters the situation's emotional significance, either by changing how one thinks about the situation itself or about one's capacity to manage its demands.

One form of cognitive change that has received particular attention is reappraisal, which refers to changing one's appraisal of a situation so as to alter emotion (Gross, 2002). To date, studies of reappraisal have focused on decreasing negative emotion. These studies have shown that reappraisal leads to decreases in negative emotion experience and expressive behavior (Dandoy & Goldstein, 1990; Gross, 1998a), as well as decreases in startle responses (Dillon & LaBar, 2005; Jackson, Malmstadt, Larson, & Davidson, 2000), neuroendocrine responses (Abelson, Liberzon, Young, & Khan, 2005), and autonomic responses (Stemmler, 1997; but see Gross, 1998a). Consistent with these behavioral and physiological findings, reappraisal in the service of emotion down-regulation is associated with decreased activation in subcortical emotion-generative regions such as the insula and amygdala, as well as increased activation in dorsolateral and medial prefrontal regions associated with cognitive control (Levesque et al., 2003; Ochsner, Bunge, Gross, & Gabrieli, 2002; Ochsner & Gross, 2004, 2008).

As the process model would predict, activations in prefrontal regions associated with the top-down control of emotion seem to occur relatively early on (in the first few seconds), whereas the down-stream consequences of decreased experience and behavior seem to last considerably longer (Goldin, McRae, Ramel, & Gross, 2008). If reappraisal occurs relatively early in the emotion-generative process, one might expect that using reappraisal would not interfere with other ongoing cognitive processes. This is just what we've found in a series of studies that have tested whether reappraisal impairs subsequent memory for information presented during the reappraisal period (Richards & Gross, 1999, 2000, 2006). Findings from these studies suggest that reappraisal does not compromise later memory for material presented while the participant was engaging in reappraisal (relative to not using reappraisal).

From a coping perspective, one dimension relevant to reappraisal is positive reinterpretation and growth (Carver et al.,

1989), which involves looking for the "silver lining" in stressful situations and trying to learn from difficulty. Gross and John (2003) found that this COPE scale was correlated with the use of reappraisal. Conceptually related constructs include optimism (Scheier & Carver, 1985, 1992), attributional style (Peterson, 1991; Peterson & Park, 2007), constructive thinking (Epstein & Meier, 1989), and psychological defenses such as denial, isolation, and intellectualization. In interpersonal contexts, the Big Five dimension of agreeableness may also provide an index of cognitive change: individuals high (vs. low) in agreeableness seem to automatically neutralize negative thoughts that would otherwise decrease interpersonal harmony (Meier, Robinson, & Wilkowski, 2006; Tobin, Graziano, Vanman, & Tassinary, 2000).

Individual differences in the use of reappraisal have been more directly assessed using the reappraisal scale from the Emotion Regulation Questionnaire (Gross & John, 2003), which includes items such as "I control my emotions *by changing the way I think* about the situation I'm in." Individuals who make frequent use of reappraisal negotiate stressful situations by taking an optimistic attitude, reinterpreting what they find stressful, and making active efforts to repair bad moods. Affectively, reappraisers both experience and express behaviorally more positive emotion and less negative emotion than those who reappraise less frequently. Reappraisers have fewer depressive symptoms and greater self-esteem, life satisfaction, and every other type of well-being we measured (Gross & John, 2003).

Response Modulation

Response modulation is the last of the emotion-regulatory families, and it is shown on the right side of Figure 28.2. As this placement indicates, it occurs late in the emotion-generative process, after response tendencies have been initiated and allowed to develop. Response modulation strategies aim to influence physiological, experiential, and/or behavioral responses in a relatively direct manner.

One of the best researched forms of response modulation is *expressive suppression*, which refers to attempts to decrease ongoing emotion-expressive behavior (Gross, 2002).

As would be expected, suppression decreases observable behavior. Interestingly, however, suppression does not change negative emotion experience, and it actually *increases* sympathetic activation of the cardiovascular system (Demaree et al., 2006; Gross, 1998a; Gross & Levenson, 1993, 1997; Harris, 2001; McCanne & Anderson, 1987; Stepper & Strack, 1993; Strack, Martin, & Stepper, 1988). Neurally, only one study to date has been conducted on expressive suppression (Goldin et al., 2008). In this study, participants were asked to suppress their ongoing emotion-expressive behavior in the scanner during 15-second-long film segments that elicited intense levels of disgust. Findings indicated that suppression led to robust increases is dorsal and medial prefrontal regions associated with cognitive control, as well as with increased activation in emotion-generative regions such as the amygdala. Importantly, as the process model of emotion regulation would predict, these activations were evident late in the induction period, suggesting that suppression was associated with ongoing cognitive activity as the participants effortfully tried to manage each of the emotional impulses as it arose throughout the course of each film.

If this conception of expressive suppression is correct, one might expect that, unlike reappraisal, we should find clear cognitive consequences of suppression. Indeed, we have found repeatedly that suppression (compared to no emotion regulation) leads to worse memory for material presented during the suppression period (Richards & Gross, 1999, 2000). Indeed, the degree of memory impairment associated with suppression was as large as when we instructed participants to distract themselves as much as possible during the presentation of information (Richards & Gross, 2006).

From a Big Five perspective, extraverts tend to freely express both positive and negative emotions (e.g., Anderson, John, Keltner, & Kring, 2001; Gross & John, 1998). By contrast, introverts are more withdrawn and are more likely to hold in their feelings and hide them from others. These predictions are consistent with findings that extraverts are much more likely than introverts to express their emotions, both positive and negative (e.g., Gross & John, 1998), even though in terms of emotion experience they differ from introverts only in terms of positive emotion experience (Gross et al., 1998; Watson & Clark, 1997). As expected, measures of extraversion correlate negatively with the tendency to suppress emotion (Gross & John, 2003). From an attachment perspective, when faced with an emotional situation they cannot avoid or escape, avoidantly attached individuals should be more likely to try to regulate their emotion via expressive suppression than nonavoidant individuals. That is, they would try to not share their emotions with others and to keep their emotions from showing in their expressive behavior. Consistent with this prediction, Gross and John (2003) found that suppression correlated positively and substantially with two different measures of attachment avoidance.

To examine individual differences in suppression, we have used the suppression scale from the Emotion Regulation Questionnaire (Gross & John, 2003), which includes items such as "I control my emotions *by not expressing them*." Individuals who make frequent use of suppression deal with stressful situations by masking their inner feelings and clamping down on their outward displays of emotion. In terms of positive affect, their efforts at suppression leave them with less positive emotion experience and expression. In terms of negative affect, they experience more negative emotions, including painful feelings of inauthenticity, than individuals who use suppression less frequently. Their suppression is partially successful, in that they express less negative emotion than they actually experience; however, in absolute terms, they still express as much as individuals who suppress less frequently. In terms of well-being, suppressors have lower levels of self-esteem, are less satisfied with life, and have more depressive symptoms (Gross & John, 2003).

SUMMARY

Emotions play a vital role in our lives, shaping everything from what we see to how we respond. In recognition of this fact, researchers in every subfield of psychology (and beyond) are at work trying to understand the biological and social bases of emotion. New complexities are emerging at every turn, and given the high level of research activity that is distributed across so many different areas, it is difficult to keep abreast of crucial developments. My goal in this chapter has been to provide a framework for organizing the literatures on emotion and emotion regulation useful to personality psychologists. In the first section, I considered what emotion is and described the modal model of emotion. In the second section, I used this model to organize a selective review of research on basic emotional processes and related individual differences. In the third section, I turned my attention to emotion regulation and described a process model of it. In the fourth section, I used this process model to organize a selective review of research on personality processes and individual differences related to emotion regulation. More specifically, I distinguished five points in the emotion-generative process at which regulation may occur: (1) selection of the situation, (2) modification of the situation, (3) deployment of attention, (4) change of cognitions, and (5) modulation of responses. Like all models, this simplifying framework is necessarily incomplete. It is my hope, however, that it will prove useful in organizing what we now know and in suggesting exciting new questions for future research.

ACKNOWLEDGMENTS

This chapter draws upon and updates previous reviews by Gross (1998b, 1999, 2001, 2007), Gross and John (2003), Gross and Thompson (2007), and John and Gross (2004, 2007). Preparation of this chapter was supported by National Institutes of Health Grant Nos. R01 MH66957, R01 MH58147, and R01 MH76074. I would like to thank Lisa Feldman Barrett and Maya Tamir for their helpful comments.

NOTES

1. Emotion scholars have long bemoaned the "conceptual and definitional chaos" that has characterized the field (Buck, 1990, p. 330). One source of confusion has been how to employ the many related terms that appear in this literature. Following Scherer (1984), I use *affect* as the superordinate category for various kinds of states that involve relatively quick good–bad discriminations. These affective states include (a) general *stress responses* to taxing circumstances, (b) *emotions* such as

anger and sadness, (c) *moods* such as depression and euphoria, and (d) *other motivational impulses* such as those related to eating, sex, aggression, or pain. I focus here on emotions. (For a more detailed treatment of these distinctions, see Gross & Thompson, 2007.)

2. These distinctions have heuristic value but should not be reified, given the permeable boundaries among categories. At present, however, the three-way distinction among emotion experience, expression, and physiology remains a useful way of organizing research on emotion.

REFERENCES

Abelson, J. L., Liberzon, I., Young, E. A., & Khan, S. (2005). Cognitive modulation of the endocrine stress response to a pharmacological challenge in normal and panic disorder subjects. *Archives of General Psychiatry, 62,* 668–675.

Allport, G. W., & Vernon, P. E. (1933). *Studies in expressive movement.* New York: Macmillan.

Anderson, A. K., & Phelps, E. A. (2001). Lesions of the human amygdala impair enhanced perception of emotionally salient events. *Nature, 411,* 305–309.

Anderson, C., John, O. P., Keltner, D., & Kring, A. (2001). Who attains social status? Effects of personality and physical attractiveness in social groups. *Journal of Personality and Social Psychology, 81,* 116–132.

Armon-Jones, C. (1986). The thesis of constructionism. In R. Harre (Ed.), *The social construction of emotion* (pp. 32–56). Oxford, UK: Blackwell.

Arnold, M. (1960). *Emotion and personality.* New York: Columbia University Press.

Aspinwall, L. G., & Taylor, S. E. (1992). Modeling cognitive adaptation: A longitudinal investigation of the impact of individual differences and coping on college adjustment and performance. *Journal of Personality and Social Psychology, 63,* 989–1003.

Averill, J. R. (1980). A constructivist view of emotion. In R. Plutchik & H. Kellerman (Eds.), *Emotion: Theory, research, and experience* (pp. 305–339). Orlando, FL: Academic Press.

Barrett, L. F. (1998). Discrete emotions or dimensions?: The role of valence focus and arousal focus. *Cognition and Emotion, 12,* 579–599.

Barrett, L. F. (2004). Feelings or words?: Understanding the content in self-report ratings of emotional experience. *Journal of Personality and Social Psychology, 87,* 266–281.

Barrett, L. F. (2006a). Emotions as natural kinds? *Perspectives on Psychological Science, 1,* 28–58.

Barrett, L. F. (2006b). Solving the emotion paradox: Categorization and the experience of emotion. *Personality and Social Psychology Review, 10,* 20–46.

Barrett, L. F., Mesquita, B., Ochsner, K. N., & Gross, J. J. (2007). The experience of emotion. *Annual Review of Psychology, 58,* 373–403.

Barrett, L. F., Ochsner, K. N., & Gross, J. J. (2007). On the automaticity of emotion. In J. Bargh (Ed.), *Social psychology and the unconscious: The automaticity of higher mental processes* (pp. 173–217). New York: Psychology Press.

Barrett, L. F., & Wager, T. D. (2006). The structure of emotion: Evidence from neuroimaging studies. *Current Directions in Psychological Science, 15,* 79–83.

Boden, J. M., & Baumeister, R. F. (1997). Repressive coping: Distraction using pleasant thoughts and memories. *Journal of Personality and Social Psychology, 73,* 45–62.

Bolger, N., & Schilling, E. A. (1991). Personality and the problems of everyday life: The role of neuroticism in exposure and reactivity to daily stressors. *Journal of Personality, 59,* 355–386.

Bowlby, J. (1969). *Attachment and loss: Attachment.* New York: Basic Books.

Brennan, K. A., Clark, C. L., & Shaver, P. R. (1998). Self-report measurement of adult attachment: An integrative overview. In J. A. Simpson & W. S. Rholes (Eds.), *Attachment theory and close relationships* (pp. 46–76). New York: Guilford Press.

Brown, G. W. (2000). Emotion and clinical depression: An environmental view. In M. Lewis & J. M. Haviland-Jones (Eds.), *Handbook of emotions* (2nd ed., pp. 75–90). New York: Guilford Press.

Brown, G. W., Andrews, B., Harris, T. O., Adler, Z., & Bridge, L. (1986). Social support, self-esteem, and depression. *Psychological Medicine, 16,* 813–831.

Buck, R. (1985). Prime theory: An integrated view of motivation and emotion. *Psychological Review, 92,* 389–413.

Buck, R. (1990). Mood and emotion: A comparison of five contemporary views. *Psychological Review, 92,* 389–413.

Bushman, B. J. (2002). Does venting anger feed or extinguish the flame?: Catharsis, rumination, distraction, anger, and aggressive responding. *Personality and Social Psychology Bulletin, 28,* 724–731.

Cacioppo, J. T., Berntson, G. G., Larsen, J. T., Poehlmann, K. M., & Ito, T. A. (2000). The psychophysiology of emotion. In M. Lewis & J. M. Haviland-Jones (Eds.), *Handbook of emotions* (2nd ed., pp. 173–191). New York: Guilford Press.

Cacioppo, J. T., Gardner, W. L., & Berntson, G. G. (1999). The affect system has parallel and integrative processing components: Form follows function. *Journal of Personality and Social Psychology, 76,* 839–855.

Cacioppo, J. T., Martzke, J. S., Petty, R. S., & Tassinary, L. G. (1988). Specific forms of facial EMG response index emotions during an interview: From Darwin to the continuous flow hypothesis of affect laden information processing. *Journal of Personality and Social Psychology, 54,* 592–604.

Canli, T., Sivers, H., Whitfield, S. L., Gotlib, I. H., & Gabrieli, J. D. E. (2002). Amygdala response to happy faces as a function of extraversion. *Science, 296,* 2191.

Canli, T., Zhao, Z., Desmond, J. E., Kang, E., Gross, J., & Gabrieli, J. D. E. (2001). An fMRI study of personality influences on brain reactivity to emotional stimuli. *Behavioral Neuroscience, 115,* 33–42.

Carver, C. S., Scheier, M. F., & Weintraub, J. K. (1989). Assessing coping strategies: A theoretically based approach. *Journal of Personality and Social Psychology, 56,* 267–283.

Caspi, A., & Roberts, B. W. (1999). Personality continuity and change across the life course. In L. A. Pervin & O. P. John (Eds.), *Handbook of personality: Theory and research* (2nd ed., pp. 300–326). New York: Guilford Press.

Caspi, A., Sugden, K., Moffitt, T. E., Taylor, A., Craig, I. W., Harrington, H., et al. (2003). Influence of life stress on depression: Moderation by a polymorphism in the 5-HTT gene. *Science, 301,* 386–389.

Cherry, E. C. (1953). Some experiments upon the recognition of speech, with one and with two ears. *Journal of the Acoustical Society of America, 25,* 975–979.

Clark, L. A., & Watson, D. (1988). Mood and the mundane: Relations between daily life events and self-reported mood. *Journal of Personality and Social Psychology, 54,* 296–308.

Clore, G. L., & Ortony, A. (1998). Cognition in emotion: Always, sometimes, or never? In L. Nadel & R. Lane (Eds.), *The cognitive neuroscience of emotion* (pp. 24–61). New York: Oxford University Press.

Cohen, M. X., Young, J., Baek, J., Kessler, C., & Ranganath, C. (2005). Individual differences in extraversion and dopamine genetics predict neural reward responses. *Cognitive Brain Research, 25,* 851–861.

Cook, E., & Turpin, G. (1997). Differentiating orienting, startle, and defense responses: The role of affect and its implications for psychopathology. In P. J. Lang, R. F. Simons, & M. T. Balaban (Eds.), *Attention and orienting: Sensory and motivational processes* (pp. 137–164). Mahwah, NJ: Erlbaum.

Costa, P. T., Jr., & McCrae, R. R. (1980). Influence of extraversion and neuroticism on subjective well-being. *Journal of Personality and Social Psychology, 38,* 668–678.

Costa, P. T., Jr., & McCrae, R. R. (1992). *NEO PI-R Professional Manual.* Odessa, FL: Psychological Assessment Resources.

Csikszentmihalyi, M. (1975). *Beyond boredom and anxiety: The experience of play in work and games.* San Francisco: Jossey-Bass.

Dandoy, A. C., & Goldstein, A. G. (1990). The use of cognitive appraisal to reduce stress reactions: A replication. *Journal of Social Behavior and Personality, 5,* 275–285.

Darwin, C. (1962). *The origin of species by means of natural selection or the preservation of favoured races in the struggle for life.* New York: Collier. (Original work published 1859)

Davidson, R. J., & Sutton, S. K. (1995). Affective neuroscience: The emergence of a discipline. *Current Opinion in Neurobiology, 5,* 217–224.

Demaree, H. A., Schmeichel, B. J., Robinson, J. L., Pu, J., Everhart, D. E., & Berntson, G. G. (2006). Up- and down-regulating facial disgust: Affective, vagal, sympathetic, and respiratory consequences. *Biological Psychology, 71,* 90–99.

Depue, R. A., & Collins, P. F. (1999). Neurobiology of the structure of personality: Dopamine, facilitation of incentive motivation, and extraversion. *Behavioral and Brain Sciences, 22,* 491–569.

Dillon, D. G., & LaBar, K. S. (2005). Startle modulation during conscious emotion regulation is arousal-dependent. *Behavioral Neuroscience, 119,* 1118–1124.

Dodge, K. A. (1991). Emotion and social information processing. In J. Garber & K. A. Dodge (Eds.), *The development of emotion regulation and dysregulation* (pp. 159–182). New York: Cambridge University Press.

Dweck, C. S. (1999). *Self-theories: Their role in motivation, personality, and development.* New York: Psychology Press.

Eibl-Eibesfeldt, I. (1975). *Ethology: The biology of behavior.* New York: Holt, Rinehart & Winston.

Ekman, P. (1972). Universals and cultural differences in facial expression of emotion. In J. Cole (Ed.), *Nebraska Symposium of Motivation* (pp. 207–283). Lincoln: University of Nebraska Press.

Ekman, P. (1994). Strong evidence for universals in facial expressions: A reply to Russell's mistaken critique. *Psychological Bulletin, 115,* 268–287.

Ekman, P., & Friesen, W. V. (1978). *Facial action coding system.* Palo Alto, CA: Consulting Psychologist Press.

Ekman, P., Friesen, W. V., & Simons, R. C. (1985). Is the startle reaction an emotion? *Journal of Personality and Social Psychology, 49,* 1416–1426.

Ekman, P., & Rosenberg, E. L. (Eds.). (1997). *What the face reveals.* New York: Oxford University Press.

Ellsworth, P. C. (1994). Some reasons to expect universal antecedents of emotion. In P. Ekman & R. J. Davidson (Eds.), *The natural of emotion: Fundamental questions* (pp. 150–154). New York: Oxford University Press.

Ellsworth, P. C., & Scherer, K. R. (2003). Appraisal processes in emotion. In R. J. Davidson, K. R., Scherer, & H. H. Goldsmith (Eds.), *Handbook of affective sciences* (pp. 572–595). New York: Oxford University Press.

Emmons, R. A., & Diener, E. (1985). Personality correlates of subjective well-being. *Personality and Social Psychology Bulletin, 11,* 89–97.

Epstein, S., & Meier, P. (1989). Constructive thinking: A broad coping variable with specific components. *Journal of Personality and Social Psychology, 57*(2), 332–350.

Erber, R., Wegner, D. M., & Therriault, N. (1996). On being cool and collected: Mood regulation in anticipation of social interaction. *Journal of Personality and Social Psychology, 70,* 757–766.

Feldman, L. A. (1995). Valence focus and arousal focus: Individual differences in the structure of affective experience. *Journal of Personality and Social Psychology, 69,* 153–166.

Freud, S. (1959). *Inhibitions, symptoms, anxiety* (A. Strachey, Trans. & J. Strachey, Ed.). New York: Norton. (Original work published 1926)

Friedman, H. S., Prince, L. M., Riggio, R. E., & DiMatteo, M. R. (1980). Understanding and assessing nonverbal expressiveness: The affective communication test. *Journal of Personality and Social Psychology, 39,* 333–351.

Frijda, N. H. (1986). *The emotions.* Cambridge: Cambridge University Press.

Frijda, N. H. (1988). The laws of emotion. *American Psychologist, 43,* 349–358.

Frijda, N. H. (1989). Aesthetic emotions and reality. *American Psychologist, 44,* 1546–1547.

Goldin, P. R., McRae, K., Ramel, W., & Gross, J. J. (2008). The neural bases of emotion regulation during reappraisal and suppression of negative emotion. *Biological Psychiatry, 63,* 577–586.

Gray, J. A. (1994). Three fundamental emotion systems. In P. Ekman & R. J. Davidson (Eds.), *The nature of emotion: Fundamental questions* (pp. 243–247). New York: Oxford University Press.

Gross, J. J. (1998a). Antecedent- and response-focused emotion regulation: Divergent consequences for experience, expression, and physiology. *Journal of Personality and Social Psychology, 74,* 224–237.

Gross, J. J. (1998b). The emerging field of emotion regulation: An integrative review. *Review of General Psychology, 2*, 271–299.

Gross, J. J. (1999). Emotion and emotion regulation. In L. A. Pervin & O. P. John (Eds.), *Handbook of personality: Theory and research* (2nd ed., pp. 525–552). New York: Guilford Press.

Gross, J. J. (2001). Emotion regulation in adulthood: Timing is everything. *Current Directions in Psychological Science, 10*, 214–219.

Gross, J. J. (2002). Emotion regulation: Affective, cognitive, and social consequences. *Psychophysiology, 39*, 281–291.

Gross, J. J. (Ed.). (2007). *Handbook of emotion regulation*. New York: Guilford Press.

Gross, J. J., & John, O. P. (1997). Revealing feelings: Facets of emotional expressivity in self-reports, peer ratings, and behavior. *Journal of Personality and Social Psychology, 72*, 435–448.

Gross, J. J., & John, O. P. (1998). Mapping the domain of emotional expressivity: Multimethod evidence for a hierarchical model. *Journal of Personality and Social Psychology, 74*, 170–191.

Gross, J. J., & John, O. P. (2003). Individual differences in two emotion regulation processes: Implications for affect, relationships, and well-being. *Journal of Personality and Social Psychology, 85*, 348–362.

Gross, J. J., & Levenson, R. W. (1993). Emotional suppression: Physiology, self-report, and expressive behavior. *Journal of Personality and Social Psychology, 64*, 970–986.

Gross, J. J., Richards, J. M., & John, O. P. (2006). Emotion regulation in everyday life. In D. K. Snyder, J. A. Simpson, & J. N. Hughes (Eds.), *Emotion regulation in couples and families: Pathways to dysfunction and health* (pp. 13–35). Washington, DC: American Psychological Association.

Gross, J. J., Sutton, S. K., & Ketelaar, T. V. (1998). Relations between affect and personality: Support for the affect-level and affective–reactivity views. *Personality and Social Psychology Bulletin, 24*, 279–288.

Gross, J. J., & Thompson, R. A. (2007). Emotion regulation: Conceptual foundations. In J. J. Gross (Ed.), *Handbook of emotion regulation* (pp. 3–24). New York: Guilford Press.

Hammen, C. (1991). Generation of stress in the course of unipolar depression. *Journal of Abnormal Psychology, 100*, 555–561.

Harmon-Jones, E. (2003). Clarifying the emotive functions of asymmetrical frontal cortical activity. *Psychophysiology, 40*, 838–848.

Harré, R. (Ed.). (1986). *The social construction of emotions*. Oxford, UK: Blackwell.

Harris, C. R. (2001). Cardiovascular responses of embarrassment and effects of emotional suppression in a social setting. *Journal of Personality and Social Psychology, 81*, 886–897.

Izard, C. E. (1977). *Human emotions*. New York: Plenum Press.

Izard, C. E. (1994). Innate and universal facial expressions: Evidence from developmental and cross-cultural research. *Psychological Bulletin, 115*, 288–299.

Izard, C. E., Libero, D. Z., Putnam, P., & Haynes, O. M. (1993). Stability of emotion experiences and their relations to traits of personality. *Journal of Personality and Social Psychology, 64*, 847–860.

Jackson, D. C., Malmstadt, J. R., Larson, C. L., & Davidson, R. J. (2000). Suppression and enhancement of emotional responses to unpleasant pictures. *Psychophysiology, 37*, 515–522.

James, W. (1884). What is an emotion? *Mind, 9*, 188–205.

James, W. (1902). *Varieties of religious experience: A study in human nature*. New York: Longmans.

John, O. P., & Gross, J. J. (2004). Healthy and unhealthy emotion regulation: Personality processes, individual differences, and lifespan development. *Journal of Personality, 72*, 1301–1334.

John, O. P., & Gross, J. J. (2007). Individual differences in emotion regulation. In J. J. Gross (Ed.), *Handbook of emotion regulation* (pp. 351–372). New York: Guilford Press.

John, O. P., & Srivastava, S. (1999). The Big Five trait taxonomy: History, measurement, and theoretical perspectives. In L. A. Pervin & O. P. John (Eds.), *Handbook of personality: Theory and research* (2nd ed., pp. 102–138). New York: Guilford Press.

Johnstone, T., & Scherer, K. R. (2000). Vocal communication of emotion. In M. Lewis & J. Haviland-Jones (Eds.), *Handbook of emotions* (2nd ed., pp. 220–235). New York: Guilford Press.

Just, N., & Alloy, L. B. (1997). The response styles theory of depression: Tests and an extension of the theory. *Journal of Abnormal Psychology, 106*, 221–229.

Kagan, J., & Snidman, N. (1991). Temperamental factors in human development. *American Psychologist, 46*, 856–862.

Keltner, D., & Ekman, P. (2000). Facial expression of emotion. In M. L. Lewis & J. M. Haviland-Jones (Eds.), *Handbook of emotions* (2nd ed., pp. 236–249). New York: Guilford Press.

Kendler, K. S., & Prescott, C. A. (2006). *Genes, environment, and psychopathology: Understanding the causes of psychiatric and substance use disorders*. New York: Guilford Press.

Knutson, B., & Bhanji, J. (2006). Neural substrates for emotional traits? In T. Canli (Ed.), *Biology of personality and individual differences* (pp. 116–132). New York: Guilford Press.

Kring, A. M., Smith, D. A., & Neale, J. M. (1994). Individual differences in dispositional expressiveness: Development and validation of the Emotional Expressivity Scale. *Journal of Personality and Social Psychology, 66,* 934–949.

Krohne, H. W. (1996). Individual differences in coping. In M. Zeidner & N. S. Endler (Eds.), *Handbook of coping: Theory, research, applications* (pp. 381–409). New York: Wiley.

Lakoff, G. (1987). *Women, fire, and dangerous things.* Chicago: University of Chicago Press.

Lane, R. D., Quinlan, D. M., Schwartz, G. E., Walker, P. A., & Zeitlin, S. B. (1990). The levels of emotional awareness scale: A cognitive-developmental measure of emotion. *Journal of Personality Assessment, 55,* 124–134.

Lang, P. J. (1995). The emotion probe. *American Psychologist, 5,* 372–385.

Larsen, R. J., & Diener, E. (1992). Promises and problems with the circumplex model of emotion. In M. S. Clark (Ed.), *Emotion: Review of personality and social psychology* (Vol. 13, pp. 25–59). Newbury Park, CA: Sage.

Lazarus, R. S. (1966). *Psychological stress and the coping process.* New York: McGraw-Hill.

Lazarus, R. S. (1991a). *Emotion and adaptation.* Oxford, UK: Oxford University Press.

Lazarus, R. S. (1991b). Progress on a cognitive–motivational–relational theory of emotion. *American Psychologist, 46,* 819–834.

Lazarus, R. S., & Folkman, S. (1984). *Stress, appraisal and coping.* New York: Springer.

LeDoux, J. E. (1993). Emotional networks in the brain. In M. Lewis & J. M. Haviland-Jones (Eds.), *Handbook of emotions* (pp. 109–118). New York: Guilford Press.

Levenson, R. W. (1992). Autonomic nervous system differences among emotions. *Psychological Science, 3,* 23–27.

Levenson, R. W. (1994). Human emotions: A functional view. In P. Ekman & R. J. Davidson (Eds.), *The nature of emotion: Fundamental questions* (pp. 123–126). New York: Oxford University Press.

Levesque, J., Fanny, E., Joanette, Y., Paquette, V., Mensour, B., Beaudoin, G., et al. (2003). Neural circuitry underlying voluntary suppression of sadness. *Biological Psychiatry, 53,* 502–510.

Lorenz, K. (1970). *Studies in animal and human behaviour: Vol. 1. The establishment of the instinct concept* (R. Martin, Trans.). London: Methuen. (Original work published 1937)

Lyubomirsky, S., & Nolen-Hoeksema, S. (1993). Self-perpetuating properties of dysphoric rumination. *Journal of Personality and Social Psychology, 65,* 339–349.

MacLean, P. D. (1949). Psychosomatic disease and the "visceral brain." *Psychosomatic Medicine, 11,* 338–353.

MacLean, P. D. (1975). Sensory and perceptual factors in emotional functions of the triune brain. In L. Levi (Ed.), *Emotions: Their parameters and measurement* (pp. 71–92). New York: Raven Press.

MacLean, P. D. (1990). *The triune brain in evolution: Role in paleocerebral functions.* New York: Plenum Press.

MacLeod, C., Mathews, A., & Tata, P. (1986). Attentional bias in emotional disorders. *Journal of Abnormal Psychology, 95,* 15–20.

Markus, H., & Kitayama, S. (1991). Culture and the self: Implications for cognition, emotion, and motivation. *Psychological Review, 98,* 224–253.

Mauss, I. B., Evers, C., Wilhelm, F. H., & Gross, J. J. (2006). How to bite your tongue without blowing your top: Implicit evaluation of emotion regulation predicts affective responding to anger provocation. *Personality and Social Psychology Bulletin, 32,* 589–602.

Mauss, I. B., Levenson, R. W., McCarter, L., Wilhelm, F. H., & Gross, J. J. (2005). The tie that binds? Coherence among emotion experience, behavior, and physiology. *Emotion, 5,* 175–190.

McCanne, T. R., & Anderson, J. A. (1987). Emotional responding following experimental manipulation of facial electromyographic activity. *Journal of Personality and Social Psychology, 52,* 759–768.

McCrae, R. R., & Costa, P. T., Jr. (1991). Adding *liebe und arbeit*: The full five-factor model and well-being. *Personality and Social Psychology Bulletin, 17,* 227–232.

McDougal, W. (1923). *Outline of psychology.* New York: Scribner.

McNair, D. M., Lorr, M., & Droppleman, L. F. (1971). *Manual: Profile of mood states.* San Diego, CA: Educational and Industrial Testing Service.

Meier, B. P., Robinson, M. D., & Wilkowski, B. M. (2006). Turning the other cheek: Agreeableness and the regulation of aggression-related primes. *Psychological Science, 17,* 136–42.

Mesquita, B., & Albert, D. (2007). The cultural regulation of emotions. In J. J. Gross (Ed.), *Handbook of emotion regulation* (pp. 486–503). New York: Guilford Press.

Meyer, G. J., & Shack, J. R. (1989). Structural convergence of mood and personality: Evidence for old and new directions. *Journal of Personality and Social Psychology, 57,* 691–706.

Miller, S. M. (1987). Monitoring and blunting: Validation of a questionnaire to assess styles of information seeking under threat. *Jour-*

nal of Personality and Social Psychology, 52, 345–353.

Mischel, W., Shoda, Y., & Rodriguez, M. L. (1989). Delay of gratification in children. Science, 244, 933–938.

Mogg, K., & Bradley, B. P. (1999). Some methodological issues in assessing attentional biases for threatening faces in anxiety: A replication study using a modified version of the probe detection task. Behavioral Research Therapy, 37, 595–604.

Mogg, K., & Bradley, B. P. (2006). Time course of attentional bias for fear-relevant pictures in spider-fearful individuals. Behavioral Research Therapy, 44, 1241–1250.

Morrow, J., & Nolen-Hoeksema, S. (1990). Effects of responses to depression on the remediation of depressive affect. Journal of Personality and Social Psychology, 58, 519–527.

Murphy, F. C., Nimmo-Smith, I., & Lawrence, A. D. (2003). Functional neuroanatomy of emotion: A meta-analysis. Cognitive, Affective, and Behavioral Neuroscience, 3, 207–233.

Niedenthal, P. M., & Kitayama, S. (Eds.). (1994). The heart's eye: Emotional influences in perception and attention. San Diego, CA: Academic Press.

Nigg, J. T., John, O. P., Blaskey, L., Huang-Pollock, C., Willcutt, E. G., Hinshaw, S. P., et al. (2002). Big Five dimensions and ADHD symptoms: Links between personality traits and clinical symptoms. Journal of Personality and Social Psychology, 83, 451–469.

Nolen-Hoeksema, S. (2000). The role of rumination in depressive disorders and mixed anxiety/depressive symptoms. Journal of Abnormal Psychology, 109, 504–511.

Nolen-Hoeksema, S., McBride, A., & Larson, J. (1997). Rumination and psychological distress among bereaved partners. Journal of Personality and Social Psychology, 72, 855–862.

Ochsner, K. N., Bunge, S. A., Gross, J. J., & Gabrieli, J. D. E. (2002). Rethinking feelings: An fMRI study of the cognitive regulation of emotion. Journal of Cognitive Neuroscience, 14, 1215–1229.

Ochsner, K. N., & Gross, J. J. (2004). Thinking makes it so: A social cognitive neuroscience approach to emotion regulation. In R. F. Baumeister & K. D. Vohs (Eds.), Handbook of self-regulation: Research, theory, and applications (pp. 229–255). New York: Guilford Press.

Ochsner, K. N., & Gross, J. J. (2005). The cognitive control of emotion. Trends in Cognitive Sciences, 9, 242–249.

Ochsner, K. N., & Gross, J. J. (2008). Cognitive emotion regulation: Insights from social cognitive and affective neuroscience. Current Directions in Psychological Science, 17, 153–158.

Ochsner, K. N., Ray, R. R., Cooper, J. C., Robertson, E. R., Chopra, S., Gabrieli, J. D. E., et al. (2004). For better or for worse: Neural systems supporting the cognitive down- and up-regulation of negative emotion. NeuroImage, 23, 483–499.

Ohman, A., & Mineka, S. (2001). Fears, phobias, and preparedness: Toward an evolved module of fear and fear learning. Psychological Review, 108, 483–522.

Panksepp, J. (1991). Affective neuroscience: A conceptual framework for the neurobiological study of emotions. In K. T. Strongman (Ed.), International review of studies of emotion (pp. 53–99). Chichester, UK: Wiley.

Panksepp, J. (1998). Affective neuroscience: The foundations of human and animal emotions. Oxford, UK: Oxford University Press.

Papez, J. W. (1937). A proposed mechanism of emotion. Archives of Neurology and Psychiatry, 38, 725–743.

Peterson, C. (1991). The meaning and measurement of explanatory style. Psychological Inquiry, 2, 1–10.

Peterson, C., & Park, N. (2007). Explanatory style and emotion regulation. In J. J. Gross (Ed.), Handbook of emotion regulation (pp. 159–179). New York: Guilford Press.

Phan, K. L., Wager, T. D., Taylor, S. F., & Liberzon, I. (2002). Functional neuroanatomy of emotion: A meta-analysis of emotion activation studies in PET and fMRI. NeuroImage, 16, 331–348.

Phelps, E. A. (2006). Emotion and cognition: Insights from studies of the human amygdala. Annual Review of Psychology, 57, 27–53.

Plutchik, R. (1962). The emotions: Facts, theories, and a new model. New York: Random House.

Plutchik, R. (1994). The psychology and biology of emotion. New York: HarperCollins.

Ray, R. D., Ochsner, K. N., Cooper, J. C., Robertson, E. R., Gabrieli, J. D., & Gross, J. J. (2005). Individual differences in trait rumination and the neural systems supporting cognitive reappraisal. Cognitive, Affective, and Behavioral Neuroscience, 5, 156–168

Ray, R. D., Wilhelm, F. H., & Gross, J. J. (2008). All in the mind's eye?: Anger rumination and reappraisal. Journal of Personality and Social Psychology, 94, 133–145.

Richards, J. M., & Gross, J. J. (1999). Composure at any cost?: The cognitive consequences of emotion suppression. Personality and Social Psychology Bulletin, 25, 1033–1044.

Richards, J. M., & Gross, J. J. (2000). Emotion regulation and memory: The cognitive costs of keeping one's cool. Journal of Personality and Social Psychology, 79, 410–424.

Richards, J. M., & Gross, J. J. (2006). Personality and emotional memory: How regulating emotion impairs memory for emotional events. *Journal of Research in Personality, 40,* 631–651.

Rinn, W. E. (1984). The neuropsychology of facial expression: A review of the neurological and psychological mechanisms for producing facial expressions. *Psychological Bulletin, 95,* 52–77.

Rottenberg, J., Ray, R. D., & Gross, J. J. (2007). Emotion elicitation using films. In J. A. Coan & J. J. B. Allen (Eds.), *Handbook of emotion elicitation and assessment* (pp. 9–28). New York: Oxford University Press.

Russell, J. A. (1980). A circumplex model of affect. *Journal of Personality and Social Psychology, 39,* 1161–1178.

Russell, J. A. (1994). Is there universal recognition of emotion from facial expression?: A review of the cross-cultural studies. *Psychological Bulletin, 115,* 102–141.

Russell, J. A. (2003). Core affect and the psychological construction of emotion. *Psychological Review, 110,* 145–172.

Russell, J. A., & Barrett, L. F. (1999). Core affect, prototypical emotional episodes, and other things called emotion: Dissecting the elephant. *Journal of Personality and Social Psychology, 76,* 805–819.

Sabini, J., & Schulkin, J. (1994). Biological realism and social constructivism. *Journal for the Theory of Social Behavior, 24,* 207–217.

Scheier, M. F., & Carver, C. S. (1985). Optimism, coping, and health: Assessment and implications of generalized outcome expectancies. *Health Psychology, 4,* 219–247.

Scheier, M. F., & Carver, C. S. (1992). Effects of optimism on psychological and physical well-being: Theoretical overview and empirical update. *Cognitive Therapy and Research, 16,* 201–228.

Scherer, K. R. (1984). On the nature and function of emotion: A component process approach. In K. R. Scherer & P. E. Ekman (Eds.), *Approaches to emotion* (pp. 293–317). Hillsdale, NJ: Erlbaum.

Scherer, K. R. (1986). Vocal affect expression: A review and a model for future research. *Psychological Bulletin, 99,* 143–165.

Scherer, K. R. (1994). Emotion serves to decouple stimulus and response. In P. E. Ekman & R. J. Davidson (Eds.), *The nature of emotion: Fundamental questions* (pp. 127–130). New York: Oxford University Press.

Scherer, K. R., Schorr, A., & Johnstone, T. (2001). *Appraisal processes in emotion: Theory, methods, research.* New York: Oxford University Press.

Scherer, K. R., Summerfield, A. B., & Wallbott, H. G. (1983). Cross-national research on antecedents and components of emotion: A progress report. *Social Science Information, 22,* 355–385.

Scherer, K. R., & Wallbott, H. G. (1994). Evidence for universality and cultural variation of differential emotion response patterning. *Journal of Personality and Social Psychology, 66,* 310–328.

Schwartz, C. E., Wright, C. I., Shin, L. M., Kagan, J., & Rauch, S. L. (2003). Inhibited and uninhibited infants "grown up": Adult amygdalar response to novelty. *Science, 300,* 1952–1953.

Shaver, P. R., & Mikulincer, M. (2007). Adult attachment strategies and the regulation of emotion. In J. J. Gross (Ed.), *Handbook of emotion regulation* (pp. 446–465). New York: Guilford Press.

Siegle, G. J., Steinhauer, S. R., Thase, M. E., Stenger, A., & Carter, C. S. (2002). Can't shake that feeling: An event-related fMRI assessment of sustained amygdala activity in response to emotional information in depressed individuals. *Biological Psychiatry, 51,* 693–707.

Simon, H. A. (1967). Motivational and emotional controls of cognition. *Psychological Review, 74,* 29–39.

Spasojevic, J., & Alloy, L. B. (2001). Rumination as a common mechanism relating depressive risk factors to depression. *Emotion, 1,* 25–37.

Spielberger, C. D., & Sydeman, S. J. (1994). State–Trait Anger Inventory and State–Trait Anger Expression Inventory. In M. E. Maruish (Ed.), *The use of psychological testing for treatment planning and outcome assessment* (pp. 292–321). Hillsdale, NJ: Erlbaum.

Srivastava, S., McGonigal, K. M., Richards, J. M., Butler, E. A., & Gross, J. J. (2006). Optimism in close relationships: How seeing things in a positive light makes them so. *Journal of Personality and Social Psychology, 91,* 143–153.

Stemmler, G. (1997). Selective activation of traits: Boundary conditions for the activation of anger. *Personality and Individual Differences, 22,* 213–233.

Stepper, S., & Strack, F. (1993). Proprioceptive determinants of emotional and nonemotional feelings. *Journal of Personality and Social Psychology, 64,* 211–220.

Strack, F., Martin, L. L., & Stepper, S. (1988). Inhibiting and facilitating conditions of the human smile: A nonobtrusive test of the facial feedback hypothesis. *Journal of Personality and Social Psychology, 54,* 768–777.

Sutton, R. I. (1991). Maintaining norms about expressed emotions: The case of bill collectors. *Administrative Science Quarterly, 36,* 245–268.

Tamir, M. (2005). Don't worry, be happy?: Neuroticism, trait-consistent affect regulation, and performance. *Journal of Personality and Social Psychology, 89,* 449–461.

Tamir, M., John, O. P., Srivastava, S., & Gross, J. J. (2007). Implicit theories of emotion: Affective and social outcomes across a major life transition. *Journal of Personality and Social Psychology, 92,* 731–744.

Tamir, M., Mitchell, C., & Gross, J. J. (2008). Hedonic and instrumental motives in anger regulation. *Psychological Science, 19,* 324–328.

Taylor, G. J., Bagby, R. M., & Parker, J. D. A. (1997). *Disorders of affect regulation: Alexithymia in medical and psychiatric illness.* Cambridge, UK: Cambridge University Press.

Taylor, J. A. (1953). A personality scale of manifest anxiety. *Journal of Abnormal and Social Psychology, 48,* 285–290.

Tellegen, A. (1985). Structures of mood and personality and their relevance to assessing anxiety, with an emphasis on self-report. In A. H. Tuma & J. D. Maser (Eds.), *Anxiety and the anxiety disorders* (pp. 681–706). Hillsdale, NJ: Erlbaum.

Tobin, R. M., Graziano, W. G., Vanman, E. J., & Tassinary, L. G. (2000). Personality, emotional experience, and efforts to control emotions. *Journal of Personality and Social Psychology, 79,* 656–669.

Tomkins, S. S. (1962). *Affect, imagery, consciousness: The positive affects* (Vol. 1). New York: Springer.

Tracy, J. L., & Robins, R. W. (2004). Show your pride: Evidence for a discrete emotion expression. *Psychological Science, 15,* 194–197.

Tsai, J. L., Knutson, B., & Fung, H. H. (2006). Cultural variation in affect valuation. *Journal of Personality and Social Psychology, 90,* 288–307.

Wallace, J. F., & Newman, J. P. (1997). Neuroticism and the attentional mediation. *Cognitive Therapy and Research, 21,* 135–156.

Watson, D., & Clark, L. A. (1984). Negative affectivity: The disposition to experience aversive emotional states. *Psychological Bulletin, 96,* 465–490.

Watson, D., & Clark, L. A. (1992). Affects separable and inseparable: On the hierarchical arrangement of the negative affects. *Journal of Personality and Social Psychology, 62,* 489–505.

Watson, D., & Clark, L. A. (1994). *The PANAS-X: Manual for the Positive and Negative Affect Schedule—Expanded Form.* Unpublished manuscript, University of Iowa, Iowa City.

Watson, D., & Clark, L. A. (1997). Extraversion and its positive emotional core. In R. Hogan, J. Johnson, & S. Briggs (Eds.), *Handbook of personality psychology* (pp. 767–793). New York: Academic Press.

Watson, D., Clark, L. A., & Tellegen, A. (1988). Development and validation of brief measures of positive and negative affect: The PANAS scales. *Journal of Personality and Social Psychology, 54,* 1063–1070.

Watson, D., Wiese, D., Vaidya, J., & Tellegen, A. (1999). The two general activation systems of affect: Structural findings, evolutionary considerations, and psychobiological evidence. *Journal of Personality and Social Psychology, 76,* 820–838.

Zuckerman, M. (1979). *Sensation seeking: Beyond the optimal level of arousal.* Hillsdale, NJ: Erlbaum.

Zuckerman, M., & Lubin, B. (1985). *Manual for the MAACL-R: The Multiple Affect Adjective Checklist—Revised.* San Diego, CA: Educational and Industrial Testing Service.

CHAPTER 29

Self-Regulatory Processes, Stress, and Coping

Charles S. Carver
Michael F. Scheier
Daniel Fulford

This chapter addresses three topics: stress, coping, and a portion of the self-regulatory structure that underlies personality. The topics of stress and coping typically go hand-in-hand, but it's less common to see them discussed jointly with self-regulation. What exactly does self-regulation have to do with stress and coping? In our view, a great deal. We think that coping essentially constitutes efforts at self-regulation in times of duress (Carver, 2007).

At their core, self-regulatory models of action are organized around people's efforts to create and maintain desired conditions in their lives. These desired conditions can be relatively static (e.g., a house set up the way you want it, good health, a coherent picture of a predictable world). They can also be much more dynamic. Examples of dynamic desired conditions include developing a career, fostering a child's growth into a responsible adult, and taking an interesting and revitalizing vacation. Whether the person's goal is to maintain a stable picture or to make something happen, the process by which the goal is realized is a process of self-regulation.

Self-regulatory efforts often run smoothly, unimpeded by external impediments or personal shortcomings. Sometimes, however,

people encounter difficulties in doing what they want to do, being what they want to be, or keeping their reality ordered in the way they want it. Self-regulatory models also address what happens in situations of that sort.

In this chapter we explore what self-regulation models tell us about the experience of stress and the processes of coping. We begin by describing some orienting assumptions and principles embedded in models of self-regulation. In so doing, we focus on constructs we have found useful in our own work. After presenting orienting principles, we move to a more explicit consideration of how the principles relate to models of stress and coping, and then how stress arises from the experiences of life. The final section of the chapter describes a few of the findings that have emerged from the attempt to integrate the literatures on stress, coping, and self-regulation.

BEHAVIORAL SELF-REGULATION

A common view among contemporary personality psychologists is that human behavior is organized around an ongoing pursuit of goals (Austin & Vancouver, 1996; Elliott

& Dweck, 1988; Pervin, 1989). The contents of most human goals appear to be relatively stable across cultures (Grouzet et al., 2005). Because of differences in emphasis, theorists use different terms to refer to goals, including "current concerns" (Klinger, 1975), "personal strivings" (Emmons, 1986), and "possible selves" (Markus & Nurius, 1986). Although these various constructs differ in ways that are not trivial, what's important at present is their similarities.

We should also reiterate that although some goals have a static quality, others are quite dynamic. The goal of taking a vacation isn't to be sitting in your driveway at the end of 2 weeks, but to actively experience the range of events that have been planned for the vacation. The goal of having a professional career isn't entirely a matter of finally being "established." It's the pathway of steps involved in getting there.

Self-regulation is the process of reaching one's goals. The processes entailed in reaching goals can be conceptualized in diverse ways. Thinking about the processes involved in attaining goals raises a number of issues. Several of them are addressed in the following sections.

Self-Regulatory Feedback Processes

Goals lead to actions. But how are goals used in acting? We take the position that goals serve as reference values for feedback processes. A feedback loop is an organization of four elements (Miller, Galanter, & Pribram, 1960): an input function, a reference value, a comparator, and an output function. An input function is a sensor, a source of information about what now exists. For our purposes this function is perception. The reference value is a second source of information. In the kinds of feedback loops we discuss here, reference values are equivalent to goals. The comparator is a mechanism for comparisons between input and reference value. The comparison always yields one of two outcomes: either the values being compared are discriminably different from each other or they're not.

Following the comparison is an output function. For our purposes, this is equivalent to behavior, though sometimes the behavior is internal. If the comparison yields a "no difference," the output function remains whatever it was: no output, or continuing

an ongoing output at its current level. If the comparison yields "discrepancy," the output function changes.

There are two kinds of feedback loops, which have two different effects (Carver & Scheier, 1998, 1999). In a discrepancy reducing loop, the output function acts to diminish any difference detected between input and reference value. The attempt to make input conform to the standard is seen in attempts to approach or attain valued or desired goals.

The second kind of loop is a discrepancy enlarging loop. The value here isn't one to match, but one to avoid. It may be convenient to think of it as an "anti-goal" (Carver & Scheier, 1998) or a threat. Intuitive examples include getting a speeding ticket and experiencing a humiliating interpersonal rejection. A discrepancy enlarging loop senses present conditions, compares them to the anti-goal, and tries to enlarge the discrepancy between the two. As an example, Cuban Americans in Miami who want to avoid any appearance of sympathy with Castro compare their opinions with the positions of Castro's government and try to make their own opinions as different from those positions as they can (Carver & Humphries, 1981).

The action of discrepancy enlarging processes is typically constrained in some way by discrepancy reducing processes (Carver, Lawrence, & Scheier, 1999; Carver & Scheier, 1998). To put it differently, avoidance behaviors often lead into approach behaviors. An avoidance loop increases distance from the anti-goal. Eventually the behavior enters the sphere of influence of an approach loop, which then pulls behavior into its orbit. For example, people who want to avoid seeming like Castro may become active in anti-Castro organizations.

Hierarchical Organization

Goals vary in many ways. As just noted, some are approach goals, others are avoidance goals. Goals also differ in their level of abstraction (Carver & Scheier, 1998). A man might have the goal, at a high level of abstraction, of being a good father. He may also have the goal, at a lower level of abstraction, of taking his son to soccer practice. The first goal is to be a particular kind of *person*, the second concerns completing particular kinds of *action*. You can also imagine goals that are even more concrete than the latter ones, such as the goal of turning left to park the car. Such goals are closer to specifications of individual acts than were the second, which was more a summary statement about the desired outcome of intended action patterns.

These examples of concrete goals link directly to our example of an abstract goal. This helps us make the point that goals can be connected in a hierarchy. Remember that our focus here is on goals as elements in feedback loops. If goals can be organized hierarchically, so should feedback loops. Long ago, Powers (1973) made precisely that argument. He proposed that in a hierarchy of feedback systems, the output of a high-level system consists of resetting reference values at the next lower level. To put it differently, higher-order systems "behave" by providing goals to the systems just below them. Each level monitors input at the level of abstraction of its own functioning, and each level adjusts output to minimize its discrepancies. Structures at various levels handle their concerns simultaneously.

Powers (1973) focused on low levels of abstraction and said little about the levels of most interest to personality psychologists, except to suggest labels for several levels whose existence makes intuitive sense. "Programs" are activities involving conscious decisions at various points. "Sequences," the next level down, are sets of acts that run off directly, once cued. The level above programs is "principles," qualities that are abstracted from (or implemented by) programs. These are the kinds of qualities that are represented by trait terms. Powers gave the cumbersome name "system concepts" to a higher level that would include the idealized overall sense of self, of a close relationship, or of a group identity.

The nature of the hierarchical model has some interesting implications. It implies that moving toward a lower goal contributes to the attainment of a higher goal (or even several at once). It implies that a higher goal often can be attained by diverse action possibilities at lower levels. This implication permits one to address the fact that people sometimes shift radically the manner in which they try to reach a goal, when the goal itself has not changed. This idea also implies that a given lower-level action can be done

in the service of diverse higher-level goals. Thus, a given act can have strikingly different meanings, depending on the purpose it's intended to serve. This is an important subtheme of this view: Behavior can be understood only by identifying the goals to which it is addressed.

Another point made by the notion of hierarchical organization is that goals differ in importance. The higher you go in the organization, the more fundamental to the overriding sense of self are the qualities encountered. Thus, goal qualities at higher levels would tend to be more important, by virtue of their closer links to the core sense of self, than those at lower levels. Even two goals at a lower level aren't necessarily equivalent in importance, though. The more directly the attainment of a concrete goal contributes to the attainment of a valued abstract goal, the more important is the concrete goal.

Feelings

Another very important aspect of human functioning is feelings. We (Carver & Scheier, 1990, 1998) suggested that feelings arise through the operation of a second layer of feedback process. This second process operates simultaneously with behavior guidance and in parallel to it. One way to characterize what this second process does is to say that it checks continuously on how well the behavior system is doing its job. Thus, the input for the affect-creating loop is a representation of the *rate of discrepancy reduction in the action system over time*.

This "velocity" input cannot create affect by itself, because a given rate of progress has different affective consequences in different circumstances. As in any feedback system, this input is compared against a reference value (cf. Frijda, 1986, 1988): an acceptable or desired (or expected) rate of behavioral discrepancy reduction. The comparison checks for a deviation from the standard. We (Carver & Scheier, 1990, 1998) suggested that the outcome of the comparison at the heart of this loop (the error signal from the comparator) is a hazy and nonverbal sense of confidence or doubt, and affective valence—a sense of positiveness or negativeness. A number of studies have now yielded evidence that is consistent with this view (e.g., Affleck et al., 1998; Baumeister & Bratslavsky, 1999; Brunstein, 1993; Brunstein, Schultheiss, & Grässmann, 1998; Hsee & Abelson, 1991; Hsee, Abelson, & Salovey, 1991; Laurenceau, Troy, & Carver, 2005; Lawrence, Carver, & Scheier, 2002).

Earlier we said that goals and anti-goals promote approach and avoidance tendencies, respectively. The view of affect we just described rests on the idea that positive feelings arise when an action system is doing well at *doing what it's organized to do.* Approach systems are organized to reduce discrepancies. When they are making good progress toward desired goals, positive affect is experienced. When satisfactory progress isn't being made, affect turns more negative. Avoidance systems function to enlarge discrepancies. If avoidance systems are doing well at what they're organized to do—distancing the person from anti-goals—positive affect should result. If they are doing poorly, the affective experience should be negative.

This much would seem to be the same across the two types of systems. On the other hand, we believe there is also a difference in the specific affects involved (Carver & Scheier, 1998). Drawing in part on work by Higgins (1987, 1996), we assume that an affect dimension relating to approach runs (in its purest form) from depression to elation (via anger and other assorted feelings; Carver, 2004). An affect dimension relating to avoidance runs (in its purest form) from anxiety to relief or contentment. Although it is beyond the scope of this chapter, it has been argued that the affects play an important role in priority management (see Carver, 2003; Carver & Scheier, 2008).

Interface between Affect and Action

The two-layered viewpoint outlined in the preceding sections implies a natural relation between affect and action. That is, if the input function of the affect loop is a sensed rate of progress in action, the output function of the affect loop must be a change in rate of that action. Thus, the affect loop has a direct influence on what occurs in the action loop.

Some changes in rate output are straightforward. If you are lagging behind, you try harder. Some changes are less straightforward. The rates of many "behaviors" are defined not by pace of physical action but in terms of choices among potential actions or entire programs of action. For example, increasing your rate of progress on a project at work may mean choosing to spend a weekend working rather than playing with family and friends. Increasing your rate of being kind means choosing to perform an act that reflects kindness when an opportunity arises. Thus, change in rate must often be translated into other terms, such as concentration or allocation of time and effort. In any case, it should be apparent that the action system and the rate system must work in concert with one another. Both are involved in the flow of action. They influence different *aspects* of the action, but both are always involved.

Confidence and Doubt

In describing the processes underlying affect, we suggested that one mechanism yields two subjective readouts: affect, and a sense of confidence versus doubt. We turned first to affect, but the affect and expectancies that are generated as behavior unfolds are intertwined. Thus, what we've said about affect applies equally well to the vague sense of confidence or doubt that also accompanies action.

This hazy sense of confidence or doubt does not operate in a psychological vacuum, however. When people experience adversity in trying to move toward goals, they periodically interrupt their efforts to assess in a more deliberative way the likelihood of a successful outcome (Carver & Scheier, 1981, 1990, 1998). In effect, people suspend the behavioral stream, step outside it, and evaluate the likelihood of success in a more thoughtful way than occurs while acting. This interruption may happen once or often. It may be brief or prolonged. In this assessment people presumably use memories of prior outcomes in similar situations, while considering such factors as additional resources they might bring to bear or alternative approaches to the problem.

How do these thoughts influence people's subsequent expectancies? In some cases, when people retrieve "chronic" expectancies from memory, the information already *is* expectancies. These chronic expectancies may simply substitute for those derived from immediate experience, or they may blend with and color those immediate expectancies to a greater or lesser degree.

In some cases, however, people think more expansively about possibilities for the situation's evolution. For such possibilities to influence expectancies, their consequences must be evaluated. They probably are played through mentally as behavioral scenarios (Taylor & Pham, 1996), leading to conclusions that affect the expectancy: For example, "If I try approaching it this way instead of that way, it should work better"; or "This is the only thing I can see to do, and it will just make the situation worse." It seems reasonable that mental simulation engages the mechanism that creates the sense of affect and confidence during actual behavior. Playing through a scenario that leads to a positive outcome yields faster perceived progress. The confidence loop thus yields a more optimistic outcome assessment. If the scenario is negative and hopeless, it indicates a further loss of progress, and the confidence loop yields further doubt.

Efforts and Giving Up

Whatever their source, expectancies influence behavior. If expectations for the desired outcome are favorable enough, the person renews effort toward the goal. If doubts are strong enough, the result is an impetus to disengage from further effort, and even from the goal itself. Sometimes the disengagement is overt. Sometimes it is mental—off-task thinking, daydreaming, wishful thinking, and so on. Often mental disengagement cannot be sustained, as situational cues force a reconfrontation of the obstacle. In such cases, the result is repetitive negative rumination, which often focuses on self-doubt and perceptions of inadequacy. This experience is both unpleasant and performance impairing.

These two classes of responses to adversity appear to form a behavioral "watershed" (Carver & Scheier, 1981, 1998). That is, one set of responses involves continued comparisons between present state and goal and continued efforts at movement forward. The other set consists of avoidance of comparisons, and quitting (Klinger, 1975; Wortman & Brehm, 1975). Just as rainwater falling on a mountain ridge ultimately flows to one side of the ridge or the other, so do be-

haviors ultimately flow to one or the other of these two classes. This theme—divergence in responses as a function of expectancies—is an important one, applying to a surprisingly broad range of literatures (Carver & Scheier, 1998, 1999).

Expectancies Vary in Specificity

The fact that goals vary in specificity—from very general, to those pertaining to a particular domain of life, to very concrete and specific—suggests that people have a comparable range of variations in expectancies (Armor & Taylor, 1998; Carver & Scheier, 1998). You can be confident or doubtful about having an interesting life, about avoiding boring people, about being able to speak clearly in public, or about buttoning your shirt.

Which of these sorts of expectancies matter? Probably all of them. Expectancy-based theories often hold that behavior is predicted best when the specificity of the expectancy matches that of the behavior. Sometimes it's argued that prediction is best when taking into account several levels of specificity. But many outcomes in life have multiple causes, people often face situations they've never experienced before, and situations unfold and change over time. It's been suggested that in circumstances such as these, generalized expectations are particularly useful in predicting behavior and emotions (Scheier & Carver, 1985).

The same principles that apply to focused confidence also apply to the generalized sense of optimism versus pessimism. When we talk about variables such as optimism and pessimism, the sense of confidence that's at issue is just more diffuse and broader in scope. Thus, when confronting a challenge (presumably any type of challenge), optimists should tend to be confident and persistent, assuming that the adversity can be handled in one way or another. Pessimists should be more doubtful and hesitant, more ready to anticipate disaster.

Scaling Back Goals as Limited Disengagement

Sometimes when people give up trying to reach a goal, they quit and that's the end of it. Sometimes, however, something else happens. In some cases when things are going poorly and expectancies of success are dim, people want to quit, but they don't quit altogether. Rather, they trade the threatened goal for a less demanding one. This is a kind of limited disengagement. They've given up on the first goal at the same time as they're adopting a lesser one. This limited disengagement has an important positive consequence: By doing this, people remain engaged in the general domain they'd wanted to quit (or felt the need to quit). By scaling back (giving up in a small way), they keep trying to move ahead (thus *not* giving up, in a larger way).

As an example, a student who wants an A in a course but who's struggling ineffectually may decide that an A is out of the question and lower his sights to a B or even C. Given the change in goal, exam scores in the B or C range will represent better progress than they would have represented in relation to the initial goal. The result is that the student keeps plugging along, completes the course adequately instead of dropping it, and may feel satisfied with a C.

Another example comes from research on couples in which one partner is dying from AIDS (Moskowtiz, Folkman, Collette, & Vittinghoff, 1996). Some healthy subjects had the goal of overcoming their partners' illness and continuing to have active lives together. As the illness progresses, however, and it becomes apparent that this goal can't be met, the healthy partners often scale back their aspirations. Now the goal is to do more limited activities during the course of a day, for example. Choosing a goal that's more limited and manageable ensures that it will be possible to move successfully toward it. The result is that even in these circumstances, the person experiences more positive feeling than would otherwise be the case and stays engaged behaviorally with efforts to move forward with this aspect of life.

The relationship between scaling back goals and well-being has been shown in other cases. One study examined goal disengagement and reengagement among college undergraduates, younger adults, older adults, parents of children with cancer, and parents of medically healthy children (Wrosch, Scheier, Miller, Schulz, & Carver, 2003). In all groups, individual differences in goal disengagement and goal reengagement predicted subjective well-being. Reengaging in

new goals predicted well-being even above and beyond the ease of abandoning goals that were unattainable.

We believe that this principle of scaling back—partial disengagement without complete abandonment of the domain—is a very important one. Both giving up on potentially attainable goals and failing to disengage in pursuit of unattainable goals can yield adverse outcomes. As we indicate later, keeping the person engaged in goal pursuits in particular domains keeps the person engaged in *living.*

SELF-REGULATION AND STRESS MODELS

The model of self-regulation sketched in the preceding pages was intended to characterize the structure and processes of everyday behavior. Although many examples used to illustrate the ideas came from achievement- or task-related contexts, the model is not one of achievement per se, or even of "task" behavior. Rather, the principles apply to human behavior in general. Some goals are highly valued and subjectively important to the people who hold them. Other goals are mundane, even trivial—the maintenance activities of daily life (e.g., doing laundry, brushing your teeth). Some goals concern professional achievement, others concern the nourishment of human relationships. We believe, however, that the actions linked to these disparate goals have a common structure, and that the structure is partially captured by the principles outlined above.

Although this model is about behavior in general, we believe it provides an interesting window on the experiences of stress and coping. From the self-regulatory viewpoint, stress is a particular class of experiences, and coping is the responses that follow from these experiences (Carver, 2007). From this viewpoint, stress occurs when people encounter obstacles to attaining desired goals or avoiding anti-goals. Coping involves efforts to create conditions that foster continued movement toward desired goals (or away from anti-goals) or efforts to disengage from goals that are seen as no longer attainable.

Although it may not be completely apparent, this line of thought has resemblances to several conceptual analyses that were devised explicitly to address stress and coping per se (Carver, 2007). In this section we briefly consider three of those approaches and their relations to these principles of self-regulation.

Stress and Coping: Lazarus and Folkman

Most contemporary views of stress and coping can be traced, in one way or another, to the work of Lazarus and Folkman and their colleagues (e.g., Lazarus, 1966; Lazarus & Folkman, 1984). The model they developed assumes that stress exists when people confront circumstances that tax or exceed their ability to manage them. This conceptualization places the experience of stress squarely in the domain of behavior in which obstacles or difficulties are being confronted. When people find themselves hard-pressed to deal with some impediment or some looming threat, the experience is stressful.

The Lazarus and Folkman model incorporates several themes. One is that stress entails the perception (appraisal) of threat, loss, or challenge (though *challenge* has held up less well in this respect than the other two). Threat is the perception of the impending occurrence of something bad or harmful. Loss is the perception that something bad or harmful has already happened. A challenge appraisal, in contrast, is the perception that one can gain or grow from what nonetheless will be a demanding encounter.

In conditions of threat or loss, impediments to desired conditions are either looming or already in place. Although work in the Lazarus and Folkman tradition has not always emphasized this point, threats and losses are conditions that prevent or impede maintenance or attainment of desired goal values. Loss prevents the continued existence of a desired state of affairs (e.g., death of a spouse prevents the continued relationship). Threat suggests imminent interference with continued pursuit of desired activities or conditions (e.g., serious illness threatens one's life goals, one's golf game, and one's perception of reality).

We framed this statement in terms of interference with desired goals. It should be obvious, however, that the principles apply just as well to the avoidance of anti-goals. Conditions that imply the imminent occurrence of an anti-goal condition (e.g., pain; Affleck, Tennen, Pfeiffer, & Fifield, 1987), or

suggest the inability to escape from such a condition, will be stressful.

Another point of similarity between self-regulation models and the Lazarus–Folkman model concerns the dynamic, continuous evaluation of the situation and one's responses to it. In the Lazarus–Folkman model, people don't always respond to stressful encounters in a reflexive, automatic way. Rather, they often weigh various options and consider the consequences of those options before acting. Decisions about how to cope depend partly on confidence or doubt about the usefulness of a particular strategy of responding. Thus, issues of confidence and doubt, as well as the disruption of intended courses of behavior, are embedded in this theoretical model.

Conservation of Resources: Hobfoll

Another view on the experience of stress, developed by Hobfoll (1989), begins with the idea that people have an accumulation of resources that they try to protect, defend, and conserve. Resources can be physical (e.g., a house, car, clothing), they can be conditions of one's current life (e.g., friends and relatives, stable employment, sound marriage), they can be personal qualities (e.g., a positive view of the world, work skills, social prowess), or they can be energy resources (e.g., money, credit, or knowledge). Resources are anything the person values.

This theory holds that people try to sustain the resources that they have and acquire further resources. From this viewpoint, stress occurs when resources are threatened or lost, or when people invest their resources and don't receive an adequate return on the investment. Hobfoll (1989) argues that loss is the central experience in stress (see also Hobfoll, Freedy, Green, & Solomon, 1996). Threat is an impending loss. One might think of the failure to receive an adequate return on investment of resources as the loss of an anticipated new resource.

Hobfoll (1989) has argued that this theory differs in important ways from other models of stress (and he has generated hypotheses that might not be as readily derived from other models). However, we want to emphasize the resemblances. This theory uses an economic metaphor for human experience. People acquire resources, defend them, and use them to acquire more resources. Stress occurs when the market has a downturn in the value of their resources or when an event of some sort wipes out part of their resource base.

We would argue that it's important to step back from a consideration of those resources and ask what their usefulness is. In our view (and nothing about this view intrinsically contradicts Hobfoll's position), these resources matter to a person inasmuch as they facilitate the person's movement toward desired goals (or avoidance of anti-goals). What use is a car? It can take you places and it can make an impression on other people. What use are friends? They can help you feel better when you're upset, and you can engage in activities of mutual enjoyment with them. What use is a positive life view? It keeps you moving toward a variety of goals. Work skills permit you to complete projects, achieve things, and hold a job that fosters continued movement toward goals. Money and influence are means to a variety of ends.

In short, for most people, resources are intimately bound up in the continuing pursuit of goals. Thus, any attempt to conserve resources occurs in the implicit service of eventual continued goal attainment. A loss of resources represents a threat to that continued goal attainment. Once again there is a strong implicit connection to principles of self-regulation.

Bereavement and Loss: Stroebe and Stroebe

Another view on stress to which we would like to devote some attention is that of Stroebe, Stroebe, and their colleagues (e.g., M. S. Stroebe, Stroebe, & Hansson, 1993). Their work has been conducted within the context of grieving over loss—particularly bereavement. Their theoretical perspective assumes two focuses on the part of the bereaved. The first is on the person who has been lost and the relationship of the bereaved with that person. The second focus is on potential relationships with other persons.

Traditionally, many approaches to bereavement have held that the task of the bereaved is to disengage from the lost relationship and move on to new attachments (e.g., Worden, 1991). This sequence is not unlike that described more generally in self-regulatory models as a disengagement

of commitment to one incentive to take up another incentive (Klinger, 1975). From this view, the key to successful adaptation for the bereaved person is finalizing the past well enough to make a start toward a future of involvement with others.

There's no question that movement forward is important. M. S. Stroebe (1994) reviewed the literature on bereavement and mortality and found that people who die after bereavement tend to lack contact with others during the bereavement period, compared to those who survive the bereavement process. Those vulnerable to dying do not remarry, they don't have people to talk to on the phone, they live alone, and they feel isolated. The general picture of those at risk that Stroebe uncovered is one of loneliness and little integration with other people.

The Stroebes and their colleagues have argued, however, that the optimal solution is not always to completely disengage psychologically from the person who's been lost (cf. Bowlby, 1980). Rather, it may be better for some people to reconfigure the psychological bond with that person into something different from what it was, something that remains positive but is more restricted than it was. Thus the person can continue to draw on that connection psychologically, in smaller ways than was once the case, but in ways that nevertheless provide benefits to the person (see Klass, Silverman, & Nickman, 1996). People may differ in whether it is more beneficial to retain a bond with the person who has been lost or to move on (W. Stroebe, Schut, & Stroebe, 2005).

This reconfiguration of the sense of the lost relationship resembles the scaling-back process of the self-regulation model. By letting go and stopping attempts to reach the unreachable (a continuation of life as it was), the bereaved person becomes free for potential attachments to others. By disengaging only partly, the person retains a sense of connection with the disrupted relationship. To the extent that the positive value of the disrupted relationship can be used by the bereaved as a psychological resource, the residual sense of attachment might help the bereaved person return to activities and connections with other people. If the limited disengagement did *not* return the person to an active life, the resolution would not be adaptive.

THREAT, LOSS, DISRUPTION, AND NORMAL LIFE PROCESSES

In the first section of this chapter we outlined a set of principles as a model of self-regulation. In the second section we indicated some broad similarities between that model and three views on the coping process. We now turn to a different point: although it is certainly possible to think of stress and coping in terms of such events as natural disasters, life-threatening illnesses, and human-inflicted cruelties, not all stress is so distinct from the normal flow of behavior. Much of the stress in life arises from being boxed into corners or experiencing conflict within oneself. These experiences have the same structure as we earlier argued underlies stress in general. That is, in each case there is an impediment to forward movement toward desired goals or away from threatening anti-goals.

As a way of illustrating the breadth of applicability of this idea, in this section we consider several sorts of impediments that originate fairly readily within the flow of ordinary behavior. We do so within the framework of self-regulation outlined earlier (Carver & Scheier, 1998; for related views, see Baumeister & Heatherton, 1996; Baumeister, Heatherton, & Tice, 1994; Baumeister & Vohs, 2004).

Problems as Conflicts among Goals

One way in which stress can arise derives from the fact that the goal structures that people hold often contain the potential for conflict. Conflict occurs when a person is committed to two or more goals that can't be attained easily at the same time (e.g., being a successful physician while being an involved wife and mother; having a close relationship while being emotionally independent). The bind here resembles that of role conflict. You can't do two mutually exclusive things at once. The very act of devoting strong efforts to attaining one goal can constitute an impediment to attaining the other goal. Given this impediment, the person experiences stress.

There's evidence that conflict among goals does create stress. Emmons and King (1988) had subjects report the personal strivings that motivate their lives and then make some further ratings about those strivings. These included ratings of the extent to which success in one striving tended to create problems for another one. The researchers found that conflicts between personal strivings were tied to psychological distress and physical symptoms. In contrast, people who valued their strivings and saw them as important expressed greater satisfaction with their lives (see also Emmons, 1986; Lecci, Okun, & Karoly, 1994).

Given the distress produced by goal conflict, people might try to engage in tactics to avoid its occurrence. One strategy is to alternate between conflicting goals, addressing first one, then the other. Jumping back and forth can be exhausting, however. It's also hard to keep the conflict from re-emerging. Another solution is to decide that one goal matters more to one's higher-order values than the other, and to reorganize or "reweight" one's hierarchy accordingly. But this isn't easy to do either. The self as an organization of values is relatively stable. Still, although reorganization of the self is hard and painful (and thus resisted), it does sometimes happen (cf. Crocker & Major, 1989; Heatherton & Nichols, 1994; Kling, Ryff, & Essex, 1997).

Automatic Doubts

Another source of stress is the residue of doubt that can build up in people's minds over extended experiences of adverse outcomes in some domain. As noted earlier in the chapter, encountering difficulty while acting induces a hazy sense of doubt, which may promote a more conscious deliberation on the likelihood of success. If the person has had a lot of experience in some domain, memories from those experiences are encoded with a great deal of redundancy. When things get difficult in that domain, people often rely heavily on those memories to inform them about the likely outcome of what's happening now.

Although this sometimes works to people's advantage (if the memories are mostly successes), all too often the residual sense is one of doubt or inadequacy. If that residual sense is strong enough or redundantly encoded enough, the person will experience an impulse to give up at the first signs of adversity. When doubts are deeply ingrained, people may not even attend well to what's *going on* in the current situation. Being convinced that the situation will end badly, people fail to realize that the difficulty they're experiencing is minor and easily resolved. They give up trying, and the doubt strengthens further. This progression can eventuate in a tendency to "catastrophize," which is a particularly problematic response among pain patients, for example (Turk & Rudy, 1992).

This automatic overreliance on heavily encoded doubts might be viewed as a case in which people bring "stress readiness" to the situation. There are many situations in life in which real but minor impediments arise. The person who brings this heavy burden of doubt into the situation is creating further impediments that needn't be there. These further impediments constitute a source of stress for some people in situations that aren't stressful for others.

Premature Disengagement of Effort

Consider further the consequences of doubt. Doubt can cause people to scale back on goals or to give up on goals entirely. It can be bad for this to happen too readily. A person who gives up whenever things get difficult will have trouble reaching any goal in life. Disengaging too fast keeps people from trying their best, and it short-circuits potential successes (cf. Steele, 1997). Sometimes the result is a repetitive pattern of quitting and going on to something else. Such a lack of persistence, moving the person endlessly from goal to goal, can be a serious problem. It's not clear that this pattern involves great stress, however. If people really can put the failures behind them and move on, the stress of failure should be brief. Only if the recurring lack of commitment serves as a source of problems in and of itself will stress be maintained.

There's also a more subtle pattern associated with premature disengagement. It involves disengagement of *effort*, but a continued commitment to the goal. This person is no longer trying but hasn't gotten the goal out of mind. This combination may be reflected in rumination, efforts at self-distraction, off-task thinking, temporarily leaving the scene of the behavior, or cognitive interference (Sarason, Pierce, & Sarason, 1996). Despite these goal-irrelevant activities, the goal hasn't been abandoned. But any attempt to

move toward it is sporadic, disrupted repeatedly.

The process seems to go like this: Difficulty leads to an interruption, and the person's doubts prompt disengagement, which is deflected into mental disengagement. However, this mental disengagement can't be maintained because the person hasn't given up the goal. Then there is a reengagement of effort, which may quickly lead to renewed doubts and a renewed impulse to disengage (McIntosh & Martin, 1992; Wine, 1971, 1980). Because there's continued commitment to the goal but no movement toward it, the person also experiences distress (Carver & Scheier, 1990, 1998; Klinger, 1975; Pyszczynski & Greenberg, 1992).

Premature disengagement of effort is another case of an impediment to movement toward a goal. The impediment in this case is the lack of effort, which stems from doubt. This situation could be made less stressful either by renewing effort or by abandoning the goal or scaling it back to something more attainable.

Struggling Too Long toward Unattainable Goals

If there are drawbacks to withdrawing effort too quickly from goals that might be attained, it's also bad to keep struggling toward goals that are unattainable. Giving up is an indispensable part of self-regulation; people need to be able to retrace their steps, back out of corners, free themselves to go elsewhere. Continued commitment to a goal that's unattainable wastes resources in futile efforts. If the futile efforts are extensive, so is the waste of resources.

Continued commitment to an unattainable goal shares two consequences with the case just considered: premature disengagement of effort while retaining commitment. In both instances, the person is prevented from taking up new, viable goals because he or she is prevented from noticing, recognizing, or responding to new opportunities (Baumeister & Scher, 1988; Feather, 1989; Janoff-Bulman & Brickman, 1982). Both also cause distress. The person who's unable to move forward but is unable to let go is condemned to suffer. These consequences suggest how important it can be to accept the reality of a permanent change in one's situation (Carver et al., 1993; Scheier & Carver, 2001).

Pursuit of the unattainable is another case of an impediment to forward movement. The impediment in this case is real, because the goal is truly out of reach. Thus, stress can arise both from lack of effort (stemming from doubt) or from commitment to a goal that's impossible to attain. In the former case there are two ways to reduce the stress, in the latter only one. If the goal is attainable, renewed effort can potentially reduce the stress. This won't happen for an unattainable goal. Whether the goal is truly attainable or not, disengagement from it (or scaling it back to something that's clearly attainable) will have the effect of reducing stress.

Hierarchical Organization and Importance Can Impede Disengagement

There is an important qualification on that last statement, however. There are many reasons why a person might find it hard to disengage. A key reason follows from the idea that goals are hierarchically arranged. Recall that goals are more important and central to the self as one moves from lower to higher levels of a goal hierarchy. Also recall that lower-order goals vary in how strongly they connect to higher-order goals. It seems likely that disengaging from higher-order goals is always troublesome. Disengaging from a higher-order goal means giving up on a core element of the self, which people resist (Greenwald, 1980). Less obvious is that disengagement from concrete goals is also hard if those concrete goals are closely linked to higher-order goals. Under such circumstances, giving up on a lower-order goal means more than simply abandoning the action in question. It also means creating a problem for the higher-order goals to which the lower goal is linked. As a result, disengagement from the concrete goal is more difficult.

Thus, the emergence of stress in people's lives is determined partly by the nature of the organization among their goals and values. It can be easy to step away from a particular unattained goal, in and of itself. But sometimes the relationship of that goal to core values of the self make it harder to do so. The attempt to give up and step away then induces stress, because it creates an impedi-

ment to the attainment or maintenance of the higher value.

When Is Disengagement the Correct Response?

It will be apparent from the foregoing that a critical question in life is when to keep trying and when to give up, when it's right to keep "hanging on" and when "letting go" is the right response (Pyszczynski & Greenberg, 1992). On the one hand, disengagement (at some level, at least) is a necessity. Disengagement is a natural and indispensable part of self-regulation (Wrosch, Scheier, Carver, & Schulz, 2003). If we are ever to turn away from efforts at unattainable goals, if we're ever to back out of blind alleys, we must be able to disengage—to give up and start over somewhere else.

The importance of disengagement is particularly obvious regarding concrete, low-level goals: People must be able to remove themselves from literal blind alleys and wrong streets, give up plans that have been disrupted by unexpected events. The tendency is also important, however, with regard to some higher-level goals. A large literature attests to the importance of moving on with life after the loss of close relationships, even if the moving on doesn't imply a complete putting aside of the old (e.g., Cleiren, 1993; Orbuch, 1992; M. S. Stroebe et al., 1993). People sometimes must be willing even to give up values that are deeply embedded in the self, if those values create too much conflict and distress in their lives. Remaining stuck in the past instead of moving on has been found to create problems for people who've experienced a variety of life traumas (Holman & Silver, 1998).

Giving up is a functional and adaptive response *when it leads to the taking up of other goals*, whether these are substitutes for the lost goal or simply new goals in a different domain. By permitting the pursuit of alternative goals, giving up provides the opportunity to reengage and move ahead again (Carver & Scheier, 1998; Scheier & Carver, 2001). In such cases, giving up occurs in service to the broader function of returning the person to an engagement with life. This depiction appears to apply to goal values and doubts that extend fairly deeply into the sense of self. People need multiple paths to such values. If one path is barricaded, people need to be able to jump to another one.

It seems likely that substituting a new path for an obstructed one is made easier by having clarity about one's goals at the abstract level. For example, if a person who has valued a sense of connectedness in a close marital relationship loses his or her spouse, the sense of connection can be experienced in different ways. A person in this situation who understands that his or her core desire is to *experience closeness* can more readily recognize that there are many ways to do this than can someone who's less clear about the nature of the higher-level goal. Similarly, it seems likely that a person who already recognizes the multiple paths that exist to a given goal will be better prepared to make such shifts, as necessary.

In any case, it seems apparent that the ability to shift to a new goal or to a new path to a continuing goal is an important part of remaining goal-engaged. What happens if there's no alternative to take up? There is no shift, because there's nothing to shift *to*. This is the worst situation: where there's nothing to pursue, nothing to take the place of what's seen as unattainable (cf. Moskowitz et al., 1996). Commitment to the unattainable goal means distress. Waning commitment, in this case, means emptiness.

COPING RESEARCH REVEALING SELF-REGULATORY PRINCIPLES

An important theme in discussing self-regulatory models is that expectations play a pivotal role in people's responses to adversity. When impediments are encountered (and stress commences), what happens depends on whether the person feels the obstacles can be overcome, the problems solved or circumvented. When people expect to succeed (given the opportunity for further effort), they keep trying and even try harder. When people see success as out of reach, they withdraw effort, even give up completely the attempt to reach the goal.

Structure of Coping

These self-regulatory principles have important implications for conceptualizing coping

activities. Indeed, the disjunction between effort and giving up is deeply embodied in current views of coping. It is common to refer to three classes of responses: (1) Problem-focused coping consists of attempts to remove the obstacle or to minimize its impact. (2) Emotion-focused coping consists of attempts to reduce the distress emotions caused by the obstacle (either by reappraisal of the obstacle or management of the emotions; Gross, 1998). (3) Avoidance coping is a class of responses that appear to be aimed either at avoiding any acknowledgment that the problem exists (via, e.g., self-distraction, denial, substance use, wishful thinking) or at giving up the attempt to do anything about the problem (via, e.g., substance use, or giving up goals that are being interfered with).

The self-regulatory principles also have important implications for thinking about individual differences in coping. It follows from our emphasis on expectancies as an influence on self-regulation that these classes of coping responses should occur differentially as a function of people's expectancies. There is considerable evidence that this is so, and we describe a little of it in the next sections. We focus on research in which expectancies were operationalized in terms of generalized optimism versus pessimism. This is by no means an exhaustive review of these studies, but rather a few examples to illustrate the broader themes.

Optimism, Pessimism, and Coping

Differences in coping responses used by optimists and pessimists have been found in a number of studies (Carver & Scheier, 2003; Scheier & Carver, 1992). One early project (Scheier, Weintraub, & Carver, 1986) asked undergraduates to recall their most stressful event of the previous month and rate a list of coping responses with respect to that event. Optimism predicted problem-focused coping, especially when the situation was seen as controllable. Optimism also related to positive reframing and (when the situation was seen as uncontrollable) with the tendency to accept the reality of the situation. In contrast, optimism related negatively to the use of denial and the attempt to distance oneself from the problem.

The fact that optimists and pessimists differed in their use of problem-focused coping is entirely consistent with the self-regulation model. Not directly predicted, however, was the fact that optimists and pessimists also differed on other responses, including accepting the reality of difficult situations and putting the situations in the best possible light. In retrospect, however, the findings make sense within the self-regulation framework. That is, it may be easier to accept the reality of a negative situation if one is confident of favorable eventual outcomes.

This general pattern of effects has continued to emerge in work on optimism and coping. For example, in research on dispositional coping styles (Carver, Scheier, & Weintraub, 1989; Fontaine, Manstead, & Wagner, 1993), optimists reported a tendency to rely on active, problem-focused coping, and to be planful when confronting stressful events. Pessimists reported a tendency to disengage from the goals with which the stressor was interfering. Optimists also reported accepting the reality of stressful events and trying to see the best in bad situations and to learn something from them. Pessimists reported tendencies toward overt denial and substance abuse—strategies that lessened their awareness of the problem.

Other projects have studied relationships between optimism and coping strategies in specific contexts. For example, Strutton and Lumpkin (1992) studied coping at work and found that optimists used problem-focused coping more than pessimists. Pessimists used avoidant coping (self-indulgent escapism, including sleeping, eating, and drinking) more than optimists. A study focusing on managerial women (Long, Kahn, & Schutz, 1992) found that optimists perceived problems at work to be less threatening to the attainment of their goals than did pessimists. Optimistic women were also more likely to use active, problem-focused coping strategies in dealing with problems, and less likely to use disengagement coping. Finally, optimistic women were more likely than pessimistic women to use preventive coping strategies (i.e., strategies to promote personal well-being and reduce the likelihood of problems).

In another study, dispositional optimism was examined among middle-age men undergoing coronary artery bypass surgery (Scheier et al., 1989). Information relating to rate of physical recovery, mood, and quality of life was assessed before and after surgery. Dispositional optimism related to more problem-focused coping, faster physical recovery and discharge from the hospital, and overall quality of life at 6 months postsurgery.

Optimism, Coping, and Emotional Well-Being

The studies just described establish that optimists cope in different ways than do pessimists. Other work has gone a step further to link such differences in coping to differences in emotional outcomes. One study followed women undergoing breast biopsy (Stanton & Snider, 1993). Optimism, coping, and mood were assessed the day before biopsy; women receiving a cancer diagnosis were reassessed 24 hours before surgery and 3 weeks after surgery. Pessimists used more cognitive avoidance in coping with the upcoming diagnostic procedure than did optimists. This reaction contributed significantly to distress prior to biopsy, and it also predicted postbiopsy distress among women with positive diagnoses.

Another study of cancer patients examined how women cope with treatment for early-stage breast cancer across the first year after treatment (Carver et al., 1993). Optimism, coping (with the diagnosis of cancer), and mood were assessed the day before surgery, 10 days postsurgery, and at three follow-up points. Both before and after surgery, optimism was associated with a pattern of coping tactics that revolved around accepting the reality of the situation, placing as positive a light on it as possible, trying to relieve the situation with humor, and (at presurgery only) taking active steps to do whatever there was to be done. Pessimism was associated with denial and behavioral disengagement (giving up) at each measurement point.

These coping tactics also related strongly to subjects' distress. Positive reframing, acceptance, and the use of humor all related inversely to distress, both before surgery and after. Denial and behavioral disengagement related positively to distress at all measurement points. Not unexpectedly, given the pattern of the correlations, the effect of optimism on distress was largely indirect through coping, particularly at postsurgery.

Another study examined the emotional adjustment of breast cancer survivors (Trunzo & Pinto, 2003). Women who had completed treatment within a year prior to the study were recruited. Optimism and mood were assessed at baseline and 6- and 12-month follow-ups. At each measurement point, optimism was a negative predictor of mood disturbance, suggesting that optimists were less vulnerable to emotional distress.

Other studies have also found that coping mediates the relationship between optimism and well-being in circumstances that are stressful but more normative. For example, Aspinwall and Taylor (1992) tracked undergraduates as they settled into college. Coping, optimism, and well-being were measured when students arrived on campus. Outcome measures were assessed again at the end of the semester. Initial optimism predicted lower levels of distress at the end of the semester (independent of other personality factors and baseline mood). Optimists were also more likely than pessimists to use active coping and less likely to use avoidance coping. Avoidance coping related to poorer adjustment, and active coping (separately) related to better adjustment. Finally, the beneficial effects of optimism seemed to operate at least partly through the coping differences.

Another study with a similar design examined optimism, stress, depression, and the development of social support among college freshmen (Brissette, Scheier, & Carver, 2002). Coping, depression, and perceptions of social networks were assessed at the end of the semester. Optimism predicted lower stress and depression throughout the semester. In addition, those who were more optimistic at the beginning of the semester displayed greater increases in their social support networks by semester's end. The findings of this study suggest that the better emotional outcomes of optimists may be fostered partly by their ability to recruit social support networks. Another study lends additional support to that interpretation. This study found that the relationship partners of optimists see them as being more supportive in resolving conflicts than is true of partners of pessimists (Srivastava, McGonigal, Richards, Butler, & Gross, 2006).

Summary

As these examples indicate, optimists differ from pessimists in their stable coping tendencies, in the kinds of coping reactions they generate when confronting stress, and in the emotional well-being that results. In general, optimists tend to use more problem-focused coping strategies than pessimists. When problem-focused coping is not a possibility, optimists turn to adaptive emotion-focused coping strategies such as acceptance, use of humor, and positive reframing. These are strategies that keep them engaged with the effort to move forward with their lives. Pessimists tend to cope through overt denial and by disengaging from the goals with which the stressor is interfering. Moreover, these differences in coping responses appear to be at least partially responsible for differences between optimists and pessimists in the emotional well-being they experience. Findings of this sort serve to link elements of self-regulation models of behavior with the literature of coping responses and their consequences.

It may be particularly noteworthy that optimists report acceptance, whereas pessimists tend toward denial. Denial and acceptance differ in important ways. Denial (the refusal to accept the reality of the stressful situation) means attempting to adhere to a worldview that is no longer valid. Acceptance implies a restructuring of one's experience to come to grips with the reality of the situation that one confronts. Acceptance thus may involve a deeper set of processes, in which the person actively works through the experience, attempting to integrate it into an evolving worldview.

The attempt to come to terms with the existence of problems may confer special benefit to acceptance as a coping response. We should be very clear, however, about what we mean. The acceptance measured in these studies is a willingness to admit that a problem exists or that an event has happened—even an event that may irrevocably alter the fabric of the person's life. We are *not* talking about stoic resignation, that is, fatalistic acceptance of negative outcomes. The latter response does not confer a benefit and may even be detrimental (Greer, Morris, & Pettingale, 1979; Greer, Morris, Pettingale, Haybittle,1990; Pettingale, Morris, & Greer, 1985; Reed, Kemeny, Taylor, Wang,

& Visscher, 1994; for further discussion of this issue, see Scheier & Carver, 2001).

CONCLUDING COMMENT

In this chapter we have tried to point to links between a model of the self-regulation of action and the experiences of stress and coping. This effort was far from exhaustive. Our intent was only to provide some illustrations of how the concepts can be integrated. In the preceding sections we pointed to conceptual links between the elements of the self-regulation model and three conceptualizations of various aspects of stress; to a series of ways in which stress can arise in the course of ordinary behavior; to distinctions among aspects of coping that seem to flow readily from the self-regulation model; and to a few findings that reveal both the divergent self-regulatory functions involved in coping (effort and disengagement) and individual differences in the manner in which people cope with adverse circumstances. Although space constraints prevent a deeper discussion of the stress literature, we believe many more aspects of that literature also fit this picture.

In closing, we make one last point about the links among stress, coping, and self-regulation. This point is surely not unique to the perspective we've take here, but it seems to be implied with particular clarity by it. The point is that stress is not an all-or-none phenomenon, and that coping is not fundamentally different in kind from other behavior. Disruptions in life fall along a continuum, ranging from minor frustrations to devastating losses. All disruptions raise issues that need to be resolved by the people involved. The approach taken here suggests that the underlying structure of those issues is the same regardless of whether the disruption is due to some minor frustration or a devastating loss. This is not to say that how the issues are resolved is the same for such disparate cases, only that the decision points are the same. Thus, a confrontation with adversity (regardless of its source) can be seen as the origin of stress, whether mild or severe. The person's effort to dissolve the adversity, to dampen its subjective impact, or to accommodate to the new life situation that the adversity brings with it, are the essence of coping—and of self-regulation.

ACKNOWLEDGMENTS

Preparation of this chapter was facilitated by Grant Nos. CA64710, CA78995, CA84944, and by additional funding to the Pittsburgh Mind–Body Center at the University of Pittsburgh and Carnegie Mellon University (Grant Nos. HL65111, HL65112, HL076852, and HL076858).

REFERENCES

Affleck, G., Tennen, H., Pfeiffer, C., & Fifield, J. (1987). Appraisals of control and predictability in adapting to a chronic disease. *Journal of Personality and Social Psychology, 53,* 273–279.

Affleck, G., Tennen, H., Urrows, S., Higgins, P., Abeles, M., Hall, C., et al. (1998). Fibromyalgia and women's pursuit of personal goals: A daily process analysis. *Health Psychology, 17,* 40–47.

Armor, D. A., & Taylor, S. E. (1998). Situated optimism: Specific outcome expectancies and self-regulation. In M. Zanna (Ed.), *Advances in experimental social psychology* (Vol. 29, pp. 309–379). San Diego, CA: Academic Press.

Aspinwall, L. G., & Taylor, S. E. (1992). Modeling cognitive adaptation: A longitudinal investigation of the impact of individual differences and coping on college adjustment and performance. *Journal of Personality and Social Psychology, 61,* 755–765.

Austin, J. T., & Vancouver, J. B. (1996). Goal constructs in psychology: Structure, process, and content. *Psychological Bulletin, 120,* 338–375.

Baumeister, R. F., & Bratslavsky, E. (1999). Passion, intimacy, and time: Passionate love as a function of change in intimacy. *Personality and Social Psychology Review, 3,* 46–67.

Baumeister, R. F., & Heatherton, T. F. (1996). Self-regulation failure: An overview. *Psychological Inquiry, 7,* 1–15.

Baumeister, R. F., Heatherton, T. F., & Tice, D. M. (1994). *Losing control: Why people fail at self-regulation.* San Diego, CA: Academic Press.

Baumeister, R. F., & Scher, S. J. (1988). Self-defeating behavior patterns among normal individuals: Review and analysis of common self-destructive tendencies. *Psychological Bulletin, 104,* 3–22.

Baumeister, R. F., & Vohs, K. D. (Eds.). (2004). *Handbook of self-regulation: Research, theory, and applications.* New York: Guilford Press.

Bowlby, W. J. (1980). *Attachment and loss: Vol. 3. Loss: Sadness and depression.* London: Hogarth Press.

Brissette, I., Scheier, M. F., & Carver, C. S. (2002). The role of optimism in social network development, coping, and psychological adjustment during a life transition. *Journal of Personality and Social Psychology, 82,* 102–111.

Brunstein, J. C. (1993). Personal goals and subjective well-being: A longitudinal study. *Journal of Personality and Social Psychology, 65,* 1061–1070.

Brunstein, J. C., Schultheiss, O. C., & Grässmann, R. (1998). Personal goals and emotional well-being: The moderating role of motive dispositions. *Journal of Personality and Social Psychology, 75,* 494–508.

Carver, C. S. (2003). Pleasure as a sign you can attend to something else: Placing positive feelings within a general model of affect. *Cognition and Emotion, 17,* 241–261.

Carver, C. S. (2004). Negative affects deriving from the behavioral approach system. *Emotion, 4,* 3–22.

Carver, C. S. (2007). Stress, coping, and health. In H. S. Friedman & R. C. Silver (Eds.), *Foundations of health psychology* (pp. 117–144). New York: Oxford University Press.

Carver, C. S., & Humphries, C. (1981). Havana daydreaming: A study of self-consciousness and the negative reference group among Cuban Americans. *Journal of Personality and Social Psychology, 40,* 545–552.

Carver, C. S., Lawrence, J. W., & Scheier, M. F. (1999). Self-discrepancies and affect: Incorporating the role of feared selves. *Personality and Social Psychology Bulletin, 25,* 783–792.

Carver, C. S., Pozo, C., Harris, S. D., Noriega, V., Scheier, M. F., Robinson, D. S., et al. (1993). How coping mediates the effect of optimism on distress: A study of women with early stage breast cancer. *Journal of Personality and Social Psychology, 65,* 375–390.

Carver, C. S., & Scheier, M. F. (1981). *Attention and self-regulation: A control-theory approach to human behavior.* New York: Springer-Verlag.

Carver, C. S., & Scheier, M. F. (1990). Origins and functions of positive and negative affect: A control-process view. *Psychological Review, 97,* 19–35.

Carver, C. S., & Scheier, M. F. (1998). *On the self-regulation of behavior.* New York: Cambridge University Press.

Carver, C. S., & Scheier, M. F. (1999). A few more themes, a lot more issues: Commentary on the commentaries. In R. S. Wyer, Jr. (Ed.), *Perspectives on behavioral self-regulation: Advances in social cognition* (Vol. 12, pp. 261–302). Mahwah, NJ: Erlbaum.

Carver, C. S., & Scheier, M. F. (2003). Optimism. In C. R. Snyder & S. J. Lopez (Eds.), *Coping: The psychology of what works.* New York: Oxford University Press.

Carver, C. S., & Scheier, M. F. (2008). Feedback processes in the simultaneous regulation of ac-tion and affect. In J. Y. Shah & W. L. Gardner (Eds.), *Handbook of motivation science* (pp. 308–324). New York: Guilford Press.

Carver, C. S., Scheier, M. F., & Weintraub, J. K. (1989). Assessing coping strategies: A theoretically based approach. *Journal of Personality and Social Psychology, 56,* 267–283.

Cleiren, M. (1993). *Bereavement and adaptation: A comparative study of the aftermath of death.* Washington, DC: Hemisphere.

Crocker, J., & Major, B. (1989). Social stigma and self-esteem: The self-protective properties of stigma. *Psychological Review, 96,* 608–630.

Elliott, E. S., & Dweck, C. S. (1988). Goals: An approach to motivation and achievement. *Journal of Personality and Social Psychology, 54,* 5–12.

Emmons, R. A. (1986). Personal strivings: An approach to personality and subjective well-being. *Journal of Personality and Social Psychology, 51,* 1058–1068.

Emmons, R. A., & King, L. A. (1988). Conflict among personal strivings: Immediate and long-term implications for psychological and physical well-being. *Journal of Personality and Social Psychology, 54,* 1040–1048.

Feather, N. T. (1989). Trying and giving up: Persistence and lack of persistence in failure situations. In R. C. Curtis (Ed.), *Self-defeating behaviors: Experimental research, clinical impressions, and practical implications* (pp. 67–95). New York: Plenum Press.

Fontaine, K. R., Manstead, A. S. R., & Wagner, H. (1993). Optimism, perceived control over stress, and coping. *European Journal of Personality, 7,* 267–281.

Frijda, N. H. (1986). *The emotions.* Cambridge, UK: Cambridge University Press.

Frijda, N. H. (1988). The laws of emotion. *American Psychologist, 43,* 349–358.

Greenwald, A. G. (1980). The totalitarian ego: Fabrication and revision of personal history. *American Psychologist, 35,* 603–618.

Greer, S., Morris, T., & Pettingale, K. W. (1979). Psychological response to breast cancer: Effect on outcome. *Lancet, 2,* 785–787.

Greer, S., Morris, T., Pettingale, K. W., & Haybittle, J. L. (1990). Psychological response to breast cancer and 15-year outcome. *Lancet, 1,* 49–50.

Gross, J. J. (1998). Antecedent- and response-focused emotion regulation: Divergent consequences for experience, expression, and physiology. *Journal of Personality and Social Psychology, 74,* 224–237.

Grouzet, F. M., Kasser, T., Ahuvia, A., Dols, J. M., Kim, Y., Lau, S., et al. (2005). The structure of goal contents across 15 cultures. *Journal of Personality and Social Psychology, 89,* 800–816.

Heatherton, T. F., & Nichols, P. A. (1994). Personal accounts of successful versus failed attempts at life change. *Personality and Social Psychology Bulletin, 20,* 664–675.

Higgins, E. T. (1987). Self-discrepancy: A theory relating self and affect. *Psychological Review, 94,* 319–340.

Higgins, E. T. (1996). Ideals, oughts, and regulatory focus: Affect and motivation from distinct pains and pleasures. In P. M. Gollwitzer & J. A. Bargh (Eds.), *The psychology of action: Linking cognition and motivation to behavior* (pp. 91–114). New York: Guilford Press.

Hobfoll, S. E. (1989). Conservation of resources: A new attempt at conceptualizing stress. *American Psychologist, 44,* 513–524.

Hobfoll, S. E., Freedy, J. R., Green, B. L., & Solomon, S. D. (1996). Coping in reaction to extreme stress: The roles of resource loss and resource availability. In M. Zeidner & N. S. Endler (Eds.), *Handbook of coping: Theory, research, applications* (pp. 322–349). New York: Wiley.

Holman, E. A., & Silver, R. C. (1998). Getting "stuck" in the past: Temporal orientation and coping with trauma. *Journal of Personality and Social Psychology, 74,* 1146–1163.

Hsee, C. K., & Abelson, R. P. (1991). Velocity relation: Satisfaction as a function of the first derivative of outcome over time. *Journal of Personality and Social Psychology, 60,* 341–347.

Hsee, C. K., Abelson, R. P., & Salovey, P. (1991). The relative weighting of position and velocity in satisfaction. *Psychological Science, 2,* 263–266.

Janoff-Bulman, R., & Brickman, P. (1982). Expectations and what people learn from failure. In N. T. Feather (Ed.), *Expectations and actions: Expectancy-value models in psychology* (pp. 207–237). Hillsdale, NJ: Erlbaum.

Klass, D., Silverman, P. R., & Nickman, S. L. (Eds.). (1996). *Continuing bonds: New understandings of grief.* Washington, DC: Taylor & Francis.

Kling, K. C., Ryff, C., & Essex, M. J. (1997). Adaptive changes in the self-concept during a life transition. *Personality and Social Psychology Bulletin, 23,* 981–990.

Klinger, E. (1975). Consequences of commitment to and disengagement from incentives. *Psychological Review, 82,* 1–25.

Laurenceau, J-P., Troy, A. B., & Carver, C. S. (2005). Two distinct emotional experiences in romantic relationships: Effects of perceptions regarding approach of intimacy and avoidance of conflict. *Personality and Social Psychology Bulletin, 31,* 1123–1133.

Lawrence, J. W., Carver, C. S., & Scheier, M. F. (2002). Velocity toward goal attainment in immediate experience as a determinant of af-

fect. *Journal of Applied Social Psychology, 32,* 788–802.

Lazarus, R. S. (1966). *Psychological stress and the coping process.* New York: McGraw-Hill.

Lazarus, R. S., & Folkman, S. (1984). *Stress, appraisal, and coping.* New York: Springer.

Lecci, L., Okun, M. A., & Karoly, P. (1994). Life regrets and current goals as predictors of psychological adjustment. *Journal of Personality and Social Psychology, 66,* 731–741.

Long, B. C., Kahn, S. E., & Schutz, R. W. (1992). Causal model of stress and coping: Women in management. *Journal of Counseling Psychology, 39,* 227–239.

Markus, H., & Nurius, P. (1986). Possible selves. *American Psychologist, 41,* 954–969.

McIntosh, W. D., & Martin, L. L. (1992). The cybernetics of happiness: The relation of goal attainment, rumination, and affect. In M. S. Clark (Ed.), *Review of personality and social psychology: Vol. 14. Emotion and social behavior* (pp. 222–246). Newbury Park, CA: Sage.

Miller, G. A., Galanter, E., & Pribram, K. H. (1960). *Plans and the structure of behavior.* New York: Holt, Rinehart & Winston.

Moskowitz, J. T., Folkman, S., Collette, L., & Vittinghoff, E. (1996). Coping and mood during AIDS-related caregiving and bereavement. *Annals of Behavioral Medicine, 18,* 49–57.

Orbuch, T. L. (Ed.). (1992). *Close relationship loss: Theoretical approaches.* New York: Springer-Verlag.

Pervin, L. A. (Ed.). (1989). *Goal concepts in personality and social psychology.* Hillsdale, NJ: Erlbaum.

Pettingale, K. W., Morris, T., & Greer, S. (1985). Mental attitudes to cancer: An additional prognostic factor. *Lancet, 1,* 750.

Powers, W. T. (1973). *Behavior: The control of perception.* Chicago: Aldine.

Pyszczynski, T., & Greenberg, J. (1992). *Hanging on and letting go: Understanding the onset, progression, and remission of depression.* New York: Springer-Verlag.

Reed, G. M., Kemeny, M. E., Taylor, S. E., Wang, H. Y., & Visscher, B. R. (1994). Realistic acceptance as a predictor of decreased survival time in gay men with AIDS. *Health Psychology, 13,* 299–307.

Sarason, I. G., Pierce, G. R., & Sarason, B. R. (Eds.). (1996). *Cognitive interference: Theories, methods, and findings.* Hillsdale, NJ: Erlbaum.

Scheier, M. F., & Carver, C. S. (1985). Optimism, coping and health: Assessment and implications of generalized outcome expectancies. *Health Psychology, 4,* 219–247.

Scheier, M. F., & Carver, C. S. (1992). Effects of optimism on psychological and physical well-being: Theoretical overview and empirical update. *Cognitive Therapy and Research, 16,* 201–228.

Scheier, M. F., & Carver, C. S. (2001). Adapting to cancer: The importance of hope and purpose. In A. Baum & B. L. Andersen (Eds.), *Psychosocial interventions for cancer* (pp. 15–36). Washington, DC: American Psychological Association.

Scheier, M. F., Matthews, K. A., Owens, J. F., Magovern, G. J., Sr., Lefebvre, R. C., Abbott, R. A., et al. (1989). Dispositional optimism and recovery from coronary artery bypass surgery: The beneficial effects on physical and psychological well being. *Journal of Personality and Social Psychology, 57,* 1024–1040.

Scheier, M. F., Weintraub, J. K., & Carver, C. S. (1986). Coping with stress: Divergent strategies of optimists and pessimists. *Journal of Personality and Social Psychology, 51,* 1257–1264.

Srivastava, S., McGonigal, K. M., Richards, J. M., Butler, E. A., & Gross, J. J. (2006). Optimism in close relationships: How seeing things in a positive light makes them so. *Journal of Personality and Social Psychology, 91,* 143–153.

Stanton, A. L., & Snider, P. R. (1993). Coping with breast cancer diagnosis: A prospective study. *Health Psychology, 12,* 16–23.

Steele, C. M. (1997). A threat in the air: How stereotypes shape intellectual identity and performance. *American Psychologist, 52,* 613–629.

Stroebe, M. S. (1994). The broken heart phenomenon: An examination of the mortality of bereavement. *Journal of Community and Applied Social Psychology, 4,* 47–61.

Stroebe, M. S., Stroebe, W., & Hansson, R. O. (Eds.). (1993). *Handbook of bereavement: Theory, research, and intervention.* Cambridge, UK: Cambridge University Press.

Stroebe, W., Schut, H., & Stroebe, M. S. (2005). Grief work, disclosure, and counseling: Do they help the bereaved? *Clinical Psychology Review, 25,* 395–414.

Strutton, D., & Lumpkin, J. (1992). Relationship

between optimism and coping strategies in the work environment. *Psychology Reports, 71,* 1179–1186.

Taylor, S. E., & Pham, L. B. (1996). Mental stimulation, motivation, and action. In P. M. Gollwitzer & J. A. Bargh (Eds.), *The psychology of action: Linking cognition and motivation to behavior* (pp. 219–235). New York: Guilford Press.

Trunzo, J. J., & Pinto, B. M. (2003). Social support as a mediator of optimism and distress in breast cancer survivors. *Journal of Consulting and Clinical Psychology, 71,* 805–811.

Turk, D. C., & Rudy, T. E. (1992). Cognitive factors and persistent pain: A glimpse into Pandora's box. *Cognitive Therapy and Research, 16,* 99–122.

Wine, J. D. (1971). Test anxiety and direction of attention. *Psychological Bulletin, 76,* 92–104.

Wine, J. D. (1980). Cognitive–attentional theory of test anxiety. In I. G. Sarason (Ed.), *Test anxiety: Theory, research, and application* (pp. 349–378). Hillsdale, NJ: Erlbaum.

Worden, W. J. (1991). *Grief counseling and grief therapy: A handbook for the mental health practitioner* (2nd ed.). New York: Springer-Verlag.

Wortman, C. B., & Brehm, J. W. (1975). Responses to uncontrollable outcomes: An integration of reactance theory and the learned helplessness model. In L. Berkowitz (Ed.), *Advances in experimental social psychology* (Vol. 8, pp. 277–336). New York: Academic Press.

Wrosch, C., Scheier, M. F., Carver, C. S., & Schulz, R. (2003). The importance of goal disengagement in adaptive self-regulation: When giving up is beneficial. *Self and Identity, 2,* 1–20.

Wrosch, C., Scheier, M. F., Miller, G. E., Schulz, R., & Carver, C. S. (2003). Adaptive self-regulation of unattainable goals: Goal disengagement, goal reengagement, and subjective well-being. *Personality and Social Psychology Bulletin, 29,* 1494–1508.

CHAPTER 30

Personality and Psychopathology

Thomas A. Widiger
Gregory T. Smith

The importance of personality to psychopathology has been recognized since the beginnings of medicine. Hippocrates (in the fourth century B.C.) distinguished between four fundamental dispositions (i.e., sanguine, melancholic, phlegmatic, and choleric) that were thought to provide a vulnerability to a variety of physical and psychological disorders (Maher & Maher, 1994). Much has been learned since his time, including a healthy appreciation for how little is, in fact, known.

We include within our consideration of personality both maladaptive personality functioning, as described within the American Psychiatric Association's (2000) *Diagnostic and Statistical Manual of Mental Disorders* (DSM-IV-TR) as well as normal personality traits, as described within dimensional models of general personality structure. Whether one considers personality traits or personality disorders, the interplay of personality and psychopathology continues to be a scientifically and clinically significant yet challenging focus of investigation (Ball, 2005; Bank & Silk, 2001; Clark, 2007; Dolan-Sewell, Krueger, & Shea, 2001; Krueger & Tackett, 2006; Mulder, 2002; Rosenbluth, Kennedy, & Bagby, 2005; Trull, Sher, Minks-Brown, Durbin, & Burr, 2000). If one considers just the co-occurrence of personality disorders with other forms of psychopathology (i.e.,

excluding the additional literature concerning the relationship of general personality to psychopathology), Clark (2007) indicated that her computer search crossing "personality disorder(s)" with "comorbidity/co-occurrence" yielded over 1,500 citations from 1985 through 2005, with more than half of them appearing since the year 2000.

Within this chapter we distinguish between three fundamental forms of potential interplay involving personality and psychopathology: (1) Personality and psychopathology can influence the presentation or appearance of one another (pathoplastic relationships); (2) they can share a common, underlying etiology (spectrum relationships); and (3) they can have a causal role in the development or etiology of one another. Each of these relationships has significant theoretical and practical implications, and each is considered in turn.

PATHOPLASTIC RELATIONSHIPS

The influence of personality and psychopathology on the presentation, appearance, or expression of each is typically characterized as a "pathoplastic relationship." This pathoplastic relationship is bidirectional, as psychopathology can vary in its appearance depending on a person's premorbid personality traits, and the appearance or presentation of personality can similarly be affected by the presence of a comorbid psychopathology. Both directions of relationship are considered in turn.

Pathoplastic Effects of Personality on Psychopathology

"Personality" is the characteristic manner in which one thinks, feels, behaves, and relates to others. Mental disorders are clinically significant impairments in one or more areas of psychological functioning, including (but not limited to) one's thinking, feeling, eating, sleeping, and other important areas (American Psychiatric Association, 2000). It would be surprising if the presentation, course, or treatment of an impairment in a psychologically important component of thinking or feeling (a disorder) were not significantly affected by a person's characteristic manner of thinking and feeling (i.e., the individual's personality). Mental disorders occur within the context of a premorbid personality structure that often has a profound effect on their presentation, course, or treatment (Millon et al., 1996).

Appearance and Presentation of a Disorder

The symptomatology shown by persons with the same mental disorder tends to be extremely heterogeneous (Rosenbluth et al., 2005; Widiger & Clark, 2000). This heterogeneity is a significant problem for diagnosis and treatment. An important contribution to this heterogeneity is variation in personality structure. For example, central to both anorexia nervosa and bulimia nervosa (the two fundamental forms of eating disorder) is the pathology of a preoccupation with body shape, weight, or appearance (American Psychiatric Association, 2000). Persons with either of these eating disorders desire intensely to lose weight. Their thoughts and concerns throughout the day are often devoted to this goal. However, prototypic cases of anorexia and bulimia nervosa can appear to be quite different, supporting the existence within DSM-IV of two separate, distinct diagnoses. On the other hand, anorexia and bulimia are also highly comorbid, concurrently and longitudinally (Polivy, Herman, & Boiven,

2004). The primary distinction between persons with anorexia nervosa and those with bulimia nervosa is perhaps simply that the former are pathologically successful in the effort to maintain a low body weight (i.e., are grossly underweight), whereas persons with bulimia nervosa are relatively unsuccessful, due partly to their binge eating and inadequate (but still excessive) compensatory behaviors. This fundamental distinction could be driven, in large part, by premorbid personality differences.

There is empirical support for an association of perfectionistic and compulsive personality traits with anorexia, particularly the restrained subtype, as well as personality traits of impulsivity with bulimic symptomatology (Cassin & von Ranson, 2005; Claes, Vandereycken, & Vertommen, 2005; Fischer, Anderson, & Smith, 2004; Fischer, Smith, & Anderson, 2003; Sansone, Levitt, & Sansone, 2005; Smith, Fischer, et al., 2007; Wonderlich et al., 2005). Much of this research is concerned with the contribution of personality traits to the etiology of an eating disorder. However, even if personality traits do not contribute to the development of the pathology of an eating disorder (e.g., the preoccupation with body shape or appearance), personality traits might contribute to the form or appearance in which the eating disorder appears (i.e., bulimic vs. anorexic). Both anorexia and bulimia tend to emerge during late adolescence and are preceded by significant negative body image and a variety of more nonspecific psychological dysfunctions (Polivy & Herman, 2002). It is possible that those who go on to develop anorexia are characterized in part by premorbid personality traits of very high conscientiousness (or constraint), one of the fundamental individual differences included within the well-validated five-factor model (FFM; McCrae & Costa, 2003; see also John, Naumann, & Soto, Chapter 4, this volume; McCrae & Costa, Chapter 5, this volume) of general personality structure. Persons high in conscientiousness have considerable self-discipline (the ability to begin and carry through tasks to completion), competence (capability, effectiveness, and prudence, the most extreme variant of which is perfectionism), and achievement striving (Costa & McCrae, 1992)—precisely the attributes that would be necessary to achieve the weight loss of a person suffering from anorexia. From this perspective, anorexia nervosa would not be due to excessive conscientiousness, but the presence of a pathological preoccupation with losing weight in a person with high conscientiousness may contribute to the development of excessive weight loss. In contrast, persons low in conscientiousness (or constraint) might in turn be prone to the impulsive dyscontrol characteristic of binge eating and bulimia.

There is also, of course, heterogeneity within the structure of personality. The FFM consists of the five broad domains of neuroticism versus emotional stability, extraversion versus introversion, openness versus closedness to experience, agreeableness versus antagonism, and conscientiousness (John et al., Chapter 4, this volume; McCrae & Costa, Chapter 5, this volume). Costa and McCrae (1992) further differentiate each of these broad domains into more specific facets, based on their development of and research with the NEO Personality Inventory—Revised (NEO-PI-R; e.g., facets of neuroticism are anxiousness, depressiveness, angry hostility, self-consciousness, vulnerability, and impulsiveness). It is worth noting briefly here how one specific aspect of this heterogeneity bears on the relationship of personality structure to eating (and other mental) disorders. The relationship of low constraint (or low conscientiousness) with bulimic symptomatology has not been consistently supported due, in part, perhaps, to the complexity of the construct of impulsivity. Impulsivity is of considerable interest to psychopathology researchers, but the term "impulsivity" is used in this research often with quite different meanings. Whiteside and Lynam (2001) use the FFM, as assessed by the NEO-PI-R, to distinguish between four different variants of impulsivity. Low self-discipline (or low perseverance) and low premeditation (the tendency to act hastily and fail to consider the consequences of one's actions) are both NEO-PI-R facets of conscientiousness. However, impulsivity is also described or assessed within the clinical and research literature as excitement seeking or stimulus seeking (an aspect of extraversion; a disposition to take risks and seek exciting, stimulating, and even dangerous activity), and also as urgency, or what is referred to as a neurotic "impulsivity" within the NEO-

PI-R. This neurotic variant of impulsivity refers to a disposition to experience strong impulses and urges, particularly under conditions of negative affect (Whiteside, Miller, Lynam, & Reynolds, 2005). In sum, urgency, self-discipline, and perseverance can each contribute to the form an eating disorder takes. Urgency may do so through an etiological relationship (Fischer et al., 2004; Fischer, Smith, & Anderson, 2003; Stice, 2002), whereas self-discipline and perserverance may do so through a pathoplastic relationship.

There are, of course, a multitude of other possible ways in which premorbid personality structure can alter the presentation or appearance of a mental disorder. For example, a number of studies have suggested subtypes of various anxiety disorders, depending on a person's characteristic manner of interpersonal relatedness (e.g., Eng & Heimberg, 2006; Kachin, Newman, & Pincus, 2006). Similarly, dyscontrolled drug usage within a person characterized by high levels of negative affectivity (neuroticism) may serve primarily to suppress or mitigate anxiety, depression, or anger, whereas dyscontrolled usage within persons characterized by high levels of positive affectivity may be primarily intended for stimulation and arousal. Negative-mood-based and positive-mood-based drug users clearly differ in an important personality precursor to use. To further complicate matters, they may also share other personality precursors, such as some form of disinhibition (Fischer, Smith, Spillane, & Cyders, 2005). Finally, depression is likely to be experienced differently depending on a person's vulnerabilities and sources of self-esteem (Rosenbluth et al., 2005). Depression within a dependent (sociotropic) person is characterized by feelings of deprivation, loss, loneliness, and unlikeability; depression within a narcissistic (autonomous, self-critical) person is characterized by feelings of defeat, failure, withdrawal, and self-blame (Blatt, 2004; Blatt & Shahar, 2005).

Treatment and Course of a Disorder

An additional way in which personality traits can have a pathoplastic effect on psychopathology is the manner or degree to which persons respond to a particular course of treatment. Maladaptive personality traits were given a special status within the 1980 edition of the American Psychiatric Association's DSM by being placed on a separate "axis" that would then require that clinicians assess for the presence of maladaptive personality traits (i.e., a personality disorder) in virtually every patient. Personality disorders were placed on Axis II, whereas most of the other mental disorders (e.g., anxiety, mood, and substance use) were placed on Axis I. "This [decision] arises from accumulating evidence that the quality and quantity of preexisting personality disturbance may indeed influence the predisposition, manifestation, course, and response to treatment of various Axis I conditions" (Frances, 1980, p. 1050).

The American Psychiatric Association (2000) currently identifies 10 distinct personality disorders that are placed (somewhat arbitrarily; Sheets & Craighead, 2007) within three different clusters: paranoid, schizoid, and schizotypal (odd–eccentric cluster); borderline, antisocial, narcissistic, and histrionic (dramatic–emotional cluster); and avoidant, dependent, and obsessive–compulsive (anxious–fearful cluster). Quite a bit of research has suggested that the presence of one or more of these Axis II personality disorders contributes to a decrease in the effectiveness of, or the response to, Axis I treatment (Ball, 2005; Dolan et al., 2001; Millon et al., 1996; Rosenbluth et al., 2005)—although questions have also been raised with respect to the consistency of these findings (Mulder, 2002).

In clinical practice it is routine to conduct a personality assessment at the beginning of treatment, because the personality of a patient could have a significant impact on treatment responsivity. Harkness and Lilienfeld (1997) stated quite boldly that "the last 40 years of individual differences research require the inclusion of personality trait assessment for the construction and implementation of any treatment plan that would lay claim to scientific status" (p. 349). Nevertheless, systematic research on the use or impact of personality traits on treatment planning and outcome is remarkably sparse (Lima et al., 2005), other than to simply indicate that the existence of maladaptive personality traits generally undermines treatment responsivity (Dolan et al., 2001).

An additional limitation of the existing research is the inability to provide empirically based information concerning personality traits that could also contribute to treatment adherence, compliance, or engagement (Cohen, Ross, Bagby, Farvolden, & Kennedy, 2004; Quilty et al., in press). The American Psychiatric Association diagnostic system is confined to the classification of personality disorder. The psychiatric diagnostic manuals used in other countries do include the recognition and consideration of normal, adaptive personality traits (e.g., the diagnostic manuals for Cuba and China). The inclusion of adaptive personality traits within the diagnostic system would allow for the provision of a more comprehensive description of a patient's entire personality functioning and might also help to identify personality traits that contribute to treatment responsivity (Widiger & Simonsen, 2005a). For example, moderate elevations within the FFM domain of conscientiousness are likely to predict a willingness and reliability to maintain the rigors of a demanding clinical regimen; moderate levels of agreeableness suggest an increased likelihood to establish a therapeutic rapport and engage with the therapist in interpersonal models of therapy; and moderate levels of openness would likely suggest an interest in, and motivation to question, existing cognitive schemas or engage in a dynamic exploration of unconscious conflicts. A number of clinical papers support these speculations (e.g., Chard & Widiger, 2005; Sanderson & Clarkin, 2002). An important line of investigation for future personality research would be to determine empirically the potential impact and clinical utility of normal (as well as abnormal) personality traits on treatment selection and outcome.

Pathoplastic Effects of Psychopathology on Personality

One of the more heavily researched and well-documented relationships between personality and psychopathology are the pathoplastic effects of episodes of psychopathology on the appearance, presentation, or perception of personality (Clark & Harrison, 2001; Farmer, 2000; Vitousek & Stumpf, 2005; Widiger & Samuel, 2005b). Just as premorbid personality traits can alter the appearance or expression of an Axis I disorder, an Axis I disorder can alter the appearance or expression of premorbid personality traits. This pathoplastic effect of an Axis I disorder is particularly problematic for studies attempting to assess and identity causal and spectrum relationships between personality (or personality disorder) and Axis I psychopathology. Clinicians (and at times researchers) assess a patient's personality during an initial intake procedure, yet this is perhaps the worst time to do so (Widiger & Boyd, in press). Persons who are very anxious, depressed, angry, or distraught will often fail to provide an accurate description of their general personality traits (i.e., their usual way of thinking, feeling, behaving, and relating to others). Distortion in self-image is a well-established symptom of mood disorder (American Psychiatric Association, 2000), and it should not be surprising to find that persons who are depressed provide inaccurate descriptions of their usual way of thinking, feeling, and relating to others. Once their mood, anxiety, or other mental disorder is successfully treated, their self-description changes accordingly.

A revealing demonstration of the pathoplastic effects of psychopathology on self-image was provided by Piersma (1987). He reported substantial changes in self-report inventory assessments of personality disorder across a very brief inpatient hospitalization. Twenty-five percent of 151 patients were diagnosed with borderline personality disorder at admission, only 7.3% at discharge; 12% were diagnosed with schizotypal personality disorder at admission, only 4% at discharge. Test–retest kappa was only .11 for the borderline diagnosis, .09 for compulsive, .01 for passive–aggressive, and .27 for schizotypal. On the basis of this study one could conclude that clinical treatment resulted in significant changes to personality functioning because personality disorders are responsive to treatment (Leichsenring & Leibing, 2003; Perry, Banon, & Ianni, 1999; Salekin, 2002; Sanislow & McGlashan, 1998). However, inconsistent with this hypothesis was the fact that the treatment was quite brief and was focused on mood, anxiety, or other forms of psychopathology. Perhaps most problematic to the hypothesis of a valid change in personality was the additional finding of significant increases in the histrionic and narcissistic personality disorder scales (Piersma, 1989). If the inpatient hospitalization did, in fact, contribute to a remission of borderline and compulsive personality disorder, it should

perhaps take responsibility as well for contributing to the creation of histrionic and narcissistic personality traits. Piersma (1989) concluded instead that the initial self-report inventory assessment at intake was "not able to measure long-term personality characteristics ('trait' characteristics) independent of symptomatology ('state' characteristics)" (p. 91).

Semistructured interviews have the potential to be relatively more impervious to the distorting effects that mood states can have on the expression of personality (e.g., self-image), but they are not immune (Farmer, 2000; Widiger & Boyd, in press). An interviewer can easily fail to appreciate the extent to which a patient's self-description is being distorted by mood, anxiety, distress, or other situational factors. In fact, results equivalent to those reported by Piersma (1987, 1989) were obtained in a study that was purportedly documenting the resilience of semistructured interviews to mood state distortions. Loranger and colleagues (1991) compared semistructured interview assessments obtained at the beginning of an inpatient admission to those obtained 1 week to 6 months later and reported "a significant reduction in the mean number of criteria met on all of the personality disorders except schizoid and antisocial" (p. 726). On the basis of the finding that the changes in personality disorder scores were not correlated with changes in anxiety or depression, the researchers argued that the reduction was not due to an initial inflation of scores secondary to depressed or anxious mood. However, an alternative perspective is that the study lacked sufficiently sensitive or accurate measures to explain why there was a substantial decrease on 10 of the 12 personality disorder scales. It is unlikely that 1 week to 6 months of treatment, focused largely on mood, anxiety, and other forms of psychopathology, resulted in the extent of changes to personality that were claimed (the change scores also failed to correlate with length of treatment). In fact, comparable to the findings of Piersma (1989), twice as many patients (eight) were diagnosed with a histrionic personality disorder at discharge than were diagnosed with this personality disorder at admission.

Similar findings continue to be reported within the personality disorder literature, yet a predominant view is that the findings reflect actual change in personality functioning (Shea & Yen, 2003; Zanarini, Frankenburg, Hennen, Reich, & Sik, 2006). Consider, for example, temporal stability findings reported in the highly published, multisite Collaborative Longitudinal Study of Personality Disorders (CLPS; Skodol et al., 2006). Twenty-three of 160 persons (14%) who met DSM-IV-TR diagnostic criteria for borderline personality disorder (BPD) at CLPS's baseline assessment had no more than two diagnostic criteria just 6 months later (Gunderson et al., 2003). Eighteen sustained this reduction from 6 months to 1 year. This is perhaps a rather sudden and remarkable change in adults who purportedly evidenced borderline personality traits in a temporally stable fashion for many years throughout their adult lives prior to entry into the study.

Gunderson and colleagues (2003) provided details concerning the recent history for many of the 18 borderlines they described as experiencing sudden, dramatic remissions within the first 6 months of the study. For one of the participants, the symptoms were attributed to the use of a stimulant for weight reduction during the year prior to the beginning of the study: "The most dramatic improvement following a treatment intervention occurred when a subject discontinued a psychostimulant she had used the year prior to baseline for purposes of weight loss. ... Discontinuation was followed by a dramatic reduction of her depression, panic, abandonment fears, and self-destructiveness" (Gunderson et al., 2003, p. 116). Five of the 18 remissions "had the dramatic reduction of BPD criteria at the same time as the remission of a coexisting Axis I disorder" (Gunderson et al., 2003, p. 114). "In these five cases, the remission of the Axis I disorder was judged to be the most likely cause for the sudden BPD improvement" (p. 114). For eight cases, "the changes involved gaining relief from severely stressful situations they were in at or before the baseline assessment" (p. 115). "For example, one subject (case 16) reported that the stress of an unexpected divorce and custody struggle led to anger, substance abuse, and the revival of early abandonment trauma" (Gunderson et al., 2003, p. 115). With the resolution of the stress of the divorce, the "borderline" symptoms abated.

In sum, it does seem reasonable to suggest that many of these 18 cases of appar-

ent changes in personality might have represented instead questionable diagnoses due to the pathoplastic effects of Axis I psychopathology (as well as situational stressors) on the appearance or perception of personality traits. Personality traits can fluctuate with situational changes, and actual changes to personality can also occur, particularly if the person is receiving clinical treatment (Leichsenring & Leibing, 2003; Perry et al., 1999; Sanislow & McGlashan, 1998). However, behaviors that are secondary to the use of a diet medication, behaviors that are readily attributable to the presence of an Axis I mood disorder, behaviors that are secondary to the stress of an unexpected divorce, and behaviors that are attributed to being involved with very intense and perhaps even abusive partners, might be best understood as temporary fluctuations secondary to unstable, stressful situations and Axis I pathoplastic effects rather than being indicative of a personality trait. The CLPS project has provided findings that are helpful in understanding the longitudinal course of personality and personality disorder (Skodol et al., 2006), but it may also be helpful in alerting researchers studying the relationship between personality and psychopathology to the tremendous difficulty in assessing (and distinguishing between) these constructs, particularly when both are present.

SPECTRUM RELATIONSHIPS

Much of the effort of the authors of the APA manual for the diagnosis of psychopathology is given to modifying, clarifying, and narrowing diagnostic criterion sets in order to improve differential diagnosis (First, Frances, & Pincus, 2002). The assumption of the diagnostic manual is that the categories refer to distinct clinical entities, each with its own distinguishable etiology, pathology, and treatment (Widiger & Mullins-Sweatt, 2007). To the extent to which this is true, it is quite meaningful to study the possibility that a personality disorder (or trait) contributes to the etiology of an Axis I disorder (or vice versa), or that a personality disorder (or trait) has a pathoplastic effect on the expression, course, or presentation of an Axis I disorder (or vice versa). However, the identification and differentiation of pathoplastic and etiological relationships of personality and psychopathology are complicated by the possibility that personality and psychopathology may themselves fail, in some instances, to be distinct entities. They may instead exist along a common spectrum of functioning. For example, rather than contributing to the etiology of depression, neuroticism may itself be a form of a depression (e.g., early-onset dysthymia; American Psychiatric Association, 2000). There are a number of ways in which general personality traits, personality disorders, and Axis I psychopathology can be integrated within a common hierarchical model, including (1) the integration of the DSM-IV-TR personality disorders with general personality traits, (2) the integration of personality disorders within Axis I mental disorders, and (3) the integration of Axis I mental disorders within general personality traits. Each of these variants of spectrum relationships is discussed in turn.

Personality on a Spectrum with Personality Disorders

The conceptualization of personality disorders in DSM-IV-TR "represents the categorical perspective that Personality Disorders are qualitatively distinct clinical syndromes" (American Psychiatric Association, 2000, p. 689), distinct from each other and from general personality structure (Shedler & Westen, 2004; Skodol et al., 2006). However, arguing against the validity of the categorical distinctions are their excessive diagnostic co-occurrence, unstable and arbitrary diagnostic boundaries, inadequate coverage, and heterogeneity among persons sharing the same diagnosis (Clark, 2007; First et al., 2002; Livesley, 2003; Trull & Durrett, 2005; Widiger & Mullins-Sweatt, 2005). The categorical model of classification has become so problematic that a Research Planning Work Group for DSM-V concluded that it will be "important that consideration be given to advantages and disadvantages of basing part or all of DSM-V on dimensions rather than categories" (Rounsaville et al., 2002, p. 12). The group suggested, in particular, that the first section of the diagnostic manual to be converted to a dimensional classification might be the personality disorders. "If a dimensional system of personality performs well and is acceptable to clinicians, it might

then be appropriate to explore dimensional approaches in other domains" (Rounsaville et al., 2002, p. 13). The American Psychiatric Association subsequently cosponsored a series of international conferences devoted to further enriching the empirical database in preparation for the eventual development of DSM-V (a description of this conference series can be found at www.dsm5.org). The first conference was devoted to setting a research agenda that would be the most useful and effective in leading the field toward a dimensional classification of personality disorder (Widiger & Simonsen, 2005b; Widiger, Simonsen, Krueger, Livesley, & Verheul, 2005).

Very few studies examine the contribution of general personality traits to the etiology of personality disorders (e.g., the contribution of introversion to the etiology of schizoid personality disorder, or the contribution of impulsivity or neuroticism to the etiology of borderline personality disorder), as it would appear more likely that personality disorders are on a spectrum with general personality structure. A number of dimensional models of general personality structure that have been proposed for, or related to, the DSM-IV-TR personality disorders include Eysenck's (1987) three dimensions of neuroticism, extraversion, and psychoticism; Harkness and McNulty's five factors of positive emotionality/extraversion, aggressiveness, constraint, negative emotionality/neuroticism, and psychoticism (Harkness, McNulty, & Ben-Porath, 1995); Tellegen's (1982) three dimensions of negative affectivity, positive affectivity, and constraint; Millon's six polarities of self, other, active, passive, pleasure, and pain (Millon et al., 1996); the interpersonal circumplex dimensions of agency and communion (Pincus & Gurtman, 2006); Zuckerman's (2002) five dimensions of sociability, activity, aggression-hostility, impulsive sensation seeking, and neuroticism-anxiety; Cloninger's (2000) seven factors of novelty seeking, harm avoidance, reward dependence, persistence, self-directedness, cooperativeness, and self-transcendence; and the FFM dimensions of neuroticism, extraversion, openness, conscientiousness, and agreeableness (Costa & McCrae, 1990). Much of the empirical research has focused on the FFM of Costa and McCrae (1990) and the seven-factor model of Cloninger.

Markon, Krueger, and Watson (2005) considered a joint structural model of the constructs assessed with the Dimensional Assessment of Personality Pathology—Basic Questionnaire (DAPP-BQ; Livesley & Jackson, in press; a dimensional measure of personality disorder symptomatology), the Eysenck Personality Questionnaire (Eysenck, 1987), the Multidimensional Personality Questionnaire (MPQ; Tellegen, 1982), the NEO-PI-R (Costa & McCrae, 1992), and the Temperament and Character Inventory (TCI; Cloninger, 2000). Markon and colleagues first used a meta-analytic approach to assemble a matrix of correlations among the 44 scales derived from all of these inventories obtained from 52 prior studies. Structural modeling indicated that no more than five major factors underlie variation in the 44 scales. These five factors strongly resembled the domains of the FFM. Further analyses, however, supported the existence of meaningful factors above the level of the five; specifically, the four-factor level resembled four-factor models often articulated in the personality and psychopathology literature (e.g., Livesley, 2003; B. P. O'Connor & Dyce, 1998; Watson, Clark, & Harkness, 1994). The three-factor level resembled the three factors of Eysenck (1987) and Tellegen (1982), with the dimensions of negative emotionality, disinhibition (a combination of disagreeableness and unconscientiousness), and positive emotionality. Finally, the two-factor model resembled the two-factor model of Digman (1990), with one factor (alpha) combining neuroticism, agreeableness, and conscientiousness, and the other factor (beta) combining extraversion and openness. In sum, the alternative dimensional models of personality and personality disorder can be subsumed within a common, hierarchical model (Trull & Durrett, 2005; Widiger & Simonsen, 2005a). However, Markon and colleagues also emphasized that their "results indicate that the Big Five [or FFM] traits occupy an important, unique position in the hierarchy, in that the other Big Trait models can be derived from the Big Five in some way" (p. 154). "Our results reinforce the position that the Big Five represent a crucial level of analysis for normal personality research and extend this position to include psychopathology research as well" (Markon et al., 2005, p. 154).

Each of the DSM-IV-TR personality disorders can, in fact, be readily understood as a maladaptive or extreme variant of the domains and facets of the FFM (Widiger & Trull, 2007). For example, DSM-IV-TR obsessive–compulsive personality disorder (OCPD; American Psychiatric Association, 2000) can be understood as largely a maladaptive variant of FFM conscientiousness. FFM conscientiousness (as assessed by the NEO-PI-R) includes such facets as order (OCPD preoccupation with details, rules, lists, and order), achievement striving (OCPD excessive devotion to work and productivity), dutifulness (OCPD overconscientiousness and scrupulousness about matters of ethics and morality), competence (OCPD perfectionism), and deliberation (OCPD rumination). DSM-IV-TR schizoid personality disorder (SZD) is largely a disorder of extreme introversion, particularly the facets of low gregariousness (social withdrawal and isolation), low warmth (indifference to social relationships), and low positive emotionality (anhedonic inability to experience pleasure). Avoidant personality disorder (AVD) also includes low gregariousness (social withdrawal) but is distinguished from SZD (in part) by the extraversion facets of low assertiveness (inhibited and restrained within interpersonal relationships) and low excitement seeking, as well as the neuroticism facets of anxiousness, self-consciousness (fears of criticism, disapproval), and vulnerability (feelings of inferiority and inadequacy). Dependent personality disorder (DPD) includes facets of neuroticism similar to AVD (anxiousness, self-consciousness, and vulnerability) but is distinguished (in part) by the inclusion of facets of agreeableness, such as compliance (difficulty expressing disagreement), altruism (sacrificing own needs for someone else), and modesty (relying on the advice and reassurance from others). DPD, AVD, and histrionic personality disorder (HPD) all include the extraversion facet of warmth (excessive attachment), but HPD also involves (in part) additional facets of extraversion, such as high gregariousness (convivial, many friends, seeking of social contact), assertiveness, excitement seeking (sensation seeking), active (energetic, exhibitionistic), and positive emotionality (high spirited, buoyant, and joyful). Borderline personality disorder (BPD) is largely a disorder of neuroticism (or negative affectivity), involving the highest levels of angry hostility (inappropriate or intense anger), anxiousness, depressiveness (suicidal ideation), self-consciousness (identity disturbance), impulsivity (self-mutilation, drug usage, bulimia), and vulnerability (helplessness, frantic efforts to avoid abandonment). (More complete descriptions of the DSM-IV-TR personality disorders are provided in Lynam & Widiger, 2001; Samuel & Widiger, 2004; Widiger, Trull, Clarkin, Sanderson, & Costa, 2002.)

Empirical support for conceptualizing the DSM-IV-TR personality disorders as maladaptive variants of the domains and facets of the FFM is extensive (Clark, 2007; B. P. O'Connor & Dyce, 1998; Saulsman & Page, 2004). Widiger and Costa (2002) identified over 50 studies that have addressed explicitly an understanding of personality disorders from the perspective of the FFM. These studies used a wide variety of measures and sampled a diverse array of clinical and nonclinical populations. In addition, many more supportive studies have since been published (Clark, 2007; Mullins-Sweatt & Widiger, 2006; B. P. O'Connor, 2005; Widiger & Lowe, 2007).

This research has been important in confirming the hypothesis that the DSM-IV-TR personality disorders can be understood as maladaptive variants of FFM personality structure. It is necessary for addressing the validity of the FFM of personality disorder, as well as for reassuring personality disorder clinicians and researchers, to document that the useful and valid information included within the diagnostic categories can be recovered by the FFM. On the other hand, the ultimate goal of an FFM of personality disorder would not be simply to reproduce the DSM-IV diagnostic categories, particularly the aspects that are fatally flawed (Clark, 2007; Widiger & Lowe, 2007).

Consider, for example, discriminant validity. Morey and colleagues (2002) demonstrated that the FFM was not successful in providing unique FFM profile descriptions of persons diagnosed with DSM-IV-TR personality disorders. Much of the profile overlap, however, could be due to the qualitatively *in*distinct categories of the DSM-IV-TR personality disorders. If individuals are not being accurately described by the DSM-IV-TR personality disorder diagnoses due to the het-

erogeneity of their personality structure, the overlap among the diagnostic categories, and the absence of distinct boundaries, it is unclear how successful the FFM should, in fact, be in distinguishing among persons provided with these diagnoses. Quite a bit of research has documented the overlap of, and excessive diagnostic co-occurrence among, the DSM-IV-TR categories (Bornstein, 1998; First et al., 2002; Livesley, 2003; Trull & Durrett, 2005; Widiger & Mullins-Sweatt, 2005), and both the overlap and co-occurrence have themselves been well explained in terms of the FFM (Lynam & Widiger, 2001; B. P. O'Connor, 2005; B. P. O'Connor & Dyce, 1998).

A four-step procedure for clinicians to use to diagnose a personality disorder from the perspective of the FFM (Widiger, Costa, & McCrae, 2002) has been proposed. The first step is to obtain a comprehensive assessment of personality functioning with an existing measure of the FFM (e.g., De Raad & Perugini, 2002; John et al., Chapter 4, this volume). The second step is to identify the social and occupational impairments and distress associated with the individual's characteristic personality traits. A misconception of the FFM is that low neuroticism, high extraversion, high openness, high agreeableness, and high conscientiousness always imply adaptive personality functioning (Coker, Samuel, & Widiger, 2002). Widiger and colleagues (2002) identify common impairments associated with all 60 poles of the 30 facets of the Costa and McCrae (1992) description of the FFM. McCrae, Lockenhoff, and Costa (2005) have provided a further expansion of likely impairments and problems in living associated with FFM elevations—a list that goes well beyond the limited coverage provided by the existing diagnostic categories (Westen & Arkowitz-Westen, 1998). The third step is to determine whether the dysfunction and distress reach a clinically significant level of impairment.

The fourth and final step is a quantitative matching of the individual's personality profile to prototypic profiles of diagnostic constructs. The extent to which an individual's FFM profile matches the FFM profile for a prototypic case be used as a quantitative indication of the likelihood that a person fits the profile for that construct, as demonstrated empirically for BPD (Trull, Widiger,

Lynam, & Costa, 2003) and for psychopathy (J. D. Miller & Lynam, 2003). An advantage of the FFM method of diagnosis relative to DSM-IV-TR is that clinicians and researchers interested in studying diagnostic constructs that are outside of the existing nomenclature (e.g., the successful psychopath) can use the FFM to provide a reasonably specific description of the construct and use the prototypal matching methodology to empirically study it. However, it should also be emphasized that the purpose of an FFM of personality disorder is not simply to provide another means with which to return to a single diagnostic label (Clark, 2007; Widiger & Lowe, 2007). In most cases the quantitative matching will serve primarily to indicate the extent to which any single construct (e.g., borderline) is inadequately descriptive of the individual person. In the vast majority of cases, the optimal description would be provided by the actual FFM profile of the person rather than a profile of a hypothetical prototype or the extent to which the person's FFM profile resembles this prototype.

Personality Disorders on a Spectrum with Axis I Mental Disorders

A spectrum relationship may also exist for personality disorders and Axis I mental disorders. In fact, a proposal for DSM-V is to abandon the classification of personality disorder altogether and subsume most of them into an existing Axis I disorder (First et al., 2002; Siever & Davis, 1991). At first blush this would appear to be a radical proposal. However, it has support from a variety of sources.

A strong precedent for such a shift in conceptualization and classification is DSM-IV-TR schizotypal personality disorder. Schizotypal personality disorder is genetically related to schizophrenia, most of its neurobiological risk factors and psychophysiological correlates are shared with schizophrenia (e.g., eye tracking, orienting, startle blink, and neurodevelopmental abnormalities), and the treatments that are effective in ameliorating schizotypal symptoms overlap with treatments used for persons with Axis I schizophrenia (Parnas, Licht, & Bovet, 2005; Raine, 2006). In fact, the World Health Organization's (WHO) International Classification of Diseases—Tenth Edition (ICD-10; World Health Organization, 1992), the par-

ent classification to the American Psychiatric Association's diagnostic manual, does not recognize the existence of schizotypal personality disorder, providing instead a diagnosis of schizotypal disorder that is included within the section of the manual for disorders of schizophrenia.

There also does not currently appear to be a meaningful distinction between avoidant personality disorder and generalized social phobia (American Psychiatric Association, 2000; Tyrer, 2005; Widiger, 2003), and some suggest that the best solution is to simply abandon the personality disorder diagnosis in favor of the generalized anxiety disorder (Schneider, Blanco, Anita, & Liebowitz, 2002). Liebowitz and colleagues (1998) state: "We believe that the more extensive evidence for syndromal validity of social phobia, including pharmacological and cognitive-behavioral treatment efficacy, make it the more useful designation in cases of overlap with avoidant personality" (p. 1060). The reference to treatment efficacy by Liebowitz and colleagues falls on receptive ears for many clinicians who struggle to obtain insurance coverage for the treatment of maladaptive personality functioning. It is often reported that a personality disorder diagnosis is stigmatizing, due in large part to its placement on a distinct axis that carries the implication of being an untreatable, lifetime disorder (Frances et al., 1991; Kendell, 1983). The Assembly of the American Psychiatric Association (which has authoritative governance over the approval of revisions to the diagnostic manual) has repeatedly passed resolutions to explore proposals to move personality disorders to Axis I (and to change the name of borderline) in large part to address the stigma and lack of reimbursement for their treatment.

A similar fate could befall other personality disorders (First et al., 2002). Just as the schizotypal and avoidant personality disorders could be readily subsumed within an existing section of Axis I, depressive personality disorder could be classified as an early-onset dysthymia; borderline personality disorder as an affective dysregulation and/or impulse dyscontrol disorder; schizoid personality disorder as an early-onset and chronic variant of the negative (anhedonic) symptoms of schizophrenic pathology (M. B. Miller, Useda, Trull, Burr, & Minks-Brown, 2001; Parnas et al., 2005); paranoid personality disorder by an early-onset, chronic, and milder variant of a delusional disorder; obsessive–compulsive personality disorder by a generalized and chronic variant of obsessive–compulsive anxiety disorder (although there is, in fact, only weak evidence to support a close relationship between the obsessive–compulsive anxiety and personality disorders; Costa, Samuels, Bagby, Daffin, & Norton, 2005); and antisocial personality disorder by an adult variant of conduct (disruptive behavior) disorder.

A concern with reformulating personality disorders as early-onset and chronic Axis I disorders, beyond the fundamental consideration that the diagnostic manual would no longer recognize the existence of maladaptive personality functioning, is that it might create more problems than it solves. It does appear to be true that persons have constellations of maladaptive personality traits that are not well described by just one or even multiple personality disorder diagnoses (Bornstein, 1998; Clark, 2007; Trull & Durrett, 2005; Widiger & Samuel, 2005). These constellations of maladaptive personality traits would be even less well described by multiple Axis I diagnoses across broad classes of anxiety, mood, impulsive dyscontrol, delusional, disruptive behavior, and schizophrenic disorders. In addition, simply because a personality disorder (or trait) shares some genetic foundation with an Axis I disorder does not then indicate that it is an Axis I disorder. For example, inconsistent with the ICD-10 classification of schizotypal personality disorder as a form of schizophrenia is that it is far more comorbid with other personality disorders than it is with psychotic disorders; persons with schizotypal personality disorder rarely go on to develop schizophrenia; and schizotypal symptomatology is seen in quite a number of persons who appear to lack a genetic association with schizophrenia and would not be at all well described as being schizophrenic (Raine, 2006).

Axis I on a Spectrum with Personality

A perspective that is complementary to a proposal to subsume personality disorders within existing Axis I disorders is to revise the Axis I classification to recognize the presence of temperaments that may provide an underlying foundation for many of the Axis I disorders. Excessive diagnostic comorbid-

ity is not unique to the personality disorders. Concurrent diagnostic comorbidity is the norm rather than the exception throughout many of the DSM-IV-TR Axis I disorders, with the rate dramatically increasing if one considers lifetime comorbidity (Brown, Campbell, Lehman, Grisham, & Mancill, 2001). Quite a few previously published reviews have documented this concern (e.g., Clark, 2005; Krueger & Markon, 2006a; Krueger, Markon, Patrick, & Iacono, 2005; Watson, 2005; Widiger & Clark, 2000; Widiger & Samuel, 2005b). There are many instances in which the presence of multiple diagnoses do suggest the presence of distinct yet comorbid psychopathologies; however, perhaps in just as many instances one has instead the presence of a single, common, underlying diathesis. "Comorbidity may be trying to show us that many current treatments are not so much treatments for transient 'state' mental disorders of affect and anxiety as they are treatments for core processes, such as negative affectivity, that span normal and abnormal variation as well as undergird multiple mental disorders" (Krueger, 2002, p. 44).

Kendler, Prescott, Myers, and Neale (2003) applied multivariate genetic analyses to 10 mental disorders (major depression, generalized anxiety, phobia, panic, animal phobia, situational phobia, alcohol dependence, drug abuse/dependence, adult antisocial personality, and conduct disorder) as assessed in more than 5,600 members of male–male and female–female twin pairs from a population based registry. Kendler and colleagues concluded that the pattern of genetic and environmental risk factors were similar in men and women, and "the patterns of comorbidity of these disorders (internalizing vs. externalizing, and within internalizing, anxious misery vs. fear) is driven largely by genetic factors" (p. 936).

Krueger and his colleagues have been particularly productive in identifying the presence of two fundamental dimensions of internalization and externalization underlying the mood, anxiety, substance use, and personality disorders, using a variety of clinical, twin, and community samples (Krueger & Markon, 2006a, 2006b). These two fundamental dimensions of adult psychopathology replicate well the two dimensions of internalization and externalization identified by Achenbach (1966) many years ago within childhood psychopathology.

The two broad domains of internalization and externalization also map well onto fundamental personality temperaments (Clark, 2005; Krueger & Tackett, 2003; Watson, 2005; Watson, Gamez, & Simms, 2005; see also Clark & Watson, Chapter 9, this volume), with internalization paralleling closely the broad five-factor domain of neuroticism or the temperament of negative affectivity, and externalization paralleling low conscientiousness or the temperament of low constraint. From this perspective, low constraint (or impulsivity) represents a broad endophenotypic risk factor for the development of a variety of Axis I disorders, including, for instance, substance use disorder and/or antisocial personality disorder, depending on additional, more specific genetic and environmental factors. Of course, externalization or low constraint may combine with internalization/negative affectivity to produce variants of some of these disorders. For example, some cases of substance use disorder appear to stem from both negative affectivity and externalizing tendencies, whereas other cases appear not to include a negative affectivity component (Windle & Scheidt, 2004).

The neuroticism and positive affective temperaments also relate closely (empirically and conceptually) to the heavily researched behavioral inhibition system (BIS) and behavioral activation system (BAS) of Gray (1987). BAS is said to be an approach-related, positive-incentive motivational system, and BIS an inhibiting sensitivity to cues of threat (Depue & Collins, 1999). At the most simplistic level, high levels of BIS would provide a neurobiological disposition to anxiety disorders, and low levels of BAS, to depressive mood disorders (Kasch, Rottenberg, Arnow, & Gottlib, 2002). Higgins (2000) has similarly researched two closely related constructs he labeled prevention focus (an orientation toward security and a sensitivity to possible negative outcomes) and promotion focus (an orientation toward accomplishment and a sensitivity to possible positive outcomes). Ultimately, prevention and treatment of psychopathology would perhaps be most effective if they addressed the endophenotypic vulnerabilities. Given the recent effort to integrate the childhood temperament research with the FFM domains (Caspi, Roberts, & Shiner, 2005; Mervielde,

De Clercq, De Fruyt, & Van Leeuwen, 2005) and a growing body of evidence demonstrating the contribution of temperament to child psychopathology (Muris & Ollendeck, 2005; Mervielde et al., 2005; Rothbart & Posner, 2006), it might be of interest for future research to explore the contribution of other temperaments, beyond positive affectivity, negative affectivity, and constraint, to additional adult Axis I disorders. Such research, though, will be limited partly by the absence of much recognition within the American Psychiatric Association diagnostic manual of disorders of dysregulated or dyscontrolled aggression (Widiger & Sankis, 2000).

ETIOLOGICAL (CAUSAL) RELATIONSHIPS

Of primary concern to many personality, personality disorder, and psychopathology researchers (and clinicians) is the etiological (causal) relationship between personality and psychopathology. This causal relationship is again bidirectional: One's characteristic way of thinking, feeling, behaving, and relating to others can result in, or contribute to, the development of a mental disorder, just as a severe or chronic mental disorder can itself contribute to fundamental changes in personality. Both directions of relationship are considered in turn.

Causal Effects of Psychopathology on Personality

Personality can change (Caspi et al., 2005; Roberts & DelVecchio, 2000; Srivastava, John, Gosling, & Potter, 2003; see also Roberts, Wood, & Caspi, Chapter 14, this volume) for the better or for the worse, and it is conceivable that the experience of having suffered from a severe mental disorder, such as a psychosis or a major depression, might have a fundamental and lasting effect on one's characteristic manner of thinking, feeling, and relating to others. This alteration to personality functioning, often referred to as a "scar" of the Axis I disorder, need not represent simply a continuing subthreshold manifestation of the Axis I pathology (e.g., a residual phase of schizophrenia appearing to be schizotypal personality traits) but may even represent the development of new personality traits due to the occurrence or experience of the psychopathology (e.g., dependent personality traits resulting from an experience of recurrent panic attacks or psychotic episodes).

The ICD-10 (World Health Organization, 1992) contains a number of mental disorder diagnoses that concern maladaptive changes to personality functioning occurring within adulthood, including enduring personality change secondary to a catastrophic experience, personality change resulting from another mental disorder, and personality change secondary to a physical disorder. However, only the last of those three is recognized in DSM-IV-TR (American Psychiatric Association, 2000). The American Psychiatric Association recognizes the occurrence of changes to personality secondary to a brain injury or a physical disease, and even identifies specific variants of such change that resemble closely many of the current personality disorder diagnoses (i.e., labile, disinhibited, aggressive, apathetic, and paranoid; American Psychiatric Association, 2000), but it does not recognize changes to personality secondary to severe or sustained psychosocial experiences, including prolonged torture, confinement, or victimization (Shea, 1996), or changes to personality secondary to psychopathology (Triebwasser & Shea, 1996). Even the changes resulting from brain injury or disease are not actually classified as personality disorders.

The reluctance of the American Psychiatric Association to recognize the potential existence of changes to personality resulting from experiences of psychopathology is understandable, as there is little empirical research to document the reliability or validity of such personality change. For example, Shea and colleagues (1996) attempted to document the occurrence of lasting personality changes resulting from episodes of major depression, using a subset of the data provided by the longitudinal National Institute of Mental Health (NIMH) Collaborative Program on the Psychobiology of Depression. Their pool of subjects consisted of 556 persons who had no prior or current mental disorder at the time of intake into the study, and who were reassessed 6 years later. Twenty-eight of these individuals suffered their first episodes of major depression during the 6-year period. However, "none of the scales for which negative change would be predicted by the scar hypothesis (increased neuroticism, emotional reliance, and lack of social self confidence; decreased ascendance/domi-nance, sociability, and extroversion) showed such change" (Shea et al., 1996, p. 1409). The personality scale scores remained largely stable across the 6 years. These findings were good news for the validity of personality assessment, because they documented the stability of test scores across a substantial period of time and across episodes of a severe mental disorder, but they were bad news for the scar hypothesis.

The ICD-10 diagnosis of personality change secondary to catastrophic experience (World Health Organization, 1992) does bear a close relationship to a construct that is receiving considerable clinical and research attention: complex posttraumatic stress disorder (PTSD). Complex PTSD is a more pervasive reaction than PTSD to severe (often sustained) interpersonal stress (e.g., abuse, battering, or torture) that includes "impaired affect modulation; self-destructive and impulsive behavior; dissociative symptoms; feeling permanently damaged; a loss of previously sustained beliefs; hostility; social withdrawal; feeling constantly threatened; impaired relationships with others; or a change from the individual's previous personality characteristics" (American Psychiatric Association, 2000, p. 465). Complex PTSD was considered for inclusion in DSM-IV-TR but is currently only described as an associated feature of the more narrowly defined PTSD (Ebert & Dyck, 2004). Persons who evidence significant personality change following severe and sustained exposure to stress but fail to evidence the more specific sequelae of PTSD cannot be given the PTSD diagnosis.

Complex PTSD bears a close relationship to a diagnosis of borderline personality disorder and can, in fact, be considered "an attempt to collapse the conceptual space between the DSM-IV-TR Axis I and II diagnoses of PTSD and borderline personality disorder" (McLean & Gallop, 2003, p. 369). Complex PTSD clearly involves personality changes (Allen, Coyne, & Huntoon, 1998; Ebert & Dyck, 2004; Simon, 2002; World Health Organization, 1992). However, most advocates for the inclusion of the construct in a future edition of the diagnostic manual prefer that it be classified as an anxiety disorder rather than as a disorder of personality change, due to a number pejorative connotations: (1) the potential implications that the victim might have been somehow vulnerable to this disorder due to deficits or inadequacies within the premorbid personality structure (i.e., blaming the victim); (2) inadequate emphasis on the source or cause of the disorder (i.e., a diagnosis of PTSD makes an explicit reference to the existence of a stressor, which in this case is often a human perpetrator); and (3) an implication of low or absent amenability to treatment (McLean & Gallop, 2003; Webster & Dunn, 2005).

Causal Effects of Personality on Psychopathology

The contribution of personality to the development of psychopathology has always been of central theoretical and clinical importance (Maher & Maher, 1994). Much of the vast literature on the relationship of personality or personality disorder with psychopathology is concerned with the potential contribution of personality or personality disorder to the onset or etiology of Axis I psychopathology, and there is little doubt that one's characteristic manner of thinking, feeling, behaving, and relating to others can contribute to the development of a variety of mental disorders. The possibility that personality influences one's response to external events may help explain why some people collapse under life stresses whereas others seem resilient in the face of traumatic circumstances such as severe illness, the death of loved ones, extreme poverty, natural disasters, or war. After all, surprisingly large numbers of people mature into normal, successful adults despite stressful, disadvantaged, or even abusive childhoods. For others, seemingly minor losses and rebuffs can be devastating, sometimes even precipitating severe mental disorder. Perhaps those individuals' personalities predispose them to greater emotion vulnerability (Basic Behavioral Science Task Force of the National Advisory Mental Health Council, 1996).

It is, of course, true that a fundamental task for personality researchers is to understand how personality traits combine with experiences to influence behavior patterns and future choices. Researchers investigating personality's causal role in psychopathology have played a leading role in developing and testing theoretical models of this process (Caspi, 1993; Caspi & Roberts, 2001; Moffitt, 2005; Shiner & Caspi, 2003). In this way, the study of psychopathology has contributed extensively to the basic science of personality. We next review this work, referred

to as personality–environment transaction theory, and the important role neuroticism likely plays in influencing negative interactions with the environment. We then consider the study of the etiological contribution of dependency, which can readily be understood from the transaction theory perspective.

Caspi and colleagues, perhaps following Scarr and McCartney's (1983) discussion of gene–environment interactions, have described three kinds of person–environment transactions likely to influence future behavior patterns (see also Roberts et al., Chapter 14, this volume). "Reactive person–environment transactions" refer to the recognition that there are individual differences in how individuals react to, or construe, environmental events. Self theory (Epstein, 1990), personal script theory (Tomkins, 1986), and personal construct theory (Kelly, 1955) all hold that two individuals exposed to a common event may construe it differently, and thus have a different psychological experience of the event. With respect to psychopathology, an individual high in neuroticism may tend to respond to unfriendly interactions with higher levels of distress, anxiety, and hurt than would someone low in neuroticism. Over time, those two individuals are likely to depart further in their ongoing experience of subjective distress.

"Evocative person–environment transactions" refer to the phenomenon that different individuals evoke different reactions from others. An antagonistic individual is more likely to evoke unfriendly responses from others than is an agreeable person. In a very real sense, those two individuals end up living in different psychological worlds: In one world, others tend to be hostile and mean; in the other world, others tend to be warm and friendly. In this way, initial personality differences are maintained and even enhanced via differential responses from the environment (Caspi & Roberts, 2001), perhaps in ways that alter risk for dysfunction.

"Proactive person–environment transactions" refer to the tendency for individuals to choose environmental settings in which they are comfortable. An introverted individual may choose a career that minimizes interactions with others and a lifestyle that avoids regular socializing. That person's introversion is thus maintained and perhaps even increased in a way that increases risk for disorders such as social phobia.

Empirical Support for Person–Environment Transaction Theory

A number of longitudinal studies have provided findings consistent with this model. Caspi, Elder, and Bem (1987) argued that transactions of these kinds help facilitate the continuity of maladaptive behavior. They found that ill-tempered 8- to 10-year-old boys tended to become men who experienced downward mobility, erratic work lives, and likely divorce. Ill-tempered 8- to 10-year-old girls tended to become women who married men with low occupational status, were likely to divorce, and tended to be ill-tempered mothers. Caspi and colleagues felt that these trajectories likely resulted, in part, from proactive, evocative, and reactive transactions between those individuals and their environments. Their study was limited in that they did not measure the specific person–environment transactions, but their findings were consistent with predictions based on the transactional perspective.

T. G. O'Connor, Deater-Deckard, Fulker, Rutter, and Plomin (1998) found evidence consistent with evocative person–environment transactions in an adoption study. Late childhood/early adolescent children with genetic liability for antisocial behavior tended to engage in more externalizing behavior and thus elicited higher levels of guilt induction, hostility, and withdrawal from their adoptive parents than did other adopted children. At least in part, these children may have evoked a different and more high-risk environment than did other children. Similarly, Wong, Zucker, Puttler, and Fitzgerald (1999) found that the influence of temperaments characterized by high reactivity and low attention at ages 3–5 on externalizing behavior at age 8 was mediated by parents' negative interactions with those children. Ge and colleagues (1996) found that psychiatric disorders of biological parents were related to the antisocial and hostile behaviors of their adopted-out children, which were related, in turn, to negative parenting practices by adoptive mothers: a process that suggests evocative reactions in the adoptive family.

Theoretical Advances in Person–Environment Transaction Theory

As Rutter and colleagues (1997) noted, little has been done to identify the proximal processes by which individual differences in traits lead to differences in responses to stressors. One possible approach to this problem is to apply a psychosocial learning perspective. Consider reactive person–environment transactions. To the degree that humans engage in reactive transactions, an objectively common learning event may not be experienced in the same way by two individuals (Hartup & Van Lieshout, 1995). It follows that two individuals may learn different things from the same event. If so, one should be able to show differential learning to a common event as a function of preexisting personality traits.

A specific demonstration of this process may have been provided by Smith, Williams, Fister, Cyders, and Kelley (2006). They taught business students how to invest in the stock market. The students then practiced investing with pretend accounts. Unbeknownst to them, all students received the exact same rate of return over five investing sessions. Despite their common outcome, growth-curve analyses of their expectancies for their future investing showed that disinhibited individuals formed more positive expectancies and inhibited individuals formed more negative expectancies than did typical individuals. It thus appears that one mechanism by which personality may influence subsequent behavioral choices is by shaping learning. Consistent with this finding, several studies of risk for alcohol abuse have found that the influence of disinhibition on drinking appears to be mediated by positive expectancies of the effects of drinking (Anderson, Smith, & Fischer, 2003; Barnow et al., 2004; McCarthy, Kroll, & Smith, 2001; McCarthy, Miller, Smith, & Smith, 2001). One can likely use psychosocial learning concepts to further understand the mechanisms of evocative and proactive transactions as well.

Neuroticism Contributes to Maladaptive Person–Environment Transactions

Person–environment transaction theory may illuminate the role of personality in risk for psychopathology beyond traditional conceptualizations of diathesis and stress. High levels on certain personality traits, such as neuroticism, can contribute to both diathesis and stress. For example, it is now perhaps well established that the broad domain of neuroticism (or negative affectivity) provides a personality disposition or vulnerability to a wide range of psychopathology (i.e., personality as diathesis; Clark, 2007; Watson et al., 2005). Neuroticism likely influences vulnerability to psychopathology through both reactive and evocative person–environment transactions. The former was considered above: A tendency to react to events with high levels of distress, anxiety, and worry likely increases risk for various forms of psychopathology. The latter may occur when one's frequent expressions of upset, worry, and vulnerability produce negative reactions from others, thus reinforcing and increasing the original distress (i.e., personality as causing stress). Within this general context, the particular mental disorder a person high in neuroticism develops will likely be due in part to other contributing variables. For example, gender, social–cultural context, other genetic vulnerabilities, and specific psychosocial learning histories can either direct the person toward a preferred method of coping (e.g., bulimic, dissociative, or substance use behavior) or reflect an additional vulnerability (e.g., for a sexual dysfunction, sleep, or somatoform disorder).

Dependency

One of the more heavily researched personality dispositions for the development of depressive episodes is the personality trait of dependency, studied within the general personality literature, using a variety of alternative measures (Blatt, 2004; Bornstein, 2005; Zuroff, Mongrain, & Santor, 2004). Extreme forms of dependency are even diagnosed as a mental disorder, included within DSM-IV-TR as a dependent personality disorder (American Psychiatric Association, 2000), defined as "a pervasive and excessive need to be taken care of that leads to submissive and clinging behavior and fears of separation" (American Psychiatric Association, 2000, p. 721).

The self-esteem of a person with a dependent personality disorder requires substantial maintenance from a supportive and nurturant relationship (Blatt, 2004; Bornstein, 2005), yet these intense needs for reassurance can have the paradoxical effect of driving the needed person away. The dependent person's worst fears are then realized (i.e., he or she is abandoned and alone), and his or her sense of self-worth, meaning, or

value is then furthered injured, perhaps even crushed by the rejection. The dependent person might then indiscriminately select a readily available but unreliable, undependable, and perhaps even abusive person simply to be with someone. This partner would again reaffirm the person's worst fears through abuse, derogation, and denigration (i.e., conveying to the dependent person that he or she is indeed undesirable and unlovable, and that the relationship is again tenuous). Such a combination of evocative, reactive, and then proactive transactions with the environment are the means by which a dependent personality style can lead to depression.

Quite a few studies have supported the hypothesis that dependency-based traits, cognitions, and behaviors contribute to the development of depressed mood in response to interpersonal loss or rejection. Santor and Zuroff (1997), for example, reported how dependent persons were excessively concerned about maintaining interpersonal relatedness, adopted the responses of friends who outperformed them, praised the people who criticized them, and minimized their disagreements. Joiner and Metalsky indicated how persons characterized by excessive reassurance seeking can contribute to their own worst fears of interpersonal rejection: "A dysphoric individual who seeks excessive reassurance in response to perceived threat in one domain (e.g., fear of being fired) may, by excessive reassurance seeking, generate stress in another domain (e.g., his or her spouse may withdraw after failing to assuage the individual's worries)" (2001, p. 378).

The concept of excessive reassurance seeking was developed historically as an alternative to a personality vulnerability model for depression (Joiner & Metalsky, 1995), but this interpersonal style is also central to a dependent person's behavioral repertoire (Blatt, 2004). Beck, Robbins, Taylor, and Baker (2001) demonstrated empirically that dependency is indeed related to excessive reassurance seeking and that the latter mediated the effects of dependency on depression. Shahar, Joiner, Zuroff, and Blatt (2004) further explored both moderating and mediating relationships between dependency, life stress, and depression. They suggested that dependent individuals appear to "invest considerable energy in avoiding confrontations so as 'not to rock the boat'" (Shahar et al.,

2004, p. 1592), and "when this yearned-for harmony is thwarted (as indicated by the presence of stressful events) ... these individuals become depressed" (p. 1592).

Hammen and colleagues (1995) obtained 6-month and 12-month follow-up assessments of 129 high school girls. They conducted multiple regression analyses to predict depression on the basis of dependency cognitions, prior interpersonal stress, and the interaction between them, controlling for initial levels of depression. All of these young women experienced stressful life events during this period of their lives, including moving away from home, separation from an important relationship, and loss of a romantic partner, but most of them did not become depressed. "It was the women with cognitions about relationships representing concerns about rejection or untrustworthiness of others who were especially challenged by normative changes" (Hammen et al., 1995, p. 441). Hammen and colleagues concluded that "overall, the results suggest that dysfunctional attachment cognitions contribute to both onset and severity of symptomatology" (p. 441).

Ayduk, Downey, and Kim (2001) conducted a 6-month longitudinal study of college women and reported that the women high in rejection sensitivity (i.e., disposition to anxiously expect, readily perceive, and overreact to rejection) became more depressed when they experienced a partner-initiated break-up during the follow-up period than women low in rejection sensitivity. No differences were obtained when they experienced a self-initiated or mutually initiated break-up, or when the stressor was not interpersonal in nature.

Mazure, Raghavan, Maciejewski, Jacobs, and Bruce (2001) used a multivariate approach to test how adverse life events and cognitive personality style (including need for approval) were related to an onset of depression. They reported that the "results of our study indicated that depression was nine times more likely after a major adverse event and was almost three times more likely in the presence of cognitive perceptual characteristics that emphasized either concern about disapproval or need for control" (Mazure et al., 2001, pp. 900, 901). Mazure and colleagues subsequently reported that need for approval (as well as autonomy) "were strong

predictors of depressive status independent of the occurrence of stressful life events" (p. 215).

Sanathara, Gardner, Prescott, and Kendler (2003) studied excessive emotional reliance on another person within a multiwave population-based twin study involving 7,174 participants. They reported that dependency scores were strongly associated with a lifetime risk for major depressive episodes. Premorbid dependency scores were also predictive of future onsets of depression, females obtained substantially higher dependency scores than males, and sex differences in risk for depression were explained largely by individual differences in dependency. They concluded that "these results suggest that a non trivial proportion of the gender differences in risk for major depression might result from gender differences in interpersonal dependency" (Sanathara et al., 2003, p. 930).

Dependency research, however, is not without fundamental concerns (Coyne, Thompson, & Whiffen, 2004). An important focus of future research on the contribution of dependency to depression will be a further articulation of the precise process or mechanism through which this association occurs. From the perspective of the FFM, dependency includes facets of neuroticism (more specifically, anxiousness, depressiveness, and feelings of vulnerability) as well as agreeableness (excessive compliance, trust, gullibility, and meekness) and extraversion (excessive needs for warmth and attachment) (Bagby & Rector, 1998; Bagby et al., 2001; Dunkley, Blankstein, Zuroff, Lecce, & Hui, 2006; Haigler & Widiger, 2001; Lynam & Widiger, 2001; Mongrain, 1993; Pincus, 2002; Zuroff, 1994). One implication of this FFM reformulation is that the basis for a dependent person's vulnerability to depressive mood disorders may not be specific to attachment needs but may reflect instead a more general emotional instability or insecurity (e.g., neuroticism) that is shared with other disorders of personality (Bagby et al., 2001; Bornstein & Cecero, 2000; Mongrain, 1993; Zuroff, 1994), along with high levels of agreeableness and extraversion. Thus, it may be more precise to consider a set of person–environment transactions that include (1) insecure reactions to events, (2) evocation of rejection through expression of one's insecurity, (3) a tendency to react to others in a compliant, agreeable way, and (4) a tendency to proactively pursue warmth and attachment.

The predominant view is that dependency contributes to the development of mood disorders through pathological cognitions (e.g., Hammen et al., 1995) and/or interpersonal mechanisms (Pettit & Joiner, 2006). However, in some instances it may be that maladaptively extreme temperaments both provide an affective underpinning to the risk and contribute to the cognitive and interpersonal difficulties. Complicating the existing research is the possibility that some measures of dependency are predominated by indicators of neuroticism, whereas other measures place more emphasis within the domains of agreeableness (compliance, gullibility, meekness) and extraversion (attachment and warmth). It will be useful for future research to dismantle the components of dependency to further isolate the specific mechanisms that contribute to the development of depressive mood disorders in response to rejection and loss (e.g., Bagby & Rector, 1998; Dunkley et al., 2006; Pincus, 2002; Shahar et al., 2004).

An additional concern for future research is the potential contribution of the interpersonal context to the development of the dependent person's sense of vulnerability. In theory, dependent personality traits contribute to the instability of intimate and supportive relationships through the expression of excessive needs for reassurance, premorbid emotional instability, and/or pathogenic cognitions. However, it is also possible that the emotional instability and pathological attitudes are themselves the result of unstable interpersonal relationships. Coyne and Whiffen (1995) noted that some self-report measures of dependent personality traits include items that concern the stability of recent relationships. These measures could then be assessing the actual instability of the relationships rather than dependent perceptions of the relationships. "Intimate relationships that are insecure or have an uncertain future may engender dependency and reassurance seeking" (Coyne & Whiffen, 1995, p. 367).

Dependency is a personality disposition that is seen much more often in women than in men (Bornstein, 1996), and many of

the dependency studies have been confined entirely to women (e.g., Ayduk et al., 2001; Hammen et al., 1995). A broader and more provocative reformulation of dependency in women is that the apparent feelings of insecurity may say less about the women than the persons with whom the women are involved. "Men and women may differ in what they seek from relationships, but they may also differ in what they provide to each other" (Coyne & Whiffen, 1995, p. 368). In other words, "women might appear (and be) less dependent if they weren't involved with such undependable men" (Widiger & Anderson, 2003, p. 63).

Personality disorder diagnoses can be used to inappropriately or inaccurately blame women for the troubles in their lives (Webster & Dunn, 2005; Widiger, Mullins-Sweatt, & Anderson, 2005). Coolidge and Anderson (2002) reported a significantly higher rate of dependent personality disorder in women with a history of multiple abusive relationships. However, many current victims of abuse who seem unwilling or unable to extricate themselves from a relationship could be acting realistically in response to threats of physical harm and to the absence of a safe or meaningful alternative (Bybee & Sullivan, 2005; Koepsell, Kernic, & Holt, 2006). It can be very difficult to leave a relationship in which one has a significant emotional involvement, and it may even seem preferable to suffer occasional assaults than to be perpetually harassed, stalked, and perhaps eventually killed. Bornstein (2005) provided arguments and empirical support for the hypothesis that it may, in fact, be emotional dependency in male perpetrators of abuse, coupled with an economic dependency of the women, that is most lethal for the occurrence of spousal abuse (see, however, Holtzworth-Munroe & Meehan, 2004, for an emphasis on borderline personality traits within male perpetrators). Future studies concerned with the contribution of dependent personality traits to depression in women should include an objective assessment of the contribution of the women's partners to the depression and to the dependent personality traits (Besser & Priel, 2003).

Longitudinal studies that explore the relationship of personality to marital instability and dissatisfaction would be particularly informative. There have been a number of cross-sectional and longitudinal studies exploring the intrapersonal and interpersonal effects of "normal" personality traits on marital happiness. Not surprisingly, who you are can have predictive value (e.g., high levels of neuroticism predict future unhappiness), as well as who you are with (e.g., high levels of antagonism and impulsivity predict future marital instability and/or lower happiness in the partner) (Donnellan, Conger, & Bryant, 2004; Donnellan, Larsen-Rife, & Conger, 2005; Kelly & Conley, 1987; Robins, Caspi, & Moffitt, 2002).

It is thus important to consider both maladaptively extreme temperaments and dysfunctional external environments as contributors to the emergence of psychopathology. Perhaps maladaptive temperaments cause some individuals to proactively select dysfunctional partners, whereas encountering a dysfunctional partner may contribute to personality psychopathology in the absence of extreme temperaments in other individuals. Evidence for the presence of one process does not rule out the presence of the other. Indeed, in light of the inevitably interactive nature of person–environment relations, it is perhaps most often the case that personality and environmental influences are reciprocal: Personality influences one's transactions with one's environment, and one's environment influences one's personality functioning. In any individual case, it may be very difficult to determine whether personality or environment played more of an initiating role in the interactive, reciprocal process.

Personality's Influence on How One Responds to What One Has Learned

The foregoing considered ways in which one's personality may help create one's environmental context, whether through choosing different environments, eliciting different environmental reactions, or interpreting environmental events in unique ways. We have also considered ways in which one's environment may influence changes in one's personality. There may be another way in which personality plays a causal role in dysfunction. It may be the case that even when individuals learn similar things from their environment, individual differences in personality cause them to use that information differently. Recently, a focus on individual differences in

personality may have helped to clarify findings in the psychosocial learning risk literature. In the case of risk for problem drinking, learned expectancies that alcohol facilitates social success appear to relate to problem drinking only for those high in extraversion. In studies conducted prior to awareness of this interaction, expectancies were found to relate only moderately to problem drinking. It now appears that those early moderate correlations effectively averaged a strong correlation among those high in extraversion with a weak correlation among those low in the trait (Fischer, Smith, Anderson, & Flory, 2003). Similarly, learned expectancies for punishment from drinking predicted reduced consumption among low-impulsive individuals much more strongly than among high-impulsive individuals (Finn, Bobova, Wehmer, Fargo, & Rickert, 2005). In the case of eating disorders, learned expectancies that eating helps alleviate negative affect predict subsequent bulimic symptoms (Smith, Simmons, Annus, Flory, & Hill, 2007), but that effect may be present only for individuals high in one form of impulsivity (Fischer et al., 2004). To the degree that individual differences in personality lead individuals to make different uses of what is learned, personality must be integrated with psychosocial learning models of risk for psychopathology.

CONCLUSIONS

One basic observation of the research on the relationship of personality and psychopathology is its vibrancy. All aspects of the various relationships between personality and psychopathology (pathoplastic, spectrum, and causal) are the focus of a number of highly productive, sophisticated, and informed research programs. Disentangling the forms of relationship from one another, however, is a formidable task. Cross-sectional studies can and do provide quite informative results, but it is also evident that the most telling findings are obtained from longitudinal studies. Personality and psychopathology affect and alter one another over time in a complex, unfolding interaction. Of most interest will be prospective studies of persons with a particular personality disposition that begin at the time of the onset of the disposition. Many vulnerability studies have used samples of convenience (e.g., persons already in treatment for the respective disorder) for which the differentiation among pathoplastic, spectrum, and causal relationships can, at times, be impossible to disentangle. Even if the study is conducted after the remission of the respective disorder, one is still faced with the complication of the scar hypothesis. Entrance into the causal sequence after a significant amount of interaction between personality, psychopathology, and life events has already occurred complicates substantially the interpretation of a study's findings, particularly if the participants have already had a history of suffering from the pathologies of interest. One approach to addressing this problem has been to exclude persons with any prior history of the respective disorder, but this exclusion effectively eliminates the very persons for whom the personality disposition would be most relevant. If personality traits do, in fact, provide a disposition to the development of a disorder, then it is quite possible, if not likely, that the persons with a prior history of the disorder are precisely those persons with the predisposition.

It may also be important to track closely the unfolding interaction of personality traits, events, and pathologies through experience sampling methodologies. A substantial amount of interaction and influence between a personality trait, a life event, and an episode of psychopathology can occur even within just 1 day. Their interactive influence upon one another will become increasingly difficult to understand and disentangle as each day passes and one relies on a retrospective description of this interaction. Any particular cross-sectional period of time may present only an arbitrary and unrepresentative slice along a continuously interacting and mutually reaffirming sequence of events.

In sum, personality continues to provide a compelling theoretical model for understanding the etiology, presentation, course, and treatment of psychopathology. All aspects of possible relationships between personality and psychopathology—pathoplastic, spectrum, and etiological—continue to be actively studied. The relationship of personality to psychopathology is complex, and it is through the dismantling of this complexity that continued progress will be made.

REFERENCES

Achenbach, T. M. (1966). The classification of children's psychiatric symptoms: A factor analytic study. *Psychological Monographs*, 80(615).

Allen, J. G., Coyne, L., & Huntoon, J. (1998). Complex posttraumatic stress disorder in women from a psychometric perspective. *Journal of Personality Assessment*, 70, 277–298.

American Psychiatric Association. (2000). *Diagnostic and statistical manual of mental disorders* (4th ed., text rev.). Washington, DC: Author.

Anderson, K. G., Smith, G. T., & Fischer, S. (2003). Women and acquired preparedness: Personality and learning implications for alcohol use. *Journal of Studies on Alcohol*, 64, 384–392.

Ayduk, O., Downey, G., & Kim, M. (2001). Rejection sensitivity and depressive symptoms in women. *Personality and Social Psychology Bulletin*, 27, 868–877.

Bagby, R. M., Gilchrist, E. J., Rector, N. A., Dickens, S. E., Joffe, R., Levitt, A., et al. (2001). The stability and validity of the sociotropy and autonomy personality dimensions as measured by the Revised Personal Style Inventory. *Cognitive Therapy and Research*, 25, 765–779.

Bagby, R. M., & Rector, N. A. (1998). Self-criticism, dependency, and the five factor model of personality in depression: Assessing construct overlap. *Personality and Individual Differences*, 24, 895–897.

Ball, S. A. (2005). Personality traits, problems, and disorders: Clinical applications to substance use disorders. *Journal of Research in Personality*, 39, 84–102.

Bank, P. A., & Silk, K. R. (2001). Axis I and Axis II interactions. *Current Opinion in Psychiatry*, 14, 137–142.

Barnow, S., Schultz, G., Lucht, M., Ulrich, I., Preuss, U., & Freyberger, H. J. (2004). Do alcohol expectancies and peer delinquency/substance use mediate the relationship between impulsivity and drinking behavior in adolescence? *Alcohol and Alcoholism*, 39, 213–219.

Basic Behavioral Science Task Force of the National Advisory Mental Health Council. (1996). Basic behavioral science research for mental health: Vulnerability and resilience. *American Psychologist*, 51, 22–28.

Beck, R., Robbins, M., Taylor, C., & Baker, L. (2001). An examination of sociotropy and excessive reassurance seeking in the prediction of depression. *Journal of Psychopathology and Behavioral Assessment*, 23, 101–105.

Besser, A., & Priel, B. (2003). A multisource approach to self-critical vulnerability to depression: The moderating role of attachment. *Journal of Personality*, 71, 515–555.

Blatt, S. J. (2004). *Experiences of depression: Theoretical, clinical, and research perspectives.* Washington, DC: American Psychological Association.

Blatt, S. J., & Shahar, G. (2005). A dialectic model of personality development and psychopathology: Recent contributions to understanding and treating depression. In J. Corveleyn, P. Luyten, & S. Blatt (Eds.), *The theory and treatment of depression: Towards a dynamic interactionism model* (pp. 137–162). Mahwah, NJ: Erlbaum.

Bornstein, R. F. (1996). Sex differences in dependent personality disorder prevalence rates. *Clinical Psychology: Science and Practice, 3,* 1–12.

Bornstein, R. F. (1998). Reconceptualizing personality disorder diagnosis in the DSM-V: The discriminant validity challenge. *Clinical Psychology: Science and Practice, 5,* 333–343.

Bornstein, R. F. (2005). *The dependent patient: A practitioner's guide.* Washington, DC: American Psychological Association.

Bornstein, R. F., & Cecero, J. J. (2000). Deconstructing dependency in a five-factor world: A meta-analytic review. *Journal of Personality Assessment, 74,* 324–343.

Brown, T. A., Campbell, L. A., Lehman, C. L., Grisham, J. R., & Mancill, R. B. (2001). Current and lifetime comorbidity of the DSM-IV anxiety and mood disorders in a large clinical sample. *Journal of Abnormal Psychology, 110,* 585–599.

Bybee, D., & Sullivan, C. M. (2005). Predicting re-victimization of battered women three years after exiting a shelter program. *American Journal of Community Psychology, 38,* 85–96.

Caspi, A. (1993). Why maladaptive behaviors persist: Sources of continuity and change across the life course. In D. C. Funder, R. D. Parke, C. Tomlinson-Kersey, & K. Widaman (Eds.), *Studying lives through time: Personality and development* (pp. 343–376). Washington, DC: American Psychological Association.

Caspi, A., Elder, G. H., & Bem, D. J. (1987). Moving against the world: Life-course patterns of explosive children. *Developmental Psychology, 23,* 308–313.

Caspi, A., & Roberts, B. W. (2001). Personality development across the life course: The argument for change and continuity. *Psychological Inquiry, 12,* 49–66.

Caspi, A., Roberts, B. W., & Shiner, R. L. (2005). Personality development: Stability and change. *Annual Review of Psychology, 56,* 453–484.

Cassin, S. E., & von Ranson, K. M. (2005). Personality and eating disorders: A decade in review. *Clinical Psychology Review, 25,* 895–916.

Chard, K. M., & Widiger, T. A. (2005). Abuse, coping, and treatment. *Journal of Psychotherapy Integration, 15,* 74–88.

Claes, L., Vandereycken, W., & Vertommen, H. (2005). Impulsivity-related traits in eating disorder patients. *Personality and Individual Differences, 39,* 739–749.

Clark, L. A. (2005). Temperament as a unifying basis for personality and psychopathology. *Journal of Abnormal Psychology, 114,* 505–521.

Clark, L. A. (2007). Assessment and diagnosis of personality disorder: Perennial issues and an emerging reconceptualization. *Annual Review of Psychology, 58,* 227–257.

Clark, L. A., & Harrison, J. A. (2001). Assessment instruments. In W. J. Livesley (Ed.), *Handbook of personality disorders: Theory, research, and treatment* (pp. 277–306). New York: Guilford Press.

Cloninger, C. R. (2000). A practical way to diagnoses personality disorders: A proposal. *Journal of Personality Disorders, 14,* 99–108.

Cohen, N. L., Ross, E. C., Bagby, R. M., Farvolden, P., & Kennedy, S. H. (2004). The 5-factor model of personality and antidepressant medication compliance. *Canadian Journal of Psychiatry, 49,* 106–113.

Coker, L. A., Samuel, D. B., & Widiger, T. A. (2002). Maladaptive personality functioning within the Big Five and the FFM. *Journal of Personality Disorders, 16,* 385–401.

Coolidge, F. L., & Anderson, L. W. (2002). Personality profiles of women in multiple abusive relationships. *Journal of Family Violence, 17,* 117–131.

Costa, P. T., Jr., & McCrae, R. R. (1990). Personality disorders and the five-factor model of personality. *Journal of Personality Disorders, 4,* 362–371.

Costa, P. T., Jr., & McCrae, R. R. (1992). *Revised NEO Personality Inventory (NEO-PI-R) and NEO Five-Factor Inventory (NEO-FFI): Professional manual.* Odessa, FL: Psychological Assessment Resources.

Costa, P. T., Jr., Samuels, J., Bagby, M., Daffin, L., & Norton, H. (2005). Obsessive–compulsive personality disorder: A review. In M. Maj, H. S. Akiskal, J. E. Mezzich, & A. Okasha (Eds.), *Personality disorders* (pp. 405–439). New York: Wiley.

Coyne, J. C., Thompson, R., & Whiffen, V. (2004). Is the promissary note of personality as vulnerability to depression in default?: Reply to Zuroff, Mongrain, and Santor (2004). *Psychological Bulletin, 130,* 512–517.

Coyne, J. C., & Whiffen, V. E. (1995). Issues in personality as diathesis for depression: The case of sociotropy dependency and autonomy self-criticism. *Psychological Bulletin, 118,* 358–378.

Depue, R. A., & Collins, P. F. (1999). Neurobiology of the structure of personality: Dopamine facilitation of incentive motivation and extraversion. *Behavioral and Brain Sciences, 22,* 491–569.

De Raad, B., & Perugini, M. (Eds.). (2002). *Big five assessment.* Bern, Switzerland: Hogrefe & Huber.

Digman, J. M. (1990). Personality structure: Emergence of the five-factor model. *Annual Review of Psychology, 41,* 417–440.

Dolan-Sewell, R. T., Krueger, R. F., & Shea, M. T. (2001). Co-occurrence with syndrome disorders. In W. J. Livesley (Ed.), *Handbook of personality disorders. Theory, research, and treatment* (pp. 84–104). New York: Guilford Press.

Donnellan, M. B., Conger, R. D., & Bryant, C. M. (2004). The Big Five and enduring marriages. *Journal of Research in Personality, 38,* 481–504.

Donnellan, M. B., Larsen-Rife, D., & Conger, R. D. (2005). Personality, family history, and competence in early adult romantic relationships. *Journal of Personality and Social Psychology, 88,* 562–576.

Dunkley, D. M., Blankstein, K. R., Zuroff, D. C., Lecce, S., & Hui, D. (2006). Neediness and connectedness and the five-factor model of personality. *European Journal of Personality, 20,* 123–136.

Ebert, A., & Dyck, M. J. (2004). The experience of mental death: The core features of complex posttraumatic stress disorder. *Clinical Psychology Review, 24,* 617–635.

Eng, W., & Heimberg, R. G. (2006). Interpersonal correlates of generalized anxiety disorder: Self versus other perception. *Journal of Anxiety Disorders, 20,* 380–387.

Epstein, S. (1990). Cognitive–experiental self-theory. In L. Pervin (Ed.), *Handbook of personality: Theory and research* (pp. 165–192). New York: Guilford Press.

Eysenck, H. J. (1987). The definition of personality disorders and the criteria appropriate for their description. *Journal of Personality Disorders, 1,* 211–219.

Farmer, R. F. (2000). Issues in the assessment and conceptualization of personality disorders. *Clinical Psychology Review, 20,* 823–851.

Finn, P. R., Bobova, L., Wehmer, E., Fargo, S., & Rickert, M. E. (2005). Alcohol expectancies, conduct disorder, and early-onset alcoholism: Negative alcohol expectancies are associated with less drinking in non-impulsive versus impulsive subjects. *Addiction, 100,* 953–962.

First, M. B., Bell, C. B., Cuthbert, B., Krystal, J. H., Malison, R., Offord, D. R., et al. (2002). Personality disorders and relational disorders: A research agenda for addressing crucial gaps in DSM. In D. J. Kupfer, M. B. First, & D. A. Regier (Eds.), *A research agenda for DSM-V* (pp. 123–199) Washington, DC: American Psychiatric Association.

First, M. B., Frances, A. J., & Pincus, H. A. (2002). *DSM-IV-TR handbook of differential diagnosis.* Washington, DC: American Psychiatric Association.

Fischer, S., Anderson, K. G., & Smith, G. T. (2004). Coping with distress by eating or drinking: The role of trait urgency and expectancies. *Psychology of Addictive Behaviors, 18,* 269–274.

Fischer, S., Smith, G. T., & Anderson, K. G. (2003). Clarifying the role of impulsivity in bulimia nervosa. *International Journal of Eating Disorders, 33,* 406–411.

Fischer, S., Smith, G. T., Anderson, K. G., & Flory, K. (2003). Expectancies influence the operation of personality and behavior. *Psychology of Addictive Behaviors, 17,* 108–114.

Fischer, S., Smith, G. T., Spillane, N. S., & Cyders, M. A. (2005). Urgency: Individual differences in reaction to mood and implications for addictive behaviors. In A. V. Clark (Ed.), *The psychology of mood* (pp. 85–108). New York: Nova Science.

Frances, A. J. (1980). The DSM-III personality disorders sections: A commentary. *American Journal of Psychiatry, 137,* 1050–1054.

Frances, A. J., First, M. B., Widiger, T. A., Miele, G., Tilly, S. M., Davis, W. W., et al. (1991). An A to Z guide to DSM-IV conundrums. *Journal of Abnormal Psychology, 100,* 407–412.

Ge, X., Conger, R. D., Cadoret, R. J., Neiderhiser, J. M., Yates, W., Troughton, E., et al. (1996). The developmental interface between nature and nurture: A mutual influence model of child antisocial behavior and parent behaviors. *Developmental Psychology, 32,* 574–589.

Gray, J. A. (1987). The neuropsychology of emotion and personality. In E. C. Goodman, S. M. Stahl, & S. D. Iversen (Eds.), *Cognitive neurochemistry* (pp. 171–190). New York: Oxford University Press.

Gunderson, J. G., Bender, D., Sanislow, C., Yen, S., Rettew, J. B., Dolan Sewell, R., et al. (2003). Plausibility and possible determinants of sudden "remissions" in borderline patients. *Psychiatry, 66,* 111–119.

Haigler, E. D., & Widiger, T. A. (2001). Experimental manipulation of NEO-PI-R items. *Journal of Personality Assessment, 77,* 339–358.

Hammen, C. L., Burge, D., Daley, S. E., Davila, J., Paley, B., & Rudolph, K. D. (1995). Interpersonal attachment cognitions and predictions of symptomatic responses to interpersonal stress. *Journal of Abnormal Psychology, 104,* 436–443.

Harkness, A. R., & Lilienfeld, S. O. (1997). Individual differences science for treatment planning: Personality traits. *Psychological Assessment, 9,* 349–360.

Harkness, A. R., McNulty, J. L., & Ben-Porath, Y. S. (1995). The Personality Psychopathology

Five (PSY 5): Constructs and MMPI-2 scales. *Psychological Assessment, 7,* 104–114.

Hartup, W. W., & Van Lieshout, C. F. M. (1995). Personality development in social context. *Annual Review of Psychology, 46,* 655–687.

Higgins, E. T. (2000). Making a good decision: Value from fit. *American Psychologist, 55,* 1217–1230.

Holtzworth-Munroe, A., & Meehan, J. C. (2004). Typologies of men who are martially violent: Scientific and clinical implications. *Journal of Interpersonal Violence, 19,* 1369–1389.

Joiner, T. J., & Metalsky, G. I. (1995). A prospective test of an integrative interpersonal theory of depression: A naturalistic study of college roommates. *Journal of Personality and Social Psychology, 69,* 778–788.

Joiner, T. J., & Metalsky, G. I. (2001). Excessive reassurance seeking: Delineating a risk factor involved in the development of depressive symptoms. *Psychological Science, 12,* 371–378.

Kachin, K. E., Newman, M. G., & Pincus, A. L. (2006). An interpersonal problem approach to the division of social phobia subtypes. *Behavior Therapy, 32,* 479–501.

Kasch, K. L., Rottenberg, J., Arnow, B. A., & Gottlib, I. H. (2002). Behavioral activation and inhibition systems and the severity and course of depression. *Journal of Abnormal Psychology, 111,* 589–597.

Kelly, E. L., & Conley, J. J. (1987). Personality and compatibility: A prospective analysis of marital stability and marital satisfaction. *Journal of Personality and Social Psychology, 52,* 27–40.

Kelly, G. A. (1955). *The psychology of personal constructs.* New York: Norton.

Kendell, R. E. (1983). DSM-III: A major advance in psychiatric nosology. In R. L. Spitzer, J. B. W. Williams, & A. E. Skodol (Eds.), *International perspectives on DSM-III* (pp. 55–68). Washington, DC: American Psychiatric Association.

Kendler, K. S., Prescott, C. A., Myers, J., & Neale, M. C. (2003). The structure of genetic and environmental risk factors for common psychiatric and substance use disorders in men and women. *Archives of General Psychiatry, 60,* 929–937.

Koepsell, J. K., Kernic, M. A., & Holt, V. L. (2006). Factors that influence battered women to leave their abusive relationships. *Violence and Victims, 21,* 131–147.

Krueger, R. F. (2002). Psychometric perspectives on comorbidity. In J. E. Helzer & J. J. Hudziak (Eds.), *Defining psychopathology in the 21st century: DSM-V and beyond* (pp. 41–54). Washington, DC: American Psychiatric Association.

Krueger, R. F., & Markon, K. E. (2006a). Reinterpreting comorbidity: A model-based approach to understanding and classifying psychopathol-ogy. *Annual Review of Clinical Psychology, 2,* 111–134.

Krueger, R. F., & Markon, K. E. (2006b). Understanding psychopathology: Melding genetics, personality, and quantitative psychology to develop an empirically based model. *Current Directions in Psychological Science, 15,* 113–117.

Krueger, R. F., Markon, K. E., Patrick, C. J., & Iacono, W. G. (2005). Externalizing psychopathology in adulthood: A dimensional–spectrum conceptualization and its implications for DSM-V. *Journal of Abnormal Psychology, 114,* 537–550.

Krueger, R. F., & Tackett, J. L. (2003). Personality and psychopathology: Working toward the bigger picture. *Journal of Personality Disorders, 17,* 109–128.

Krueger, R. F., & Tackett, J. L. (Eds.). (2006). *Personality and psychopathology.* New York: Guilford Press.

Leichsenring, F., & Leibing, E. (2003). The effectiveness of psychodynamic therapy and cognitive behavior therapy in the treatment of personality disorders: A meta analysis. *American Journal of Psychiatry, 160,* 1223–1232.

Liebowitz, M. R., Barlow, D. H., Ballenger, J. C., Davidson, J., Foa, E. B., Fyer, A. J., et al. (1998). DSM-IV anxiety disorders: Final overview. In T. A. Widiger et al. (Eds.), *DSM-IV sourcebook* (Vol. 4, pp. 1047–1076). Washington, DC: American Psychiatric Association.

Lima, E. N., Stanley, S., Kaboski, B., Reitzel, L. R., Richey, A., Castro, Y., et al. (2005). The incremental validity of the MMPI-2: When does therapist access not enhance treatment outcome? *Psychological Assessment, 17,* 462–468.

Livesley, W. J. (2003). Diagnostic dilemmas in classifying personality disorder. In K. A. Phillips, M. B. First, & H. A. Pincus (Eds.), *Advancing DSM: Dilemmas in psychiatric diagnosis* (pp. 153–190). Washington, DC: American Psychiatric Association.

Livesley, W. J., & Jackson, D. (in press). *Manual for the Dimensional Assessment of Personality Pathology Basic Questionnaire.* Port Huron, MI: Sigma Press.

Loranger, A. W., Lenzenweger, M. F., Gartner, A. F., Susman, V. L., Herzig, J., Zammit, G. K., et al. (1991). Trait–state artifacts and the diagnosis of personality disorders. *Archives of General Psychiatry, 48,* 720–729.

Lynam, D. R., & Widiger, T. A. (2001). Using the five-factor model to represent the DSM-IV personality disorders: An expert consensus approach. *Journal of Abnormal Psychology, 110,* 401–412.

Maher, B. A., & Maher, W. B. (1994). Personality and psychopathology: A historical perspective. *Journal of Abnormal Psychology, 103,* 72–77.

Markon, K. E., Krueger, R. F., & Watson, D. (2005). Delineating the structure of normal and abnormal personality: An integrative hierarchical approach. *Journal of Personality and Social Psychology, 88,* 139–157.

Mazure, C. M., Raghavan, C., Maciejewski, P. K., Jacobs, S. C., & Bruce, M. L. (2001). Cognitive personality characteristics as direct predictors of unipolar major depression. *Cognitive Therapy and Research, 25,* 215–225.

McCarthy, D. M., Kroll, L., & Smith, G. T. (2001). Integrating disinhibition and learning risk for alcohol use. *Experimental and Clinical Psychopharmacology, 9,* 389–398.

McCarthy, D. M., Miller, T. L., Smith, G. T., & Smith, J. A. (2001). Disinhibition and expectancy in risk for alcohol use: Comparing black and white college samples. *Journal of Studies on Alcohol, 62,* 313–321.

McCrae, R. R., & Costa, P. T., Jr. (2003). *Personality in adulthood: A five-factor theory perspective* (2nd ed.). New York: Guilford Press.

McCrae, R. R., Lockenhoff, C. E., & Costa, P. T., Jr. (2005). A step toward DSM-V: Cataloguing personality related problems in living. *European Journal of Personality, 19,* 269–286.

McLean, L. M., & Gallop, R. (2003). Implications of childhood sexual abuse for adult borderline personality disorder and complex posttraumatic stress disorder. *American Journal of Psychiatry, 160,* 369–371.

Mervielde, I., De Clercq, B., De Fruyt, F., & Van Leeuwen, K. (2005). Temperament, personality, and developmental psychopathology as childhood antecedents of personality disorders. *Journal of Personality Disorders, 19,* 171–201.

Miller, J. D., & Lynam, D. R. (2003). Psychopathy and the five-factor model of personality: A replication and extension. *Journal of Personality Assessment, 81,* 168–178.

Miller, M. B., Useda, J. D., Trull, T. J., Burr, R. M., & Minks Brown, C. (2001). Paranoid, schizoid, and schizotypal personality disorders. In P. B. Sutker & H. E. Adams (Eds.), *Comprehensive handbook of psychopathology* (3rd ed., pp. 535–558). New York: Plenum Press.

Millon, T., Davis, R., Millon, C. M., Wenger, C. M., Van Zuilen, M. H., et al. (1996). *Disorders of personality: DSM-IV and beyond* (2nd ed.). New York: Wiley.

Moffitt, T. E. (2005). The new look of behavioral genetics in developmental psychopathology: Gene–environment interplay in antisocial behaviors. *Psychological Bulletin, 131,* 533–554.

Mongrain, M. (1993). Dependency and self-criticism located within the five-factor model of personality. *Personality and Individual Differences, 15,* 455–462.

Morey, L. C., Gunderson, J. G., Quigley, B. D., Shea, M. T., Skodol, A. E., McGlashan, T. H., et al. (2002). The representation of borderline, avoidant, obsessive–compulsive, and schizotypal personality disorders by the five-factor model. *Journal of Personality Disorders, 16,* 215–234.

Mulder, R. T. (2002). Personality pathology and treatment outcome in major depression: A review. *American Journal of Psychiatry, 159,* 359–371.

Mullins-Sweatt, S. N., & Widiger, T. A. (2006). The five-factor model of personality disorder: A translation across science and practice. In R. F. Krueger & J. L. Tackett (Eds.), *Personality and psychopathology: Building bridges* (pp. 39–70). New York: Guilford Press.

Muris, P., & Ollendick, T. H. (2005). The role of temperament in the etiology of child psychopathology. *Clinical Child and Family Psychology Review, 8,* 271–289.

O'Connor, B. P. (2005). A search for consensus on the dimensional structure of personality disorders. *Journal of Clinical Psychology, 61,* 323–345.

O'Connor, B. P., & Dyce, J. A. (1998). A test of models of personality disorder configuration. *Journal of Abnormal Psychology, 107,* 3–16.

O'Connor, T. G., Deater-Deckard, K., Fulker, D., Rutter, M., & Plomin, R. (1998). Genotype–environment correlations in late childhood and early adolescence: Antisocial behavioral problems and coercive parenting. *Developmental Psychology, 34,* 970–981.

Parnas, J., Licht, D., & Bovet, P. (2005). Cluster A personality disorders: A review. In M. Maj, H. S. Akiskal, J. E. Mezzich, & A. Okasha (Eds.), *Personality disorders* (pp. 1–74). New York: Wiley.

Perry, J. C., Banon, E., & Ianni, F. (1999). Effectiveness of psychotherapy for personality disorders. *American Journal of Psychiatry, 156,* 1312–1321.

Pettit, J. W., & Joiner, T. E. (2006). *Chronic depression: Interpersonal sources, therapeutic solutions.* Washington, DC: American Psychological Association.

Piersma, H. L. (1987). The MCMI as a measure of DSM-III Axis II diagnoses: An empirical comparison. *Journal of Clinical Psychology, 43,* 478–483.

Piersma, H. L. (1989). The MCMI-II as a treatment outcome measure for psychiatric inpatients. *Journal of Clinical Psychology, 45,* 87–93.

Pincus, A. L. (2002). Constellations of dependency within the five-factor model of personality. In P. T. Costa & T. A. Widiger (Eds.), *Personality disorders and the five-factor model of personality* (pp. 203–214). Washington, DC: American Psychological Association.

Pincus, A. L., & Gurtman, M. B. (2006). Interpersonal theory and the interpersonal circumplex: Evolving perspectives on normal and abnormal personality. In S. Strack (Ed.), *Differentiating normal and abnormal personality* (2nd ed., pp. 83–111). New York: Springer.

Polivy, J., & Herman, C. P. (2002). Causes of eating disorder. *Annual Review of Psychology, 53,* 187–213.

Polivy, J., Herman, C. P., & Boivin, M. (2004). Eating disorders. In J. E. Maddux & B. A. Winstead (Eds.), *Psychopathology: Foundations for a contemporary understanding* (pp. 229–254). Mahwah, NJ: Erlbaum.

Quilty, L. C., De Fruyt, F., Rolland J.-P., Kennedy, S. H., Rouillon, P. F., & Bagby, R. M. (in press). Dimensional personality traits and treatment outcome in patients with major depressive disorder. *Journal of Affective Disorders.*

Raine, A. (2006). Schizotypal personality: Neurodevelopmental and psychosocial trajectories. *Annual Review of Clinical Psychology, 2,* 291–326.

Roberts, B. W., & DelVecchio, W. F. (2000). The rank-order consistency of personality traits from childhood to old age: A quantitative review of longitudinal studies. *Psychological Bulletin, 126,* 3–25.

Robins, R. W., Caspi, A., & Moffitt, T. E. (2002). It's not just who you're with, it's who you are: Personality and relationship experiences across multiple relationships. *Journal of Personality, 70,* 925–964.

Rosenbluth, M., Kennedy, S. H., & Bagby, R. M. (Eds.). (2005). *Depression and personality: Conceptual and clinical challenges.* Washington, DC: American Psychiatric Association.

Rothbart, M. K., & Posner, M. (2006). Temperament, attention, and developmental psychopathology. In D. Cicchetti & D. J. Cohen (Eds.), *Developmental psychopathology: Vol. 2. Developmental neuroscience* (2nd ed., pp. 465–501). New York: Wiley.

Rounsaville, B. J., Alarcon, R. D., Andrews, G., Jackson, J. S., Kendell, R. E., & Kendler, K. (2002). Basic nomenclature issues for DSM-V. In D. J. Kupfer, M. B. First, & D. E. Regier (Eds.), *A research agenda for DSM-V* (pp. 1–29). Washington, DC: American Psychiatric Association.

Rutter, M., Dunn, J., Plomin, R., Simonoff, E., Pickles, A., Maughan, B., et al. (1997). Integrating nature and nurture: Implications of person–environment correlations and interactions for developmental psychology. *Development and Psychopathology, 9,* 335–364.

Salekin, R. T. (2002). Psychopathy and therapeutic pessimism: Clinical lore or clinical reality? *Clinical Psychology Review, 22,* 79–112.

Samuel, D. B., & Widiger, T. A. (2004). Clinicians' personality descriptions of prototypic personality disorders. *Journal of Personality Disorders, 18,* 286–308.

Sanathara, V. A., Gardner, C. O., Prescott, C. A., & Kendler, K. S. (2003). Interpersonal dependence and major depression: Aetiological interrelationship and gender differences. *Psychological Medicine, 33,* 927–931.

Sanderson, C., & Clarkin, J. F. (2002). Further use of the NEO-PI-R personality dimensions in differential treatment planning. In P. T. Costa, Jr. & T. A. Widiger (Eds.), *Personality disorders and the five-factor model of personality* (2nd ed., pp. 351–375). Washington, DC: American Psychological Association.

Sanislow, C. A., & McGlashan, T. H. (1998). Treatment outcome of personality disorders. *Canadian Journal of Psychiatry, 43,* 237–250.

Sansone, R. A., Levitt, J. L., & Sansone, L. A. (2005). The prevalence of personality disorders among those with eating disorders. *Eating Disorders, 13,* 7–21.

Santor, D. A., & Zuroff, D. C. (1997). Interpersonal responses to threats of status and interpersonal relatedness: Effects of dependency and self-criticism. *British Journal of Clinical Psychology, 36,* 521–541.

Saulsman, L. M., & Page, A. C. (2004). The five-factor model and personality disorder empirical literature: A meta-analytic review. *Clinical Psychology Review, 23,* 1055–1085.

Scarr, S., & McCartney, K. (1983). How people make their own environments: A theory of genotype–environment effects. *Child Development, 54,* 424–435.

Schneider, F. R., Blanco, C., Anita, S., & Liebowitz, M. R. (2002). The social anxiety spectrum. *Psychiatric Clinics of North America, 25,* 757–774.

Shahar, G., Joiner, T. E., Zuroff, D. C., & Blatt, S. J. (2004). Personality, interpersonal behavior, and depression: Co-existence of stress-specific moderating and mediating effects. *Personality and Individual Differences, 36,* 1583–1596.

Shea, M. T. (1996). Enduring personality change after catastrophic experience. In T. A. Widiger et al. (Eds.), *DSM-IV sourcebook* (Vol. 2, pp. 849–860). Washington, DC: American Psychiatric Association.

Shea, M. T., Leon, A. C., Mueller, T. I., Solomon, D. A., Warshaw, M. G., & Keller, M. B. (1996). Does major depression result in lasting personality change? *American Journal of Psychiatry, 153,* 1404–1410.

Shea, M. T., & Yen, S. (2003). Stability as a distinction between Axis I and Axis II disorders. *Journal of Personality Disorders, 17,* 373–386.

Shedler, J., & Westen, D. (2004). Dimensions of personality pathology: An alternative to the five-factor model. *American Journal of Psychiatry, 161,* 1743–1754.

Sheets, E., & Craighead, W. E. (2007). Toward an empirically based classification of personality pathology. *Clinical Psychology: Science and Practice, 14,* 77–93.

Shiner, R., & Caspi, A. (2003). Personality differences in childhood and adolescence: Measurement, development, and consequences. *Journal of Child Psychology and Psychiatry, 44,* 2–32.

Siever, L., & Davis, K. (1991). A psychobiologic perspective on the personality disorders. *American Journal of Psychiatry, 148,* 1647–1658.

Simon, R. I. (2002). Distinguishing trauma-associated narcissistic symptoms from posttraumatic stress disorder: A diagnostic challenge. *Harvard Review of Psychiatry, 10,* 28–36.

Skodol, A. E., Gunderson, J. G., Shea, M. T., McGlashan, T. H., Morey, L. C., Sanislow, C. A., et al. (2006). The Collaborative Longitudinal Personality Disorders Study (CLPS): Overview and implications. *Journal of Personality Disorders, 20,* 487–504.

Smith, G. T., Fischer, S., Cyders, M. A., Annus, A. M., Spillane, N. S., & McCarthy, D. M. (2007). On the validity and utility of discriminating among impulsivity-like traits. *Assessment, 14,* 155–170.

Smith, G. T., Simmons, J., Annus, A. M., Flory, K., & Hill, K. K. (2007).Thinness and eating expectancies predict subsequent binge eating and purging behavior among adolescent girls. *Journal of Abnormal Psychology, 116,* 188–197.

Smith, G. T., Williams, S., Fister, L. S., Cyders, M., & Kelley, S. (2006). Reactive personality–environment transactions and adult developmental trajectories. *Developmental Psychology, 42,* 877–887.

Srivastava, S., John, O. P., Gosling, S. D., & Potter, J. (2003). Development of personality in early and middle adulthood: Set like plaster or persistent change? *Journal of Personality and Social Psychology, 84,* 1041–1053.

Stice, E. (2002). Risk and maintenance factors for eating pathology: A meta-analytic review. *Psychology Bulletin, 128,* 825–848.

Tellegen, A. (1982). *Brief Manual for the Multidimensional Personality Questionnaire.* Unpublished manuscript, University of Minnesota, Minneapolis.

Tomkins, S. (1986). Script theory. In J. Aronoff, A. I. Rabin, & R. A. Zucker (Eds.), *The emergence of personality* (pp. 147–216). New York: Springer.

Triebwasser, J., & Shea, M. T. (1996). Personality change resulting from another mental disorder. In T. A. Widiger et al. (Eds.), *DSM-IV sourcebook* (Vol. 2, pp. 861–868). Washington, DC: American Psychiatric Association.

Trull, T. J., & Durrett, C. A. (2005). Categorical and dimensional models of personality disorder. *Annual Review of Clinical Psychology, 1,* 355–380.

Trull, T. J., Sher, K. J., Minks-Brown, C., Durbin, J., & Burr, R. (2000). Borderline personality disorder and substance use disorders: A review and integration. *Clinical Psychology Review, 20,* 235–253.

Trull, T. J., Widiger, T. A., Lynam, D. R., & Costa, P. T., Jr. (2003). Borderline personality disorder from the perspective of general personality functioning. *Journal of Abnormal Psychology, 112,* 193–202.

Tyrer, P. (2005). The anxious cluster of personality disorders: A review. In M. Maj, H. S. Akiskal, J. E. Mezzich, & A. Okasha (Eds.), *Personality disorders* (pp. 349–375). New York: Wiley.

Vitousek, K. M., & Stumpf, R. E. (2005). Difficulties in the assessment of personality traits and disorders in eating-disordered individuals. *Eating Disorders, 13*(1), 37–60.

Watson, D. (2005). Rethinking the mood and anxiety disorders: A quantitative hierarchical model for DSM-V. *Journal of Abnormal Psychology, 114,* 522–536.

Watson, D., Clark, L. A., & Harkness, A. R. (1994). Structures of personality and their relevance to psychopathology. *Journal of Abnormal Psychology, 103,* 18–31.

Watson, D., Gamez, W., & Simms, L. J. (2005). Basic dimensions of temperament and their relation to anxiety and depression: A symptom-based perspective. *Journal of Research in Personality, 39,* 46–66.

Webster, D. C., & Dunn, E. C. (2005). Feminist perspectives on trauma. *Women and Therapy, 28,* 111–142.

Westen, D., & Arkowitz Westen, L. (1998). Limitations of Axis II in diagnosing personality pathology in clinical practice. *American Journal of Psychiatry, 155,* 1767–1771.

Whiteside, S. P., & Lynam, D. R. (2001). The five-factor model and impulsivity. Using a structural model of personality to understand impulsivity. *Personality and Individual Differences, 30,* 669–689.

Whiteside, S. P., Miller, J. D., Lynam, D. R., & Reynolds, S. K. (2005). Validation of the UPPS impulsive behavior scale: A four-factor model of impulsivity. *European Journal of Personality, 19,* 559–574.

Widiger, T. A. (2003). Personality disorder and Axis I psychopathology: The problematic boundary of Axis I and Axis II. *Journal of Personality Disorders, 17,* 90–108.

Widiger, T. A., & Anderson, K. G. (2003). Personality and depression in women. *Journal of Affective Disorders, 74,* 59–66.

Widiger, T. A., & Boyd, S. (in press). Assessing personality disorders. In J. N. Butcher (Ed.),

Oxford handbook of personality assessment (3rd ed.). New York: Oxford University Press.

Widiger, T. A., & Clark, L. A. (2000). Toward DSM-V and the classification of psychopathology. *Psychological Bulletin, 126,* 946–963.

Widiger, T. A., & Coker, L. A. (2002). Assessing personality disorders. In J. N. Butcher (Ed.), *Clinical personality assessment: Practical approaches* (2nd ed., pp. 407–434). New York: Oxford University Press.

Widiger, T. A., & Costa, P. T., Jr. (2002). Five-factor model personality disorder research. In P. T. Costa, Jr. & T. A. Widiger (Eds.), *Personality disorders and the five-factor model of personality* (2nd ed., pp. 59–87). Washington, DC: American Psychological Association.

Widiger, T. A., Costa, P. T., Jr., & McCrae, R. R. (2002). A proposal for Axis II: Diagnosing personality disorders using the five-factor model. In P. T. Costa, Jr. & T. A. Widiger (Eds.), *Personality disorders and the five-factor model of personality* (2nd ed., pp. 431–456). Washington, DC: American Psychological Association.

Widiger, T. A., & Lowe, J. R. (2007). Five-factor model personality disorder assessment. *Journal of Personality Assessment, 89,* 16–29.

Widiger, T. A., & Mullins-Sweatt, S. (2005). Categorical and dimensional models of personality disorder. In J. Oldham, A. Skodol, & D. Bender (Eds.), *Textbook of personality disorders* (pp. 35–53). Washington, DC: American Psychiatric Association.

Widiger, T. A., & Mullins-Sweatt, S. (2007). Mental disorders as discrete clinical conditions: Dimensional versus categorical classification. In M. Hersen, S. M. Turner, & D. Beidel (Eds.), *Adult psychopathology and diagnosis* (3rd ed., pp. 3–33). New York: Wiley.

Widiger, T. A., Mullins-Sweatt, S., & Anderson, K. (2005). Personality and depression in women. In C. Keyes & S. Goodman (Eds.), *Handbook for the study of women and depression: Views from social, behavioral, and biomedical science* (pp. 176–198). New York: Cambridge University Press.

Widiger, T. A., & Samuel, D. B. (2005a). Diagnostic categories or dimensions: A question for DSM-V. *Journal of Abnormal Psychology, 114,* 494–504.

Widiger, T. A., & Samuel, D. B. (2005b). Evidence-based assessment of personality disorders. *Psychological Assessment, 17,* 278–287.

Widiger, T. A., & Sankis, L. (2000). Adult psychopathology: Issues and controversies. *Annual Review of Psychology, 51,* 377–404.

Widiger, T. A., & Simonsen, E. (2005a). Alternative dimensional models of personality disorder: Finding a common ground. *Journal of Personality Disorders, 19,* 110–130.

Widiger, T. A., & Simonsen, E. (2005b). The American Psychiatric Association's research agenda for the DSM-V. *Journal of Personality Disorders, 19,* 103–109.

Widiger, T. A., Simonsen, E., Krueger, R., Livesley, J., & Verheul, R. (2005). Personality disorder research agenda for the DSM-V. *Journal of Personality Disorders, 19,* 317–340.

Widiger, T. A., & Trull, T. J. (2007). Plate tectonics in the classification of personality disorder: Shifting to a dimensional model. *American Psychologist, 62,* 71–83.

Widiger, T. A., Trull, T. J., Clarkin, J. F, Sanderson, C., & Costa, P. T., Jr. (2002). A description of the DSM-IV personality disorders with the five-factor model of personality. In P. T. Costa, Jr. & T. A. Widiger (Eds.), *Personality disorders and the five-factor model of personality* (2nd ed., pp. 89–99). Washington, DC: American Psychological Association.

Windle, M., & Scheidt, D. M. (2004). Alcoholic subtypes: Are two sufficient? *Addiction, 99,* 1508–1519.

Wonderlich, S. A., Crosby, R. D., Joiner, T., Peterson, C. B., Bardone-Cone, A., Klein, M., et al. (2005). Personality subtyping and bulimia nervosa: Psychopathological and genetic correlates. *Psychological Medicine, 35,* 649–657.

Wong, M. M., Zucker, R. A., Puttler, L. I., & Fitzgerald, H. E. (1999). Heterogeneity of risk aggregation for alcohol problems between early and middle childhood: Nesting structure variations. *Development and Psychopathology, 11,* 727–744.

World Health Organization. (1992). *International classification of diseases* (10th ed.). Geneva, Switzerland: Author.

Zanarini, M. C., Frankenburg, F. R., Hennen, R., Reich, D. B., & Silk, K. R. (2006). The McLean study of adult development (MSAD): Overview and implications of the first six years of prospective follow-up. *Journal of Personality Disorders, 20,* 505–523.

Zuckerman, M. (2002). Zuckerman–Kuhlman Personality Questionnaire (ZKPQ): An alternative five-factorial model. In B. de Raad & M. Perugini (Eds.), *Big five assessment* (pp. 377–396). Seattle, WA: Hogrefe & Huber.

Zuroff, D. C. (1994). Depressive personality styles and the five-factor model of personality. *Journal of Personality Assessment, 63,* 453–472.

Zuroff, D. C., Mongrain, M., & Santor, D. A. (2004). Conceptualizing and measuring personality vulnerability to depression: Comment on Coyne and Whiffen (1995). *Psychological Bulletin, 130,* 489–511.

CHAPTER 31

Personality and Health

A Lifespan Perspective

Sarah E. Hampson
Howard S. Friedman

I t is time to bury the old models of personality and health and replace them with theories and models that employ the most modern concepts from personality psychology. It has long been understood that some individuals are more prone to illness and premature mortality than are others. Indeed, assumptions about variations in disease proneness form part of the basis for clinical judgments by medical practitioners about their individual patients, the predictions of epidemiologists and insurance companies about health trends and costs, and much targeted preventive medical screening. Yet the extant models, both implicit and explicit, of the links between individual differences and health generally have relied on primitive and incomplete conceptions.

Although some threats to a person's life and health are truly random, most of the threats to well-being are a function of various biopsychosocial characteristics of the individual. In principle, anyone may catch the flu or suffer a myocardial infarction, but individuals vary tremendously in the likelihood that they will achieve good health and longevity. That is, there is astonishing variation in whether one is vulnerable to various diseases and whether one is likely to recover quickly from any diseases that take hold. A person does not contract the flu without exposure to an influenza virus, but persons vary tremendously as to whether they are exposed to the virus, whether they are infected after exposure, and how they respond to the illness if infected. In other words, understanding the likelihood of disease for the individual is often as important as knowing the general causes of disease. Much of this variation can be captured by a concept that encapsulates the biopsychosocial nature of the individual across time, namely the modern concept of personality.

THE OUTDATED MODELS

Although the idea of ties between personality and health dates back thousands of years to the postulated four bodily humors (blood, black bile, phlegm, and yellow bile) in the writings of Hippocrates and Galen, it was not until the mid-20th century that scientific study of personality and health began in earnest (Friedman, 2007). The work of the psychosomatic theorists and physicians on the ties between specific unconscious emotional conflicts and disease (e.g., Alexander, 1950) grew out of a neoanalytic framework and provided many observations and insights linking psyche and soma; but this approach was nearly impossible to validate in a rigorous manner. For example, it could be documented that an emotionally conflicted and miserably unhappy woman would be ill more often (Dunbar, 1955), but neither the psychological predisposition nor the links to disease could be reliably assessed or explained.

Medical Syndrome Models

In response to this turbidity of psychosomatic psychiatry, some researcher–clinicians turned to a biologically and medically focused tack. A prime early example is the Type A behavior pattern. Proposed by two cardiologists in the 1950s, the Type A pattern appeared predictive of coronary disease (Rosenman et al., 1964). The idea was to view Type A as a medical syndrome of coronary proneness and avoid ambiguous psychological concepts. Yet Type A people were defined as those hostile or aggressive people involved in a constant struggle to do more and more things in less and less time, a definition that invoked psychosocial concepts (ambiguously proposed) even as it sought to avoid them. The eventual (and ironic) result was thousands of studies with seemingly contradictory findings, as researchers soon began uncoordinated efforts endeavoring to understand the measurement of Type A, the trait correlates of Type A, the subcomponents of Type A, and the behavioral and developmental aspects of Type A (Houston & Snyder, 1988). Several decades of meandering research revealed the necessity of comprehensive models and rigorous assessment if progress were ever going to be made regarding the relations of individual differences and health. We argue in this chapter that sophisticated modern notions of personality point us toward the needed refined models of personality in its relations to health.

Simple Health–Behavior Models

In health–behavior models, personality traits influence the adoption or maintenance of health-enhancing behaviors and the cessation or avoidance of health-damaging behaviors, which in turn affect health status. For example, a health–behavior model may be concerned with the influence of personality traits on behaviors such as smoking, drinking, diet, and exercise. A prominent subclass of these models speaks of a so-called addictive personality, which may be prone to alcoholism, other drug abuse, overeating, or compulsive gambling.

Unfortunately, such approaches often do not address the correlates and consequences of these behaviors. That is, the further consequences and the mechanisms by which health-related behaviors have their impact on health, the associations among various health behaviors, and the ranges of health outcomes are typically left unexamined in health–behavior research. Unhealthy behavior is not isomorphic with bad health, and there is substantial variation in what is helpful or harmful for an individual and why. For example, moderate alcohol consumption is healthy for some people but unhealthy for others. Health habits vary widely in their impact (i.e., effect size). Cigarette smoking has been documented to be much more harmful than many other behaviors considered unhealthy. Furthermore, dosage and duration can have complex and interactive effects, and health-damaging behaviors can combine synergistically to be even more detrimental (e.g., smoking and drinking alcohol). It matters how much one smokes, when, for how long, and with what accompanying behaviors and bodily responses. These complexities are often ignored in applications of simple health–behavior models.

Simple Stress-to-Disease Models

Another basic approach to personality and health uses "stress" as the key explanatory concept. It is assumed that stress is bad, that challenging environments produce stress, and that some people are poor at coping with stress. Here, the focus is usually on the associations among personality traits, individual cognitive strategies (effective and ineffective), and on the life changes (such as losing one's job) that are presumably stressful. Although it is now clear that individuals who are well adjusted and well integrated into stable social systems are generally healthier, it is also clear that there are many exceptions to this general rule and that these relations often depend on other relevant factors remaining constant. For example, many people get married, move to a new city, and start a new job (thus facing many life change stressors) but thrive anyway.

Some approaches within this stress paradigm focus on psychophysiological models—the mechanisms by which coping traits influence body systems that promote disease. These models typically spotlight the cell-damaging effects of stress and poor coping, implicating body systems such as the hypothalamic–pituitary–adrenal (HPA) axis, cardiovascular hyperreactivity, and impaired immune functioning. Prolonged states of arousal or damage to the immune system can result in disease (Kemeny, 2007). Yet almost no well-controlled studies document the full process in operation (e.g., poor coping, stress, immune dysfunction, and resultant serious disease), and such long-term prospective studies are rarely feasible.

Simple Genetic Models

In simple genetic models of personality and disease, it is proposed that some underlying third variable, often seen as genetically based, causes both a certain trait or behavioral pattern and a certain disease. Although this is sometimes the case, as, for example, with genetic diseases causing mental retardation and personality quirks as well as various health problems, it is rare that links are so simple. Shared underlying biology could give rise to spurious associations between personality and health, in which case changing personality traits or personality-driven behavior would have no effect on health. Simple genetic models are limited by the failure to consider the various environmental circumstances relevant to both personality and health.

Previous analyses of personality and health have sketched these basic models and variations (e.g., Contrada, Cather, & O'Leary, 1999; Friedman, 2007; Ouellette & DiPlacido, 2001; Smith & Gallo, 2001; Wiebe & Smith, 1997). These models each have some significant support, which suggests that all have some validity. Yet the overall field lacks a unifying paradigm and sufficient replicability. New efforts need to further elaborate and integrate the basic approaches in terms of new understandings.

MODERN REPLACEMENTS: MORE SOPHISTICATED MODELS

Sophisticated models of personality and health develop from two considerations. First, the various causal mechanisms predicted by the simpler models are often simultaneously present, and they influence and interact with each other. Second, personality and health are not static. Personality develops and changes over the lifespan, as does health (Roberts & DelVecchio, 2000; Roberts, Walton, & Viechtbauer, 2006). More sophisticated models of personality and health recognize the interplay among mechanisms and the dynamic nature of the variables involved.

The idea of transactions is a key mechanism linking personality to health, well exemplified by the selection of healthful or harmful environments. Personality traits influence situational choices, and they also have evocative effects, provoking typical patterns of responses in others (Bolger & Zuckerman, 1995; Scarr & McCartney, 1984). Selective exposure to certain types of situations (e.g., riskier ones) and selective evocation of certain patterns of behavior in others (e.g., hostility) are linked reciprocally to personality and to health through health behaviors and psychophysiology.

More sophisticated models also take into account the fact that biological changes and the experience of disease can influence personality. For example, brain damage or impairment can dramatically alter an individual's personality, and deteriorating health can affect personality as a consequence of illness-related unemployment, divorce, drug use, and depression. Not only are the relations between personality and health reciprocal, but the relations may progress and change across time. The way disease affects personality varies depending on life stage.

The Importance of Longitudinal Study

Health behaviors and individual patterns, as well as health indices (such as occlusion of the coronary arteries, blood pressure, cortisol levels, or body mass index [BMI]), are all dynamic variables. When snapshots of the association between personality and such health variables are examined in cross-sectional studies, they do not take into account the rising or falling trajectories of either personality or health variables. Cross-sectional designs do not identify reciprocal influences between personality and health, and they do not place these snapshots in the broader context of longer-term trends—biological, social, and psychological. Given that disease and disease susceptibility often develop over decades rather than days, and are influenced by mechanisms linking personality and health that unfold over the life course, we believe that models of personality and health should adopt a comparable lifespan perspective: that is, the assumption that personality, health, and the intervening mechanisms are moving targets. Hence, in this chapter, we focus primarily on prospective studies.

Modern conceptions of personality as an evolving biopsychosocial cluster of traits, motivations, abilities, and behavior patterns are well suited to this dynamic lifespan approach. As we shall see, cognitive–motivational, social–emotional, and situational–behavioral influences on clusters of dynamic outcomes are comfortable concepts in modern personality research. Yet the lifespan approach to the study of personality and health is a relatively new development (Friedman, 2000a, 2000b; Smith & Spiro, 2002). One goal of this chapter to push such theorizing a few steps further. Another goal is to demonstrate that the field is now ready to transition from studies that demonstrate prospective relations between personality and health to studies that evaluate how and why these relations are observed. Other reviews and chapters (e.g., Roberts, Wood, & Caspi, Chapter 14, this volume) document various important associations between personality and health. Here we attempt to draw inferences about the "dynamisms" and "tropisms" of the mechanisms unfolding over time that explain the observed relations between personality and health (Friedman, 2000a, 2000b). In this way, we aim to help set a more challenging agenda for future studies.

LIFESPAN APPROACHES

Developmental psychology was transformed by the adoption of a lifespan perspective (Baltes & Goulet, 1970; Baltes, Reese, & Lipsitt, 1980), and the study of personality and health is poised on the brink of a similar revolution. Ultimately, research on personal-

ity and health has two purposes. On the utilitarian side, there is a wish to find interventions for people of all ages that can promote health and longevity. On the conceptual side, there is a desire to understand better what it means to be a healthy person across time. Both goals involve illuminating the complex pathways to good health as people age.

Lifespan approaches to personality and health benefit from an infusion of ideas from other disciplines with a lifespan perspective. Therefore, we have drawn upon life-course epidemiology to develop further the theoretical underpinnings of lifespan models of personality and health (Kuh & Ben-Shlomo, 1997; Krueger, Caspi, & Moffitt, 2000; Lynch & Davey Smith, 2005; Smith & Spiro, 2002). Two models are particularly relevant to personality and health: critical period models and accumulation models.

Critical Period Models

Critical period models assert that exposure to risk factors during critical periods of development have long-lasting effects and more pronounced effects than exposure at other points in the lifespan. Timing of exposure to the risk factor is key. Take the example of the drug thalidomide, which was used in the 1950s in Europe to treat morning sickness during pregnancy in those women who complained to their physicians and were willing to take a newly prescribed medication in early pregnancy. It became apparent that when used during the first 25–50 days of gestation, thalidomide resulted in abnormal fetal limb development. Early pregnancy is a critical period for the developing fetus, during which irrevocable damage resulted from just one dose of this drug.

Some of the earliest and best-known work along these lines showed that poor nutrition during the prenatal period or infancy raises the risk of coronary heart disease decades later (Barker, 1994, 1998; Barker, Osmond, Forsén, Kajantie, & Eriksson, 2005). This work was a shock to the cardiology community because it questioned the focus on concurrent and short-to-medium-term risk factors. Such models are in striking contrast to the common assumption that one is healthy until afflicted by disease over some relatively short period of time, and even to the idea that there is a slow progression. A critical period analysis should be followed by specification of the relevant causal pathways. For example, biological alterations may initiate a long-term internal disease process; or there may be early, irreversible structural damage; or early physiological changes may result in lifelong behavioral changes damaging to heart health. Yet other pathways, or combinations of pathways, may be at work.

Critical period models of personality and health suggest that certain levels of particular traits or motivations increase the sensitivity to, or likelihood of, a risk factor during a critical period. Exposure to particular levels of the trait at certain periods in life, such as high levels of "difficult temperament" in infancy and childhood, might increase the individual's vulnerability to certain disease processes or to behaviors or environments that will eventually damage body systems. For example, especially high levels of sensation seeking in adolescence would increase vulnerability to increased risk from experimenting with drugs during this critical period (Chambers, Taylor, & Potenza, 2003). Levels of sensation seeking typically decrease with age, but by then the damage may be done.

The concept of critical periods has evolved from being defined strictly by age to looser phases that occur in a maturational sequence (Michel & Tyler, 2005). For example, there may be a critical period of adolescent neurodevelopment that promotes adaptation to adult roles but that also increases vulnerability to the addictive properties of certain drugs (Chambers et al., 2003). However, the fact that the effects of exposure to the risk factor during a critical period may only become apparent much later and only for certain people makes such effects difficult to demonstrate conclusively (Lynch & Davey Smith, 2005).

Accumulation Models

Accumulation models in lifespan epidemiology emphasize that the effects of risk exposure build progressively over the life course. Insults (e.g., x-ray exposure, the pollutants in a low-income neighborhood) build up and interact with other risk factors, gradually increasing the threat to health. A sophisticated elaboration on this idea is Caspi, Elder, and Bem's (1987) cumulative continuity model, in which childhood personality has the ef-

fect of channeling the individual into a particular set of environments, which results in an accumulation of consequences. As a variant of the model, Caspi and colleagues proposed interactional continuity: Personality traits will influence an individual's interaction style, which in turn will evoke a style of responding from others that may serve to perpetuate that style, even if it is ultimately maladaptive.

A refined type of accumulation model applied to stress is the allostasis model (McEwen, 1998). Allostasis is the ability to achieve stability through change. Throughout ongoing challenges, the body uses the autonomic nervous system, the HPA axis, and the cardiovascular, metabolic, and immune systems to respond to threats. However, repeated and relentless stress and coping results in accumulation of allostatic load that is ultimately damaging to the integrity of these systems.

The effects of critical periods and accumulation need not be independent. The consequences of exposure to risk factors may both accumulate over the life course and be greater during critical periods. However, neither critical period nor accumulation models necessarily specify the mechanisms of association between risk factors and disease in any depth. Combining these epidemiological models with the traditional models of personality and health, described above in this chapter, may provide a deeper analysis of mechanisms. In particular, it stimulates us to consider whether and how the intervening mechanisms of health behaviors, or physiological processes, or situation selection have a cumulative influence or are disproportionately influential during one or more particular life stages.

Lifespan Research

A lifespan perspective naturally draws attention to the influence of gender on health. Indeed, one of the most robust findings in epidemiology is that women outlive men. All sorts of explanations for this difference have been proposed and investigated, but none has been definitively confirmed, indicating how much we still have to learn about gender effects on health. In addition to personality- and health-relevant physiological, anatomical, and maturational differences, there are many constantly changing sociocultural differences in the lives of men and women. Therefore, gender is a central variable in any lifespan approach to personality and health. Where feasible, gender differences should always be examined, although studies devoted to testing gender-specific hypotheses in samples limited to one gender are also desirable.

We have organized our illustrative review of research by life stage (infancy, childhood and adolescence, adulthood, and old age). Within each life stage, we present studies in which personality was assessed at that stage and subsequently related to health outcomes later in life. This organizational structure emphasizes the pathways from personality to health status and brings together studies of different traits assessed at the same life stage. Alternative organizations, such as by trait or by disease, tend to overemphasize links between specific traits and specific diseases (Friedman & Booth-Kewley, 1987) and overlook key aspects from the lifespan perspective accentuated here.

Before beginning our examination of lifespan research, a word of caution is necessary. Individuals cannot be randomly assigned to a particular personality, nor can they be randomly assigned to long-term patterns of behavior. That is, research in this area must be, by necessity, correlational, with long-term prospective research designs being the most informative. Occasionally, pieces of the puzzle can be subjected to experimental analysis, such as when there are randomized trials of pharmaceuticals or behavior modification, or studies involving laboratory animals. However, such experiments rarely capture the full range of interacting influences on subsequent health. So, it is important to remain aware of the temptation to over-infer causality, even when considering longitudinal findings. Religious people are generally healthier, as are physically active people, but this does not imply that we should impose religious observance to improve health or target activity interventions indiscriminately at the whole population.

INFANCY

The brain and the rest of the nervous and neuroendocrine systems are at the center of the relations between personality and health, and their development deserves attention.

The most rapid development begins a few weeks after conception and continues until about age 4 or 5, at which point a recognizable personality and self-identity has formed. For example, by age 5 most children have a gender identity, and their personality and IQ are moderately correlated with what they will be decades later.

During infancy and toddlerhood (and probably prenatally), however, temperament (as opposed to personality traits) is key. Temperament, or individual differences in emotional responsiveness, is heavily influenced by biological differences (genetic, hormonal, environmental); it forms the basis for later personality traits and for health. Although there is less agreement on the structure of infant temperament than there is on adult personality structure, influential approaches typically have included dimensions reflecting positive emotionality, negative emotionality, impulsivity, and effortful control (e.g., Ahadi & Rothbart, 1994; Caspi, 1998). Positive emotionality, which includes sociability and activity, is expected to relate to adult traits involving extraversion, and negative emotionality is expected to relate to later levels of emotional stability (Caspi, 1998). However, any one infant temperament may relate to more than one adult trait. For example, aspects of infant effortful control may affect later agreeableness and conscientiousness, and perhaps extraversion and emotional stability, probably depending on environmental interactions. Whether and when infant temperaments develop into later personality traits or serve to modulate them is not clear. These issues of continuity and relations between infant and adult temperament/personality constructs present a challenge to lifespan approaches to personality and health.

In a prospective study of the influence of infant temperament, Caspi and colleagues (1997) related observer ratings of temperament at age 3 to self-ratings of personality at age 18 in the Dunedin study, a longitudinal study of a complete birth cohort (N = 1,037) born in the city of Dunedin on New Zealand's South Island in 1972–1973. Infant temperament, in particular undercontrolled temperament, predicted self-rated traits of negative emotionality and lack of constraint at age 18. These traits at age 18 predicted various health-risk behaviors at age 21, as did undercontrolled infant temperament.

Furthermore, the effects of infant undercontrolled temperament on age 21 health-risk behaviors were mediated by age 18 personality traits. Infant temperament shaped later personality traits, and these traits determined health-risk behaviors. As the Dunedin cohort ages, it will be possible to determine whether these health-risk behaviors predict later morbidity and mortality, directly or indirectly or not at all.

There is great potential for further study of the effects of temperament very early in life. Infancy is a critical period for numerous aspects of psychological development, but whether it is also a critical stage for associations from temperament to health remains unclear. Furthermore, infant temperament and later adult personality may be associated with subsequent disease in a manner consistent with accumulation models. A methodological challenge when relating factors in infancy to subsequent health is to adequately account for the many intervening influences on health over such long time intervals.

One intriguing aspect of the influence of personality on infant health that has not received much attention from personality psychologists is that of transgenerational effects. The life of any one individual begins in utero, but from the life-course perspective on health, there is no clear starting place. Maternal health and behavior and the mother's social context prior to and during pregnancy influence the health of the fetus, and fetal development is rich in critical periods. For example, women with high stress prenatally were substantially more likely to have a low-birth-weight infant and to deliver preterm compared to women with low stress (Lobel, Dunkel-Schetter, & Scrimshaw, 1992). Furthermore, women who were least optimistic delivered infants of significantly lower birth weight, controlling for a variety of other predictors (Lobel, DeVincent, Kaminer, & Meyer, 2000). In turn, studies in rats and other mammals document long-lasting effects of prenatal exposure to stress hormones and sex hormones. Not surprisingly, there are relatively few studies beginning prenatally or shortly after birth relating temperament to long-term health in humans. However, we foresee great value from multigenerational studies of personality and health that will enable the study of how parental character-

istics and experiences impact the personality and health of their offspring.

CHILDHOOD AND ADOLESCENCE

Childhood, starting at about the time when children begin school (age 5) and ending at early adolescence (10–12 years), is increasingly well documented as important to understanding trajectories to health and longevity decades later. Moreover, childhood personality has a surprisingly powerful influence on these trajectories. Longitudinal studies of childhood personality and later health were initiated years or decades before the contemporary dominance of the five-factor model of personality, and before the development of measures of the five-factor structure specifically for children (e.g., Measelle, John, Ablow, Cowan, & Cowan, 2005; Mervielde & DeFruyt, 2002). Accordingly, it makes sense when examining childhood personality influences on health to group studies according to broader trait categories, such as effortful control (conscientiousness), negative emotionality, and positive emotionality.

Conscientiousness (Effortful Control or Restraint)

The health significance of childhood levels of restraint and prudence as embodied in the trait of conscientiousness only became apparent relatively recently in analyses of archival data collected for the Terman Life Cycle Study. Due to extensive early measurement and lifelong follow-up, these data offer an unprecedented opportunity to examine the influence of childhood personality on longevity. Starting in 1921–1922, 1,528 California schoolchildren, of average age 11 years with IQs of 135 or greater, were recruited for a prospective study of the growing up of gifted children. Although not originally designed as a longitudinal study of personality and health, I (H. S. F.) and my colleagues were able to construct measures of childhood personality from the parent and teacher data available in the archives that were meaningful in contemporary terms of the five-factor model (Friedman et al., 1993; Martin & Friedman, 2000). The most striking finding from this study was that childhood conscientiousness predicted longevity across the lifespan and emerged as a risk factor for all-cause mortality of the same magnitude as ones that are widely accepted by the medical profession, such as serum cholesterol and elevated resting systolic blood pressure (Friedman et al., 1993; Friedman, Tucker, Schwartz, Tomlinson-Keasy, et al., 1995). The effect of conscientiousness held up even after controlling for other mortality risk factors, such as parental divorce and gender.

This work prompted a surge of interest in the relation between conscientiousness and health. The long-term effects of childhood conscientiousness on adult health, as well as its relations to unhealthy habits such as smoking in the Terman sample (Tucker et al., 1995), were confirmed in the Hawaii Personality and Health Cohort, a prospective study across 40 years. At midlife, men and women who as boys and girls were assessed by their teachers as more conscientious had better self-rated health, smoked less or not at all, and the women (but not the men) had lower BMI. The effect of childhood conscientiousness on self-rated health was found to be mediated by smoking and BMI (Hampson, Goldberg, Vogt, & Dubanoski, 2006). Childhood conscientiousness also contributed to educational attainment, which, in turn, influenced health behaviors and health status, confirming the wide-reaching effects of conscientiousness on life outcomes (Hampson, Goldberg, Vogt, & Dubanoski, 2007).

Although there is a tendency to be skeptical of relationships uncovered in any particular longitudinal sample, much follow-up research confirms the validity of the robust findings that emerge in lifespan studies. The relevance of conscientiousness to health has been confirmed in a meta-analysis of both cross-sectional and longitudinal studies demonstrating that lack of conscientiousness is related to low activity levels, excessive alcohol use, drug use, unhealthy eating, risky driving, risky sex, suicide, tobacco use, and violence (Bogg & Roberts, 2004), as well as in a nationally representative sample, which showed unconscientiousness associated with illness and likelihood of physical limitations (Goodwin & Friedman, 2006).

Why would a factor such as conscientiousness be so robust? It is likely that it is relevant to the full range of ongoing biopsychosocial processes described above in the sophisticated models of personality and health. The prospective association of conscientiousness with health behaviors and longevity suggests that a child with a higher level of conscientiousness initiates a life-course pathway that leads to less morbidity through disease and physical trauma and hence to longer life (Friedman, Tucker, Schwartz, Martin, et al., 1995). The details of this process remain speculative, but some version of a health behavior/transactional model is usually invoked: more conscientious children may establish lasting health habits early in their lives that result in cumulative beneficial consequences, and they may seek out health-enhancing environments and avoid health-damaging ones.

What about the relative benefits of higher sustained levels of conscientiousness over the lifespan versus higher levels only in adulthood? Conscientiousness, measured independently in childhood and adulthood, predicts mortality risk across the full lifespan, and the link from childhood remains robust when adult conscientiousness and certain behavioral variables are controlled (Martin, Friedman, & Schwartz, 2007). The lowest mortality risk is for those with high conscientiousness at both time points. In addition, although the physiological correlates of conscientiousness are not yet well understood, there is evidence that serotonin function may be relevant (Friedman, 2007). That is, conscientious people may develop more modulated physiological reaction patterns, or an underlying biopsychological tendency may lead both to conscientiousness and salutary reaction patterns. For example, individuals with a variant serotonin transporter might have abnormal hypothalamic–pituitary responses to stress and corresponding conscientiousness variations (Carver & Miller 2006; Wand et al., 2002).

Negative Emotionality, Negative Affect, or Neuroticism (Emotional Instability)

The study of Cardiovascular Risk in Young Finns (CRYF) is an ongoing cohort sequential study that began in 1980, when participants were ages 3–18 years (Akerblom et al., 1991). Participants were chosen at random from a national register, so the sample was representative of the general Finnish population. Follow-up studies occurred in 1983, 1986, and 2001. At each assessment, a medical examination was conducted, including a fasting blood draw, and various psychological measures were administered. The strengths of this study include the interdisciplinary approach and the population-based sample; a weakness is the rather substantial loss to follow-up over the years (20%, 30%, and 34%, over 3, 6, and 21 years, respectively).

In the CRYF study, negative emotionality and hyperactivity (restlessness and impatience) among both boys and girls ages 9–15, assessed by mothers' ratings, predicted adverse changes on indicators of the metabolic syndrome 3 years later (Ravaja & Keltikangas-Järvinen, 1995). The metabolic syndrome is a cluster of symptoms that constitute a risk factor for type 2 diabetes and cardiovascular disease, including abnormal levels of insulin, high levels of low-density lipoprotein, and overweight as defined by BMI, particularly central adiposity (i.e., the apple body type). Positive emotionality had a protective effect. Overall, the effects were stronger for boys than girls. Expanding on this study, Pulkki-Råback, Elovainio, Kivimäki, Raitakari, and Keltikangas-Järvinen (2005) examined the younger CRYF cohorts. They related maternal ratings of temperament (negative emotionality and aggression, activity, and sociability) at ages 6–12 to BMI assessed in young adulthood (ages 24–30). They found that negative emotionality had the strongest association with adult BMI, after controlling for childhood BMI and several other well-established risk factors, such as parents' obesity.

Why is childhood negative emotionality prospectively related to obesity in the CRYF sample? Consistent with transactional/interactional models, these children may evoke more stress in their lives and be more responsive to stress. Consistent with psychophysiological models, psychosocial stress in childhood is associated with weight gain in adulthood (e.g., Williamson, Thompson, Anda, Dietz, & Felitti, 2002). Transactional processes can lead to an accumulation of stress, which will take its toll on the HPA axis over time. Perceived stress is associated with higher levels of C-reactive protein, an indication of inflammation that is predictive of subsequent cardiovascular disease (McDade, Hawkley, & Cacioppo, 2006). However, childhood hyperactivity (for girls) but not negative emotionality was related to

later carotid intima media thickness (another cardiovascular risk factor), indicating that relations between childhood negative temperaments and later health are not simple and likely involve multiple traits and pathways (Keltikangas-Järvinen, Pulkki-Raback, Puttonen, Viikari, & Raitakari, 2006).

Further support for a psychosocial stress model of negative emotionality and obesity comes from the Dunedin study, in which an association was found between lower childhood socioeconomic status (SES) and higher BMI at age 26, independent of adult SES (Poulton et al., 2002). This finding hints that childhood psychosocial stress or associated behaviors may have enduring effects on health, consistent with a critical period model. Furthermore, Pine, Goldstein, Wolk, and Weissman (2001) found that children (ages 6–17 years) with major depression had significantly higher BMI as adults than a control group that was free of psychiatric disorders as children. This effect remained significant after controlling for various potentially confounding variables, including childhood BMI, and indicates that more extreme forms of negative emotionality are also related to obesity.

Hostility

Several studies have shown a prospective association between aspects of difficult temperament (hostility and aggression) in childhood and subsequent substance use, including alcohol and tobacco (e.g., Caspi et al., 1997; Gerrard, Gibbons, Stock, Houlian, & Dykstra, 2006; Jessor & Jessor, 1977). Working with data from the longitudinal Oregon Youth Substance Use Project, I (S. E. H.) and my colleagues identified a mechanism by which more hostile children adopt a pathway leading to adolescent substance use: the development of cognitive susceptibility. Using latent-growth modeling, we showed that children who were rated by their teachers as exhibiting more hostile behavior at the beginning of the study believed increasingly over the next 4 years that more of their friends and peers were smoking or drinking, and these beliefs predicted stronger intentions to smoke and drink (Hampson, Andrews, & Barckley, 2007; Hampson, Andrews, Barckley, & Severson, 2006). The children's intentions were correlated with subsequent experimentation with smoking and drinking. The effects of hostility were mediated by these normative beliefs. Hostility in childhood is a relatively stable trait, which may serve to strengthen its effects through accumulation (Hampson, Andrews, Barckley, & Peterson, 2007; Woodall & Matthews, 1993).

In an alternative approach to measuring hostility, the construct has been assessed by the Cook–Medley scale of the MMPI. This construct includes some pathologically relevant elements, such as suspiciousness and cynicism. In a study of children and adolescents, Räikkönen, Matthews, and Salomon (2003) demonstrated that hostility at baseline (measured by a modified Cook–Medley scale and by interview) predicted development of risk factors for the metabolic syndrome 3 years later, largely because of the prediction of obesity and insulin resistance. These studies illustrate how narrowly focused, short-term investigations can identify associations and mechanisms that may eventually be integrated into a more complete lifespan model.

Studies of negative emotionality in childhood predicting poorer health status lend themselves to a transactional psychosocial stress model in which negative emotionality may both heighten a child's responsiveness to stress as well as evoke negative emotionality in others. Over time, these children may experience a life path of low SES, adversity, and stress, thus creating a downward spiral. Yet stress, such as parental divorce in childhood, need not necessarily lead to negative later-life outcomes. In the Terman study, the higher mortality risk associated with parental divorce was ameliorated among individuals (especially men) who achieved a sense of personal satisfaction by midlife (Martin, Friedman, Clark, & Tucker, 2005). Clearly, potentially harmful trajectories can be deflected, and lifespan models need to accommodate such twists and turns in the pathways from personality to health outcomes.

Positive Emotionality

Positive emotionality in childhood is associated with both beneficial and detrimental long-term consequences for health. The negative consequences of positive emotionality are most starkly demonstrated in survival analyses for participants in the Terman Life

Cycle Study. Contrary to popular wisdom and a body of research on adults, the Terman study indicated that childhood cheerfulness (a combination of cheerfulness/optimism and sense of humor) increased mortality risk (Friedman et al., 1993). No simple explanation for this association was supported empirically, suggesting that cheerfulness may be a complex blend of traits associated with both health costs and benefits (Martin et al., 2002).

Extraversion in the five-factor model is aligned with aspects of positive emotionality. In children, the sociable component of extraversion can have desirable and undesirable consequences. The association between sociability and subsequent substance use is not straightforward; in some studies it is a risk factor whereas in others it appears to be protective (Tarter, Sambrano, & Dunn, 2002), probably dependent on the characteristics of one's peers and social environment. Sociability sometimes may have curvilinear associations with substance use. It may have stronger associations with socially acceptable substances (e.g., alcohol) than with illicit drugs. In the Hawaii study and the Terman study, children who were assessed as more extraverted reported drinking more alcohol at midlife (Hampson, Goldberg, et al., 2006; Tucker et al., 1995).

Another aspect of positive emotionality, sensation seeking, can accompany extraverted disinhibition (Depue & Collins, 1999), described by Zuckerman (1994) as impulsive unsocialized sensation seeking. Children with such tendencies are at risk for a cluster of problem behaviors in adolescence, including substance use, school failure, and delinquency, which in turn are risk factors for poor life outcomes. These children are also at risk for accidents, which are a major cause of morbidity and mortality in young people. Thus, all in all, positive emotionality in childhood is a double-edged sword. Outgoing and sociable children will be more likely to enjoy the benefits of friendship and popularity but also the costs associated with peer-initiated problem behaviors. Future research on the far-reaching effects of childhood positive emotionality must tackle issues of conceptual clarity (what exactly is being measured by cheerfulness, extraversion, or sociability), and consider nonlinear effects in the association between the personality measure and the outcomes. It is a good illustration of the complexity of the study of personality and health: The same childhood trait can serve as both a risk and protective factor, depending on the pathway, the health outcome, and the segment of the lifespan in which the health outcome is examined.

Intelligence

Childhood IQ is associated with longevity (Whalley & Deary, 2001), and lower childhood IQ is a risk factor for health-damaging behavior in adulthood, such as smoking, and for cardiovascular disease (Hart et al., 2004) and dementia (Deary, Whiteman, Starr, Whalley, & Fox, 2004) later in life. These findings emerged from studies of two birth cohorts in Scotland. On one day in 1932 and one day in 1947, virtually the entire population of Scottish 11-year-old children was tested for IQ. Higher childhood IQ was related to lower all-cause mortality and cardiovascular mortality after adjusting for social class and deprivation (Hart et al., 2003). Those with lower childhood IQ were more likely to die from lung and stomach cancers (Deary, Whalley, & Starr, 2003), and higher childhood IQ was related to smoking cessation by midlife (Taylor et al., 2003), suggesting that some IQ effects are mediated through modifiable risk factors (especially health behavior mechanisms). Analyses combining the two large databases showed that childhood IQ was significantly related to mortality up to and including age 65 but not after age 65, which may be attributed primarily to the higher-risk people's (i.e., the ones with lower childhood IQ) deaths before age 65 (Hart et al., 2005).

Clearly intelligence, which is highly stable from age 11 (Deary, Whalley, Lemmon, Crawford, & Starr, 2000), can have a profound influence on an individual's life course, but the precise effects depend, to some extent, on the pathways to which the intelligence leads the individual. Intelligence likely affects health outcomes through a number of different mechanisms, which need further elucidation. Interestingly, these findings tend to strengthen the findings for personality from the Terman Life Cycle study because for the Terman sample, IQ was restricted to a fairly narrow range at the high end of the distribution. However, what remains to be examined in future studies are personality and intelligence interactions in the prediction of health outcomes.

Conclusions So Far

The discovery of replicable associations between childhood traits and lifelong mortality risk has been a major development in health psychology in the past 15 years, and has contributed to the revitalization of the study of individual differences as predictors of consequential outcomes (Ozer & Benet-Martínez, 2006; Roberts et al., 2006). Traits associated with more rational processes (e.g., intelligence and conscientiousness) and with affective processes (e.g., negative and positive emotionality) are important childhood and adolescent influences on adult morbidity and mortality. The findings suggest that a dual process model, in which personality and health relations are viewed as the result of a combination of rational and affect-based pathways, may be a fruitful way for future conceptualizations of lifespan models—a way that is nicely consistent with a biopsychosocial approach to health.

Although comparative prospective studies of personality and health that are carefully focused on different ages are lacking, Bogg and Roberts (2004) observed stronger relations between conscientiousness and health-risk behaviors for people younger than 30 compared with those over 30 years of age. As noted, adolescence and early adulthood may be a critical period to incur adverse effects from low levels of conscientiousness because of experimentation with behaviors such as smoking and drinking, as well as high frequencies of potentially health-damaging risky activities (e.g., risky sex, dangerous driving, violence). This stage is also the time when mean levels of conscientiousness are at their lowest. As Bogg and Roberts observed, some of the association between conscientiousness and health behaviors may develop in a reciprocal fashion from this life stage onward: Those who perform health-protective behaviors may come to see themselves as more conscientious and hence be more inclined to maintain these healthful behavior patterns.

Adolescence may also be a critical period in terms of physical maturation and irreversible effects. Raitakari and colleagues

(2003), using CRYF data, demonstrated that cardiovascular risk factors (cholesterol, triglycerides, blood pressure, BMI) measured in adolescence (ages 12–18) were associated with the development of atherosclerosis in adulthood, measured by carotid artery intima thickness, whereas this relation was weak or absent for the same risk factors measured in childhood (ages 3–9). Moreover, adolescent risk factors predicted adult disease independent of concurrent (adult) levels on the same risk factors. They concluded that the onset of adolescence may be the turning point after which the presence of the risk factor is associated with adult disease. Thus adolescence may be a critical period for establishing physiological risk factors for cardiovascular disease.

ADULTHOOD

One of the earliest longitudinal studies of adult temperament and health followed medical students at Johns Hopkins University in the late 1940s. They were categorized as slow and solid (wary, self-reliant), rapid and facile (cool, clever), or irregular and uneven (moody, demanding). During a 30-year follow-up, about half developed some serious health problem. Most (77%) of the previously labeled "irregular and uneven" types developed a serious disorder during these 30 years, but only about a quarter of the rest suffered a major health setback. In further follow-ups, the "irregular and uneven" temperament types as well as those physicians who seemed to have social and emotional problems (were repressed loners) and held "tension in" were more likely to have developed cancer or to have died (Betz & Thomas, 1979; Graves, Mead, Wang, Liang, & Klag, 1994; Shaffer, Graves, Swank, & Pearson, 1987). This study, as well as a study of Harvard students also begun in the 1940s, illustrated the value of long-term studies of personality and heath in adulthood, as well as the power of biopsychosocial assessments of individual differences to predict key long-term outcomes (Peterson, Seligman, & Vaillant, 1988; see Friedman, 2000b, for other examples). Clearly, *something* of importance is going on here, and it is up to researchers to employ more sophisticated research designs and measures to explicate the processes.

Adulthood (approximately ages 21 to between 60 and 70) should not be regarded as monolithic; a range of distinct adult periods can be defined in terms of various major psychosocial changes (e.g., getting married, becoming parents, getting or losing a job) or physical changes (e.g., the decline in athletic ability in one's 30s, the sharp rise in cardiovascular and cancer disease risk in one's 50s, and the menopause for women). Adult personality traits are readily (reliably and validly) assessed by self-report. The childhood temperament of effortful control or restraint is replaced in adulthood by conscientiousness and related traits. Adult trait equivalents for childhood negative emotionality are commonly low agreeableness and high neuroticism, in addition to measures of negative affect and pessimism. For childhood positive emotionality, adult measures include positive affect and aspects of extraversion such as optimism and sociability. Longitudinal studies over periods of adult life, taking psychosocial changes into account, offer valuable opportunities to evaluate lifespan models of personality and health, with both constructs seen as moving targets.

Conscientiousness

The beneficial effects of conscientiousness on longevity have been observed prospectively in adulthood. In the Edinburgh Artery Study (a prospective study of a community sample of men and women), men who were low in conscientiousness were more likely to die from any cause over a 7-year follow-up (Whiteman, 2006). Studies of disease progression with patient samples also demonstrate the protective effects of being more conscientiousness. For example, renal patients low on conscientiousness were more likely to have died 4 years later, as were those high on neuroticism, after controlling for age and diabetic status (Christensen et al., 2002). A number of studies confirm a relation between conscientiousness and a range of health-enhancing behaviors among adult patient and nonpatient groups (Bogg & Roberts, 2004). For example, women with breast problems who were more conscientious were more likely to undergo mammography 2 years later, even when the effects of eight other predictors of mammography were controlled (Siegler, Feaganes, & Rimer, 1995). Adults tend to gain weight at midlife, and a study of over 3,000 participants in the North Carolina Alumni Heart Study has shown that midlife weight gain measured at four time points over 14 years was larger among men and women who were less conscientious, implying poorer eating and exercise habits (Brummett et al., 2006). These studies support health–behavior models by demonstrating that more conscientious adults have healthier lifestyles and are more adherent to disease treatment and self-management. However, the studies cannot rule out underlying biological contributions to both health and a conscientious trajectory.

The absolute level of conscientiousness may be important. For example, only high levels of conscientiousness may be protective, or only very low levels of conscientiousness may be dangerous. Brickman, Yount, Blaney, Rothberg, and Kaplan De-Nour (1996) compared adult patients with diabetes, grouped by their scores on neuroticism and conscientiousness, on renal deterioration time (presumed to be a function of treatment adherence). The combination of moderate neuroticism and high conscientiousness was the most protective. A study of the combined effects of risk perceptions and conscientiousness on subsequent desirable changes in smoking showed effects of risk perceptions only observed at higher levels of conscientiousness (Hampson, Andrews, Barckley, Lichtenstein, & Lee, 2000, 2006). Further study of such interactions, and of individuals at the extremes of trait distributions, will be valuable.

Negative Emotionality

Anger, Hostility, Anxiety, and Depression

Twenty years ago, I (H. S. F.) and Booth-Kewley (1987) proposed a generic "disease-prone personality" characterized by negative emotionality, in particular anger/hostility and depression. This construct was contrasted with the then-popular focus on narrow trait-to-disease links, such as Type A behavior and coronary heart disease. Recently, the idea of a clustering of negative emotionality traits associated with cardiovascular disease was affirmed in Suls and Bunde's (2005) review (see also Smith & Gallo, 2001). They concluded that anger, anxiety, and depression are overlapping constructs that together predict cardiovascular disease among initially healthy populations and, to a lesser extent, predict disease progression among those with cardiovascular disease. However, investigators typically examine the effects of only one aspect of negative emotionality (e.g., just hostility or just depression) and one disease; what is needed are studies where the various components are all measured so that their combined influence on cardiovascular health and general health can be assessed. There may even be synergistic effects that have hitherto gone unobserved because of the emphasis on studying single constructs.

Adult negative emotionality is associated with risk factors for cardiovascular disease. For example, suppressed hostility predicted incident hypertension among middle-age men (Zhang et al., 2005), and associations between depression, hostility, anger, and neuroticism with higher BMI and weight gain in adulthood have been demonstrated in a number of studies (e.g., Brummett et al., 2006; Faith, Flint, Fairburn, Goodwin, & Allison, 2001). Over a 5-year follow-up of the community sample participating in the Edinburgh Artery Study, hostility did not predict myocardial infarction, but submissiveness was protective, particularly for women. Hostility was associated with cardiovascular risk factors such as smoking (Whiteman, 2006; Whiteman, Deary, & Fowkes, 2000). Negative emotionality may increase BMI via health behaviors such as overeating and insufficient physical activity, and by stress-related processes. Niaura and colleagues (2000) showed that hostility was concurrently related to indicators of the metabolic syndrome, and path analysis suggested that hostility influenced BMI, which mediated the effects of hostility on lipids. This was a cross-sectional study, but it suggests a mechanism for the effects of hostility through BMI.

The Healthy Women Study (HWS) is a prospective study of changes in behavioral and biological characteristics of a population-based cohort of middle-age women during the peri- and postmenopausal years. Results show prospective relations between negative emotionality and clinical measures of health status. Women in the HWS who were more depressed, tense, and angry at baseline were at increased risk of developing the metabolic syndrome during the 7–8 years of follow-up

(Räikkönen, Matthews, & Kuller, 2002). Interestingly, this study also found reciprocal effects: Metabolic syndrome at baseline predicted increasing anger and anxiety over the follow-up period. Furthermore, women in the HWS with higher levels of trait anger at baseline showed increased carotid atherosclerosis across 3 years and increased their risk for developing the metabolic syndrome (Räikkönen, Matthews, Sutton-Tyrell, & Kuller, 2004).

The effects of negative emotionality may go beyond the artifact introduced when self-report measures of health (negatively biased by neurotics) are used. In some studies, neuroticism predicts the reporting of symptoms but not the onset of actual disease (Costa & McCrae, 1985; Feldman et al., 1999; Watson & Pennebaker, 1989). Overall, trait neuroticism (low emotional stability) has not demonstrated consistent relations with health outcomes, including mortality. For example, the Western Electric Study of middle-age men (Almada et al., 1991) did not show a relation between neuroticism and mortality, but renal patients who were high on neuroticism were more likely to have died 4 years later (Christensen et al., 2002).

One explanation for these conflicting results is that there are two quite different life paths characterized by neuroticism (Friedman, 2000a). In one case, adults who are pessimistic, resentful, and anxious will fail to adhere to treatment regimens, engage in an unhealthy lifestyle, and have a lack of social support, all of which increase the risk of poor health. The other pathway leads to better health as a consequence of neurotic vigilance and treatment adherence. Some recent research supports the idea that factors associated with neuroticism, such as self-reports of psychological distress and mental strain, can predict lower mortality risk for men (Gardner & Oswald, 2004; Korten et al., 1999). Also, as noted, the effects of neuroticism are further complicated by evocative effects: Neurotics tend to experience more negative events and to react more strongly to them (Bolger & Zuckerman, 1995). Finally, there is evidence of common genetic vulnerability to depression and coronary artery disease (McCaffery et al., 2006). In other words, to the extent that both depression and heart disease derive in part from a genetically based vulnerability in the serotonin system, interven-

tions to affect depression will not necessarily have expected effects on heart disease risk. And in fact, depression interventions for patients who have experienced a heart attack have had no impact on the likelihood of subsequent heart attacks (Writing Committee for the ENRICHD Investigators, 2003).

Pessimism

Although pessimism overlaps with other aspects of negative emotionality, particularly depression, it may also have unique components, especially in the short term. Pessimism (measured independently from optimism) predicted mortality from cancer 8 months later only for patients ages 30–59 and not for older patients, perhaps because of differences in the meaning of being pessimistic and the significance of cancer for younger versus older people (Schulz, Bookwala, Knapp, Scheier, & Williamson, 1996). Pessimistic explanatory style assessed at age 25 for participants in the Harvard Study of Adult Development predicted poor health at ages 45–60, controlling for physical and mental health at age 25 (Peterson et al., 1988). Given correlational and short-term studies reporting an association between optimism and self-reported health, it may be that pessimism is most important or relevant when there is a short-term obstacle (e.g., surgery or an acute infection) that must be faced. However, pessimism (measured on a bipolar optimism–pessimism scale) was associated with increased mortality risk over a 30-year follow-up of self-referred general medical patients (Maruta, Colligan, Malinchoc, & Offord, 2000). Pessimism is one of those constructs that should be examined along with other aspects of negative emotionality so that its truly unique contribution to health can be evaluated.

Type D personality, advanced by Denollet and colleagues, is defined as chronic emotional distress, a combination of negative affect and social inhibition, which in personality trait terms is a combination of high neuroticism, low extraversion, and low conscientiousness (De Fruyt & Denollet, 2002). This personality type has been related to cardiac events, including mortality in patients with coronary heart disease, in several prospective studies that controlled for other predictors (Denollet & Brutsaert, 1998; Denollet, Pederson, Vrints, & Conraads, 2006; Denollet, Vaes, & Brutsaert, 2000). The medical world is more comfortable with categorical than continuous variables, yet, somewhat paradoxically, there is now a continuous measure of Type D personality (Denollet, 2005). The success of Type D personality to predict cardiac events is significant conceptually because it demonstrates the value of examining combinations of traits, not just single-trait predictors of disease outcomes. However, it may prove more fruitful to employ combinations of traits, situations, and pathways, rather than return to the past problems of relying on personality "types."

Positive Emotionality

It has been hypothesized that to the extent that adults tend to experience positive emotions, they will not be exposed to the accumulation of adverse physiological stress reactions, and hence should be more likely to have long and healthy lives. Provocative evidence to support this assertion was found in a prospective study of 185 Catholic nuns (Danner, Snowdon, & Friesen, 2001), which reported an association between positive emotional content of written autobiographies at age 22 and longevity six decades later, after controlling for age and education. There was a 2.5-fold difference in the risk of dying for those in the lowest versus the highest quartiles of positive emotional expression in their writing. Whether emotional expression in these autobiographies reflected a coping style in response to stress, a pervasive disposition to experience more positive emotion, an ability to resolve negative emotions, or indeed some other mechanism, could not be determined from these data, and not all studies relating positive emotionality to mortality have found it to be protective (e.g., Janoff-Bulman & Marshall, 1982).

Although positive emotionality, in the form of a tendency to experience positive affect, may be a protective factor for adults against subsequent ill health and injury, the causal links remain murky (Cohen & Pressman, 2006; Pressman & Cohen, 2005; see also Cohen, Doyle, Turner, Alper, & Skoner, 2003). Postulated mechanisms include health practices, physiological responses, and a stress-buffering effect in which positive affect modulates the stress response (Pressman

& Cohen, 2005). It may be more relevant for older individuals who are dealing with terminal chronic illness than for younger adults, who may take risks and for whom premature death is more likely to be due to accidents and violence.

Consistent with a focus on short-term motivation, optimists recover better from medical interventions than pessimists. For example, patients who were more optimistic were less likely to be rehospitalized after coronary artery bypass graft surgery (Scheier et al., 1999); more optimistic women demonstrate better adjustment to breast cancer (Carver et al., 1993); and more optimistic patients with head and neck cancer had a greater chance of 1-year survival, controlling for sociodemographic and clinical variables (Allison, Guichard, Fung, & Gilain, 2003). Women in the HWS who were more optimistic showed less progression of carotid artery disease than did those who were chronically pessimistic (Matthews, Räikkönen, Sutton-Tyrrell, & Kuller, 2004). This diversity of evidence is compelling testament to the benefits of optimism in the short term, where likely mechanisms for the beneficial effects of optimism include coping strategies (Scheier & Carver, 2003). However, because measures of positive and negative affect may reflect how a person feels, and self-reports of health often capture affect, it is necessary to (1) institute a number of corrections, preferably including objective health outcomes (or using longevity as the outcome); (2) control for concurrent self-rated health; and (3) as emphasized, use a prospective design. More correlational studies of self-reported affect and self-reported health (or minor health fluctuations) are not needed.

Intelligence

Longevity is predicted by childhood as well as by adult intelligence, not surprisingly, given that intelligence is a stable trait. The adult association has been examined using various measures of ability. Linguistic ability in young adulthood was protective against mortality in the nun study (Snowdon, Greiner, Kemper, Nanayakkara, & Mortimer, 1999). Cognitive ability assessed at army recruitment predicted mortality between ages 22 and 40 for Australian Vietnam war veterans (O'Toole & Stankov, 1992). A study of middle-age adults who were ages 48–67 when tested for cognitive functioning were followed up, on average, for 6.3 years, and poorer functioning was related to all-cause mortality (Pavlik et al., 2003). Lower intelligence is associated with high systolic blood pressure at midlife and is a risk factor for various cardiac events (Hart et al., 2004; Starr et al., 2004).

Numerous mechanisms are likely to be involved in the relation between intelligence, health status, and longevity, including SES, common causes such as genes, and health behaviors. People with greater intellectual ability acquire more health knowledge (Beier & Ackerman, 2003) and presumably have more learning, problem-solving, and reasoning skills to apply to their health practices and self-care (Gottfredson & Deary, 2004). Central nervous system functioning has also been implicated as a mechanism. Decrement in reaction time predicted mortality in younger and older adults (although not those of middle age) over 19 years of follow-up (Shipley, Der, Taylor, & Deary, 2006). On the other hand, many cognitively talented people drink too much, get too much sun exposure, indulge gourmet tastes, and seek risky medical care. Indeed, the Terman cohort shows that a large percentage of highly intelligent individuals succumb to unhealthy behaviors and diseases in patterns that are not substantially different from many persons of average intelligence (Friedman & Markey, 2003), indicating the importance of personality traits and other factors in addition to intelligence for health outcomes. The time is ripe for research on the many biopsychosocial variables that may divert the trajectory relating intelligence to good health and longevity.

OLD AGE

When studying the relation between personality and health in older samples, an important caveat is the issue of the "survival elite"—these are individuals who have survived the other predictors of mortality (Korten et al., 1999). The relation between traditional risk factors and mortality (e.g., smoking, hypertension) can be weaker (or different) in old age, in part because of selective earlier mortality or successful treatment (Swan & Carmelli, 1996). Moreover, simple health–behavior or physiological models are less applicable in old age when insults have accumulated, physical limitations place restrictions on activities, and body chemistry has changed. Other problems for research with older samples include the distinction between normal aging and terminal decline preceding death, the presence of illness and disability, as well as social disruptions, which often may produce changes in personality and emotional well-being. Despite these challenges, a number of studies have addressed personality in old age and subsequent functioning and mortality.

Conscientiousness

Conscientiousness continues to exert an influence on longevity even into old age. Weiss and Costa (2005) evaluated all the five traits and their facets in the five-factor model as predictors of mortality in a study of a community sample of men and women ages 65–100. They confirmed protective effects of high conscientiousness on mortality over a 5-year follow-up. Also, Wilson, Mendes de Leon, Bienias, Evans, and Bennett (2004) studied personality predictors of mortality in a group of Catholic clergy members (men and women). The mean age for the group was 75 when they completed a comprehensive personality inventory, and they had no dementia at baseline. They were followed for 5 years. The risk of mortality was halved for those with high versus low conscientiousness scores, controlling for the effects of the other traits and physical health. Again, these results are all the more striking when viewed from a lifespan perspective because less conscientious individuals are more likely to die at all ages (Friedman, Tucker, Schwartz, Martin, et al., 1995; Martin et al., 2007), and hence the survivors into old age are likely to be relatively conscientious.

Negative Emotionality

Depression

Depression assessed in old age predicted mortality after controlling for other predictors, including subclinical and prevalent disease (Schulz, Martire, Beach, & Scheier, 2000). In the Religious Orders Study, internally experienced negative affect (i.e., depression and suppressed anger) was related to mortality but externally directed negative affect was not, after controlling for other personality traits, physical health, health habits, and cognitive functioning (Wilson, Bienias, Mendes de Leon, Evans, & Bennett, 2003).

Neuroticism

As discussed earlier, neuroticism is related to willingness to report symptoms and may be associated with different paths to health status; some degree of neuroticism may be protective because it motivates vigilance and adherence. The inconsistent findings persist into old age. For example, Korten and colleagues (1999) found that older men who were more neurotic were less likely to die, whereas in the Religious Orders Study, Wilson and colleagues (2004) found that the risk of mortality was nearly doubled for those with high versus low neuroticism scores. The effects of neuroticism may take time to build up (the cumulative model), in which case these effects should be strongest in old age (Wilson et al., 2004). Mroczek, Spiro, Griffin, and Neupert (2006) proposed that people who experience high levels of neuroticism throughout their lives will develop a hair-trigger response to negative emotion. According to this "kindling hypothesis," people with a life history of high levels of neuroticism have consistently reacted strongly and negatively to stress, and, over the years, this has had a cumulative, detrimental effect on the HPA axis. Mroczek and Almeida (2004) provide some support for this process in a study of older peoples' daily experiences. The relation between daily stress and negative affect was stronger for neurotics.

Using data from the Normative Aging Study, Mroczek and Spiro (2007) showed that increasing neuroticism was associated with increased mortality risk over a 10-year period (mean age 63 for the personality assessments). They used growth-curve modeling of multiple assessments of neuroticism to look at the change over time on this trait. Both the level and slope of neuroticism predicted mortality, controlling for age and physical health. An increase in neuroticism of about half a standard deviation led to a 40% increase in the risk of dying. Such a growth-curve approach may help resolve some of the conflicting findings for trait effects by evaluating whether relative change

on a particular trait, rather than absolute level, is the parameter with the most predictive power.

Positive Emotionality

Studies of older age groups have not demonstrated a reliable association between extraversion and mortality (Korten et al., 1999; Maier & Smith, 1999; Wilson et al., 2004). However, data from the Normative Aging Study indicate that extraversion predicts trajectories of life satisfaction in men (Mroczek & Spiro, 2005), and optimism was related to subsequent psychological well-being, self-rated general health, and freedom from bodily pain, but not to physical, social, and role functional status, independent of depression (Achat, Kawachi, Spiro, DeMolles, & Sparrow, 2000).

Dispositional optimism was associated with prudent health behavior (i.e., less smoking and alcohol use and more physical activity), and with self-rated health among relatively healthy older participants with a mean age of 70.5 years from the community (Steptoe, Wright, Kunz-Ebrecht, & Iliffe, 2006). The effects of optimism were mediated through health behaviors for physical, but not mental, health. This was a cross-sectional study, so reciprocal relations between optimism and health cannot be ruled out, but it is interesting to see support for a health–behavior model with these older participants.

Intelligence

Several studies have found prospective relations between lower levels of cognitive abilities assessed in old age and subsequent mortality (Bassuk, Wypij, & Berkman, 2000; Korten et al., 1999; Neale, Brayne, & Johnson, 2001). For example, Korten and colleagues (1999) studied an elderly community sample in Australia, at least 70 years old at baseline in 1991, and surviving participants were reinterviewed in 1994. A range of psychosocial, behavioral, and personality predictors were studied. After controlling for sex and physical health, poorer cognitive performance predicted mortality.

Maier and Smith (1999), like Korten and colleagues (1999), compared a variety of potential predictors of mortality in the Berlin

Aging Study (mean age 83) 3–6 years after baseline assessment. Poorer intellectual functioning was the strongest predictor of impending mortality, controlling for age. The effects were pervasive across different aspects of cognitive functioning. Maier and Smith (1999) discussed the difficulties involved in distinguishing between declines associated with normal aging versus the more rapid terminal decline immediately preceding death (Berg, 1996). However, a study by Rabbitt and colleagues (2002) demonstrated an association between poorer cognitive functioning and mortality over 11 years—a longer period than previous studies, which argues against terminal decline.

Why should poor cognitive functioning predict mortality in old age? One explanation is that it is an indicator of declining physical health, such as compromised cardiovascular and cerebrovascular function (Hassing et al., 2002). Consistent with this account, Deary and Der (2005) obtained measures of IQ and of reaction time at age 56 and followed up for mortality to age 70. The effect of IQ on mortality was no longer significant after adjusting for reaction time, suggesting that reduced efficiency of information processing—presumably a consequence of cardiovascular and cerebrovascular deterioration—may be a mechanism linking lower mental ability and earlier death.

Wilson and colleagues (2004) found no relation between openness at 75 years and subsequent mortality. However, Swan and Carmelli (1996) found that state (but not trait) curiosity (openness plus autonomy), assessed at age 71, predicted survival 5 years later in men in the Western Collaborative Group Study, controlling for other risk factors, and similarly it predicted survival for women age 69 at baseline.

The studies in which personality assessment takes place in old age tend to predict mortality and functional status, which are more salient endpoints for this age group than any particular morbidity. The role of personality on the causes of disease is probably more pertinent in previous life stages when chronic illness may be prevented or postponed. Conscientiousness and intelligence continue to play the same role in health in old age as they have across the lifespan, whereas the roles of negative and positive emotionality are less consistent.

CONCLUSIONS AND FUTURE DIRECTIONS

Because understanding the likelihood of disease for the individual is often as important as knowing the general causes of disease, personality psychology is a necessary complement to biology in understanding and promoting health and longevity. Modern conceptions of personality are already addressing many of the limitations of static conceptions of health, although these new developments are generally unknown in medical research and treatment. Personality concepts and theories are comfortable with interacting biological, psychological, and social contributions to individual differences, as well as changes as a function of maturation, environmental press, situation selection, and cultural influence. Personality psychologists are also comfortable with describing an introverted, working-class Latino American boy with genetically based hyperreactivity and slow metabolism, who grows up exposed to a high-carbohydrate diet reinforced by social gatherings and who sets himself, during adolescence, on a sociobehavioral pathway toward diabetes, whereas a physician might struggle to find which condition to "treat." Thus although there is no pill to treat this progression (and no pill to change personality), there are many positive steps that can be taken.

To illustrate the lifespan approach, we have examined the relations between personality and health at each life stage in terms of four broad domains: (1) restraint, effortful control, and conscientiousness, (2) negative emotionality, (3) positive emotionality, and (4) intelligence. All four domains are proving fruitful in the search for links between personality and health, but these are not necessarily an exhaustive or optimal categorization. Although health–behavior models tend to be invoked as mechanisms to account for the effects of the conscientiousness and intelligence domains, and stress-related psychoneuroimmunological models tend to be used to explain the effects of emotionality, more complete models will eventually integrate the various interacting forces. Such innovative models are beginning to appear. For example, Rozanski and Kubzansky (2005) focused on vitality, emotional flexibility, and coping flexibility, and others likewise have taken new tacks in trying to integrate the biological with the psychological and the social in addressing individual differences and health (Vollrath, 2006).

To test lifespan models, we need to use modern statistical techniques that can optimally analyze trajectories, such as latent-growth models and latent-transition analysis. This methodology requires multiple, reliable assessments over the longitudinal period under study. Relatedly, survival analysis is standard in epidemiology but only slowly making its way into personality psychology. These methods allow for personality change as well as changes in health status. As noted, it may prove valuable to identify life stages when both personality and health are more likely to change in regard to particular habits, behaviors, reactions, and health status. For example, when are long-term patterns of physical activity most strongly influenced? We also should look at combinations of traits and characteristics, and interactions among them, not just their main effects (e.g., Brickman et al., 1996). Trait interactions may help explain some seemingly contradictory findings.

Because the relations are dynamic and complex, there may always be severe limits on the size of the relations between personality and health, just as there are limits on the ability of personality alone to predict behavior. This limitation and complexity does not mean that personality is unimportant or of minor significance in predicting or improving health. On the contrary, because modern notions of personality are well suited to capturing complex and ongoing biopsychosocial processes relevant to health, personality may prove more valuable than traditional but relatively static measures, including traditional biological measures (e.g., serum cholesterol, which is often difficult to lower without lifelong pharmaceutical intervention), demographic measures (e.g., age or ethnicity, which are certainly relevant to health but of little meaning in isolation from other variables), social measures (e.g., marriage status, limited by the variations in the context and quality of marriage), or psychopathological measures (e.g., depression, which is better conceived as multidimensional and time varying than as a static risk factor).

The study of biopsychosocial mechanisms in long-term pathways for good health must become more sophisticated. Personality psychologists need to collaborate further with disease experts to develop testable models of these mechanisms. Our own research involves interdisciplinary teams that include physicians and epidemiologists, who are often key to solid progress. All in all, the field of personality and health needs further conceptual development, and this development can be guided by the significant progress already made by personality psychologists in understanding individual differences across the lifespan.

ACKNOWLEDGMENTS

Sarah E. Hampson's contribution to the preparation of this chapter was supported in part by Grant No. AG20048 from the National Institute on Aging and Grant No. DA10767 from the National Institute on Drug Abuse. Howard S. Friedman's contribution was supported in part by Grant Nos. AG08825 and AG027001 from the National Institute on Aging.

REFERENCES

Achat, H., Kawachi, I., Spiro, A., III, DeMolles, D. A., & Sparrow, D. (2000). Optimism and depression as predictors of physical and mental health functioning: The Normative Aging study. *Annals of Behavioral Medicine, 22*(2), 127–130.

Ahadi, S., & Rothbart, M. K. (1994). Temperament, development and the Big Five. In C. Halverson, Jr., D. Kohnstamm, & R. Martin (Eds.), *Development of the structure of temperament and personality from infancy to adulthood* (pp. 189–208). Hillsdale, NJ: Erlbaum.

Akerblom, H. K., Uhari, M., Pesonen, E., Dahl, M., Kaprio, E. A., Nuutinen, E. M., et al. (1991). Cardiovascular risk in young Finns. *Annals of Medicine, 23*, 35–40.

Alexander, F. (1950). *Psychosomatic medicine.* New York: Norton.

Allison, P. J., Guichard, C., Fung, K., & Gilain, L. (2003). Dispositional optimism predicts survival status 1 year after diagnosis in head and neck cancer patients. *Journal of Clinical Oncology, 21*(3), 543–548.

Almada, S. J., Zonderman, A. B., Shekelle, R. B., Dyer, A. R., Daviglus, M. L., Costa, P. T., Jr., et al. (1991). Neuroticism and cynicism and risk of death in middle-aged men: The Western Electric Study. *Psychosomatic Medicine, 53*, 165–175.

Baltes, P. B., & Goulet, L. R. (1970). Status and issues of a life-span developmental psychology.

In L. R. Goulet & P. B. Baltes (Eds.), *Life-span developmental psychology: Research and theory* (pp. 4–21). New York: Academic Press.

Baltes, P. B., Reese, H. W., & Lipsitt, L. P. (1980). Life-span developmental psychology. *Annual Review of Psychology, 31*, 65–110.

Barker, D. J. P. (1994). *Mothers, babies and disease in later life*. London: BMJ.

Barker, D. J. P. (1998). In utero programming of chronic disease. *Clinical Science, 95*, 115–128.

Barker, D. J. P., Osmond, C., Forsén, T. J., Kajantie, E., & Eriksson, J. G. (2005). Trajectories of growth among children who have coronary events as adults. *New England Journal of Medicine, 353*, 1802–1809.

Bassuk, S. S., Wypij, D., & Berkman, L. F. (2000). Cognitive impairment and mortality in the community-dwelling elderly. *American Journal of Epidemiology, 151*, 676–688.

Beier, M. E., & Ackerman, P. L. (2003). Determinants of health knowledge: An investigation of age, gender, abilities, personality, and interests. *Journal of Personality and Social Psychology, 84*(2), 439–448.

Berg, S. (1996). Aging, behavior and terminal decline. In J. E. Birren & K. W. Schaie (Eds.), *Handbook of psychology of aging* (4th ed., pp. 323–337). New York: Academic Press.

Betz, B., & Thomas, C. (1979). Individual temperament as a predictor of health or premature disease. *Johns Hopkins Medical Journal, 144*, 81–89.

Bogg, T., & Roberts, B. W. (2004). Conscientiousness and health-related behaviors: A meta-analysis of the leading behavioral contributors to mortality. *Psychological Bulletin, 130*, 887–919.

Bolger, N., & Zuckerman, A. (1995). A framework for studying personality in the stress process. *Journal of Personality and Social Psychology, 69*, 890–902.

Brickman, A. L., Yount, S. E., Blaney, N. T., Rothberg, S. T., & Kaplan De-Nour, A. (1996). Personality traits and long-term health status: The influence of neuroticism and conscientiousness on renal deterioration in Type-1 diabetes. *Psychosomatics, 37*(5), 459–468.

Brummett, B. H., Babyak, M. A., Williams, R. B., Barefoot, J. C., Costa, P. T., Jr., & Siegler, I. C. (2006). NEO personality domains and gender predict levels and trends in body mass index over 14 years during midlife. *Journal of Research in Personality, 40*, 222–236.

Carver, C. S., & Miller, C. J. (2006). Relations of serotonin function to personality: Current views and a key methodological issue. *Psychiatry Research, 144*, 1–15.

Carver, C. S., Pozo, C., Harris, S. D., Noriega, V., Scheier, M. F., Robinson, D. S., et al. (1993). How coping mediates the effect of optimism on distress: A study of women in early stage breast cancer. *Journal of Personality and Social Psychology, 65*, 375–390.

Caspi, A. (1998). Personality development across the life course. In N. Eisenberg (Ed.), *Handbook of child development* (pp. 311–388). New York: Wiley.

Caspi, A., Begg, D., Dickson, N., Harrington, H., Langley, J., Moffitt, T. E., et al. (1997). Personality differences predict health-risk behaviors in young adulthood: Evidence from a longitudinal study. *Journal of Personality and Social Psychology, 73*(5), 1052–1063.

Caspi, A., Elder, C. H., Jr., & Bem, D. J. (1987). Moving against the world: Life-course patterns of explosive children. *Developmental Psychology, 23*(2), 308–313.

Chambers, R. A., Taylor, J. R., & Potenza, M. N. (2003). Developmental neurocircuitry of motivation in adolescence: A critical period of addiction vulnerability. *American Journal of Psychiatry, 160*(6), 1041–1052.

Christensen, A. J., Ehlers, S. L., Woebe, J. S., Moran, P. J., Raichle, K., Ferneyhough, K., et al. (2002). Patient personality and mortality: A 4-year prospective examination of chronic renal insufficiency. *Health Psychology, 21*(4), 315–320.

Cohen, S., Doyle, W. J., Turner, R. B., Alper, C. M., & Skoner, D. (2003). Emotional style and susceptibility to the common cold. *Psychosomatic Medicine, 65*, 652–657.

Cohen, S., & Pressman, S. D. (2006). Positive affect and health. *Current Directions in Psychological Science, 15*, 122–125.

Contrada, R. J., Cather, C., & O'Leary, A. (1999). Personality and health: Dispositions and processes in disease susceptibility and adaptation to illness. In L. A. Pervin & O. P. John (Eds.), *Handbook of personality: Theory and research* (pp. 576–604). New York: Guilford Press.

Costa, P. T., Jr., & McCrae, R. R. (1985). Hypochondriasis, neuroticism, and aging: When are somatic complaints unfounded? *American Psychologist, 40*, 19–28.

Danner, D. D., Snowdon, D. A., & Friesen, W. V. (2001). Positive emotions in early life and longevity: Findings from the nun study. *Journal of Personality and Social Psychology, 80*(5), 804–813.

De Fruyt, F., & Denollet, J. (2002). Type D personality: A five-factor model perspective. *Psychology and Health, 17*, 671–683.

Deary, I. J., & Der, G. (2005). Reaction time explains IQ's association with death. *Psychological Science, 16*(1), 64–69.

Deary, I. J., Taylor, M. D., Davey Smith, G., Whalley, L. J., Starr, J. M., Hole, D. J., et al. (2005). Childhood IQ and all-cause mortality before and after age 65: Prospective observational study linking the Scottish Mental Survey 1932 and the Midspan studies. *British Journal of Health Psychology, 10,* 153–165.

Deary, I. J., Whalley, L. J., Lemmon, H., Crawford, J. R., & Starr, J. M. (2000). The stability of individual differences in mental ability from childhood to old age: Follow-up of the 1932 Scottish Mental Survey. *Intelligence, 28,* 49–55.

Deary, I. J., Whalley, L. J., & Starr, J. M. (2003). IQ at age 11 and longevity. In C. E. Finch, J.-M. Robine, & Y. Christen (Eds.), *Brain and longevity: Perspectives in longevity* (pp. 153–164). Berlin: Springer.

Deary, I. J., Whiteman, M. C., Starr, J. M., Whalley, L. J., & Fox, H. C. (2004). The impact of childhood intelligence on later life: following up the Scottish Mental Surveys of 1932 and 1947. *Journal of Personality and Social Psychology, 86*(1), 130–147.

Denollet, J. (2005). DS14: Standard assessment of negative affectivity, social inhibition, and Type D personality. *Psychosomatic Medicine, 67,* 89–97.

Denollet, J., & Brutsaert, D. L. (1998). Personality, disease severity, and the risk of long-term cardiac events in patients with decreased ejection fraction after myocardial infarction. *Circulation, 97,* 167–173.

Denollet, J., Pedersen, S. S., Vrints, C. J., & Conraads, V. M. (2006). Usefulness of Type D personality in predicting five-year cardiac events above and beyond current symptoms of stress in patients with coronary heart disease. *American Journal of Cardiology, 97,* 970–973.

Denollet, J., Vaes, J., & Brutsaert, D. L. (2000). Inadequate response to treatment in coronary heart disease: Adverse effects of Type-D personality and younger age on 5-year prognosis and quality of life. *Circulation, 102,* 630–635.

Depue, R. A., & Collins, P. F. (1999). Neurobiology of the structure of personality: Dopamine, facilitation of incentive motivation, and extraversion. *Behavior and Brain Sciences, 22,* 491–569.

Dunbar, F. (1955). *Mind and body: Psychosomatic medicine.* New York: Random House.

Faith, M. S., Flint, J., Fairburn, C. G., Goodwin, G. M., & Allison, D. B. (2001). Gender differences in the relationship between personality dimensions and relative body weight. *Obesity Research, 9,* 647–650.

Feldman, P. J., Cohen, S., Lepore, S., Matthews, K., Kamarck, T. W., & Marsland, A. L. (1999). The impact of personality on the reporting of unfounded symptoms and illness. *Annals of Behavioral Medicine, 21,* 216–222.

Friedman, H. S. (2000a). Long-term relations of personality and health: Dynamisms, mecha-

nisms, tropisms. *Journal of Personality, 68,* 1089–1108.

Friedman, H. S. (2000b). *Self-healing personality: Why some people achieve health and others succumb to illness.* New York: Henry Holt. Also available online at *www.iuniverse.com.*

Friedman, H. S. (2007). Personality, disease, and self-healing. In H. S. Friedman & R. C. Silver (Eds.), *Foundations of health psychology* (pp. 172–199). New York: Oxford University Press.

Friedman, H. S., & Booth-Kewley, S. (1987). The "disease-prone personality": A meta-analytic view of the construct. *American Psychologist, 42,* 539–555.

Friedman, H. S., & Markey, C. N. (2003). Paths to longevity in the highly intelligent Terman cohort. In C. E. Finch, J.-M. Robine, & Y. Christen (Eds.), *Brain and longevity* (pp. 165–175). New York: Springer.

Friedman, H. S., Tucker, J., Schwartz, J. E., Martin, L. R., Tomlinson-Keasey, C., Wingard, D., et al. (1995). Childhood conscientiousness and longevity: Health behaviors and cause of death. *Journal of Personality and Social Psychology, 68,* 696–703.

Friedman, H. S., Tucker, J. S., Schwartz, J. E., Tomlinson-Keasey, C., Martin, L. R., Wingard, D. L., et al. (1995). Psychosocial and behavioral predictors of longevity: The aging and death of the "termites." *American Psychologist, 50,* 69–78.

Friedman, H. S., Tucker, J., Tomlinson-Keasey, C., Schwartz, J., Wingard, D., & Criqui, M. H. (1993). Does childhood personality predict longevity? *Journal of Personality and Social Psychology, 65,* 176–185.

Gardner, J., & Oswald, A. (2004). How is mortality affected by money, marriage and stress? *Journal of Health Economics, 23,* 1181–1207.

Gerrard, M., Gibbons, F. X., Stock, M. L., Houlihan, A. E., & Dykstra, J. L. (2006). Temperament, self-regulation, and the prototype willingness model of adolescent health risk behavior. In D. T. Ridder & J. B. F. de Wit (Eds.), *Self-regulation in health behavior* (pp. 97–118). Chichester, UK: Wiley.

Goodwin, R. G., & Friedman, H. S. (2006). Health status and the five factor personality traits in a nationally representative sample. *Journal of Health Psychology, 11,* 643–654.

Gottfredson, L., & Deary, I. J. (2004). Intelligence predicts health and longevity: But why? *Current Directions in Psychological Science, 13,* 1–4.

Graves, P. L., Mead, L. A., Wang, N-Y, Liang, K-Y, & Klag, M. J. (1994). Temperament as a potential predictor of mortality: Evidence from a 41-year prospective study. *Journal of Behavioral Medicine, 17,* 111–126.

Hampson, S. E., Andrews, J. A., & Barckley, M. (2007). Predictors of development of elementary-school children's intentions to smoke cigarettes: Prototypes, subjective norms, and hostility. *Nicotine and Tobacco Control, 9*(7), 751–760.

Hampson, S. E., Andrews, J. A., Barckley, M., Lichtenstein, E., & Lee, M. L. (2000). Conscientiousness, perceived risk, and risk-reduction behaviors: A preliminary study. *Health Psychology, 19,* 496–500.

Hampson, S. E., Andrews, J. A., Barckley, M., Lichtenstein, E., & Lee, M. (2006). Personality traits, perceived risk, and risk-reduction behaviors: A further study of smoking and radon. *Health Psychology, 25,* 530–536.

Hampson, S. E., Andrews, J. A., Barckley, M., & Peterson, M. (2007). Trait stability and continuity in childhood: Relating sociability and hostility to the five-factor model. *Journal of Research in Personality, 41*(3), 507–523.

Hampson, S. E., Andrews, J. A., Barckley, M., & Severson, H. H. (2006). Personality predictors of the development of elementary-school children's intentions to drink alcohol: The mediating effects of attitudes and subjective norms. *Psychology of Addictive Behaviors, 20,* 288–297.

Hampson, S. E., Goldberg, L. R., Vogt, T. M., & Dubanoski, J. P. (2006). Forty years on: Teachers' assessments of children's personality traits predict self-reported health behaviors and outcomes at midlife. *Health Psychology, 25,* 57–64.

Hampson, S. E., Goldberg, L. R., Vogt, T. M., & Dubanoski, J. P. (2007). Mechanisms by which childhood personality traits influence adult health status: Educational attainment, healthy eating habits, and smoking. *Health Psychology, 26,* 121–125.

Hart, C. L., Deary, I. J., Taylor, M. D., MacKinnon, P. L., Davey Smith, G., Whalley, L. J., et al. (2003). The Scottish Mental Survey 1932 linked to the Midspan studies: A prospective investigation of childhood intelligence and future health. *Public Health, 117,* 187–195.

Hart, C. L., Taylor, M. D., Davey Smith, G., Whalley, L. J., Starr, J. M., Hole, D. J., et al. (2004). Childhood IQ and cardiovascular disease in adulthood: Prospective observational study linking the Scottish Mental Survey 1932 and the Midspan studies. *Social Science and Medicine, 59,* 2131–2138.

Hart, C. L., Taylor, M. D., Davey Smith, G., Whalley, L. J., Starr, J. M., Hole, D. J., et al. (2005). Childhood IQ and all-cause mortality before and after age 65: Prospective observational study linking the Scottish Mental Survey 1932 and the Midspan studies. *British Journal of Health Psychology, 10,* 153–165.

Hassing, L. B., Johansson, B., Berg, S., Nilsson, S. E., Pedersen, N. L., Hofer, S. M., et al. (2002). Terminal decline and markers of cerebro- and cardiovascular disease: Findings from a longitudinal study of the oldest old. *Journal of Gerontology B: Psychological Science and Social Science, 57*(3), P268–P276.

Houston, B. K., & Snyder, C. R. (Eds.). (1988). *Type A behavior pattern: Research, theory, and intervention.* New York: Wiley.

Janoff-Bulman, R., & Marshall, G. (1982). Mortality, well-being, and control: A study of a population of institutionalized aged. *Personality and Social Psychology Bulletin, 84,* 691–698.

Jessor, R., & Jessor, S. L. (1977). *Problem behavior and psychosocial development: A longitudinal study of youth.* New York: Academic Press.

Keltikangas-Järvinen, L., Pulkki-Raback, L., Puttonen, S., Viikari, J., & Raitakari, O. T. (2006). Childhood hyperactivity as a predictor of carotid artery intima media thickness over a period of 21 years: The Cardiovascular Risk in Young Finns study. *Psychosomatic Medicine, 68,* 509–516.

Kemeny, M. E. (2007). Psychoneuroimmunology. In H. S. Friedman & R. C. Silver (Eds.), *Foundations of health psychology* (pp. 92–116). New York: Oxford University Press.

Korten, A. E., Jorm, A. F., Jiao, Z., Letenneur, L., Jacomb, P. A., Henderson, A. S., et al. (1999). Health, cognitive, and psychological factors as predictors of mortality in an elderly community sample. *Journal of Epidemiology and Community Health, 53,* 83–88.

Krueger, R. F., Caspi, A., & Moffitt, T. E. (2000). Epidemiological personology: The unifying role of personality in population-based research on problem behaviors. *Journal of Personality, 68*(6), 967–998.

Kuh, D., & Ben-Shlomo, Y. (Eds.). (1997). *A life course approach to chronic disease epidemiology.* New York: Oxford University Press.

Lobel, M., DeVincent, C. J., Kaminer, A., & Meyer, B. A. (2000). The impact of prenatal maternal stress and optimistic disposition on birth outcomes in medically high risk women. *Health Psychology, 19,* 544–553.

Lobel, M., Dunkel-Schetter, C., & Scrimshaw, S. C. M. (1992). Prenatal maternal stress and prematurity: A prospective study of socioeconomically disadvantaged women. *Health Psychology, 11,* 32–40.

Lynch, J., & Davey Smith, G. (2005). A life course approach to chronic disease epidemiology. *Annual Review of Public Health, 26,* 1–35.

Maier, H., & Smith, J. (1999). Psychological predictors of mortality in old age. *Journal of Gerontology: Psychological Sciences, 54B,* P4–P54.

Martin, L. R., & Friedman, H. S. (2000). Comparing personality scales across time: An illustrative study of validity and consistency in life-span archival data. *Journal of Personality*, 68, 85–110.

Martin, L. R., Friedman, H. S., Clark, K. M., & Tucker, J. S. (2005). Longevity following the experience of parental divorce. *Social Science and Medicine*, 61, 2177–2189.

Martin, L. R., Friedman, H. S., & Schwartz, J. E. (2007). Personality and mortality risk across the lifespan: The importance of conscientiousness as a biopsychosocial attribute. *Health Psychology*, 26, 428–436.

Martin, L. R., Friedman, H. S., Tucker, J. S., Tomlinson-Keasey, C., Criqui, M. H., & Schwartz, J. E. (2002). A life course perspective on childhood cheerfulness and its relation to mortality risk. *Personality and Social Psychology Bulletin*, 28, 1155–1165.

Matthews, K. A., Räaikkönen, K., Sutton-Tyrrell, K., & Kuller, L. H. (2004). Optimistic attitudes protect against progression of carotid atherosclerosis in healthy middle-aged women. *Psychosomatic Medicine*, 66, 640–644.

McCaffery, J. M., Frasure-Smith, N., Dubé, M.-P., Théroux, P., Rouleau, G. A., Duan, Q., et al. (2006). Common genetic vulnerability to depressive symptoms and coronary artery disease: A review and development of candidate genes related to inflammation and serotonin. *Psychosomatic Medicine*, 68, 187–200.

McDade, T. W., Hawkley, L. C., & Cacioppo, J. T. (2006). Psychosocial and behavioral predictors of inflammation in middle-aged and older adults: The Chicago Health, Aging, and Social Relations Study. *Psychosomatic Medicine*, 68, 376–381.

McEwen, B. S. (1998). Stress, adaptation and disease: Allostasis and allostatic load. *Annals of the New York Academy of Sciences*, 840, 33–44.

Measelle, J. R., John, O. P., Ablow, J. C., Cowan, P., & Cowan, C. P. (2005). Can children provide coherent, stable, and valid self-reports on the Big Five dimensions?: A longitudinal study from ages 5 to 7. *Journal of Personality and Social Psychology*, 89, 90–106.

Mervielde, I., & De Fruyt, F. (2002). Assessing children's traits with the hierarchical personality inventory for children. In B. De Raad & M. Perugini (Eds.), *Big Five assessment* (pp. 129–142). Ashland, OH: Hogrefe & Huber.

Michel, G. F., & Tyler, A. N. (2005). Critical period: A history of the transition from questions of when, to what, to how. *Developmental Psychology*, 46(3), 156–162.

Mroczek, D. K., & Almeida, D. M. (2004). The effect of daily stress, personality, and age on daily negative affect. *Journal of Personality*, 72(2), 355–378.

Mroczek, D. K., & Spiro, A., III. (2005). Change in life satisfaction during adulthood: Findings from the Veterans Affairs Normative Aging Study. *Journal of Personality and Social Psychology*, 88(1), 189–202.

Mroczek, D. K., & Spiro, A., III. (2007). Personality change influences mortality in older men. *Psychological Science*, 18(5), 371–376.

Mroczek, D. K., Spiro, A., III, Griffin, P. W., & Neupert, S. D. (2006). Social influences on adult personality, self-regulation, and health. In L. L. Carstensen & K. W. Schaie (Eds.), *Social structures, aging, and self-regulation* (pp. 70–122). New York: Springer.

Neale, R., Brayne, C., & Johnson, A. L. (2001). Cognition and survival: An exploration in a large multicenter study of the population aged 65 years and over. *International Journal of Epidemiology*, 30, 1383–1388.

Niaura, R., Banks, S. M., Ward, K. D., Stoney, C. M., Spiro, A., III, Aldwin, C. M., et al. (2000). Hostility and the metabolic syndrome in older males: The normative aging study. *Psychosomatic Medicine*, 62, 7–16.

O'Toole, B. I., & Stankov, L. (1992). Ultimate validity of psychological tests. *Personality and Individual Differences*, 13, 699–716.

Ouellette, S. C., & DiPlacido, J. (2001). Personality's role in the protection and enhancement of health: Where the research has been, where it is stuck, how it might move. In A. Baum, T. A. Revenson, & J. Singer (Eds.), *Handbook of health psychology* (pp. 175–193). Mahwah, NJ: Erlbaum.

Ozer, D. J., & Benet-Martínez, V. (2006). Personality and prediction of consequential outcomes. *Annual Review of Psychology*, 57, 401–421.

Maruta, T., Colligan, R. C., Malinchoc, M., & Offord, K. P. (2000). Optimists vs. pessimists: Survival rate among medical patients over a 30-year period. *Mayo Clinic Proceedings*, 75, 140–143.

Pavlik, V., de Moraes, S., Szklo, M., Knopman, D., Mosley, T., Jr., & Hyman, D. (2003). Relation between cognitive function and mortality in middle-aged adults: The Athersclerosis Risk in Communities study. *American Journal of Epidemiology*, 157, 327–334.

Peterson, C., Seligman, M. E. P., & Vaillant, G. E. (1988). Pessimistic explanatory style is a risk factor for physical illness: A thirty-five-year longitudinal study. *Journal of Personality and Social Psychology*, 55, 23–27.

Pine, D. S., Goldstein, R. B., Wolk, S., & Weissman, M. M. (2001). The association between childhood depression and adulthood body mass index. *Pediatrics*, 107(5), 1049–1056.

Poulton, R., Caspi, A., Milne, B. J., Thomson, W.

M., Taylor, A., Sears, M. R., et al. (2002). Association between children's experience of socioeconomic disadvantage and adult health: A life-course study. *Lancet, 360,* 1640–1645.

Pressman, S. D., & Cohen, S. (2005). Does positive affect influence health? *Psychological Bulletin, 131*(6), 925–971.

Pulkki-Råback, L., Elovainio, M., Kivimäki, M., Raitakari, O. T., & Keltikangas-Järvinen, L. (2005). Temperament in childhood predicts body mass index in adulthood: The Cardiovascular Risk in Young Finns study. *Health Psychology, 24*(3), 307–315.

Rabbitt, P., Watason, P., Donlan, C., Mc Innes, L., Horan, M., Pendleton, N., et al. (2002). Effects of death within 11 years on cognitive performance in old age. *Psychology and Aging, 17,* 468–481.

Räikkönen, K., Matthews, K. A., & Kuller, L. H. (2002). The relationship between psychological risk attributes and the metabolic syndrome in healthy women: Antecedent or consequences? *Metabolism, 51,* 1573–1577.

Räikkönen, K., Matthews, K. A., & Salomon, K. (2003). Hostility predicts metabolic syndrome risk factors in children and adolescents. *Health Psychology, 22,* 279–286.

Räikkönen, K., Matthews, K. A., Sutton-Tyrell, K., & Kuller, L. H. (2004). Trait anger and the metabolic syndrome predict progression of carotid atherosclerosis in healthy middle-aged women. *Psychosomatic Medicine, 66,* 903–908.

Raitakari, O. T., Juonala, M., Kähönen, M., Taittonen, L., Mäki-Torkko, N., Järvisalo, M. J., et al. (2003). Cardiovascular risk factors in childhood and carotid artery intima–media thickness in adulthood: The cardiovascular risk in young Finns study. *Journal of the American Medical Association, 290,* 2277–2283.

Ravaja, N., & Keltikangas-Järvinen, L. (1995). Temperament and metabolic syndrome precursors in children: A three-year follow-up. *Preventive Medicine, 24,* 518–527.

Roberts, B. W., & DelVecchio, W. F. (2000). The rank-order consistency of personality from childhood to old age: A quantitative review of longitudinal studies. *Psychological Bulletin, 126,* 3–25.

Roberts, B. W., Walton, K. E., & Viechtbauer, W. (2006). Patterns of mean-level change in personality traits across the life course: A meta-analysis of longitudinal studies. *Psychological Bulletin, 132*(1), 1–25.

Rosenman, R. H., Friedman, M., Straus, R., Wurm, M., Kositcheck, R., Hahn, W., et al. (1964). A predictive study of coronary disease. The Western Collaborative Group study. *Journal of the American Medical Association, 189,* 103–110.

Rozanski, A., & Kubzansky, L. D. (2005). Psychologic functioning and physical health: A paradigm of flexibility. *Psychosomatic Medicine, 6,* S47–S53.

Scarr, S., & McCartney, K. (1984). How people make their own environments: A theory of genotype—environment effects. *Annual Progress in Child Psychiatry and Child Development,* pp. 98–118.

Scheier, M. F., & Carver, C. S. (2003). Self-regulatory processes and responses to health threats: Effects of optimism on well-being. In J. Suls & K. A. Wallston (Eds.), *Social psychological foundations of health and illness* (pp. 395–428). Malden, MA: Blackwell.

Scheier, M. F., Matthews, K. A., Owens, J. F., Schulz, R., Bridges, M. W., Magover, G. J., Sr., et al. (1999). Optimism and rehospitalization after coronary artery bypass graft surgery. *Archives of Internal Medicine, 159*(8), 829–835.

Schulz, R., Bookwala, J., Knapp, J. E., Scheier, M., & Williamson, G. M. (1996). Pessimism, age, and cancer mortality. *Psychology and Aging, 11*(2), 304–309.

Schulz, R., Martire, L. M., Beach, S. R., & Scheier, M. F. (2000). Depression and mortality in the elderly. *Current Directions in Psychological Science, 9*(6), 204–208.

Shaffer, J., Graves, P. L., Swank, R. T., & Pearson, T. A. (1987). Clustering of personality traits in youth and the subsequent development of cancer among physicians. *Journal of Behavioral Medicine, 10,* 441–444.

Shipley, B. A., Der, G., Taylor, M. D., & Deary, I. J. (2006). Cognition and all-cause mortality across the entire adult age range: Health and lifestyle survey. *Psychosomatic Medicine, 68,* 17–24.

Siegler, I. C., Feaganes, J. R., & Rimer, B. K. (1995). Predictors of adoption of mammography in women under age 50. *Health Psychology, 14*(3), 274–278.

Smith, T. W., & Gallo, L. C. (2001). Personality traits as risk factors for physical illness. In A. Baum, T. Revenson, & J. Singer (Eds.), *Handbook of health psychology* (pp. 139–172). Hillsdale, NJ: Erlbaum.

Smith, T. W., & Spiro, A., III. (2002). Personality, health, and aging: Prolegomenon for the next generation. *Journal of Research in Personality, 36,* 363–394.

Snowdon, D. A., Greiner, L. H., Kemper, S. J., Nanayakkara, N., & Mortimer, J. A. (1999). Linguistic ability in early life and longevity: Findings from the nun study. In J.-M. Robine, B. Forette, C. Francheschi, & M. Allard (Eds.), *The paradoxes of longevity* (pp. 103–113). Berlin: Springer-Verlag.

Starr, J. M., Taylor, M. D., Hart, C. L., Davey Smith, G., Whalley, L. J., Hole, D. J., et al.

(2004). Childhood mental ability and blood pressure at midlife: Linking the Scottish Mental Survey 1932 and the Midspan studies. *Journal of Hypertension, 22,* 893–897.

Steptoe, A., Wright, C., Kunz-Ebrecht, S. R., & Iliffe, S. (2006). Dispositional optimism and health behavior in community-dwelling older people: Associations with health ageing. *British Journal of Health Psychology, 11,* 71–84.

Suls, J., & Bunde, J. (2005). Anger, anxiety, and depression as risk factors for cardiovascular disease: The problems and implications for overlapping affective dispositions. *Psychological Bulletin, 131*(2), 260–300.

Swan, G. E., & Carmelli, D. (1996). Curiosity and mortality in aging adults: A 5-year follow-up of the Western Collaborative Group study. *Psychology and Aging, 11*(3), 449–453.

Tarter, R. E., Sambrano, S., & Dunn, M. D. (2002). Predictor variables by developmental stages: A Center for Substance Abuse Prevention multisite study. *Psychology of Addictive Behaviors, 16,* S3–S10.

Taylor, M. D., Hart, C. L., Davey Smith, G., Starr, J. M., Hole, D. J. , Whalley, L. J., et al. (2003). Childhood mental ability and smoking cessation in adulthood: Prospective observational study linking the Scottish Mental Survey 1932 and the Midspan studies. *Journal of Epidemiology and Community Health, 57,* 464–465.

Tucker, J., Friedman, H. S., Tomlinson-Keasey, C., Schwartz, J. E., Wingard, D. L., & Criqui, M. H. (1995). Childhood psychosocial predictors of adulthood smoking, alcohol consumption, and physical activity. *Journal of Applied Social Psychology, 25,* 1884–1899.

Vollrath, M. E. (2006). *Handbook of personality and health.* Chichester, UK: Wiley.

Wand, G. S., McCaul, M., Yang, X., Reynolds, J., Gotjen, D., Lee, S., et al. (2002). The mu-opioid receptor gene polymorphism (A188G) alters HPA axis activation induced by opioid receptor blockade. *Neuropsychopharmacology, 26,* 106–114.

Watson, D., & Pennebaker, J. W. (1989). Health complaints, stress, and distress: Exploring the central role of negative affectivity. *Psychological Review, 96,* 234–254.

Weiss, A., & Costa, P. T., Jr. (2005). Domain and facet personality predictors of all-cause mortality among Medicare patients aged 65–100. *Psychosomatic Medicine, 67,* 724–733.

Whalley, L. J., & Deary, I. J. (2001). Longitudinal cohort study of childhood IQ and survival up to age 76. *British Medical Journal, 322,* 819–822.

Whiteman, M. C. (2006). Personality, cardiovascular disease and public health. In M. E. Vollrath (Ed.), *Handbook of personality and health* (pp. 13–34). Chichester, UK: Wiley.

Whiteman, M. C., Deary, I. J., & Fowkes, F. G. R. (2000). Personality and health: Cardiovascular disease. In S. E. Hampson (Ed.), *Advances in personality psychology* (Vol. 1, pp. 157–198). Hove, UK: Psychology Press.

Wiebe, D. J., & Smith, T. W. (1997). Personality and health: Progress and problems in psychosomatics. In R. Hogan, J. Johnson, & S. Briggs (Eds.), *Handbook of personality psychology* (pp. 892–918). San Diego, CA: Academic Press.

Williamson, D. F., Thompson, T. J., Anda, R. F., Dietz, W. H., & Felitti, V. J. (2002). Adult body weight, obesity, and self-reported abuse in childhood. *International Journal of Obesity, 26,* 1075–1082.

Wilson, R. S., Bienias, J. L., Evans, D. A., Mendes de Leon, C. F., & Bennett, D. A. (2003). Negative affect and mortality in older persons. *American Journal of Epidemiology, 158*(9), 827–835.

Wilson, R. S., Mendes de Leon, C. F., Bienias, J. L., Evans, D. A., & Bennett, D. A. (2004). Personality and mortality in old age. *Journal of Gerontology: Psychological Sciences, 59B,* P110–P116.

Woodall, K. L., & Matthews, K. A. (1993). Changes in and stability of hostile characteristics: Results form a 4-year longitudinal study of children. *Journal of Personality and Social Psychology, 64*(3), 491–4099.

Writing Committee for the ENRICHD Investigators. (2003). Effects of treating depression and low perceived social support on clinical events after myocardial infarction: The enhancing recovery in coronary heart disease patients (ENRICHD) randomized trial. *Journal of the American Medical Association, 289,* 3106–3116.

Zhange, J., Niaura, R., Todaro, J. F., McCaffery, J. M., Shen, B., Spiro, A., III, et al. (2005). Suppressed hostility predicted hypertension incidence among middle-aged men: The Normative Aging study. *Journal of Behavioral Medicine, 28*(5), 443–453.

Zuckerman, M. (1994). Impulsive, unsocialized sensation seeking: The biological foundations of a basic dimension of personality. In J. E. Bates & T. D. Wachs (Eds.), *Temperament: Individual differences at the interface of biology and behavior* (pp. 219–255). Washington, DC: American Psychological Association.

CHAPTER 32

Personality and Subjective Well-Being

Richard E. Lucas
Ed Diener

Subjective well-being (SWB) reflects the extent to which people think and feel that their life is going well. This construct—which is often referred to more colloquially as happiness—plays somewhat of an unusual role within personality psychology. On the one hand, neither the previous two editions of this handbook (Pervin, 1990; Pervin & John, 1999) nor Hogan, Johnson, and Briggs's (1997) *Handbook of Personality Psychology* included chapters on the topic (though these handbooks did address the topic of emotion). This absence suggests that well-being research has not played a central role in personality theory. Yet on the other hand, the strong influence of personality is seen as one of the most replicable and most surprising findings to emerge from the last four decades of research on SWB. In fact, Gilovich and Eibach (2001) suggested that the relatively weak influence of situational factors and the relatively strong influence of personality factors is an important, counterintuitive finding that came as a considerable surprise to social psychologists. If the links between personality and SWB are so strong and so surprising, why hasn't SWB research played a more important role in personality theory? Furthermore, why are personality effects in the SWB domain viewed as being so surprising in the first place?

We believe that part of the answer to these questions comes when we consider the dual nature of the construct. SWB can be thought of both as an outcome for which individuals strive and as part of a functional process that helps individuals to achieve other goals. In reference to the first point, William James suggested that "how to keep, how to gain, how to recover happiness is … for most men at all times the secret motive for all they do" (1902, p. 76). We would argue that the only thing that James got wrong in this statement is the suggestion that this motive is secret. Most people agree that being happy is the ultimate goal toward which they strive. For instance, one study reported that being happy was rated to be more important than having good health, a high income, or high levels of attractiveness; and it was rated as being more important than experiencing love or meaning in life (Diener & Oishi, 2004). Thus, happiness is seen as an ultimate goal that guides individual choices and that can be achieved if the external circumstances in a person's life coincide with his or her desires (for a different view/emphasis, see Ryff & Keyes, 1995; also Ryff, Chapter 15, this volume).

When people conceptualize happiness in this way—as an outcome that can be achieved if things go well—they naturally think about it as something that can change. Not surprisingly, initial work in the area focused on identifying the external life circumstances that reliably correlate with SWB (Wilson, 1967). It was thought that these correlations could reveal basic human needs, and that by understanding these needs, psychologists could identify pathways to greater well-being. These efforts have continued over the years, and some progress has been made in identifying interventions that can lead to lasting changes in happiness (Lyubomirsky, Sheldon, & Schkade, 2005; Seligman, Steen, Park, & Peterson, 2005). In fact, psychologists and economists have increasingly advocated for the implementation of large-scale surveys of well-being so that population levels can be tracked over time (Diener, 2000; Diener & Seligman, 2004; Kahneman, Krueger, Schkade, Schwartz, & Stone, 2003). Again, the principle that underlies this suggestion is that by identifying macro-level characteristics that reliably affect well-being, policy decisions could be optimized to increase well-being for all.

If happiness is conceptualized as an outcome that reflects the conditions in a person's life, it may seem counterintuitive and even somewhat distressing when research suggests that happiness is stable over time and unresponsive to changes in life circumstances. It is this outcome-focused aspect of well-being research and theory that makes strong personality effects seem so surprising. Yet when SWB is thought of not as an outcome but as an integral part of an ongoing process, the strong effects of personality and the relatively weak effects of situations should come as no surprise. For at the heart of well-being judgments lie affective reactions (Lucas & Diener, 2008), and these emotions and moods likely play a functional role in people's lives (Fredrickson, 1998; Gross, 1999; Lyubomirsky, King, & Diener, 2005). Negative affect does not simply relay the news that something in one's life is not going well. Instead it provides the motivation and perhaps even the tools that allow for corrections. Similarly, pleasant feelings are not simply a reward for a job well done; these feelings are functional. Thus, negative emotions should not cease when a person's life circumstances become ideal, nor should pleasure endure forever when all important goals are achieved. In fact, the pleasure that

one experiences after the achievement of a goal may actually promote the desire to seek new goals (Carver, 2003; Fredrickson, 1998). If there are individual differences in these underlying affective processes, then SWB will also exhibit the characteristics of a personality trait. Thus, well-being should be play an important role in personality research.

In the current chapter, we first discuss general issues regarding the nature of SWB. We then address concerns about the measurement of well-being. Finally, we review the evidence linking personality and well-being constructs. We believe that confusion about the dualistic nature of well-being has sometimes led to the misinterpretation of existing research, particularly when it comes to questions about the impact of external circumstances and the possibility for change. Although we believe that personality processes matter, research suggests that happiness can change and that life circumstances can have important consequences.

DEFINING SWB

Although researchers sometimes discuss happiness and well-being as if they reflect a unitary construct, there is no single judgment that captures the entirety of SWB. Instead, SWB researchers divide the domain into narrower classes of constructs that tap into distinct ways in which one's life could be evaluated (see Schimmack, 2008, for a more detailed review). For instance, SWB researchers often distinguish cognitive judgments of well-being from affective experience (Diener, 1984). The cognitive components assess an individual's reflective judgment that his or her life or the circumstances of that life are going well. To assess this component, researchers often administer measures of life satisfaction or domain satisfaction—measures that ask people to consider and consciously evaluate the conditions in their lives.

This type of reflective judgment can be contrasted with the emotions and moods that individuals actually experience as they live their lives. Experience sampling studies (i.e., those studies that assess experience repeatedly over time) show that there are very few moments that are affectively neutral: People report some affective feeling almost all the time (Diener, Sandvik, & Pavot, 1991). Furthermore, one of the most basic features of these feelings is that people can tell whether they are pleasant or unpleasant (Kahneman, 1999). Thus, a life could be considered to be a good one if there were more pleasant experiences than unpleasant ones over an extended period of time. Thus, *reflective judgments* and *affective experiences* provide two distinct ways in which a person's life could be evaluated.

In addition, affective experiences themselves can be further divided into narrower categories. The study of these more precise affect variables often reveals unique information about the quality of a person's life and the processes that underlie the evaluation of that life. For instance, although it is tempting to conceptualize affective experience simply as the ratio of positive to negative, much information is lost when such an index is constructed. Two individuals who have equal amounts of positive and negative experiences may have very different lives, depending on the intensity of their experiences. In addition, because positive and negative feelings are not polar opposites, it may be inappropriate to combine them in a single index. As early as 1969, Bradburn recognized that pleasant and unpleasant affect were empirically separable. Following up on this work, Watson, Tellegen, and their colleagues suggested that positive and negative affect are distinct and orthogonal factors (Watson, Clark, & Tellegen, 1988; Watson & Tellegen, 1985; Zevon & Tellegen, 1982). Furthermore, these distinct factors often correlate with unique sets of predictors (e.g., Carver, Sutton, & Scheier, 2000; Costa & McCare, 1980; Elliott & Thrash, 2002; Tellegen, 1985). To be sure, the independence view is not without its critics (see Schimmack, 2008, for a review), but SWB researchers often recommend assessing positive and negative affect separately.

Although it is easy to understand the conceptual distinctions among the various facets of well-being, it is still important to ask how the various components interrelate, both at a theoretical and empirical level. First, it is clear that the various components are, in fact, separable. For instance, multimethod studies show that when different methods of assessment are used to measure distinct well-being components, different measures of the same construct tend to correlate more strongly than do different constructs assessed by similar methods (Lucas, Diener, & Suh, 1996). This means that at a measurement level, the various components are distinct.

However, at a theoretical level it is necessary to explain the associations among the various constructs and to develop theories about the factors that will influence each. For instance, one major debate that has implications for personality theory concerns the top-down versus bottom-up issue (Diener, 1984; Heller, Watson, & Ilies, 2004; Schimmack, 2008). According to bottom-up models, individuals construct global well-being judgments by evaluating the various characteristics in their lives. People might examine the various domains in their lives, calculate satisfaction scores for each domain, and then aggregate across domains to arrive at an overall judgment of life satisfaction. In this model (which is consonant with the SWB-as-outcome view described above), life circumstances affect intermediate judgments of domain satisfaction along with day-to-day emotional experience, and these intermediate judgments and experiences combine to affect global judgments of well-being.

Although bottom-up models are intuitively appealing, the strong forms of these models do not appear to be correct. For one thing, the amount of information that one must aggregate to calculate a global judgment of happiness is probably too large to allow for quick and efficient ratings. Reaction time studies suggest that once people are asked to evaluate relatively long periods of time (i.e., longer than a few hours), they do not search their memory for relevant information. Instead, they rely on existing beliefs about their happiness to make a global judgment (Robinson & Clore, 2002). We must caution that this finding does not necessarily mean that these quick judgments are not valid; it simply suggests that people do not conduct an exhaustive search of information about satisfaction with lower-level domains before coming up with a global judgment. This fact, combined with research showing that the associations among domain satisfaction ratings are too high to be explained by a simple bottom-up model (Schimmack, 2008), shows that well-being judgments are not constructed in a purely bottom-up manner. Instead, top-down processes likely play a role.

Top-down models posit that personality processes influence the general affective tone that a person experiences, and this general tendency colors all aspects of that person's life. A happy person will not only experience frequent positive emotions and infrequent negative emotions, but he or she will view the various aspects of life as being more positive than they really are. Thus, the moderate association between domain and life satisfaction could be explained by the tendency for happy people to be satisfied with all aspects of their lives, rather than by a causal effect of domains on global judgments. According to this top-down model, life circumstances have weak effects on happiness because personality-based processes affect how one views the world (see, e.g., Brief, Butcher, George, & Link, 1993; Feist, Bodner, Jacobs, Miles, & Tan, 1995; Judge & Watanabe, 1993; Saris, 2001; Schyns, 2001).

The final structural consideration concerns the links between the affective and cognitive components. As the evidence from discriminant validity studies shows, life satisfaction judgments do not simply reflect the sum of one's affective experiences over time (Lucas et al., 1996). Instead, these cognitive judgments and affective experiences provide different information about the quality of one's life as a whole. It appears that affective experience may provide one source of information that individuals can use to judge the overall quality of their lives. However, they may also consider additional factors, including the objective conditions in their lives or their satisfaction with narrower domains (Schimmack, 2008).

Furthermore, the role that these affective experiences play in the construction of global judgments may vary across individuals. For instance, we showed that positive and negative affect predicted life satisfaction to different degrees in different cultures (Suh, Diener, Oishi, & Triandis, 1998). Among participants from individualist cultures, affective experience was strongly correlated with life satisfaction, whereas among participants from collectivist cultures, the associations were somewhat weaker. Because people living in individualist cultures tend to view the self as an autonomous, self-sufficient entity (Markus & Kitayama, 1991), feelings and emotions weigh heavily as determinants of behavior. Collectivist cultures, on the other hand, stress harmony with family and friends rather than stressing one's autonomy from these people. Feelings about the self (including emotional reactions) weigh less heavily in these cultures. Thus, people appear to rely on their emotions when making satisfaction judgments, but the exact role that these experiences play may vary depending on the value that individuals place on these experiences (see Kim-Prieto, Diener, Tamir, Scollon, & Diener, 2005, for a more detailed discussion of the processes that link the various components of SWB).

In summary, SWB can be defined as an individual's subjective belief or feeling that his or her life is going well. There is no single judgment that can capture the diverse ways that life can be evaluated. Instead, a variety of cognitive and affective components are needed to provide a relatively complete picture of one's life as a whole. It is important to stress that each component may be affected by different predictors and may result from distinct but overlapping processes (Kim-Prieto et al., 2005). Thus, researchers who study SWB must carefully consider which components are most useful for their purposes—not all components will behave in similar ways. An important goal for ongoing and future research will be to identify and explain the links between these diverse ways of evaluating a person's life.

MEASURING SWB

Because SWB researchers place value on an individual's own opinion about his or her life, it is sometimes assumed that self-reports of well-being provide the "gold standard" measure of the construct. But this is simply not the case. Although it is true that self-reports are used quite frequently within the field, there are also reasons to be skeptical of these measures. For instance, people may not want to reveal their true level of happiness, and method factors such as scale use or acquiescence bias could overwhelm the true variance that is captured by self-report techniques. Furthermore, if certain cognitive theories are correct, people may not have the cognitive capacity to report accurately on their experiences over time (Robinson & Clore, 2002; Schwarz & Strack, 1999). Thus, the validity of self-reports must not be taken for granted simply because they have strong face validity as measures of subjective feelings. Researchers must make sure that responses to these measures make sense in a larger nomological network that includes non-self-report measures and criteria.

Research examining the psychometric properties of SWB measures has shown that self-report scales tend to be reliable and valid. For instance, multiple-item measures of life satisfaction, domain satisfaction, and positive and negative affect scales all show high reliability, regardless of whether reliability is assessed using interitem correlations or short-term test–retest correlations (Diener, Suh, Lucas, & Smith, 1999). More importantly, there is increasing evidence for the validity of these measures. Different measures of the same well-being construct tend to correlate more strongly with one another than with measures of related but theoretically distinct constructs (Lucas et al., 1996). In addition, these measures also converge with non-self-report methods of assessment. For instance, Lucas et al. showed that self-reports of life satisfaction, positive affect, and negative affect correlated between .35 and .52 with informant reports of the same constructs. Similarly, Sandvik, Diener, and Seidlitz (1993) showed that expert ratings of participants' happiness correlated approximately .50 with self-reports. Even indirect measures, such as the number of positive versus negative life events that an individual could remember and list, tend to correlate with self-report measures of happiness (Sandvik et al., 1993). Finally, well-being measures are correlated with physiological indicators, including asymmetrical hemispheric activation in the prefrontal cortex (Davidson, 2004). This evidence suggests that unwanted method variance does not overwhelm the valid variance that is captured by self-report methods of assessment.

Research also shows that self-report measures are responsive to life events and sensitive to different life circumstances. Although we review this evidence in more detail when we discuss the factors that influence well-being, it is worth noting here that well-being measures change when significant life events occur (Headey & Wearing, 1989; Lucas, 2005, 2006; Lucas, Clark, Georgellis, & Diener, 2003, 2004; Magnus, 1991; Suh, Diener, & Fujita, 1996). Furthermore,

individuals living in disadvantaged circumstances tend to report lower well-being than do those living in more ideal settings. For instance, Biswas-Diener and Diener (2001) found that individuals living in the slums of Calcutta reported life satisfaction scores that were considerably lower than individuals living in more affluent circumstances. Similarly, individuals with severe spinal cord injuries or other lasting disabilities tend to report well-being scores that are much lower than those of individuals without such injuries (Brickman, Coates, & Janoff-Bulman, 1978; Dijkers, 1997; Lucas, 2007).

In fact, even among individuals with spinal cord injuries, well-being measures are able to distinguish between those who have additional complications and those who do not. For instance, Putzke, Richards, Hicken, and DeVivo (2002) used the Satisfaction With Life Scale (SWLS; Diener, Emmons, Larsen, & Griffin, 1985) to examine life satisfaction in a cohort of 940 adults with traumatic-onset spinal cord injury. The entire sample of participants reported relatively low levels of life satisfaction ($M = 17.3$, $SD = 7.7$) when compared to adult norms, which tend to average between 23 and 27 in most samples (Pavot & Diener, 1993). But more importantly, a number of additional characteristics were significantly related to SWLS scores. For example, spinal-cord-injured patients with no additional medical complications (e.g., bladder management, ventilator use, autonomic dysreflexia, and deep vein thrombosis) were significantly more satisfied than individuals with either one or more than one complication. Similarly, individuals who had required no additional hospitalizations following injury were significantly more satisfied than individuals who had undergone one or more than one subsequent hospitalization (effect sizes were in the small to moderate range). Thus, life circumstances seem to matter, and the effects of these circumstances are reflected in SWB measures.

It is also the case that SWB measures predict relevant behaviors and outcomes. For instance, Koivumaa-Honkanen and colleagues have examined the predictive validity of self-report life satisfaction and happiness measures in a sample of over 29,000 Finnish adults (mostly twins) who were followed for up to 20 years. Their analyses show that life satisfaction prospectively predicts outcomes that include suicide (Koivumaa-Honkanen, Honkanen, Koskenvuo, & Kaprio, 2003; Koivumaa-Honkanen, Honkanen, Viinamäki, Heikkilä, Kaprio, & Koskenvuo, 2001) and the onset of depression (Koivumaa-Honkanen, Kaprio, Honkanen, Viinamäki, & Koskenvuo, 2004). Even measures of domain satisfaction predict outcomes that might be expected to occur among those who are unsatisfied with a particular area of their lives. For instance, research shows that job satisfaction measures predict absenteeism and the likelihood of changing jobs (Clark, Georgellis, & Sanfey, 1998; P. Frijters, 2000; Pelled & Xin, 1999). In other words, those who are not dissatisfied with their jobs tend to stay away from those jobs and tend to leave those jobs. These results show that people who say they are unsatisfied do things that psychologists would expect unsatisfied people to do.

Of course, this evidence does not mean that SWB measures are beyond reproach. Researchers have raised serious challenges to the validity, and these challenges must be acknowledged and addressed by any psychologist who wishes to use these measures. For instance, Schwarz, Strack, and their colleagues have argued that a variety of irrelevant contextual factors (including minor changes in instructions, setting, question wording, question order, or response options) can have a strong influence on well-being judgments and therefore that these reports should not be trusted. For instance, in a study that is often cited as evidence for the malleability of well-being reports, Strack, Martin, and Schwarz (1988) showed that simply changing the order of two questions could dramatically influence the correlation between them. In their study, when questions about satisfaction with a specific domain (e.g., relationship satisfaction) preceded a question about general life satisfaction, then the correlation between the two measures was strong. When the general life satisfaction question was asked first, however, then the two measures correlated quite weakly. This pattern of associations suggests that asking about specific life domains makes information about these domains salient when an individual is later asked to judge his or her life as a whole. It also implies that life satisfaction judgments are constructed "on the fly" and are susceptible to irrelevant contextual effects.

Schwarz and Strack have amassed an impressive body of research that provides insight into the processes that underlie self-reported judgments of well-being (see Schwarz, 1999, for a review of more general processes). Based on their review of the literature, they concluded that one might interpret this body of evidence to mean that "there is little to be learned from self-reports of global well-being" and that "what is being assessed, and how, seems too context-dependent to provide reliable information about a population's well-being" (Schwarz & Strack, 1999, p. 80). However, we believe that such statements are much too strong and are not supported by the large body of evidence showing that SWB measures are stable and valid. Experimental studies in controlled laboratory settings reveal important information about the processes that may underlie complex psychological phenomena. But it is important to remember that demonstrating that such processes exist does not reveal the extent to which these processes affect real-world judgments. Additional research is needed to determine the extent to which irrelevant contextual factors actually influence SWB measures, although existing research suggests that these influences are not strong.

For instance, Schimmack and Oishi (2005) conducted a meta-analysis of studies that had manipulated the order of life satisfaction and domain satisfaction ratings (along with five new replication studies of their own), and they showed that the item-order effect that Strack, Martin, and Schwarz (1988) identified is, on average, quite small. In addition, Schimmack and Oishi, along with Schimmack, Diener, and Oishi (2002), showed that people tend to use chronically accessible information rather than transient sources of information when constructing well-being judgments. Furthermore, contextual factors such as current mood have only a very small influence on well-being judgments that theoretically should be stable (Eid & Diener, 2004). Together, this evidence suggests that although people may be influenced by transient and irrelevant contextual information, these effects are not large.

In summary, evidence to date suggests that self-report measures of SWB are reliable and valid, sensitive to external circumstances, and responsive to change. They correlate with additional self-report measures in addition to non-self-report measures and criteria. Finally, they prospectively predict theoretically relevant behaviors and outcomes, which shows that they can be useful both in research and in practice. It is true that there may be times when contextual factors influence these judgments, but we are aware of no research that suggests that such contextual effects have a large impact on the validity of the measures. Thus, researchers can be confident that SWB can be assessed well with standard self-report measures. That being said, we also believe that self-report does not provide a gold standard, and thus alternative techniques should be used when possible. Experience sampling techniques (Scollon, Kim-Prieto, & Diener, 2003) or other self-report procedures that do not require memory for, and aggregation across, numerous events can help. In addition, non-self-report measures, including informant reports, psychophysiological measures, textual analysis, and other novel techniques, can provide important information about the extent to which a person's life is going well.

EVIDENCE FOR THE IMPORTANCE OF PERSONALITY

After decades of research on SWB researchers have often arrived at what to some seems like a startling conclusion: The most important factor in determining a person's SWB appears to be the personality with which he or she is born. Evidence for this conclusion comes from at least four lines of research. First, studies of objective life circumstances (including such factors as a person's income, age, education level, doctor-rated health, and social relationships) show that associations with such factors tend to be quite small. Second, SWB is moderately heritable, which means that some inborn factors are at work. Third, SWB is stable over time, sometimes even in the face of changing life circumstances. And finally, when effect sizes are compared directly, correlations with personality traits tend to be much larger than correlations with external circumstances. This evidence has been interpreted to mean that happiness cannot change and that individuals are stuck with a biologically determined level of happiness that is only weakly linked to the circumstances that they experience in life. In the following sections, we review evidence from these four different lines of research. Although we believe that personality plays an important role in SWB, a careful examination of the existing evidence suggests that life circumstances also matter and that there is room for change.

Associations with External Life Circumstances

People's behavior is often guided by their beliefs about the types of things that will make them happy (Gilbert, 2006). People may choose a high-paying job, an expensive house, or a short commute over other alternatives because they believe that these life circumstances will improve or maintain their happiness. Thus, one goal for psychological research is to identify the factors that actually do correlate with happiness. Through such research, people's intuitions could be tested, and practical guidance could be offered. Unfortunately, the most common conclusion from such inquiries is that very few objective life circumstances exhibit strong associations with any SWB variable. In one of the first attempts to quantify the links between SWB and a broad set of predictors, Andrews and Withey (1976) concluded that about 10% of the variance in well-being could be accounted for by demographic characteristics. In later reviews, Diener (1984) and Argyle (1999) suggested a slightly higher estimate of 15%. Below we review some of the findings from this literature, focusing not just on effect sizes but also on the practical implications of these effects.

Perhaps the most surprising finding in this line of research concerns the link between income and happiness. Many studies have been conducted, and a number of consistent findings have emerged (Diener & Biswas-Diener, 2002). Most important for the current discussion, research shows that at an individual level, correlations tend to be positive but very small. For instance, Lucas and Dyrenforth (2006) reviewed evidence from two meta-analyses (Haring, Stock, & Okun, 1984; Pinquart & Sorensen, 2000), a more recent narrative review of cross-national results (Diener & Biswas-Diener, 2002), and many waves of an annual nationally representative survey (General Social Survey; Davis, Smith, & Marsden, 2003). This review showed that the correlation between income and happiness tends to fall between .17 and .21. The typical conclusion that one draws from these data is that people overestimate the importance of money, and that once people have their basic needs met, income does not matter.

Although we do not dispute the size of the correlations that have been found in previous research, we caution that such correlations need to be interpreted carefully. For instance, a .20 correlation would mean that each additional standard deviation of income would only "buy" one-fifth of a standard deviation in happiness. However, income standard deviations tend to be quite small relative to the range of the distribution. Thus, when people's intuition suggests that money will make them happier, they may by concerned with moving closer to the endpoint of the distribution rather than just moving one or two standard deviations away from their current position. Even with a relatively weak .20 correlation, the intuition that money matters could still be correct.

To illustrate, we examined data from the most recent wave of the German Socio-Economic Panel (GSOEP) study, a long-running, nationally representative panel study that is in its 22nd year (Lucas & Schimmack, 2007). We first transformed household income scores from Euros into U.S. dollars and then computed the correlation between income and life satisfaction. Consistent with previous research, the correlation was a small .18. However, this small correlation can result from very large differences between the various income groups. For instance, those in the richest group report life satisfaction scores that are more than one-half of one standard deviation above the mean level of satisfaction and almost three-quarters of one standard deviation above the satisfaction of those living at the poverty level. We do not consider these to be small effects, even though income can only explain a very small amount of the variance in life satisfaction measures among the full sample.

Additional interpretational concerns arise when inappropriate measures of the predictor variables are used. This problem can be illustrated by examining the association between health and well-being. Correlations with health tend to be small to moderate in size. Okun, Stock, Haring, and Witter (1984)

conducted a meta-analysis of over 200 effect sizes, and they found correlations around .30. Similarly, Brief and colleagues (1993) found that subjective reports of health tended to correlate between .30 to .40 with life satisfaction. Effects of this size might suggest that health plays a reasonably important role in SWB. However, both groups of researchers have suggested that when more objective measures of health are obtained, the correlation drops close to zero. For instance, Okun and George (1984) found that physician ratings of health were not correlated with well-being, and Brief et al. found that the number of doctor visits only correlated about .10 with life satisfaction.

Although some have suggested that this type of discrepancy provides evidence that self-reports of health are not valid (e.g., Diener et al., 1999; Kahneman & Riis, 2005), there is some indication that the opposite might be true. Self-reports may in fact be more valid (at least in terms of content validity) than other objective measures. For instance, self-reports of health predict mortality over and above more objective measures (e.g., Ganz, Lee, & Siau, 1991; Mossey & Shapiro, 1982; Rumsfeld et al., 1999), and studies that have investigated the discrepancies between self- and doctor-rated health have found evidence that it may be the doctors' judgments that are wrong (e.g., Nelson et al., 1983). Finally, as was noted in the section on validity, there is considerable evidence that objective measures of specific health conditions, such as spinal cord injuries and severe disability, are associated with large and lasting differences in SWB.

The examples described above show that associations that appear to be very small can actually be quite large when alternative effect-size indexes are examined or when appropriate measures of predictor variables are used. Unfortunately, the opposite can also be true. Effects that have been considered to be very large may not be so large when examined closely. Recently, we argued that this is the case with variables related to the existence of social relationships (Lucas & Dyrenforth, 2005, 2006). When predictors of SWB are compared, variables such as the existence of strong social relationships are presented as if they were the strongest correlates to emerge from the literature (e.g., Argyle, 2001). However, reviews of this literature often focus on satisfaction with relationships or the extent to which people value relationships, rather than on the existence of relationships themselves. If these more objective measures are evaluated, the correlations are similar to, and perhaps even smaller than, the association with income.

For example, Lucas and Dyrenforth (2006) reviewed the literature on the associations between SWB and the number of friends that people have, whether individuals have a close friend to whom they can talk, the amount of time that people spend with friends, and the amount of time that people spend with family members. Existing meta-analyses (e.g., Okun et al., 1984; Pinquart & Sörensen, 2000) along with new analyses of data from nationally representative surveys showed that correlations with these variables tended to be around .15 and very rarely exceeded .20. Even marital status, which has often been held up as one of the most important demographic predictors, only correlates .14 with measures of SWB (Haring-Hidore, Stock, Okun, & Witter, 1985). Thus, at least when relatively objective measures are assessed, these associations are smaller than the effect of income or health.

We acknowledge that the same concerns about the interpretation of effect sizes that we raised for income and health may also apply to correlations with social relationship variables. A very small correlation may be meaningful, and simple count- and frequency-based measures of social relationships may not adequately capture the quality of these relationships. Furthermore, social relationships, including marriage, predict a wide variety of outcomes that include risk for mental illness, poor physical health, and even death (e.g., Berkman & Syme, 1979; House, Landis, & Umberson, 1988; House, Robbins, & Metzner, 1982). Thus, the robustness of these effects across domains may be important, even if the individual effects are quite small. However, because it is difficult to say whether an individual effect size is practically important, researchers must be careful to compare apples to apples when drawing conclusions about the relative importance of different life circumstances.

The three domains reviewed above provide just a small sample of effects from the large body of literature linking SWB to demographic characteristics and other external life circumstances. Considerable amounts of research have also investigated factors such

as age, gender, education, employment status, ethnicity, and religion. A more detailed review is beyond the scope of this chapter, though we refer the reader to other sources, including Argyle (1999; 2001) and one of our previous reviews (Diener et al., 1999) for more detailed coverage. Our goal here is to point out that although effect sizes have often been found to be quite small, these effects must be interpreted carefully. The types of characteristics reviewed in this section do not account for much variance in SWB scores, but this lack of variance does not necessarily mean that they are unimportant. Individuals who become unemployed, acquire a disability, or lose contact with a close friend may, in fact, experience lasting changes as a consequence of these losses. Thus, SWB may be more strongly influenced by life circumstances than has generally been assumed.

Heritability of SWB

The second piece of evidence for personality effects comes from behavioral genetic studies that examine the heritability of the various SWB components. In the typical design, identical and fraternal twins complete happiness measures and then the cross-twin correlations are compared. Simple additive genetic effects are implied when the cross-twin correlation for identical twins is approximately twice as large as the cross-twin correlation for fraternal twins. Nonadditive genetic effects are implied when the ratio of identical to fraternal twin correlations is higher than two (though more sophisticated designs are often required to isolate these effects). Extensions of the basic twin design can be used to examine additional questions about the heritability of happiness. For instance, the inclusion of twins who were raised in different households allows researchers to isolate shared-environment effects more precisely and to rule out alternative explanations of the results. In addition, by acquiring multiple waves of data over time, researchers can examine the genetic effects on stability and change.

A number of studies have been conducted to examine the heritability of various well-being measures, and most arrive at similar conclusions about the broad heritability of SWB. For instance, in perhaps the first such study, Tellegen and colleagues (1988) examined twins who were reared together and those who were reared apart to estimate the contribution of genes and environment to various scales from the Multidimensional Personality Questionnaire. The estimated heritabilities of the well-being facet and global positive emotionality factor were .48 and .40, respectively. The heritabilities of the stress reaction facet and negative emotionality factor were .53 and .55, respectively. These estimates suggest that about half of the variance in these well-being measures could be accounted for by shared genes. Importantly, this study also suggested that growing up in the same household played very little role in the similarity of twins. The only significant shared-environment effect was for the global positive emotionality trait, where this component accounted for 22% of the variance.

One criticism that could be raised about this study is that the assessed measures were not developed as measures of subjective well-being. Instead, they were developed to assess stable personality characteristics that have an affective core. Thus, they may not reflect "happiness" as it is typically studied by SWB researchers. However, more recent studies have replicated this basic effect using a variety of measures. For instance, Roysamb, Harris, Magnus, Vitterso, and Tambs (2002; also see Roysamb, Tambs, Reichborn-Kjennerud, Neale, & Harris, 2003) examined the heritability of a four-item global well-being measure that assessed satisfaction, happiness, nervousness, and activity level. Like Tellegen and colleagues (1988), they found that about 50% of the variance could be accounted for by a genetic component, and the shared-environment component contributed very little. Similarly, Stubbe, Posthuma, Boomsma, and DeGeus (2005) reported that 38% of the variability in the SWLS (Diener et al., 1985) was heritable.

These studies consistently show that regardless of the measure that is used, broad heritability estimates for well-being constructs tend to fall between .40 and .50. However, this does not mean that behavioral genetic research is without controversy. Perhaps the most controversial issue relates to questions regarding the heritability of the stable component of happiness. According to one prominent model of SWB, people have a setpoint level of happiness that is stable over time (Brickman & Campbell, 1971). Events and life circumstances can move peo-

ple away from this setpoint, but eventually people adapt and return to baseline. Thus, at any given moment, a person's happiness score might reflect the combined effects of the stable baseline and the temporary influence of life events. If so, the heritability of happiness might be higher if the stable baseline could be isolated from these temporary deviations.

In 1996, Lykken and Tellegen attempted to accomplish this goal using data from identical and fraternal twins who completed happiness measures on two occasions separated by approximately 10 years. Lykken and Tellegen found that the stability of well-being was about .50, meaning that approximately 50% of the variance at either of the two occasions was stable trait variance. But more importantly, they found that the cross-time, cross-twin correlation was .40 in the identical twins. Because this cross-twin, cross-time correlation is 80% as large as the stability coefficient, Lykken and Tellegen estimated that 80% of the stable component of well-being is heritable. The authors suggested that this extremely high heritability means that "trying to be happier [may be] as futile as trying to be taller" (p. 189).

There are three reasons why this conclusion may be too extreme. First, as Rutter (1997) noted, estimates of heritability "provide no unambiguous implications for theory, policy, or practice" (p. 391). In other words, even if Lykken and Tellegen's (1996) estimate of heritability is correct, this does not necessarily mean that happiness cannot be changed. Until the mechanisms by which these genetic effects work are discovered, questions about the possibility for change remain even when the heritability is known to be strong.

Second, the high heritability only refers to the part of happiness that is stable over time, and this makes up only about half of the variance at any given wave in Lykken and Tellegen's (1996) study. Furthermore, these stability estimates appear to be at the upper bound for what is typically found in longitudinal studies of SWB. As we review in the section on stability below, most studies find 10-year stabilities that are somewhat lower than that found by Lykken and Tellegen. Thus, even if the stable component was 100% heritable and completely unchangeable, there would still be considerable room for change.

Finally, Lykken and Tellegen's (1996) conclusion is based on a single study with a relatively small sample of twins. Although a more recent study has replicated these findings in a much larger sample (Nes, Roysamb, Tambs, Harris, & Reichborn-Kjennerud, 2006), a second study has not. Johnson, McGue, and Krueger (2005) presented cross-twin, cross-time correlations that suggest that 38% of the stable variance in well-being is heritable (though they did not set out to address this question and did not explicitly analyze their data in this way). The major difference between these two samples was the age of the participants. The Johnson and colleagues study included older adults, whereas the Nes and colleagues study and the original Lykken and colleagues study included a sample of participants in their 20s. Thus, with only three studies available, the replicability of this more controversial effect (along with the role that age plays in this effect) cannot be evaluated.

Stability of SWB

It is tempting to interpret heritability statistics as an index of changeability. But as noted above, there is no direct and necessary correspondence between the heritability of a characteristic and the extent to which it can change. If the process linking genes to well-being is indirect, then even characteristics with very strong heritabilities could be changed if the underlying processes were identified and effective interventions were designed. Furthermore, because even stable biological characteristics can be changed under the right circumstances (e.g., Davidson et al., 2003), even a direct link from genes to physiology to SWB does not guarantee that change cannot occur. Therefore, for researchers interested in the stability of SWB over time, it is important to address this question directly. How stable is happiness, and is there evidence that lasting changes can occur under the right circumstances?

For decades, psychologists have recognized that there is considerable stability in people's affective and cognitive evaluations of their lives. This stability is reflected both in the consistency of individuals' affective reactions to distinct situations and in the maintenance of their relative level of global happiness over time. For instance, in his early studies on the consistency of personality, Ep-

stein (1979) showed that affect during any one day correlates relatively weakly with affect on any other day. However, once affect is aggregated over multiple days, strong correlations emerge. Similarly, momentary affect was assessed across multiple situations using the experience sampling method (Diener & Larsen, 1984). Like Epstein, it was found that moment-to-moment correlations were quite weak. However, once affect ratings were aggregated within similar types of situations, average levels of affect were highly consistent over time and across situations. For instance, average positive affect at work correlated .70 with average positive affect experienced during recreation. Similarly, average negative affect at work correlated .74 with average negative affect during recreation. Thus, there are stable individual differences in the level of positive and negative affect that emerge even across diverse situations.

Of course, cross-situational consistency does not guarantee long-term stability, and therefore to determine whether happiness can change, it is necessary to conduct longitudinal studies over very long periods of time. Results of such studies show that the various SWB components exhibit moderate long-term stability. For instance, Schimmack and Oishi (2005) conducted a meta-analysis of existing studies that had examined the stability of life satisfaction measures. Not surprisingly, they found that stability decreased with increasing intervals. However, even after relatively long periods of time had elapsed, life satisfaction measures were moderately stable. For instance, the predicted 2-, 5-, and 10-year stabilities were approximately .60, .50, and .35, respectively.

More recently, Fujita and Diener (2005) and Lucas and Donnellan (2006) used data from large-scale panel studies to estimate the stability of a single-item life satisfaction measure. Fujita and Diener showed that even over a period of 17 years, the stability of life satisfaction was approximately .25. Lucas and Donnellan used the same data and an additional panel study to isolate stable trait variance from slowly changing autoregressive variance and unstable state variance. They calculated that between 34 and 38% of the variance in single-item life satisfaction measures is trait variance that is perfectly stable over time. Thus, these estimates predict that long-term stabilities should asymptote around .35.

Fewer studies have been conducted examining the long-term stability of affect measures, but the research that exists lead to comparable conclusions to those from studies of life satisfaction. For instance, Watson and Walker (1996) examined the 3-year stability of affect ratings and found correlations that ranged from .36 to .46. Lucas and colleagues (1996) found slightly higher estimates, with 3-year stabilities of .56 and .61 for positive and negative affect, respectively. They also showed that these stabilities only dropped slightly (to .42 and .45) when self-reports were used to predict informant reports 3 years later (Magnus, 1991, reported similar results for self- and informant reports of life satisfaction). Thus, like life satisfaction, positive and negative affect are moderately stable over time.

It is important to note, however, that these stabilities tend to be lower than the stability of other personality traits. For instance, Schimmack and Oishi's (2005) meta-analysis and Lucas and Donnellan's (2006) analysis of the GSOEP data suggest that the 20-year stability for life satisfaction should be around .30–.35. Roberts and DelVecchio (2000) conducted similar analyses using personality traits, and they estimated that the 20-year stability for personality traits would be around .41. However, because Roberts and DelVecchio only reported the predicted 20-year stability for the least stable group of adults in their meta-analysis (20-year-olds), this value probably underestimates the long-term stability of personality traits among a broader sample of participants. For example, Roberts and DelVecchio found that the average stability coefficient for 18- to 20-year-olds was .54, whereas the average stability coefficient for 50- to 59-year-olds was .74. Thus, these comparisons show that SWB variables, while moderately stable over long periods of time, tend to be less stable than other established personality traits (also see Vaidya, Gray, Haig, & Watson, 2002).

Examination of stability coefficients provides one important piece of information about the extent to which personality can change. However, there are alternative techniques for investigating change that go beyond simply assessing rank-order stability. For instance, stability coefficients alone cannot distinguish stochastic change (where a variety of factors causes random changes that accumulate over time) from systematic change resulting from major life events (Fraley & Roberts, 2005). To assess the reasons for change, more sophisticated designs are required.

Recently, we have turned to the analysis of large-scale, long-running, nationally representative panel studies to determine whether major life events have lasting effects on SWB. These studies allow us to examine long-term levels of SWB both before and after events occur. This means that preexisting differences between those who experienced a particular life event and those who did not can be separated from true longitudinal change. Three important conclusions can be drawn from these studies (for a review see Diener, Lucas, & Scollon, 2006).

First, life events can have important effects on long-term levels of SWB. Divorce (Lucas, 2005), unemployment (Lucas et al., 2003), and the onset of a long-term disability (Lucas, 2007) are all associated with lasting changes in life satisfaction, and the effects can sometimes be quite large. For instance, the onset of a lasting disability was associated with more than a half a standard deviation drop in life satisfaction. The effects of severe disabilities were even larger, with effect sizes over a full standard deviation.

Second, there is no single answer to the question of whether people adapt to major life events. Very little adaptation occurred following the onset of disability, even over very long periods of time (Lucas, 2006). For events such as unemployment and divorce, on the other hand, some amount of adaptation occurred, but this adaptation was incomplete (Lucas, 2005; Lucas et al., 2004). Finally, for events such as marriage and widowhood, a great deal of adaptation occurred, with average levels of happiness returning to pre-event levels (Lucas et al., 2003).

Finally, there are considerable individual differences in the amount of change that occurs following life events. Because pre-event levels of SWB are known in these studies, it is possible to examine both average change as well as variability around this average level. Analyses show that the amount of variability is often quite large. For instance, Lucas and colleagues (2003) showed that on average, people adapt to marriage. Within approximately 2 or 3 years after marriage, participants who got married were no happier than they were before they got married. However, the amount of variability in the change scores was almost as great as the variability that existed in pre-event baseline levels. Thus, many people reported lasting positive changes in happiness following the marriage, but there were also many people who reported lasting negative changes. Importantly, results showed that those people who had very positive initial reactions to marriage were also still far from baseline many years later. Thus, the fact that happiness levels are not greater after marriage than they were before marriage does not mean that adaptation is inevitable. Instead, the results from this study of marriage show that the same event may affect individuals in different ways, and these differential reactions may hide the amount of true change that occurs.

Associations with Personality Traits

The final piece of evidence we review concerns the empirical links between personality and SWB. In 1967, Warner Wilson published one of the first reviews of the literature on the correlates of what he called "avowed happiness." Although this review was based on a fairly small body of evidence, Wilson's conclusions foreshadowed modern research quite well. Although some external circumstances were judged to be important, many of the most reliable findings concerned individuals' characteristic outlook on life. For instance, his summary suggests that the happy person is "extraverted, optimistic, worry-free" and has high self-esteem and modest aspirations (p. 294). The research conducted since Wilson published this review confirms that personality characteristics often exhibit moderate to strong correlations with well-being variables.

The personality characteristics that have been most frequently studied in relation to SWB are extraversion and neuroticism (Diener & Lucas, 1999). As early as the 1930s, researchers had linked characteristics such as social interest and the tendency to worry to reports of subjective well-being (e.g., Jasper, 1930; see Wilson, 1967, for a review). Research on these characteristics continued in the years that followed, but the modern focus on these two traits is often traced to a landmark study by Costa and McCrae (1980). These researchers argued that the broad trait

of extraversion influenced feelings of positive affect, the trait of neuroticism influenced negative affect, and together these two components of emotional well-being influenced overall feelings of life satisfaction. In support of this hypothesis, Costa and McCrae found that extraversion was correlated with feelings of positive affect, and neuroticism was correlated with negative affect. Although the correlations in their study were actually quite weak (e.g., rs around .20), the fact that they were stable over time led Costa and McCrae to suggest that stable individual differences were important for well-being. The basic pattern of results that Costa and McCrae identified has been replicated often (Emmons & Diener, 1985; Headey & Wearing, 1989; Magnus, Diener, Fujita, & Pavot, 1993) and has been found using non-self-report measures of personality and subjective well-being (Lucas & Fujita, 2000).

Yet in a comprehensive meta-analysis of the literature on personality and SWB, DeNeve and Cooper (1998) found that the associations between these two personality traits and SWB were not particularly strong. For instance, the correlation between extraversion and SWB was only .17, and the correlation for neuroticism was only .22. These correlations were significantly different from zero, but surprisingly weak. In addition, they were approximately the same size as the correlations that emerged from meta-analyses of demographic predictors of well-being. Thus, DeNeve and Cooper's review suggested that once meta-analytic techniques were used, the correlations that had been emphasized in narrative reviews were not so large after all.

Although the scope of DeNeve and Cooper's (1998) meta-analysis is impressive, there are also reasons to interpret these results cautiously. As with all meta-analyses, decisions must be made about which studies to include and which predictors and outcomes are similar enough to be treated as equivalent. If trait measures that do not really tap the dimension in question are included in the analysis, then the average correlation with well-being may be diluted. Similarly, if correlations with different forms of SWB are aggregated even when those different components are only weakly correlated with one another, then the meta-analytic averages may not accurately reflect the associations with the individual components themselves.

There is some evidence that these factors contributed to the surprisingly weak correlations found in DeNeve and Cooper's (1998) meta-analysis. For instance, it was suggested that the correlation between extraversion and positive affect would be higher if only established extraversion scales were assessed (Lucas & Fujita, 2000). Furthermore, it was argued that existing theory would predict that the association between extraversion and positive affect should be stronger than the correlation with the other components of SWB. Thus, this link should be examined separately. An updated meta-analysis was conducted that focused only on established extraversion scales and the positive affect component of SWB and a meta-analytic average correlation of .37 was found—considerably higher than the estimate found by DeNeve and Cooper.

This finding has been confirmed in a larger meta-analysis that focused specifically on the associations between SWB and the personality trait measures from three widely used personality inventories: the NEO Personality Inventory—Revised (NEO-PI-R; Costa & McCrae, 1992), the Eysenck Personality Inventory (EPI; H. J. Eysenck & Eysenck, 1968), and the Eysenck Personality Questionnaire (EPQ; S. B. J. Eysenck & Eysenck, 1975). Shultz, Schmidt, and Steel's (2008) analysis shows that when results from only established scales are used, correlations are much higher than those found by DeNeve and Cooper (1998). For instance, the correlations between extraversion and positive affect were .44 for the NEO, .35 for the EPQ, and .25 for the EPI (Lucas & Fujita, 2000, also found that the EPI exhibited weaker correlations, probably because of the inclusion of an impulsivity component). The correlations between neuroticism and negative affect were .54 for the NEO, .53 for the EPQ, and .46 for the EPI. These results confirm the importance of extraversion and neuroticism as predictors of SWB.

Both DeNeve and Cooper's (1998) and Shultz, Schmidt, and Steel's (2006) meta-analyses also show that extraversion and neuroticism are not the only traits that matter. For instance, Shultz et al. showed that correlations between agreeableness and SWB constructs were consistently significantly different from zero and ranged from .12 for positive affect to .30 for happiness. Similarly, correlations with conscientiousness ranged from −.21 for negative affect to .40 for overall quality of life. DeNeve and Cooper (1998) found that repressiveness–defensiveness, trust, hardiness, and some forms of locus of control and self-esteem also exhibited relatively high correlations (though many of these correlations were derived from a very small number of studies). Finally, personality traits such as optimism and self-esteem reflect general positive views about the self and the world, and they too have been shown to correlate with well-being (e.g., Lucas et al., 1996; Schimmack & Diener, 2003).

Explanations for these associations generally take one of two forms. McCrae and Costa (1991) suggested that *instrumental theories* posit an indirect link from personality to SWB through choice of situations or the experience of life events. For example, extraverts may enjoy and participate in social activities, which may in turn affect the amounts of positive affect that they experience. These instrumental theories can be contrasted with *temperament theories*, which posit a direct link from the trait to the outcome in question. According to temperament theories, the association does not flow through life choices, life events, or life experiences.

The most widely studied temperament theories link extraversion and neuroticism to affect through two basic motivational systems that have been proposed and investigated by Gray (1970, 1981, 1991; see also Elliot & Thrash, 2002; Tellegen, 1985). According to Gray, much of the variability in personality can be explained by three fundamental systems: the behavioral activation system (BAS), which regulates reactions to signals of conditioned reward and nonpunishment; the behavioral inhibition system (BIS), which regulates reactions to signals of conditioned punishment and nonreward; and the fight–flight system (FFS), which regulates reactions to signals of unconditioned punishment and nonreward. Extraverts are though to be higher in BAS strength, and thus, they should be more sensitive to signals of reward. This reward sensitivity should be expressed in the form of enhanced information processing and increased positive emotions when exposed to positive stimuli. Similarly, the neuroticism dimension is thought to reflect individual differences in BIS strength. Thus, neurotics should be more sensitive than stable people to signals of punishment.

Tests of these hypotheses have proceeded either by ruling out instrumental explanations of the associations (e.g., by determining whether social activity mediates the association between extraversion and positive affect; e.g., Lucas, Le, & Dyrenforth, in press) or by examining possible direct links between the constructs. For instance, Larsen and Ketelaar (1991) showed that extraverts are more sensitive than introverts to laboratory-based positive mood induction procedures and that neurotics are more sensitive than stable individuals to negative mood induction procedures (though, see Lucas & Baird, 2004, for meta-analytic evidence suggesting that the extraversion effect is not reliable). Other researchers have used paradigms that assess attention to and memory for positive and negative events (e.g., Derryberry & Reed, 1994; Rusting, 1998). Finally, researchers have linked these individual differences and affective reactions through specific psychophysiological processes (e.g., Canli, 2004; Depue & Collins, 1999; Depue & Morrone-Strupinsky, 2005). Theoretical progress on the links between these traits and well-being outcomes have advanced rapidly in recent years.

It is also important to note that personality traits are not the only personality constructs that have been studied in relation to SWB. Other stable individual differences have also been shown to be associated with well-being. For instance, Wilson's (1967) suggestion that aspirations affect well-being has been supported by more recent research. A number of studies show that the goals held by individuals are reliably associated with happiness constructs. For instance, Emmons (1986) showed that distinct characteristics of people's goals correlate with the various SWB components in different ways. Positive affect was associated with past fulfillment of goals and the degree of effort that the goal required, whereas negative affect was associated with lower perceived probability of success and high conflict between goals. Other personality researchers have examined stable individual differences in cognitive factors (e.g., Robinson & Compton, 2008) or emotion regulation strategies (e.g., John & Gross, 2004) that may play a role in SWB. A goal for future research will be to understand the processes that underlie the various characteristics that are related to well-being and to determine which are most important in driving this highly valued outcome.

SUMMARY

The research reviewed in this chapter shows that when studying SWB, personality matters. Happiness, like most personality characteristics, is moderately heritable and moderately stable over time. In addition, happiness has been linked to specific personality traits and processes. In fact, the correlations between SWB and personality characteristics such as extraversion and neuroticism are stronger than correlations with any demographic predictor or major life circumstance that has been studied so far. Thus, a theory of well-being that fails to incorporate personality characteristics would be incomplete, and much of what we know about well-being comes from taking a personality perspective on the construct.

That being said, some caution is warranted when interpreting the evidence that has been presented in support of personality effects. For instance, it is important not to interpret strong heritabilities as evidence that happiness cannot change. Until researchers understand the processes that underlie stable individual differences in SWB, questions about the possibility for change remain unanswered. In addition, our review suggests that researchers should be careful not to dismiss effects that may appear to be quite small at first, but that have important implications for individual experience. Income may only account for about 5% of the variance in happiness, but this relatively small effect can hide the fact that the wealthy are considerably happier than individuals who live at the poverty level and below. Finally, although the stability of SWB over long periods of time is impressive, it appears that at most about 35% of the variance reflects a stable trait component that does not change over time (though the percentage of reliable variance is probably higher). In addition, the study of major life events shows that significant changes in life circumstances can have large and lasting effects on happiness. Thus, well-being is responsive to life events and changing life circumstances—which leaves hope that it can be improved.

Researchers and practitioners hoping to use SWB in applied settings are sometimes dismayed by the effects described in this chapter. But it is important to realize that even if there is a reasonable amount of stability and strong personality effects, attempts to improve overall levels of SWB can still be a worthwhile goal. As an analogue, we can consider physical health. If it was possible to construct a purely objective index of overall physical health, it is likely that this index would be moderately to strongly stable over time, moderately heritable, and at least somewhat related to personality traits. Yet these facts alone would probably not persuade medical researchers to give up their quest to improve levels of health. Instead, research on the stability and personality correlates of this construct would be incorporated into broad theories that explain the processes that underlie these stable individual differences in physical health. This should also be true of research on SWB. Much of what we know about the construct comes from studies that investigate the personality predictors of the trait. This research can be used to develop broad theories that explain both stability and change in happiness over time.

REFERENCES

Andrews, F. M., & Withey, S. B. (1976). *Social indicators of well-being.* New York: Plenum Press.

Argyle, M. (1999). Causes and correlates of happiness. In D. Kahneman, E. Diener, & N. Schwarz (Ed.), *Well-being: The foundations of hedonic psychology* (pp. 353–373). New York: Sage Foundation.

Argyle, M. (2001). *The psychology of happiness* (2nd ed.). New York: Routledge.

Berkman, L. F., & Syme, S. L. (1979). Social networks, host resistance, and mortality: A nine-year follow-up study of Alameda county residents. *American Journal of Epidemiology, 109*(2), 186–204.

Biswas-Diener, R., & Diener, E. (2001). Making the best of a bad situation: Satisfaction in the slums of Calcutta. *Social Indicators Research, 55,* 329–352.

Brickman, P., & Campbell, D. T. (1971). Hedonic relativism and planning the good society. In M. H. Appley (Ed.), *Adaptation level theory: A symposium* (pp. 287–302). New York: Academic Press.

Brickman, P., Coates, D., & Janoff-Bulman, R. (1978). Lottery winners and accident victims: Is happiness relative? *Journal of Personality and Social Psychology, 36,* 917–927.

Brief, A. P., Butcher, A. H., George, J. M., & Link, K. E. (1993). Integrating bottom-up and top-down theories of subjective well-being: The case of health. *Journal of Personality and Social Psychology, 64*(4), 646–653.

Canli, T. (2004). Functional brain mapping of extraversion and neuroticism: Learning from individual differences in emotion processing. *Journal of Personality, 72,* 1105–1132.

Carver, C. S. (2003). Pleasure as a sign you can attend to something else: Placing positive feelings within a general model of affect. *Cognition and Emotion, 17*(2), 241–261.

Carver, C. S., Sutton, S. K., & Scheier, M. F. (2000). Action, emotion, and personality: Emerging conceptual integration. *Personality and Social Psychology Bulletin, 26,* 741–751.

Clark, A., Georgellis, Y., & Sanfey, P. (1998). Job satisfaction, wage changes and quits: Evidence from Germany. *Research in Labor Economics, 17,* 95–121.

Costa, P. T., Jr., & McCrae, R. R. (1980). Influence of extraversion and neuroticism on subjective well-being: Happy and unhappy people. *Journal of Personality and Social Psychology, 38,* 668–678.

Costa, P. T., Jr., & McCrae, R. R. (1992). *Revised NEO Personality Inventory (NEO PI-R) and NEO Five-Factor Inventory (NEO-FFI): Professional manual.* Odessa, FL: Psychological Assessment Resources.

Davidson, R. J. (2004). Well-being and affective style: Neural substrates and biobehavioural correlates. *Philophical Transactions of the Royal Society of London B, 359,* 1395–1411.

Davidson, R. J., Kabat-Zinn, J., Schumacher, J., Rosenkranz, M., Muller, D., Santorelli, S. F., et al. (2003). Alterations in brain and immune function produced by mindfulness meditation. *Psychosomatic Medicine, 65*(4), 564–570.

Davis, J. A., Smith, T. W., & Marsden, P. V. (2003). *General social surveys, 1972–2002.* Ann Arbor, MI: Inter-University Consortium for Political and Social Research. Available at *www.webapp.icpsr.umich.edu/GSS/.*

DeNeve, K. M., & Cooper, H. (1998). The happy personality: A meta-analysis of 137 personality traits and subjective well-being. *Psychological Bulletin, 124,* 197–229.

Depue, R. A., & Collins, P. F. (1999). Neurobiology of the structure of personality: Dopamine, facilitation of incentive motivation, and extraversion. *Behavioral and Brain Sciences, 22,* 491–569.

Depue, R. A., & Morrone-Strupinsky, J. V. (2005). A neurobehavioral model of affiliative bonding: Implications for conceptualizing a human trait of affiliation. *Behavioral and Brain Sciences, 28,* 313–395.

Derryberry, D., & Reed, M. A. (1994). Temperament and attention: Orienting toward and away from positive and negative signals. *Journal of Personality and Social Psychology, 66,* 1128–1139.

Diener, E. (1984). Subjective well-being. *Psychological Bulletin, 95,* 542–575.

Diener, E. (2000). Subjective well-being: The science of happiness and a proposal for a national index. *American Psychologist, 55*(1), 34–43.

Diener, E., & Biswas-Diener, R. (2002). Will money increase subjective well-being? A literature review and guide to needed research. *Social Indicators Research, 57*, 119–169.

Diener, E., Emmons, R. A., Larsen, R. J., & Griffin, S. (1985). The Satisfaction with Life Scale. *Journal of Personality Assessment, 49*(1), 71–75.

Diener, E., & Larsen, R. J. (1984). Temporal stability and cross-situational consistency of affective, behavioral, and cognitive responses. *Journal of Personality and Social Psychology, 47*, 871–883.

Diener, E., & Lucas, R. E. (1999). Personality and subjective well-being. In D. Kahneman, E. Diener, & N. Schwarz (Eds.), *Well-being: The foundations of hedonic psychology* (pp. 213–229). New York: Sage Foundation.

Diener, E., Lucas, R. E., & Scollon, C. (2006). Beyond the hedonic treadmill: Revising the adaptation theory of well-being. *American Psychologist, 61*, 305–314.

Diener, E., & Oishi, S. (2004). Are Scandinavians happier than Asians?: Issues in comparing nations on subjective well-being. In F. Columbus (Ed.), *Asian economic and political issues* (Vol. 10, pp. 1–25). Hauppauge, NY: Nova Science.

Diener, E., Sandvik, E., & Pavot, W. (1991). Happiness is the frequency, not the intensity, of positive versus negative affect. In F. Strack, M. Argyle, & N. Schwarz (Eds.), *Subjective well-being: An interdisciplinary perspective* (pp. 119–139). Elmsford, NY: Pergamon Press.

Diener, E., & Seligman, M. E. P. (2004). Beyond money: Toward an economy of well-being. *Psychological Science in the Public Interest, 5*, 1–31.

Diener, E., Suh, E. M., Lucas, R. E., & Smith, H. L. (1999). Subjective well-being: Three decades of progress. *Psychological Bulletin, 125*, 276–302.

Dijkers, M. (1997). Quality of life after spinal cord injury: A meta analysis of the effects of disablement components. *Spinal Cord, 35*, 829–840.

Eid, M., & Diener, E. (2004). Global judgments of subjective well-being: Situational variability and long-term stability. *Social Indicators Research, 65*, 245–277.

Elliot, A. J., & Thrash, T. M. (2002). Approach–avoidance motivation in personality: Approach and avoidance temperaments and goals. *Journal of Personality and Social Psychology, 82*, 804–818.

Emmons, R. A. (1986). Personal strivings: An approach to personality and subjective well-being.

Journal of Personality and Social Psychology, 51(5), 1058–1068.

Emmons, R. A., & Diener, E. (1985). Personality correlates of subjective well-being. *Personality and Social Psychology Bulletin, 11*(1), 89–97.

Epstein, S. (1979). The stability of behavior: I. On predicting most of the people much of the time. *Journal of Personality and Social Psychology, 37*, 1097–1126.

Eysenck, H. J., & Eysenck, S. B. G. (1968). *Manual of the Eysenck Personality Inventory*. San Diego, CA: Education and Industrial Testing Service.

Eysenck, S. B. J., & Eysenck, H. J. (1975). *Manual of the Eysenck Personality Questionnaire*. London: Hodder & Stoughton.

Feist, G. J., Bodner, T. E., Jacobs, J. F., Miles, M., & Tan, V. (1995). Integrating top-down and bottom-up structural models of subjective well-being: A longitudinal investigation. *Journal of Personality and Social Psychology, 68*(1), 138–150.

Fraley, R. C., & Roberts, B. W. (2005). Patterns of continuity: A dynamic model for conceptualizing the stability of individual differences in psychological constructs across the life course. *Psychological Review, 112*(1), 60–74.

Fredrickson, B. L. (1998). What good are positive emotions? *Review of General Psychology: New Directions in Research on Emotion, 2*(3), 300–319.

Frijters, P. (2000). Do individuals try to maximise general satisfaction? *Journal of Economic Psychology, 21*, 281–304.

Fujita, F., & Diener, E. (2005). Life satisfaction set point: Stability and change. *Journal of Personality and Social Psychology, 88*, 158–164.

Ganz, P. A., Lee, J. J., & Siau, J. (1991). Quality of life assessment: An independent prognostic variable for survival in lung cancer. *Cancer, 67*, 3131–3135.

Gilbert, D. (2006). *Stumbling on happiness*. New York: Knopf.

Gilovich, T., & Eibach, R. (2001). The fundamental attribution error where it really counts. *Psychological Inquiry, 12*(1), 23–26.

Gray, J. A. (1970). The psychophysiological basis of introversion–extraversion. *Behaviour Research and Therapy, 8*, 249–266.

Gray, J. A. (1981). A critique of Eysenck's theory of personality. In H. J. Eysenck (Ed.), *A model for personality* (pp. 246–276). New York: Springer-Verlag.

Gray, J. A. (1991). Neural systems, emotion, and personality. In J. Madden (Ed.), *Neurobiology of learning, emotion, and affect* (pp. 273–306). New York: Raven Press.

Gross, J. J. (1999). Emotion and emotion regulation. In L. A. Pervin & O. P. John (Eds.), *Handbook of personality: Theory and research* (2nd ed., pp. 525–552). New York: Guilford Press.

Haring, M., Stock, W. A., & Okun, M. A. (1984). A research synthesis of gender and social class as correlates of subjective well-being. *Human Relations, 37,* 645–657.

Haring-Hidore, M., Stock, W. A., Okun, M. A., & Witter, R. A. (1985). Marital status and subjective well-being: A research synthesis. *Journal of Marriage and the Family, 47*(4), 947–953.

Headey, B., & Wearing, A. (1989). Personality, life events, and subjective well-being: Toward a dynamic equilibrium model. *Journal of Personality and Social Psychology, 57,* 731–739.

Heller, D., Watson, D., & Ilies, R. (2004). The role of person versus situation in life satisfaction: A critical examination. *Psychological Bulletin, 130,* 574–600.

Hogan, R., Johnson, J. A., & Briggs, S. R. (Eds.). (1997). *Handbook of personality psychology.* San Diego, CA: Academic Press.

House, J. S., Landis, K. R., & Umberson, D. (1988). Social relationships and health. *Science, 241*(4865), 540–545.

House, J. S., Robbins, C., & Metzner, H. L. (1982). The association of social relationships and activities with mortality: Prospective evidence from the Tecumseh Community Health Study. *American Journal of Epidemiology, 116*(1), 123–140.

James, W. (1902). *Varieties of religious experience: A study in human nature.* New York: Longmans, Green.

Jasper, H. H. (1930). The measurement of depression–elation and its relation to a measure of extraversion–introversion. *Journal of Abnormal and Social Psychology, 25,* 307–318.

John, O. P., & Gross, J. J. (2004). Healthy and unhealthy emotion regulation: Personality processes, individual differences, and life span development. *Journal of Personality, 72*(6), 1301–1334.

Johnson, W., McGue, M., & Krueger, R. F. (2005). Personality stability in late adulthood: A behavioral genetic analysis. *Journal of Personality, 73*(2), 523–551.

Judge, T. A., & Watanabe, S. (1993). Another look at the job satisfaction–life satisfaction relationship. *Journal of Applied Psychology, 78*(6), 939–948.

Kahneman, D. (1999). Objective happiness. In D. Kahneman, E. Diener, & N. Schwarz (Eds.), *Well-being: The foundations of hedonic psychology* (pp. 3–25). New York: Sage Foundation.

Kahneman, D., Krueger, A. B., Schkade, D., Schwarz, N., & Stone, A. (2003). Toward national well-being accounts. *American Economic Review, 94,* 429–434.

Kahneman, D., & Riis, J. (2005). Living and thinking about it: Two perspectives on life. In F. A. Huppert, N. Baylis, & B. Keverne (Eds.),

The science of well-being (pp. 285–304). New York: Oxford University Press.

Kim-Prieto, C., Diener, E., Tamir, M., Scollon, C. N., & Diener, M. (2005). Integrating the diverse definitions of happiness: A time-sequential framework of subjective well-being. *Journal of Happiness Studies, 6*(3), 261–300.

Koivumaa-Honkanen, H., Honkanen, R., Koskenvuo, M., Kaprio, J., & Alcohol Research. (2003). Self-reported happiness in life and suicide in ensuing 20 years. *Social Psychiatry and Psychiatric Epidemiology, 38*(5), 244–248.

Koivumaa-Honkanen, H., Honkanen, R., Viinamäki, H., Heikkilä, K., Kaprio, J., & Koskenvuo, M. (2001). Life satisfaction and suicide: A 20-year follow-up study. *American Journal of Psychiatry, 158*(3), 433–439.

Koivumaa-Honkanen, H., Kaprio, J., Honkanen, R., Viinamäki, H., & Koskenvuo, M. (2004). Life satisfaction and depression in a 15-year follow-up of healthy adults. *Social Psychiatry and Psychiatric Epidemiology, 39*(12), 994–999.

Larsen, R. J., & Ketelaar, T. (1991). Personality and susceptibility to positive and negative emotional states. *Journal of Personality and Social Psychology, 61,* 132–140.

Lucas, R. E. (2005). Time does not heal all wounds: A longitudinal study of reaction and adaptation to divorce. *Psychological Science, 16,* 945–950.

Lucas, R. E. (2007). Long-term disability has lasting effects on subjective well-being: Evidence from two nationally representative panel studies. *Journal of Personality and Social Psychology, 92,* 717–730.

Lucas, R. E., & Baird, B. M. (2004). Extraversion and emotional reactivity. *Journal of Personality and Social Psychology, 86,* 473–485.

Lucas, R. E., Clark, A. E., Georgellis, Y., & Diener, E. (2003). Reexamining adaptation and the set point model of happiness: Reactions to changes in marital status. *Journal of Personality and Social Psychology, 84,* 527–539.

Lucas, R. E., Clark, A. E., Georgellis, Y., & Diener, E. (2004). Unemployment alters the set point for life satisfaction. *Psychological Science, 15,* 8–13.

Lucas, R. E., & Diener, E. (2008). Subjective well-being. In M. Lewis & J. M. Haviland (Eds.), *Handbook of emotions* (3rd ed., pp. 471–484). New York: Guilford Press.

Lucas, R. E., Diener, E., & Suh, E. (1996). Discriminant validity of well-being measures. *Journal of Personality and Social Psychology, 71*(3), 616–628.

Lucas, R. E., & Donnellan, M. B. (2007). Can happiness change?: Using the STARTS model to estimate the stability of subjective well-being. *Journal of Research in Personality, 41,* 1091–1098.

Lucas, R. E., & Dyrenforth, P. S. (2005). The

myth of marital bliss? *Psychological Inquiry*, *16*(2–3), 111–115.

Lucas, R. E., & Dyrenforth, P. S. (2006). Does the existence of social relationships matter for subjective well-being? In K. D. Vohs & E. J. Finkel (Eds.), *Self and relationships: Connecting intrapersonal and interpersonal processes* (pp. 254–273). New York: Guilford Press.

Lucas, R. E., & Fujita, F. (2000). Factors influencing the relation between extraversion and pleasant affect. *Journal of Personality and Social Psychology*, *79*, 1039–1056.

Lucas, R. E., Le, K., & Dyrenforth, P. S. (in press). Explaining the extraversion/positive affect relation: Sociability cannot account for extraverts' greater happiness. *Journal of Personality*.

Lucas, R. E., & Schimmack, U. (2007). *Money matters*. Manuscript in preparation, Michigan State University.

Lykken, D., & Tellegen, A. (1996). Happiness is a stochastic phenomenon. *Psychological Science*, *7*, 186–189.

Lyubomirsky, S., King, L., & Diener, E. (2005). The benefits of frequent positive affect: Does happiness lead to success? *Psychological Bulletin*, *131*, 803–855.

Lyubomirsky, S., Sheldon, K. M., & Schkade, D. (2005). Pursuing happiness: The architecture of sustainable change. *Review of General Psychology*, *9*, 111–131.

Magnus, K. B. (1991). *A longitudinal analysis of personality, life events, and subjective well-being*. Unpublished manuscript, University of Illinois.

Magnus, K. B., Diener, E., Fujita, F., & Pavot, W. (1993). Extraversion and neuroticism as predictors of objective life events: A longitudinal analysis. *Journal of Personality and Social Psychology*, *65*, 316–330.

Markus, H. R., & Kitayama, S. (1991). Culture and the self: Implications for cognition, emotion, and motivation. *Psychological Review*, *98*, 224–253.

McCrae, R. R., & Costa, P. T., Jr. (1991). Adding *Liebe und Arbeit*: The full five-factor model and well-being. *Personality and Social Psychology Bulletin*, *17*, 227–232.

Mossey, J. M., & Shapiro, E. (1982). Self-rated health: A predictor of mortality among the elderly. *American Journal of Public Health*, *72*, 800–808.

Nelson, E., Conger, B., Douglass, R., Gephart, D., Kirk, J., Page, R., et al. (1983). Functional health status levels of primary care patients. *Journal of the American Medical Association*, *249*, 3331–3338.

Nes, R. B., Roysamb, E., Tambs, K., Harris, J. R., & Reichborn-Kjennerud, T. (2006). Subjective well-being: Genetic and environmental contributions to stability and change. *Psychological Medicine*, *36*(7), 1033–1042.

Okun, M. A., & George, L. K. (1984). Physician- and self-ratings of health, neuroticism and subjective well-being among men and women. *Personality and Individual Differences*, *5*, 533–539.

Okun, M. A., Stock, W. A., Haring, M. J., & Witter, R. A. (1984). Health and subjective well-being: A meta-analysis. *International Journal of Aging and Human Development*, *19*, 111–132.

Pavot, W., & Diener, E. (1993). Review of the Satisfaction with Life Scale. *Psychological Assessment*, *5*(2), 164–172.

Pelled, L. H., & Xin, K. R. (1999). Down and out: An investigation of the relationship between mood and employee withdrawal behavior. *Journal of Management*, *25*, 875–895.

Pervin, L. A. (Ed.). (1990). *Handbook of personality: Theory and research*. New York: Guilford Press.

Pervin, L. A., & John, O. P. (Eds.). (1999). *Handbook of personality: Theory and research* (2nd ed.). New York: Guilford Press.

Pinquart, M., & Sörensen, S. (2000). Influences of socioeconomic status, social network, and competence on subjective well-being in later life: A meta-analysis. *Psychology and Aging*, *15*(2), 187–224.

Putzke, J. D., Richards, J. S., Hicken, B. L., & DeVivo, M. J. (2002). Predictors of life satisfaction: A spinal cord injury cohort study. *Archives of Physical Medicine and Rehabilitation*, *83*, 555–561.

Roberts, B. W., & Del Vecchio, W. F. (2000). The rank-order consistency of personality traits from childhood to old age: A quantitative review of longitudinal studies. *Psychological Bulletin*, *126*, 3–25.

Robinson, M. D., & Clore, G. L. (2002). Belief and feeling: Evidence for an accessibility model of emotional self-report. *Psychological Bulletin*, *128*(6), 934–960.

Robinson, M. D., & Compton, R. J. (2008). The happy mind in action: The cognitive basis of subjective well-being. In M. Eid & R. J. Larsen (Eds.), *The science of subjective well-being* (pp. 220–238). New York: Guilford Press.

Roysamb, E., Harris, J. R., Magnus, P., Vitterso, J., & Tambs, K. (2002). Subjective well-being: Sex-specific effects of genetic and environmental factors. *Personality and Individual Differences*, *32*(2), 211–223.

Roysamb, E., Tambs, K., Reichborn-Kjennerud, T., Neale, M. C., & Harris, J. R. (2003). Happiness and health: Environmental and genetic contributions to the relationship between subjective well-being, perceived health, and somatic illness. *Journal of Personality and Social Psychology*, *85*(6), 1136–1146.

Rumsfeld, J. S., McWhinney, S., McCarthy, M., Jr., Shroyer, A. L. W., VillaNueva, C. B., O'Brien, M., et al. (1999). Health-related quality of life as a predictor of mortality following coronary artery bypass graft surgery. *Journal of the American Medical Association, 281,* 1298–1303.

Rusting, C. L. (1998). Personality, mood, and cognitive processing of emotional information: Three conceptual frameworks. *Psychological Bulletin, 124,* 165–196.

Rutter, M. L. (1997). Nature–nurture integration: The example of antisocial behavior. *American Psychologist, 52,* 390–398.

Ryff, C. D., & Keyes, C. L. M. (1995). The structure of psychological well-being revisited. *Journal of Personality and Social Psychology, 69,* 719–727.

Sandvik, E., Diener, E., & Seidlitz, L. (1993). Subjective well-being: The convergence and stability of self-report and non-self-report measures. *Journal of Personality, 61*(3), 317–342.

Saris, W. E. (2001). The relationship between income and satisfaction: The effect of measurement error and suppressor variables. *Social Indicators Research, 53*(2), 117–136.

Schimmack, U. (2008). The structure of subjective well-being. In M. Eid & R. J. Larsen (Eds.), *The science of subjective well-being* (pp. 97–123). New York: Guilford Press.

Schimmack, U., & Diener, E. (2003). Predictive validity of explicit and implicit self-esteem for subjective well being. *Journal of Research in Personality, 37*(2), 100–106.

Schimmack, U., Diener, E., & Oishi, S. (2002). Life-satisfaction is a momentary judgment and a stable personality characteristic: The use of chronically accessible and stable sources. *Journal of Personality, 70*(3), 345–384.

Schimmack, U., & Oishi, S. (2005). The influence of chronically and temporarily accessible information on life satisfaction judgments. *Journal of Personality and Social Psychology, 89*(3), 395–406.

Schwarz, N. (1999). Self-reports: How the questions shape the answers. *American Psychologist, 54*(2), 93–105.

Schwarz, N., & Strack, F. (1999). Reports of subjective well-being: Judgmental processes and their methodological implications. In D. Kahneman, E. Diener, & N. Schwarz (Eds.), *Well-being: The foundations of hedonic psychology* (pp. 61–84). New York: Sage Foundation.

Schyns, P. (2001). Income and satisfaction in Russia. *Journal of Happiness Studies, 2*(2), 173–204.

Scollon, C., Kim-Prieto, C., & Diener, E. (2003). Experience sampling: Promises and pitfalls, strengths and weaknesses. *Journal of Happiness Studies, 4,* 5–34.

Seligman, M. E. P., Steen, T. A., Park, N., & Peter-son, C. (2005). Positive psychology progress: Empirical validation of interventions. *American Psychologist, 60,* 410–421.

Steel, P., Schmidt, J., & Shultz, J. (2008). Refining the relationship between personality and subjective well-being. *Psychological Bulletin, 134,* 138–161.

Strack, F., Martin, L. L., & Schwarz, N. (1988). Priming and communication: Social determinants of information use in judgments of life satisfaction. *European Journal of Social Psychology, 18,* 429–442.

Stubbe, J. H., Posthuma, D., Boomsma, D. I., & De Geus, E. J. C. (2005). Heritability of life satisfaction in adults: A twin-family study. *Psychological Medicine, 35*(11), 1581–1588.

Suh, E., Diener, E., & Fujita, F. (1996). Events and subjective well-being: Only recent events matter. *Journal of Personality and Social Psychology, 70*(5), 1091–1102.

Suh, E. M., Diener, E., Oishi, S., & Triandis, H. (1998). The shifting basis of life satisfaction judgments across cultures. *Journal of Personality and Social Psychology, 70,* 1091–1102.

Tellegen, A. (1985). Structures of mood and personality and their relevance to assessing anxiety, with an emphasis on self-report. In A. H. Tuma & J. D. Maser (Eds.), *Anxiety and the anxiety disorders* (pp. 681–706). Hillsdale, NJ: Erlbaum.

Tellegen, A., Lykken, D. T., Bouchard, T. J., Wilcox, K. J., Segal, N. L., & Rich, S. (1988). Personality similarity in twins reared apart and together. *Journal of Personality and Social Psychology, 54*(6), 1031–1039.

Vaidya, J. G., Gray, E. K., Haig, J., & Watson, D. (2002). On the temporal stability of personality: Evidence for differential stability and the role of life experiences. *Journal of Personality and Social Psychology, 83,* 1469–1484.

Watson, D., Clark, L. A., & Tellegen, A. (1988). Development and validation of brief measures of positive and negative affect: The PANAS scales. *Journal of Personality and Social Psychology, 54,* 1063–1070.

Watson, D., & Tellegen, A. (1985). Toward a consensual structure of mood. *Psychological Bulletin, 98*(2), 219–235.

Watson, D., & Walker, L.-M. (1996). The long-term stability and predictive validity of trait measures of affect. *Journal of Personality and Social Psychology, 70,* 567–577.

Wilson, W. (1967). Correlates of avowed happiness. *Psychological Bulletin, 67,* 294–306.

Zevon, M. A., & Tellegen, A. (1982). The structure of mood change: An idiographic/nomothetic analysis. *Journal of Personality and Social Psychology, 43*(1), 111–122.

Author Index

Subject Index

Page numbers followed by *f* indicate figures; *n*, note; and *t*, table.

Intimacy motive, 609, 619–620,
   622. *See also* Affiliative
   motive
Intrapsychic conflict, 87–88
Intrinsic motivation
   cognitive evaluation theory,
      660–661
   extrinsic motivation distinction,
      660
   and life goals, 667–669
   reward effects on, 660–661
   in self-determination theory, 656
   well-being link, 668
Introversion
   balanced selection for, 53
   and creativity, 684
   expressive suppression, 716
   in identity negotiation, 458–459
   schizoid personality disorder
      variant, 750
   subjective well-being, 809
Intuition
   implicit processes, 589
   in personality perceptions,
      226–228
Ipsative continuity, 381–382
   correlates, 381–382
   maturity effects, 382
IQ
   genius definition, 681–682
   health outcome, 780, 784–787
   positive parenting benefits, 353,
      367
Italian study, Big Five taxonomy,
   123
Item-order effect, self-report
   inventories, 800

James–Lange formulation, 592
James's self theory, 424–426
Japanese
   depression label, 550
   facial recognition, 549
   self-esteem studies, 552
   values, 554
Jealousy
   adaptive patterning, 47–48
   evolutionary psychology, 43–44,
      47–48
   individual differences, 47–48
   sex differences, 44
Job performance/satisfaction
   Big Five link, 142
   Big Three correlates, 275
   identity-congruent appraisals
      effect, 462
   self-report measures, 800
*Journal of Abnormal and Social
   Psychology*, 6

K-factor, evolutionary theory, 52–53
Knowability assumption, five-factor
   theory, 161
Knowledge activation, motivated
   bias, 187–188
Koreans, self-concept consistency,
   553

Laboratory animals, well-being, 343
Landscape preferences, evolutionary
   explanation, 37–38
Lang's emotion theory, 592–593
Latent class techniques, 559
Latent content, dreams, 63
Lay theories, of personality, 227
Learned expectancies, 761
Learning, implicit processes,
   586–587, 619–620
Lesch–Nyhan syndrome, 434
Lexical approach
   Big Five discovery, 117–118, 145
   Big Five facets, 126t, 145
   circumplex method, 121
   five-factor theory, 169–170
   personality traits agnostic stance,
      145, 160
Libido
   Freud's model, 64
   motivation role, 71–72
Life events
   emotion antecedent, 704
   self-report measures, 799
   and subjective well-being,
      806–807
Life experiences, personality
   change, 382
Life satisfaction.
   and aging, 402–404, 407
   general issues, 796–798
   personality factors, 407
   self-report measures, 799–800
   stability, 805–806
   See also Subjective well-being
Life stories, 242–262
   adaptations in, 248–250, 249f
   as autobiographical project, 243
   cultural influences, 246–247
   evolutionary aspects, 248
   identity model, 243
   integrative function, 244–245
   narrative identity emergence,
      250–252
   negative events, 252–256
   nomothetic and idiographic
      research, 256–257
   personal meaning in, 343
   personality development effects,
      246
   personality traits in, 248–250,
      249f
   psychological quality of, 247–
      248
   redemptive self theme, 255–256
   self-transformation, 252–256
   as situated performance, 243
   six principles, 244–248
   social relational principle,
      245–246, 251
   temporal instability, 246
Life stress, *5-HTT* alleles
   interaction, 321–322,
      340–341, 521–522
Life transitions, narrative studies,
   254–255
Limbic system, and emotion, 709

Linkage studies, definition, 312
Longevity
   Big Five prediction, 141–142
   conscientiousness predictor, 777,
      781, 785
   intelligence predictor, 784–785
   and optimism, 784
   See also Mortality
Longitudinal studies, health,
   772–773
Loss, stress model, 731–732
Lymph nodes, and sociability,
   nonhuman primates, 342

Macaque species
   ecological pressures effect, 339
   personality differences, 338–339
Main genetic effects
   versus gene × environment
      interactions, 303–304
   personality traits, 301–304
Malnutrition, and self-regulation,
   482
Manifest content, dreams, 63
MAO-A gene, environmental
   interdependence, 303, 354
Marital satisfaction/status
   and identity-disconfirming events,
      462
   person–environment interactions,
      761
   personality traits, 760–761
   and subjective well-being, 803
Marlowe–Crowne scale, 500–502
Marriage
   personality change factor,
      387–388
   and subjective well-being, 803,
      806–807
Master narrative positioning, 245
Maternal sensitivity, and attachment
   behavior, 521
Mating behavior/motivation
   and adaptive self-assessment, 49
   evolutionary context, 42–43,
      48–49
   frequency dependence, 51–52
   niche specialization, 48
   shy–bold continuum, 335–336
Maturity principle, 376t
   ipsative longitudinal study, 382
   personality mean level stability,
      279
   personality trait change, 379–380
"Me" phenomenon, 425
Mean differences, in person–
   situation research, 570
Mean-level personality change,
   379–380
   longitudinal studies, 379–380,
      400–402
   setpoint theory, 380
   sex differences, 379
Medial prefrontal cortex
   Self-referential processes, 435
   sense of self study, 433
Mental hygiene movement, 6